D1690721

Dr. med. Michael Pruggmayer
Dipl. Biol.
Frauenarzt - Medizinische Genetik
Zytogenetisches Labor
Bahnhofstr. 5 - Tel. (0 51 71) 37 **75**
D-31224 Peine

Multiple pregnancy

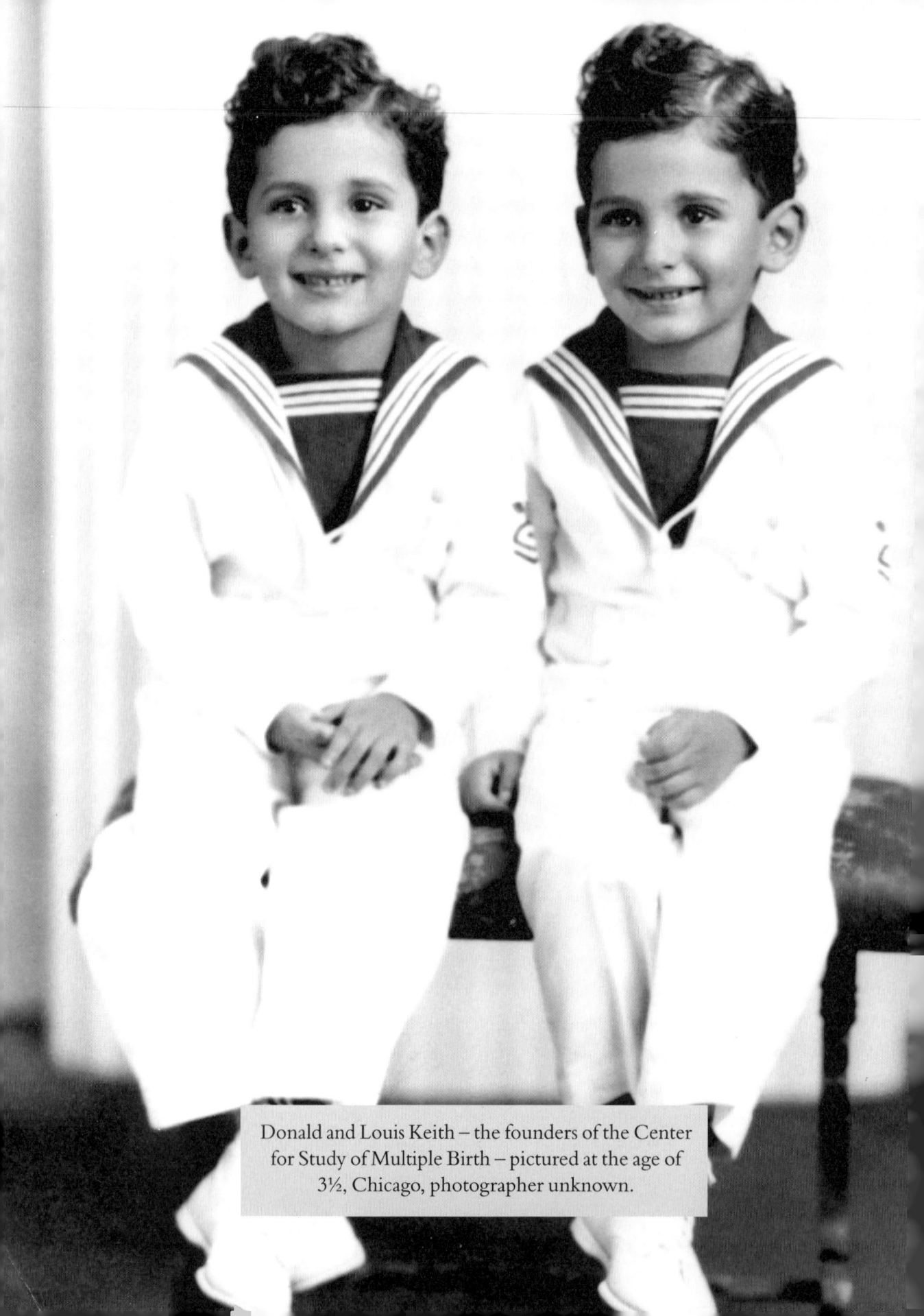

Donald and Louis Keith – the founders of the Center for Study of Multiple Birth – pictured at the age of 3½, Chicago, photographer unknown.

Multiple pregnancy

Epidemiology, Gestation & Perinatal outcome

Edited by

Louis G. Keith,
Northwestern University Medical School, Chicago

Emile Papiernik
Université Réné Descartes, Paris

Donald M. Keith
The Center for Study of Multiple Birth, Chicago

Barbara Luke
University of Michigan Medical School, Ann Arbor, Michigan

With a Foreword by John J. Sciarra
Northwestern University Medical School, Chicago

Special photography by David Teplica
University of Chicago, Chicago

The Parthenon Publishing Group
International Publishers in Medicine, Science & Technology

NEW YORK   LONDON

British Library Cataloguing in Publication Data
Multiple Pregnancy: Epidemiology, Gestation and
Perinatal Outcome
  I. Keith, Louis G.
  618.25

ISBN 1-85070-666-2

Library of Congress Cataloging-in-Publication Data
Multiple pregnancy : epidemiology, gestation &
  perinatal outcome / edited by Louis G. Keith . . .
  (et al.) : with a foreword by John J. Sciarra : special
  photography by David Teplica.
      p.   cm.
  Includes bibliographical references and index.
  ISBN 1-85070-666-2 (hardback)
  1. Multiple pregnancy. I. Keith, Louis G.
  [DNLM: 1. Pregnancy, Multiple. 2. Fetal
  Monitoring. WQ 235 M961   1995]
RG567.M85   1995
618.2'5—dc20
DNLM/DLC
for Library of Congress   95-11481

Published in the UK and Europe by
The PARTHENON Publishing Group
Casterton Hall, Carnforth
Lancs. LA6 2LA, UK

Published in North America by
The Parthenon Publishing Group Inc.
One Blue Hill Plaza
PO Box 1564, Pearl River
New York 10965, USA

Copyright © 1995 Parthenon Publishing Group Ltd

First published 1995

No part of this book may be reproduced in any form without
permission from the publishers, except for the quotation of brief
passages for the purposes of review.

All photographs by David Teplica, MD, MFA are
copyright 1995. They may not be reproduced without
prior written permission from The Collected Image,
806, Monroe St., Evanston, IL 60202, USA.

Typeset in 10/12 Baskerville by Martin Lister Publishing
Services, Carnforth, UK
Printed by Butler & Tanner Ltd, Frome and London, UK

Contents

Photographic plates ... ix

List of contributors ... xi

Foreword ... xvii

Preface ... xix

Acknowledgements ... xxi

Dedication ... xxiii

Section I Introduction

1. The role of research in twin medicine ... 3
   L. Gedda

2. The twin method ... 9
   P. Parisi

Section II Biology

3. The mechanism of monozygosity and double ovulation ... 25
   O. Bomsel-Helmreich and W. Al Mufti

4. The frequency and survival probability of natural twin conceptions ... 41
   C.E. Boklage

5. Documenting the vanishing twin by pathological examination ... 51
   K. Yoshida

6. The vanishing twin ... 59
   H.J. Landy and B.M. Nies

7. Congenital anomalies and pregnancy loss ... 73
   C. Meyers, S. Elias and P. Arrabal

8. Conjoined twins ... 93
   M. Creinin

9. Placentation ... 113
   R. Derom, C. Derom and R. Vlietinck

Section III Epidemiology

10 Demographic trends in twin births: USA 133
    S.M. Taffel

11 The epidemiology of multiple births in Europe 145
    R. Derom, J. Orlebeke, A. Eriksson and M. Thiery

12 The role of birth weight, gestational age, race and other infant characteristics 163
    in twin intrauterine growth and infant mortality
    W.F. Powers, J.L. Kiely and M.G. Fowler

13 The impact of assisted reproductive technology on the incidence of multiple 175
    gestation
    B.R. Hecht

Section IV Diagnosis and general considerations

14 Ultrasound scanning techniques 195
    R. Bessis

15 Population ultrasound: the Swedish experience 205
    H. Rydhström and L. Grennert

16 Pregnancy dating and evaluation by ultrasonography 215
    R.E. Sabbagha

17 Diagnosis of fetal congenital anomalies by ultrasonography 239
    R.E. Sabbagha

18 Maternal adaptation to multifetal pregnancy 269
    S.N. MacGregor and R.K. Silver

19 Maternal clinical and biochemical changes 279
    A.M. Peaceman

20 Psychophysiological adaptation to multiple pregnancy 289
    E. Noble

21 Maternal characteristics and prenatal nutrition 299
    B. Luke

Section V Assessment and management of fetal well-being

22 Prenatal genetic diagnosis: amniocentesis and chorionic villus sampling 313
    E. Pergament

23 Biophysical assessment 325
    J.A. Lopez-Zeno

24 Intrauterine behavior 331
    B. Arabin, U. Gembruch and J. van Eyck

25	The natural history of grand multifetal pregnancies and the effect of pregnancy reduction L. Lynch and R.L. Berkowitz	351
26	Multifetal pregnancy reduction and selective second-trimester termination M.I. Evans, N.B. Isada, P.G. Pryde and J.C. Fletcher	359
27	The twin–twin transfusion syndrome: vascular anatomy of monochorionic placentas and their clinical outcomes G.A. Machin and K. Still	367
28	The twin–twin transfusion syndrome: three-dimensional modelling of the 'common villous district' A. Schoenfeld, M. Hod, J. Ovadia and R. Amir	395
29	The twin–twin transfusion syndrome: treatment of chorioangiopagus and asymmetry J.E. De Lia	399
30	The intrauterine demise of one fetus J.A. Lopez-Zeno and J. Navarro-Pando	407

Section VI   Antepartum considerations

31	The physiology of preterm labor R.E. Besinger and N.J. Carlson	415
32	Normal and abnormal patterns of labor E.A. Friedman	427
33	Reducing the risk of preterm delivery E. Papiernik	437
34	Assessment of cervical change R.B. Newman, R.K. Godsey and J.M. Ellings	453
35	Ambulatory tocolysis F. Lam and P.J. Gill	471
36	The optimum route of delivery F.A. Chervenak	491
37	Labor and delivery L.G. Keith, T.R.B. Johnson, J.A. Lopez-Zeno and M. Creinin	503
38	Analgesic and anesthetic considerations H. Cohen and E.A. Brunner	517
39	Clinical management of monoamniotic twins M. Motew and N.A. Ginsberg	527
40	Management of triplet and higher-order pregnancies J.-C. Pons, Y. Laurent, D. Selim and E. Papiernik	535

Section VII Postpartum considerations

41	Breast feeding multiples *J.M. Wilton*	553
42	Bonding and attachment *R. Theroux and J.F. Tingley*	563
43	Psychiatric considerations after the birth of multiples *K.E. Merenkov*	573

Section VIII Childhood growth and development

44	Fetal brain and pulmonary adaptation in multiple pregnancy *C. Amiel-Tison and L. Gluck*	585
45	Factors affecting developmental outcome *M.C. Allen*	599
46	The long-term development of twins: anthropometric factors and cognition *F. Falkner and A.P. Matheny, Jr*	613
47	Postnatal zygosity determination *E. Pergament*	625

Section IX Parental concerns

48	The parent–doctor relationship *D.M. Keith*	637
49	Ethical considerations *M.W. Gallagher*	645
50	National Organization of Mothers of Twins Clubs, Inc. *M.M. Eicker*	655
51	Parenting twins: a pediatrician's point of view *E.M. Bryan*	659
52	Parents of multiples clubs and clinics: the United Kingdom experience *E.M. Bryan*	663
	Appendix: Resources	667
	Index	681

Photographic Plates by David Teplica, MD, MFA

All photographs opening sections of this text were produced as part of an ongoing body of work exploring the physical and psychological bonds between identical twins. The series was begun as the thesis project presented to the School of the Art Institute of Chicago by Dr Teplica, Clinical Assistant Professor of Surgery at the University of Chicago, in fulfilment of the requirements for the degree of Master of Fine Arts. This work was produced with the support of Professional Imaging, Eastman Kodak Company, Rochester, New York.

Images were obtained with a Nikon FM camera and a 24 mm, 50 mm or 105 mm lens. Technical Pan Film was utilized for image capture. Negatives were processed in Technidol and gelatin silver prints were produced with Kodak paper and chemistry. Exhibition prints were processed archivally and toned with Kodak Selenium Toner. The work has been exhibited widely in the United States, the former Soviet Union and in Taiwan.

Use of the images in this book was coordinated by Jerri Zbiral, The Collected Image, Evanston, Illinois.

Location	Title, names, size and credit	Location	Title, names, size and credit
Front Cover	Untitled, 1990 Alexandra and Jaclyn Payto, age 3, Brecksville, Ohio 8 × 12 in The Art Institute of Chicago	Section III page 130	The Reed Twins, 1990 Vicky and Valerie Reed, age 24, Brook Park, Ohio 16 × 20 in Collection of Gary C. Burget, MD, Chicago, Illinois
Section I page xxiv	The Awakening, 1989 Sarah and Christina Schell, age 12, New Preston, Connecticut 8 × 10 in The Art Institute of Chicago	Section IV page 192	The Dworkin Twins, 1990 Joel and Steven Dworkin, age 25, Nashville, Tennessee and Austin, Texas 11 × 14 in The Smart Museum, University of Chicago
Section II page 22	Untitled, 1994 Tim and Todd Derma, age 20, Itasca, Illinois 11 × 14 in Collection of the Artist	Section V page 310	The Schell Twins, 1990 Sarah and Christina Schell, age 13, New Preston, Connecticut 5 × 9 in Palmer Museum of Art, University Park, Pennsylvania

Location	Title, names, size and credit	Location	Title, names, size and credit
Section VI page 412	Refusion, 1991 Joel and Steven Dworkin, age 25, Nashville, Tennessee and Austin, Texas 16 × 20 in Collection of Harry Drake, Minneapolis, Minnesota	Section IX page 634	The Bossolt Twins, 1990 Kathi and Karen Bossolt, age 21, Upper Saddle River, New Jersey 11 × 14 in The Collected Image, Evanston, Illinois
Section VII page 550	Monozygotic Fusion, 1989 Sarah and Christina Schell, age 12, New Preston, Connecticut 11 × 14 in Collection of Lisa Jackley Dayton, Minneapolis, Minnesota	Appendix page 666	Repose, 1990 Joel and Steven Dworkin, age 25, Nashville, Tennessee and Austin, Texas 20 × 24 in The Center for Study of Multiple Birth, Chicago, Illinois
Section VIII page 582	Difference, 1990 Alexandra and Jaclyn Payto, age 3, Brecksville, Ohio 16 × 20 in Collection of Jane and Stephen Lorch, Boston, Massachusetts		

List of contributors

Marilee C. Allen, MD
Associate Professor of Pediatrics
The Johns Hopkins Hospital School of
  Medicine
Baltimore, MD 21287-3200
USA

Widad Al Mufti, MD
Unité INSERM 187
Hôpital Antoine Béclère
92141 Clamart
France

Claudine Amiel-Tison, MD
Associate Professor of Pediatrics
Clinique Universitaire Baudelocque
Hôpital Cochin
75014 Paris
France

Reuven Amir, PhD
IBM Corporation
Tel Aviv
Israel

Birgit Arabin, MD, PhD
Perinatologist
Assistant Professor
Sophia Ziekenhuis
8025 AB Zwolle
The Netherlands

Pedro Arrabal, MD
Associate Professor of Obstetrics and
  Gynecology
University of Maryland School of Medicine
Baltimore, MD 21201
USA

Richard L. Berkowitz, MD
Professor of Obstetrics, Gynecology and
  Reproductive Science
Mount Sinai Medical Center
New York, NY 10029
USA

Richard E. Besinger, MD
Associate Professor of Obstetrics and
  Gynecology
Loyola University Medical Center
Maywood, Illinois 60153
USA

Roger Bessis, MD
Obstetrics and Gynecology
Departement Baudelocque Port Royal
75014 Paris
France

Charles E. Boklage, PhD
Professor and Director
Laboratory of Behavioral and Developmental
  Genetics
East Carolina University School of Medicine
Greenville, NC 27858-4354
USA

O. Bomsel-Helmreich, DSc
Department of Obstetrics and Gynecology
Hôpital Antoine Béclère
92141 Clamart
France

Edward A. Brunner, MD, PhD
James E. Eckenhoff Professor and Chairman
Department of Anesthesia
Northwestern University Medical School
Chicago, IL 60611
USA

Elizabeth M. Bryan, MD
Institute of Obstetrics and Gynecology Trust
Queen Charlotte's and Chelsea Hospital
London W6 OXG
UK

Nancy J. Carlson, MD
Assistant Professor of Obstetrics and
  Gynecology
Loyola University Medical Center
Maywood, IL 60153
USA

Frank A. Chervenak, MD
Professor of Obstetrics and Gynecology
The New York Hospital-Cornell Medical
  Center
New York, NY 10021
USA

Harry Cohen, MD
Professor of Clinical Anesthesia
Northwestern University Medical School
Chicago, IL 60611
USA

Mitchell Creinin, MD
Assistant Professor of Obstetrics, Gynecology
  and Reproductive Sciences
University of Pittsburgh School of Medicine
Pittsburgh, PA 15213-3180
USA

Julian E. De Lia, MD
Associate Professor of Obstetrics and
  Gynecology
Medical College of Wisconsin
Milwaukee, WI 53226
USA

C. Derom, PhD
Research Associate
Department of Human Genetics
Katholieke Universiteit Leuven
B-3000 Leuven
Belgium

Robert Derom, MD, PhD, FRCOG
Professor Emeritus of Obstetrics and
  Gynecology
University of Gent, and
Research Associate
Department of Human Genetics
Katholieke Universiteit Leuven
B-3000 Leuven
Belgium

Martha M. Eicker
Executive Vice-President
National Organization of Mothers of Twins
  Clubs, Inc. (NOMTC)
Albuquerque, NM 87192-1188
USA

Sherman Elias, MD
Professor of Obstetrics and Gynecology/
  Molecular and Human Genetics
Baylor College of Medicine
Houston, TX 77030
USA

Janna M. Ellings, CNM
PO Box 309
Tuba, AZ 86045
USA

A. Eriksson
Fulkshalsan Population Genetics Unit
Topeliusgatan 20
Fin 00101 Hensingfors
Finland

Mark I. Evans, MD
Professor and Vice-Chief of Obstetrics and
  Gynecology/Medicine and Molecular
  Genetics
Wayne State University School of Medicine
Detroit, MI 48201
USA

Frank Falkner, MD, FRCP
Professor Emeritus Maternal and Child
  Health/Pediatrics
University of California, Berkeley, and
  San Francisco
Berkeley, CA 94708
USA

John C. Fletcher, PhD
Director for the Center for Biomedical Ethics
Health Science Center
University of Virginia
Charlottesville, VA 22908
USA

Mary Glenn Fowler, MD, MPH
Chief, Perinatal Transmission and Pediatric
 Section
Efficacy Trials Branch
Division of AIDS, NIAID, NIH
Rockville, MD 20852
USA

Emanuel A. Friedman, MD
Professor Emeritus, Obstetrics and Gynecology
Harvard University Medical School
New York, NY 10023
USA

Michael W. Gallagher, MD
Staff Perinatalogist
Department of Obstetrics and Gynecology
National Naval Medical Center
Bethesda, MD 20889-5600
USA

Luigi Gedda
Director, The Mendel Institute
Piazza Galeno, 5
Rome 00161
Italy

Ulrich Gembruch, MD
Perinatologist
Associate Professor
University of Lübeck
D-23538 Lübeck
Germany

Pamela J. Gill, RN, MSN
Assistant Clinical Professor of Nursing
University of California, San Francisco
San Francisco, CA 94143
USA

Norman A. Ginsberg, MD
Assistant Professor of Obstetrics and
 Gynecology
Northwestern University Medical School
Chicago, IL 60611
USA

Louis Gluck, MD
Professor of Pediatrics and Obstetrics
University of California College of Medicine
Orange, CA 92668
USA

Raleigh K. Godsey, MD
Bradford Clinic
Matthews, NC 28105
USA

Lars Grennert, MD
Associate Professor of Obstetrics and
 Gynecology
Malmö General Hospital
Malmö
Sweden

Bryan R. Hecht, MD
Associate Professor of Obstetrics and
 Gynecology
North Eastern Ohio Universities College of
 Medicine
Canton, OH 44710
USA

Moshe Hod, MD
Director, Diabetes in Pregnancy Center
Beilinson Medical Center
Petah Tiqva and Sackler Faculty of Medicine
Tel Aviv University
Petah Tiqva 49100
Israel

Nelson B. Isada, MD
Associate Professor of Obstetrics and
 Gynecology
Eastern Virginia Medical School
Norfolk, VA 23507-1912
USA

Timothy R.B. Johnson, MD
Professor and Chairman Department of
 Obstetrics and Gynecology
University of Michigan Medical School
Ann Arbor
MI 48109
USA

Donald M. Keith, MBA, LTC, USA (Ret.)
The Center for Study of Multiple Birth
333 East Superior St., Suite 464
Chicago, IL 60611
USA

Louis G. Keith, MD
Professor of Obstetrics and Gynecology
Northwestern University Medical School
Chicago, IL 60611
USA

John L. Kiely, PhD
Chief, Infant and Child Health Studies Branch
 at National Center for Health Statistics
Centers for Disease Control and Prevention
Hyattsville, MD 20728
USA

Fung Lam, MD
Assistant Clinical Professor of Obstetrics and
 Gynecology
University of California San Francisco
San Francisco, CA 94143
USA

Helain J. Landy, MD
Associate Professor of Obstetrics and
 Gynecology
University of Miami School of Medicine
Miami, FL 33101
USA

Yvon Laurent, MD
Service de Gynéco-Obstétrique
Centre hospitalier d'Avranches
50303 Avranches Cedex
France

José A. Lopez-Zeno, MD
Assistant Professor of Obstetrics and
 Gynecology
Georgetown University Medical Center
Washington, DC 20007
USA

Barbara Luke, ScD, MPH
Associate Professor
University of Michigan Medical School
Ann Arbor
MI 48109
USA

Lauren Lynch, MD
Assistant Professor of Obstetrics and
Gynecology
Mt. Sinai Medical Center
One Gustave Levy Place
New York, NY 10029
USA

Scott N. MacGregor, DO
Associate Professor of Obstetrics and
 Gynecology
Evanston Hospital
Evanston, IL 60201
USA

Geoffrey A. Machin, MD, PhD, FRCP(C)
Professor of Pediatric Pathology
University of Alberta Hospitals
Edmonton T6G 297
Canada

Adam P. Matheny, Jr, PhD
Professor of Pediatrics
University of Louisville School of Medicine
Louisville, MY 40292
USA

Kimberly E. Merenkov, MD
Clinical Instructor of Psychiatry
Northwestern University Medical School
Chicago, IL 60611
USA

Carole Meyers, MD
Assistant Professor of Obstetrics and
 Gynecology
University of Maryland School of Medicine
Baltimore, MD 21201
USA

Martin Motew, MD
Assistant Professor of Clinical Obstetrics and
 Gynecology
Northwestern University Medical School
Chicago, IL 60602
USA

José Navarro-Pando, MD, PhD
Departmento de Obstetricia y Ginecologia
Hospital de Municipalidad
Murcia
Spain

List of contributors

Roger B. Newman, MD
Associate Professor of Obstetrics and Gynecology
Medical University of South Carolina
Charleston, SC 29425-2233
USA

Barbara M. Nies, MD
Assistant Professor of Obstetrics and Gynecology
George Washington University Medical Center
Washington, DC 20037
USA

Elizabeth Noble, BA, PT
Director, Women's Health Resources
Cape Cod, MA
USA

J. Orlebeke, PhD
Professor of Physiological Psychology
Free University
1081 HV Amsterdam
The Netherlands

Jardena Ovadia, MD
Associate Professor and Chairman
Department of Obstetrics and Gynecology
Beilinson Medical Center
Petah Tiqva and Sackler Faculty of Medicine
Tel Aviv University
Petah Tiqva 49100
Israel

Emile Papiernik, MD
Professeur et Directeur Gynécologie et Obstétrique
Université Réné Descartes
75674 Paris
France

Paolo Parisi, MD
Dip. Sanità Pubblica
University of Rome – Tor Vergata
00173 Rome
Italy

Alan M. Peaceman, MD
Assistant Professor
Department of Obstetrics and Gynecology
Northwestern University Medical School
Chicago, IL 60611
USA

Eugene Pergament, MD, PhD, FACMG
Associate Professor of Obstetrics and Gynecology
Northwestern University Medical School
Chicago, IL 60611
USA

Jean-Claude Pons, MD
Maternité de Port Royal
123 boulevard de Port Royal
75014 Paris
France

William F. Powers, MD, MHS
Director of Special Care Nursery
Joint Program in Neonatalogy
Winchester Hospital
Winchester, MA 01890
USA

Peter G. Pryde, MD
Perinatalogist/Geneticist
Parinatal Associates of Northern California
Sacramento, CA 95819
USA

Hakan Rydhström, MD, PhD
Professor of Obstetrics and Gynecology
University Hospital
S-2121 85 Lund
Sweden

Rudy E. Sabbagha, MD
Professor of Obstetrics and Gynecology
Northwestern University Medical School
Chicago, IL 60611
USA

A. Schoenfeld, MD
Associate Professor
Deputy Chairman of Obstetrics and Gynecology
Beilinson Medical Center
Petah-Tiqva and Sackler School of Medicine
Tel-Aviv University
Petah Tiqva 49100
Israel

John J. Sciarra, MD, PhD
Thomas J. Watkins Professor and Chairman of Obstetrics and Gynecology
Northwestern University Medical School
Chicago, IL 60611
USA

Madame Dagmar Selim
Maternité de Port Royal
123 boulevard de Port Royal
75014 Paris
France

R.K. Silver, MD
Associate Professor of Obstetrics and Gynecology
Evanston Hospital
Evanston, IL 60201
USA

K. Still, MD, FRCS
Associate Professor of Obstetrics and Gynecology
University of Alberta Hospital
Edmonton T6G 297
Canada

Selma M. Taffel
Statistician, Division of Vital Statistics
National Center for Health Statistics
Hyattsville, MD 20782
USA

David Teplica, MD, MFA
Clinical Assistant Professor of Surgery
Section of Plastic and Reconstructive Surgery
The University of Chicago
Chicago, IL 60637
USA

Rosemary Theroux, RN, MS
30 Summer Hill Road
Medway, MA 02053
USA

Michel Thiery, MD, PhD, FRCOG
Professor Emeritus of Obstetrics and Gynecology
University of Gent
B-9000 Gent
Belgium

Josephine F. Tingley, RN, BSN
101 South Street
Westboro, MA 01581
USA

Jim van Eyck, MD
Perinatologist
Department of Obstetrics and Pediatrics
Sophia Ziekenhuis
8025 AB Zwolle
The Netherlands

R. Vlietinck, MD, PhD
Professsor of Human Genetics
Katholieke Universiteit Leuven
B-3000 Leuven
Belgium

Paul J. Weinbaum, MD
Associate Professor of Obstetrics and Gynecology
The Albany Medical College
Albany, NY 12208
USA

Jeanne M. Wilton, RN, MS, IBCLC
OB/GYN Nurse Practitioner
All Saints OB/GYN
Racine, WI 53404
USA

Keiji Yoshida, MD
Professor of Obstetrics and Gynecology
Tokyo Medical College
Kasumigaura Hospital
Ibaraki 300-03
Japan

Foreword

I am very pleased to introduce this important new text under the editorship of Professors Keith and Papiernik, Lt. Col. Donald Keith and Dr Barbara Luke. This volume is a significant contribution to the study of twins and multiple pregnancies. It is the first major contribution on multiple pregnancy prepared after the widespread recognition that multiple births are presently more common than they had been, even in the recent past. It was also written after physicians and scientists realized that advances in neonatal care generally led to the survival of much smaller infants and the higher probability of these infants being handicapped. The authors and editors have provided a full discussion of these and other important problems.

This text is unique in a number of ways. Unlike others, of which there are notably few, it has an international rather than a parochial scope. This is especially important to me because, as Past President of the International Federation of Gynecology and Obstetrics (FIGO) and Editor of the *International Journal of Gynecology and Obstetrics*, I have had the opportunity to obtain first-hand knowledge of the health concerns of women and their families throughout the world, and of the numerous attempts by health care providers and organizations to respond to these needs. As the problems associated with multiple births are worldwide and growing, it is vital that the international community understands the issues relating to multiple pregnancy and their implications for health care.

This book is by far the most comprehensive and up-to-date source on multiple pregnancy. It discusses cutting-edge opinions and technologies, and covers subjects not mentioned in other monographs on twins. Specifically, it describes the vanishing twin and its causes, congenital defects, selective reduction procedures, the use of ultrasound, and the twin-to-twin transfusion syndrome. Additionally, it provides an extensive discussion of epidemiology, which makes use of governmental data sources from the USA and Europe. An important section on the childhood growth and development of twins is also included. Finally, thorough consideration is given to parental needs both in the antepartum and the postpartum periods. The volume concludes with a special section on support organizations.

Multiple Pregnancy: Epidemiology, Gestation and Perinatal Outcome benefits from the combined input of its editors. Dr Louis Keith was able to draw upon his own personal experience as an identical twin and as a member of numerous important national and international organizations catering to multiples, as well as his experience as an obstetrician/gynecologist, in determining the organization and content of the book. Dr Papiernik, who is the head of the Clinique Universitaire Baudelocque at the Hôpital Cochin, an important maternity unit in Paris, and an international authority on maternity care, offered advice and collaboration on content and potential authors. Lt. Col. Donald Keith, who has extensive experience in the world of twins and has collaborated with his twin brother, Louis, on many occasions, was able to help with many of the logistical tasks that required solution before a volume of this magnitude could be brought together. Dr Luke provided valuable assistance on organizational matters and epidemiological issues and concerns.

It is my sincere hope that this textbook will serve as the basis for the continued discussion and study of the many complex medical and social issues surrounding the care of mothers with multiple pregnancy. The varied content of *Multiple Pregnancy: Epidemiology, Gestation and Perinatal Outcome* should act as a source of stimulation for clinicians, investigators, and others involved in either the care of these patients or in research in this important and fascinating area of medicine. The four editors have provided comprehensive and thought-provoking information destined to serve as the classic reference work for years to come.

Thomas J. Watkins Professor and Chairman of
  Obstetrics and Gynecology
and Past-President of FIGO
Northwestern University Medical School, Chicago

John J. Sciarra

Preface

The need for this unique text becomes increasingly obvious with each passing year. Although other monographs on twins are available in English, their scope tends to be limited to obstetric problems or to specific, albeit large and well-studied, groups of patients. Today, anyone who attempts to study the broad area of multiple gestation (described as that branch of science known as 'Gemellology' – see comments by Professor Luigi Gedda in Chapter 1) soon realizes that he or she must simultaneously consider three distinct topics: first, the worldwide 'explosion' in the number of multiples; second, the phenomenal advances in maternal and neonatal care that help reduce neonatal morbidity and mortality; and finally, the core subject matter.

Our intention from the beginning was to provide readers with a truly comprehensive overview of the entire field along with classic and recent references. We deliberately included topics overlooked or barely discussed in standard textbooks of obstetrics. Thus, we began with introductory chapters dealing with the science of twinning. These precede the section on the biology of twinning (including an indepth exposition of one of the Center for Multiple Birth's early contributions – the vanishing twin syndrome) and an extensive discussion of various aspects of the epidemiology of twinning. These sections are followed by the 'core' of the book which separately discusses diagnosis and general considerations, assessment and management of fetal well-being and antepartum considerations. These latter concerns form the nucleus of what normally is expected in a book devoted solely to multiple pregnancy. The book concludes with sections on postpartum considerations, childhood growth and development and parental concerns. An appendix of resources, books and organizations or groups for those involved or interested in multiple births concludes the volume.

The decision to surround the central portion of the book with related subject matter was based upon the experience of the Center for Study of Multiple Birth, where annually hundreds of questions are received from physicians, parents and the media. These individuals have told us repeatedly of their vain struggles to find one reference source for all of their needs. We sincerely hope that a broad point of view will lighten the burden of any reader who wants to know more than other texts provide about multiples.

This volume may contain some overlaps, as occasional subjects are addressed by two or more authors. Hopefully, subject overlap will only rarely equate with content overlap. Differing points of view may also be apparent regarding topics for which there is no consensus. Nevertheless, the authors of almost every chapter have provided the reader with liberal references for their statements and opinions.

We are publishing this book for an international audience. The editors, two obstetricians, one twin brother, and a renowned reproductive epidemiologist, believe that our work will fill a void in the literature on multiple pregnancy. The four of us, as well as the staff of the Parthenon Publishing Group, have taken pains to provide readers with a uniform linguistic style without destroying the integrity of each author's voice. By remaining true to the voices of specialists with expertise in numerous areas of medicine, we also serve the interests of parents and their children, be they unborn or newly born.

Chicago — *Louis Keith, MD*
Paris — *Emile Papiernik, MD*
Washington — *Donald Keith, MBA (Lt. Col. USA Ret.)*
Ann Arbor — *Barbara Luke, ScD, MPH*

Acknowledgements

A book of this magnitude results from the combined efforts of numerous individuals and organisations.

First and foremost, the editors wish to thank the Department of Obstetrics and Gynecology at Northwestern University Medical School and the Prentice Women's Hospital and Maternity Center of Northwestern Memorial Hospital in Chicago for providing an academic affiliation to the Center for the Study of Multiple Birth during the past 15 years. We also thank Professor Sciarra for writing the Foreword.

We are grateful to a number of organisations which graciously provided partial funding for the vast task of assembling and collating the manuscript: in Chicago, the Department of Obstetrics and Gynecology of Northwestern University Medical School, the Jeanette Kennelly Kroch Center for Twin Studies of the Northwestern Memorial Hospital, and the Center for the Study of Multiple Birth: and in Paris, the Association for the Prevention of Birth Accidents. The final grant for pre-publication costs was provided by the Celia Porter Charitable Trust.

The cover photographs, as well as the photographs that enhance each section divider, were selected from the comprehensive body of work on twins by David Teplica, MD, MFA of the Faculty of Medicine at the University of Chicago. Dr Teplica's photographs are provided through the courtesy of The Collected Image in Evanston, Illinois.

In our experience, no publisher has been easier to work with and more deserving of recognition than Mr David Bloomer of the Parthenon Publishing Group. For this, he merits a true accolade. He and his staff worked with us for several months before a contract was signed. Rarely indeed, in these times, is business conducted in the old English manner with 'a wink, a handshake and a nod'. We also wish to extend special thanks to Mrs Jean Wright, herself the mother of dizygotic twins, who is the International Managing Editor of Parthenon Publishing and who acted as the *de facto* editor of this book. Mrs Wright willingly acceded to all our requests regarding copy-editing, selection of typeface and page style. It was she who supervised the myriad details required to move a book from manuscript to hard-bound copy in a relatively short time.

Great praise must be given to Abi Bloomer, who served as the graphic designer for this project. The Directors of the Center for Study of Multiple Birth were overwhelmed upon seeing her proposals for the cover and the advertising materials. Of greater importance was Dr Teplica's reaction when he saw how his work had been utilized to provide a truly aesthetic component to an otherwise scientific book. Dr Teplica has always been a staunch advocate of enhancing science with art, and he was completely enchanted with the book's marriage of text and image.

We especially wish to thank Ms Paula Hamilton of Tiburon, California. This book could not have been completed without her redoubtable efforts as Project Coordinator, *'sans pareil'*. We know of no one else who could have dealt with so many authors in a comparable manner, even managing to keep the Senior Editor in line. This book is the latest in a collaboration of nearly 20 years, beginning in Chicago and continuing in San Francisco, on many projects requiring individualized expert editorial handling.

Our final debt of gratitude goes to all the authors who worked so hard for so long. This is a monumental work written by individuals residing all over the world, organized and edited in several locations, finally coming together in an exceptional transatlantic cooperation.

Louis Keith, MD
Emile Papiernik, MD
Donald Keith, MBA (Lt. Col. USA Ret.)
Barbara Luke, ScD, MPH

Dedication

From Louis Keith

- to Emile for proposing the book
- to Barbara for expanding its horizons
- to Donald for making it all happen

From Donald Keith

- to my wife Phyllis for your patience and understanding of the many long hours spent away from you in the world of multiples and, above all, for your love
- to my daughters Nina and Paula for the stolen time from you for this and all of my work

From Emile Papiernik

- to Martine who has supported this and all my other work

From Barbara Luke

- to all our children, whether born alone or in pairs, from those of us who love and care for them

From Louis Keith and Donald Keith

- to our parents Myron and Jannette who gave us the precious gift of our very special identity, an awareness of self
- to our Aunt, Celia Bersk Porter, for endowing the Center for Study of Multiple Birth

The Center for Study of Multiple Birth wishes to thank Mr Jeffrey Grossman for the initial grant which brought the Center into being

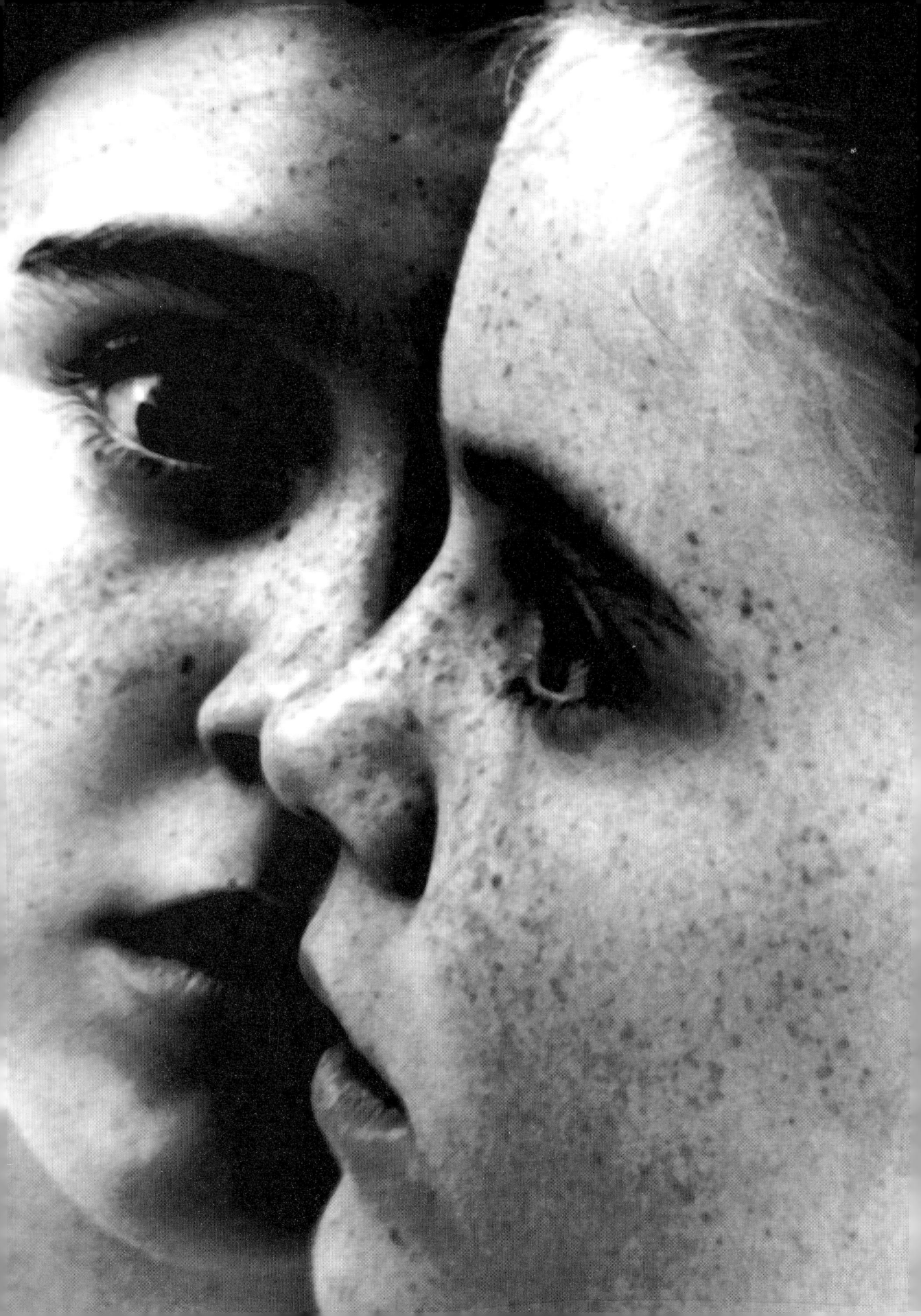

section I
Introduction

The Awakening

David Teplica, 1989,
The Art Institute of Chicago

The role of research in twin medicine

L. Gedda

Introduction

This book comes at an opportune moment. It is particularly necessary as interest in gemellology (the science of twins) is expanding, not only in human genetics but also in obstetrics and gynecology. This interest was amply demonstrated in August, 1989, during the *VI International Congress of Twin Studies* held in Rome under the auspices of the International Society of Twin Studies (ISTS) whose proceedings were published in the official journal of the Association, *Acta Geneticae Medicae et Gemellologiae*. The first of these congresses was held in Rome in 1974, when I founded the Society. Subsequent congresses were held in Washington (1977), Jerusalem (1980), London (1983), Amsterdam (1986), Rome (1989) and Tokyo (1992).

It was not by accident that the ISTS was created in Rome, because it was in this city that the Gregor Mendel Institute of Medical Genetics and Gemellology was founded in 1953. The Institute used the term 'gemellology' intentionally to indicate that it represented a medical branch of the discipline of genetics, previously founded by Gregor Mendel. As Director of the Mendel Institute and promoter of the International Society for Twin Studies, I warmly thank Professors Louis Keith and Emile Papiernik, Col. Donald Keith and Dr Barbara Luke, the editors of this book, for their initiative, because it extends the knowledge of gemellology to the fundamental and immense fields of obstetrics and perinatology.

My gratitude is based on two fundamental points. The first is that the concerns surrounding the conception, antenatal period and birth of twins are heightened today, thanks to a growing awareness of the numerous opportunities to avoid some of the risks which often accompany multiple pregnancy. The second is that obstetricians can learn from and collaborate with geneticists in the specific areas of heredity, the mechanism of conception and the phenomenon involving the genotype of twins.

Monozygotic twinning

A primary area of research in which obstetricians can collaborate with geneticists concerns monozygotic (MZ) twinning and the question of how two identical genomes yield two identical phenotypes. The historical basis of such endeavors often begins with a reconstruction of the genealogical tree of a family with MZ twins. Virtually always, careful search of the families of twins studied at the Mendel Institute documented the presence of other MZ twins. In addition, in a small percentage of cases, dizygotic (DZ) twins were found as well. We believe that obstetricians are in a particularly favorable position to record familial manifestations of the twinning phenomena, whose mechanism of transmission is not yet clear. For now, it is apparent that the gemellogenetic zygote contains a hereditary factor that, in certain conditions, induces cloning, that is, replicating its genes in two like examples.

The duplication of hereditary material in MZ twins occurs after amphimixis, or before metaphase which produces the first two cells of the morula, or before the blastocyst's content assumes the characteristics of bilateral symmetry by which the genes controlling the left and right parts of the organism are distinguished. If, on the other hand, gemellogenetic duplication occurs belatedly, the phenomenon of inverse laterality is produced. In this case, one of the MZ twins can be right-handed and the other left-handed. Indeed, one could hypothesize that left-handed singletons originally may have been MZ twins, with a co-twin that was unable to develop, and thus became a 'vanishing twin'[1].

Inverse laterality of MZ twins occasionally takes on pathological peculiarities, as occurred in a case I studied with some colleagues some years ago. These gentlemen were specialists in pain relief and were called to treat a MZ twin pair in which one presented with neuralgia of the right facial nerve and the other of the left. It is generally not possible to make a diagnosis of inverse laterality during the neonatal period unless, as sometimes happens, warts or other skin lesions are present on the right side of one twin and on the left side of the co-twin. Inverse laterality generally becomes apparent in later years, when one twin loses a tooth from a specific site and the co-twin loses the same tooth on the opposite side of the mouth.

The blastocyst evolves to produce two discoblastulas; in this phase, the ovular appendages of the amnion and chorion appear. As in every pregnancy, these are designed to protect the products of amphimixis which, in this case, are double or plural. As a geneticist, I believe it important to remember that these structures are not crucial for life; in the MZ twins this structure (the amnion) can be monoamniotic or diamniotic, and the diagnosis of monoamniotic twins or monochorionic twins does not always coincide with that of MZ twins.

Monozygotism, which means identicalness of the hereditary patrimony and, consequently, identicalness of the phenotype, is a twinning phenomenon of extraordinary interest, not only for twin studies but also for studies of general genetics, medical genetics and biology. However, one must not confuse the term 'twin identicalness' with that of 'twin identity'. These two concepts are not only different but actually opposite, as I will discuss later in this chapter.

What matters to me is to emphasize the great value of the phenomenon of identical hereditary patrimony in MZ twins. This genetic identicalness in the phase of the zygote and, even more in its phase of ontogenetic evolution, makes it possible to single out in the phenotype that which depends on heredity and that which is dependent on the environment. In this regard, twins are unique and frequently have been used to determine the effect that natural or artificial phenomena bear on equivalent organisms. In this manner, for example, American and Swedish researchers used twins to establish the effect produced by smoking on the organism and its functions[2]. It is likely that future ecological studies of the environment will also find the study of twins a reliable reference. Regardless of the nature of such a study, it will always be necessary to ensure that the natural situation is respected and that the twins are not used as objects for experiment. For experimental utilization, one can always have recourse to twin animals.

Genetic considerations

The study of MZ twins has recently enriched the field of genetics, and it is useful to mention this development as it relates to the practice of obstetrics. Obstetricians are essentially phenotypists, from the Greek word *faino*, which means 'to let see'. Stated another way, they are doctors who base their diagnoses and therapy on what is seen directly and/or indirectly of the human body. The phenotype also forms the basis of the diagnosis and treatment of hereditary diseases.

It is up to geneticists to probe beyond the visible level of the phenotype to the level of the genotype found in the nucleus of each cell. In fact, it is in the genome that one finds the 70 000 or so 'genes' (called 'elements' by Mendel) that determine the existence of those particulars of the phenotype called 'characters'. A gene, or group of genes called the genotype, corresponds in the innermost part of the organism to every character that falls under the eye of the clinician.

Genetics, by extending its observations from Mendel's careful scrutiny of this hidden labyrinth of the human body, was able to ascertain that when the cell reproduces, the hereditary material of its nucleus, which includes all the genes, divides in a specific way (and one that is characteristic of every species) into a certain number of little colored bodies, hence called chromosomes, which comprise certain genes and always the same ones.

The branch of genetics concerned with the hereditary material during this reproductive phase is called cytogenetics. Cytogeneticists, taking as a basis the number and form of chromosomes, have thus far been able to distinguish more than 100 hereditary diseases which appropriately are called chromosomal mutations. Of the numerous examples that come to mind, Down's syndrome is perhaps the most widely appreciated. In this condition, instead of the 46 chromosomes characteristic of the human species, 47 are found as a result of the presence of a small additional acrocentric chromosome 21. Other examples abound. For instance, the 'cri du chat' syndrome has 46 chromosomes but has lost a trait (p) of chromosome 5. The 'cat's eye' syndrome has an additional trait (q) of chromosome 22. Turner's syndrome is characterized by 45 chromosomes, due to the presence of a single sex chromosome (X). In contrast, Klinefelter's syndrome has 47 chromosomes because of the interrelated presence of three sex chromosomes (XXY). The list could go on and on.

At the time of twin births, obstetricians can assume that a chromosomal aberration is present if the twins are different not only in some normal characters (for example, sex, in the case of DZ twins) but also in evident anatomic malformations. In these cases, the obstetrician should advise the parents to have both twins examined by a cytogenetically trained physician.

Genetics has probed even deeper into the study of hereditary material, passing from cytogenetics to molecular genetics or the study of the great double helix molecule upon which the genes are located. Numerous investigations have shown, and continue to show, the genes' structure and their number and position regarding the individual genotypes of a certain character. However, this complicated and very delicate type of scientific study can in turn be surpassed in depth and complexity by a study of genes and genotypes that Gianni Brenci and I introduced into the framework of genetics many years ago and have chosen to characterize as chronogenetics[3]. Chronogenetics studies the stability of the genes or the genotypes with regard to the length of their activity or their lifetime.

Chronogenetics

I asked the editors if I could deal with this research as a part of the introduction to the present book for two reasons: first, because we have arrived at our present level of knowledge about the gene (or genotype) only after studying twins from a genetic point of view; and second, because chronogenetics is of practical use to phenotypists in a manner that perhaps has not been well appreciated.

Just as the seeds of the *Pisum sativum* (vegetal twins) were the material that allowed Gregor Mendel to establish the laws of heredity in plants and animals, so are human MZ twins the material which enabled Brenci and myself to establish the value of time in the study of the gene. What strikes doctor and layman alike when confronted with so-called 'real twins' is their identicalness. This differs completely from the phenomenon of 'doubles', not only because the latter are born of different mothers but also because the resemblance is temporary and accidental. In the case of MZ twins, this identicalness continues over time to the point that the parents (and others) may occasionally take Remus for Romulus and Romulus for Remus. The question that requires an answer is: does this permanent identicalness, which involves and survives the changes produced by development and the environment, exist?

In the past, this question was simplistically answered by declaring that the phenomenon of identicalness related to the fact that these twins were derived from a single zygote, that is, from the cloning of one zygote. No one, however, had previously appreciated the mechanism of this genetic identicalness as a dynamic characteristic of ontogenesis.

Our reply to this question has been simple, yet fruitful. The dynamic identicalness of twins is due to the fact that the genes controlling their specific characteristics have an identical temporal potential. This genetic parameter is not evident in singletons, because no means of comparison exists. In contrast, MZ twins have enabled us to affirm the existence of an identical temporal potential and to understand its mechanism.

In the study of chronogenetics, we stated that the longevity of genetic action depends on the stability of the gene, and that this stability, and consequently its time, depends both on the environment in which the life of the individual is lived, and on his or her hereditary patrimony[3].

If environment is identical, the identicalness of MZ twins continues. If not, the identicalness diminishes, as we have shown in our study of twins who separate because of marriage. This study demonstrates that correlation goes from the values of: 0.96 for height in cohabitants to 0.84 in non-cohabitants; 0.94 for weight in cohabitants to 0.87 in non-cohabitants; 0.84 for systolic blood pressure in cohabitants to 0.58 in non-cohabitants; and finally, 0.63 for diastolic blood pressure in cohabitants to 0.46 in non-cohabitants.

The gene's temporal dimension is important not only from a theoretical point of view, in that it allows us to study the nature and efficiency of the tie that binds the four constitutive bases of an individual, but also from a clinical point of view, in that it is a function of preventive medicine. In this regard, the so-called 'family history' becomes a panorama of life that the doctor must carefully piece together and interpret, because, as the time of the gene is hereditary, both the appearance of the normal characters of the phenotype, as well as the pathological characters of hereditary diseases, repeat themselves in the offspring in accordance with the laws of Mendelian and post-Mendelian genetics.

Preventive medicine today not only is able to forecast those medical circumstances that are due to heredity and environment, but also is able to forecast the appearance of a pathological process due initially to the diminution and subsequently to the absence of the gene's effect. In the doctrine of chronogenetics, we gave the name *ergon* to the degree of the gene's stability and the name *chronon* to the period of time that the ergon assures its effect for a particular environment[3].

In the chronogenetic study of the family, the age of the individuals affected by a hereditary disease is normally repetitive, as is likewise the age of death. It is further noted that the gene's stability does not disappear suddenly but lessens gradually, so that the genetic product is supplied to the corresponding phenotypic character in lesser amounts and more slowly. This phenomenon was pointed out long ago by Alexis Carrel in his book *L'homme c'est inconnu*, albeit without chronogenetic interpretation. During World War I Carrel stated that young soldiers recovered faster than older soldiers, given equal conditions of damage to tissues.

The greater slowness and fragility of information produced by a progressive exhaustion of the ergon may be of particular interest to obstetricians, because remaining in the uterus during the last weeks of gestation can, in our opinion, represent a period which, if shortened, subjects the ergon not only to the limited activity in endouterine life but also to conditions of increasing stress that precociously exhaust the stability of many genes. This hypothesis interests those taking care of mothers of multiples, in that these pregnancies frequently are complicated by preterm delivery and the fetuses are deprived of the terminal period of living within the mother.

Twin identity

I now wish to clarify my earlier statement that the concept of identicalness in MZ twins does not coincide with the concept of identity. Identicalness simply means that the physical phenotype of these twins, with the exception of cases of inverse laterality, is identical and particularly obvious in the period of prepubertal development. Identity, on the other hand, means something quite different. Each twin has his or her own personality that serves to distinguish that individual from his or her twin. Stated another way, each MZ twin, like every singleton, is from a certain point of view absolutely unique (or different from its co-twin). That this is true has been shown by study of the psychology of MZ twins[4].

The most revealing of the tests we conducted over the years concerns twins of preschool age (5 to 6 years) living in the same environment. We studied graphic expression, as the children did not yet know how to read or write. A pair of preliterate MZ twins was asked to perform a creative test which consisted of representing, by means of a drawing, a family scene (for example, having lunch together) or a memory test (for example, drawing a group of dolls shown to them for a few minutes). Each twin was given an identical set of coloring pencils and some sheets of white paper and asked to make a drawing of the family scene previously mentioned or of the dolls they had just seen. The twins were then each placed in different rooms so they could not communicate with each other.

The spontaneous drawings were made very willingly and extremely seriously by each of the twins. The surprising and revealing result was that each child selected pencils of different colors, executed the drawing on a different part of the paper, pictured the personages in diverse numbers and attitudes, and finally added some details to the creative or memorized sketch that were absolutely individual. This was true for every other parameter that the person in charge of the testing wanted to explore and compare.

These tests demonstrate quite convincingly that the physical identicalness of MZ twins does not imply psychic identicalness. When a twin's mind is able to express itself freely, he or she reveals the existence of a unique personal identity. Despite the truth of this statement, it is also true that to a greater or lesser degree, behavioral solidarity is common in MZ twins, as is the case of the so-called secret language they voluntarily speak with each other or in the exceptional cases of contemporaneous suicide. In a case recently reported from Udine, Italy, twin 19-year-old girls killed themselves by hooking up an automobile exhaust pipe to a shack in which they had shut themselves. Analogous phenomena have occurred in Italy on the part of singletons as well, but these instances represent cases of behavioral suggestion in which the uniformity characteristic of MZ twin pairs only plays a secondary role.

At the same time, the individual identity of each MZ twin, shown by the previously described test, is a suitable explanation for a phenomenon described by various authors in which the twin represents a small but distinct society. In this society the answers to questions and initiatives directed toward the exterior environment are mainly performed by one twin, who is characterized by Bracken as *Aussenminister* (Minister of Foreign Affairs)[5]. In considering this proposal, we realized that another differentiation could also exist relative to the control of the uniform behavior of the twin couple. This activity is taken by a single twin who can be described as the *leader* twin. Obviously, spontaneous attributions such as these have their genesis in the psychological identity of the twin who is more qualified or suited to perform the task of Minister of Foreign Affairs or be the leader twin.

On occasion, the task of representing the twin pair to the outside world is not assumed by the same twin, but rather alternates between the co-twins. This latter phenomenon speaks for a greater similarity in the individual psychological identities.

Twins, science and ethics

It seems to me at the present moment that the study of twins is particularly useful to science because of the significance that the product of conception, that is, the zygote, assumes in the case of MZ twinning.

As you well know, owing to insemination *in vitro* and the noteworthy production of the products of conception that are nourished or preserved outside the body, the opinion that the beginnings of true human life take place some days after conception has gained ground, and that this extraordinary event is preceded by an undifferentiated period in which the products of conception are called a pre-embryo that can be the object of experimentation and destroyed, since it does not deal with true human life.

This theory, which has no objective reference, evidently collides with our experience in that we know the zygote does not produce an anodyne pre-embryo but divides into two secondary zygotes capable of producing two somatically identical individuals, though endowed with differentiated psychic personalities.

My thoughts concerning the unique identity of each individual twin, even in the case of MZ twins, are in accord with the spoken message of His Holiness John Paul II to the participants of the *VI International Congress of Twin Studies* (Rome, August 28, 1989), some of which I quote in the following passage:

'Indeed, twinning has proven to be a rich source of new biological data regarding the beginnings of human life. The comparison of biological processes present in twins has helped to clarify the extent to which both heredity and environment affect human life. As a result, the numerous developments within the field of Twin Studies serve to increase our knowledge, not only of questions concerned with the specific phenomenon of twinning: its appearance, as well as the problems it raises in terms of physiology, psychology and family or social adjustment.

The study of multiple pregnancy also tends to strengthen the conviction that *the defense of life and the dignity of the human person must be of paramount concern in all scientific research*. Similarly, recent developments in our understanding of the phenomenon of twinning have helped curtail a certain tendency which considered the termination of pregnancy a justifiable medical procedure. Such developments have also demonstrated the unacceptability in moral as well as in strictly scientific terms of all forms of genetic manipulation.'

References

1. Landy, H.S., Weiner, S., Corson, S.L. *et al.* (1986). The vanishing twin: ultrasonographic assessment of fetal disappearance in the first semester. *Am. J. Obstet. Gynecol.*, **155**, 14
2. Crumpacker, D.W., Cederlöf, L., Friberg, W.J. *et al.* (1979). A twin methodology for the study of genetic and environmental control of variation in human smoking behavior. *Acta Genet. Med. Gemellol.*, **23**, 173
3. Gedda, L. and Brenci, G. (1978). *Chronogenetics. The Inheritance of Biological Time.* (Springfield, IL: Charles C. Thomas)
4. Gedda, L. (1948). Psicologia della società intrageminale. *Riv. Psicol.*, **44**, 4
5. Bracken, H. (1939). Das Schreibtempe von zwillingen und den sozialenpsychologischen Fehlerquellen der zwilling forschung. *Ztshr. Menschl. Vererb. Konstitutionslehre*, **23**, 278

The twin method

P. Parisi

Introduction

Twins have been the object of great interest and a specific subject of enquiry since ancient times. Hippocrates and other Greek and Roman scholars discussed the twinning phenomenon at length, and their ideas were reiterated during the many centuries dominated by the Arabic and Salernitan schools of medicine down through modern times[1]. This interest, however, was confined to the etiology of twinning and to the clinical hazards of plural births, of which 19th century obstetricians were particularly aware, as documented by Duncan's early observations[2].

It was not until the second half of the 19th century that twins ceased to be regarded simply as a natural wonder and started to be considered as a possible subject for scientific research. The discipline of twin research is usually characterized as having begun in 1875, when the famous British scientist, Francis Galton, published in *Fraser's Magazine* what is now regarded as a classic paper entitled: 'The History of Twins, as a Criterion of the Relative Powers of Nature and Nurture'. This subject had already been treated in a cursory manner in Galton's 1874 book, *English Men of Science*, and the 1875 article was in turn followed by a revised version which appeared in 1876 in the *Journal of the Anthropological Institute*[3].

Galton is usually credited as the first to outline what then became universally known as 'the twin method'. Close review, however, shows that this is not really so. This issue has been examined in detail by Rende *et al.*[4], who noted that Galton only envisioned testing the power of the environment to change twins, by making initially similar twins different and initially different twins similar. The twin method, as we now call it, was in fact developed much later.

Galton's publications were not followed by additional studies until 1905, when Thorndike reported twin resemblances in cognitive tests. Thorndike, however, did not compare identical and non-identical twins, which is the essence of the twin method. He was in fact convinced that all twins were of the same kind – a view supported by the great biometrician Ronald A. Fisher in his 1919 paper on the genesis of twins. Not until the 1920s did it become obvious that, contrary to previous beliefs, twins were of two different kinds. Until then, the twin method was probably only 'in the air', but had not yet been truly developed and even lacked its theoretical basis.

The twin method finally materialized in 1924, when an article by the American psychologist Curtis Merriman and a book by the German dermatologist Hermann Siemens independently provided its first explicit description. These writings set the basis for the actual comparison of identical vs. non-identical twins that began to be made in the late 1920s[4].

Initially confined to the realm of psychology, and particularly to the study of the inheritance of intelligence, the twin method was soon applied to other areas in human biology. It was enthusiastically hailed as an easy means to overcome the natural limitations inherent in studies on humans, at least in terms of experimentation. Twinning represented, in a way, an experiment carried out by nature, which scientists could easily exploit.

From the 1930s and through the late 1950s, the twin method was applied to the study of widely differing human traits and conditions.

It contributed heavily to the early development of the new discipline of human genetics, for which it came to represent the method of election. The twin method is extremely well documented in Gedda's monumental handbook which reviewed more than five thousand references on the study of twins as of 1951. It was originally published in Italian, but was later translated into English, though unfortunately only in part[1].

Inevitably, perhaps, oversimplifications, indiscriminate applications, ill-designed studies and uncritical conclusions appeared in the literature. Moreover, in the cultural climate of the 1930s, profoundly influenced by hereditarian theories and ideologies, particularly in Europe, the study of twins, and more generally the implications of human genetic studies, were partly distorted in order to provide a basis for racial discrimination policies. Thus, following the end of World War II, when the ideological climate rapidly shifted towards the opposite extreme, a criticism of the twin method was raised, and doubts were cast on some of its basic assumptions[5]. As these doubts were emerging in scientific circles, starting with the late 1950s, the developments of cytogenetic, biochemical and molecular techniques permitted *direct* genetic analyses in humans and thus reduced the usefulness of the indirect approach provided by the twin method. As a result, the latter became much less popular and was considered obsolete by many.

As frequently happens, however, the crisis was beneficial, in that it stimulated a careful revision of the classic design and of its basic assumptions. Limitations and pitfalls were identified and corrected, and new approaches and methodologies were developed. By the mid-1970s, the scientific study of twins had entered a new stage of development, and a vast array of new applications became possible. These developments have already been described by the present author in a 1980 review[6] and in later accounts (see, for example, reference 7), of which this chapter represents in part an update.

Today, the study of twins represents a method of election in behavior genetics, developmental studies, matched-pair experimental designs and epidemiology[8]. At the same time, important applications are found in an increasing number of areas, particularly in psychology and psychiatry, medical genetics, reproductive biology and, of course, obstetrics and neonatology. In order to better understand the current implications and potentialities of the twin method, it is useful to re-examine its basic aspects, as well as its evolution and extensions.

The classic twin method and its basic assumptions

The classic twin method is based on a number of fundamental assumptions that stem from the nature of the twinning phenomenon and the different mechanisms by which it can occur.

As is well known, identical twins originate when, at some stage during the first 2 weeks following fertilization, the early embryo splits into two parts that subsequently develop separately and eventually give rise to two individuals. Because these two siblings originate from one and the same zygote, they are called monozygotic (MZ) twins. Clearly, these twins are genetically identical, which, in formal genetic terms, is enunciated by stating that, for any given gene, the probability, p, that it be identical in the two co-twins of any given MZ pair is $p = 1.00$. This implies that any difference existing between MZ co-twins must necessarily originate from environmental influences (where by *environment* one should understand *any* factor other than the specific gene under consideration). This is the first, and most fundamental assumption of the twin method.

The second recognized mechanism of twinning is polyovulation and consequent multiple fertilization. This phenomenon results in the simultaneous development of at least two embryos, and eventually in the birth of twins (or higher order multiples) that have originated from different zygotes. These siblings are therefore called dizygotic (DZ) in the case of twins, or polyzygotic in the case of higher order multiples. Genetically, these individuals are no more similar than any other pair of full siblings. Although it is frequently stated that these non-identical or 'fraternal' twins share 50% of their genes, that is not totally correct. Indeed, the similarity between two DZ twins can vary widely, and 50% genetic similarity should only be taken as an average. Once again, in classical genetic terms, for any given gene, the probability, p, that it be identical in the two co-twins of any given DZ pair is $p = 0.5$. Again, this is a probability, not a frequency.

Under these circumstances, whereas two MZ co-twins normally differ only as a result of environmental effects, two DZ co-twins can differ as a result of either genetic or environmental factors, or both, exactly as happens in non-twin siblings. On the other hand, precisely because they are also twins, DZ co-twins share with MZ co-twins a number of conditions that a pair of non-twin siblings would not share. In fact, DZ as well as MZ co-twins are always of the same age and have always been simultaneously exposed to the same prenatal environment. Moreover, they continue to share the same environment, at least to a large extent, in their postnatal life and for a considerable number of years.

The classic twin method assumes that the extent to which any given morphological, biochemical, functional or behavioral trait or condition exhibits a higher average within-pair similarity in MZ than DZ co-twins is a reflection of the extent to which that particular variable is under genetic control. For this assumption to hold general value, however, the method must further assume that, at least for the variable under study, genotypic and environmental variances in twins are the same as those in singletons, that is, that twins are representative of the general population.

These are the basic assumptions of the twin method. As previously noted, however, some of them have been questioned in the past and considered to represent possible sources of bias, so that the issue of the validity of these assumptions will now be addressed in some detail.

A revision of the assumptions

Mechanisms of twinning and possible genetic bias

It has frequently been asserted that the assumption that twins are either MZ or DZ may not be true because non-identical twins may not necessarily be DZ, but also possibly arise through other twinning mechanisms. Such twins would result from the double fertilization of ova that are not independent (as is true of DZ twinning), but have developed in one of the following ways: (1) from the same primary oocyte; (2) from the same secondary oocyte as a result of an equal, rather than the usual unequal, first or second meiotic division; or (3) from a subdivision of the ovum immediately before its fertilization. The resulting twins, collectively characterized as dispermatic or 'third-type' twins, would be genetically more similar than the usual DZ twins, and their presence in the twin sample would bias any comparison between MZ and DZ twins.

Although some evidence suggests that dispermatic twins might in fact occasionally occur in various animal groups, the possibility that they exist in humans is still little more than a speculation. In a classic monograph written in 1970, Bulmer noted that 'several lines of investigation have failed to reveal any evidence of the existence of a third type of twinning in man', and concluded that 'such twins must be very rare if they occur at all'[9]. No evidence has been produced since these comments were made that could substantially modify Bulmer's conclusion, in my opinion.

Regardless, even if dispermatic twins existed in humans to any appreciable extent, their effect would most probably be minimal. In fact, as a result of the genetic recombination occurring in the course of meiosis, hypothetical dispermatic co-twins would, after all, not be considerably more similar than DZ co-twins[9–11]. More specifically, co-twins originating from the simultaneous fertilization of the ovum and of a second gamete derived from the first polar body would be genetically *less* similar than two DZ twins, whereas co-twins originating from the simultaneous fertilization of two gametes derived from the second polar body would only be slightly more similar. In formal genetic terms, the probability that a given gene would be identical in two dispermatic twins varies as a function of its specific distance from the centromere (because of the different probability of crossing over); this probability will only rarely approach its upper limit at $p=0.75$, and will, as a rule, not very much exceed the value of $p=0.5$, or even be lower.

Two additional mechanisms of twinning are theoretically possible, though presumably uncommon, and should also be considered in this context for the sake of completeness. These are *superfecundation*, consisting in the fertilization of simultaneously released ova by sperms released in different coital acts, and *superfetation*, consisting in the fertilization of ova released in different menstrual cycles.

The resulting twins may differ in gestational age, but will be genetically as similar as any other pair of DZ twins. That may not be true in the event of twins of different fathers, however, as may happen if the mother had intercourse with two different men within a short period of time. In this case, the probability of identical genes in the two twins would be lowered to $p=0.25$. The presence of such twins (realistically unlikely) in any given sample of DZ twins would somewhat balance the equally hypothetical effect of possible dispermatic twins, thereby eventually confirming the value of $p=0.5$, a figure generally assumed to be the probability of identical genes in any sample of non-MZ twins.

These and related aspects of the biology of twinning have been dealt with at length in the literature, both in the past and in recent years (see, for example, references 9 and 12, as well as Chapters 3 and 4 in this book).

Possible antenatal bias and the problem of representativeness

Following publication of Bronson Price's widely quoted paper in 1950, 'Primary biases in twin studies'[5], it has become increasingly clear that the twin condition presents certain peculiarities that prevent a strict comparison of twins to singletons, and suggest that twins are not necessarily representative of the general population. Accordingly, it has been claimed that the results obtained through various applications of the twin method do not necessarily hold true.

For example, many complications of the twin pregnancy, aside from the associated high rate of prenatal and early postnatal mortality, affect the survivors in a variety of ways. For example, although twins generally experience a delay in mental and physical development as compared to singletons, longitudinal studies, and particularly the long-term follow-up of about 1000 twins from birth into adulthood carried out by the Louisville Twin Study, have consistently indicated that twins show a remarkable tendency to recover immediately after birth and eventually to catch up, after a few years, in most developmental variables[13].

A more specific problem related to twinning stems from the alterations in the placental circulation experienced by monochorionic twins. This anatomic aberration often results in the twin–twin transfusion syndrome. This antenatal condition has serious implications for development and survival and can produce important alterations in the twins' original constitution that may in turn bias the results of later twin comparisons. Because this problem only involves monochorionic twins, who represent about two-thirds of all MZ twins, theoretically all one has to do in order to avoid such bias is to isolate the monochorionic twins from the rest of the sample and analyze them separately[14]. However, the severity of the condition varies enormously and clearly not all traits are likely to be influenced by it to the same extent; in fact, many may not be influenced at all. Fortunately, the effects of many of these antenatal alterations are usually temporary, because longitudinal studies clearly show that these differences are rapidly overcome in the course of early postnatal development[13]. (Editor: A comprehensive discussion of the twin–twin transfusion syndrome is presented in Chapters 27–29.)

Regardless, in order to avoid any bias deriving from the possible peculiarities of the twins, it is useful to ascertain that the twins are indeed comparable to singletons with respect to the trait or condition under study. A similar procedure can be adopted in order to check the comparability of twin subsamples, such as monochorionic vs. dichorionic. Simple tests, based on comparisons of sample means and variances, have been designed to that effect[15].

In this way, when the necessary caution is used, the problem of representativeness can be overcome, the various comparisons can be instituted, and the conclusions reached by applying the twin method can be generalized.

The problem of the common environment

Another fundamental objection to the twin method, particularly as applied to the study of psychological and behavioral variables, refers to the problem of a possible environmental bias stemming from the common environment the twins share in their postnatal life. It has been claimed that environmental influences, and particularly parental behavior, tend to stress similarity between MZ co-twins, whereas in DZ co-twins dissimilarity is favored. If true, this behavioral variation would bias similarity measures and overestimate genetic effects.

Such an argument has frequently been used to cast doubt on the results of twin studies that indicate a relevant role of inheritance in traits such as intelligence, personality and other psychological or behavioral measures. Given the considerable sensitivity of such delicate areas of human variability, and considering the simplistic character of some of these studies, it is not surprising that some psychologists and educators, perhaps greatly influenced by 'progressive' ideologies and inclined to consider the human mind and behavior as primarily or solely influenced by culture and society[16], may have somewhat uncritically endorsed this point of view and even harshly rejected[17] the results of decades of twin studies consistently giving the same picture. However, this claim has never been substantiated to any meaningful degree and, even assuming that some parental bias might actually occur, the existing evidence seems to indicate that its effects would be unlikely to play any relevant role.

First of all, the physical appearance of the twins at birth may be misleading. Within-pair correlations for weight and size, for instance, are higher in DZ than in MZ co-twins[13]. The effects of the twin–twin transfusion syndrome can initially mask the genetic resemblance of MZ co-twins, and additional confounding effects can be produced by the frequent occurrence of birth trauma and other complications. Thus, similarity may take some time to become evident. In this respect, it is interesting to note that, whereas the choice of the twins' names appears to be influenced by zygosity, this is not in the manner critics would expect. In reality, the similarity of names appears to be higher in DZ than in MZ and opposite-sex twins[18].

Early infant care and child-rearing practises are unlikely to be more similar for MZ than for DZ co-twins. The few reports supporting differential treatment might actually be biased, having been obtained by interviewing parents long after the birth of their twins, when their impressions might be influenced by the similarities or differences that have meanwhile become apparent. As for adult MZ co-twins, they are indeed more similar than DZ co-twins in terms of having the same friends, studying together, etc., but it is questionable whether this is due to parental behavior and/or other environmental influences, or whether it results from individual tendencies of a genetic nature.

At any rate, speculations on the existence and effects of such forms of environmental bias have been overcome by the results of two studies that have clarified the issue experimentally[19,20]. A measure supposedly very much exposed to potential bias was taken into account, that is, the intelligence quotient (IQ), and within-pair IQ differences were compared in pairs correctly and incorrectly classified by their parents in terms of zygosity. The result was that the pairs erroneously classified provided results similar to those of the pairs correctly classified, showing that, even assuming differential parental treatment, this clearly had not affected within-pair similarity. It was concluded that 'Until strong evidence shows that parental bias results in an exaggeration of differences between identical and fraternal twins, the rejection of data accruing from the study of twins does not seem warranted on empirical grounds'[20]. This conclusion still holds true today and has not been challenged.

Twin data ascertainment

Samples and populations

The first problem one has to face in order to conduct a twin study consists, of course, in finding the twins. This is a very delicate process, and it is fairly easy and common to incur various forms of ascertainment bias which may then invalidate the entire study.

Any process of ascertainment must be conducted in such a way as to obtain a sample that, although necessarily selected with respect to a number of criteria stemming from the study design (age, sex, condition, etc.), must otherwise be random with respect to all other variables, making it representative of the specific population to which the results of the study should apply (such as the population of all the subjects affected by a given condition). Ascertaining a twin sample may present a double problem, in that the twins may have to be referred to the population of all twins, as well as to the population of all the subjects with the specific condition under study. The definition of the reference population(s) is therefore very important and must be clearly made when the study is designed.

As previously noted, it is always desirable to make sure that the twins are indeed representative of the reference population by instituting specific comparisons, both with respect to the general population and between subsamples, such as monochorionic vs. dichorionic twin pairs[15].

Other, somewhat more general criteria must also be considered in the process of ascertainment. Samples collected through announcements and similar procedures are usually non-random, because of the presumably higher motivation of the respondents that may in turn be related to specific problems or peculiarities that may make them not representative of the general population. Samples from hospital populations are also subject to bias, because of the specific risks related to the twin condition, among other reasons. Obviously, for many research purposes, some selection may be necessary, and in other cases it may be irrelevant and introduce no bias.

Clearly, when one combines the prevalence of the condition under study with the prevalence of twins and the need to subdivide them into subsamples (by sex, zygosity, etc.), it may prove difficult to end up with a truly random sample of sufficient size. The problem can be solved if the ascertainment is based on sufficiently large and representative strata of the general population (such as school students, military conscripts, and the like), or better, on population-based twin registers, as are now available in many areas of the world (for examples, see references 21–23).

Zygosity determination

An important problem related to ascertainment is the necessary subdivision of the sample into classes, usually by sex combination and zygosity (and sometimes placentation, age, or other variables). This necessarily requires the assessment of zygosity. Opposite-sex pairs are obviously DZ and, in most cases it is desirable to consider them in a separate class (MF). Monochorial pairs can be considered as MZ and should, whenever possible, also be considered separately (MC). In many cases, however, the information on placentation may either not be available or not be fully reliable. If so, not only the dichorial (DC), but also all the same-sex pairs (MM and FF) need to be classified. The subject of twin zygosity determination will be examined in detail in later chapters of this book, but a few general comments are in order none the less.

Essentially, zygosity can be determined, through *objective* or *subjective* criteria. The former consist in the analysis of blood groups and/or other genetic polymorphisms in all same-sex pairs: the higher the number of systems tested, the higher the probability that DZ pairs be detected because of discordance(s). Concordant pairs, however, are not necessarily MZ, because there always remains a probability (however slight) that two DZ co-twins be concordant for all the genetic polymorphisms tested. Thus, a diagnosis of monozygosity is always problematic to some degree, and its probability of error (that is, the probability that the pair be actually DZ) declines as the number of concordant polymorphisms observed increases. Cost-efficiency should be considered in selecting the systems of zygosity detection, because not all of them have the same power. Most recently, the application of DNA fingerprinting techniques has made objective zygosity determination easier and more reliable[24]. Its use, however, is not yet widespread. (See Chapter 47.)

As for subjective criteria, these now essentially consist in the use of specific questionnaires, validated against objective methods[25]. However, the application of these criteria should be restricted to large samples, such as are frequently used in studies of an epidemiological nature.

Finally, in the case of population data (vital statistics, large registers, etc.), the well-known Weinberg's method can be used. Because in the general population the departure from equality of the two sexes at birth is not large, the four sex combinations possible for DZ pairs (MM, FF, MF, FM) are assumed to be equally probable at $p = 0.25$. Let d and m be the estimates of DZ and MZ pairs, respectively, and $U = MF + FM$ be the number of unlike-sex pairs, and the equations will be: $d = 2U$ and $m = 1 - d$. In other words, the number of DZ pairs is estimated by doubling the number of opposite-sex pairs (on the assumption that an equal number of DZ pairs be of the same sex), whereas the number of MZ pairs is estimated by difference (total number of pairs minus estimated number of DZ pairs). Hence the name of 'difference method' given to this approach. Although its validity has frequently been questioned[10], Weinberg's method still appears to give sufficiently reliable results with large numbers.

Twin data analysis

Once the twin sample has been collected and each twin has been examined with respect to the trait or condition under consideration, the data are typically analyzed in terms of comparison of within-pair similarity in MZ vs. DZ pairs. These measures are then used to derive an estimate of the importance of hereditary factors in the determination of the trait under consideration. Various formulas were developed in the past to that effect; however, doubt has been cast on the actual value and theoretical background of these heritability estimates, so that corrections and somewhat more complex approaches have been introduced in recent years.

Concordance studies (qualitative analysis)

If the study is concerned with a categorical, all-or-none variable, such as a disease or other qualitative condition, the analysis essentially considers the number of pairs in which both partners show the condition (*concordant pairs*) vs. those in which only one twin shows it (*discordant pairs*), and the rate of concordance (number of concordant pairs/total number of pairs) is then compared in the two zygosity classes.

Concordance studies, particularly those concerned with specific diseases, require that problems of ascertainment be very carefully considered. As extensively discussed by Allen and Hrubec[26], two stages may be required to correctly estimate twin concordance rate. The first stage, involving the ascertainment of the condition in the general population or population sample, is likely to underestimate the actual number of concordant pairs, so that further investigation of pairs found to be discordant on primary ascertainment is required. Secondary ascertainment usually leads to the discovery of additional concordant pairs. This two-stage sequential model has recently been challenged by Kendler and Eaves[27] who proposed instead a model based on survival analysis as a more realistic approach to the problems of ascertainment bias in twin concordance studies.

When reliable measures of concordance have been obtained, heritability estimates can be derived. An easy formula was classically used to that effect:

$$HC = (CMZ - CDZ)/(1 - CDZ) \quad (Eq.\ 1)$$

where HC is the heritability estimate and CMZ and CDZ are the proportions of concordant pairs in the two zygosity classes.

Smith[28] later developed a transformation table of proband concordance rate into an index of genetic determination, G, that frequently yields unrealistic values, larger than 1. For that reason, Allen[29] proposed to use the revised formula,

$$H'C = (CMZ - CDZ)/CMZ$$
$$= 1 - CDZ/CMZ \quad (Eq.\ 2)$$

except when $CMZ + CDZ > 1$, in which case Eq. 1 may still be preferable.

The twin correlations in liability to illness (r) calculated through Smith's approach[28] have more recently been used[27] to estimate the heritability of liability to disease (h^2), the effect of common environment (c^2) and the effect of random environment (e^2), according to the following formulas:

$$h^2 = 2(rMZ - rDZ) \quad (Eq.\ 3)$$
$$c^2 = rDZ - rMZ \quad (Eq.\ 4)$$
$$e^2 = 1 - (h^2 + c^2) \quad (Eq.\ 5)$$

Continuous variables (quantitative analysis)

The analysis of twin data for continuous variables has classically consisted in the calculation of within-pair correlations or variance and the subsequent estimation of some coefficient describing the relative importance of genetic vs. environmental factors in the determination of the trait under study. In addition to the original heritability estimates introduced by Holzinger in 1929[30],

$$H_1 = (varDZ - varMZ)/varDZ \quad (Eq.\ 6)$$
$$H_2 = (rMZ - rDZ)/(1 - rDZ) \quad (Eq.\ 7)$$

a number of revisions have been suggested over the years[31–33], e.g.:

Falconer (1960)[31]:
$$h^2 = 2(rMZ - rDZ) \quad (Eq.\ 8)$$

Nichols (1965)[32]:
$$HR = 2(rMZ - rDZ)/rMZ = h^2/rMZ \quad (Eq.\ 9)$$

Vandenberg (1965)[33]:
$$F = varDZ/varMZ = 1/(1 - H_1) \quad (Eq.\ 10)$$

Further improvements were suggested in the late 1960s by Jensen[34] and Elston and Gottesman[35], among others. In the same years, a more comprehensive approach was developed by Cattel[36,37] and improved by Loehlin[38], the Multiple Abstract Variance Analysis (MAVA). This was based on the comparison of within- and between-family variances of full and half-sib families, as well as MZ and DZ twin pairs, and was useful in assessing not only the importance of genetic vs. environmental factors, but also the correlation between the two. The MAVA approach was a considerable improvement, because many of the past criticisms of the twin method concerned the controversial nature of heritability estimates because of the highly composite nature of the total variance. Let us examine this issue somewhat closer, so that the more recent developments of the biometric genetic analysis of twin data can be better appreciated.

The partitioning of variance Given a specific trait, or phenotype (P), total variance (V_P) can be partitioned into one component determined by genetic factors (V_G) and one determined by environmental factors (V_E), according to the classic formulation,

$$V_P = V_G + V_E \quad (Eq.\ 11)$$

The ratio, V_G/V_P ($\times 100$), giving the percentage of variance determined by genetic factors, is precisely what allows investigators to derive a heritability estimate that typically tends to 1 (implying 100% genetic determination) when V_E tends to 0, whereas heritability tends to 0 (implying 100% environmental determination) when V_G tends to 0.

This approach, however, is somewhat simplistic. In fact, G and E are not necessarily alternative forces but can interact and/or be correlated to some extent. Therefore, Eq. 11 should be rewritten as follows:

$$V_P = V_G + V_E + V_{GE} + V_{G \times E} \qquad (Eq.\ 12)$$

where V_{GE} indicates the interactions, and $V_{G \times E}$ the correlations, between genetic and environmental factors.

It should then be noted that both the genetic and the environmental variances can in turn be partitioned into a variety of components, not all of which are easy to estimate. In particular, the total genetic variance consists of one basic component resulting from the sum total of the effects of each individual gene, and therefore called additive variance (V_A), as well as in additional components. The latter derive from gene interactions, on account of dominance effects (D) and of the effects of the interactions of all other genes with the specific gene(s) under consideration (I). Therefore, the genetic variance should actually be partitioned as follows:

$$V_G = V_A + V_D + V_I \qquad (Eq.\ 13)$$

Modern approaches to the quantitative analysis of twin data One reason for some of the past criticism of the twin method is that the classical heritability coefficients can estimate only the additive portion of the genetic variance, whereas the effects of dominance and gene interactions, as well as of genotype × environment correlations and interactions, remain unknown.

This problem has, however, been solved in recent years following a classic paper by Jinks and Fulker[39], who extended Fisher's biometric genetic analysis to the quantitative analysis of twin data, with a general approach in which the classic estimates and the MAVA approach were included as special cases. These techniques, increasingly developed and extended since the late 1970s by a number of authors[40–43], allow a general treatment of the different variance components, providing specific estimates for dominance, gene interaction, shared environment and other effects.

Essentially, the within-pair and between-pair mean squares are calculated for the MZ and DZ twins, or even other subsamples, and their values are interpreted in terms of a theoretical model describing the different contributions to the total variation. Model-based estimates of the various parameters are obtained and the fit of the model to the actual data can then be assessed by the likelihood ratio χ^2 test. In this way, best-fitting procedures provide maximum likelihood estimates of additive genetic variation as well as shared family environment, individual environment, or other variance components. Alternative models postulating different sources of variability can be tested and the most adequate and parsimonious model can thus be identified. Specific computer programs have been developed to that effect, such as LISREL-VI (analysis of linear structural relationships by maximum likelihood, instrumental variables and least squares methods). A number of accounts and applications of this program, and more generally of model-fitting procedures, can be found in the recent literature[44–46].

Conclusions

The past two decades have witnessed a general process of revision of the twin method, the results of which have gone far beyond its original aims. Essentially intended to address various criticisms to which the twin method had been exposed, particularly with respect to the potential bias in its basic assumptions the revision has not only served to reject unwarranted contentions as well as identify and correct past limitations and pitfalls, but has, in addition, extended to the development of new and highly powerful methodologies for twin data analysis. At the same time, a number of variations of the classic twin study design have been developed or implemented.

These include, in particular, the study of twins reared apart (see references 47 and 48, for reviews of past studies, and 22 for an account of the more recent Minnesota Twin Study), or of the offspring of MZ co-twins (half-sib method[49]), as powerful means to control for shared environment effects. The incorporation of other family members in twin data analysis can also add greater efficiency to the estimation of the different genetic and non-genetic effects.

A completely different approach, essentially experimental in nature, is the so-called *co-twin control study*, in which MZ pairs are broken so as to have one twin in the experimental sample and the other twin in the control sample. This is a very powerful approach to the testing of the actual effect of any kind of variable (a treatment, a drug, a habit such as smoking or drinking, etc.), all other factors in the exposed and the non-exposed MZ co-twins being equal, and thus controlled for. (For a detailed treatment, see reference 50.)

As already noted[6,8], the study of twins is far from obsolete, as its critics had sometimes contended, and has particularly flourished in the past couple of decades. Today, twin studies have come to represent the most incisive technique in human behavior genetics and to provide substantial contributions in the most varied areas of human biology, medicine and psychology.

Also, thanks to the advent of high-speed computers, elegant techniques have been developed for the multivariate analysis of twin and family data, as well as the detection of developmental changes in gene expression through the analysis of longitudinal data. Powerful techniques have also been applied to the analysis of variables of clinical interest, particularly in relation to cardiovascular disease. Clinical conditions of great relevance, such as coronary heart disease, diabetes, obesity, mental illness, cancer, ageing processes, etc., are being studied with increasing success. Meanwhile, the development of molecular genetic techniques should eventually provide powerful new approaches to the use of twins in the assessment of the contribution of any given portion of the human genome to the genetic variation of any measurable phenotype. Even the study of the twinning phenomenon per se (see, for example, reference 20) is proving of great importance to many aspects of reproductive biology, embryology and teratology.

The study of twins has been the object of a growing literature over the past couple of decades and appears to represent today an active field of research, increasingly characterized by relevant achievements and promising perspectives for further developments and applications.

References

1. Gedda, L. (1961). Studio dei Gemelli. Roma: Orizzonte Medico, 1951. English translation of first part: *Twins in History and Science*, pp. 21–24. (Springfield, IL: Charles C. Thomas)
2. Duncan, J.M. (1865). On the comparative frequency of twin bearing in different pregnancies. *Edinburgh Med. J.*, **10**, 928
3. Galton, F. (1876). The history of twins, as a criterion of the relative powers of nature and nurture. *Fraser's Magazine*, Nov. 1875. Reprinted, with revisions and additions, in *J. Anthropol. Inst.*, **5**, 391
4. Rende, R.D., Plomin, R. and Vandenberg, S.G. (1990). Who discovered the twin method? *Behav. Genet.*, **20**, 227
5. Price, B. (1950). Primary biases in twin studies. *Am. J. Hum. Genet.*, **2**, 293
6. Parisi, P. (1980). Methodology of twin studies: a general introduction. In Johnston, F.E., Roche, A.F. and Susanne, C. (eds.) *Human Physical Growth and Maturation: Methodologies and Factors*, pp. 243–63. (New York and London: Plenum Press)
7. Parisi, P. (1990). L'étude des jumeaux dans la recherche scientifique. In Papiernik, E. and Pons, J.C. (eds.) *L'Etude des Jumeaux dans la Recherche Scientifique*, pp. 411–22. (Paris: Editions Doin)
8. Nance, W.E. and Parisi, P. (1987). New approaches in twin research: applications in genetic epidemiology. In Vogel, F. and Sperling, K. (eds.) *Human Genetics*, pp. 390–3. (Berlin, Heidelberg, New York: Springer Verlag)
9. Bulmer, M.G. (1970). *The Biology of Twinning in Man.* (Oxford: Clarendon Press)

10. Elston, R.C. and Boklage, C.E. (1978). An examination of fundamental assumptions of the twin method. In Nance, W.E., Allen, G. and Parisi, P. (eds.) *Twin Research*, Part A, pp. 189–99. (New York: Alan R. Liss)
11. Goldgar, D.E. and Kimberling, W.J. (1981). Genetic expectations of polar body twinning. *Acta Genet. Med. Gemellol.*, **30**, 257
12. Parisi, P. (1989). Biology of twinning. In Meisami, E. and Timiras, P. (eds.) *Handbook of Human Growth and Developmental Biology*, pp. 207–28. (Boca Raton, FL: CRC Press)
13. Wilson, R.S. (1986). Genetic influence on growth and maturation. In Malina, R.M. and Bouchard, C. (eds.) *Sports and Human Genetics*. (Champaign, IL: Human Kinetics)
14. Corey, L.A., Nance, W.E., Kang, K.W. and Christian, J.C. (1979). Effects of type of placentation on birthweight and its variability in monozygotic and dizygotic twins. *Acta Genet. Med. Gemellol.*, **28**, 41
15. Christian, J.C. (1979). Testing twin means and estimating genetic variance. Basic methodology for the analysis of quantitative twin data. *Acta Genet. Med. Gemellol.*, **28**, 35
16. Kamin, K. (1974). *The Science and Politics of IQ*. (New York: John Wiley)
17. Hirsch, J. (1981). To unfrock the charlatans. *Sage Race Relations Abst.*, **6**, 1
18. Vandenberg, S.G. (1976). Twin studies. In Kaplan, A.R. (ed.) *Human Behavior Genetics*, pp. 90–150. (Springfield, IL: Charles C. Thomas)
19. Scarr, S. (1968). Environmental bias in twin studies. *Eugen. Q.*, **15**, 34
20. Matheny, A.P. (1979). Appraisal of parental bias in twin studies: ascribed zygosity and IQ differences in twins. *Acta Genet. Med. Gemellol.*, **28**, 155
21. Kaprio, J., Koskenvuo, M. and Rose, R.J. (1990). Population-based twin registries: illustrative applications in genetic epidemiology and behavior genetics from the Finnish Twin Cohort Study. *Acta Genet. Med. Gemellol.*, **39**, 427
22. Lykken, D.T., Bouchard, T.J., McGue, M. and Tellegen, A. (1990). The Minnesota Twin Family Registry: some initial findings. *Acta Genet. Med. Gemellol.*, **39**, 35
23. Pedersen, N.L., McClearn, G.E., Plomin, R. *et al.* (1991). The Swedish adoption twin study of aging: an update. *Acta Genet. Med. Gemellol.*, **40**, 7
24. Machin, G.A. (1990). Definitive methods of zygosity determination in twins: relevance to problems in the biology of twinning. *Acta Genet. Med. Gemellol.*, **39**, 459
25. Kasriel, J. and Eaves, L.J. (1976). The zygosity of twins: further evidence on the agreement between diagnosis by blood groups and written questionnaires. *J. Biosoc. Sci.*, **8**, 263
26. Allen, G. and Hrubec, Z. (1979). Twin concordance: a more general model. *Acta Genet. Med. Gemellol.*, **28**, 3
27. Kendler, K.S. and Eaves, L.J. (1989). The estimation of probandwise concordance in twins: the effect of unequal ascertainment. *Acta Genet. Med. Gemellol.*, **38**, 253
28. Smith, C. (1974). Concordance in twins: methods and interpretations. *Am. J. Hum. Genet.*, **26**, 454
29. Allen, G. (1979). Holzinger's Hc revised. *Acta Genet. Med. Gemellol.*, **28**, 161
30. Holzinger, K.J. (1929). The relative effect of nature and nurture on twin differences. *J. Educ. Psychol.*, **20**, 241
31. Falconer, D.S. (1960). *Introduction to Quantitative Genetics*. (Edinburgh: Oliver & Boyd)
32. Nichols, R.C. (1965). The National Merit Twin Study. In Vandenberg, S.G. (ed.) *Methods and Goals in Human Behavior Genetics*. (New York: Academic Press)
33. Vandenberg, S.G. (1965). Multivariate analysis in twin differences. In Vandenberg, S.G. (ed.) *Methods and Goals in Human Behavior Genetics*. (New York: Academic Press)
34. Jensen, A.R. (1970). IQs of identical twins reared apart. *Behav. Genet.*, **1**, 133
35. Elston, R.C. and Gottesman, I.I. (1968). The analysis of quantitative inheritance simultaneously from twin and family data. *Am. J. Hum. Genet.*, **20**, 512
36. Cattel, R.B. (1960). The Multiple Abstract Variance Analysis. Equations and solutions for nature–nurture research on continuous variables. *Psychol. Rev.*, **67**, 353
37. Cattel, R.B. (1965). Methodological and conceptual advances in evaluating hereditary and environmental influences and their interactions. In Vandenberg, S.G. (ed.) *Methods and Goals in Human Behavior Genetics*. (New York: Academic Press)
38. Loehlin, J.C. (1965). Some methodological problems in Cattel's Multiple Abstract Variance Analysis. *Psychol. Rev.*, **72**, 156
39. Jinks, J.L. and Fulker, D.W. (1970). Comparison of the biometrical, genetical, MAVA, and classical approaches to the analysis of human behavior. *Psychol. Bull.*, **73**, 311

40. Eaves, L.J., Last, K., Martin, N.G. and Jinks, J.L. (1977). A progressive approach to non-additivity and genotype–environmental covariance in the analysis of human differences. *Br. J. Math. Stat. Psychol.*, **30**, 1
41. Eaves, L.J., Last, K.A., Young, P.A. and Martin, N.G. (1978). Model-fitting approaches to the analysis of human behaviour. *Heredity*, **41**, 249
42. Fulker, D.W. (1978). Multivariate extensions of a biometrical model of twin data. In Nance, W.E., Allen, G. and Parisi, P. (eds.) *Twin Research*, Part A, pp. 217–36. (New York: Alan R. Liss)
43. Fulker, D.W. (1982). Extensions of the classical twin method. In Bonné-Tamir, B. (ed.) *Human Genetics*, Part A. (New York: Alan R. Liss)
44. Heath, A.C., Neale, M.C., Hewitt, J.K., Eaves, L.J. and Fulker, D.W. (1989). Testing structural equation models for twin data using LISREL-VI: hypothesis testing. *Behav. Genet.*, **19**, 9
45. Neale, M.C., Heath, A.C., Hewitt, J.K., Eaves, L.J. and Fulker, D.W. (1989). Fitting genetic models with LISREL: hypothesis testing. *Behav. Genet.*, **19**, 37
46. Hewitt, J.K., Stunkard, A.J., Carroll, D., Sims, J. and Turner, J.R. (1991). A twin study approach towards understanding genetic contributions to body size and metabolic rate. *Acta Genet. Med. Gemellol.*, **40**, 133
47. Shields, J. (1979). MZA twins: their use and abuse. In Nance, W.E., Allen, G. and Parisi, P. (eds.) *Twin Research*, Part A, pp. 79–93. (New York: Alan Liss)
48. Farber, S.L. (1981). *Identical Twins Reared Apart: A Reanalysis.* (New York: Basic Books)
49. Nance, W.E. (1976). Genetic studies of the offspring of identical twins. A model for the analysis of quantitative inheritance in man. *Acta Genet. Med. Gemellol.*, **25**, 103
50. Hrubec, Z. (1981). Methodologic problems in matched-pair studies using twins. In Gedda, L., Parisi, P. and Nance, W.E. (eds.) *Twin Research 3*, Part C, pp. 1–7. (New York: Alan R. Liss)

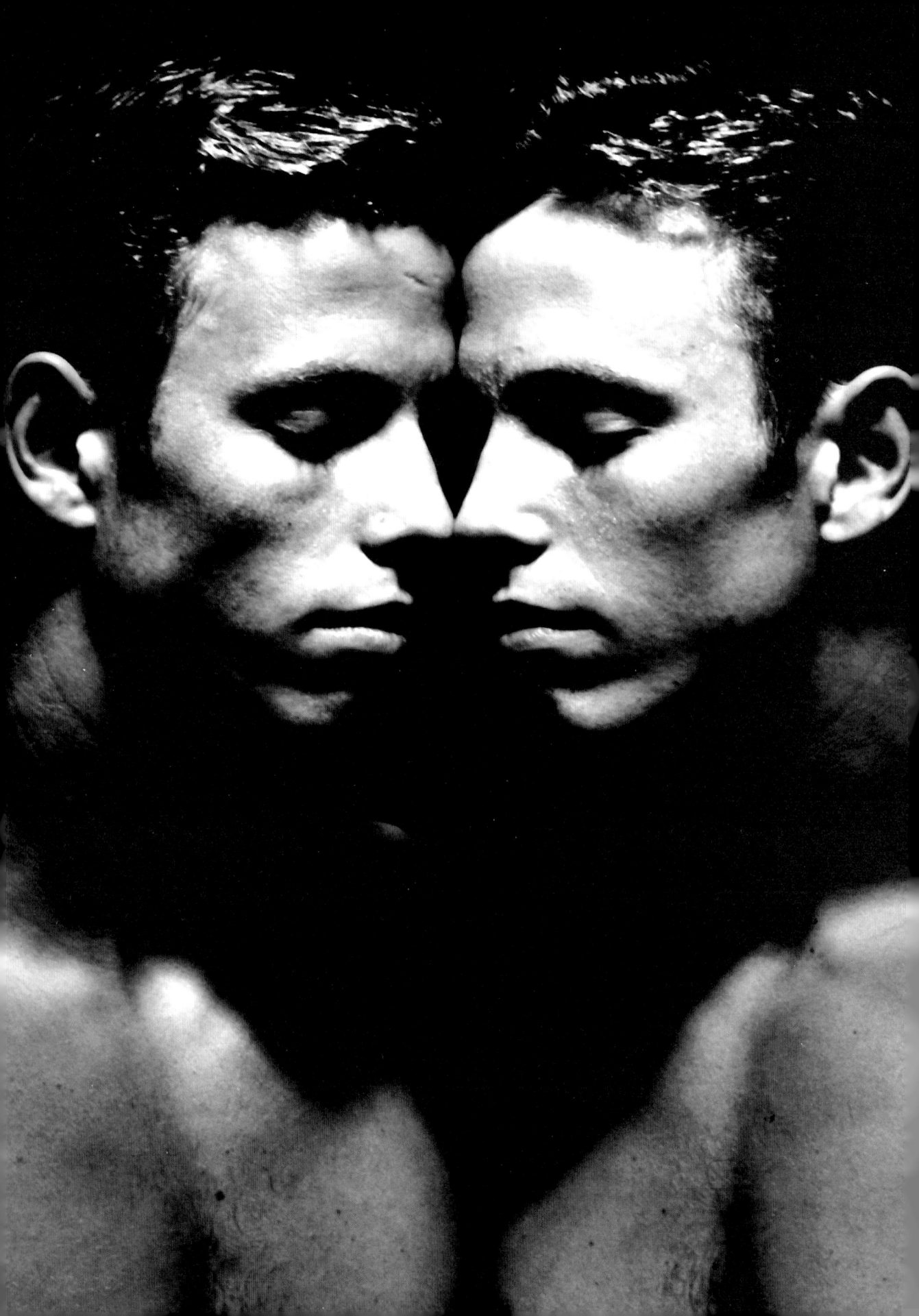

section II
Biology

Untitled

David Teplica, 1994,
Collection of the Artist, Chicago, Illinois

The mechanism of monozygosity and double ovulation

O. Bomsel-Helmreich and W. Al Mufti

Introduction

Multifetal pregnancies are associated with various ante- and perinatal conditions that justifiably characterize them as high risk; however it is not generally appreciated that the biologic mechanisms underlying twinning are particularly complex. For the most part, they begin prior to fertilization. This chapter will review those factors known or thought to influence the early embryonic division that leads to monozygotic (MZ) twins and the growth of two ovulatory follicles in the same cycle, a process that leads to dizygotic (DZ) twins.

Monozygotic twinning

Monozygotic twins result from the division of one embryo. Both halves carry the same genetic heritage and hence are of the same sex. In mammals, the MZ condition is rare. Its frequency is about one per thousand. In contrast, the di- or polyzygotic condition is the rule in most species that bear more than one offspring per conception.

In humans, the frequency of MZ twins ranges from 3.5 to 5.0 per thousand. The figure of 4.0 per thousand is most often quoted and probably is close to the median. Regardless, this frequency corresponds to about one third the number of DZ twins. Because of the high incidence of malformation, the probability of antenatal mortality among MZ twins is much higher than it is among either DZ twins or singletons. In addition, major malformations are found in 2.3% of MZ twins compared to 1% of singletons, and minor malformations are found in 4.1% of MZ twins compared to 2.5% in singletons[2]. Thirty-five per cent of MZ twins are left-handed, a rate which is double that in the general population; speech laterality is five times more frequent[1]. The most vulnerable type of MZ twin is monoamniotic, monochorionic (MC–MA); in addition, male–male pairs fare less well than female–female pairs[2].

Definition

The division of a single embryo into two equal halves must in reality be described as an accident. The actual division takes place during the first 14 days following fertilization. The timing of the separation can be deduced from a later study of the membranes. In 18% to 36% of cases, separation occurs between the zygote and morula stage, that is, up to 120 h postfertilization. Such embryos are dichorionic–diamnionic (DC–DA). When the division occurs later, as it does in 60–70% of cases at the blastocyst stage from D5 to D7, the resulting embryos are monochorionic–diamnionic (MC–DA). Separation rarely occurs (1%) after D8, and these embryos are monochorionic–monoamniotic (MC–MA) (see Chapter 9).

Conjoined twins represent the rarest type of MZ twins and the result from division at a much later stage. Their frequency generally is 1 in 200 MZ pairs or 1 per 33 000 births, although some geographic variations in this frequency exist. In the USA, for example, the frequency of conjoined twins is 1 in 200 000; in Japan it is 1 in 100 000, in India 1 in 2800, and in Uganda 1 in 4200[3]. Possibly the abnormally high frequency of these latter two countries does not correspond to the real incidence, as only deliveries registered in hospitals are recorded. Regardless of parentage, 70% of conjoined twins are females, most likely because the higher general vulnerability of male twins leads to their earlier demise and elimination via spontaneous abortion.

Experimental production of MZ twins in mammals

The experimental production of MZ twins in mammals represents the ideal means for studying the differential effect of heredity vs. environment, because until a certain stage, embryonic cells are toti- or equipotential. Stated another way, they retain their ability to create a normal individual. This stage represents the optimal time for separation of blastomeres. A review of some experimental animal work follows.

As early as 1952, Seidel[4] destroyed one blastomere of a rabbit embryo at the two-cell stage and transferred the remaining blastomere to a host rabbit. It continued to develop as a normal embryo. Somewhat later, Tarkowski[5] performed the same type of experiment in the mouse. He destroyed one blastomere and re-implanted the remaining one with equally positive results. During the last 10 years, monozygotic twins have been produced in larger mammals by bisection of even more advanced embryos, i.e. morulas or blastocysts. Willadsen[6] separated blastomeres from embryos of sheep, cattle and horses varying from the two-cell to the morula stage. After transfer, he obtained a number of multiples. Moore et al.[7] transferred one blastomere of an eight-cell rabbit embryo and obtained a newborn. Taken as a group, these experiments support the concept that blastomeres retain their totipotentiality at the eight-cell stage in the mammal.

Once the compaction (morula) stage is reached, the cells, by their topographical position, differentiate into external or internal cells that eventually become trophectoderm and the inner cell mass, respectively. Until the 32-cell stage, however, compensatory crossing from external into internal cells (or vice versa) is possible. In other words, until blastocyst formation, embryonic cell differentiation is not fixed[8]. This long duration of totipotentiality explains the later division of some twins at the inner cell mass stage, and the possibility of more or less equal divisions because of compensatory mechanisms.

Totipotentiality notwithstanding, experimental separation of blastomeres, even at an early stage, occasionally fails to produce identical individuals. After separation and transfer of all cells of a four-cell mare embryo into four different mothers, only two ponies were obtained[9]. The fact that they were born 23 days apart and had different birth weights was related to the surrogate mother in each instance. However, the different hide markings of the two animals suggests that the embryonic micromanipulation may have altered the normal genetic expectation to some unknown degree.

Patterns of separation in the human

Early separation

The existence of DC–DA monozygotic twins provides proof of separation in the first 5 days after fertilization. The existence of MZ twins with different karyotypes provides another confirmation. One of them always has one chromosome less than the other, e.g. one is $2n$, the other is a trisomic 21. The zygote is necessarily trisomic 21; at the first cleavage division which is followed by the twinning separation of the two blastomeres, one chromosome, the supplementary 21, is lost from the mitotic spindle so that it is lacking in one of the blastomeres. The most striking case is the one described by Turpin et al.[10], a monozygotic twin pair with different sex: one a boy XY; the other a girl, XO. Since these individuals were not mosaic, separation should have taken place at the two-cell stage of an originally XY zygote with an error of mitotic division.

The existence of natural quintuplets provides evidence that some embryos are able to divide repeatedly at very early stages. Sixty cases of spontaneous quintuplets were recorded between the beginning of the last century and 1950[11]. Of these, only two sets survived beyond adolescence, one in Canada (Dionne, 1935) and the other in Argentina (Deligentis, 1943). The Argentine quintuplets originated in a double ovulation: one XY oocyte divided once, and one XX oocyte divided twice, so that two MZ boys and three MZ girls were born. The Dionne quintuplets apparently started as MZ twins that underwent three consequent divisions; a sixth embryo was dead *in utero*. The last pair (by division) was the least similar to the others. Despite improvement of perinatal care since the 1950s and consequently an increase of MZ twins[12], only one other case where all MZ quintuplets have survived has been reported[13]. Since the middle 1960s, more surviving quintuplets were born but mostly after ovulation induction; in consequence, they are most probably polyzygotic.

Late separation

MC–MA twins separate late, i.e. after 8 days. However, neither the moment nor the manner of this separation is well understood, especially in MZ twins with mirror image differences for handedness or hair whorls[1]. The perfect, albeit rare, example of internal mirror imaging is the situs inversus observed in MZ and particularly in conjoined twins[14]. Numerous MZ twins are discordant for anomalies or diseases, e.g. anencephaly or diabetes. Loevy *et al.*[15] reported MZ twins who both exhibited trisomy 21 but were discordant for other major anomalies. The phenomenon of regularly occurring later separation and discordancy is best illustrated in animals, however. For example, the polyembryonic armadillo produces up to ten monozygotic embryos with discordance of phenotypic and biochemical markers[16].

Another hypothesis of the origin of discordance in MZ twins is suggested by the random unequal X inactivation. As this occurs very early in embryonic development, depending on the number of cells present, gene expression might differ during somatic development so that phenotypic differences may exist between the twins. Examples are numerous: glucose-6-phosphate dehydrogenase deficiency, color blindness, muscular dystrophy, etc. Genome imprinting (genes inherited from either parent do not always behave the same way) may be an additional source of variation in gene activity between twins: e.g. the Beckwith–Wiedemann syndrome and even more so autoimmune disorders, where environmental stressors or viruses can interfere. This explains the high rate (70–75%) of discordance of autoimmune diseases among MZ twins[17]. Indeed, MZ twins are highly similar but not identical.

Discordant twins and etiology of MZ twinning

Abnormal unequal inactivation of the X chromosome has been associated with MZ twinning and neural tube defects[18]. Unequal X inactivation exists when, instead of random inactivation of one of the X chromosomes of a female embryo, distinct cellular clusters of two different types are seen. In one cluster, one specific X chromosome is inactivated, in the second cluster, only the other. In reality, this type of segregation might actually cause separation of these two groups of cells, and thus MZ twinning (see Chapter 7).

Possibly, there is a triple link between twinning, neural tube anomalies and unequal X chromosome inactivation. However, this type of induction of twinning would concern only female MZ and, as a result, the number of female MZ twins should be higher than the number of males. Data established by James[19] show indeed that if the sex ratio (SR) is normal (0.571) in early formed (DC– and MC–DA) twins, later separations (MC–MA, SR 0.416) and, even more so, conjoined twins (SR 0.229) are related with a higher proportion of females. This hypothesis, plus the suggestion of Hall[20], who showed the relation between neural tube defects and anomalous X inactivation, could explain the excess of anencephaly in MZ but not in DZ twins and the increase of anencephaly with late separations of MZ. In contrast, spina bifida, which occurs much later in embryogenesis, is to a lesser degree sex linked[19]. Jongbloet[21] disputes the cause and effect of abnormal X-chromosome inactivation and the occurrence of MZ twins, and suggests that the error is in the ovum itself (ovopathy).

A possible synthesis of these two hypotheses is that early twinning is linked to ovopathy relative to aging of the oocyte and evidenced by heterokaryotic MZ twins; for late separation, the hypothesis of Burn et al.[18] of unequal X inactivation related to twinning is an interesting alternative. Heredity may also play a role in inducing monozygosity[22], but its effect apparently is plurigenic. The moment of separation could depend on factors other than accidental, such as genetic or nutritional considerations.

Unfortunately, these diverse considerations are insufficient to explain the phenomenon of MZ twinning in humans. In experimental models, induced delay of ovulation leads to ovopathy, chromosomal anomalies, congenital malformations and twinning. These effects have been obtained repeatedly in the rabbit[23,24]. In these experiments, the incidence of MZ twins was 6% and 3.2% at the blastocyst and postimplantation stages, respectively, whereas the usual incidence is 0.1%. In similar experiments in the rat, MZ and conjoined twins resulted[25]. Kaufman[26] observed two pairs of MC–MA twins after mouse blastocysts were aged in culture.

In the human, similar phenomena, e.g. chromosomal aberrations, congenital malformations and twinning often appear together. Nance and Uchida[27] highlighted the frequency of chromosomal anomalies (XO, trisomy 21) in MZ twins and their relatives. If oocyte aging leads to ovopathy and its consequences, it is logical to expect this to happen more frequently in humans than in animals. Whereas in mammals, fecundity is limited to the estrus period corresponding to ovulation, in humans, sexual intercourse occurs without regard to cycle day. As a result, there is a higher possibility of temporal dissociation between oocyte maturation and fertilization.

Experimental work in mammals has shown that postovulatory aging of the oocyte (delayed fertilization) can lead to chromosomal aberrations and abortions, and MZ twinning. Thus, delayed fertilization can be accepted as one etiological factor for monozygous twinning. In the human, the prolonged length of the follicular phase and the changes in hormonal levels enhance the probability of postovulatory aging. Bomsel-Helmreich and Papiernik[28] have shown that although the incidence of DZ twins and, to a certain extent, MZ twins increases with maternal age, the incidence of MZ twins also peaks in young mothers. Both periods correspond to the extremes of reproductive life, and both are associated with hormonal imbalance. In this regard, mothers of MZ twins have an earlier menopause[29].

The influence of *in vitro* fertilization (IVF) and ovulation induction

The introduction of IVF has provided a unique opportunity to observe very early stages of embryonic development and so to consider additional aspects of twinning in the human. In 1986, Edwards et al.[30] were the first to note that, among infants born after IVF in which several embryos were transferred, the number of MZ twins was abnormally high. Of the 600 infants included in their study, 1.3% were MZ twins, instead of the expected 0.4%. All transfers had been at the 2- to 4-cell stage. Because two of the twin pairs were DC–DA, it was presumed that early separation had taken place in these cases. Salat-Baroux et al.[31] reported a case of monoamniotic triplets together with diamniotic twins after *in vitro* fertilization in a patient with a strong family history of twinning (see Chapter 13 for additional discussion).

A possible explanation for this finding comes from animal work. Longo[32] had previously demonstrated that the zona pellucida of mouse oocytes hardens in culture. If, during hatching of the blastocyst, there was an insufficient rupture of a 'hardened zona', the inner cell mass might get squeezed and divided and hence produce monozygotic twins.

Edwards et al.[30] also observed that during the culture of human blastocysts, 70% are unable to escape from the zona and 10% get out only partially. These authors suggested that, whereas this mechanism might explain late-separated MZ twins, it clearly did not apply to the DC–DA monozygotics of early separation. Malter and Cohen[33] more recently suggested that lesions of the zona pellucida at the time of ovulation may interfere with normal hatching and thus lead to division of the blastocyst into two portions. Cohen et al.[34] used the technique of 'assisted hatching' to make a small incision in the zona pellucida; these authors proposed it to facilitate the escape of the blastocyst, but it also induced MZ twins who were MC–MA[34]. Nijs et al.[35] reported the birth of MZ twins after a transfer of a blastocyst to which rubbing of zona pellucida was used to assist hatching.

Multiple births conceived after hormonal stimulation of follicular growth have been particularly well studied in the East Flanders Prospective Twin Study[36]. Zygosity was ascertained by all available methods. The study sample included 972 multiple births over a 7-year period. MZ twins represented 1% of the total sample, instead of the expected 0.4%. Of the induced monozygotic twins, 54% were DC–DA vs. 37% in patients who conceived twins without the benefit of hormonal induction. Corson et al.[35] also described MZ twins occurring after gamete intrafallopian tube transfers. Clinical observations such as these raise many questions about hitherto unknown effects of ovulation inducers. As asynchrony of oocyte maturation has been demonstrated[38], the possibility of some ovopathy cannot be excluded.

Intermediary (half-identical) twinning

Some observations, especially the rare occurrence of discordance between monozygotic twins, suggest the existence of a third type of twinning. It has been shown that aging of oocytes, whether intrafollicular or postovulatory, can induce twinning, aneuploidy and embryonic mortality, together or separately. Attention has focused on the earliest separation occurring at the two-cell stage. In rodents, one effect of oocyte aging is the migration of the spindle of the first or second meiotic metaphase from its usual peripheral position to the interior of the cytoplasm. This central migration is a common occurrence in aged human oocytes[39]. In this manner, a more or less equal sharing of the cytoplasm occurs between oocyte and polar body once division takes place. This phenomenon represents the immediate cleavage state of the oocyte[40]. Under these circumstances, a large 'polar body' is formed. Boklage has characterized this structure as a tertiary oocyte[41]. In theory, fertilization of these two 'gametes' by two different sperms is possible. However, Boklage has emphasized the difficulty of distinguishing between this theoretical type of twinning and true monozygotic twinning. Although the two embryos are inside the same zona pellucida, in reality the ensuing twins will be somehow dizygotic as the result of fertilization of 'two' oocytes (the oocyte proper and the teriary oocyte) by two sperms.

Gartler et al.[42] were first to point out the possibility of this double fertilization giving rise to chimeras. A few other cases have been described since then[43,44]. Since oocyte aging can induce this form of immediate cleavage, this process could eventually lead to separation rather than aggregation of the two fertilized cells.

Immediate cleavage substituting for the expulsion of either the first or the second polar body has also been observed in super-ovulated mice[45] (Figure 1). Van de Leur and Zeilmaker[46] recently described a human zygote

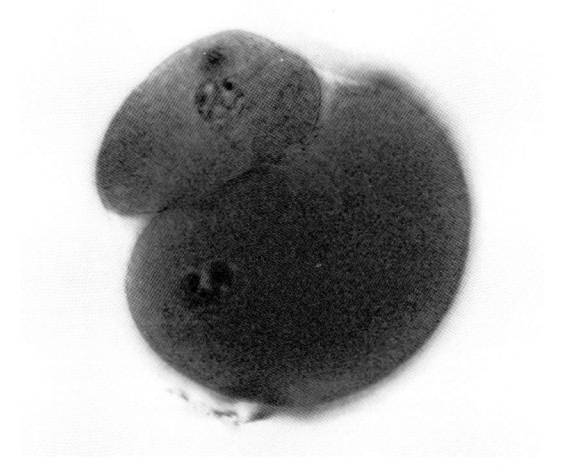

Figure 1 Abnormally large second polar body in mouse zygote aged *in vivo*, 15 h postovulation. Courtesy of Dr M.L. Boerjan, Agricultural University, Wageningen

with two cells both fertilized, which they suggest resulted from an immediate cleavage of a metaphase-II oocyte. This is comparable to the second meiotic division (expulsion of the second polar body). They mention two similar cases among 11 000 oocytes. Intrafollicular aging is the most probable cause for the abnormal cleavage observed in their case (Editor: These diverse observations give support to the existence of the intermediate type of twinning but they shed no light on the frequency of its occurrence, either in the natural state or in the case of twins which have followed IVF–ET).

Chimeras

The chimera is an individual with different cell populations derived from more than one fertilized egg[47]. It differs from mosaicism in that the different cell populations arise during development by mutation or mitotic non-disjunction. An individual who is XX/XO is mosaic, but one who is XX/XY must be a chimera. Two types can be distinguished:

(1) Primary: genetically different cell populations present from the very early stages of embryogenesis; and

(2) Secondary: a later occurrence resulting from common circulation between the mother and fetus or between both twins.

Most chimeras reported in man show ambiguous external genitalia or other manifestation of hermaphroditism.

By comparing the blood groups of the chimeric individual and those of his parents, it is possible to demonstrate the participation of either parent or both. The most usual situation is the finding of two paternal contributions. Sometimes two maternal as well as two paternal contributions can be demonstrated.

Primary chimerism with two separate contributions from the father means involvement of two separate sperm in the fertilization of:

(1) Two separate eggs which then aggregate;

(2) Two haploid products of precocious division of an unfertilized ovum;

(3) The ovum and the second polar body;

(4) The ovum and the first polar body; and finally,

(5) A secondary oocyte and its first polar body.

A chimera with two maternal contributions arises from the fusion of the second polar body with a normal diploid mitotic product of the first cleavage division giving rise to a diploid cell line and a triploid cell line as well.

Biologically speaking, the most likely mechanism is the double fertilization of an ovum and its second polar body. This mechanism was demonstrated by Braden[40] in the mouse, as noted earlier. Other factors affect this process as well, and will be discussed in the section that follows.

Despite the numerous observations of oocytes during IVF, none of the possibilities suggested above have been observed up to now. The hypothesis of fertilization of a polar body adds to the possibility of existence of intermediary (half-identical) twins.

Traits shared by twins

Various observations point out that factors other than zygosity may be connected with development of twins. In rodents, asymmetry of behavior can be induced by sex hormones; a female embryo implanted between two males or with a majority of males would change its behavioral phenotype in a masculine direction[48]. A similar effect exists in human DZ twins manifest by dental diameter asymmetries linked to sex pairing more than to zygosity[41,48]. A masculinizing effect on the auditory system appears in females having a co-twin of the opposite sex[49]. In addition, embryonic mortality in twins is linked more to sex than to zygosity. Male mortality is reduced by 60% if the other twin is female, whereas for females it is reduced by only 33% if the other twin is male (Table 1). Further, an excess of malformations is present in children or mothers of twins, whether MZ or DZ. This process involves a familial link between malformations and

Table 1 Twin fetal mortality in sex-pairing and zygosity groups (after Boklage[95])

	White		Black	
	M	F	M	F
Observed MZ fetal mortality	0.141	0.039	0.060	0.031
Estimated same-sex DZ fetal mortality	0.092	0.038	0.131	0.064
Observed other-sex fetal mortality	0.065	0.044	0.054	0.071

Note: For males SS DZ and especially Black males, the fetal mortality was much higher than for other-sex males

twinning without relation to zygosity. Children with anomalies often have left-handed parents[1,50]. Moreover, Klinefelter's syndrome is more frequent in DZ twins and their relatives than in singletons[51], whereas Turner's syndrome is more frequent in MZ and their relatives than in singletons[52]. Despite this, both syndromes are caused by chromosomal non-disjunction.

Dizygotic twinning

Etiology

DZ twinning results from the fertilization of two different oocytes arising in two distinct follicles. The growth and maturation of ovarian follicles is dependent on the level of gonadotropin secretion. As early as 1964, Milham[53] postulated that the high number of DZ twins in African populations was due to higher levels of follicle stimulating hormone (FSH). Since that time, other investigators working on different continents and with different racial groups have attempted to clarify this premise.

Among the earliest investigations were those of Nylander[54] who studied women of the Yoruba tribe in Nigeria. The Yoruba are distinguished by a very high incidence of DZ twins. Nylander found that during the 8 days around ovulation the level of FSH was much higher in mothers of twins than in mothers of singletons. These high levels were even more pronounced in women who had given birth to twins on more than one occasion. In contrast, the level of luteinizing hormone (LH) was not different. Soma et al.[55] compared levels of gonadotropin in Japanese and Nigerian women and found both FSH and LH levels higher in the Nigerian population. This is not surprising, in view of the low rates of twinning in Asian countries.

Martin et al.[56] demonstrated that the levels of FSH in Australian mothers in the early follicular phase and estradiol in the mid-follicular phase were significantly higher in mothers of DZ twins than in mothers of singletons or MZ twins, thus denoting the presence of more than one dominant follicle.

Similar findings have been found in some mammals. McNatty et al.[57] studied sheep during the luteal phase preceding conception and determined that the FSH levels were 20–40% higher in those animals with twins compared to those with singletons. The effect of the quantity of FSH is perhaps best illustrated in marmoset monkeys. These primates are peculiar in that they always carry DZ twins. When unilaterally ovariectomized, the remaining ovary continues to produce two ovulations because of the high level of FSH. The role of LH is less obvious, although when high doses of human chorionic gonadotropins (hCG) with LH effect are administered to polyovular mammals, this medication increases the number of ovulations[58,59].

Dizygotic twins arise from two different follicles, but no precise information concerning their growth is available. According to Hodgen[60], during spontaneous cycles the dominant follicle (by size) is selected from a cohort of follicles of comparable maturity on the fifth day of the cycle: it continues to grow until ovulation about 10 days later. Only the dominant follicle reaches pre-ovulatory size, and under its influence the other follicles become atretic.

In a study of the growth and maturation of multiple follicles after induction of ovulation, Bomsel-Helmreich et al.[38] demonstrated that the size of induced follicles was variable and that maturation of specific follicles was asynchronous. To our knowledge, the only study of follicle growth in spontaneous cycles was carried on 19 cycles by Dervain[61]. In nine cycles, evidence of asynchronous growth was found for two or three dominant follicles that eventually reached 16 mm in size. Nevertheless, in all these cases only one follicle underwent ovulation. Thus, the question remains open whether or not more than one follicle is selected at the same moment, as defined by Hodgen[60]. If so, it remains to be determined if growth is synchronous, resulting in equal degrees of maturity and healthiness, and if simultaneous ovulation takes place. Because strict chronology of maturation is crucial for producing a healthy oocyte and successful pregnancy, these distinct elements are essential.

Using sonography, Hackeloer et al.[62] were the first investigators to observe the presence of more than one dominant follicle prior to ovulation. This phenomenon occurs in 6–10% of all spontaneous cycles. Dominant follicles were noted in both ovaries, but which follicle ovulated or became atretic was not predictable.

Queenan et al.[63] described two cases illustrating this point. In one, the two oocytes were released the same day; in the other, the second ovulation took place between 24 and 48 h after the first. In the latter case, a twin pregnancy resulted, but one embryo aborted at 9 weeks. Although it is possible to postulate that some deficiency in the second oocyte resulting from delay in ovulation might explain the loss, it is not possible to ascertain the fate of each oocyte vis-à-vis the loss. It is equally possible that the abortion was the product of the first ovulation.

Triplets can result from fertilization of one, two, or three oocytes or two oocytes with subsequent division of one of them leading to a mixed DZ and MZ multifetal pregnancy. If two eggs were fertilized and one divided, the result would be a triplet set with MZ twins and one DZ triplet. This is often the case in high-order multifetal pregnancies, and points to the issue of the quality of a specific oocyte, because division into two indicates a degree of vulnerability of the egg. If three eggs are fertilized, the result is TZ triplets (trizygotic).

Incidence of twins

The exact frequency of DZ and MZ twins varies widely within the world, even among populations that are supposedly genetically homogeneous (see Chapter 11). Accurate zygosity determination requires precise recording of sex, placentation and membrane state at birth and should be complemented by other tests, such as blood groups, chromosomal analysis, enzymes and DNA (see Chapters 9 and 47).

All too frequently, the simplistic hypothesis proposed by Weinberg[64] is used to analyze demographic data in which zygosity was not determined at birth. The Weinberg formula proposes that the sex ratio is equal among DZ twins, a supposition which is contrary to fact. With this formula, the number of dizygotic twins within a population is obtained by multiplying by two the number of male/female pairs, and the number of monozygotic twins is determined by subtracting the DZ twins from the total number of twin births. Thus, the total twins – total DZ (1 FF + 2MF + 1 MM) = MZ (see Chapters 2 and 4).

This formula had been strongly criticized by many authors, because both zygosity and sex distribution influence the rates of early pregnancy loss and of congenital abnormalities. Both conditions also clearly influence the types and sex of twins who survive till birth. Weinberg considered the sex ratio in the beginning of pregnancy to be the same as it is at birth, although this is clearly not the case[65] (Table 1). On the average, the frequency of spontaneous twinning at birth is 1:80, but this ratio neither indicates the incidence of double ovulation nor the fate of double fertilization.

Sonography has clarified this issue somewhat. Robinson and Caines[66] followed twin gestations from the first trimester in 30 women; only 14 gave birth to twins, 11 delivered singletons and five aborted twins. Other authors have confirmed early embryonic loss (see Chapter 6 for full references). Landy et al.[67] examined the world literature and found that disappearance rates ranged from 0 to 78% in various publications. From this report, Boklage[68] identified 325 twin pregnancies that continued to term. Only 61 ended as twins (18.8%), 125 as singletons (38.5%) and 139 (42.8%) as complete loss. Kelly et al.[69] studied hormonal levels of early twin pregnancies, and determined that one twin was resorbed in 13 out of 40 twin pregnancies (32.5%) during the first 52 days of pregnancy.

Livingston and Poland[70] approached this subject from a different point of view. They studied spontaneous abortion before 18 weeks' gestation and found the incidence of twins to be 2.9%, a figure that is about three times the incidence of twins at birth. Of these twin abortions, 47% occurred before 8 weeks, thus corroborating a high rate of early embryonic loss. Uchida et al.[71] studied twinning rate in abortions: twins were deduced when two cell lines were ascertained in the products of the abortion. They estimated the true rate of twins to be about 1/30. Both these reports concluded that the frequency of twins among abortions is three times the frequency of twins at birth.

Boklage[68] analyzed a number of data sets to derive a mathematical estimate of twinning. Taking into account the high embryonic loss in the rates reported in the publications reviewed, he estimated that the true rate of twin conception is 1/8. Based upon this analysis, he postulated that for every live-born twin pair, there are at least six singletons who represent the survivors of twin conceptions (see Chapter 4 for details).

A decline in DZ twinning unrelated to decrease in parity has been observed in Western countries. In Aberdeen (Scotland), the frequency dropped from 9.4 per thousand in 1948 to 7.2 per thousand in 1968, probably due to decreased endogamy. In Sweden and Finland, where accurate population records existed for many centuries, the downward trend began toward the middle of this century. At the same time, however, the estimated rate of MZ twinning remained rather constant. Of equal interest, in Sweden in the 1960s, the twinning rate was half what it was 200 years ago; the decline in the numbers of triplets and quadruplets was even greater, to a quarter of what it was centuries ago[72].

Factors predisposing to double ovulation

The main factor leading to the natural as opposed to induced maturation of two follicles in a given cycle is a high level of FSH secretion. Other factors affect this process as well, however, and these will be discussed in the section that follows.

Heredity and race

In contrast to the incidence of MZ twinning which is relatively constant between 3.5 and 5.0 per thousand, the incidence of DZ twinning varies widely from a low note of 3 per thousand in Orientals, to 8 per thousand in Caucasians, to 16 per thousand in Africans, irrespective of their geographic localization. Different isolated populations within the same ethnic group also show some variation[73], and although American Blacks are not genetically a pure population, the incidence of DZ twinning in this population is similar to that of their African ancestors[74]. Amerindians have a twinning rate intermediate between that of Asians and Caucasians[75].

Clinical observations such as these strongly indicate that Weinberg's formula[64] is obsolete and that its continued use leads to confusion. The variations between racial groups are due to the variations in frequency of DZ twins. The

African population is a case in point. When Nylander[76] originally assessed twin frequency in the Yoruba population, he found twins occurring in every 22 births. This meant for all practical purposes that one Yoruba in 11 was a twin; the number of triplets was also high, presumably because of increased levels of FSH. However, the rate of MZ twins among the Yoruba was almost the same as in Europe, i.e. 3.8 per thousand. Later studies from Nigeria document a substantial degree of variation in the twinning rates among other tribal groups[77]. In addition to genetic considerations, part of this variation may be bound to social habits and economic status. The Yoruba live in the countryside and their staple nutrition is a particular species of yam, *Dioscorea rotundata (Discoreaceae)* (in Yoruba, *omi funfun* = mother of yam), a plant containing substances with estrogen-like effects that in some way may be inducers of ovulation through secretion of high levels of FSH[78]. In the last two or three decades, as a result of economic necessity, many Yoruba have left the countryside to live in cities and of necessity have changed their diets. Among these urban Yoruba, the rate of twinning has declined. Interestingly, the original finding by Hardman[78] has not been followed by studies using more modern methods to determine hormone levels (Editor: The Yoruban cultural attitude toward twins is unique and has been the object of discussion in numerous text and treatises over the years. Of particular interest are the 'Ibeji' (Figure 2)).

Ovulation induction, as used since the 1960s, generally produces dizygotic multiple ovulation. These therapies have been used in Japan since 1967. From 1951 to 1974, the rate of multiple births was low and almost constant. Since 1975, however, a remarkable increase in multiple births was observed. Imaizumi[79] studied the trends of higher-order multiple births in Japan during two periods, 1955 to 1967 and 1974 to 1988. For triplets the incidence rose from 53 per million to 109 per million; for quadruplets the rate increased from 1 per million to 9 per million.

Between 1955 and 1967, Imaizumi and Inouye[80] found that the majority of spontaneous triplets and quadruplets were MZ. In Japan, MZ triplets were twice as frequent as in England, USA, Italy or Australia; DZ triplets 3–4 times less frequent; and TZ triplets 6–13 times less frequent. The same situation holds with regard to quadruplets. Low zygosity is a characteristic feature of Asian populations. Only subsequent to the use of ovulation induction, and the multiple transfers of embryos after IVF in the 1980s, has the rate of DZ twins or higher-order multiples increased.

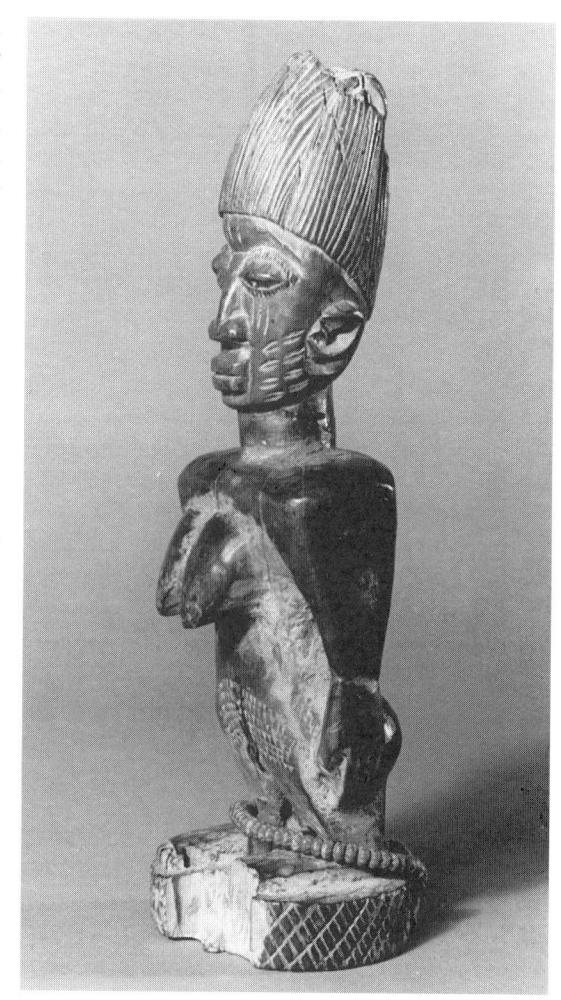

Figure 2 Twins play an important role in the cultural life of the Yoruba. A wooden statue called 'Ibeji' (two are born) representing an adult takes the place of one twin, if it dies in infancy, and as such is carried, fed and cared for like the surviving twin. Photograph by: Philippe Delangle, CNRS, Meuden, France

Parity and maternal age

Mothers of DZ twins are at times considered to be more fecund than mothers of singletons[81]. Although mothers of DZ twins have a higher average age than that of singletons (29.3 vs. 27.9 years), the influence of parity is not conclusive. The probability of having DZ twins increases with maternal age, most likely due to increasing FSH secretion leading to double ovulation. In contrast, after 37 years of age this rate declines. Bulmer[82] suggested that this decline was due to a diminishing number of previable follicles, but this explanation does not fit the physiological reality. Lazar *et al.*[83] suggested that the decrease in twinning after age 37 was related to an increase in spontaneous abortions in older women that would affect singletons as well as twins. It is thus possible that the decrease in twinning is reflective of reduced fertility in older women.

Seasonality, nutrition and environment

Seasonality appears to act through the effect of the length of daylight. FSH secretion depends on photoperiods. This is particularly evident in northern countries. Twin birth rates are the highest in Northern Finland and show clearly the effect of long summer days on the conception rate. There is a peak of conception of DZ twins in July and a nadir in January. The same phenomenon is seen in the northern part of Japan[84].

Nutrition also affects incidence of DZ twins. A decrease occurs in periods of malnutrition, as was the case during the famine of Rotterdam in 1945, whereas the relative incidence of MZ twins did not change[85].

Environmental factors affect twinning in different ways. Industrial development and urbanization have been shown to have a negative effect on twin frequency[86]. Toxic substances in the food or water can also affect human reproduction. Nelson and Bunge[87] reported a decrease in the average sperm count that might be due to dietary stilbestrol in beef and poultry. Low sperm count might not impair fatherhood in general but could decrease the possibility of fertilization of two ova in the same cycle. On the other hand, Lloyd *et al.*[88] observed an increase in twinning from 3% to 16–20% in regions polluted with polychlorinated hydrocarbons. It is possible that some of these pollutants might have estrogen-like effects.

Special categories of DZ twinning

Superfecundation

The simultaneous fertilization by two different fathers of two oocytes ovulated at the same time is very rare, although such a case was described in the first medical thesis published in the USA in 1810. One infant was white, the other mulatto[89]. Other cases have been described in ensuing years, but were suspect until the advent of sophisticated blood analyses and HLA typing. No criterion for paternity other than differences in skin color at birth was used in early reports. Moreover, skin color at birth cannot be assumed to correlate completely with skin color of childhood or later life, when environmental influences exert their effect. (Editor: Skin color can also differ markedly in cases of twin–twin transfusion syndrome.) Since the advent of HLA typing, however, this phenomenon has been documented conclusively[90].

Superfetation

In recent years superfetation has been expanded to include ovulation of two follicles at different dates in the same cycle or in successive cycles leading to twin pregnancy. This expanded definition led to the description of cases of a few days' or even one month's difference in birth dates. However, this expanded definition only confuses the issue. The definition does not, in reality, rest upon differences in birth dates, but rather upon a temporal dissociation between the times of conception of the twins. Thus, in the case described by Queenan *et al.* in 1980[63], the extrusion of the dominant follicle of each ovary was separated by more than 24 h. Because the phenomenon of timing of double ovulation has been insufficiently studied, it remains possible that such delays are entirely normal. On the other hand, because a 24-h delay is sufficient to induce overripeness and ovopathy (*vide supra*), the fact that one member of Queenan's twin pair was aborted at 9 weeks and the other born at term speaks for the presence of a blighted ovum (first or second).

Similarly, the three cases cited by Cabau and Bessis in 1981[91] fail to meet the definitional criteria. In this report, following induction of ovulation, several follicles were observed by sonography in each of the three cases. After two doses of hCG given at 48-h intervals, a number of follicles disappeared and multifetal pregnancies ensued with twins, triplets and quadruplets. Once again, our knowledge of the timing of polyovulation is so scant that it would be imprudent to state that these cases failed to represent the norm.

Scrimgeour and Baker[92] and Rhine and Nance[93] reported pedigrees of familial twinning, in which there was a consistently large weight difference among the newborn twins and in which the twinning tendency appeared to be transmitted through the twins' father. According to each pair of authors, both families may have had a genetic endocrine defect in the placenta that may possibly have permitted the pituitary to continue to elaborate its hormones for at least 1 month (these inferences gain support from the clinical observation of patients who report having menses during part or all of their pregnancy). Exceptionally, pregnancy does not seem completely to block the maturation of additional follicles if gonadotropin stimulation is used. In a case reported by Lefebvre *et al.*[94], from an IVF program, healthy fertilizable oocytes were obtained after inadvertent stimulation of a patient in the early stages of pregnancy. These oocytes eventually underwent cleavage and the spontaneous pregnancy continued to term.

In the human, only a small percentage of follicles (0.1–2.4%) contain more than one oocyte, especially the small preantral follicles. Whether these follicles reach the preovulatory stage is not certain. In animals, however, preovulatory polyovular follicles have been observed, along with some delay in oocyte growth which may indicate a deleterious effect on the subsequent growth of the embryo[95].

Telfer and Gosden[96] reported a 14% incidence of polyovular follicles in young bitches compared to a 5% incidence in older ones. In young bitches, all stages of preantral follicles were found, whereas only early stages were seen in the older ones, indicating a decreased viability during growth and subsequent selection. Two reports describing aspiration of two oocytes from the same follicle have been published in the IVF literature[97,98]. The fact remains, however, that during aspiration it is technically difficult to say with certainty if both oocytes come from the same follicle.

Conclusion

Despite a great deal of investigation in the last 20 years, the causes of twinning are still unclear. None the less, advances in fertility investigation and treatment, together with the progress in experimental biology, have widened our appreciation of very early development. Confirmation of the susceptibility of ova to early division in case of monozygosity and the role of gonadotropin in multiovulation have been demonstrated. The origin of MZ twins appears to be closely related to an abnormal chronology of oocyte maturation and fertilization processes (the phenomenon of over-ripeness). The origin of DZ twins is evidently double ovulation, but at present we know little about the uniformity (or lack thereof) of growth of the two follicles as they mature. In my opinion, further progress in this field will depend on the fulfilment of certain requirements:

(1) Clear definition of zygosity and avoidance of the use of general terms. In many articles, the term 'twinning' is used without specifying the type and, as such, the term is of little value.

(2) Investigation of physiological phenomena with state-of-the-art technology: sonography around the time of ovulation; hormonal measurements, especially FSH; investigation of the effect of nutrition and pollution in various populations.

(3) The use of experimental embryology to explain the origin of MZ twins. The production of MZ twins in mammals, and especially in primates, is possible today with available technology.

(4) In the human, where ethical problems must always be considered, studies of oocytes after failure of IVF can yield much information about ovopathy.

Such physiological investigations should clarify many unanswered questions in this field.

References

1. Boklage, C.E. (1987). Twinning, non-righthandedness and fusion malformations: evidence for heritable causal elements held in common. *Am. J. Med. Genet.*, **28**, 67
2. Cameron, A.H. (1968). The Birmingham twin survey. *Proc. R. Soc. Med.*, **61**, 229
3. Imaizumi, Y. (1988). Conjoined twins in Japan 1979–1985. *Acta Genet. Med. Gemellol.*, **37**, 227
4. Seidel, F. (1952). Bissektion von Mausezweizelleiern. *Naturwissenschaften*, **39**, 355
5. Tarkowski, A.K. (1959). Experiments on the development of isolated blastomeres of mouse eggs. *Nature (London)*, **184**, 1286
6. Willadsen, S.M. (1979). A method for culture of micromanipulated sheep embryos and its use to produce monozygotic twins. *Nature (London)*, **277**, 298
7. Moore, M.W., Adams, C.E. and Rowson, L.E.A. (1968). Developmental potential of single blastomeres of the rabbit egg. *J. Reprod. Fertil.*, **17**, 527
8. Rossant, J. and Vishk, M. (1980). Ability of outside cells from preimplantation mouse embryos to form inner cell mass derivatives. *Dev. Biol.*, **76**, 475
9. Allen, W.R. and Pashen, R.L. (1984). Production of monozygotic (identical) horse twins by embryo micromanipulation. *J. Reprod. Fertil.*, **71**, 607
10. Turpin, R., Lejeune, J., LaFourcade S. *et al.* (1961). Présumption de monozygotisme en dépit d'un dimorphisme sexuel. Sujet masculin XY et sujet neutra haplo X. *C.R. Acad. Sci. III*, **252**, 2945
11. Lawrence, A.C., Paterson, N.J. and Pauli, A.J. (1951). Quintuplet pregnancy. *J. Med. Soc. N.J.*, **48**, 547
12. Nylander, P.P.S. (1971). Biosocial aspects of multiple births. *J. Biosoc. Sci.* (Suppl) 3, **29**
13. Berbos, J.N., King, B.F., Janusz, A. (1964). Quintuple pregnancy. *J. Am. Med. Assoc.*, **188**, 813
14. Fankalsrud, E.W. (1966). Abdominal manifestations of situs inversus in infants and children. *Arch. Surg.*, **192**, 779
15. Loevy, H.T., Miller, M. and Rosenthal, I.M. (1985). Discordant MZ twins with trisomy 13. *Acta Genet. Med. Gemellol.*, **34**, 185, 1985
16. Storrs, E.E. and Williams, R.J. (1968). A study of monozygous quadruplet armadillos in relation to mammalian inheritance. *Proc. Natl. Acad. Sci. USA*, **60**, 910
17. Gregersenn, P.R. (1993). Discordance for autoimmunity in monozygotic twins: are identical twins really identical? *Arth. Rheum.*, **36**, 1185
18. Burn, J., Povey, S., Boyd, Y. *et al.* (1986). Duchenne muscular dystrophy in one of MZ twin girls. *J. Med. Genet.*, **23**, 494
19. James, W.H. (1988). Anomalous X chromosome inactivation: the link between female zygotes, monozygotic twinning and neural tube defect? *J. Med. Genet.*, **25**, 213
20. Hall, J.G. (1986). Neural tube defects, sex ratios and X inactivation. *Lancet*, **2**, 1334
21. Jongbloet, P.H. (1988). Duchenne muscular dystrophy in one of MZ twin girls. *J. Med. Genet.*, **25**, 214
22. Parisi, P., Gatti, M., Prinzi, G. *et al.* (1983). Familial incidence of twinning. *Nature (London)*, **304**, 626
23. Bomsel-Helmreich, O. (1972). Effets de l'ovulation retardée sur le développement des blastocystes de la lapine. *VIIème Congrès Int. Reprod. Anim. Féc. Artif.*, **1**, 205
24. Al Mufti, W. and Bomsel-Helmreich, O. (1979). Etude expérimentale de la surmaturité ovocytaire et ses conséquences chez les rongeurs. *Contracept. Fertil. Sexual.*, **7**, 845
25. Butcher, R.L., Blue, J.O. and Fugo, N.W. (1969). Overripeness and the mammalian ova. III. Fetal development at midgestation and at term. *Fertil. Steril.*, **20**, 223

26. Kaufman, M.H. (1982). Two examples of monoamniotic MZ twinning in diploid parthenogenetic mouse embryos. *J. Exp. Zool.*, **224**, 277
27. Nance, W.E. and Uchida, I. (1964). Turner's syndrome, twinning and an unusual variant of glucose 6-phosphate dehydrogenase. *Am. J. Human. Genet.*, **16**, 380
28. Bomsel-Helmreich, O. and Papiernik, E. (1976). Delayed ovulation and monozygotic twinning. *Acta Genet. Med. Gemellol.*, **25**, 73
29. Philippe, P. and Roy, R. (1989). Conception delays of twin-prone mothers; a demographic epidemiologic approach. *Hum. Biol.*, **61**, 599
30. Edwards, R.G., Mettler, L. and Walters, D.E. (1986). Identical twins and *in vitro* fertilization. *J. In Vitro Fert. Embryo Transfer*, **3**, 114
31. Salat-Baroux, J., Alvarez, S. and Antoines, M. (1994). A case of triple monamniotic pregnancy combined with a biamniotic twinning after *in vitro* fertilization. *Hum. Reprod.*, **9**, 374
32. Longo, F.J. (1981). Changes in the zone pellucida and plasmalemma of aging mouse eggs. *Biol. Reprod.*, **25**, 399
33. Malter, H.E. and Cohen, J. (1989). Blastocyst formation and hatching *in vitro* following zona drilling of mouse and human embryos. *Gamete Res.*, **24**, 67
34. Cohen J., Elsner, C., Kort, H. *et al.* (1990). Impairment of the hatching process following IVF in the human and improvement of implantation by assisting hatching using micromanipulation. *Hum. Reprod.*, **5**, 7
35. Nijs, M., Vanderzwalmen, P., Segal-Bertin, G. *et al.* (1993). A monozygotic twin pregnancy after application of zona rubbing on a frozen-thawed blastocyst. *Hum. Reprod.*, **8**, 127
36. Derom, C., Vlietinck, R., Derom, R. *et al.* (1987). Increased MZ twinning rate after ovulation induction. *Lancet*, **1**, 1236
37. Corson, S.L., Dickey, R.P., Gocial, B. *et al.* (1989). Outcome in 242 *in vitro* fertilization–embryo replacement or gamete intrafallopian transfer-induced pregnancies. *Fertil. Steril.*, **51**, 644
38. Bomsel-Helmreich, O., Vu. N. Huyen, L., Durand-Gasselin, I. *et al.* (1987). Mature and immature oocytes in large and medium follicles after clomiphene citrate and human menopausal gonadotropin without human chorionic gonadotropin. *Fertil. Steril.*, **48**, 596
39. Van Wissen, B., Bomsel-Helmreich, O. Debey, P. *et al.* (1991). Fertilization and aging processes in non-divided human oocytes after GnRHa treatment: an analysis of individual oocytes. *Hum. Reprod.*, **6**, 879
40. Braden, A.W.H. (1957). Variation between strains in the incidence of various abnormalities of egg maturation and fertilization in the mouse. *J. Genet.*, **55**, 476
41. Boklage, C.E. (1987). The organization of the ovocyte and embryogenesis in twinning and fusion malformations. *Acta Genet. Med. Gemellol.*, **36**, 421
42. Gartler, S.M., Waxman, S.H. and Giblett, E. (1962). An XX/XY human hermaphrodite resulting from double fertilization. *Proc. Natl. Acad. Sci.*, **48**, 332
43. Zuelzer, W.W., Beatty, K.M. and Reismann, L.E. (1964). Generalized unbalanced mosaicism attributable to dispermy and probable fertilization of a polar body. *Am. J. Hum. Genet.*, **16**, 38
44. Goldar, D.E. and Kimberling, W.J. (1981). Genetic expectations of polar body twinning. *Acta Genet. Med. Gemellol.*, **30**, 257
45. Boerjan, M.L. and de Boer, P. (1990). First cell cycle of zygotes of the mouse derived from oocytes aged postovulation *in vivo* and fertilized *in vivo*. *Mol. Reprod. Dev.*, **25**, 155
46. Van de Leur, S.S.C.M. and Zeilmaker, G.H. (1990). Double fertilization *in vitro* and the origin of human chimerism. *Fertil. Steril.*, **54**, 539
47. McLaren, A. (1976). *Mammalian Chimaeras*. (Cambridge: Cambridge University Press)
48. Denenberg, V.H. (1984). Behavioral asymmetry. In Geschwind, N. and Galaburda, A. (eds.) *Cerebral Dominance: The Biological Foundations*, pp. 114–33. (Cambridge, MA: Harvard University Press)
49. Fadden, D. (1993). A masculinizing effect on the auditory systems of human females having male co-twins. *Proc. Natl. Acad. Sci. USA*, **90**, 11900
50. Boklage, C.E. (1981). On the distribution of nonrighthandedness among twins and their families. *Acta Genet. Med. Gemellol.*, **30**, 167
51. Hoefnagel, D. and Benirschke, K. (1962). Twinning in Klinefelter syndrome. *Lancet*, **2**, 1282
52. Carothers, A.D., Prackiewicz, A. and De Mey, R. (1980). A collaborative study of the etiology of Turner's syndrome. *Ann. Hum. Genet.*, **43**, 355
53. Milham, S. Jr (1964). Pituitary gonadotropin and dizygotic twinning. *Lancet*, **2**, 566

54. Nylander, P.P.S. (1973). Serum levels of gonadotropins in relation to multiple pregnancy in Nigeria. *J. Obstet. Gynaecol. Br. Commonw.*, **80**, 651
55. Soma, H., Takayama, M. and Kiyokawa, T. (1975). Serum gonadotropin levels in Japanese women. *Obstet. Gynecol.*, **46**, 311
56. Martin, N.G., Beaini, J.L., Olsen, M.E. *et al.* (1984). Gonadotropin levels in mothers who have had two sets of twins. *Acta Genet. Med. Gemellol.*, **33**, 131
57. McNatty, K.P., Hudson N., Gibb, M. *et al.* (1985). FSH influences follicle viability, oestradiol synthesis and ovulation rate in Romney ewes. *J. Reprod. Fertil.*, **75**, 121
58. Dukelow, W.R. (1979). Human chorionic gonadotrophin: induction of ovulation in the squirrel monkey. *Nature (London)*, **206**, 234
59. Bomsel-Helmreich, O., Vu, N. Huyen, L. and Durand-Gasselin, I. (1989). Effects of varying doses of hCG on the evolution of preovulatory rabbit follicles and oocytes. *Hum. Reprod.*, **4**, 636
60. Hodgen, G.D. (1982). The dominant follicle. *Fertil. Steril.*, **38**, 281
61. Dervain, I. (1980). *Etude échographique de la croissance du follicule ovarien normal et détection de l'ovulation.* Thèse de Médecine, Université Louis Pasteur, Strasbourg
62. Hackeloer, B.J., Fleming, R., Robinson, H.P. *et al.* (1979). Correlation of ultrasonic and endocrinologic assessment of human follicular development. *Am. J. Obstet. Gynecol.*, **135**, 122
63. Queenan, J.T., O'Brien, G.D., Bains, LM. *et al.* (1980). Ultrasound scanning of ovaries to detect ovulation in women. *Fertil. Steril.*, **34**, 99
64. Weinberg, W. (1902). Beiträge zur physiologie und pathologie der mehrlingsgeburten beim menschen. *Pflueger Arch. Ges. Physiol.*, **88**, 346
65. Boklage, C.E. (1987). Race, zygosity and mortality among twins: interaction of myth and method. *Acta Genet. Med. Gemellol.*, **36**, 275
66. Robinson, H.P. and Caines, J.S. (1977). Sonar evidence of early pregnancy failure in patients with twin conceptions. *Br. J. Obstet. Gynaecol.*, **84**, 22
67. Landy, H.J., Keith, L. and Keith, D. (1982). The vanishing twin. *Acta Genet. Med. Gemellol.*, **31**, 179
68. Boklage, C.E. (1990). Survival probability of human conceptions from fertilization to term. *Int. J. Fertil.*, **35**, 75
69. Kelly, M.P., Molo, M.W., Maclin, V.M. *et al.* (1991). Human chorionic gonadotropin rise in normal and vanishing twin pregnancies. *Fertil. Steril.*, **56**, 221
70. Livingston, J.E. and Poland, B.J. (1980). A study of spontaneously aborted twins. *Teratology*, **21**, 139
71. Uchida, I.A., Freeman, V.C.P., Gedeon, M. *et al.* (1983). Twinning rate in spontaneous abortions. *Am. J. Hum. Genet.*, **35**, 987
72. Eriksson, A.W., Eskola, M.R. and Fellman, J.O. (1976). Retrospective studies on the twinning rate in Scandinavia. *Acta Genet. Med. Gemellol.*, **25**, 29
73. Eriksson, A.W. (1973). Human twinning in and around the Aland Islands. *Commentationes Biol.*, **64**, 159
74. Parkes, A.S. (1969). Multiple births in man. *J. Reprod. Fertil.*, (Suppl) **6**, 105
75. Allen, G. (1984). Multiple births. In Bracken. M. (ed.) *Epidemiology of Perinatal Disorders*, p. 153–68. (Oxford: Oxford University Press)
76. Nylander, P.P.S. (1969). The frequency of twinning in a rural community in western Nigeria. *Ann. Hum. Genet.*, **33**, 41
77. Creinin, M. and Keith, L.G. (1989). The Yoruba contribution to our understanding of the twinning process. *J. Reprod. Med.*, **34**, 379
78. Hardman, R. (1969). Pharmaceutical products from plant steroids. *Trop. Sci.*, **11**, 196
79. Imaizumi, Y. (1990). Triplets and higher order multiple births in Japan. *Acta Genet. Med. Gemellol.*, **39**, 295
80. Imaizumi, Y. and Inouye, E. (1982). Analysis of multiple birth rates in Japan. VI. Quadruplets: birth and stillbirth rates. *Jpn. J. Hum. Genet.*, **27**, 227
81. Philippe, P. and Roy, R. (1989). Conception delays of twin-prone mothers; a demographic epidemiologic approach. *Hum. Biol.*, **61**, 599
82. Bulmer, M.G. (1970). *The Biology of Twinning in Man.* (Oxford: Clarendon Press)
83. Lazar, P., Hemon, D. and Berger, C. (1978). Twinning rate and reproduction failures. In Nance, W.E., Allen, G. and Parisi, P. (eds.) *Twin Research: Biology and Epidemiology*, pp. 125–32. (New York: Alan R. Liss)
84. Timonen, S. and Carpen, E. (1968). Multiple pregnancies and photoperiodicity. *Ann. Chir. Gynaecol. Fenn.*, **57**, 135
85. Eriksson, A.W., Bressers, W.M.A., Kostense, P.J. *et al.* (1988). Twinning rate in Scandinavia, Germany and the Netherlands during years of privation. *Acta Genet. Med. Gemellol.*, **37**, 277
86. Parisi, P. and Caperna, G. (1981). The changing incidence of twinning: one century of

87. Nelson, C.M.K. and Bunge, R.G. (1974). Semen analysis: evidence for changing parameters of male fertility potential. *Fertil. Steril.*, **25**, 503
88. Lloyd, O.D., Lloyd, M.M., Williams, F.L.R. *et al.* (1988). Twinning in human populations and in cattle exposed to air pollution from incinerators. *Br. J. Ind. Med.*, **45**, 556
89. Archer, J. (1810). Observations showing that a white woman, by intercourse with a white man and a Negro man, conceive twins, one of which shall be white and the other mulatto. *Med. Repository*, **3d, Hexade 1**, 319
90. Majsky, A. (1991). HLA antigen typing in paternity disputes – analysis of results. *Cas-Lek-Cesk*, **130**, 367
91. Cabau, A. and Bessis, R. (1981). Monitoring of ovulation induction with human menopausal gonadotrophin and human chorionic gonadotrophin by ultrasound. *Fertil. Steril.*, **36**, 178
92. Scrimgeour, J.B. and Baker, T.G. (1974). A possible case of superfetation in man. *J. Reprod. Fertil.*, **36**, 69

Italian statistics. In Gedda, L., Parisi, P. and Nance, W.E. (eds.) *Twin Research 3: Twin Biology and Multiple Pregnancy*, pp. 35–48 (New York: Alan R. Liss)

93. Rhine, S.A. and Nance, W.E. (1976). Familial twinning: a case for superfetation in man. *Acta Genet. Med. Gemellol.*, **25**, 66
94. Lefebvre, G., Vauthier, D., Gonzales, J. *et al.* (1990). Assisted reproductive technology and superfetation: a case report. *Fertil. Steril.*, **53**, 1100
95. Al Mufti, W., Bomsel-Helmreich, O. and Christides, J.P. (1988). Ovocyte size and intrafollicular position in polyovular follicles in rabbits. *J. Reprod. Fertil.*, **82**, 15
96. Telfer, E. and Gosden, R.G. (1987). A quantitative cytological study of polyovular follicles in mammalian ovaries with particular reference to the domestic bitch (canis familiaris). *J. Reprod. Fertil.*, **81**, 137
97. Zeilmaker, G.H., Alberda, A. Th. and Van Gent, I. (1983). Fertilization and cleavage of ovocytes from a binovular human ovarian follicle: a possible cause of dizygotic twinning and chimerism. *Fertil. Steril.*, **40**, 841
98. Simonetti, S., Veeck, L. and Jones, H.W. (1985). Correlation of follicular fluid volume with ovocyte morphology from follicles stimulated by human menopausal gonadotropin. *Fertil. Steril.*, **44**, 177

The frequency and survival probability of natural twin conceptions

C.E. Boklage

Introduction

Most human pregnancies never reach term, as they fail before clinical recognition. The same is true for twin pregnancies. Optimized projections using available data indicate term survival of no more than one in four natural conceptions, and no more than one in 50 natural twin pairs. These projections also indicate that more than one pregnancy in eight begins as twins, and that, for every liveborn twin pair, 10–12 twin pregnancies result in single births. Using these estimates, 12–15% of all live births are products of twin embryogenesis.

Twin pregnancy ends with a single birth more often than with twins; the concept of the 'vanishing twin syndrome' (or phenomenon) has attracted considerable attention over the past several years[1–4]. In reality, however, losing one or both offspring from a twin pregnancy is too common to be called phenomenal, and occurs for too many different reasons to qualify as a syndrome. The concept found its present name in 1980, at the *Third International Congress on Twin Studies* in Jerusalem. Elizabeth Noble, who went on to explore the psychology of surviving the early loss of a twin[4], asked the question that provoked the discussion. One or both of the Keith twins interjected the term 'vanishing twins'. Their later paper with Landy[2], assaying the scope of the problem and labelling the event for the literature, followed from that discussion. The actual quantitation of losses from twin pregnancies remains, however, a relatively small part of a more general problem, for which we recently published a plausible statistical approach[5].

The causes, frequency and timing of prenatal losses are of interest at several levels, none of which is unique to twins. Despite this, understanding these processes can help clarify the epidemiology and developmental biology of twinning and numerous anomalies of human reproduction associated with twinning either in individuals or in families[6]. If, for example, the risk of prenatal death for the individual member of a multiple pregnancy were identical to that for a single pregnancy, multiple pregnancies appear to suffer greater losses for the simple reason that more lives are at risk. Although this likelihood must be considered in any proper analysis, considerable data indicate that multiple pregnancies are in fact at greater risk from a variety of sources[3]. The nature and extent of the excess risks for each or both twin(s) are difficult to define precisely, but remain worthy of our best efforts at understanding[5,7–9].

Before proceeding further, it is important to understand the importance of twin prenatal mortality in the broader perspective of human reproduction and developmental biology. In the persistent hope of clarifying a deeply rooted misunderstanding, I must emphasize that the excess mortality of twins is *not* confined to monozygotic (MZ) twins, even though it is indeed concentrated in same-sex (SS) pairs. There is every reason to believe that the same is true of excess malformations and other morbidity so long attributed exclusively to MZ twins when the 'Weinberg difference method' was used. Simply stated, to reach a useful understanding, one must relinquish the assumption that opposite-sex pairs and same-sex dizygotics are developmentally equivalent.

The Weinberg approach

Conclusions drawn from the Weinberg approach provide the only basis for the general assertion that the excess anomalies associated with twinning arise exclusively from MZ twins. The notion that a same-sex excess of an anomaly is by definition an MZ excess is so deeply ingrained in the literature and in the minds of clinicians that a same-sex pair in which either member is malformed or stillborn is simply assumed to be MZ. I have heard this logic defended as if challenging it demonstrated florid psychosis in the questioner. In one blatant example, I reviewed a paper in which a malformed same-sex pair was called MZ despite difference in the blood antigen *N*. Granted, the twins matched for a complex DNA polymorphism. However, the authors were unaware that this specific polymorphism, in spite of its complexity, represents a single DNA locus with a 25% chance of matching in a random sib pair. Even if the twins had matched for a multi-locus fingerprint, the probability that they were MZ was no greater than the probability that the *N* antigen difference was in error, a possibility that was not retested. That the authors tested zygosity at all represented substantial progress; that they ignored results contradicting their prior assumption represents the enduring problem.

The Weinberg method of estimating zygosity fractions, in its simplest form, calculates the MZ fraction of any sample of twins as the excess of SS over OS pairs (SS – OS = MZ). Adjustment of the expected number of DZ–SS pairs for the usual deviation of sex fractions from 0.5 is minor. Even at a sex ratio as extreme as 1.5, the expected fraction of opposite-sex pairs would be reduced only to 48%.

Applicability to anomalous twin births

The method has been proven basically sound for a large population-based sample of white, normal twins with accurate genotyping[10]. It is, however, based on two simplistic assumptions which make its applicability among *anomalous* twin births extremely doubtful. In particular, it is unsound for estimation of zygosity fractions among dead or malformed twins, or any other subset in which departures from these assumptions may be concentrated. The assumptions necessary for use of the Weinberg method are:

(1) That the binomial assortment of sex in DZ pairs at fertilization remains the same at birth; and

(2) That opposite-sex (OS) twins are developmentally representative of all DZ twins.

Both assumptions ignore clear contradictory evidence that males and members of same-sex pairs incur substantially greater prenatal and neonatal mortality. The usual escape allowing the second assumption to persist is to assume that the extra problems of same-sex pairs are concentrated in MZ pairs. It should be obvious that this is flawed logic, attempting to use a statement as its own proof.

An example will be helpful at this point. I once reanalyzed the zygosity vs. mortality distribution among the twins of the National Collaborative Perinatal Project, using three alternative approaches not requiring the standard assumptions. All three produced similar numbers and the same answer. By each of the alternative estimations, same-sex DZ twins pooled over race and sex suffer at least as much prenatal and neonatal mortality as MZs. The single exception is fetal mortality among white males: 0.141 MZ, 0.092 SSDZ, 0.065 OS. Without exception, neonatal mortality is higher for SSDZs than for MZs[7,8]. Given those results, I felt compelled to conclude that OS twinning is not developmentally representative of all DZ twinning. Clear overall sex differences in correlation structure of craniofacial development are also absent among OS twins. A set of dental measures that identifies gender with over 95% accuracy in singletons or same-sex twins via discriminant function analysis gives no better than random results among OS twins[7,8].

For the same conceptual reasons, the Weinberg method is highly unlikely to prove sound among malformed twins, if ever a database suitable for proper analysis (with accurate diagnosis of both zygosity and malformations, and statistically useful sample sizes) might be accumulated. Aside from mortality itself, twins suffer an excess of numerous difficulties associated with excess mortality. For example, twins, and also their siblings and offspring, suffer an excess of midline fusion malformations. Twinning and fusion malformations both concentrate in families with non-righthanded parents. Twins are more symmetrical than singletons in dental diameters. These relationships involve MZ and DZ twins and their families about equally, and all involve the mechanisms of embryogenic body symmetry determination[6]. Until recently, no significant zygosity-related difference had been reported for any of these familial associations. For neural tube defects (NTD), the excess of twins among the parents of affected children was shown to be due to DZs (not MZs) in Brittany[11]. Fraser and Garabedian[12] confirmed the excess of twins among the parents of children with NTD (cephalic and thoracic, but not lumbar), and extended the observations to cleft lip (CL) and cleft palate (CL/CP) families. The excess twinning in the population studied by Fraser and Garabedian was primarily SS among the NTD families and OS among the CLP families. It is not reasonable to suppose that those differences represent zygosity differences without additional information. Even if such differences should prove to be zygosity-dependent, the possible discrepancy between distributions at the time of occurrence and at the time of observation at birth does not allow a safe conclusion that a causal relationship exists.

A chronic problem underlying the general inability to address these questions has been the difficulty and expense of accurate genotyping for zygosity diagnosis, particularly with dead or dying babies. As demonstrated by Derom et al.[13], presently available technology can overcome the technical limitations of blood typing. Resolution of these problems can be expected soon after the decision is made that understanding these aspects of human developmental biology will provide enduring health care value worth paying for.

Unusual asymmetry of craniofacial development, midline malformations and twinning (both zygosities) share some heritable part of their causes[6]. It is appropriate to consider all these issues in this present context. Given the excess anomalies associated with twinning and with first-degree relationships to twins, the prospect that sole survivors of twin pregnancies may greatly outnumber those born as twins carries with it serious implications for the epidemiology of all anomalies associated with twinning. If, as it seems, more than one natural human pregnancy in eight begins as twins, and there are at least six single-born survivors for each liveborn twin pair[5], such numbers make it entirely possible that most non-righthanded individuals and every midline malformation are products of pregnancies which began as twins.

Fundamental questions

For all of the reasons cited above, the study of 'the vanishing twin' raises questions of fundamental biological importance. The loss of one member of a twin pair can be understood quite simply as part of the highly imperfect biology of human reproduction. Most human conceptions fail before birth. It is no different and no more mysterious for twins, except for two things: first, twins are more vulnerable to prenatal death than singletons; and second, some fraction of twins cannot die independently. If the lethal defect is genetic, there is some risk of concordance in any affected pair of siblings. Also, with few if any exceptions, monochorionic pairs share placental circulation to some extent, so that death of one for any reason may lead to death of the other through emboli, disseminated intravascular coagulation, passage of toxic products of autolysis or other mechanisms. The reasons for the failure of most pregnancies and for the excess of such losses among twins are not fully understood. Proper quantitation of the losses, and their distribution in time over pregnancy, may assist in that understanding.

Analyzing available data

Data sets suitable for analyses of the type required here are rare. To assure useful size for statistical purposes and an appropriate level of detail is difficult, time-consuming and expensive. It is possible to make progress with available data, given a proper combination of creativity and caution. Assuming honesty on the part of previous investigators, various results have common points to derive useful information. In this chapter, I used original data from several publications which presented results in a form that allowed comparison on common points. A description of these disparate sources follows. Examples of these sources include the microfilm files on the 616 twin pairs from the National Collaborative Perinatal Project, and from over 600 000 North Carolina 1979–85 birth records.

Another source was Landy et al.[2] who provided an early review of the literature on the frequency of vanishing twins. They collected a number of studies in which twin pregnancy had been discovered by ultrasound, in some cases as early as the first trimester. From 325 twin pregnancies with identified birth outcomes, there were 61 (18.8%) twin births, 125 (38.5%) singletons, and 139 (42.8%) pregnancies completely lost. Of that constructed cohort of 325, 81.3% suffered at least one loss, and the overall individual survival rate was 38%. In only two of the studies cited by Landy et al.[2] were the number of twin pregnancies sorted according to the time of discovery. From those two studies, 75 twin pairs identified between 6 and 10 weeks of gestation resulted in ten twin pairs, 36 single births, and 29 complete losses, for 37.3% individual survival. Thirty-four pairs identified between 10 and 14 weeks produced 17 twin pairs, 13 single births, and four complete losses, for 69.1% individual survival. There were 168 pairs discovered after 14 weeks, of which all but one survived to term as twins.

Still another source was Layde et al.[14] who studied 208 699 pregnancies in metropolitan Atlanta from 1969 to 1976. They reported 17.9% of all twins as stillbirths, a figure much higher than reported elsewhere. At my request they reviewed their records. For the twins only, the published numbers in fact represented all prenatal deaths from 8 weeks to term. Their database is unusual in that recording of miscarriage losses between 8 and 18 weeks is required by Georgia law.

In contrast, Livingston and Poland[15] collected tissues from 2222 spontaneous abortions; 1886 (84.9%) were morphologically distinct conceptuses. They found 53 anatomically distinct twin pairs (2.8%), more than three times the frequency of twins among live births in their Canadian sampling area (1: 108). The aborted twins included 25 pairs of less than 8 weeks' estimated gestation ('embryos'), 26 pairs of 8–18 weeks' gestation ('fetuses'), and two with one fetus and one embryo. Respectively, 58% of the 1833 single abortuses and 51% of the aborted twins had failed in the first two of the 12 weeks between the usual time of clinical pregnancy recognition and 18 weeks. These results make clear the higher rate of loss in early stages of pregnancy, and show no significant difference between twins and singletons in the distribution of losses between the embryonic and fetal periods of gestation.

Uchida et al.[16] also collected tissue from 661 spontaneous abortions, to be exact. They identified eight twin pairs as morphologically distinct conceptuses and seven more by the presence of two distinct cell lines on cytogenetic examination (both also clearly distinct from maternal cells). These authors excluded from the twin sample 30 specimens with two cell lines in which they could not rule out a maternal origin of the second cell line (of the seven pairs included without two distinct specimens, five were of opposite sex). They also counted as singletons nine specimens they considered to be mosaic (two cell lines with no clear difference beyond a single chromosome anomaly). The frequency of twins among spontaneous abortions was therefore at least one in

44 (they estimated it to be closer to one in 30), vs. one per 103 live births in their population.

These two Canadian reports do not differ significantly in the frequency of twins among spontaneous complete abortions. Their average, 2.67%, is 3.14 times the twin frequency among live births. This figure suggests a 32% survival of twin pairs from the time of clinical recognition to term. If the fraction of aborted twins occurring as distinct conceptuses should be the same between the two samples, Livingston and Poland may have missed at least half the twins in their sample. Apart from two distinct specimens, Uchida's cytogenetic approach cannot detect MZ twins or SS-DZ pairs which happen not to differ in informative cytogenetic variants. Karyotypically discordant MZ twins (due to somatic mutation by mitotic nondisjunction or the 'splitting' of a 'mosaic' embryo) would be seen as a 'mosaic', as would DZ twins with only one cytogenetically detectable difference. These studies should be repeated, or the samples reanalyzed using DNA fingerprinting. It is virtually certain that both studies underestimated the frequency of twins among spontaneous abortions, and it is likely that the degree of underestimation was substantial. Since these two reports constitute the majority of the earliest cases considered in this chapter, the effect of this bias will be to minimize estimates of the frequency of twins at conception.

Additional information was available from the Collaborative Perinatal Project of the National Institute of Neurological Disease and Stroke. This study followed some 55 000 pregnancies from first prenatal visit to term at multiple clinic locations in the United States over a period of nearly 20 years. We previously reanalyzed those data with respect to prenatal and perinatal mortality of twins[7,8]. Most abortions and miscarriages were lost to follow-up; few were examined in such a way as to identify twin pregnancies, making this study an unrepresentative and unreliable sample with respect to the number of twin abortions and miscarriages identified. Not so with stillbirths, however. A total of 1203 twin fetuses were identified among deliveries with recorded ages beyond 20 weeks of gestation. Of those, 73 were stillborn – a loss rate of 6.1% from 20 weeks to term.

The final source of data for the present work comes from birth records of 614 606 infants delivered beyond 20 weeks of gestation in North Carolina from 1979 through 1985. Of these, 12 906 were twins. Of these twins, 486 (3.77%) are recorded as stillbirths vs. 0.93% among singletons. Individual twins represent 8.1% of all stillbirths vs. 2.1% of all live births.

The mathematics of exponential decay provides an appropriate logical framework for quantitation of pregnancy loss over gestational time[5]. While not a part of ordinary clinical conversation, this mathematics is not particularly difficult to understand. It is rather like negative compound interest. Instead of increasing the amount of money in an account by a certain percentage of the present value per unit time, there is a reduction in number of surviving pregnancies by a certain fraction per unit time. The value of that fraction, and the timing of any change in that fraction, can provide the information we need.

The survival probability of twin pregnancies

Figure 1 shows the available data for total natural pregnancies from several sources plotted as a fraction of exposed cycles with a pregnancy in progress at each time point. As previously noted[5], the studies included in this figure differed in sensitivity and timing of their hCG assays, in the age distribution of the mothers, and in the fraction of patients having proven fertility. They were not controlled with respect to the distribution of inseminations within the exposed cycles. The desired denominator, that is, the number of fertilizations, is unknown in every instance. Sample variation in fecundity might therefore explain a sizeable portion of the apparent differences among results. It is clear in every study that the rate of pregnancy loss differs before and after clinical recognition.

Useful integration of these data requires two steps. The first is to estimate the fraction of fertilizations resulting in clinical pregnancy. This provides a means to translate the various

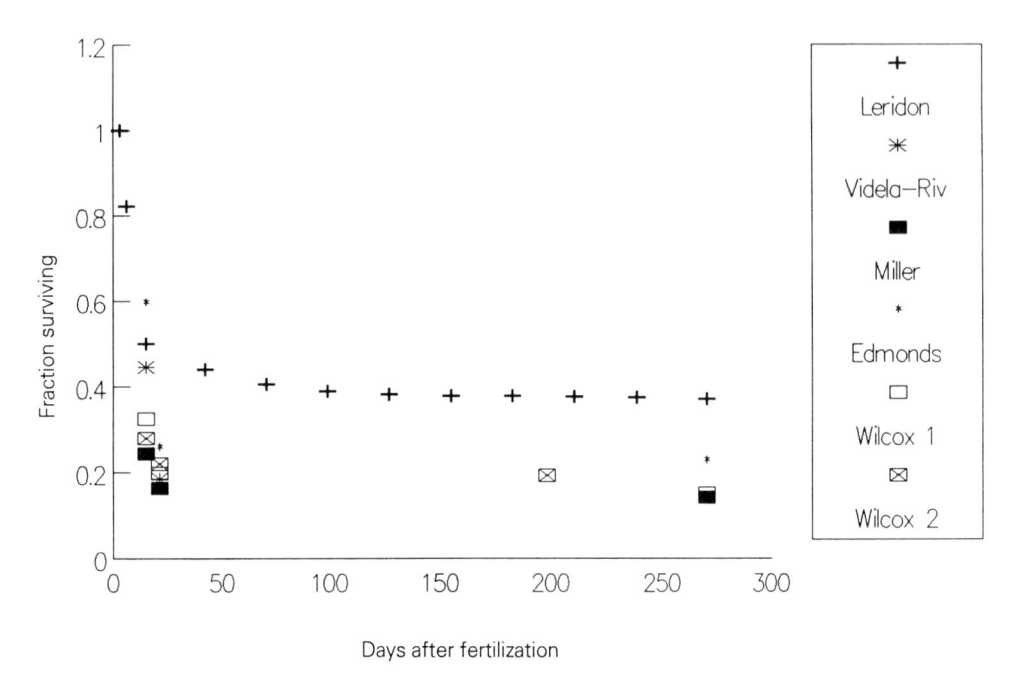

Figure 1 Results from various studies of total natural pregnancies, with early detection via hCG assay, compared to Leridon's study[25], which combined Hertig's hysterectomy results for early detection[26] with data from a large population observed from first missed period[27]. hCG results collected from references 18–20, 28 and 29, plotted as pregnancies in progress per exposed cycle. Figure redrawn from reference 5.

studies to a reasonable uniform scaling. The results in Table 1 (retabulated from reference 17) arise from 1898 cycles in couples of proven fertility, with no chemical or mechanical contraception, with daily records of menstruation and coitus, and with a clear shift in basal body temperature as evidence of ovulation. A missed period was considered evidence of conception. The calculations in Table 1 yield an estimate of 28.7% probability of clinical pregnancy per optimally timed insemination. This value agrees well with the authors'[17] estimate of 30% from applying logistic regression to calculate the expected results of daily coitus throughout the fertile period.

It is reasonable to assume that the clinicians who provided the results in Figure 1 accurately recognized clinical pregnancies. I am willing to suppose that survival from fertilization to clinical pregnancy was more or less uniform over those studies. This estimate of 28.7% clinical pregnancy per optimally timed fertilization is probably high for a general population not selected for proven fertility. However, it provides a reasonable basis for uniform rescaling of the results in Figure 1 on a per-fertilization basis. In Figure 2, I have replotted each point from Figure 1 as its ratio to the number of pregnancies at clinical recognition. The two studies from Wilcox et al.[18,19], especially the second, appear to have been executed about as well as could be done. The study by Miller et al.[20], the second largest and second most thorough sampling, provides the result most similar to those of Wilcox. The sample sizes alone allow these studies the greatest weight in drawing the theoretical curve. The equation defining that curve is:

$$P_t = 0.73\, e^{-0.155t} + 0.27\, e^{-0.0004t}$$

where t is time in days postfertilization, P_t is the time-dependent probability of pregnancy survival, and e the base of natural logarithms. Seventy-three per cent of all fertilizations constitute

Table 1 Probability of clinical pregnancy vs. cycle day of insemination

| Cycle day vs. basal T° shift | Inseminations | | Daily relative conception risk[†] | χ^2 | Pregnancies distributed by relative risk[‡] | Probability of clinical pregnancy per coitus** |
	In pregnant cycles*	In non-pregnant cycles*				
−9	22	233	1.716	1.907	2.107	0.0083
−8	20	201	1.808	2.35	2.018	0.0091
−7	25	156	2.912	15.315	4.063	0.0224
−6	22	115	3.476	19.724	4.268	0.0312
−5	25	71	6.398	57.366	8.927	0.0930
−4	29	59	8.932	96.2	14.456	0.1643
−3	28	58	8.773	91.224	13.709	0.1594
−2	36	52	12.58	162.562	25.275	0.2872
−1	26	66	7.159	68.124	10.388	0.1129
T° shift 0	26	82	5.762	52.234	8.361	0.0774
1	18	151	2.166	4.671	2.176	0.0129
2	21	411	0.928	1.661	1.088	0.0025
3	14	548	0.464	13.579	0.363	0.0006
4	18	557	0.587	9.753	0.59	0.0010
5	17	595	0.519	12.715	0.492	0.0008
6	11	554	0.361	17.68	0.222	0.0004
7	10	615	0.295	22.699	0.165	0.0003
8	9	576	0.284	21.79	0.143	0.0002
9	10	528	0.344	17.503	0.192	0.0004
Total inseminations	387	5628			99.003	
Total cycles	99	1799				

*Data retabulated from Barrett and Marshall[17]; [†]fraction of pregnant cycles with insemination on a given day ÷ fraction of non-pregnant cycles inseminated the same day; [‡]99 times daily fraction of total (relative risk times inseminations in pregnant cycles); **pregnancies per insemination

one group which loses 1550 per 10 000 (15.5%) of its remaining members each day (half-life 4.5 days), with less than 10^{-18} probability of surviving 270 days. The remaining 27% constitute a second group which loses only four per 10 000 remaining members (0.04%) daily (half-life 1733 days), with about 90% probability of surviving to term. The inflection point appears to represent the successful completion of embryogenesis and organogenesis.

With no useful idea of the number of twin pregnancies present at the onset of gestation, I worked back from birth, plotting twins as a fraction of total pregnancies identified at each stage, in proportion to the fraction of twins at term. For scaling and curve-fitting, the late-phase decay constant can be computed directly from losses beyond 6–8 weeks postfertilization when early losses are complete. Extrapolation of the late-loss curve to time zero, and subtraction of its predicted values from the observed early numbers, provides values from which to compute the early-loss curve. The ratio of the two time-zero intercepts defines the proportional representation of the two populations. The equation of the fitted curve for naturally-occurring twins is:

$$P_t = 0.9726\, e^{-0.10344 t} + 0.0274\, e^{-0.001072 t}$$

where P_t is the probability of survival. By the resulting estimate, at $t = 270$ days, about 2% of all twin pregnancies survive to term, with over 97%

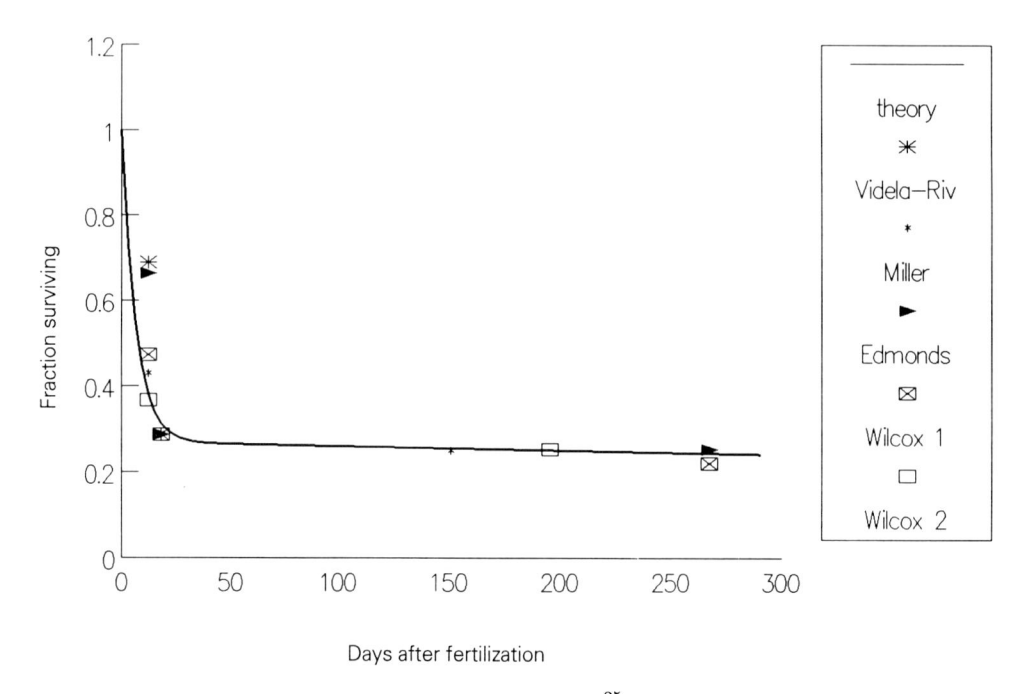

Figure 2 Results of Figure 1, minus results from Leridon[25], adjusted to uniform 0.287 survival from fertilization to clinical pregnancy (21 days postfertilization, 5 weeks post-LMP), with weighted-average theoretical curve. Equation of theoretical curve explained in text. Figure from reference 5

having suffered at least one loss before clinical recognition. Figure 3 shows the result, with the singleton theoretical curve for comparison.

According to these results, twin deliveries among live births represent 2.05% of twin conceptions, and total live births represent 24.24% of all fertilizations. Given that twins constitute about one in 90 live births, then

$$[(1/90) \times (1/0.0205)/(1/0.2424)] = 0.1313$$

indicating that more than one pregnancy in eight begins as twins. If early losses of twins are under-counted, as was inferred above, these estimates are low for the frequency of twins at conception and for the fraction lost before recognition, and high for the fraction surviving to term.

Estimation of the frequency of individual twin survival ('vanishing twins' or sole survivors) requires more complex consideration, because some co-twins cannot die independently. Some obviously share genetic reasons for dying. Monochorionic pairs at least nearly always share some placental circulation in such a way that death of either member may cause the death of the other. Using data from Landy et al.[2], concerning pregnancies identified by ultrasound after at least 6 weeks' gestation, Boklage[5] calculated the fraction of all twin pairs for whom independent survival is possible to be 0.81625. Assuming independence of viability in 0.81625 of all twin pairs, individual twin survival probability can be calculated as the square root of joint independent survival ($\sqrt{(0.81625 \times 0.0205)} = 0.1294$). The fraction of twin pregnancies with a single survivor is thereby estimated to be $2 \times 0.1294 \times (1 - 0.1294) = 0.2252$. That would represent 11 sole survivors of twin gestations for every liveborn twin pair. On that basis, more than one-eighth of all live births are products of twin embryogenesis. Because of conservative use of the available data and the likelihood of undercounting previously mentioned, these figures are likely to represent minimum estimates.

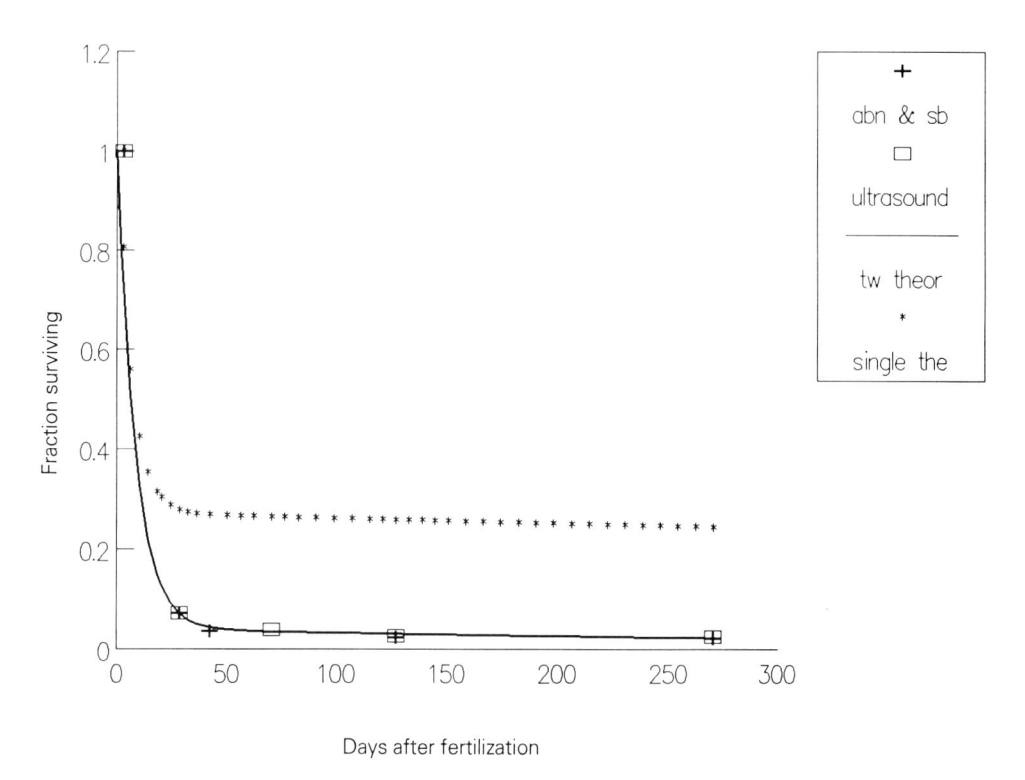

Figure 3 Survival of twins as pairs, from stillbirth, spontaneous abortion and ultrasound studies. Computed as a fraction of twins among pregnancies detected at various stages, proportional to twin fraction at birth; adjusted to surviving fraction of total twins present at conception

Looking forward

The increasing use of transvaginal ultrasonography should provide earlier detection of multiple pregnancy as well as better viability prognosis[21]. Its use, combined with serial assay of hCG[22–24], should make it possible to detect twin pregnancies at least nearly as early as single pregnancies. Application of these techniques in a sample of sufficient size should provide much more straightforward and more accurate answers to all of these present questions.

There is little room to doubt that the question of vanishing twins and sole survivors of twin gestation represents issues of broad and fundamental importance. The numbers estimated here for the frequency of twinning at conception and the prevalence of sole survivors of twin gestations are little short of astonishing at first consideration, and they are conservative, perhaps even minimum, estimates. To expect significant improvement in these estimates will require obstetricians in the field to collect sound data using early non-invasive means with careful documentation, so that we may calculate these rates with improved confidence.

Acknowledgements

We appreciate partial support for this work from NIH grant HD22507, the provision of original birth record data from the North Carolina State Center for Health Statistics, access to original records of the Collaborative Perinatal Project courtesy of Dr Ntinos Myrianthopoulos and NINCDS, and review of original records of the Metropolitan Atlanta Congenital Defects Program by Dr Arthur Falek of the Georgia Mental Health Institute and Drs David Erickson and Brian McCarthy of the Bureau of Epidemiology, Center for Disease Control.

References

1. Alexander, T.P. (1987). *Make Room for Twins.* (New York: Bantam Books)
2. Landy, H.J., Keith, L.G. and Keith, D. (1982). The vanishing twin. *Acta Genet. Med. Gemellol.*, **31**, 179
3. MacGillivray, I., Campbell, D.M. and Thompson, B. (1988). *Twinning and Twins.* (New York: John Wiley & Sons)
4. Noble, E. (1991). *Having Twins*, 2nd edn. (Boston: Houghton Mifflin)
5. Boklage, C.E. (1990). Survival probability of human conceptions from fertilization to term. *Int. J. Fertil.*, **35**, 75
6. Boklage, C.E. (1987). Twinning, non-righthandedness, and fusion malformations. Evidence for heritable causal elements held in common. *Am. J. Med. Genet.*, **28**, 67
7. Boklage, C.E. (1987). Race, zygosity and mortality among twins: interaction of myth and method. *Acta Genet. Med. Gemellol.*, **36**, 275
8. Boklage, C.E. (1985). Interactions between opposite-sex dizygotic fetuses and the assumptions of Weinberg difference method epidemiology. *Am. J. Hum. Genet.*, **37**, 591
9. Bryan, E.M. (1986). The intrauterine hazards of twins. *Arch. Dis. Child.*, **61**, 1044
10. Vlietinck, R.F. (1986). *Determination of the Zygosity of Twins*, Doctoral dissertation. (Leuven: Katholieke Universiteit)
11. Journel, H. and Le Marec, B. (1989). Letter to the editor: dizygotic twinning in mothers of spina bifida. *Am. J. Med. Genet.*, **32**, 257
12. Fraser, F.C. and Garabedian, B. (1991). Schisis malformations and twinning: a familial association. *Proceedings, 8th International Congress of Human Genetics*, Abstr. 915, p. 173
13. Derom, C., Vlietinck, R.F., Derom, R. *et al.* (1991). Genotyping macerated stillborn fetuses. *Am. J. Obstet. Gynecol.*, **164**, 797
14. Layde, P.M., Erickson, J.D., Falek, A. *et al.* (1980). Congenital malformations in twins. *Am. J. Hum. Genet.*, **32**, 69
15. Livingston, J.E. and Poland, B.J. (1980). A study of spontaneously aborted twins. *Teratology*, **21**, 139
16. Uchida, I.A., Freeman, V.C.P., Gedeon, M. *et al.* (1983). Twinning rate in spontaneous abortions. *Am. J. Hum. Genet.*, **35**, 987
17. Barrett, J.C. and Marshall, J. (1969). The risk of conception on different days of the menstrual cycle. *Population Stud.*, **23**, 455
18. Wilcox, A.J., Weinberg, C.R., Wehmann, R.E. *et al.* (1985). Measuring early pregnancy loss: laboratory and field methods. *Fertil. Steril.*, **44**, 366
19. Wilcox, A.J., Weinberg, C.R., O'Connor, J.E. *et al.* (1988). Incidence of early loss of pregnancy. *N. Engl. J. Med.*, **319**, 189
20. Miller, J.F., Williamson, E., Glue, J. *et al.*, (1980). Fetal loss after implantation. *Lancet*, **2**, 554
21. Pampiglione, J.S. and Mason, B.A. (1988). Fetal viability in multiple pregnancy. *Lancet*, **2**, 183
22. Thiery, M., Dhont, M. and Vandekerckhove, D. (1977). Serum HCG and HPL in twin pregnancies. *Acta Obstet. Gynecol. Scand.*, **56**, 495
23. Bernaschek, G., Rudelstorfer, R. and Csaicsich, P. (1988). Vaginal sonography versus serum human chorionic gonadotropin in early detection of pregnancy. *Am. J. Obstet. Gynecol.*, **158**, 608
24. Kelly, M.P., Molo, M.W., Maclin, V.M. *et al.* (1991). Human chorionic gonadotropin rise in normal and vanishing twin pregnancies. *Fertil. Steril.*, **56**, 221
25. Leridon, H. (1977). *Human Fertility: The Basic Components.* (Chicago: University of Chicago Press)
26. Hertig, A.T. (1967). The overall problem in man. In Benirschke, K. (ed.) *Comparative Aspects of Reproductive Failure*, pp. 11–41. (New York: Springer-Verlag)
27. French, F.E. and Bierman, J.E. (1962). Probabilities of fetal mortality. *Pub. Health Rep.*, **77**, 835
28. Edmonds, D.K., Lindsay, K.S., Miller, J.F. *et al.* (1985). Early embryonic mortality in women. *Fertil. Steril.*, **38**, 447
29. Videla-Rivero, L., Etchepareborda, J.J. and Kesseru, E. (1987). Early chorionic activity in women bearing inert IUD, copper IUD and levonorgestrel-releasing IUD. *Contraception*, **36**, 217

Documenting the vanishing twin by pathological examination

K. Yoshida

Introduction

Early documentation of fetal loss in multiple pregnancies was rarely possible prior to the development of obstetric ultrasonography. With this technique, however, in recent years more twin pregnancies have been detected *in utero* compared to the number of twin births. Disappearance rates vary widely, depending to some degree on the timing of ultrasonographic procedures and the techniques available to the obstetrician[1]. Despite widespread clinical and academic interest in this subject, morphological evidence of the vanishing twin has been described in only a few reports[2,3].

It usually is difficult to find evidence of the vanishing twin, because the fetus typically has been resorbed or has degenerated as pregnancy advances. Notwithstanding, at the time of birth, attempts to document residual evidence of the vanishing twin should begin with a careful examination of the placenta and membranes delivered with the co-twin. The confirmatory or suspected pathological evidence of a vanishing twin can often be recognized on the placental plate or in the membranes adjacent to the placental margin.

This chapter reviews our experience documenting the vanishing twin. The data in our files are particularly rich, because of the tendency of Japanese women to have monozygous (MZ) twins and monochorionic placentation. Our interest in this subject has resulted in several publications[4-6].

Between February 1961 and December 1991, at the Tokyo Medical College Hospital, we were able to examine the placentas from 147 monochorionic twin pregnancies macroscopically shortly after birth. These pregnancies represented 60.2% of all our twin deliveries

Table 1 Vascular anastomoses in monochorionic twin placentae and fetal outcome

Types of anastomosis	Cases (n)	Survivors		
		Both	One	None
Artery–artery	56	49	4	3
Artery–artery and artery–vein	11	9	2	0
Artery–artery and vein–vein	27	9	9	9
Vein–vein and artery–vein	2	1	0	1
Vein–vein	3	0	1	2
Artery–vein	12	6	2	4
Unknown or none	36	11	19	6
Total (n)	147	85	37	25
(%)		57.8	25.2	17.0

MULTIPLE PREGNANCY

Table 2 Clinical data of vanishing twin gestations

Case no.	Gestational complications	Sonographic disappearance of FHM	Gestational complications and age of liveborn twin	Placental findings (umbilical cord insertion)
1	1st trimester bleeding and abd. pain (6–8 weeks)	8 weeks	none M: 3532 g (41 weeks)	thin accessory lobe, fibrinoid degeneration (marginal)
2	1st trimester bleeding (7–8 weeks)	9 weeks	mild toxemia M: 4090 g (41 weeks)	marginal infarction (velamentous)
3	1st trimester bleeding (8–9 weeks)	9 weeks	none M: 3010 g (40 weeks)	normal (marginal)
4	1st trimester bleeding (5–6 weeks)	5–6 weeks	proteinuria F: 3194 g (39 weeks)	retroplacental hematoma (central)

FHM, fetal heart movements; M, male; F, female

Table 3 Suspected evidence of vanishing twins

Case no.	Gestational complications	Sonographic findings	Liveborn	Placental findings
5	1st trimester bleeding and abdominal pain (5–12 weeks)	1 sac, FHM (+) 1 sac, FHM (−), deformed	F: 3331 g (39 weeks)	subchorionic fibrin, circumvallate, intervillous thrombosis, marginal hemorrhage
6	1st trimester bleeding (6–10 weeks)	1 sac, FHM (+) 1 sac, FHM (−), deformed	F: 2999 g (40 weeks)	subchorionic fibrin, accessory lobe, decidual necrosis

FHM, fetal heart movements; F, female

during this period. Thirty-nine cases were also evaluated microscopically. Table 1 shows that in 37 pairs (25.2%), one fetus had died during the pregnancy, both twins had died in 25 pairs (17.0%) and both twins survived in 85 pairs (57.8%). Differing degrees of evidence of the vanished twin were found in 15 cases in the first trimester. The text, tables and figures that follow describe the cases in detail.

Confirmed cases

In four cases, one of the two fetal heart movements had disappeared by 9 weeks of gestation (Table 2). When the placentas of these cases were examined, three exhibited a yellowish-white thickening plaque on the membranes adjacent to the placental margin. The fourth revealed a 5.4 × 5.4 cm cyst on the placental chorionic plate containing amorphous material connected to the membranes by a slender string, which appeared as if it were a blighted umbilical cord. Two additional cases in which sonographic findings were abnormal during the first trimester are shown in Table 3. The following reports are illustrative of these cases.

Case 1

A 25-year-old woman, gravida 1, para 0, had her last menstrual period on February 1, 1986. It lasted 6 days. She visited our clinic on March

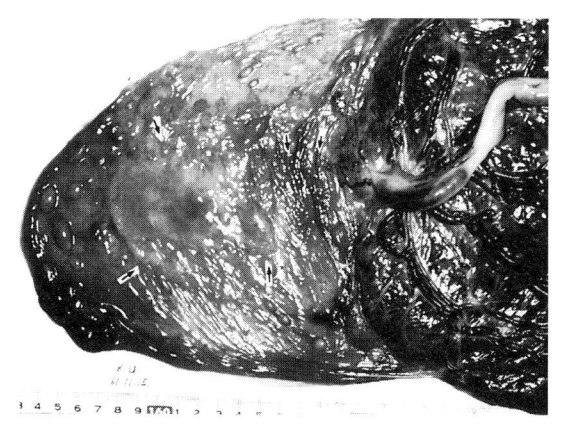

Figure 1 A thickened area (arrows) of the membranes in case 1

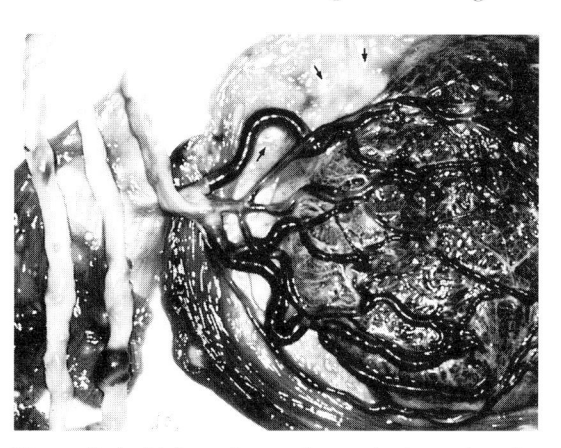

Figure 3 A thickened area (arrows) along the placental margin in case 2

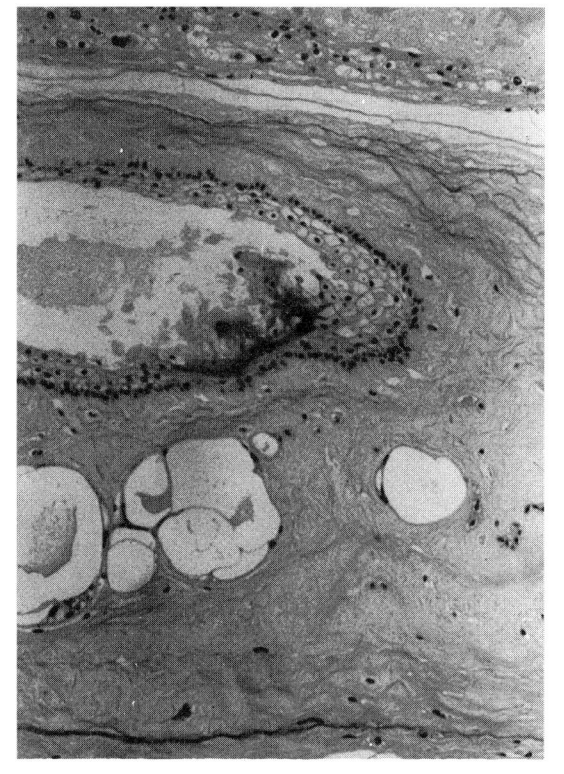

Figure 2 The remnants of vanished embryonic somites in case 1 (HE × 80)

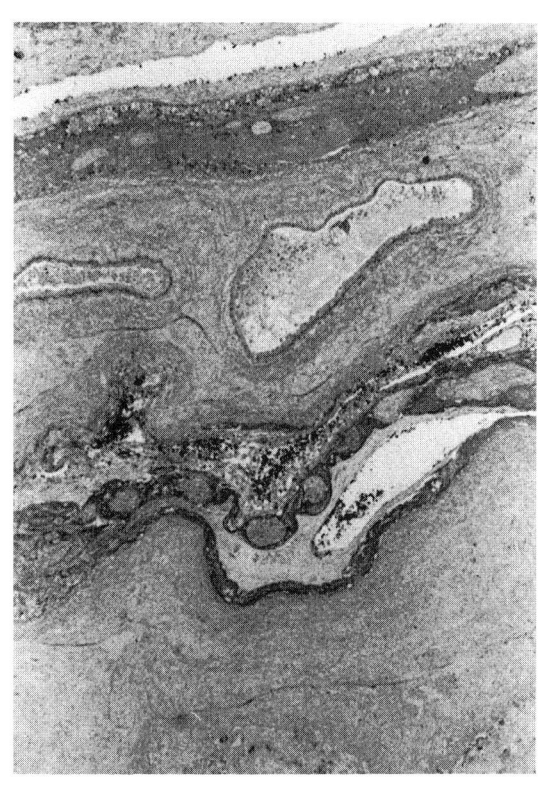

Figure 4 The remnants of the embryonic tissue in case 2 (HE × 17)

13 and was diagnosed as having a pregnancy of 5 weeks' duration. A week later, however, she returned, complaining of abdominal pain and slight vaginal bleeding. She was admitted for treatment of threatened abortion. At that time, two gestational sacs, each with a fetus having fetal heart movements, were detected by ultrasonography. The patient's complaints disappeared and she was discharged a week later. On her next visit (at 8 weeks of gestation) only one of two fetal heart movements was recognized. After that, the surviving fetus developed

uneventfully up to term. On November 15, she delivered a 3532 g male infant by vacuum extraction with an Apgar score of 9 at 1 min. A 450 g ovoid placenta (21×17×1.8 cm) followed. The insertion of the umbilical cord was marginal. The fetal and maternal surfaces of the placenta revealed normal color and consistency, but the membranes showed a thickened yellowish-white area (8×7×0.3 cm) adjacent to the small accessory lobe of the placental margin (Figure 1). Histological findings of the thickened area suggested the remnants of vanished embryonic somites between membranes (Figure 2).

Case 2

A 37-year-old woman, gravida 4, para 2, had her last menstrual period on July 15. It lasted 6 days. She first visited our clinic at 7 weeks of gestation and she was diagnosed as having myomata uteri. Two gestational sacs were visualized by ultrasonography. Each contained a fetus with fetal heart movements. At her next visit, the patient complained of persistent vaginal spotting for two weeks. A repeat sonographic examination showed that fetal heart movements were not present in one fetus. As the pregnancy advanced, the live fetus grew uneventfully, and the dead fetus disappeared. On May 3, 1988, the patient delivered a 4090 g male infant at 41 weeks of gestation with an Apgar score of 9 at 1 min. A 440 g ovoid placenta (19×18×1.8 cm) followed. The insertion of the umbilical cord was velamentous. The fetal membranes were slightly stained with meconium and a thickened yellowish-white area with dimensions of 4×2×0.3 cm was present along the placental margin (Figure 3). Histological findings of the thickened area featured the remnants of the embryonic tissue between two rows of ghost villi of the membranes (Figure 4).

Case 3

A 26-year-old primigravida visited our clinic complaining of vaginal bleeding; she was found on ultrasonography to have an 8-week twin gestation. At 9 weeks, the fetal heart movements of one fetus disappeared, but the pregnancy continued unremarkably to term. The patient delivered a 3010 g male infant uneventfully at 40 weeks of gestation. A 350 g ovoid placenta (20×17×1.7 cm) was also delivered. The insertion of the umbilical cord was marginal, and a thickened yellowish-white area (10×4×0.5 cm) was present on the fetal membranes along the placental margin. Traces of fetal vessels could be followed on the thickened area (Figure 5). Histologically, the thickened area showed amorphous material and retromembranous hemorrhage, but no embryonic remnants were found (Figure 6).

Suspected cases

Table 3 shows data from two cases associated with first-trimester bleeding of several weeks' duration in which ultrasonography revealed a normal amniotic cavity containing a fetus with regular heart movements and an anembryonic deformed amniotic cavity. In the postpartum placental examination of these two cases, only patchy subchorionic fibrin was recognized on the respective chorionic plates. Although the histological findings showed degenerated amorphous tissue, no specific embryonic remnants could be identified. The following case is illustrative.

Case 5

A 33-year-old woman, gravida 2, para 1, had been referred from a clinic. She complained of persistent vaginal spotting with slight lower abdominal pain. The presumptive diagnosis was a 12-week gestation and threatened abortion. On ultrasound scan, both a normal amniotic sac containing a fetus with regular heart movements and an anembryonic amniotic sac were demonstrated (Figure 7). After 2 weeks, her complaints disappeared and the pregnancy proceeded uneventfully to term. The patient delivered a 3331 g healthy baby girl at 39 weeks of gestation. Careful examination of the placenta revealed a 2×1.5 cm yellowish-white fleck on the placental margin contiguous with

Documenting the vanishing twin

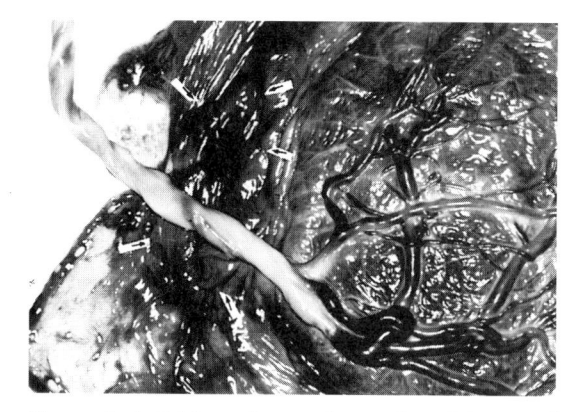

Figure 5 A thickened area (arrows) and traces of the fetal vessels in the membranes in case 3

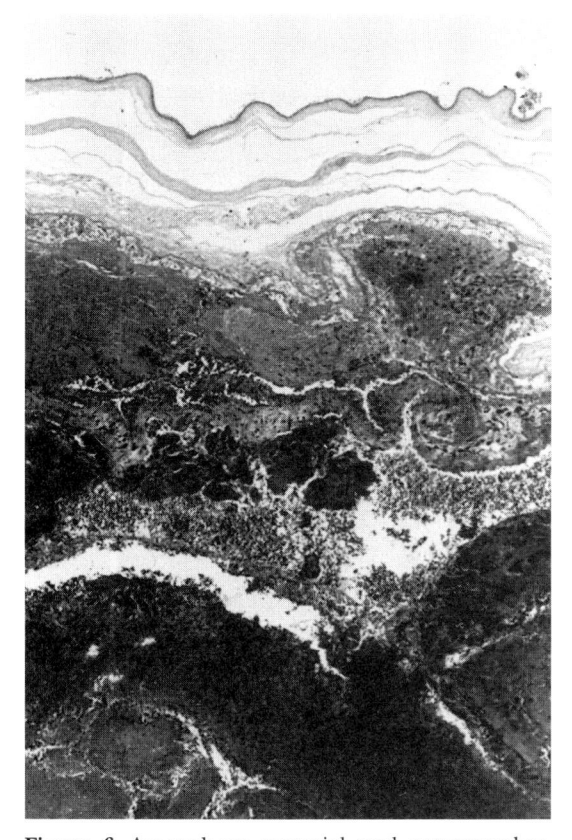

Figure 6 Amorphous material and retromembranous hemorrhage in the membranes in case 3 (HE × 8)

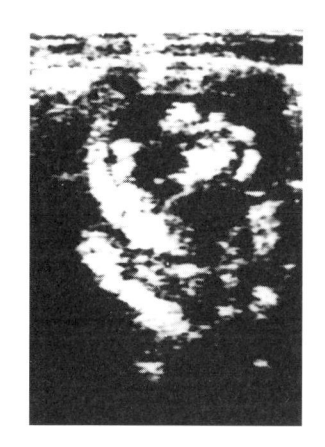

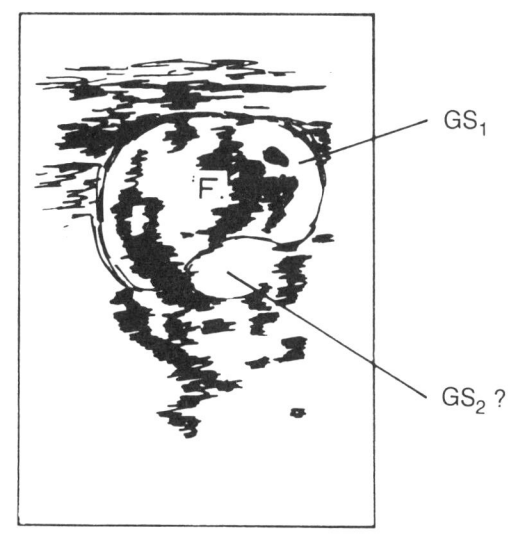

Figure 7 A normal (GS$_1$) and a deformed gestational sac (GS$_2$) in case 5

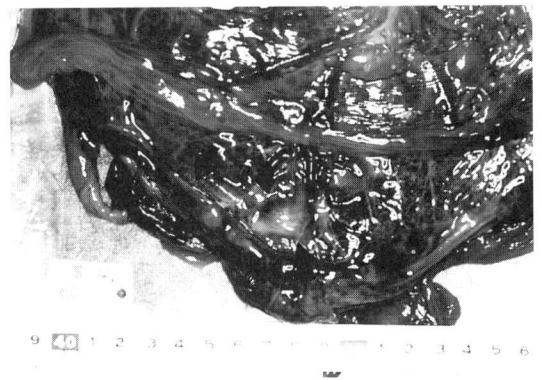

Figure 8 A yellowish-white fleck and circumvallate membranes with marginal hemorrhage of the placenta in case 5

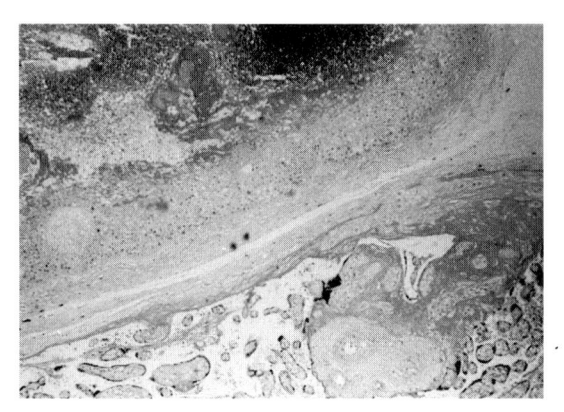

Figure 9 Amorphous material, ghost villi and degenerated membranes on the viable membranes in case 5 (HE × 6)

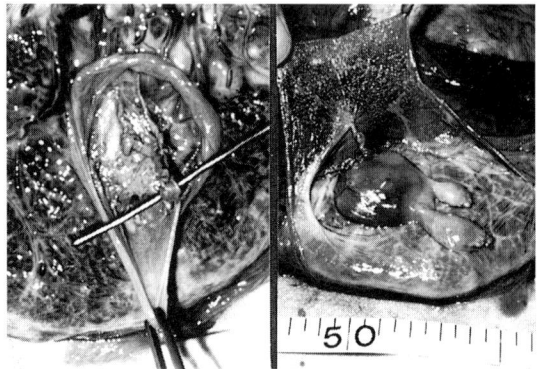

Figure 10 Amorphous material in the cystic tumor on the chorionic plate (left) and a fetus papyraceus of acardiac monster (right)

a circumvallate membrane and marginal hemorrhage (Figure 8). Histological examination of this area demonstrated amorphous material, degenerated chorionic villi and degeneration of membranes juxtaposed against viable membranes (Figure 9). Although no embryonic remnants could be found, these observations are highly suggestive of an early demise of a blighted embryo. The other case of suspected vanishing twin listed in Table 3 demonstrated similar histological features on the chorionic plate.

Doubtful cases

Table 4 presents data from nine cases with doubtful evidence of the vanishing twin syndrome suspected or recognized by placental examination alone, because ultrasonographic examinations were not available. On gross examination of the placentas from these nine cases, all were noted to have a cystic tumor on the chorionic plate. Maximum dimensions varied from 2.8 to 6 cm. Contents of the cysts varied and included in one case degenerated embryonic tissues and a blighted umbilical cord in brownish serous fluid.

As shown in Figure 10, these findings are similar to the case associated with the death of a co-twin in the second trimester, which was identified as a fetus papyraceus in the cyst on the right half of the picture. However, if death of one twin occurs in the first trimester, the dead fetus might be resorbed or highly degenerated, resulting only in amorphous material as pregnancy advances. Therefore, it is not possible to find evidence of the dead fetus, which is only observed as doubtful evidence on the chorionic plate, as shown on the left half of the picture (Figure 10).

On histological examination, amorphous materials surrounded by degenerated chorionic villi and the viable amniochorionic membranes were present in the placental sections in most cases listed in Table 4. In some cases, however, degenerated amorphous tissues were barely visible, whereas well-delineated perivillous fibrin deposition was present in a section of placental marginal region. In reality, amorphous materials and fibrin deposition on placental sections may represent findings of the vanished twin, but in many cases these findings are overlooked. Despite the death of one twin, the surviving co-twin with unaffected placental tissues continued to grow until term in all cases and was born without any complication, except that in one case, the liveborn fetus had congenital heart disease.

Comment

Resorption of one or more fetuses during pregnancy was commonly observed in experimental animals. In humans, however, it was not possible to prove the existence of a vanishing twin until the advent of ultrasonography.

Table 4 Doubtful evidence of vanishing twins

Case no.	Gestational complications Live-born infant	Placental weight Size of cyst	Placental findings
7	1st trimester bleeding F: 3250 g (39 weeks)	435 g 4 × 3 cm	subchorionic fibrin; fetus papyraceus? (5 g)
8	1st trimester bleeding F: 3300 g (40 weeks)	435 g 4 × 3.3 cm	subchorionic fibrin; amorphous material (cord?)
9	1st trimester bleeding F: 3730 g (40 weeks)	580 g 5 × 3 cm	amorphous material
10	1st trimester bleeding F: 2748 g (39 weeks)	420 g 5 × 3 cm	circum-marginate; fetus papyraceus? (7 g)
11	1st trimester bleeding F: 3258 g (41 weeks)	510 g 3 × 2 cm	marked subchorionic fibrin; intervillous thrombi
12	1st trimester bleeding F: 3510 g (39 weeks)	525 g 6 × 4 cm	marked subchorionic fibrin; intervillous thrombi; amorphous material
13	1st trimester bleeding M: 3803 g (41 weeks)	495 g 5 × 4.6 cm	circum-marginate; amorphous material
14	1st trimester bleeding F: 3017 g (40 weeks)	380 g 2.8 × 2 cm	subchorionic fibrin; intervillous thrombosis; accessory lobe
15	1st trimester bleeding M: 2934 g (39 weeks) heart anomaly	400 g 5 × 5 cm	subchorionic fibrin; circum-marginate; amorphous material

After Levi initially reported that only 28.6% of women with twin pregnancies diagnosed using ultrasound before 10 weeks of gestation gave birth to twin babies[7], other reports on the vanishing twin have also been published[1,8,9].

Sulak and Dodson[2] first presented pathological confirmation of the vanishing twin and Jauniaux et al.[3] provided histological evidence of this phenomenon. In 1982, Landy et al. reported that disappearance rates of one or more fetuses in multiple pregnancies ranged from 0 to 70%. One of the reasons why disappearance rates range so widely is that pathological confirmation has rarely been accomplished.

Of the 15 cases in our series, the four cases summarized in Table 2 exhibited two fetal heart movements by ultrasonography before 9 weeks of gestation and in each case, one of two fetal heart movements disappeared one or two weeks later. In two cases (cases 1 and 2), embryonic remnants were histologically identified in a thickened area of the membranes. These placental lesions were associated with remnants consisting of embryonic somites. In the other two cases (cases 3 and 4), no embryonic tissues were identified, but marked retromembranous hemorrhage containing amorphous material and well-delineated plaques of perivillous fibrin deposition were found between the chorionic and basal plates in case 3. In case 4, amorphous material and marked fibrin deposition were observed in a sac on the chorionic plate. The macroscopic and microscopic features of these four cases represent confirmatory evidence of the vanished twin, though not all cases are as clear.

Two cases in Table 3 revealed single fetal heart movements in a normal sac that adjoined another deformed anembryonic sac. At the postpartum placental examination, subchorionic fibrin deposition was present as a gross finding and amorphous material was found on microscopy at the chorionic plate of the placental margin. These observations suggest an early demise of a blighted embryo.

Nine cases with a cystic tumor on the chorionic plate are summarized in Table 4. All were found prior to the availability of the ultrasound technique for diagnosis of pregnancy. Robinson and Caines[8] reported that of 30 patients who were diagnosed by ultrasonography as having twins in the first trimester, only 14 gave birth to twins. Of the remaining 16 patients, ten gave birth to singleton infants and six aborted electively or spontaneously. One patient's placenta revealed a flattened empty sac on the fetal surface, but no histological findings of tissue were described.

The combination of ultrasonography and histopathological examination demonstrates that the second sac of a twin gestation sometimes remains on the fetal surface of the placenta until the time of delivery, without complete resorption. This phenomenon can be confirmed histologically by the findings of embryonic remnants and perivillous fibrin deposition. Further studies are needed to determine whether the finding of amorphous materials and fibrin deposition alone or together are confirmative evidence of the vanishing twin syndrome.

References

1. Landy, H.J., Keith, L. and Keith, D. (1982). The vanishing twin. *Acta Genet. Med. Gemellol.*, **31**, 195
2. Sulak, L.A. and Dodson, M.G. (1986). The vanishing twin; pathologic confirmation of an ultrasonographic phenomenon. *Obstet. Gynecol.*, **68**, 811
3. Jauniaux, E., Elkazen, N., Leroy, F. *et al.* (1988). Clinical and morphologic aspects of the vanishing twin phenomenon. *Obstet. Gynecol.*, **72**, 577
4. Yoshida, K. and Soma, H. (1986). Outcome of the surviving cotwin of a fetus papyraceus or of a dead fetus. *Acta Genet. Med. Gemellol.*, **35**, 91
5. Yoshida, K. and Matayoshi, K. (1990). A study on prognosis of surviving cotwin. *Acta Genet. Med. Gemellol.*, **39**, 383
6. Yoshida, K. (1992). Management and prognosis in intrauterine death of one twin in twin pregnancy. *Treatment Obstet. Gynecol.*, **65**, 55 (in Japanese)
7. Levi, S. (1976). Ultrasonic assessment of the high rate of human multiple pregnancy in the first trimester. *J. Clin. Ultrasound.*, **4**, 3
8. Robinson, H.P. and Caines, J.S. (1977). Sonar evidence of early pregnancy failure in patients with twin conceptions. *Br. J. Obstet. Gynaecol.*, **84**, 22
9. Finberg, H.J. and Birnholz, J.C. (1979). Ultrasound observations in multiple gestation with first trimester bleeding: the blighted twin. *Radiology*, **132**, 137

The vanishing twin

H.J. Landy and B.M. Nies

Introduction

Early fetal loss in multiple gestations, long recognized clinically, has been confirmed and characterized with the evolution of sonography. Indeed, even before sonography, animal studies had illustrated the loss of fetuses from litters, possibly related to lack of intrauterine space or crowding[1]. With improvements in sonographic techniques, the 'vanishing twin' phenomenon, first documented in the earlier days of ultrasound, has become widely accepted. Using sonography, many reports have demonstrated (1) 'disappearance' of at least one of multiple sacs among human conceptions; and (2) fewer twins observed at delivery than were previously identified in the first trimester.

The first suggestion that the conception rate of multiple gestations was higher than the multiple birth rate was made in 1945 by Stoeckel[2]: 'It thus appears that twins are more often conceived than born; not only in addition to the evidence of foeti papyracei, it may be that twin material is reabsorbed due to early death, without leaving any trace.'. Since the advent of ultrasound, Stoeckel's hypothesis has been proven.

In 1982, we reviewed the world literature on the vanishing twin phenomenon[3]; nine papers in the obstetric and radiologic literature between 1973 and 1981 documented fetal disappearance in multiple gestations[4–12]. Since that publication, numerous other reports have elaborated the sonographic, clinical, pathological and laboratory characteristics of the vanishing twin[13–35].

Commentary prior to 1982

Hellman et al.[4] reported the earliest sonographic demonstration of the vanishing twin in 1973. These authors described sonographic abnormalities in 140 patients, 114 of whom ultimately miscarried. Twenty-two patients had double gestational sacs. All 13 patients who had conceived spontaneously and had two sacs miscarried; this group presumably represented monozygous twins. In nine patients given medication to induce ovulation, presumably conceiving dizygous twins, five sets of twins and three singletons were delivered. The authors commented: 'Presumably... one twin was absorbed.'. The frequency of monozygous twinning, almost 10% in this group of patients, was approximately 25 times higher than the expected rate.

In 1974, Kohorn and Kaufman[5] prospectively evaluated 65 patients scanned in the first trimester. The initial scans of three patients revealed two sacs; all delivered singletons.

In 1976, Levi's study[6] described 6990 women, each of whom had at least ten sonographic evaluations; of these, 118 had multiple sacs. The data were divided, based on timing of initial scan; follow-up was available for 101 patients. The smallest number of twin pairs were delivered among those patients scanned the earliest: only four sets of twins (28.6%) were delivered of the 14 patients scanned before 10 weeks. As gestation advanced, however, the sonographic diagnosis of multiple gestation became more predictive. Among eight patients scanned between 10 and 15 weeks, three sets of twins (37.5%) were born; 78 sets of multiples and one case of fetus papyraceus coexisting with a singleton were seen among the 79 patients scanned before 15 weeks. Levi cited a 71% 'disappearance' rate when twins were diagnosed before 10 gestational weeks and explained this high 'disappearance' rate as being due to diagnostic errors. (The concept of sonographic overdiagnosis of multiple gestation was further elaborated by Defoort et al.[13] in a 1976 publication in which three sources of false positive errors were identified: (1) simple technical artifacts; (2) sonographic echoes derived from fetal movement; and (3) error from off-center scanning of a single hourglass-shaped sac.)

Thirty women with twins identified by first-trimester ultrasound were described in a 1977 report by Robinson and Caines[7]. All 14 patients with sonographic evidence of normal twins delivered twins. The remaining 16 cases (four cases of blighted ovum/blighted ovum, one blighted ovum/missed abortion, and 11 cases of blighted ovum/normal pregnancy) ended as six spontaneous abortions and ten singleton deliveries. Repeat scans showed that the second sac became smaller and ultimately disappeared in several patients. The first published evidence of pathological confirmation of the vanishing process was presented in this report: a flattened empty 3-cm sac on the fetal surface of the placenta was identified after delivery in one patient whose scan had previously shown a blighted ovum coexisting with a normal pregnancy.

The following year, Levi and Reimers published a study in the French literature describing 143 of 159 patients with multiple sacs observed in first-trimester scans[8]. The likelihood that the sonographic findings represented a normal twin gestation was considered in dividing the patients into 'certain', 'probable, and 'doubtful' diagnostic groups. Of 47 patients scanned between 4 and 9 weeks (34 'certain', eight 'probable' and five 'doubtful') among whom follow-up had been obtained for 32 patients, only six multiple births resulted. In contrast, 14 multiples resulted from 23 patients scanned between 10 and 14 weeks (ten 'certain', six 'probable' and seven 'doubtful') for whom follow-up was possible in 22 instances. Confirming the concept that later scans were more reliable, all 89 patients scanned after 14 weeks and in whom the diagnosis was 'certain' in all instances, delivered multiples. The authors proposed a 78% fetal disappearance rate when a 'certain' diagnosis was made before 10 weeks and a 1.9% incidence of multiple pregnancy. False positive errors (lack of continuity from scan to scan and artifacts from the developing embryo) and false negative errors (erroneous diagnosis of singleton rather than multiple pregnancy from insufficient scanning) were discussed, as well as the importance of the sonographer's experience in minimizing interpretative errors.

In 1979, four related papers appeared in obstetric and radiological journals. Varma described 30 cases of multiple pregnancy in the first trimester in the *British Journal of Obstetrics and Gynaecology*[9]. Four sonographic findings were described: (1) multiple sacs (15 patients); (2) blighted ovum/normal pregnancy (seven patients); (3) missed abortion/missed abortion (three patients); and (4) blighted ovum/blighted ovum (five patients). Fourteen multiples (46.7%) resulted. Vaginal bleeding occurred in 12 patients (40%), 11 of whom eventually miscarried. The frequency of multiple gestation was cited as one in 50.

Finberg and Birnholz[10] described 22 patients, 19 with first-trimester bleeding, who were scanned before 15 weeks of gestation and in whom an abnormal region was seen adjacent to a normally progressing fetus. The separate anechoic or hypoechoic area identified within the uterus was thought to represent a coexistent 'blighted twin' or anembryonic pregnancy. Three distinct patterns were outlined: (1) a second sac; (2) a crescent of fluid surrounding a normal sac; and (3) septal division of the amniotic cavity with one empty compartment. Of 14 patients with double sacs, there were ten singleton deliveries, three elective terminations and one spontaneous loss at 22 weeks. Two instances of pathology were described: a 'collection of 30 milliliters of dark brown altered blood' initially obtained during the termination of one pregnancy was thought to represent a second hemorrhagic sac identified sonographically. In addition, a patient who had had a spontaneous abortion with 'pathologic confirmation of an intact six-week fetus' was found to have a normal single 12-week fetus on sonogram 6 weeks later.

Only eight singletons were delivered from a group of 41 patients with abnormal first-trimester multiple pregnancies studied by Kurjak and Latin[11]. Sonographic findings included blighted ovum/normal pregnancy (20 patients), blighted ovum/blighted ovum (nine patients), blighted ovum/missed abortion (two patients), missed abortion/missed abortion (two patients), twin embryonic echoes with development and delivery of a singleton (three patients), normal fetus/anencephalic fetus (one patient), normal fetus/fetus papyraceus (two patients) and normal fetus/two fetuses papyraceus (two patients).

Schneider et al.[14] reported a high rate of early ovular resorption in both spontaneous and ovulation-induced multiple gestations in 1979. There were 54 spontaneous and 24 induced twin pregnancies (clomiphene citrate in 11 cases, gonadotropins in 12 cases and cyclofenil in one case) scanned in early pregnancy. The overall disappearance rate was 50%, occurring in 41 of 78 cases; however, early ovular resorption (a phrase not further defined) occurred in 63% of spontaneous and 29% of induced twin conceptions. Only those pregnancies induced with clomiphene citrate demonstrated ovular resorption (64%); this phenomenon was not observed with the other agents. The suggestion was made that the recognized differences in twinning rates following clomiphene citrate and gonadotropin therapy may depend more on differences in the vanishing rates than on individual drug characteristics. (Editor: To our knowledge, this suggestion has languished in the literature.)

The 1981 paper by Jeanty and colleagues from the French journal, Ultrasons, described 23 of 300 patients scanned before 14 weeks in whom multiple gestations were diagnosed[12]. Of 21 sets of twins diagnosed sonographically, 18 singletons and three twin pairs resulted; one set of triplets progressed to normal twins; and, finally, one set of diagnosed quadruplets resulted in a singleton delivery. The authors stressed that 'only six pregnancies were seen for the first time as normal twin gestations'. Three sonographic findings specific to the vanishing twin were described: (1) a smaller sac; (2) a crescent-shaped sac; and (3) a small echogenic spot. These authors postulated that early embryonic disappearance could result sonographically in an echogenic spot, whereas later disappearance could produce a crescent-shaped sac that might grow or regress. Although the methods of statistical analyses were not elaborated, a high rate of multiple pregnancies ($7.6 \pm 3.9\%$) was reported.

Finally, a Japanese study from 1981[15] described the sonographic findings of 18 patients with multiple pregnancies scanned between 7 and 12 weeks. Nine cases (50%) demonstrated a decrease in the number of sacs and two cases (11%) showed a decrease in the number of fetuses. Based on the number of gestational sacs, fetal wastage occurred in 30–70% of pregnancies; the critical period for the continuation of multiple gestation was 14 weeks. A Canadian investigator described three patients with vanishing twins in 1982[16]. Each case report was detailed, as all patients experienced vaginal bleeding.

Commentary 1982–89

Nine of the 13 communications cited above were reviewed in our paper on the vanishing twin presented at the 1982 *Workshop on Multiple Pregnancies of the International Society for Twin Studies* in Paris[3]. After examining data from these reports, it became clear that, whereas the vanishing twin phenomenon was real, an extremely wide range of disappearance had been reported (0 to 78%). We then sought to determine a more accurate incidence of fetal disappearance by studying 1000 viable first-trimester pregnancies[17]. Fifty-four patients with suspected multiple gestations were identified, 26 of whom delivered 26 sets of multiples and 28 of whom had a vanishing fetus. The latter 28 cases were separated into three groups: (1) 'documented' diagnoses in seven pregnancies in which fetal heart motion was seen in two sacs and the subsequent scan showed only one viable fetus; (2) 'suspected' diagnoses in 17 pregnancies in which an empty or abnormal sac was seen adjacent to one or more viable gestations with the resultant number of viable fetuses being one less than the number of sacs originally seen; and (3) 'doubtful' diagnoses in four pregnancies in which a viable fetus was present within a bilobed gestational sac and the possibility of a twin gestation could not be excluded. Considering only those patients with a documented diagnosis of twin gestation, the overall disappearance rate for one fetus was 21.2%; inclusion of patients with suspected and doubtful diagnoses increased the frequency to 48% and 51.8%, respectively. First-trimester bleeding occurred in 25% of pregnancies with a vanishing fetus. Using the most conservative estimate possible for this prospective series, the postconception incidence of multiple gestation was 3.29%.

Additional studies have been published since then. Four pregnancies with at least one empty gestational sac in viable multiple gestations were reported by Gindoff and co-workers in 1986[18]. In each case, resorption of the empty sacs was documented. Vaginal bleeding occurred in three of four patients. Steptoe et al.[19] described 767 clinical pregnancies after in vitro fertilization (IVF). A total of 91 patients had multiple sacs in first-trimester scans. Vanishing fetuses were identified in 'approximately 18%' of pregnancies: 26 of 74 patients with two sacs lost one or two fetuses and eight of 17 patients with three sacs lost more than one fetus. (Independent calculation of these data reveal 35.1% and 47.1% frequencies of vanishing fetuses and sacs, respectively.)

Two studies in 1986 provided pathological confirmation of the vanishing process. The report by Sulak and Dodson[20] described a triplet gestation following IVF, in which only a singleton was delivered. The placenta contained a thickened 4 cm area composed of degenerated chorionic villi with two additional distinct layers of chorion that formed a well-defined 1.1-cm sac-like structure. The authors commented that 'the chorion-lined sac containing amorphous (nonvillous) material... was seen to represent the histologic remnants of an early gestational sac. Because no fetal remnants could be identified, ...the histologic findings suggested an early degenerate blighted ovum, which became compressed against the viable amnion–chorion of the surviving twin'. Interestingly, however, no histological evidence for the third sac was found. Yoshida and Soma examined 189 twin placentas[21]. Of 115 monochorionic pregnancies, 21 were complicated by the *in utero* death of a fetus, nine in the first trimester. In all nine cases with vanishing twins, careful examination of the fetal surface of the placenta after term delivery revealed a chorionic cyst-like sac that often contained a stunted embryo. In one case, the authors described a sac (7×7 cm) which upon opening revealed 'a strand of umbilical cord-like tissue and a highly compressed embryo'.

Indirect evidence of early fetal wastage can also be derived through studies evaluating diverse aspects of ultrasound and obstetrics. In 1987, Belfrage's group described 2054 patients scanned between 10 and 14 weeks to assess the benefit of routine vs. selective ultrasound examinations[22]. Although 19 patients had multiple gestations, only two had vanishing twins. In presenting data on a successful IVF program, Meldrum and colleagues[23] described 22 clinical pregnancies with multiple sacs (20 twins, one triplet, one quadruplet). Six pregnancies (27%) resulted in delivery of a singleton. A *Lancet* article by Stabile and associates[24] detailed the results of high-resolution transabdominal scans of 624 women presenting with bleeding and/or pain. Of 406 pregnant patients, 16 (3.9%) had a normal pregnancy and a second smaller empty sac. Weekly scans showed the smaller sac to decrease in size. Although the patients continued to experience intermittent painless vaginal bleeding, none miscarried.

Jauniaux's group evaluated clinical and histological aspects of ten pregnancies with a vanishing twin[25]. Vaginal bleeding occurred in seven pregnancies in the first trimester and in one triplet pregnancy in the early second trimester; in all cases, bleeding coincided with sonographically identified fetal disappearance. Intrauterine growth retardation was present in three infants, and one stillbirth occurred at 20 weeks. Pathological confirmation consisting of well-delineated plaques of perivillous fibrin deposition was noted in five cases; in one case, embryonic remnants were also seen. The authors commented that '*This focal degenerative change of the placental mass, which also exists in about 25% of placentas from uncomplicated term pregnancies, may be the only clue to the disappearance of one conceptus*'. (Editor: Emphasis added.)

Three patients presenting with abdominal cramping and vaginal bleeding in early pregnancy were described by Saidi in 1988[26]. All cases revealed twin gestations on sonogram. In one patient, a folded gestational sac containing serosanguinous fluid was found when the placenta was ultimately examined.

A Danish article demonstrated the vanishing twin phenomenon in a private practice[27]. Sonography revealed two sacs in 12 patients who ultimately delivered singletons and one case of triplets in which twins resulted. Ultrasound findings of the gestations with two sacs included normal pregnancy/blighted ovum (two patients), normal pregnancy/missed abortion (nine patients), and normal pregnancy/anencephalic pregnancy (one patient). The twin conception rate was reported as one in 51 (1.96%), although only one in 106 produced viable twins (0.94%).

Goldman and colleagues described vanishing fetuses in 17 cases of higher order multiples at the Sherman Fertility Institute in Israel[28]. Twelve patients conceived after ovulation induction, five after IVF. Vaginal bleeding occurred in 13 patients (76.5%). No fetal disappearance occurred beyond 14–16 weeks.

In a case report by Tharapel and colleagues, the vanishing twin phenomenon was postulated to explain discrepant chromosome results[29]. Transabdominal chorionic villus sampling performed at 10.5 weeks when sonography indicated a single intrauterine pregnancy revealed 47,XX,+16 karyotype. Ten days later, sonography showed the pregnancy to be progressing normally. Amniocentesis performed at 16 weeks yielded a normal 46,XX karyotype. At delivery, a 1.5×1.3×0.4 cm placental nodule was identified, the karyotype of which revealed 46,XX/47,XX,+16. Chromosomal evaluation of the fetal membranes and the infant's blood were both 46,XX. This interesting example suggests that fetuses may disappear without exhibiting the characteristic sonographic or clinical manifestations already described.

Commentary after 1990

The advent of transvaginal ultrasound represents advance that affords detailed sonographic information much earlier in gestation than traditional transabdominal methods. A 1990 study by Bateman and associates[30] described vaginal sonography applied in 74 women with intrauterine pregnancies, 18 with spontaneous abortions and 34 with ectopic gestations. Seven patients had multiple sacs, two of whom had normal multiple gestations (one set each of twins and triplets), and five who subsequently had disappearance of a sac. The ultrasound findings of one patient continued to show evidence of three extra sacs adjacent to a normally progressing intrauterine pregnancy.

Dickey and colleagues described the outcome of 227 twin, 45 triplet and five quadruplet gestations diagnosed sonographically in the first trimester after a variety of infertility treatments[31,33]. Maternal age was found to be a significant factor in the resorption process with a 30.2% chance of one sac being resorbed after finding twin sacs in women under 30 years of age and a 34.2% chance in those 30 and older; the risk of both sacs resorbing was 6.7% and 14.8%, respectively in these two age groups. After documentation of viable twins, there was a 90% chance of delivery of two infants in patients younger than 30 years of age and 84% in those older than 30 years of age. When three sacs were seen, triplet delivery was observed in 45% of younger and 17% of older patients, respectively. When three viable embryos were present, the chance of having a triplet birth was 90% for women under 30 and only 44% for those 30 and older.

Another 1990 study evaluated 27 multiple pregnancies conceived after IVF and embryo transfer at Yale University School of Medicine[33]. Four 'vanishing sacs' were described resulting in two twin and two singleton pregnancies.

An interesting Japanese study[34] suggested a seasonality to fetal loss among multiple gestations. Vanishing twins, occurring in two of six cases with two fetal heart beats seen initially, and in seven of eight cases in which sonography revealed echo-free spaces (considered to represent an empty gestational sac), occurred between January and May. In further reporting that all six women with twins delivered during these months, these authors postulate a seasonality to 'twin-prone and abortion-prone characteristics'. To our knowledge, no other studies have addressed this issue regarding twinning in general or the vanishing twin phenomenon in particular.

Human chorionic gonadotropin (hCG) levels in twin gestations were studied by Kelly and associates in 1991[35]. The rise in hCG was compared in vanishing twin and normally progressing twin pregnancies by obtaining serial levels (up to three times per week) during the early part of the first trimester. Of the 40 patients studied, resorption of one twin occurred in 13 (32.5%): seven (54%) vanished when an early fetal pole was observed and six (46%) resorbed after fetal heart activity had been detected sonographically. These data also showed that the rate of rise of hCG was significantly slower in vanishing twin pregnancies than in normally progressing twin pregnancies throughout the study period.

Two 1991 reports explain karyotype discrepancies by the occurrence of vanishing twins. In the report by Callen et al.[36], a normal 46,XX infant was associated with a predominantly triploid 69,XXY placenta, the latter presumably originating from a vanishing twin. Reddy and colleagues[37] postulated that the vanishing twin was the most likely cause of a descrepant karyotype obtained via chorionic villus sampling. A third article[38] describes a vanishing twin pregnancy in which tetraploidy was associated with degenerated chorionic villi found in a thickened area opposite the main placenta, whereas a diploid karyotype was found in association with most of the placental cells.

Kapur and associates reported an interesting case of sirenomelia occurring in the surviving co-twin from a vanishing twin pregnancy[39]. This case represents the only published anomaly occurring in conjunction with a vanishing twin; the authors further elaborated on the frequent association between sirenomelia, a rare congenital malformation, and monozygotic twinning.

An Australian study examined the outcome of 126 twin pregnancies identified sonographically between 6 and 16 weeks, 59 patients having conceived after IVF and embryo transfer[40]. When viable twins were detected prior to 7 weeks, a 29% fetal disappearance rate was reported, compared to pregnancies between 7 and 9 weeks, in which 16% of pregnancies had associated vanishing twins. The fetal disappearance rate was similar for IVF and non-IVF gestations.

A 1992 Israeli study evaluated 88 multiple gestations established after ovulation induction and diagnosed by transvaginal sonography between 5 and 6 weeks[41]. After detection of 54 viable twin gestations, 51 resulted in the birth of singletons and three ended in spontaneous abortions in 50 of these 54 twin pregnancies, a vanishing twin was detected before 13 weeks; one patient had an intrauterine fetal demise of one twin at 25 weeks. Pathological identification of the resorbed fetus was confirmed in three pregnancies. Of the 26 viable triplet gestations, fetal resorption occurred in 14 pregnancies, 12 resulting in delivery of twins and two in spontaneous abortions; the remaining 12 pregnancies ended in the birth of singletons. Fetal disappearance was described before 13 weeks in all except one case in which fetal demise was detected at 17 weeks. Pathological confirmation of fetal resorption was identified in one pregnancy. Quadruplet pregnancies, identified in five patients, resulted in fetal resorption to triplet gestations in three patients, twins in two women and a singleton in one patient. There were three quintuplet pregnancies, all with spontaneous fetal disappearance: two fetuses resorbed in one patient and one fetus in two patients. The latter two patients also underwent selective fetal reduction, ultimately delivering triplets in one case and twins in the other. The authors recommended delaying iatrogenic fetal reduction in higher order multiple gestations until after 12 weeks.

Pathologic confirmation of vanishing twins was reported in two European articles[42,43]. Placental examination in 15 cases of vanishing twins was reported in a German article[42]. Ten cases revealed remnants of a second gestation identified at the placental margin or within the amniotic membranes, ranging from macerated, but recognizable, fetal tissues to distinct, empty gestational sacs. Observing a 'plurichorionic placenta' in all cases, the authors discussed the vanishing twin phenomenon as a possible cause of development of isoimmunization in subsequent pregnancies. Gavriil and colleagues[43] investigated 100 placentas from pregnancies conceived with IVF and embryo transfer; ten multiple pregnancies were associated with vanishing twins and an additional five multiple pregnancies underwent selective reduction. First-trimester bleeding, the only clinical finding related to fetal disappearance, was not observed in those pregnancies selectively reduced.

The outcomes of 68 sonographically viable first-trimester twin pregnancies were reported by Benson and associates[44]. Conception occurred with assisted reproductive techniques in 40% and spontaneously in 60% of pregnancies. Loss of one fetus with subsequent singleton delivery occurred in 12% of patients; an additional 9% of pregnancies were complicated by loss of the entire twin gestation. The authors reported a 16% loss rate among dichorionic twins from 6 to 7.9 weeeks compared to a 4% loss rate after 8–13 weeks. Disappearance of one twin with survival of its co-twin was seen only in twins identified at 6–7.9 weeks; when twins were diagnosed 8–13 weeks, either both or neither were liveborn. A better prognosis was seen for dichorionic compared to monochorionic twins, worse outcomes being associated with advanced maternal age (≥ 35 years) and assisted conception[44]. These same investigators published another article in 1994 in which they tried to determine those clinical and sonographic characteristics which could aid in developing formulas for calculating probabilities of twin prgnancies resulting in two, one, or no liveborn infants[45]. The population included 137 viable first-trimester twin pregnancies (56.9% spontaneously occurring and 43.1% through assisted conception); although not clearly delineated, it seems likely that this study incorporates information from the 68 twin pregnancies described in the 1993 paper. The 1994 data indicate that 8.8% of pregnancies resulted in singletons and 10.9% produced no liveborn infants. Paradoxically, all 18 patients who underwent early sonography because of symptoms of bleeding or pain delivered liveborn twins. In contrast to the earlier report, this study concluded that maternal age and method of conception were not significant prognostic factors; using logistic regression analysis, gestational age at the time of sonography was the single best characteristic to correlate with pregnancy outcome.

Cytogenetic and molecular analysis of a clomiphene-induced pregnancy in which two cell lines were detected after chorionic villus sampling is reported by Falik-Borenstein and colleagues[46]. The two cell lines that were discovered were 46,XX (in 94% of cells cultured) and 47,XY,+9 (in 6%). Chimerism was suspected and the most likely etiology for the autosomal trisomy was a vanishing twin. The pertinent details and cytogenetic literature review are suggested for the interested reader.

Observations

Early fetal loss in multiple gestation, first suspected and described clinically in 1945 and later confirmed sonographically beginning in the early 1970s, is an established entity in both animal and human pregnancies. Figures 1–4 show examples of vanishing twins: Figures 1 and 2, from the same patient, show 5-week twins (Figure 1) and a 9.5-week viable singleton (Figure 2); Figures 3 and 4, from another patient, show a viable triplet pregnancy at 6 weeks (Figure 3)

MULTIPLE PREGNANCY

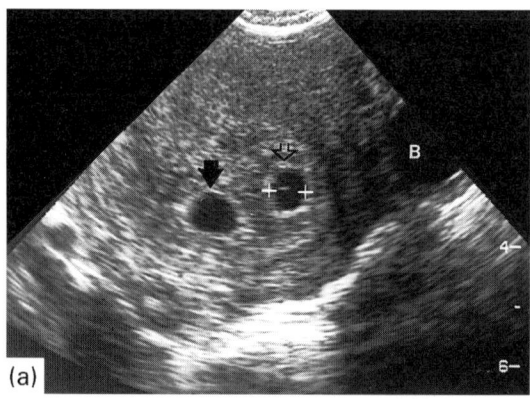

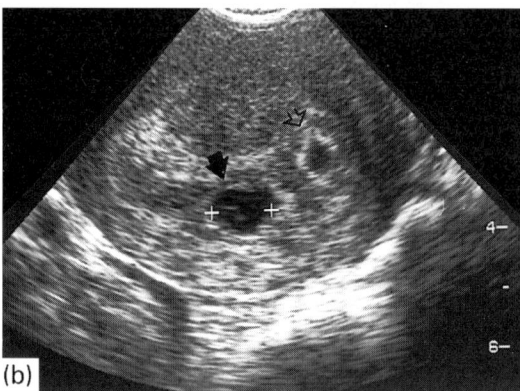

Figure 1 Twin intrauterine pregnancy at 5 weeks. Two gestational sacs were identified, each containing a yolk sac. No fetal pole or fetal heart motion was seen in either sac. (a) and (b): Right sac, 7 mm (open arrows); left sac, 9 mm (closed arrows); B, bladder

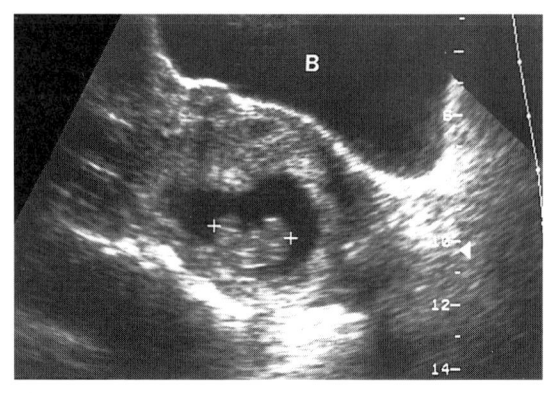

Figure 2 Sonogram in same patient as in Figure 1, indicating the 'vanishing twin' phenomenon. At 9.5 weeks, a viable singleton pregnancy was present; no evidence of the second sac was seen. B, bladder

ultimately becoming viable twins by 12.5 weeks (Figure 4); in both examples, there was no evidence of the additional gestational sac by the time of the second sonogram.

The incidence of this condition remains difficult to assess; based on data presented in the studies reviewed above, frequencies range from 10.5% to 100%. These figures are misleading, however, because each study involves different patient populations, sonographic criteria, and follow-up data. Review of these reports makes it clear that gestational sacs, often seen earlier in pregnancy, disappear more frequently than do well-defined fetuses observed after 6 or 7 gestational weeks. Interestingly, despite improved sonographic technology, early fetal disappearance rates do not differ when studies performed in the 1970s are compared to more recent investigations.

Perhaps more important than establishing a reliable vanishing rate, sonographic assessment in early pregnancy has provided clear insights into numerous aspects of the multifetal pregnancy *per se*. For example, a major benefit has been the ability to revise the purported incidence of human multiple gestation. As Table 1 shows, multiple gestations may occur as frequently as 9.5% of pregnancies. Indeed, analytical data presented in a 1990 paper suggest that multiple pregnancies may constitute over 12% of all conceptions[47] (Editor: See Chapter 4 for further details and amplification of these comments.)

Explanations for this sonographic phenomenon include physiological disappearance, as well as artifactual and interpretative error. The physiological process of early fetal disappearance may involve resorption, formation of a blighted ovum or of a fetus papyraceus; the latter is more commonly seen with later fetal death. Over-diagnosis of multiple pregnancies can occur early in gestation by incorrectly interpreting normal embryological and anatomical structures or sonographic artifacts. Structures such as the amniotic cavity, chorionic sac, yolk sac and extraembryonic coelom, normally present in early pregnancy, must not be misinterpreted as evidence of a twin gestation[3]. Physiological conditions, such

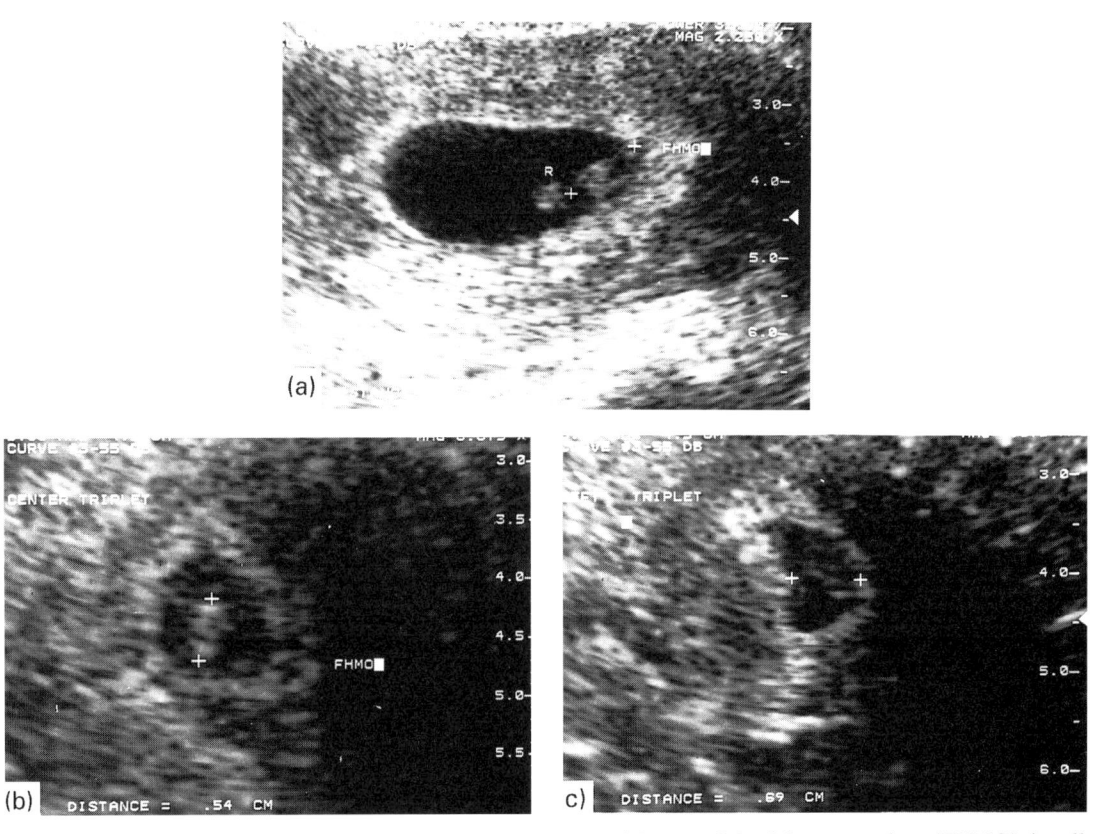

Figure 3 Triplet intrauterine pregnancy at 6 weeks with evidence of fetal heart motion (FHMO) in all three fetuses. Calipers measure fetal poles. (a) Right fetus; (b) center fetus; (c) left fetus

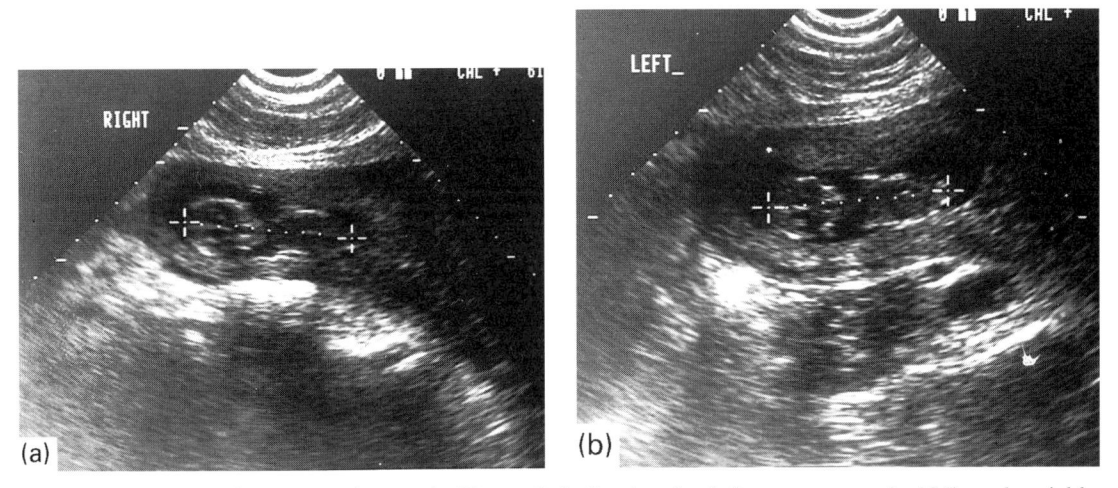

Figure 4 Sonogram in same patient as in Figure 3, indicating fetal disappearance. At 12.5 weeks, viable twins were seen; no evidence of the third gestational sac was present. Calipers measure crown–rump length. (a) Right twin, (b) left twin

Table 1 Reported range of incidence of multiple gestation using first-trimester sonography

Reference	Multiple gestation (%)
Belfrage et al. (1987)[22]	0.9
Levi (1976)[6]	1.7
Robinson and Caines (1977)[7]	1.7
Gerdts (1989)[27]	2.0
Varma (1979)[9]	2.0
Levi and Reimers (1978)[8]	2.2
Blumenfeld et al. (1992)[41]	2.3
Landy et al. (1986)[17]	3.3
Kohorn and Kaufman (1974)[5]	4.6
Jeanty et al. (1981)[12]	7.6
Hellman et al. (1973)[4]	9.3
Bateman et al. (1990)[30]	9.5

Table 2 Reported range of incidence of first-trimester bleeding with the vanishing twin

Reference	First-trimester bleeding (%)
Yoshida and Soma (1986)[21]	7.8
Gavriil et al. (1993)[43]	10.0
Bateman et al. (1990)[30]	20.0
Landy et al. (1986)[17]	25.0
Jeanty et al. (1981)[12]	26.1
Varma (1979)[9]	40.0
Meldrum et al. (1987)[23]	55.0
Saidi (1988)[26]	66.7
Gindoff et al. (1986)[18]	75.0
Goldman et al. (1989)[28]	76.5

as a collection of blood at the site of the trophoblast in a singleton pregnancy or in an abnormally progressing gestation[15], hydropic change in chorionic villi[15], or a decidual reaction in a second horn of a bicornuate uterus[12] also must be recognized as independent processes and not mistaken to be multiple pregnancies. Similarly, artifacts inherent in the technique of sonography must be recognized as such to avoid an erroneous over-diagnosis of multiple gestation. The relative contribution of artifactual over-diagnosis vs. the true vanishing twin phenomenon cannot be assessed when reviewing older literature; over-diagnosis due to artifact theoretically should be minimized with advances in sonographic technology.

The prognosis for continuing a pregnancy associated with the vanishing twin phenomenon is good. Except for rare descriptions of subsequent stillbirth or intrauterine growth retardation in the surviving co-twin, no detrimental effects occur in association with fetal disappearance. The single case of sirenomelia reported in a pregnancy with vanishing twins[39] is pertinent for the association of this rare congenital abnormality with the twinning process in general, rather than with the vanishing twin phenomenon in particular. In the case of monochorionic twins, however, the theoretical potential for passage of necrotic tissue through placental vascular connections exists, albeit at a frequency that is not possible to calculate. This situation conceivably could result in complications in the survivor. It is important to note that the complications that are described in the latter part of pregnancy[48–50], have never been described with the vanishing twin.

The only apparent pregnancy complication associated with vanishing is vaginal bleeding, which has been shown to coincide with the sonographic disappearance of a gestational sac or fetus in the first trimester. Reports indicate a wide range of bleeding frequency (i.e. from 7.8 to 76.5%) (Table 2). With these data in mind, the utility of a sonographic examination in the presence of first trimester bleeding cannot be overemphasized, because immediate patient management depends on which diagnosis is assigned: multiple pregnancy or incomplete abortion.

The study by Nakamura's group[34] has suggested a seasonality to twin loss or twin birth; however, no other reports before or since have confirmed this. Since this report is based only on six cases and in a particular geographic locality, a much larger study in different areas would be required to further corroborate this finding.

Prior to the early 1990s, a relative paucity of pathological confirmation of the vanishing phenomenon has been reported. Finberg and Birnholz[10] interpreted a collection of old blood at the time of pregnancy termination to represent a sonographic finding of a second sac as well as a persistent viable gestation 6 weeks after the pathologically confirmed spontaneous abortion of a 6-week fetus. Later investigators described more convincing histology on the fetal surface of the placenta: well-defined sacs or cysts[7,20,21,26,36,42], areas of degenerated chorionic villi[20,38], well-delineated areas of perivillous fibrin deposition[25,39], placental nodules[29,46] and stunted embryos[21,25,41,42]. In one respect, given the reported high frequencies of vanishing twins, more confirmatory evidence at delivery might be expected. In another, however, the early time of disappearance in gestation provides ample time for the body's mechanisms of resorption to remove any histological remnants.

The fascinating case report by Tharapel and colleagues[29] was the first to suggest a vanished twin as the explanation for discrepant chromosome results obtained through chorionic villus sampling and amniocentesis; the presence of a placental nodule and confirmatory chromosomal evaluation of this area support their hypothesis. Since this report, others[36–38,46] have confirmed that prenatal diagnoses yeilding discrepant genetic abnormalities are most likely the result of a vanishing twin. Similarly, it has been proposed that some cases of isoimmunization during pregnancy could result from a disappearing Rh-positive fetus in an unsensitized Rh-negative mother[17,42].

Final thoughts

Available data support the occurrence of the vanishing twin in human pregnancy. Vaginal bleeding may be the only sign in a high percentage of women experiencing this phenomenon. No other complications have been described consistently. Prognosis for the surviving co-twin is generally good, although stillbirths or intrauterine growth retardation have been reported rarely. The incidence of fetal disappearance is still difficult to estimate, in spite of major advances in sonography.

The following recommendations are suggested in the clinical management of patients with vanishing twins:

(1) Recognition of vaginal bleeding as a frequent occurrence with the vanishing phenomenon;

(2) Serial sonographic evaluation of the pregnancy to follow progression of the vanishing process and confirm viability and continued growth in the remaining twin;

(3) Reassurance of a good prognosis for the remainder of the pregnancy;

(4) Careful evaluation of the placenta and membranes after delivery for confirmatory evidence of the vanishing process; and

(5) For higher order multiple gestations in which selective reduction is a consideration, delay in performing the procedure until after 12 weeks.

Acknowledgement

The authors wish to acknowledge Dr Michael B. Hill for his assistance in providing the photographs of the sonograms for this manuscript.

References

1. Wu, M.C., Hentzel, M.D and Dziuk, P.J. (1988). Effect of stage of gestation, litter size and uterine space on the incidence of mummified fetuses in pigs. *J. Anim. Sci.*, **66**, 3202
2. Stoeckel, W. (1945). *Lehbuch der Geburtschilfe.* (Jena: Gustav Fischer) (Quoted in reference 6)
3. Landy, H.J., Keith, L. and Keith, D. (1982). The vanishing twin. *Acta Genet. Med. Gemellol.*, **31**, 179
4. Hellman, L.M., Kobayshi, M. and Cromb, E. (1973). Ultrasonic diagnosis of embryonic malformations. *Am. J. Obstet. Gynecol.*, **115**, 615
5. Kohorn, E.I. and Kaufman, M. (1974). Sonar in the first trimester of pregnancy. *Obstet. Gynecol.*, **44**, 473
6. Levi, S. (1976). Ultrasonic assessment of the high rate of human multiple pregnancy in the first trimester. *J. Clin. Ultrasound*, **4**, 3
7. Robinson, H.P. and Caines, J.S. (1977). Sonar evidence of early pregnancy failure in patients with twin conceptions. *Br. J. Obstet. Gynaecol.*, **84**, 22
8. Levi, S. and Reimers, M. (1978). Démonstration échographique de la fréquence relativement élevée des grossesses multiple humaines pendant la période embryonnaire. In du Mesnil du Buisson, F., Psychoyos, A. and Thomas, K. (eds.) *L'Implantation de L'Oeuf*, pp. 295–307. (Paris: Masson)
9. Varma, T.R. (1979). Ultrasound evidence of early pregnancy failure in patients with multiple conceptions. *Br. J. Obstet. Gynaecol.*, **86**, 290
10. Finberg, H.J. and Birnholz, J.C. (1979). Ultrasound observations in multiple gestation with first trimester bleeding: the blighted twin. *Radiology*, **132**, 137
11. Kurjak, A. and Latin, V. (1979). Ultrasound diagnosis of fetal abnormalities in multiple pregnancy. *Acta Obstet. Gynecol. Scand.*, **58**, 153
12. Jeanty, P., Rodesch, F., Verhoogen, C. *et al.* (1981). The vanishing twin. *Ultrasons*, **2**, 25
13. Defoort, P., Van Eyck, J., DeSchryver, D. *et al.* (1976). Early diagnosis of twin pregnancy by ultrasonography – sources of false positive errors. *Reprod. Obstet. Gynecol.*, **4**, 166
14. Schneider, L., Bessis, R. and Simonnet, T. (1979). The frequency of ovular resorption during the first trimester of twin pregnancy. *Acta Genet. Med. Gemellol.*, **29**, 271
15. Nakano, H., Kubota, S., Koyanagi, T. *et al.* (1981). The prognosis of multiple pregnancy assessed by ultrasonic tomography. *Acta Obstet. Gynaecol. Jpn.*, **35**, 839
16. Brown, B. St J. (1982). Disappearance of one gestational sac in the first trimester of multiple pregnancies – ultrasonographic findings. *J. Can. Assoc. Radiol.*, **33**, 273
17. Landy, H.J., Weiner, S., Corson, S.L. *et al.* (1986). The 'vanishing twin': ultrasonographic assessment of fetal disappearance in the first trimester. *Am. J. Obstet. Gynecol.*, **155**, 14
18. Gindoff, P.R., Yeh, M.-N. and Jewelewicz, R. (1986). The vanishing sac syndrome: ultrasound evidence of pregnancy failure in multiple gestations, induced and spontaneous. *J. Reprod. Med.*, **31**, 322
19. Steptoe, P.C., Edwards, R.G. and Walters, D.E. (1986). Observations on 767 clinical pregnancies and 500 births after human *in-vitro* fertilization. *Hum. Reprod.*, **1**, 89
20. Sulak, L.E. and Dodson, M.G. (1986). The vanishing twin: pathologic confirmation of an ultrasonographic phenomenon. *Obstet. Gynecol.*, **68**, 811
21. Yoshida, K. and Soma, H. (1986). Outcome of the surviving cotwin of fetus papyraceus or of a dead fetus. *Acta Genet. Med. Gemellol.*, **35**, 91
22. Belfrage, P., Fernstrom, I. and Hallenberg, G. (1987). Routine or selective ultrasound examinations in early pregnancy. *Obstet. Gynecol.*, **69**, 747
23. Meldrum, D.R., Chetkowski, R., Steingold, K.A. *et al.* (1987). Evolution of a highly successful *in vitro* fertilization–embryo transfer program. *Fertil. Steril.*, **48**, 86
24. Stabile, I., Campbell, S. and Grudzinskas, J.G. (1987). Ultrasonic assessment of complications during first trimester of pregnancy. *Lancet*, **2**, 1237
25. Jauniaux, E., Elkazen, N., Leroy, F. *et al.* (1988). Clinical and morphologic aspects of the vanishing twin phenomenon. *Obstet. Gynecol.*, **72**, 577
26. Saidi, M.H. (1988). First trimester bleeding and the vanishing twin: a report of three cases. *J. Reprod. Med.*, **33**, 831
27. Gerdts, E. (1989). [Ultrasonic diagnosis in abortion of one twin. The vanishing twin

phenomenon]. *Tidsskr-Nor-Laegeforen*, **109**, 3328

28. Goldman, G.A., Dicker, D., Feldberg, D. *et al.*, (1989). The vanishing fetus. A report of 17 cases of triplets and quadruplets. *J. Perinat. Med.*, **17**, 157

29. Tharapel, A.T., Elias, S., Shulman, L.P. *et al.* (1989). Resorbed co-twin as an explanation for discrepant chorionic villus results: non-mosaic 47,XX,+16 in villi (direct and culture) with normal (46,XX) amniotic fluid and neonatal blood. *Prenat. Diagn.*, **9**, 467

30. Bateman, B.G., Nunley, W.C., Kolp, L.A. *et al.* (1990). Vaginal sonography findings and hCG dynamics of early intrauterine and tubal pregnancies. *Obstet. Gynecol.*, **75**, 421

31. Dickey, R.P., Olar, T.T., Curole, D.N. *et al.* (1990). The probability of multiple births when multiple gestational sacs or viable embryos are diagnosed at first trimester ultrasound. *Hum. Reprod.*, **5**, 880

32. Dickey, R.P., Olar, T.T., Curole, D.N. *et al.* (1992). The vanishing pregnancy? (letter). *Fertil. Steril.*, **57**, 1140

33. Hershlag, A., Floch, J.A., DeCherney, A.H. *et al.* (1990). Comparison of singleton and multiple pregnancies in *in vitro* fertilization (IVF) and embryo transfer (ET). *J. In Vitro Fertil. Embryo Trans.*, **7**, 157

34. Nakamura, I., Uno, M., Io, Y. *et al.* (1990). Seasonality in early loss of one fetus among twin pregnancies. *Acta Genet.*, **39**, 339

35. Kelly, M.P., Binor, Z., Molo, M.W. *et al.* (1991). Human chorionic gonadotropin rise in normal and vanishing twin pregnancies. *Fertil. Steril.*, **56**, 221

36. Callen, D.F., Fernandez, H., Hull, Y.J. *et al.* (1991). A normal 46,XX infant with a 46,XX/69,XXY placenta: a major contribution to the placenta is from a resorbed twin. *Prenat. Diagn.*, **11**, 437

37. Reddy, K.S., Petersen, M.B., Antonarakis, S.E. *et al.* (1991). The vanishing twin: an explanation for discordance between chorionic villus karyotype and fetal phenotype. *Prenat. Diagn.*, **11**, 679

38. Rudnicki, M., Vejerslev, L.O. and Junge, J. (1991). The vanishing twin: morphologic and cytogenetic evaluation of an ultrasonographic phenomenon. *Gynecol. Obstet. Invest.*, **31**, 141

39. Kapur, R.P., Mahony, B.S., Nyberg, D.A. *et al.* (1991). Sirenomelia associated with a 'vanishing twin'. *Teratology*, **43**, 103

40. Sampson, A. and de Crespigny, L.Ch. (1992). Vanishing twins: the frequency of spontaneous fetal reduction of a twin pregnancy. *Ultrasound Obstet. Gynecol.*, **2**, 107

41. Blumenfeld, Z., Dirnfeld, M., Abramovici, H. *et al.* (1992). Spontaneous fetal reduction in multiple gestations assessed by transvaginal ultrasound. *Br. J. Obstet. Gynaecol.*, **99**, 333

42. Nerlich, A., Wisser, J. and Krone, S. (1992). [Placental findings in 'vanishing twins'] [German]. *Gerburtshilfe Frauenheildkd.*, **52**, 230

43. Gavriil, P., Jauniaux, E. and Leroy, F. (1993). Pathologic examination of placentas from singleton and twin pregnancies obtained after *in vitro* fertilization and embryo transfer. *Pediatr. Pathol.*, **13**, 453

44. Benson, C.B., Doubilet, P.M. and Laks, M.P. (1993). Outcome of twin gestations following sonographic demonstration of two heart beats in the first trimester. *Ultrasound Obstet. Gynecol.*, **3**, 343

45. Benson, C.B., Doubilet, P.M. and David, V. (1994). Prognosis of first-trimester twin pregnancies: polychotomous logistic regression analysis. *Radiology*, **192**, 765

46. Falik-Borenstein, T.C., Korenberg, J.R. and Schreck, R.R. (1994). Confined placental chimerism: prenatal and postnatal cytogenetic and molecular analysis, and pregnancy outcome. *Am. J. Med. Genet.*, **50**, 51

47. Boklage, C.E. (1990). Survival probability of human conceptions from fertilization to term. *Int. J. Fertil.*, **35**, 75

48. Benirschke, K. (1961). Twin placenta in perinatal mortality. *NY State J. Med.*, **61**, 1499

49. Melnick, M. (1977). Brain damage in survivor after *in utero* death of monozygous co-twin. *Lancet*, **2**, 1287

50. Moore, C.M., McAdams, A.J. and Sutherland, J. (1969). Intrauterine disseminated intravascular coagulation: a syndrome of multiple pregnancy with a dead twin fetus. *J. Pediatr.*, **74**, 523

Congenital anomalies and pregnancy loss

C. Meyers, S. Elias and P. Arrabal

Introduction

Twins and congenital anomalies have interested physicians for centuries. Indeed, the scientific study of congenital malformations in twins has been important to our understanding of the various etiologies of several congenital malformations. In particular, twin studies have been used to elucidate the contribution of genetic factors to normal phenotypic variation, behavior, and many diseases. This chapter reviews four topics related to congenital anomalies and pregnancy loss in twins: (1) the nosology of congenital anomalies; (2) congenital anomalies that are unique to twins; (3) the usefulness of twin studies to determine the contribution of genetic factors to the etiology of particular anomalies; and finally (4) the frequency of spontaneous abortions in twin pregnancies.

Definitions

The term 'anomaly'

No standard definition of 'anomaly' exists. In general, an anomaly is an abnormality of structure or function. Although this definition appears reasonably precise, attempts to classify specific anomalies along this broad line soon meet with difficulty. For example, many structural malformations such an anencephaly or thanatophoric dwarfism are clearly anomalies. Other anomalies, such as single vertebra spina bifida occulta or retrognathia, are more subtle and might arguably be regarded as normal variants rather than anomalies. In addition, some specific disorders, such as congenital tumors, are considered anomalies by some investigators and not by others, whereas inherited metabolic disorders meet some, but not all, definitions of anomaly because they are abnormalities of enzyme function. In general, phenotypic abnormalities resulting from underlying metabolic disorders are considered as anomalies, but the metabolic disorder itself is not. Thus, a female infant with ambiguous genitalia due to 21-hydroxylase deficiency has an anomaly, but a phenotypically normal female with 21-hydroxylase deficiency does not. Additional problems of precisely defining anomalies will be discussed in the section on ascertainment biases.

Anomalies can be classified as major or minor, single or multiple, hereditary or non-hereditary. Major anomalies are those that interfere with normal function, are of serious cosmetic consequence or generally require treatment. Minor anomalies, if isolated, are generally harmless, although their presence may indicate the need for a more detailed search for other anomalies that may not be immediately apparent. Pre-auricular pits, for example, represent a minor earlier anomaly, but they are often associated with renal anomalies which are not visible to the naked eye. The recognition of patterns of anomalies is particularly important for detecting underlying malformation syndromes, in determining prognosis, and in counselling parents regarding the risks of recurrence.

A useful classification scheme separates anomalies into three types (Figure 1): malformations resulting from abnormal formation of

```
                    Types of problems in
                       MORPHOGENESIS
                              |
                              v
Poor formation         Unusual forces           Breakdown
  of tissue           on normal tissue        of normal tissue
       \                    |                       |
        v                   v                       v
  MALFORMATION          DEFORMATION              DISRUPTION
       or                   or                       or
Malformation sequence  Deformation sequence   Disruption sequence
```

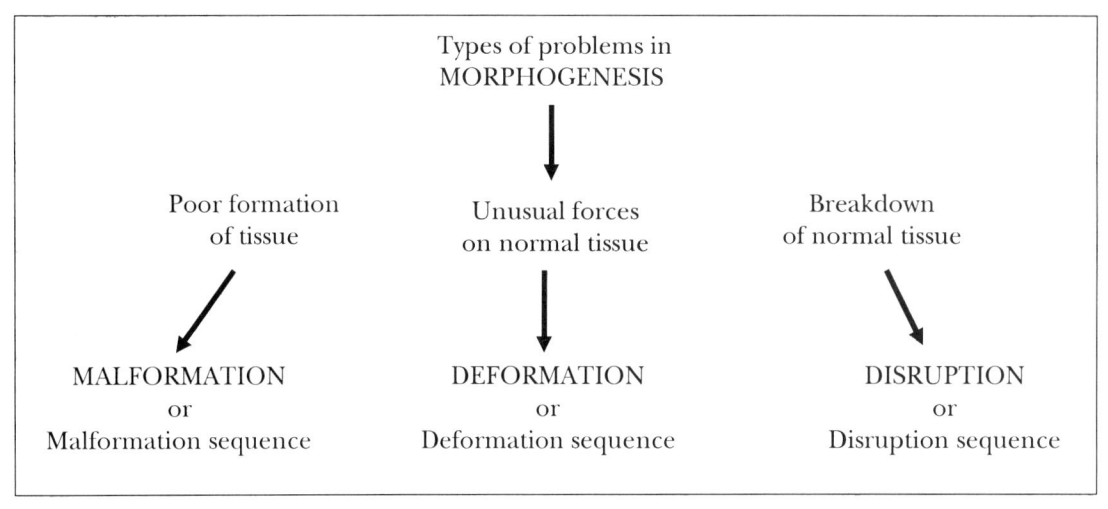

Figure 1 Three types of structural defects that can result in a chain of defects (sequence) by the time of birth. (Reproduced with permission. Jones, K.L. (1988). *Smith's Recognizable Patterns of Human Malformation*, 4th edn. Philadelphia: W.B. Saunders Company)

a structure (e.g. anencephaly); deformations caused by external mechanical forces, acting on originally normal structures, resulting in altered morphogenesis, usually of the molding type; and some deformations resulting from impingement on the volume of the uterine cavity (e.g. large submucosal fibroid, bicornuate uterus, multiple gestation) or from fetal malpresentation (e.g. congenital hip dislocation secondary to breech presentation). Finally, disruptions are those abnormalities caused by physical interference during the time potentially normal tissue is developing (e.g. limb amputation secondary to amniotic band syndrome).

The term 'congenital'

It is far too simplistic to categorically state that congenital anomalies only include those anomalies present at birth. Clearly, many anomalies are present at birth, but are not or cannot be detected until later in life (e.g. ovarian agenesis). Other problems concerning the 'congenital' nature of anomalies will be discussed later in this chapter in relation to the difficulty in determining population frequencies of specific anomalies.

Whereas the etiology of many congenital anomalies is well known and has been understood for decades, there are many others for which an explanation as to cause, and therefore the recurrence risk, is still unclear. Thus, whenever the clinician is faced with a fetus or newborn with congenital anomalies, it is important to obtain all relevant information to help establish a definitive diagnosis and assist in providing appropriate counselling. At the minimum, data collection should include family and medical histories, photographs, a detailed physical description, radiographs, tissue for chromosome analysis and autopsy data when appropriate. Additional studies, such as DNA testing, enzyme analysis or histological studies should also be performed when indicated. Consultation with geneticists should be sought whenever the clinician feels unable to explain the nature of an anomaly, its origins and consequences, its potential risks to the infant's health, or the risk of recurrence.

Congenital anomalies unique to twins

Monozygotic twins

Monozygotic twinning may arguably be thought of as a specific type of congenital anomaly, because the separation of human blastomeres into two distant zygotes does not represent the normal course of embryological development. Experimental animal evidence regarding the influence of environmental and teratogenic factors on monozygotic twinning rates lends credence to this point of view. For example, delayed fertilization of the rabbit ovum[1], vincristine sulfate administration in mice[2] and alterations in oxygenation tension and temperature in Atlantic minnows[3] all induce monozygotic twinning. (Editor: See Chapter 3 for full discussion.) To date, however, no evidence for the teratogenic induction of monozygotic twinning has been found in humans.

Conjoined twins

The incidence of conjoined twins is variably described as in 1/33 000 to 1/165 000 deliveries[4]. Incomplete separation of a 15 to 17 day embryo (primitive streak stage) is the most likely etiology of conjoined twins. This concept is supported by concordance for sex in all cases. Chromosome abnormalities have not been reported in human conjoined twins. Teratogens can induce this phenomenon in hamsters[5] and zebra fish[6], and have been postulated to play a similar role in humans[7]. Hypothetically, the fusion of early blastocysts with chimera formation might cause dizygotic conjoined twins. However, dizygotic conjoined twins have not been described nor induced experimentally.

Conjoined twins are classified by the anatomical site of juncture. Thoracopagus twins, joined at the chest, are most common. Craniopagus twins, joined at the head, and ischiopagus twins, joined at the hip, also occur. Figure 2 shows thoracopagus twins with extensive cranial fusion. Sirenomelic twins are distinguished by fusion of the lower abdomen and lower extremities. (Editor: The reader is referred to Chapter 8 for a full discussion.)

Congenital anomalies of other organs are commonly reported in conjoined twins[8,9]. Mohr found an overall incidence of 50% of additional malformations in one or both of the conjoined twins[9]. Even after exclusion of cardiac defects,

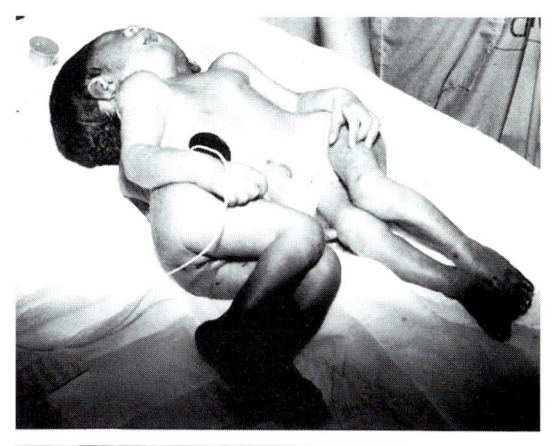

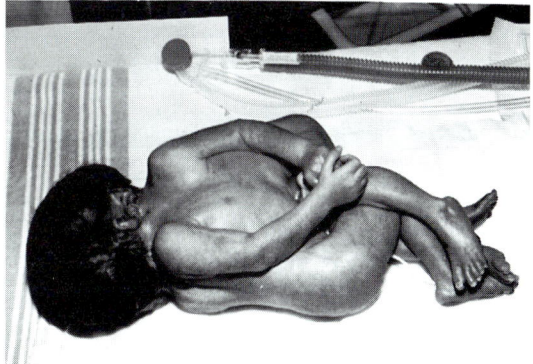

Figure 2 Unusual thoracopagus twins with extensive fusion of craniums. (Photograph courtesy of Dr David Shaver, University of Tennessee, Memphis)

the incidence was still increased to 10 to 20%[9]. Figure 3 shows sirenomelic conjoined twins discordant for anencephaly and cleft lip. Internal malformations, particularly of a cardiac nature, have obvious implications in conjoined twins if surgical separation is considered. Survival depends on the extent of shared vital organs and presence of associated anomalies.

Diagnosis of conjoined twins was previously only made at delivery, often following the diagnosis of dystocia. Today, the diagnosis may be made antenatally with ultrasonograhy. Figure 4 shows a 13-week conjoined twin pair with one body and two heads. Although the diagnosis may be difficult to establish with lesser degrees of joining, it may be suspected if fetal positions remain constant relative to one another over time. Obstetric management for delivery should be individualized, but in many cases, Cesarean section is indicated[10,11].

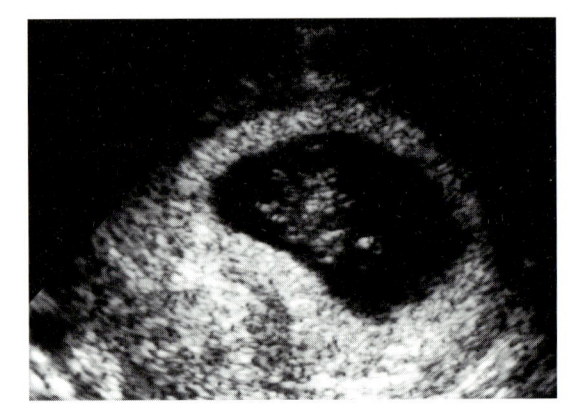

Figure 4 Scan of 13-week sirenomelic twins diagnosed prenatally by ultrasound. (Photograph courtesy of Dr Donald Emmerson, University of Tennessee, Memphis)

Kimmel et al.[12] reported a case of a 19-day-old infant with hydrocephaly in whom a tumor was found containing representative parts of five additional fetuses. In another instance[13], a right upper quadrant mass was noted in a 5-month-old female and a plain abdominal radiograph demonstrated an apparent vertebral column within the mass. This mass was located in the retroperitoneal space and was connected to the infant's abdominal aorta by two small vessels. These very rare situations have been reviewed by Grosfeld et al.[14].

The pathogenesis of the fetus-in-fetu is controversial. Differentiation between fetus-in-fetu and teratoma is a source of both pathological and radiological debate. Some authors propose that these masses are examples of well-differentiated teratomas[15], whereas others suggest that this situation occurs after the incorporation of a monozygotic twin very early in fetal development[13]. This latter concept often is misrepresented in the lay press as an example of intrauterine cannibalism of one twin by its co-twin.

Acardiac malformation

Acardia is a particular congenital malformation unique to monozygotic multiple gestations. In acardia, one fetus is present without a well-defined cardiac structure and is kept alive through placental anastomoses to the circulatory system

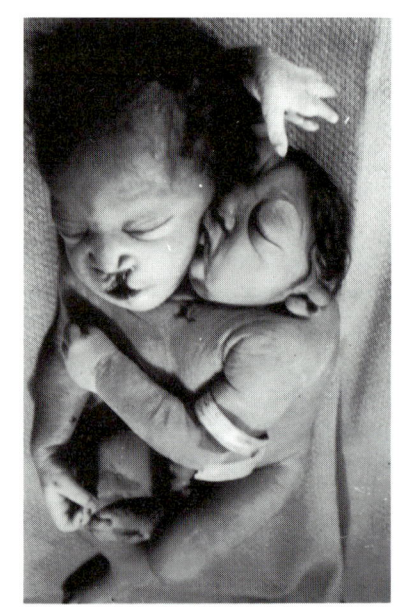

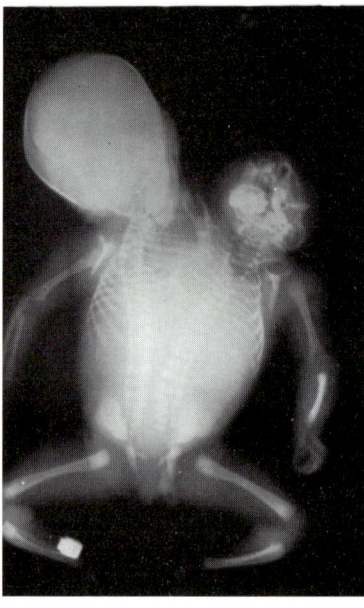

Figure 3 Sirenomelic twins discordant for anencephaly and cleft lip. X-rays confirm the presence of two spines, but only one set of lower extremities. (Photograph courtesy of Dr Sherman Elias, Baylor University, Houston)

Fetus-in-fetu

The fetus-in-fetu is a rare finding of evidence of an abnormally developed fetus in an aberrant location within the body of an individual.

of the viable fetus. Cardiac anomalies are present in all acardiac twins; these range from the total absence of cardiac tissue to the presence of a cardiac-like structure consisting of a folded muscular mass with a common chamber and a truncus arteriosis[16–18]. Less than 20% of acardiac fetuses have identifiable cardiac tissue[19,20]. The frequency of this sporadic malformation is 1/35 000 deliveries, or not more than 1/100 monozygotic deliveries[21–23].

The first recorded description of an acardiac malformation was by Benedetti in 1553[24]. Cases of triplet, quadruplet and quintuplet pregnancies complicated by an acardiac malformation have also been described[22,25–34]. Higher order monozygotic multiple births show a threefold increased incidence of this abnormality. The acardiac and its normal co-twin are always of the same sex and the female gender predominates[21,22,34–36]. Pregnancies complicated by an acardiac anomaly are most often monoamniotic[34]. This condition is uniformly fatal for the affected twin. The incidence of fetal malformations in the normal co-twin is approximately 10%[37–44]. Because of this, a careful structural survey of the non-acardiac twin should always be performed.

Acardiac twins differ greatly in their morphology and degree of organogenesis. Detailed classification systems are based on anatomical descriptions[20,27,37,45], but these add little to our understanding of the pathogenesis of the disorder. Indeed, many authors recommend that all classifications be abandoned[23,25,46].

Most acardiac twins have a central trunk or portion of a central trunk with lower limbs. In addition to the cardiac malformation, absent or partially absent structures include the head, limbs, pancreas, lungs, liver and upper intestines[37]. Rudimentary and hypoplastic evidence of many structures may be found. Normal kidneys are often present, but may be non-functional and result in oligohydramnios secondary to low arterial perfusion pressures and hypoxemic blood.

The vast majority of acardiac twin pairs are normal from a cytogenetic point of view. Thus, chromosomal abnormalities are unlikely to be the primary etiology of this defect, although abnormal karyotypes which are discordant from the normal co-twin[47–50] have occasionally been reported. Chromosomal mosaics have been observed in two cases[51,52].

The most popular theory regarding the pathogenesis of acardiac twinning suggests that the formation of placental vascular anastomoses in monochorionic placentas is followed by reversal of blood flow in the future acardiac twin and that this process subsequently leads to abnormal cardiac development[16,17,27,46,47,53,54]. Because normal cardiac development is dependent on critical blood flows and pressures early in embryogenesis, the reversal of the normal circulation interferes with the proper enfolding of the embryonic cardiac tube. Alterations in blood pressure and flow may also lead to early arrest of cardiac development or possibly degeneration of those cardiac structures present earlier in development. Subsequent hemodynamic and cardiovascular changes result in the passive circulation of suboptimally oxygenated blood at subnormal pressure in the acardiac fetus. Thus, low pressure, deoxygenated blood enters the umbilical arteries and follows a course through the iliac arteries to preferentially perfuse the caudal rather than the cephalad structures of the fetus and provide the basis of inadequate development and growth of the cephalad fetal structures. Alternative theories have also been proposed, including: (1) a primary defect in cardiac development[55]; (2) unequal splitting of the embryos[56]; (3) teratomatous malformations[57]; and (4) immunological factors[58]. To date, no hypothesis is totally satisfactory and the true etiology may be heterogeneous.

The major differential diagnostic consideration is a teratoma. Teratomas contain elements originating from the three germinal layers and may be found at any location along the umbilical cord. The following criteria distinguish a teratoma from an acardiac twin: (1) the acardiac twin has a separate, although rudimentary, umbilical cord; (2) the twin cannot be entirely intrafunicular; and (3) the twin shows some evidence of body organization

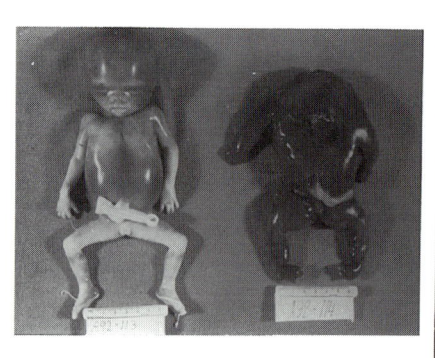

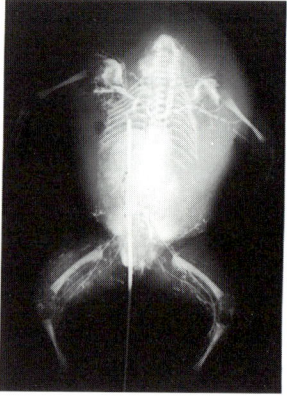

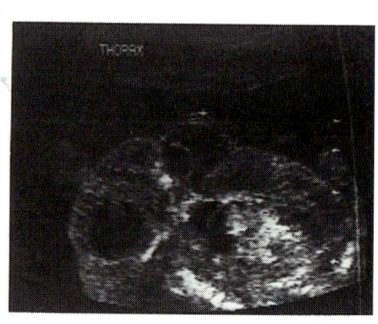

Figure 5 Acardiac twin pregnancy diagnosed by ultrasound. Both twins were found to be non-viable at 18 weeks. (Photograph and radiograph courtesy of Dr Chen-chih Sun, University of Maryland, Baltimore. Ultrasound scan courtesy of Dr Roger Sanders, Ultrasound Institute of Baltimore, Baltimore)

(e.g. cranium, spine), whereas the tissues in teratomas are completely disorganized.

Formerly, the diagnosis of an acardiac twin was made only at delivery. Today, the diagnosis can be made antenatally by ultrasonography. The first report of an *in utero* diagnosis of acardiac twinning appeared in 1978[36]. Figure 5 shows an acardiac twin in which the diagnosis was made prenatally. *In utero* demise of both twins was diagnosed at 18 weeks.

Moore *et al.* found an overall perinatal mortality of 55% in a series of 49 pregnancies involving acardiac fetuses[21]. This increased mortality was primarily due to preterm delivery, which was strongly associated with development of congestive heart failure and hydramnios in the normal twin.

Various therapeutic regimens have been advocated. These include expectant management, serial amniocentesis when polyhydramnios is present in the normal twin[59], administration of inotropic agents such as digoxin to treat heart failure in the normal twin[60], and elective termination of the entire pregnancy. Selective termination by placement of thrombogenic coils has also been attempted, but with generally disappointing results[61]. Selective delivery of the acardiac twin by hysterotomy has been reported in several cases with apparent benefit to the remaining twin[62–64]. However, this approach commits the mother to two major abdominal operations, an initial hysterotomy to remove the acardiac fetus and a subsequent Cesarean section for delivery of the normal co-twin. Selective delivery should be regarded as an investigational therapeutic approach and attempted only in centers experienced in treating these patients.

Anomalies associated with demise of a monozygotic co-twin

Fetal death of one or both twins occurs in 0.5–6.8% of all twin gestations, and death of one fetus occurs three times more often in monochorionic twin gestations[65–69]. Following a demise of one twin, 82% of co-twins survive[68]. However, the surviving twin is at substantial risk for having anomalies at birth.

A variety of anomalies have been reported in surviving monochorionic co-twins. These include hydrancephaly[37,70,71], spina cord transection[71], porencephaly[37,70,72], microcephaly[37,72–74], intestinal atresia[37,71,72,75,76,77], multicystic encephalomalacia[78], renal cortical damage[65,79], and skin defects[67,68,80]. Most of these cases were either associated with an obvious macerated dead co-twin or a fetus papyraceus. Figure 6 shows an infant with cutis aplasia congenita in which a fetus papyraceus was also identified at delivery. Dichorionic gestations do not appear to be at increased risk of these complications.

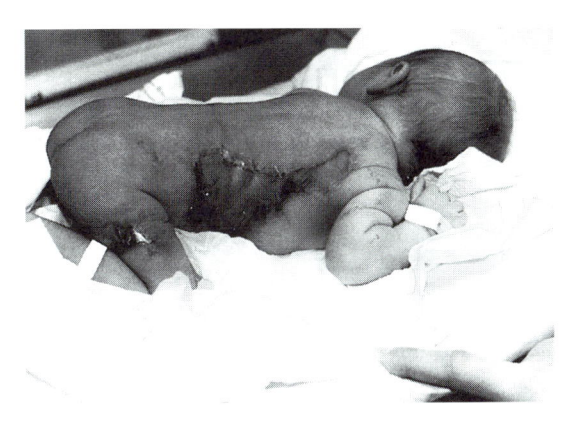

Figure 6 Infant with cutis aplasia congenita. Fetus papyraceus of a co-twin was found at delivery. (Photograph courtesy of Dr Sherman Elias, University of Tennessee, Memphis)

The pathogenesis of damage to the surviving twin is not fully understood. In 1961, Benirschke postulated that it is based on a coagulopathy secondary to transfer of thromboplastin-rich blood from a dead to a living monochorionic twin through placental vascular anastomoses, followed by embolization and infarction of various organs[65]. Because this circumstance only occurs in monochorionic pregnancies with placental vascular anastomoses, the hypothesis of embolization from the dead to the living twin seems plausible. However, there are no documented cases of disseminated intravascular coagulation among survivors either *in utero* or at birth, as might be expected with this hypothesis. The importance of the gestational age at the time of the demise also remains unclear. However, survivors with anomalies have been reported after deaths in all trimesters[72,75,81].

Although vascular disruption or infarction seem plausible causes for some anomalies, congenital cardiac and neural tube defects may not be explained by this mechanism, because their development is complete very early in gestation. Consideration of the genetic aspects of these anomalies may provide an alternative explanation for some cases. Monozygotic twins are more likely to be concordant for genetically influenced anomalies (e.g. polygenic/multifactorial), although expression of the anomaly may differ between the fetuses. Given a monozygotic twin pair in which both twins are affected with an anomaly, one would predict a higher rate of fetal loss than a gestation with non-anomalous twins. Because twins may not be affected equally for various reasons (environmental influences, for example), one twin may die as a result of being more severely affected or subject to different environmental effects. In these cases, the anomaly in the surviving twin would be unrelated to the demise of the first. Rather, the demise was due to the anomaly, and not vice versa.

Recently, Fusi *et al.* proposed acute hemodynamic changes at the time of intrauterine death of the co-twin (i.e. hypotension and subsequent ischemia in the surviving fetus) resulting from twin–twin transfusion as a possible factor leading to the anomalies[82]. In one case, they observed the surviving co-twin to have spontaneous fetal heart rate decelerations at the time of death of the other twin. Fetal blood sampling of the surviving fetus showed normal blood gases and clotting screen, but hemoglobin was 6.5 g/dl. The fetal heart rate decelerations disappeared and the pregnancy was then allowed to continue. However, repetitive fetal heart rate decelerations recurred two days later and delivery was accomplished by Cesarean section at 27 weeks' gestation. Cord blood gases showed a mild acidosis and severe anemia (hemoglobin 5.8 g/dl) with a normal coagulation profile. The liveborn twin died from hyaline membrane disease and renal failure. At autopsy, the kidneys showed a combination of acute and established infarction and the brain showed bilateral parietal lobe infarcts with secondary hemorrhage. The placenta was found to have one major vein-to-vein anastomosis. This observation suggests that if intervention is proposed to prevent neurological sequelae in the surviving twin, it must be carried out before the death of the first twin. A similar mechanism was proposed previously by Larroche *et al.* in 1990 in a series of monochorionic twins with hypoxic-ischemic or hemorrhagic cerebral lesions[83]. Acknowledging that the pathogenesis was not fully understood, these authors suggested that blood pressure instability or severe hypotension could lead to brain and visceral lesions in surviving twins.

Management is dependent on the gestational age at which fetal death occurs. When fetal death is diagnosed early in the second trimester, management primarily involves an extensive sonographic study of the surviving twin for evidence of injury. The finding of such injury may or may not lead to consideration of pregnancy termination. Maternal coagulopathy is a rare complication if fetal death occurs at this early gestational age, but should still be considered[84].

When fetal death occurs later in pregnancy, other antepartum tests of fetal well-being (e.g. biophysical profile) should also be performed. Conservative management has been recommended for gestations less than 34 weeks with delivery at term or at the time maturity is documented[81,85]. Although such a management scheme may not avoid anomalies due to vascular complications, it will decrease the risk of additional morbidity due to prematurity. However, one study has shown a 70% incidence of abnormal antepartum fetal heart rate testing with a 37% Cesarean section rate for fetal distress, a 76% preterm delivery rate, a 42% incidence of small for gestational age infants, and a 74% incidence of hyperbilirubinemia. All these rates are greater than is usual in multiple gestations of similar gestational age[81]. The delivery method should be chosen on the basis of obstetric considerations.

After birth, a systematic evaluation of the living neonate is indicated. This should include neurological assessment, appropriate intracranial studies and evaluation of the gastrointestinal and renal systems[72]. Whereas a careful inspection of the placenta is important in all twin pregnancies, it is even more so in those complicated by the death of one twin. The chorionicity of the placenta should be carefully investigated, because placental vascular connections appear to be a necessary component in the pathogenesis of this condition, whether due to coagulopathy and embolization or hypotension at the time of the demise.

The occurrence of an anomalous fetus with a dead co-twin has important implications for counselling about recurrence risks. The risk of recurrence would only be increased if the mother became pregnant with another monochorionic twin gestation. Monozygotic twin gestations are rarely familial, except possibly in the Yoruba tribe in Nigeria. However, a complete family history must be obtained to assess the possibility of the malformation occurring as part of a syndrome unrelated to twinning.

Congenital anomalies not unique to twins – nature vs. nurture

The existence of two types of twins, monozygotic and dizygotic, make twin studies particularly useful for studying the 'nature vs. nurture' or the genetic vs. the environmental components of specific phenotypes, including congenital anomalies. Monozygotic twins arise from the same zygote and theoretically possess identical genotypes. In contrast, dizygotic twins occur because of multiple ovulations and have the genetic relationship of siblings. Both types of twins theoretically share a common intrauterine environment, regardless of their zygosity, whereas singleton siblings share neither identical genotypes nor common intrauterine environments. Therefore, comparisons of phenotypes of monozygotic twins vs. dizygotic twins vs. singleton siblings is a useful tool to elucidate the genetic contribution to a given phenotype. If the phenotype under study is controlled exclusively by genetic factors, concordance should be expected in monozygotic twins, whereas dizygotic twins and singletons would be concordant only as often as expected by mode of inheritance. Conversely, if the phenotype under study is produced exclusively by environmental factors, one would expect that all twins, monozygotic and dizygotic, would be concordant and singleton siblings discordant. These expectations are both theoretic and simplistic, however, as the following discussion will show that monozygotic twins are not necessarily genetically identical, nor is the intrauterine environment always uniform. Despite this, twin studies continue to be of importance in the study of the etiology of congenital anomalies. Below, we review the

Table 1 Chance of concordance for chromosome abnormalities in dizygotic twins. These numbers are for illustration only and assume that each non-disjunctional event is independent

Chromosome abnormality	First twin	Second twin	Sex	Chance of concordance in dizygotic twins
Trisomy 21	1/660	1/660	1/2	1/871 200
Trisomy 18	3/10 000	3/10 000	1/2	1/22 222 222
Trisomy 13	1/5000	1/5000	1/2	1/50 000 000

expectations for concordance of congenital anomalies in monozygotic and dizygotic twins, and the significance of deviations from these expectations, according to the underlying etiological mechanism.

Chromosome abnormalities

Disconcordance for chromosome abnormalities is the expectation for dizygotic twins. Dizygotic twins are concordant for chromosome abnormalities as often as non-twin siblings. Therefore, the rarer the chromosomal abnormality, the less likely the individuals are to be dizygotic if both twins are concordant for the cytogenetic abnormality. Additionally, for cytogenetic concordance, sex of the individuals must be identical (Table 1). Equally rare are twins with different chromosome abnormalities, for example one with trisomy 21 and the other with trisomy 18. The exact probabilities for such situations are difficult to calculate, because of the confounding effects of maternal age and possible genetic or environmental predisposition to recurrent aneuploidy.

Because the incidence of twinning and early spontaneous loss of one twin is not known with certainty, dizygotic twin discordance for chromosome abnormalities may be more common in early gestations than in livebirths. The early loss rate of chromosomally abnormal conceptions is high. Perhaps this is the explanation for some cases of a vanishing twin. The phenomenon of discordant dizygotic twins with demise of the chromosomally abnormal twin is also suggested by the finding of confined placental mosaicism in some chorionic villus samples; the prior demise of a co-twin is believed to be an explanation for some of these cases[86].

The expectation for chromosome complements in monozygotic twins is concordance. Thus, identical cytogenetic abnormalities are often interpreted as evidence of monozygosity, because of the rarity of concordance in dizygotic twins as illustrated earlier in Table 1. While this is undoubtedly true in the majority of instances, discordance could occur in monozygotic twins as a result of post-zygotic errors. Beginning with a chromosomally normal zygote, two events must occur to result in cytogenetically discordant, monozygotic twins: the early cell mass must split, forming monozygotic twins and then a cytogenetic error must occur. Given the complexity of each of the events necessary for the creation of cytogenetically discordant monozygotic twins, the finding of such twin pairs is extremely rare.

A variety of types of cytogenetic discordances might occur depending upon the timing and the type of cytogenetic errors (Figures 7–9). If the original conception is trisomic (a result of meiotic non-disjunction), anaphase lag at the time of the first cell division, concurrent with separation of the two blastocysts could result in a trisomic twin and a chromosomally normal twin (Figure 7). If the original conception is 47,XXY and loss of the Y chromosome occurs by anaphase lag, the result would be monozygotic twins of opposite sex: a 47,XXY male and 46,XX female. If anaphase lag occurs during a mitosis *after* blastomere separation of an originally trisomic conception, the result would be a trisomic twin and a disomic/trisomic mosaic twin (Figure 8). The phenotype of mosaic individuals varies

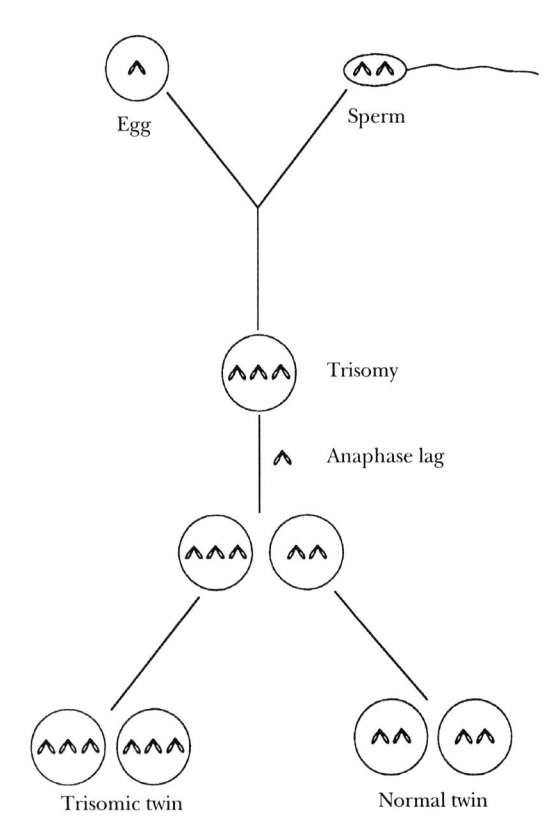

Figure 7 Anaphase lag in a trisomic zygote occurring at the time of blastomere separation, resulting in one trisomic and one cytogenetically normal twin

depending on the extent and distribution of the abnormal cell line. These types of post-zygotic errors have been given as the explanation for monozygotic twins discordant for trisomy 21[87,88].

Chromosomally normal conceptions can also undergo mitotic non-disjunction or anaphase lag. If the original conception is 46,XY and loss of the X-chromosome occurs by anaphase lag at the time of blastomere separation, monozygotic twins of opposite sex would result: a 46,XY male and a 45,X female. Such twins have been reported[89]. However, if a mitotic error occurs prior to division of the early embryo into twins, it is possible that the two cell lines would not be distributed evenly between the resulting twins, and possibly lead to varying degrees of mosaicism. Variations in phenotype would be expected if the distribu-

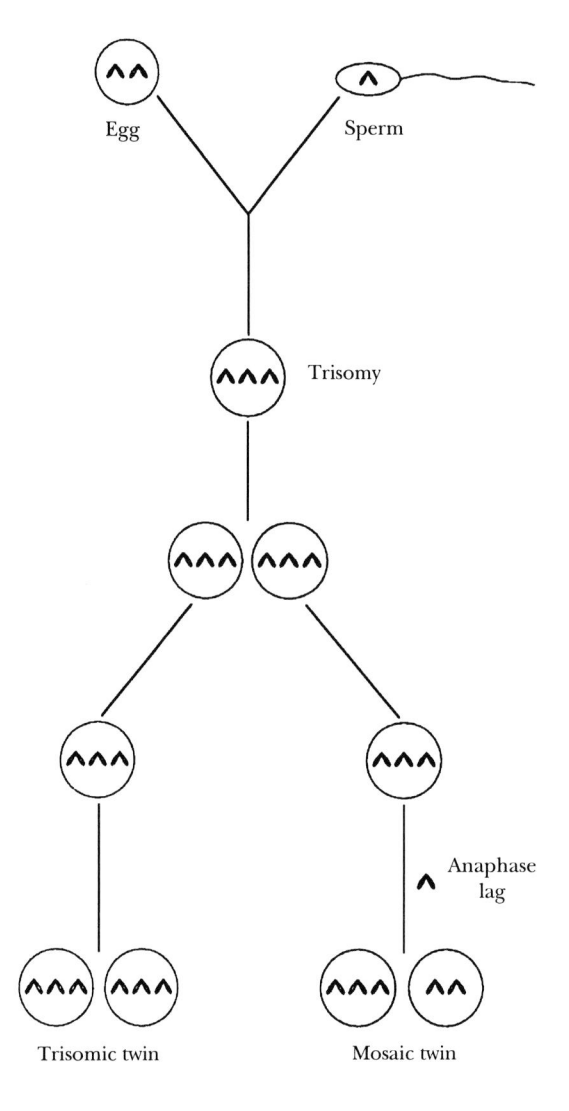

Figure 8 Anaphase lag in a trisomic zygote occurring after blastomere separation, resulting in one trisomic and one mosaic twin. For alternative explanation of the origination of mosaicism, see text

tion of cytogenetically abnormal cells were unequal. Sex discordance in monozygotic twins and triplets may have resulted from this mechanism[90–94]. Alternatively, mosaicism in monozygotic twins could be due to chimerism after post-zygotic cytogenetic errors. Vascular connections are frequent in monozygotic placentas and exchange of cytogenetically different cell lines could occur. These mechanisms were proposed to explain a pair of 45,X/46,XY monozygotic twins discordant for sex[95] and

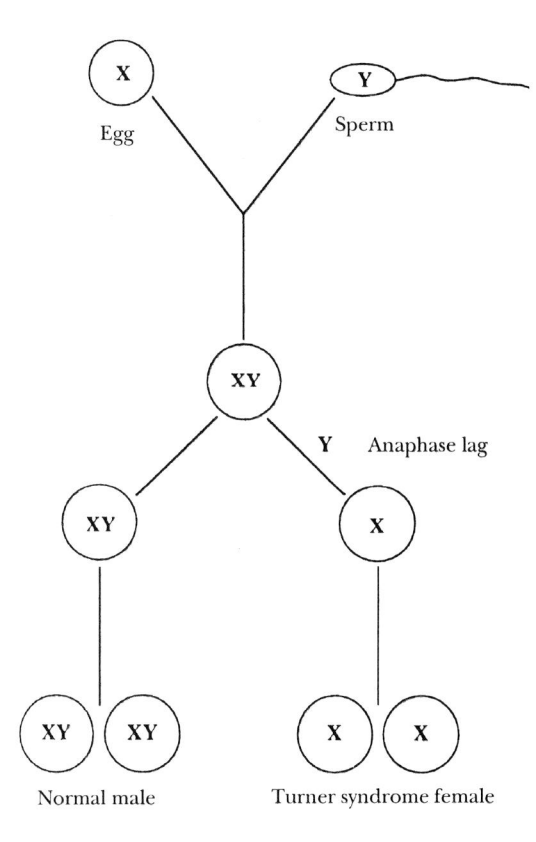

Figure 9 Anaphase lag of Y-chromosome in cytogenetically normal conception occurring at the time of blastomere separation, resulting in a normal male and a Turner syndrome female, i.e. monozygotic twins discordant for sex

monozygotic twins discordant for Turner phenotype[96]. Anaphase lag or non-disjunction of autosomes probably occurs, but the monosomic cell line is lethal. The result is a single surviving cell line which is trisomic for the autosome involved.

Finally, there are monozygotic twins concordant for chromosome abnormalities (i.e. trisomy 13 or 18), but discordant for major anomalies[97,98]. These situations help clarify the interaction of environment and genetic background with a particular genotype (see discussion below).

Mendelian disorders

Monozygotic and dizygotic twins are expected to follow classical genetic inheritance patterns for Mendelian disorders. Monozygotic twins should be genetically identical, and therefore, concordant. Dizygotic twins are as genetically related as non-twin siblings, and therefore concordance is predicted by the type of inheritance.

Contrary to expectations, however, phenotypic discordance is rather frequent in monozygotic twins. Several newly described genetic mechanisms attempt to explain observations which conflict with classical genetics teachings. One of these, mitotic crossing over was reviewed by Coté and Gyftodimou in 1991 as a mechanism to explain many cases of monozygotic twin discordance[99]. They postulated that post-zygotic mitotic crossing over in one twin may result in discordance from uniparental homozygosity (the equivalent of loss of heterozygosity), disruption of normal parental imprinting, unequal crossing over, or disruption of closely-linked DNA *cis*-sequences. Mitotic crossing over is hypothesized to explain discordance of X-linked diseases, such as Duchenne muscular dystrophy, which typically have been thought to result from skewed X-inactivation or asymmetric splitting of the inner cell mass[100–102]. Kastern and Kryspin-Sorensen reviewed a variety of potential somatic cell DNA alterations, such as DNA rearrangements, mobile genetic elements, extrachromosomal DNA and fragile sites, all of which may affect phenotype[103]. Hall has extensively reviewed existing hypotheses regarding the phenotypic effects of somatic mosaicism[104]. The types of somatic mosaicism that may act as mechanisms for discordance include cytogenetic (see above), single gene mutations, and uniparental disomy. A later paper by Hall postulated a connection between genetically abnormal cells and the twinning process, whereby genetically discordant cells are expelled from the inner cell mass and subsequently form a monozygotic twin, albeit one with non-identical DNA[105].

Environmental disorders

It is evident from a review of monozygotic twins reported with the same genetic disorder

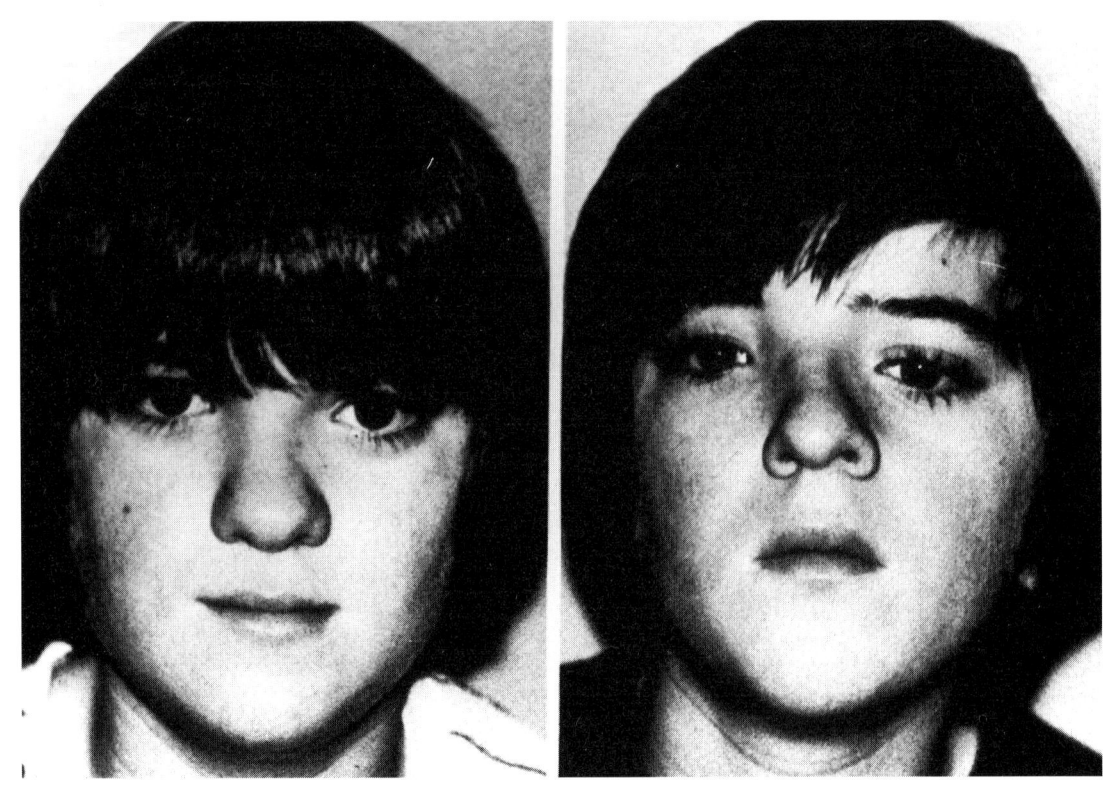

Figure 10 Monozygotic twins with permanent deformation due to varying degrees of head molding *in utero*. (Photograph reproduced with permission. Graham, J.M. (1988). *Smith's Recognizable Patterns of Human Deformation*, (2nd edn). Philadelphia: W.B. Saunders Company)

and differences in phenotype that other factors must also influence phenotype. All genetic disorders show variation in expression. This phenomenon is usually thought to be due to differences in genetic background or the *in utero* or postnatal environment. As should be evident from the discussion above, neither environment nor genotype is likely to be completely identical and expression of all genetic disorders is probably influenced by environmental differences and variations in genetic background. Discordance for congenital rubella syndrome[106], fetal alcohol syndrome[107], and fetal hydantoin syndrome[108] are examples where concordance is expected, but discordance has been reported. Figure 10 demonstrates permanent differences in head shape in monozygotic twins due to *in utero* head molding, a purely environmental effect.

Frequency of congenital anomalies in twins

Ascertainment biases

It is important to review relevant ascertainment biases before discussing studies that estimate the incidence of congenital anomalies in twins. Particular biases apply to some studies but not others, and additional biases result from the nature of congenital anomalies or the study of twins in general.

A myriad of ascertainment biases are present in studies of congenital anomalies. These include: (1) the skill and interest of the examiner – an increasing number of congenital anomalies are detected by physical examination if the examination is performed by an obstetrician, pediatrician, or dysmorphologist, respectively; (2) the extent of investigation used to ascertain the presence of congenital anomalies – an increased number of congenital anomalies will be detected if extensive evaluations such as radiological studies or autopsy are performed; (3) the length of time that a population is followed for the presence of congenital anomalies – studies that look at the incidence of anomalies at a fixed point in time, e.g. at birth or the first month of life, underestimate the actual incidence of congenital anomalies compared to studies that follow populations over years; and (4) many studies do not control for ethnic background, although it is well known that certain anomalies are much more common among particular ethnic groups.

Often the determination of the incidence of congenital anomalies is based on a review of birth records. Under these circumstances, congenital anomalies in stillbirths are not included. Clerical errors in data coding frequently influence studies utilizing vital statistic or medical records, and rarer anomalies are occasionally coded erroneously because of coder inexperience. Moreover, in many medical records, the number of diagnoses that can be entered is limited, and minor anomalies and even some major anomalies may not be coded at all. This may be particularly relevant in twin gestations, in which prematurity and its complications are frequent.

Ascertainment biases that are specific to twin studies are also of importance. For example, in studies of congenital anomalies or genetics, determination of zygosity is often based on the proportion of like-sexed twin pairs (see discussion on Weinberg formula in Chapter 4). Thus, concordance of anomalies might be interpreted falsely as evidence of monozygosity. As is the case with all pregnancies complicated by congenital anomalies, multiple pregnancies with anomalies are more likely to end in spontaneous abortion or fetal death. This fact leads to a gross underestimation of the incidence of twin pregnancies in studies that are restricted to live births. Although the diagnosis of an anomaly in one twin often leads to a more detailed examination of the second, anomalies in the second twin ascertained in this manner create a bias towards an increased incidence in twin pregnancies.

Compounding the problems cited above are those that occur in any study of two rare events that occur simultaneously. Because of the small numbers of twins with congenital anomalies, it is virtually impossible to obtain a large enough sample to adequately investigate any question that might be posed. To address the problem of inadequate sample size, many investigators either survey records of several large centers or focus on data obtained from twin registries to increase the number of individuals available for study. In large population surveys, for example, concentration of particular anomalies into specialized centers is common, and this phenomenon may either result in under- or over-reporting of their incidences. Virtually all studies of congenital anomalies and/or twins are performed by review of medical records. This method is based on two assumptions: (1) that medical care is available; and (2) that all affected individuals present for care. For some individuals, referral to multiple medical specialists may be indicated. This circumstance makes it more likely that this individual will be included in a study, and also increases the chance that he or she may be included more than one time. Studies requiring enrolment of twin pairs often fail to detect twins if a congenital anomaly has resulted in the death of one or both twins. For detailed discussions of ascertainment biases relevant to studies of twins and congenital anomalies, the reader is referred to several reviews[109–112].

Incidence of specific anomalies in twins

Many studies report the incidence of specific congenital anomalies in twin as compared to singleton pregnancies. Caution must be used in interpreting results, however, because of significant, albeit unavoidable, ascertainment biases. Statistical analyses are often not performed, and the significance of a reported difference may be uncertain.

In most studies, congenital heart defects are increased in twins compared to singletons[113–125]. Like-sexed twins make a disproportionate contribution to all studies. In one population-based study of the incidence of congenital cardiovascular malformations, a higher incidence of twins was found in cases than in controls[126]. Interestingly, the proportion of monozygotic twins was the same in both the cases and the controls. The apparent susceptibility of the developing heart to malformations may be due to extreme sensitivity to very early disturbances of pressure, flow, or laterality, perhaps associated with the monozygotic twinning process (see above).

Although one might also expect that the developing central nervous system would be extremely sensitive to early developmental insults, the data on this point are less clear than for congenital cardiac anomalies. Some studies report an increase in open neural tube defects[114,116,127], whereas others do not[117,118,121,128,129]. Those which do report an increase demonstrate a larger contribution to the overall rate from like-sexed pairs than from unlike-sexed pairs. Windham et al.[130] reported an increase in anencephaly in twins as compared to singletons, but not in spina bifida. The increase in hydrocephalus reported by some authors[114,116,117,120] may be due to complications of prematurity, rather than from early developmental disturbances.

Spontaneous abortion in twin gestation

Any review of existing studies of the frequency of spontaneous pregnancy loss is necessarily hampered by methodological problems resulting from the changing definitions of pregnancy based upon increasing sensitivity of biochemical tests and earlier diagnosis by ultrasound. Methodological problems in the determination of fetal loss rates are beyond the scope of this chapter, but are reviewed elsewhere[131]. Although the more frequent use of ultrasound had identified twin pregnancies at earlier gestational ages, what remains unclear is the frequency of dizygotic twin conceptions or of monozygotic twinning in which only one of the embryos develops to the point at which it can be detected by ultrasound. These rates will probably never be known with certainty (see Chapter 4). Information presented elsewhere in this volume discusses the early disappearance of one fetus, i.e. a vanishing twin (see Chapter 6). Accordingly, we will limit our discussion to identifiable twin gestations that end in spontaneous abortion of both fetuses.

Estimates of the rate of spontaneous abortion in twin gestations are derived from two major sources: pathological study of spontaneous abortions (i.e. the incidence of twin gestations in spontaneous abortions) and outcome information regarding twin gestations diagnosed by ultrasound (i.e. the incidence of spontaneous abortions in twin gestation). Not unexpectedly, the results obtained by those different methods are not directly comparable.

Reports by Benirschke[65], and Livingston and Poland[132] acknowledge underestimating the incidence of twins in spontaneous abortions of less than 20 weeks' gestational age, because only specimens in which an intact embryo or fetus was identified were included. Therefore, pregnancies lacking development of an embryo or fetus were excluded. The number of twin gestations in these excluded pregnancies is unknown, but might be disproportionately high. More importantly, with dichorionic twins, one fetus may be identified and the other missed or lost prior to clinical evaluation. In these cases, a twin pregnancy would be included as a singleton. Not surprisingly, a preponderance of monozygotic twins has been identified in spontaneous abortion specimens. This finding is consistent with the high mortality rate observed in monozygotic twins in later pregnancy.

Uchida et al. reported a twinning rate among first-trimester spontaneous abortions of 1/44 based on findings of chromosomal mosaicism for Q-band variants[133]. However, correcting for the frequency of monozygotic pairs that would not have been detected, an incidence as high as 1/30 may be possible. This incidence of twins assumes the rate of monozygotic twinning in the study group to be the same in livebirths, undoubtedly further underestimating the true frequency. These findings are comparable to an earlier study by Kajii et al.[134] which reported 1/51 first-trimester spontaneous abortions to be a twin pregnancy.

Table 2 Rate of twin gestation in spontaneous abortions

Author	Rate	MZ	DZ	Unknown zygosity	Ascertainment
Benirschke (1961)[65]	1/223	6/7	1/7	0/7	pathological study of spontaneous abortions at <20 weeks' gestation
Creasy et al. (1976)[135]	1/50	—	—	—	cytogenetic study of spontaneous abortions at <28 weeks' gestation
Livingston and Poland (1980)[132]	1/35	35/37	2/37	16/53	pathological study of spontaneous abortions at <20 weeks' gestation
Kajii et al. (1980)[134]	1/51	—	—	—	cytogenetic study of spontaneous abortions at <13 weeks' gestation
Uchida et al (1983)[133]	1/44	4/15	10/15	1/15	unselected 1st-trimester abortions

Table 3 Rate of spontaneous abortion in twin pregnancies

Author	Frequency of spontaneous abortion	Ascertainment
Hellman et al. (1973)[136]	14/22 (64%)	twin gestational sacs
Levi (1976)[137]	20/28 (71%)	twin pregnancy <10 weeks
Robinson and Caines (1977)[138]	6/30 (20%)	twin pregnancy diagnosed in first trimester
Varma (1979)[139]	11/30 (37%)	multiple gestational sacs

Interestingly, Creasy et al.[135] found the same incidence of twins (1/50) in a study of predominantly second-trimester spontaneous abortions. A summary of these studies is found in Table 2.

An alternative method for assessing the relationship of spontaneous abortion and twin gestation is determination of the frequency of spontaneous abortion in known twin pregnancies identified by ultrasound. Studies reporting the frequency of spontaneous abortion in this group of individuals are summarized in Table 3. The wide range in observed frequency of spontaneous abortion is undoubtedly due to variations in the resolution of ultrasound and inclusion criteria for each study. Obviously, pregnancies spontaneously aborting prior to ultrasound would not have been included.

References

1. Bomsel-Helmreich, O. (1974). Delayed ovulation and monozygotic twinning in the rabbit. *Acta Genet. Med. Gemellol.*, **23**, 19
2. Kaufman, M.H. and O'Shea, K.S. (1978). Induction of monozygotic twinning in the mouse. *Nature (London)*, **276**, 707
3. Stockard, C.R. (1921). Developmental rate and structural expression: an experimental study of twins, 'double monsters', and single deformities and the interaction among embryonic organs during their origin and development. *Am. J. Anat.*, **28**, 115
4. Benirschke, K. and Kim, C.K. (1973). Multiple pregnancy (second of two parts). *N. Engl. J. Med.*, **288**, 1329
5. Ferm, V.H. (1969). Conjoined twinning in mammalian teratology. *Arch. Environ. Health*, **19**, 353
6. Ingalls, T.H., Philbrook, F.R. and Majima, A. (1969). Conjoined twins in zebra fish. *Arch. Environ. Health*, **19**, 344
7. Tan, K.L., Tock, E., Dawood, M.Y. *et al.* (1971). Conjoined twins in a triplet pregnancy. *Am. J. Dis. Child.*, **122**, 455
8. Bergsma, D. (ed.) (1967). *Conjoined Twins*, Birth Defects Original Article Series, vol. 3, no. 1. (New York: The National Foundation)
9. Mohr, H.P. (1972). Abnormalities in twins. *Ergeb. Inn. Med. Kinderheilkd.*, **33**, 1
10. Vaughn, T.C. and Powell, L.C. (1979). The obstetrical management of conjoined twins. *Obstet. Gynecol.*, **53**, 67S
11. Sakala, E.P. (1986). Obstetric management of conjoined twins. *Obstet. Gynecol.*, **67**, 21S
12. Kimmel, D.L., Moyer, E.K., Peale, A.R. *et al.* (1950). A cerebral tumor containing five human fetuses. A case of fetus-in-fetu. *Anat. Rec.*, **106**, 141
13. Yasuda, Y., Mitomori, T., Matsuura, A. *et al.* (1985). Fetus-in-fetu: report of a case. *Teratology*, **31**, 337
14. Grosfeld, J.L., Stepita, D.S., Nance, W.E. *et al.* (1974). Fetus-in-fetu. *Ann. Surg.*, **180**, 80
15. Alpers, C.E. and Harrison, M.R. (1985). Fetus-in-fetu associated with an undescended testis. *Ped. Path.*, **4**, 37
16. Benirschke, K. and Des Roches Harper, V. (1977). The acardiac anomaly. *Teratology*, **15**, 311
17. Hein, P.R., van Groeninghen, J.C. and Puts, J.J.G. (1985). A case of acardiac anomaly in the cynomolgus monkey (*Macaca fascicularis*): a complication of monozygotic monochorial twinning. *J. Med. Primatol.*, **14**, 133
18. Warkany, J. (1971). Cardiovascular malformations. In *Congenital Malformations: Notes and Comments*, pp. 473–5. (Chicago: Yearbook Medical Publishers)
19. Frutiger, P. (1969). Zum Problem der Akardie. *Acta Anat.*, **74**, 505
20. Simonds, J.P. and Gowen, G.A. (1925). Fetus amorphus. *Surg. Gynecol. Obstet.*, **41**, 171
21. Moore, T.R., Gale, S. and Benirschke, K. (1991). Perinatal outcome of forty-nine pregnancies complicated by acardiac twinning. *Am. J. Obstet. Gynecol.*, **163**, 907
22. Gillim, D.L. and Hendricks, C.H. (1953). Holoacardius: review of the literature and case report. *Obstet. Gynecol.*, **2**, 647
23. Benirschke, K. and Kim, C.K. (1973). Multiple pregnancy (first of two parts). *N. Engl. J. Med.*, **288**, 1276
24. Benedetti, A. (1553). *De Morborum a Capite ad Pedis Signis. Habes Lector Studioso Hox Volumine*
25. Landy, H.J., Larsen, J.W. Jr, Schoen, M. *et al.* (1988). Acardiac fetus in a triplet pregnancy. *Teratology*, **37**, 1
26. Ilberg, G. (1939). Thoracopagus with cor biloculare: case in triplets. *Z. Geburtsh. Gynaek.*, **119**, 369
27. McNeil, R.J. Jr, Crowther, H.L. and Paxson, N.F. (1941). Siamese twins (thoracopagus) complicating triplet pregnancy. *Am. J. Obstet. Gynecol.*, **41**, 337
28. Messinger, R.F. and Shryock, E.H. (1943). Conjoined fetuses (thoracopagus disymmetros) occurring in a set of monozygotic triplets: report of a case. *Am. J. Clin. Pathol.*, **13**, 215
29. Foster, P.M. (1948). Conjoined fetuses (thoracopagus) in a dizygotic triplet pregnancy. *Am. J. Obstet. Gynecol.*, **56**, 799
30. Mazumdar, L.B. (1956). Conjoined twins in a case of triplets. *J. Indian Med. Assoc.*, **26**, 313
31. Pepper, H. and Lindsay, S. (1958). Gasteropagus in a triplet pregnancy. *Arch. Pathol.*, **65**, 63

32. Franklin, A.W., Tomkinson, J.S. and Williams, E.R. (1958). A triplet pregnancy with craniopagus twins. *Lancet.*, **2**, 683
33. Ganzau, H. and Stein, F. (1962). Thoracopagus in unidentical triplet pregnancy. *Munchen. Med. Wshr.*, **104**, 1475
34. James, W.H. (1977). A note on the epidemiology of acardiac monsters. *Teratology*, **16**, 211
35. Napolitani, F.H. and Schreiber, I. (1960). The acardiac monster: a review of the world literature and presentation of 2 cases. *Am. J. Obstet. Gynecol.*, **80**, 582
36. Lehr, C. and DiRe, J. (1978). Rare occurrence of a holoacardius acephalic monster: sonographic and pathologic findings. *J. Clin. Ultrasound*, **6**, 259
37. Schinzel, A., Smith, D.W. and Miller, J.R. (1979). Monozygotic twinning and structural defects. *Pediatrics*, **95**, 921
38. Dugal, D. (1914). Description of a specimen of allantoidoangiopagus twins. *J. Obstet. Gynaecol. Br. Emp.*, **26**, 42
39. Onykoswova, Z., Dolezal, A. and Jedlicka, V. (1970). The frequency and the character of malformation in multiple births. *Acta Univ. Carol. [Med. Monogr.] (Praha)*, **16**, 333
40. Osathanondh, R., Driscoll, S.G. and Naftolin, F. (1975). Discordant severe cranial defects in monozygotic twins. *Am. J. Obstet. Gynecol.*, **122**, 301
41. Fries, H. (1959). Acardius amorphus. *Zentrabl. Gynaekol.*, **81**, 676
42. Panse, F. and Gierlich, J. (1948). Zur Frange der Anencephalic (auf Grand der Untersuchung eines Akardiers und seines Paarlings). *Virchows Arch. (Pathol. Anat.)*, **316**, 135
43. Kermauner, F. (1906). Uber Missbildungen mit Storungen des Korperverschlusses. *Arch. Gynakol.*, **78**, 221
44. Funikura, T. and Wellings, S.R. (1964). A teratoma-like mass on the placenta of a malformed infant. *Am. J. Obstet. Gynecol.*, **89**, 842
45. Das, K. (1902). Acardiacus anceps. *J. Obstet. Gynaecol. Br. Emp.*, **2**, 341
46. Gewolb, I.R., Freedman, R.M., Kleinman, C.S. *et al.* (1983). Prenatal diagnosis of a human pseudoacardiac anomaly. *Obstet. Gynecol.*, **61**, 657
47. Bieber, F.R., Nance, W.E., Morton, C.C. *et al.* (1981). Genetic studies of an acardiac monster: evidence of polar body twinning in man. *Science*, **213**, 775
48. Nance, W.A. (1981). Malformations unique to the twinning process. In Gedda, L., Parisi, P. and Nace, W.E. (eds.) *Twin Research 3: Part A, Twin Biology and Multiple Pregnancy*, pp. 123–38. (New York: Alan R. Liss)
49. Scott, J.M. and Ferguson-Smith, M.A. (1973). Heterokaryotypic monozygotic twins and the acardiac monster. *J. Obstet. Gynaecol. Br. Commonw.*, **80**, 52
50. Rehder, H., Geisler, M., Kleinbrecht, J. *et al.* (1978). Monozygotic twins with 47,XXY karyotype and discordant malformations. *Teratology*, **17**, 50a
51. Rashad, M.N. and Kerr, M.G. (1966). Observations on the so-called holoacardius amorphus. *J. Anat.*, **100**, 425
52. Turpin, R., Bocquet, L. and Grasset, J. (1967). Etude d'une couple monozygote: fille normale – monster acardiaque feminin. Considerations anatomo-pathologiques et cytogenetiques. *Ann. Genet.*, **10**, 107
53. Kaplan, C. and Benirschke, K. (1979). The acardiac anomaly new case reports and current status. *Acta Genet. Med. Gemellol.*, **28**, 51
54. Van Allen, M.I., Smith, D.W. and Shepard, T.H. (1983). Twin reversed arterial perfusion (TRAP) sequence: a study of 14 twin pregnancies with acardius. *Semin. Perinatol.*, **7**, 285
55. Severn, C.B. and Holyoke, E.A. (1973). Human acardiac anomalies. *Am. J. Obstet. Gynecol.*, **116**, 358
56. Ketchum, J. and Motyloff, L. (1957). Chorioangiopagus parasiticus (Schwalbe). *Am. J. Obstet. Gynecol.*, **73**, 1349
57. Fox, H. and Butler-Manuel, R. (1964). A teratoma of the placenta. *J. Pathol. Bacteriol.*, **88**, 137
58. Wilson, E.A. (1972). Holoacardius. *Obstet. Gynecol.*, **40**, 740
59. Simpson, P.C., Trudinger, B.J., Walker, A. *et al.* (1983). The intrauterine treatment of fetal acardiac failure in a twin pregnancy with an acardiac, acephalic monster. *Am. J. Obstet. Gynecol.*, **147**, 842
60. Platt, L.D., DeVore, G.R., Bieniarz, A. *et al.* (1983). Antenatal diagnosis of acephalus acardia: a proposed management scheme. *Am. J. Obstet. Gynecol.*, **146**, 857
61. Porreco, R.P., Barton, S.M. and Haverkamp, A.D. (1991). Occulusion of umbilical artery in acardiac, acephalic twin. *Lancet*, **337**, 326
62. Ginsberg, N.A., Applebaum, M., Rabin, S.A. *et al.* (1992). Term birth after midtrimester hysterotomy and selective delivery of an acardiac twin. *Am. J. Obstet. Gynecol.*, **167**, 33
63. Robie, G.F., Payne, G.G. and Morgan, M.A. (1989). Selective delivery of an acardiac, acephalic twin. *N. Engl. J. Med.*, **320**, 512

64. Fries, M.H., Goldberg, J.D. and Golbus, M.S. (1992). Treatment of acardiac-acephalus twin gestations by hysterotomy and selective delivery. *Obstet. Gynecol.*, **79**, 601
65. Benirschke, K. (1961). Twin placenta in perinatal mortality. *NY State J. Med.*, **61**, 1499–508
66. Hanna, J.H. and Hill, J.M. (1984). Single intrauterine fetal demise in multiple gestation. *Obstet. Gynecol.*, **63**, 126
67. D'Alton, M.E., Newton, E.R. and Cetrulo, C.L. (1984). Intrauterine fetal demise in multiple gestation. *Acta Genet. Med. Gemellol.*, **33**, 43
68. Eubom, J.A. (1985). Twin pregnancy with intrauterine death of one twin. *Am. J. Obstet. Gynecol.*, **152**, 424
69. Litschgi, M. and Stucki, D. (1980). Course of twin pregnancies after death *in utero*. *Z. Geburtschilfe Perinatol.*, **184**, 227
70. Jung, J.H., Graham, J.M., Schultz, N. *et al.* (1984). Congenital hydranencephaly/porencephaly due to vascular disruption in monozygotic twins. *Pediatrics*, **73**, 467
71. Hoyme, H.E., Higginbottom, M.C. and Jones, K.L. (1981). Vascular etiology of disruptive structural defects in monozygotic twins. *Pediatrics*, **67**, 288
72. Anderson, R.L., Golbus, M.S., Curry, C.J.R. *et al.* (1990). Central nervous system damage and other anomalies in surviving fetus following second trimester antenatal death of co-twin. *Prenat. Diagn.*, **10**, 513
73. Durkin, M.V., Kaveggia, E.G., Pendelton, E. *et al.* (1976). Analysis of etiological factors in cerebral palsy with severe mental retardation. I. Analysis of gestational, parturitional and neonatal data. *Eur. J. Pediatr.*, **123**, 67
74. Melnick, M. (1977). Brain damage in survivor after death of monozygotic co-twin. *Lancet*, **2**, 1287
75. Yoshida, K. and Matayoshi, K. (1990). A study on prognosis of surviving cotwin. *Acta Genet. Med. Gemellol.*, **39**, 383
76. Confalonieri, C. (1951). Gravidanza gemellare monocoriale biamniotica con feto papiraceo ed atresia intestinale congenita nell'altro feto. *Riv. Ost. Ginec. Prac.*, **33**, 199
77. Saier, F., Burden, L. and Cavanagh, D. (1975). Fetus papyraceus: an unusual case with congenital anomaly of the surviving fetus. *Obstet. Gynecol.*, **45**, 217
78. Yoshioka, H., Kadomoto, Y., Mino, M. *et al.* (1979). Multicystic encephalomalacia in liveborn twin with a stillborn macerated co-twin. *J. Pediatr.*, **95**, 798

79. Moore, C.M., McAdams, A.J. and Sutherland, J. (1969). Intrauterine disseminated intravascular coagulation: a syndrome of multiple pregnancy with a dead twin fetus. *J. Pediatr.*, **74**, 523
80. Mannino, F.L., Jones, K.L. and Benirschke, K. (1977). Congenital skin defects and fetus papyraceus. *J. Pediatr.*, **91**, 559
81. Carlson, N.J. and Towers, C.V. (1989). Multiple gestation complicated by the death of one fetus. *Obstet. Gynecol.*, **73**, 685
82. Fusi, L., McParland, P., Fisk, N. *et al.* (1991). Acute twin–twin transfusion: a possible mechanism for brain-damaged survivors after intrauterine death of a monochorionic twin. *Obstet. Gynecol.*, **78**, 517
83. Larroche, J.C., Droulle, P., Delezoide, A.L. *et al.* (1990). Brain damage in monozygous twins. *Biol. Neonate*, **57**, 261
84. Romero, R., Duffy, T.P., Berkowitz, R.L. *et al.* (1984). Prolongation of a preterm pregnancy complicated by death of a single twin *in utero* and disseminated intravascular coagulation. *N. Engl. J. Med.*, **310**, 772
85. Puckett, J.D. (1988). Fetal death of second twin in second trimester. *Am. J. Obstet. Gynecol.*, **159**, 740
86. Tharapel, A.T., Elias, S., Shulman, L.P. *et al.* (1989). Resorbed co-twin as an explanation for discrepant chorionic villus results: nonmosaic 47,XX+16 in villi (direct and culture) with normal (46,XX) amniotic fluid and neonatal blood. *Prenat. Diagn.*, **9**, 467
87. deWolff, E., Scharer, K. and Lejeune, J. (1962). Contribution a l'étude des jumeaux mongoliens. Un cas de monozygotisme ketercaryote. *Helvet. Paediat. Acta*, **17**, 301
88. Fanconi, V.G. (1962). Weitere Falle von wahrscheinlich eineiigen Zwillingen, von denender eine gesund ist, der andere einen Mongolismus zeight. *Helvet. Paediat. Acta*, **17**, 490
89. Turpin, R., Lejeune, J., Lafoureade, J. *et al.* (1961). Présomption de monozygotisme en dépit d'un dimorphisme sexuel: sujet masculin XY et sujet neutre haplo X. *Compt. Rend. Acad. Sci.*, **252**, 2945
90. Dallapiccola, B., Stomeo, C., Ferranti, G. *et al.* (1985). Discordant sex in one of three monozygotic triplets. *J. Med. Genet.*, **22**, 6
91. Edwards, J.H., Dent, T. and Kahn, J. (1966). Monozygotic twins of different sex. *J. Med. Genet.*, **3**, 117
92. Russell, A., Moschos, A., Butler, L.J. *et al.* (1966). Gonadal dysgenesis and its unilateral

variant with testis in monozygotic twins: related to discordance in sex chromosome status. *J. Clin. Endocrinol.*, **26**, 1282
93. Karp, L., Bryant, J.L., Tagatz, G. et al. (1975). The occurrence of gonadal dysgenesis in association with monozygotic twinning. *J. Med. Genet.*, **12**, 70
94. Schmidt, R., Sobel, E.H., Nitowsky, H.M. et al. (1976). Monozygotic twins discordant for sex. *J. Med. Genet.*, **13**, 64
95. Reindollar, R.H., Byrd, J.R., Hahn, D.H. et al. (1987). A cytogenetic and endocrinologic study of a set of monozygotic isokaryotic 45,X/46,XY twins discordant for phenotypic sex: mosaicism versus chimerism. *Fertil. Steril.*, **47**, 626
96. Kaplowitz, P.B., Bodurtha, J., Brown, J. et al. (1991). Monozygotic twins discordant for Ullrich–Turner syndrome. *Am. J. Med. Genet.*, **41**, 78
97. Loevy, H.T., Miller, M. and Rosenthal, I.M. (1985). Discordant monozygotic twins with trisomy 13. *Acta Genet. Med. Gemellol.*, **34**, 185
98. Mulder, A.F., van Eyck, J., Groenendaal, F. et al. (1989). Trisomy 18 in monozygotic twins. *Hum. Genet.*, **83**, 300
99. Coté, G.B. and Gyftodimou, J. (1991). Twinning and mitotic crossing-over: some possibilities and their implications. *Am. J. Hum. Genet.*, **49**, 120
100. Nance, W.E. (1990). Invited Editorial: Do twin lyons have larger spots? *Am. J. Hum. Genet.*, **46**, 646
101. Lupski, J.R., Garcia, C.A., Zoghbi, H.Y. et al. (1991). Discordance of muscular dystrophy in monozygotic female twins: evidence supporting asymmetric splitting of the inner cell mass in a manifesting carrier of Duchenne Dystrophy. *Am. J. Med. Genet.*, **40**, 354
102. Richards, C.S., Watkins, S.C., Hoffman, E.P. et al. (1990). Skewed X inactivation in a female MZ twin results in Duchenne muscular dystrophy. *Am. J. Hum. Genet.*, **46**, 672
103. Kastern, W. and Kryspin-Sorensen, I. (1988). Penetrance and low concordance in monozygotic twins in disease: are they the results of alterations in somatic genomes? *Mol. Reprod. Develop.*, **1**, 63
104. Hall, J.G. (1988). Review and hypotheses: somatic mosaicism: observations related to clinical genetics. *Am. J. Hum. Genet.*, **43**, 355
105. Hall, J.G. (1992). New theory on the phenomenon of identical twins. Presented at the *Bar Harbor-Jackson Laboratories Seminar*, Bar Harbor, Maine, July
106. Wang, L.N., Wang, Y.F., Horne, C.C. et al. (1990). Congenital rubella infection: escape of one monozygotic twin with two amnions, one chorion, and single placenta. *Taiwan I Hsueh Hui Ts'a Chih (Taiwan)*, **89**, 30
107. Chasnoff, I.J. (1985). Fetal alcohol syndrome in twin pregnancy. *Acta Genet. Med. Gemellol.*, **34**, 229
108. Phelan, M.C., Pellock, J.M. and Nance, W.E. (1982). Discordant expression of fetal hydantoin syndrome in heteropaternal dizygotic twins. *N. Engl. J. Med.*, **307**, 99
109. Allen, G. (1965). Twin research: problems and prospects. In Steinberg, A.G. and Bearn, A.G. (eds.) *Progress in Medical Genetics*, (4th edn), pp. 242–69. (New York: Grune & Stratton)
110. Warkany, J. (1971). *Congenital Malformations: Notes and Comments.* (Chicago: Year Book Medical Publishers)
111. Kendler, K.S. and Holm, N.V. (1985). Differential enrollment in twin registries: its effect on prevalence and concordance rates and estimates of genetic parameters. *Acta Genet. Med. Gemellol.*, **34**, 125
112. Little, J. and Carr-Hill, R.A. (1984). Problems of ascertainment of congenital anomalies. *Acta Genet. Med. Gemellol.*, **33**, 97
113. Kallen, B. (1986). Congenital malformations in twins: a population study. *Acta Genet. Med. Gemellol.*, **35**, 167
114. Hay, S. and Wehrung, D.A. (1970). Congenital malformations in twins. *Am. J. Hum. Genet.*, **22**, 662–78
115. Burn, J. and Corney, G. (1984). Congenital heart defects and twinning. *Acta Genet. Med. Gemellol.*, **33**, 61
116. Stevenson, A.C., Johnston, H.A., Stewart, M.I.P. et al. (1966). Congenital malformations: a report of a study of series of consecutive births in 24 centres. *Bull. WHO*, **34**, (Suppl.), 1
117. Edwards, J.H. (1968). The value of twins in genetic studies. *Proc. R. Soc. Med.*, **61**, 227
118. Myrianthopolous, N.C. (1975). Congenital malformations in twins. Epidemiologic survey. *Birth Defects Orig. Art. Ser. XI*, **8**, 1
119. Windham, S.C. and Bjerkedal, T. (1984). Malformations in twins and their siblings, Norway, 1967–79. *Acta Genet. Med. Gemellol.*, **33**, 87
120. McKeown, T. and Record, R.G. (1960). Malformations in a population observed for five years after birth. In Wolstenholme, G.E.W. and O'Connor, C.M. (eds.) *CIBA Foundation Symposium on Congenital Malformations*, pp. 2–21. (Boston: Little, Brown)

121. Little, J. and Nevin, N.C. (1989). Congenital anomalies in twins in Northern Ireland III: anomalies of the cardiovascular system, 1974–1978. *Acta Genet. Med. Gemellol.*, **38**, 27
122. Layde, P.M., Erickson, J.D., Falek, A. *et al.* (1980) Congenital malformations in twins. *Am. J. Hum. Genet.*, **32**, 69
123. Mitchell, S.C., Sellmann, A.H., Westphal, M.C. *et al.* (1971). Etiological correlates in a study of congenital heart disease in 56 109 births. *Am. J. Cardiol.*, **28**, 653
124. Kenna, A.P., Smithells, R.W. and Fielding, D.W. (1975). Congenital heart disease in Liverpool: 1960–69. *Q. J. Med.*, **154**, 17
125. Camerson, A.H., Edwards, J.H., Derom, R. *et al.* (1994). The value of twin surveys in the study of malformations. *Eur. J. Obstet. Gynaecol.*, in press
126. Berg, K.A., Astemborski, J.A., Boughman, J.A. *et al.* (1989). Congenital cardiovascular malformations in twins and triplets from a population-based study. *Am. J. Dis. Child.*, **143**, 1461
127. James, W.H. (1976). Twinning and anencephaly. *Ann. Hum. Biol.*, **3**, 401
128. Elwood, J.M. and Elwood, J.H. (1980). *Epidemiology of Anencephalus and Spina Bifida*, pp. 205–21 (Oxford: Oxford University Press)
129. Little, J. and Nevin, N.C. (1989). Congenital anomalies in twins in Northern Ireland II: neural tube defects, 1974–1979. *Acta Genet. Med. Gemellol.*, **38**, 17
130. Windham, G.C., Bjerkedal, T. and Sever, L.E. (1982). The association of twinning and neural tube defects: studies in Los Angeles, California, and Norway. *Acta Genet. Med. Gemellol.*, **31**, 165
131. Simpson, J.L. and Mills, J.L. (1985). Methodologic problems in determining fetal loss rates: relevance to chorionic villus sampling. In Fraccaro, M., Simon, G., Brambati, B. (eds.) *First Trimester Fetal Diagnosis*, pp. 321–33. (Berlin: Springer-Verlag)
132. Livingston, J.E. and Poland, B.J. (1980). A study of spontaneously aborted twins. *Teratology*, **21**, 148
133. Uchida, I.A., Freeman, V.C.P., Gedeon, M. *et al.* (1983). Twinning rate in spontaneous abortions. *Am. J. Hum. Genet.*, **35**, 987
134. Kajii, T., Ohama, K., Nikawa, N. *et al.* (1973). Banding analysis of abnormal karyotypes in spontaneous abortion. *Am. J. Hum. Genet.*, **25**, 539
135. Creasy, M.R., Crolla, J.A. and Alberman, E.D. (1976). A cytogenetic study of human spontaneous *bortions using banding techniques. *Hum. Genet.*, **31**, 177
136. Hellman, L.M., Kobayashi, M. and Cromb, E. (1973). Ultrasonic diagnosis of embryonic malformations. *Am. J. Obstet. Gynecol.*, **115**, 615
137. Levi, S. (1976). Ultrasonic assessment of the high rate of human multiple pregnancy in the first trimester. *J. Clin. Ultrasound*, **4**, 3
138. Robinson, H.P. and Caines, J.S. (1977). Sonar evidence of early pregnancy failure in patients with twin conceptions. *Br. J. Obstet. Gynaecol.*, **84**, 22
139. Varma, T.R. (1979). Ultrasound evidence of early pregnancy failure in patients with multiple conceptions. *Br. J. Obstet. Gynaecol.*, **86**, 290

Conjoined twins

M. Creinin

Introduction

The term 'conjoined twins' is used to describe those infants intimately united at some point in their anatomy. For centuries, conjoined twins have fascinated physicians and laymen alike. Some of the earliest illustrations of this condition are found in Egyptian tombs and on Roman coins. Today, the birth or successful surgical separation of conjoined twins is widely reported in the popular press, and the medical literature contains numerous case reports that also review the world literature.

One of the earliest documented cases of surviving conjoined twins was that of the Biddenden twins born in England in AD 1100. These women lived to the age of 34 joined at the hips. Perhaps the most famous conjoined twins were Chang and Eng Bunker, born in Siam (now Thailand) in 1811. These twins, who gave rise to the popular term 'Siamese twins', were joined at the umbilicus by a firm band of tissue; each individual, however, was able to lead a full and productive life. Chang and Eng arrived in the USA at the age of 18 and soon after began touring the country in the circus of P.T. Barnum. After amassing a considerable sum of money from their circus activities, they married two sisters and retired to a farm in North Carolina. During their lives, they fathered 22 children, none of whom were twins. They died at the age of 63, only hours apart of each other.

Several more sets of conjoined twins have survived into adulthood, especially in the last half of this century as resuscitative measures have improved. Although it can be said that such individuals may lead productive lives, one can only wonder about their isolation from society and the severe restrictions placed on their daily living activities that inevitably result from their congenital deformity.

The incidence of conjoined twinning varies among countries, most likely due to racial differences in overall twinning rates as well as ascertainment biases. The overall incidence approximates 1/50 000–1/100 000 births[1] and 1/546 twin births[2]. Conjoined twinning is an uncommon event in humans as compared to lower animals. The veterinary literature contains numerous reports of conjoined twinning among such diverse species as the hamster, guinea pig, goat, cow, mouse, chicken and buffalo. The relative infrequency of this anomaly in humans may be explained by the fact that it represents a teratogenic occurrence that generally terminates in spontaneous abortion.

The most commonly accepted theory regarding the etiology of conjoined twinning assumes that the fetuses are derived from a single ovum; normal fission produces identical monozygotic (MZ) twins, and abnormal fission produces conjoined twins. Indeed, conjoined twinning occurs in a relatively constant ratio of 1 per 400 pairs of MZ twins[2], and all sets of conjoined twins join individuals of the same sex; these findings support the single ovum theory. Although commonly associated with the lowest order of multiple gestation, conjoined twinning has been reported to occur in association with triplet[2-7] and quadruplet[8] pregnancies as well.

Adapted and revised from Ellis, J.W., Keith, L. and Keith, D.M. (1983). Conjoined twins. In *Current Problems in Obstetrics and Gynecology*, vol. VI, no. 8, pp. 55–80. (Chicago: Year Book Medical Publishers) (With permission)

Female conjoined twins occur more commonly than males in a ratio of approximately 1.6 to 1[3,7,9,10]. Interestingly, all conjoined chickens are female[11]. The explanation for this female preponderance is unclear. Perhaps, as suggested by Potter and Craig, incomplete division of the embryonic plate occurs more often in females, conjoined twinning is more lethal in males, or some of the phenotypically female twins are in fact an XO portion of an improperly divided XY zygote[12].

This chapter reviews the concepts of etiology, diagnosis, and obstetric and surgical management of conjoined twinning.

Classification of conjoined twins

The many types of conjoined twins may be broadly classified as either equal or unequal. The equal forms (*duplicatas completa*) show equal or nearly equal duplication of structures. The unequal forms, belonging to the category *duplicatas incompleta*, include the parasitic variety in which there is unequal duplication of structures. In these cases, only part of the anatomical structure of the fetus is duplicated.

Classification of conjoined twins is typically based on the fused anatomic region followed by the Greek suffix '-pagus', to indicate fastened. The following classification of equal and unequal types of conjoined twinning has been proposed by Potter and Craig[12].

I. *Diplopagus* Conjoined twins in which the components, or component parts, are equal and symmetrical.

  A. Each component is complete, or nearly so.

  (1) *Thoracopagus, sternopagus, xiphopagus* and *sternoxiphopagus*: connection in or near the sternal region, usually median, and the components are face to face (Figure 1).

  (2) *Pygopagus*: connection at the sacrum and the components are back to back (Figure 2).

  (3) *Craniopagus*: connection by the heads, usually median (Figure 3).

  (4) *Ischiopagus*: connection in the lower pelvic region with the axes of the bodies extending in a straight line in opposite directions (Figure 4).

  B. The two components equal each other but each is less than an entire individual.

  (1) Duplication beginning in the cranial region.

    (a) *Monocephalus diprosopus* (single head)
      1. Partial duplication of frontal region and nose (Figure 5A);
      2. Partial duplication of frontal region, nose and mouth (Figure 5B and 5C);
      3. Duplication of the face either complete or with one eye of each face fused into a common median orbit (Figure 5D).

    (b) *Dicephalus* (two heads, one body)
      1. *Dicephalus dipus dibrachius:* two arms and legs with partial duplication of the spine and varying degrees of duplication of the median shoulder (Figure 6);
      2. *Dicephalus dipus tribrachius:* similar to dibrachius but with a median third arm or arm rudiment (Figure 7);
      3. *Dicephalus dipus tetrabrachius:* components united at the pelvis with varying degrees of fusion of the upper parts of the trunk but each component having a head and a pair of arms. The pelvis is partially duplicated but only two legs are present (Figure 8).

  (2) Duplication originating in the caudal region (*dipygus*).

    (a) *Monocephalus tripus dibrachius:* partial duplication of the pelvis with a third median leg that may be rudimentary or complete.

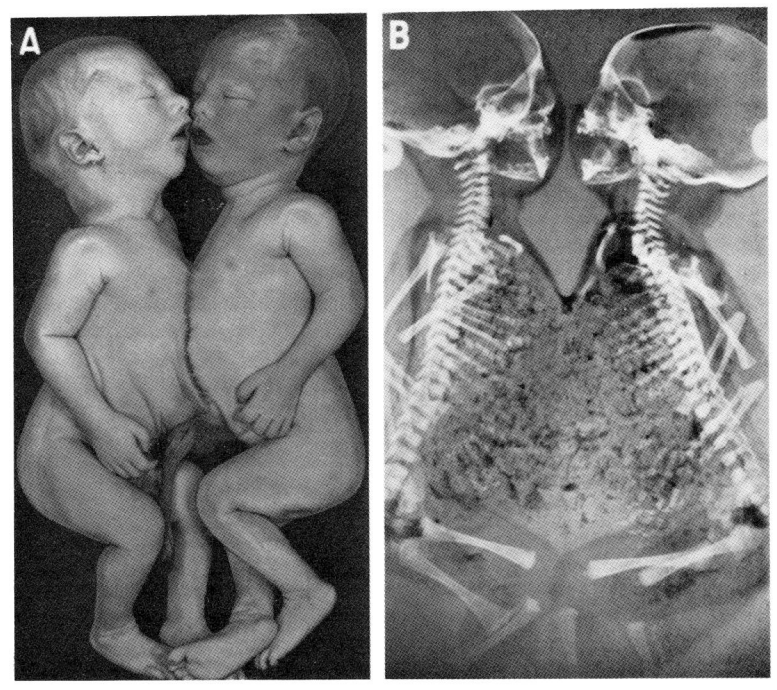

Figure 1 Thoracopagus twins. Male twins joined by thorax and upper abdomen. Umbilical cord contained four arteries and two veins. Hearts and liver were joined and only partially duplicated. Gastrointestinal tracts were separate. A, external view; B, roentgenogram. (Reproduced from Potter, E.L. and Craig, J.M.[12] with permission)

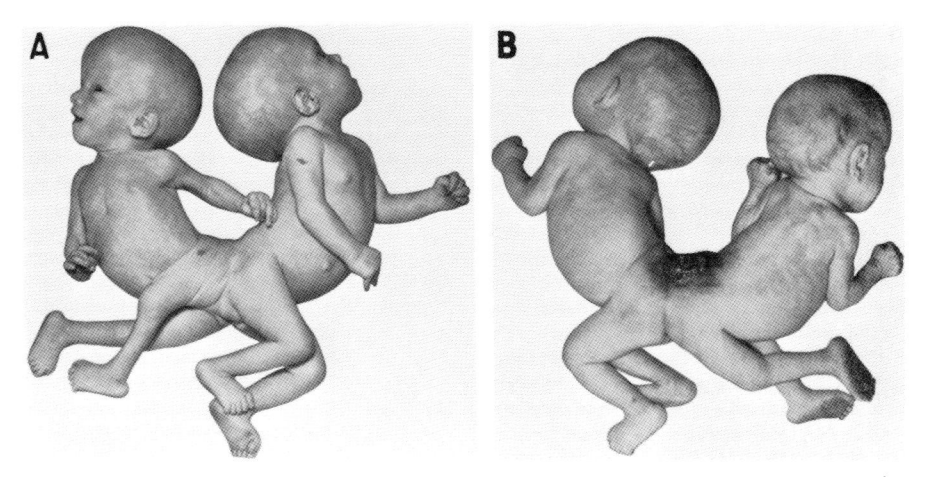

Figure 2 Pygopagus female twins. Infants joined by sacral areas, each of which was the site of a spina bifida. External genitalia were partially fused and common vaginal and anal orifices were divided by septa separating the two orifices of the two twins. Bladders and all organs were duplicated except the kidneys, of which there were only three. A, anterior view; B, posterior view. (Reproduced from Potter, E.L. and Craig, J.M.[12] with permission)

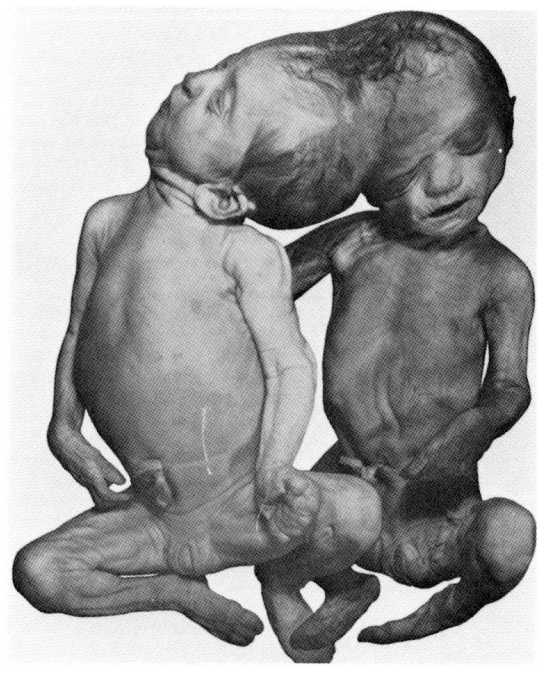

Figure 3 Craniopagus twins. Median parietal area of right twin is united with right frontoparietal area of left twin. (Reproduced from Potter, E.L. and Craig, J.M.[12] with permission)

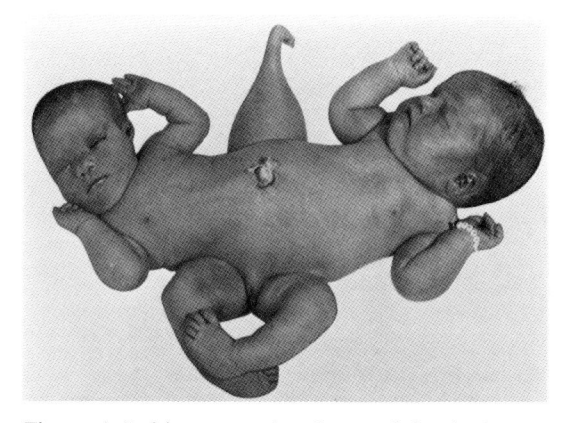

Figure 4 Ischiopagus twins. Lower abdominal areas are fused and extremities consequently displaced laterally. One pelvis is present with single normal external genitalia located between right leg of left twin and left leg of right twin. The legs are normal except for clubfoot. Opposite legs are fused into a single composite limb. Viscera of one was in situs inversus position. Aortas were fused. The heart of one twin was hypoplastic and circulation through that twin was in reverse direction through arteries and veins. (Reproduced from Potter, E.L. and Craig, J.M.[12] with permission)

  (b) *Monocephalus tetrapus dibrachius*: partial or complete duplication of the pelvis with four legs, the pair belonging to one member often being fused in a sirenomelic limb (Figure 9).
  (c) *Cephalothoracopagus*: two nearly complete components joined front to front over more or less the trunk region, but with a single neck and with heads more or less completely fused into a single compound mass.
    1. *Deradelphus*: one face with two ears and a single normally formed cerebrum;
    2. *Syncephalus*: one face with four ears, two on the back of the head. The cerebrum is single or partially duplicated (Figure 10);
    3. *Janiceps*: two faces on opposite sides of the head with half of each belonging to each component (Figure 11).
 (3) Duplication of both cranial and caudal regions (*Dicephalus dipygus*).
  (a) *Dicephalus tripus tribrachius*: two members with a common trunk but with two heads, two or three arms and three legs (Figure 12).
  (b) Similar to tripus tribrachius but with either upper or lower extremities or both completely duplicated.
  (c) Complete duplication of head, arms and legs with anterior or lateral fusion of the trunk area.
II. *Heteropagus* Unequal and symmetrical conjoined twins in which one component is smaller and dependent on the other. Two members with very unequal degrees of development, the one (autosite) being normal or nearly so and the other (parasite) being incomplete and attached to the first as a dependent growth, usually attached at some point on the ventral surface.

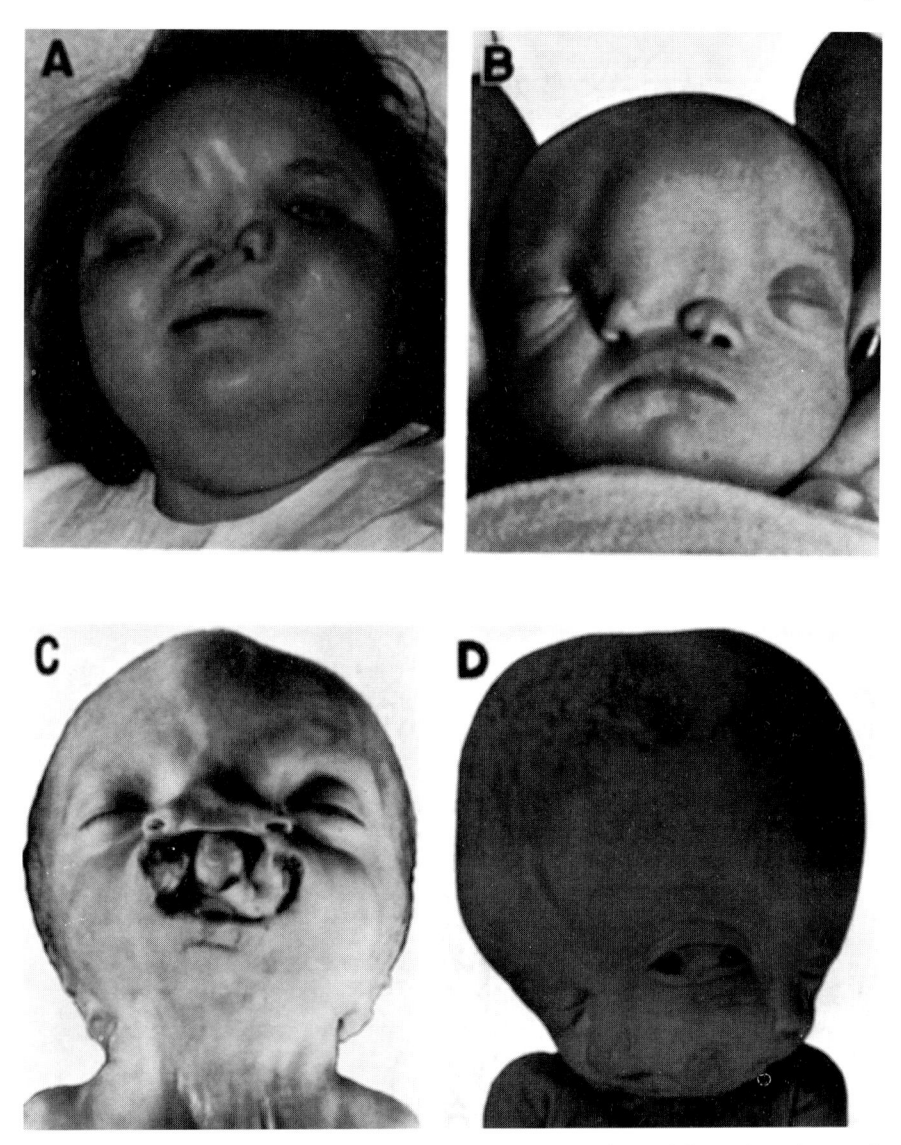

Figure 5 Monocephalus diprosopus. A, partial duplication of frontal region and nose; B, partial duplication of frontal region, nose and palate with increase in width of mouth; C, widening of frontal region with duplication of mouth and nose, harelip and cleft palate; D, duplication of face with a common median orbit. (Reproduced from Potter, E.L. and Craig, J.M.[12] with permission)

A. Parasite attached to the visible surface of the autosite.

   (1) Parasite having arms, or a head and arms, usually attached to the autosite at or near the epigastrium.

   (2) Parasite having legs and varying portions of abdomen usually attached at or near the epigastrium (Figure 13).

   (3) Parasite having arms and legs with or without a head with attachment at or near the epigastrium.

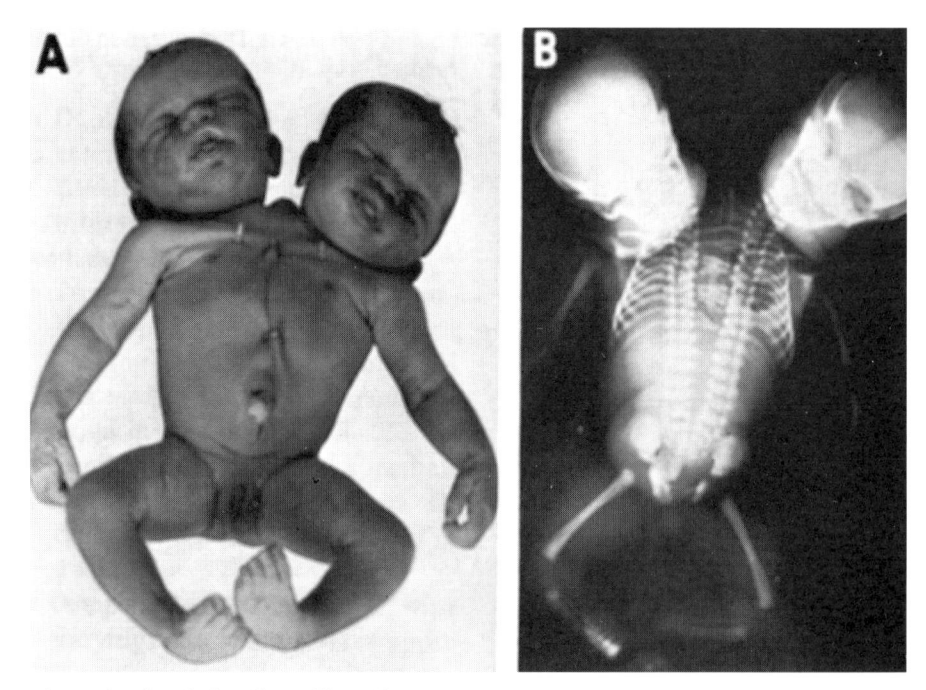

Figure 6 Dicephalus dipus dibrachius. A, external surface; B, roentgenogram. (Reproduced from Potter, E.L. and Craig, J.M.[12] with permission)

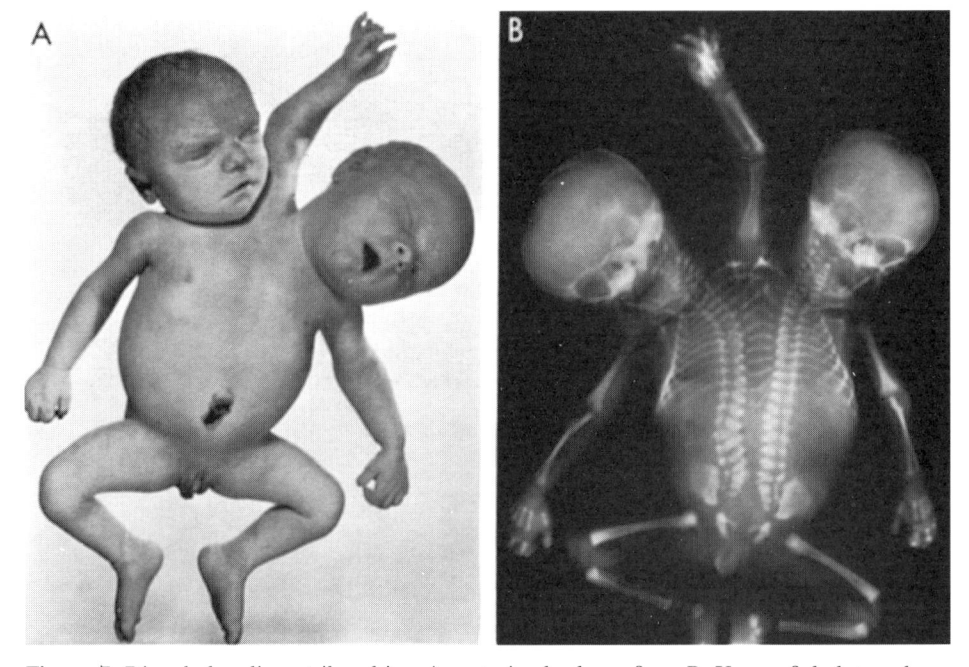

Figure 7 Dicephalus dipus tribrachius. A, anterior body surface; B, X-ray of skeleton showing common arm with fused humerus and three bones in forearm. (Reproduced from Potter, E.L. and Craig, J.M.[12] with permission)

Conjoined twins

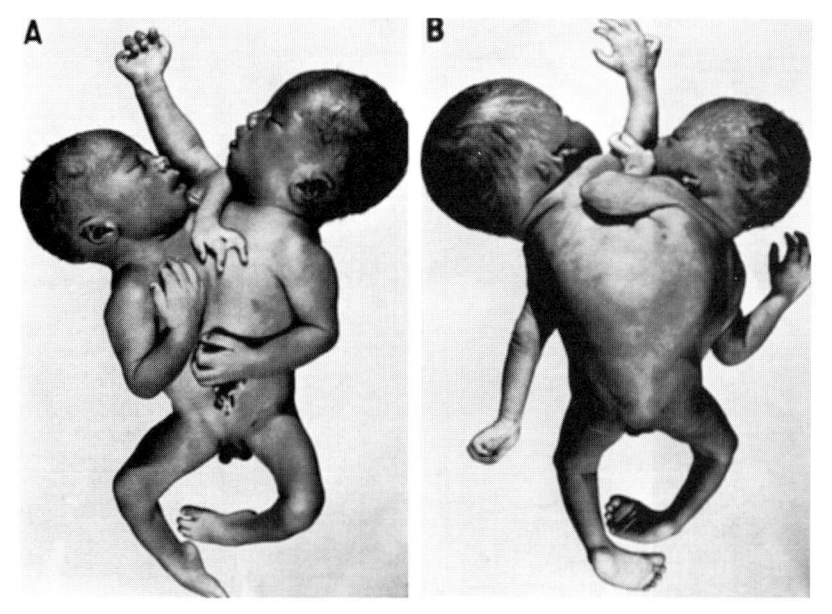

Figure 8 Dicephalus dipus tetrabrachius. A, anterior view; B, posterior view. (Reproduced from Potter, E.L. and Craig, J.M.[12] with permission)

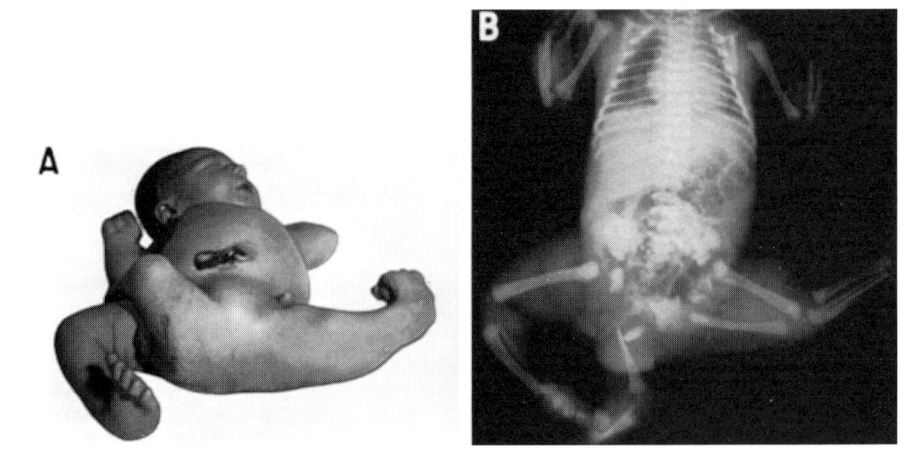

Figure 9 Monocephalus tetrapus dibrachius. The two legs on one side are fused into a sirenomelic limb belonging to the left-hand component. This is to be distinguished from a median composite limb made up of components from both twin members in a tripus abnormality. A, exterior view; B, roentgenogram. (Reproduced from Potter, E.L. and Craig, J.M.[12] with permission)

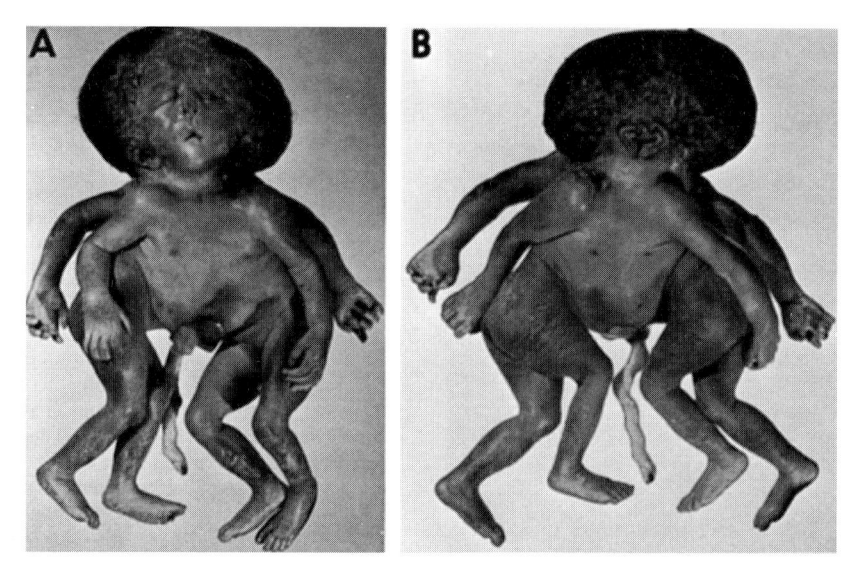

Figure 10 Cephalothoracopagus syncephalus. A, anterior view; B, posterior view. (Reproduced from Potter, E.L. and Craig, J.M.[12] with permission)

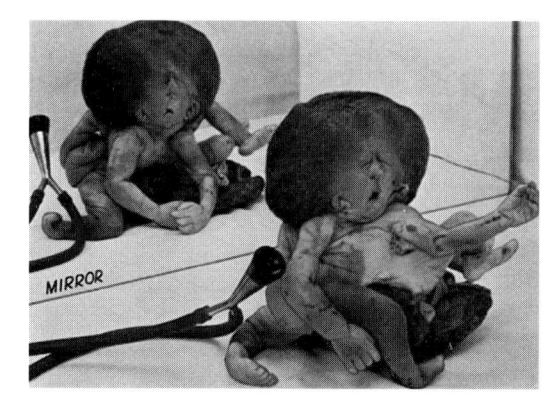

Figure 11 Cephalothoracopagus janiceps. Fetus has two faces, one of which is visible in the mirror. (Reproduced from Potter, E.L. and Craig, J.M.[12] with permission)

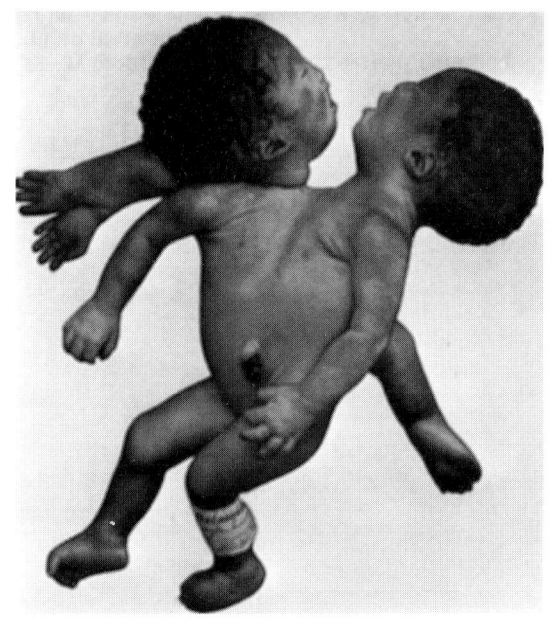

Figure 12 Dicephalus tripus tribrachius. Upper composite limb is a result of fusion of soft tissues and bones of the two medial arms. Lower medial limb has a common femur, tibia and great toe. (Reproduced from Potter, E.L. and Craig, J.M.[12] with permission)

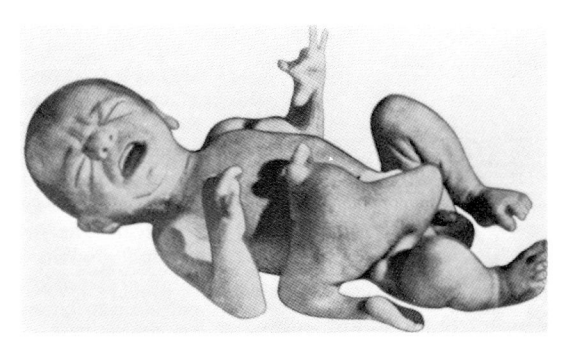

Figure 13 Parasitic fetus composed of fairly well-developed legs, rudimentary pelvis and one finger attached to epigastrium of an otherwise normal male infant. (Reproduced from Potter, E.L. and Craig, J.M.[12] with permission)

(4) Parasite attached to the head of the autosite.

(5) Parasite attached to the palate of the autosite.

(6) Parasite attached to the back, sacrum, or pelvis of the autosite.

B. Parasite developed in the autosite, usually in the thoracic or abdominal cavity, but occasionally in other regions (usually classified as tumors) (see Chapter 7).

(1) Fetus-in-fetu. Well-differentiated parasitic growth showing some degree of internal symmetry and cranial caudal differentiation.

(2) Teratomas. Amorphous growth derived from three germ layers and lacking differentiation.

Other attempts have been made to standardize terminology of conjoined twins. Cuq and Woronoff[13] proposed a classification that divides the types of conjoined twinning into orders, suborders, tribes, families, genera and varieties. The more simplified classification proposed by Guttmacher and Nichols (Table 1)[14] is also used by some authors.

The most common type of conjoined twinning, comprising approximately 59% of all cases, involves conjunction in the mid-body (thoracopagus, xiphopagus, omphalopagus, or some combination thereof). In contrast, unequal conjoined twins are rare, accounting for less than 10% of cases[3,9].

Table 1 Types of conjoined twins

Inferior conjunction
Diprosopus – two faces with one head and body
Dicephalus – two heads and one body
Ischiopagus – inferior sacrococcygeal fusion
Pygopagus – posterolateral sacrococcygeal fusion

Superior conjunction
Dipygus – two pelves and four legs
Syncephalus – facial + thoracic fusion
Craniopagus – cranial fusion

Mid conjunction
Thoracopagus – thoracic fusion
Omphalopagus – fusion from umbilicus to xiphoid cartilage
Rachipagus – vertebral fusion above sacrum

Adapted from Guttmacher, A.F. and Nichols, B.L. (1967). Teratology of conjoined twins. In Bergsma, D. (ed.) *Birth Defects Original Article Series: Conjoined Twins*. (New York: The National Foundation – March of Dimes)

Etiology

Numerous theories have been proposed over the centuries to explain conjoined twinning. In ancient times, 'evil' prenatal influences were generally believed to be responsible for all congenital anomalies including 'double monsters'. In *The Cosmology*, written in 1552, Sebastian Munster proposed that abnormal twinning was caused by prenatal influences or 'maternal impressions'. He cited the example of two women who accidentally hit their heads together, one later delivering craniopagus twins. During the 18th century, the prevailing theory centered around the fertilization of one egg by two sperm. During the 19th century, it was proposed that conjoined twins result from the fusion of separate twins.

The precise etiology of conjoined twinning remains unknown; the prevailing theory is that the same influences that cause MZ twinning are responsible for cases of abnormal twinning. The causes of MZ twinning are reviewed in Chapter 3.

The embryology of conjoined twinning has been discussed in depth by Potter and Craig[12] and Zimmermann[15]. Conjoined twins are a rare complication of MZ twinning whereby fission of the inner cell mass is delayed following the 14th day after fertilization. Because fission begins after formation of the germinal disc, separation cannot be complete. The chorion and amnion are already formed, resulting in monochorionic/monoamniotic placentation. The three derivatives of the germinal disc (ectoderm, mesoderm and endoderm), the yolk sac and the body stalk are all typically shared. However, there are rare examples of selective involvement of these components, most notably two cases of mono- chorionic/diamniotic conjoined twins[15,16]. These two cases may, in fact, be examples of MZ twins with inadequate spatial separation following fission, thereby resulting in overlap fusion of tissue domains[16].

The cause of this delayed fission is not known; however, several reasonable theories have been proposed. One such theory proposes that development is retarded or stopped at a critical period of susceptibility, thus inducing abnormal fission or budding of the embryonic disc[17]. Another hypothesis stresses the development of two or more centers of axial growth. The critical period for this event is thought to occur soon after the formation of the rudimentary amniotic sac in the blastocyst stage[12,17,18].

Benirschke and Temple[19] proposed the theory of 'twinning impetus', which claims that certain factors are capable of affecting reproduction at random. This impetus results in normal MZ twins during the first 2 weeks after fertilization, before the embryo has completed its axiation. During the 13th to 15th days after ovulation, however, this 'impetus' may be responsible for a variety of twinning anomalies ranging from minimally to extensively fused twins. The point of connection or the degree and nature of an organ duplication depends on the areas affected by the deleterious twinning event.

Wedberg et al.[20] proposed that, based on the mechanism of somite development, the poles of the embryo are able to duplicate themselves later than the more central areas. This theory is supported by the observation that conjoined twins are more frequently fused in the mid-axial rather than in the proximate or distal areas.

At present, few proponents of the so-called 'collision theory' remain. This hypothesis suggests that conjunction may result from the fusion of separate blastomeres of dizygotic (DZ) twins[21]. Since conjoined twins are always fused in identical areas on each twin, only rare and unusual cases provide support for this theory.

Conjoined twinning occurs more commonly in the lower mammalian orders, an observation that may reflect the increased incidence of multiple gestation in these animals[22–25] (see Chapter 7). Many experiments have induced conjoined twinning in the laboratory. In 1921, Stockard[18] produced a variety of anomalies, including conjoined twinning, by exposing zygotes to hypoxia, heat change and other environmental insults. Ingalls[26] produced conjoined twins in zebra fish by applying a combination of heat and hypoxia to the fertilized eggs near the time of gastrulation. He suggested that similar principles governing the formation of such deformities operate widely in nature and may be involved in the production of human deformity. The work of Ferm[27] also supports the concept that conjoined twins may be experimentally induced by manipulation of the microclimate of the young embryo at a susceptible stage of its development.

In human gestations, however, no factors have been consistently linked to the incidence of conjoined twinning. In the majority of instances, the prenatal course was uneventful, with no history of exposure to teratogens or environmental hazards.

As with MZ twinning in general, the incidence of conjoined twinning is independent of maternal age[9,28,29], race, parity and heredity. Milham[30] reported on 22 sets of conjoined twins born in New York and proposed a possible seasonal effect on incidence and a possible time–space clustering of cases. Occasional geographic and seasonal clusterings have also been observed. These observations have not been reported with consistency by other investigators, however.

Moreover, no evidence has yet been presented to support a genetic etiology for conjoined twinning. Only one instance of a second set of conjoined twins within a family has been reported[31]. Cytogenetic studies using peripheral lymphocytes have revealed normal chromosomal patterns in conjoined twins. Kim et al.[32] studied both peripheral lymphocytes and connective tissue in one case and reported a normal chromosome pattern.

Anatomy of conjoined twins

Many reports describe the gross anatomy of conjoined twins, although most of these data are based on postmortem findings. The internal anatomy of conjoined twins generally depends on the site and extent of the union. In some, organs may be shared or just connected. In others, the union may only be a thin bridge of skin and muscle with no shared or connected organs. Conjoined twinning is additionally associated with a high incidence of congenital anomalies; frequently, these anomalies are not obviously associated with the site of conjoining.

Craniopagus

Craniopagus twins may be united in the vertex, occiput, or parietal areas and in varying degrees of facial orientation and rotation. Asymmetry may occur to the extent that the vertex of one twin may be joined to the parietal region of the other.

The classification of craniopagi, as proposed by Winston[33], is divided into four types according to the deepest shared structure:

Type A: scalp is shared but each brain has its own dura mater;

Type B: dura is shared but an intact plane of dura separates the brains;

Type C: pia or arachnoid are shared but the brains are still discrete;

Type D: brains are contiguous.

This classification relates to the chance for survival after separation: A = 75%, B = 50%, and C and D = 30%[34]. When a Type D junction is present, the cerebral hemispheres are always involved.

Thoracopagus, sternopagus, xiphopagus

Organs are usually disymmetrical with the extent of sharing dependent on the degree of fusion. The condition of the heart(s) is crucial for the determination of survival and the feasibility of separation, especially in thoracopagus twins[35–37]. The pericardium is shared in 90% of cases[38] and, in 75%, the hearts are so extensively joined that surgical separation is precluded[35]. Possible abnormalities are known to include atrial fusion with or without an atrial septal defect (ASD), ventricular fusion with or without a ventricular septal defect (VSD), atrial and ventricular fusion, a single atrioventricular valve, truncus arteriosus, and fusion of the great vessels[39].

The pleural, pericardial and peritoneal cavities can be in open communication. Generally, the liver is shared to some degree and a common gastrointestinal tract is found in 50% of cases[39].

Omphalopagus

The area of fusion involves the abdomen between the xiphoid process and the umbilicus. Approximately 40–50% of omphalopagus twins do not have concomitant thoracic fusion[40]. Conjoined structures can include any portion of the gastrointestinal tract, liver or biliary system, and bladder. Omphaloceles occur in one-third of omphalopagus twins but are infrequent (<10%) when the fusion involves the xiphoid process. Gastroschisis is generally not found in omphalopagus or xiphopagus twins but does occur with thoracopagus. A recent report, however, detailed a case of omphalopagus twins joined by gastroschisis[40].

Pygopagus

In cases of pygopagus twinning, the areas of fusion may occur anywhere along the dorsal surface of the body but generally are limited to the pelvic region. Internal anatomy is variable, the sacrum and coccyx are usually shared, while the free portions of the vertebral columns are generally complete[12]. The digestive tracts of the twins usually unite to form a single rectum and anus. There is most commonly a single bladder and urethra, although there may be two, three, or four kidneys. Considerable variation exists in the genital structures; both one and two vaginas and uteri have been reported.

Ischiopagus

The bodies of ischiopagus twins are fused in the region of the pelvis as far as the level of the common umbilicus; above this, each infant is normally developed[12]. The sacrum and pelvis are often combined, with associated abnormalities of the lower spines. The extremities are subsequently displaced laterally. Vaginal, urethral and anal orifices may open between each pair of legs or, if a tripus (fused leg) is present, only one genital opening will be present. There may be an associated aortic fusion, common systemic circulation, or shared gastrointestinal systems. The intestinal tract is usually joined at the terminal ileum, which then empties into a single colon. Four kidneys and two bladders are usually present; one ureter from each twin may be found to empty into the other's bladder. Regardless of the degree of fusion of the genital systems, four gonads are usually present.

Associated anomalies

Congenital malformations occur in almost all sets of conjoined twins. These malformations most likely result from the factors associated with the etiology of conjoining as well as crowding *in utero*. Although the majority of these malformations are associated with the site(s) of fusion, 60–70% of reported cases also have anomalies not associated with the area of fusion. Most commonly these include neural tube defects and orofacial clefts[7,9]. Overall, the most common malformations involve the cardiovascular system.

Discordance of the malformation is common when it involves the site of joining[41]. However, true primary discordance, where the malformations are discordant in non-joined organs, are rare. This type of discordance most likely occurs because one twin has a greater liability to dysmorphogenetic events[42].

The diagnosis of conjoined twins

Accurate antepartum diagnosis of conjoined twins will minimize maternal morbidity and enhance the chances of fetal survival. In particular, early diagnosis and precise characterization of the malformation can provide adequate time to formulate an obstetric plan, assemble the appropriate pediatric and surgical team (if desired), and prepare the parents for the birth of anomalous twins. Additionally, an accurate diagnosis at a previable stage of pregnancy would give the parents the option to request pregnancy termination.

Techniques useful in the diagnosis of conjoined twins include plane radiography, sonography, computed tomography (CT) and magnetic resonance imaging (MRI). In 1950, Gray *et al.*[43] proposed the following radiographic criteria for diagnosing ventrally fused twins: (1) fetal heads at the same level and body plane; (2) unusual extension of the fetal spines; (3) unusual proximity of the fetal spines; and (4) no change in the relative position of the fetuses after movement, manipulation, or the passage of time. These criteria recognize that most conjoined twins are joined ventrally and face each other. However, with the advent of modern real-time ultrasound, CT and MRI, plane radiography has lost its importance as a diagnostic tool.

During the pre-ultrasound era, prenatal diagnosis of conjoined twins occurred at best only 50–75% of the time. Today, in countries in which ultrasound is routinely available, the majority of conjoined twin pregnancies are diagnosed antenatally by ultrasound. The diagnosis of conjoined twins can be excluded with the finding of two placentas or a dividing membrane. A thorough description of modern techniques for the antenatal diagnosis of conjoined twinning has been provided by Barth et al.[44], including the use of transabdominal and transvaginal sonography and CT. Using transvaginal sonography, the diagnosis was made as early as 9 weeks' gestation for a set of dicephalus twins and 11 weeks' for a set of thoraco-omphalopagus twins.

The ultrasonographic criteria associated with a diagnosis of conjoined twins were summarized by Koontz et al. in 1983[45].

(1) Lack of a separating membrane suggesting monoamniotic twins (5–10% of monoamniotic twins are conjoined);
(2) Inseparable fetal bodies and skin contours;
(3) Bibreech and less commonly bicephalic presentation;
(4) Detection of fetal anomalies;
(5) Single umbilical cords with more than three vessels; and
(6) Ultrasonographic findings consistent with Gray's radiographic criteria (see above).

Other important findings include polyhydramnios and shared organs. In older series of conjoined twins, polyhydramnios was found in 50–75% of cases[28,46] compared to 10% of normal twin and 2% of normal singleton pregnancies. However, since the diagnosis of conjoined twins is more commonly made today in the first or second trimester, the incidence of polydramnios more closely approximates that of normal twin pregnancies[44].

Most of the criteria mentioned above are not applicable to craniopagus twins. Sonographic findings suggestive of craniopagus twins mainly include constant positions of the fetal head(s) relative to each other and/or a non-separable continuous skin contour[47]. For prognosis, it is important to distinguish fusion involving only the skull from that involving the cerebral structures. If brain fusion is present, it is almost impossible to determine sonographically if the two cerebral hemispheres are separated by dura or pia mater, a distinction important for prognosis[34]. Perhaps MRI or color flow Doppler (to detect vascular connections) may prove beneficial in the future.

It is important to understand the pitfalls and limitations of ultrasound when attempting to diagnose conjoined twins[44]. First, inseparable skin contours must be a persistent finding at the same level. Second, a discordant presentation does not preclude the diagnosis of conjoined twins, particularly in xiphopagus twins. Cephalic-breech presentation is the most common presentation for xiphopagus twins[17], because the joining bridge is commonly thin and pliable, allowing rotation to occur. Third, the diagnosis of conjoined twins can be overlooked in a bicephalic presentation in which one head is engaged and the second head is higher in position and apparently separate. Finally, with extensive fusion, the twins may be melded into a mass of tissue that, sonographically, may appear to be a singleton pregnancy with malformations. This error can be avoided by carefully searching for duplication of any fetal structures.

Two reports in the literature detail the use of MRI as an adjunct to sonography in the diagnosis of conjoined twins[48,49]. As is the case with MRI of normal pregnancies, studies performed in the third trimester, when fetuses are larger and fetal movement is decreased, are superior to studies performed earlier in pregnancy. In one of the reports, the fetuses were paralyzed for a MRI evaluation during the second trimester using pancurorium directly injected into the umbilical vein. The MRI provides more detailed information about the extent of fusion of internal organs, allowing a better evaluation of prognosis.

In the event that conjoined twins had not been identified prior to the onset of labor, several observations during the course of labor may suggest this diagnosis. Since conjoined twins always develop within a single amniotic sac, palpation of a second sac after rupture of the first will rule out conjoined twins. On the other hand, multiple fetal limbs in close approximation, failure of traction on the first twin to effect delivery after complete dilatation, and inability to move one twin without moving the other all suggest conjoined twins. The diagnosis can be confirmed when vaginal examination demonstrates a bridge of tissue between the fetuses.

Antepartum and obstetric management

Once the diagnosis of conjoined twins has been made, appropriate counselling is necessary. The nature of such counselling may vary with gestational age, potential viability and parental desires. If the pregnancy is pre-viable, termination is an option. If termination is not an option, it is important to follow a clear plan for continued antenatal assessment and to determine the most feasible route of delivery. As Herbert et al.[50] have noted, 'the goals of antepartum assessment are to: (1) define the type and extent of union; (2) detect and describe associated anomalies; (3) determine the optimal time, method, and details of delivery; (4) make arrangements for neonatal care; (5) manage intercurrent complications of the pregnancy; and (6) provide support for the family'. Sonographic examinations every 1–2 weeks and/or MRI during the third trimester may help define earlier impressions of the extent of the union as well as the presence or absence of associated anomalies. Fetal echocardiography is important for thoracopagus twins for whom the prevalence of congenital heart disease is high and is related to the extent of the union[51]. Since cardiac malformations may exist in the absence of cardiac fusion, fetal echocardiography should be performed in all cases of thoracopagus twins[44]. Still, when anomalies are present, the echocardiographic findings tend to underestimate their severity[44].

Biophysical profile (BPP) can be performed 1–2 times/week beginning in the third trimester because of the risk of stillbirth; its use in conjoined twins has not been studied. At 36–37 weeks' gestation, amniocentesis can be performed for determination of fetal lung maturity.

The following points should be considered when determining the least traumatic route of delivery:

(1) The possibility of survival of the infants;
(2) Their combined size;
(3) The site and extent of the union;
(4) Fetal presentation;
(5) The attitudes of the family; and
(6) Other obstetric factors, including the adequacy of the pelvis, the presence of a uterine scar, etc.

In many instances, the chances of survival of the infants cannot be accurately predicted. Some associated anomalies, such as anencephaly, obviously preclude survival. However, in recent years increasingly sophisticated diagnostic methods and improved surgical and postoperative care have substantially increased the chances of separation and survival. The welfare of the twins should be considered unless there is an anomaly incompatible with life.

In the series reported by Rudolph et al. in 1967[28], the mean birth weight of the conjoined twins was 4112 g; the highest recorded weight was 7258 g. In most cases, the combined birth weight does not exceed 5000 g[52] although a report from 1912 details the delivery of thoracopagus twins weighing 14 pounds[53]. The typically low combined birth weight is probably secondary to preterm delivery as well as poor fetal growth due to malformations. In the series reported by Rudolph et al., the mean gestational age at the time of delivery was 36.4 weeks[28]. Milham[30] reported an average gestational age of 33 weeks in 22 cases and Métneki and Czeizel[3] reported an average of 34.7 weeks in 36 cases.

The site and extent of the union between the fetuses obviously affects the plausibility of a vaginal delivery. In many cases, the joining bridge is pliable, allowing considerable movement and enabling vaginal delivery with or without manipulation or forceps. Extensive bony fusion, however, as is frequently present in cases of thoracopagus twins, may preclude movement and prevent vaginal delivery.

Abnormal presentations commonly occur in twin gestations. In cases of conjoined twins diagnosed before delivery, the incidence of bi-breech presentation and transverse lie is increased.

Once the above factors have been determined and evaluated, three modes of delivery can be considered: (1) Cesarean section; (2) vaginal delivery with the twins intact; or (3) vaginal delivery with a destructive procedure. In the past when destructive procedures were part of the standard obstetric armamentarium, reports described vaginal delivery with intrauterine separation[54,55]. Their success was predicated on a pliable soft-tissue union between the twins. Because of the potential for serious maternal injury, however, intrauterine separation cannot be recommended today. Any planned destructive procedures performed at the time of delivery should be reserved for pregnancy termination (dilatation and evacuation) at a previable gestation. Still, destructive procedures may become necessary during a vaginal or Cesarean delivery if the conjoined twins have not been diagnosed antenatally.

Cesarean section

Cesarean section is the method of choice for delivery in most diagnosed cases of conjoined twinning. Most authors recommend elective Cesarean section as soon as the diagnosis has been confirmed and the fetal lungs have reached maturity. Maternal injury is thereby obviated and the best chances for survival are secured for the twins. Even when the fetuses have died, Cesarean section has been advised to avoid maternal injury[56,57]. If the twins are quite small, however, a trial of labor may be allowed.

When Cesarean section is performed, a vertical incision is recommended for skin and uterine incisions to provide maximal exposure[50]. The uterine incision is begun in the lower segment and can be carried upward if difficulty with delivery is encountered.

If the presentation is cephalic/cephalic, each head should be delivered one after another followed by both trunks simultaneously. If the presentation is breech/breech, all of the lower extremities should be delivered first followed by the trunks and heads. If the presentation is a combination of cephalic and breech, the pliability of the union should allow for delivery by the most logical means. Should the union between the twins limit adequate mobility, regardless of presentation, delivery as a single unit is least traumatic. The main goal at delivery by Cesarean section is to proceed slowly and carefully so as to minimize maternal and fetal trauma[50]. Only in rare instances will intrauterine separation or destructive procedures be necessary during Cesarean section.

Vaginal delivery

Patients may choose to attempt a vaginal delivery if antepartum assessment indicates non-viable twins or in the case of extreme prematurity. The older literature contains many descriptions of successful vaginal deliveries[58–61], usually possible because of tissue pliability and prematurity. No reports detail a critical fetal weight or size after which vaginal delivery is inadvisable.

Dystocia is relatively common during labor[3,56]. As such, maternal and fetal morbidity are definitely increased with vaginal delivery. An unanticipated obstruction to delivery may lead to spontaneous uterine rupture or severe maternal soft tissue injury after intrauterine manipulation. Fetal morbidity and mortality are increased, as is the case with delivery of twins in general.

Conjoined twins frequently present as a bi-breech presentation; this facilitates vaginal delivery by extraction. Roddie[61] discusses these manipulations in detail. When all four lower extremities are within reach, simultaneous traction on all of them effect delivery. In other instances, especially small thoracopagus twins, the entire bulk of the conjoined trunk may be delivered simultaneously. With larger twins, a large episiotomy is important to facilitate delivery and avoid maternal trauma. Assuming there is sufficient mobility at the site of the union, the trunks may be delivered simultaneously and the heads separately. As the trunks are delivered, the body of the fetuses is flexed over the mother's abdomen. The posterior head is delivered first and the second head generally follows without difficulty. If complete delivery cannot be effected after expulsion of the trunk, a destructive procedure becomes the only alternative.

A vertex presentation usually leads to more difficulties. Assuming that there is a loose union between the twins, the infants may be delivered simultaneously in parallel by sliding the body of one over the other, fixing the head of one over the chin of the other so as to allow both to engage together[28]. This technique is most effective in the delivery of xiphopagus and omphalopagus twins. In these instances it may also be possible to deliver one twin as a breech and the second as a vertex.

Destructive procedures are indicated when a part of the fused twins has been expelled and no further progress can be accomplished by ordinary obstetric procedures[28]; destructive procedures generally include evisceration or amputation of body parts.

Survival and separation of conjoined twins

The incidence of stillbirth of conjoined twins ranges from 40 to 60%[3,9,28,29]; these figures have decreased in recent years because of early detection and termination. For liveborn sets, survival depends on the type and extent of fusion. Any consideration of separation requires a sophisticated and knowledgeable team approach throughout the preoperative, intraoperative and postoperative phases.

The success of a separation procedure depends upon many factors, including the degree and nature of the communication between the twins, their general health and the experience and degree of preparedness of the medical staff. Once the decision has been made to attempt surgical separation, the timing of the separation and detailed aspects of anesthetic, operative and postoperative management must be considered. A definite management plan must be established prior to surgery, and all possible problems should be anticipated.

Preoperative evaluation

It is generally acknowledged that the results of attempts to separate conjoined twins depend upon the completeness of preoperative evaluation of each infant and upon a precise knowledge of the nature and degree of organ sharing. In some instances, poor health or the sharing of vital organs, such as the heart, preclude any attempt whatsoever at separation.

A plane radiograph is a simple procedure that can be performed within a short time after delivery; it often can provide important basic information regarding anatomy. Later, angiography, CT, MRI, radionuclide scanning and sonography are required to fully assess the extent of the union and other anomalies.

The preoperative evaluation of thoracopagus twins has been well described in the literature. The nature and degree of the shared cardiovascular system is the critical factor in these twins. Cardiovascular evaluation should be directed at establishing whether there is: (1) pericardial union only; (2) atrial connection with separate ventricles; or (3) ventricular connection usually associated with multiple cardiac anomalies[62]. Echocardiography[63] and angiography[33,64,65] allow full assessment of the heart, pulmonary vasculature and the systemic arterial circulation. Leachman *et al.*[35] suggested a systematic approach to cardiac evaluation based on the findings of single or separate QRS complexes on the ECG. However, Izukawa *et al.*[62] and Patel *et al.*[37] point out the pitfalls of this approach and advocate the importance of cardiac catheterization and angiography in addition to ECG evaluation before separation is considered.

In cases where gastrointestinal communication is suspected, upper and lower gastrointestinal series are useful[66]. Passage of nasogastric tubes can be easily and quickly performed in the early neonatal period to assess patency of the upper gastrointestinal tract.

Timing of the surgical separation

The majority of authors recommend delaying any attempt at separation until late infancy.

Mulcare et al.[67] cited two reasons to delay surgery: (1) to allow the fetuses to develop pulmonary and immunological maturity and increased tolerance to surgical trauma; and (2) to minimize the physiological, anesthetic and technical problems of neonatal surgical care. Just as importantly, it allows for a thorough preoperative evaluation. In some cases, however, emergent surgical separation may be necessary during the neonatal or early infancy periods. Bankole et al.[68] have described two *absolute indications* for emergent surgical separation: (1) when one twin is stillborn or its critical condition threatens the other; and (2) the presence of any lesion that ordinarily indicates immediate operation in either infant (e.g. intestinal obstruction, ruptured omphalocele). Eighteen such cases have been reported: five with bowel obstruction, five with 'poor condition' of one or both twins, four for the removal of a stillborn, two with trauma to the conjoined tissue, one for a thin omphalocele membrane, and one with a conjoining gastroschisis[41].

Anesthetic management

The anesthetic management of the separation of conjoined twins has been described[69–71]. The presence of two separate anesthetic teams, however, each managing a single infant, is absolutely mandatory. The difficulty in estimating blood loss and subsequent fluid requirements for each infant has been emphasized by all authors. Technical problems, such as intubation of thoracopagus twins in a face-to-face position, may require a preoperative simulation practice session.

Operative management

A detailed discussion of the operative management for separation of conjoined twins is beyond the scope of this chapter. Each case should be approached individually based on the type(s) and extent of the union. If time permits, a thorough preoperative evaluation will allow the best estimate of survival and sufficient time to plan and develop the necessary operative interventions. A dress rehearsal including surgeons, anesthesiologists, nurses and radiologists may be very helpful.

Postpartum ethical considerations

Although the outlook is favorable for increasing success in separating even the most complex of conjoined twins, three alternative management plans are possible: (1) support may be withdrawn and the twins allowed to die; (2) the twins may be raised maintaining their conjoined status; (3) surgical separation may be attempted with the knowledge that one twin may be sacrificed so that the other may live.

These moral dilemmas are difficult to contemplate; all must be considered in cases of conjoined twinning. A complete discussion of these issues is beyond the scope of this chapter; other authors have addressed these problems[72,73].

References

1. Little, J. and Bryan, E.M. (1988). Congenital anomalies. In MacGillivray, I., Campbell, D.M. and Thompson, B. (eds) *Twinning and Twins*, pp. 207–40. (Chichester: John Wiley & Sons)
2. Tan, K.L., Goon S.M., Salmon, Y. *et al.* (1971). Conjoined twins. *Acta Obstet. Gynecol. Scand.*, **50**, 373
3. Métneki, J. and Czeizel, A. (1989). Conjoined twins in Hungary, 1970–1986. *Acta Genet. Med. Gemellol.*, **38**, 285
4. Foster, P.M. (1948). Conjoined fetuses (thoracopagus) in a dizygotic triplet pregnancy. *Am. J. Obstet. Gynecol.*, **56**, 799

5. Pepper H. and Lindsay, S. (1958). Gasteropagus in a triplet pregnancy. *Arch. Pathol.*, **65**, 63
6. Michaels, J.P. (1967). The conjoined twins of Orlando (I, II and III). In Bergsma, D. (ed.) *Birth Defects Original Article Series: Conjoined Twins*, pp. 145–7. (New York: The National Foundation – March of Dimes)
7. The International Clearinghouse for Birth Defects Monitoring Systems. (1991). Conjoined twins – an epidemiological study based on 312 cases. *Acta Med. Gemellol.*, **40**, 325
8. Ripman, H.A. (1958). Conjoined twins as an obstetric problem. *Guy's Hosp. Rep.*, **107**, 173
9. Edmonds, L.D. and Layde, P.M. (1982). Conjoined twins in the United States, 1970–1977. *Teratology*, **25**, 301
10. Imaizumi, Y. (1988). Conjoined twins in Japan. *Acta Genet. Med. Gemellol.*, **37**, 339
11. Munro, S.S. (1965). Are monovolar avian twins always female? *J. Hered.*, **56**, 285
12. Potter, E.L. and Craig, J.M. (1975). *Pathology of the Fetus and the Infant.* (Chicago: Year Book Medical Publishers)
13. Cuq, P. and Woronoff, M. (1980). Proposition for the classification and nomenclature of double monstrosities. *Anat. Histol. Embryol.*, **9**, 108
14. Guttmacher, A.F. and Nichols, B.L. (1967). Teratology of conjoined twins. In Bergsma, D. (ed.) *Birth Defects Original Article Series: Conjoined Twins*, pp. 3–9. (New York: The National Foundation – March of Dimes)
15. Zimmermann, A.A. (1967). Embryologic and anatomic considerations of conjoined twins. In Bergsma. D. (ed.) *Birth Defects Original Article Series: Conjoined Twins*, pp. 18–27. (New York: The National Foundation – March of Dimes)
16. Weston, P.J., Ives, E.J., Honore, R.L.H. *et al.* (1990). Monochorionic diamniotic minimally conjoined twins: a case report. *Am. J. Med. Genet.*, **37**, 558
17. Harper, R.G., Kenigsberg, K., Sia, C.G. *et al.* (1980). Xiphopagus conjoined twins: a 300 year review of the obstetric, morphopathologic, neonatal and surgical parameters. *Am. J. Obstet. Gynecol.*, **137**, 617
18. Stockard, E.R. (1921). Developmental rate and structural expressivity: experimental study of twins. *Am. J. Anat.*, **28**, 115
19. Benirschke, K. and Temple, W.W. (1977). Conjoined twins: nosology and congenital malformations. Presented at *Birth Defects Conference*, Memphis, TN, July 9
20. Wedberg, R., Kaplan, C., Leopold, G. *et al.* (1979). Cephalothoracopagus (janiceps) twinning. *Obstet. Gynecol.*, **54**, 392
21. Aird, I. (1959). Conjoined twins – further observations. *Br. Med. J.*, **1**, 1313
22. Selby, L.A., Khalili, A., Stewart, R.W. *et al.* (1973). Pathology and epidemiology of conjoined twinning in swine. *Teratology*, **8**, 1
23. Chai, C.K. and Crary, D.D. (1971). Conjoined twinning in rabbits. *Teratology*, **4**, 433
24. Kaplun, A., Shamir, B. and Kuttin, E.S. (1972). A case of guinea pig conjoined twins. *Lab. Animal Sci.*, **22**, 581
25. Leipold, H.W., Dennis, S.M. and Huston, K. (1972). Embryonic duplications in cattle. *Cornell Vet.*, **62**, 572
26. Ingalls, T.H. (1969). Conjoined twins in zebra fish. *Arch. Environ. Health*, **19**, 353
27. Ferm, V.H. (1969). Conjoined twinning in mammalian teratology. *Arch. Environ. Health*, **19**, 353
28. Rudolph, A.J., Michaels, J.P. and Nichols, B.L. (1967). Obstetric management of conjoined twins. In Bergsma, D. (ed.) *Birth Defects Original Article Series: Conjoined Twins*, pp. 28–37. (New York: The National Foundation – March of Dimes)
29. Viljoen, D.L., Nelson, M.M. and Beighton, P. (1983). The epidemiology of conjoined twinning in Southern Africa. *Clin. Genet.*, **24**, 15
30. Milham, S. (1986). Symmetrical conjoined twins. *J. Pediatr.*, **69**, 642
31. Hamon, A. and Dinno, N. (1978). Dicephalus dipus infant. In Summitt, R.L. and Bergsma, D. (eds.) *Birth Defects: Original Article Series: Cell Surface Factors, Immune Deficiencies, Twin Studies*, pp. 213–18. (New York: Alan R. Liss)
32. Kim, C.K., Barr, R.J. and Benirschke, K. (1971). Cytogenetic studies of conjoined twins. *Obstet. Gynecol.*, **38**, 877
33. Winston, K.R. (1987). Carniopagi: anatomical characteristics and classification. *Neurosurgery*, **21**, 769
34. Winston, K.R., Rockoff, M.A., Mulliken, J.B. *et al.* (1987). Surgical division of craniopagi. *Neurosurgery*, **21**, 782
35. Leachman, R.D., Latson, J.R., Kohler, C.M. *et al.* (1967). Cardiovascular evaluation of conjoined twins. In Bergsma, D. (ed.) *Birth Defects Original Article Series: Conjoined Twins*, pp. 52–62. (New York: The National Foundation – March of Dimes)
36. Sanders, S.P., Chin, A.J. and Parness, I.A. (1985). Prenatal diagnosis of congenital heart

defects in thoracoabdominally conjoined twins. *N. Engl. J. Med.*, **313**, 370
37. Patel, R., Fox, K., Dawson, J. *et al.* (1977). Cardiovascular anomalies in thoracopagus twins and the importance of preoperative cardiac evaluation. *Br. Heart J.*, **39**, 1254
38. Nichols, B.L., Blattner, R.J. and Rudolph, A.J. (1967). General clinical management of thoracopagus twins. In Bergsma, D. (ed.) *Birth Defects Original Article Series: Conjoined Twins*, pp. 38–51. (New York: The National Foundation – March of Dimes)
39. Edwards, W.D., Hagel, D.R., Thompson, J. *et al.* (1977). Conjoined thoracopagus twins. *Circulation*, **56**, 491
40. Walton, J.M., Gillis, D.A., Giacomantonio, J.M. *et al.* (1991). Emergent separation of conjoined twins. *J. Pediatr. Surg.*, **26**, 1337
41. Ornoy, A., Navbot, D., Menashi, M. *et al.* (1980). Asymmetry and discordance for congenital anomalies in conjoined twins. *Teratology*, **22**, 145
42. Seller, M.J. (1990). Conjoined twins discordant for cleft lip and palate. *Am. J. Med. Genet.*, **37**, 530
43. Gray, C.N., Nix, N.G. and Wallace, A.J. (1950). Thoracopagus twins: prenatal diagnosis. *Radiology*, **54**, 398
44. Barth, R.A., Filly, R.A., Goldberg, J.D. *et al.* (1990). Conjoined twins: prenatal diagnosis and assessment of associated malformations. *Radiology*, **177**, 201
45. Koontz, W.L., Herbert, W.N.P., Seeds, J.W. *et al.* (1983). Ultrasonography in the antepartum diagnosis of conjoined twins. A report of two cases. *J. Reprod. Med.*, **28**, 627
46. Strauss, S., Tamarkin, M., Engelberg, S. *et al.* (1987). Prenatal sonographic appearance of diprosopus. *J. Ultrasound Med.*, **6**, 93
47. Abrams, S.L., Callen, P.W., Anderson, R.L. *et al.* (1985). Anencephaly with encephalocele in craniopagus twins: prenatal diagnosis by ultrasonography and computed tomography. *J. Ultrasound Med.*, **4**, 485
48. Turner, R.J., Hankins, G.D.V., Weinreb, J.C. *et al.* (1986). Magnetic resonance imaging and ultrasonography in the antenatal evaluation of conjoined twins. *Am. J. Obstet. Gynecol.*, **255**, 645
49. Zoppini, C., Vanzulli, A., Kusterman, A., Rizzuti, T., Selicorni, A. and Nicolini, U. (1993). Prenatal diagnosis of anatomical connections in conjoined twins by use of contrast magnetic resonance imaging. *Prenat. Diagnosis*, **13**, 995–9
50. Herbert, W.N.P., Cefalo, R.C. and Koontz, W.L. (1983). Perinatal management of conjoined twins. *Am. J. Perinatol.*, **1**, 58
51. Little, J. and Bryan, E. (1986). Congenital anomalies in twins. *Semin. Perinatol.*, **10**, 50
52. Freedman, H.L., Tafeen, C.H. and Harris, J. (1962). Conjoined thoracopagus twins. *Am. J. Obstet. Gynecol.*, **84**, 1904
53. Ligat, D. (1912). Cesarean section for double monstrosity. *Lancet*, **1**, 896
54. Dwyer, P.J., Ripman, H.A. and Williams, P.L. (1959). Delivery of thoracopagus twins after intrauterine separation. *J. Obstet. Gynaecol. Br. Emp.*, **66**, 437
55. Graber, E.A. (1945). Thoracopagus twins: X-ray diagnosis. *Am. J. Obstet. Gynecol.*, **49**, 276
56. Compton, H.L., Conjoined twins. (1971). *Obstet. Gynecol.*, **37**, 27
57. Vaughn, T.C. and Powell, L.C. (1979). The obstetrical management of conjoined twins. *Obstet. Gynecol.*, **53** (Suppl), 67
58. Rawlings, E.E. and Marick, R. (1951). A case of conjoined twins. *J. Obstet. Gynaecol. Br. Emp.*, **58**, 452
59. Lu, T.L. and Lee, K.H. (1967). Obstetric management of conjoined twins. *J. Obstet. Gynaecol. Br. Commonwlth.*, **74**, 757
60. Aird, I. (1954). The conjoined twins of Kano. *Br. Med. J.*, **1**, 831
61. Roddie, T.S. (1957). A case of conjoined twins. *Br. Med. J.*, **1**, 1163
62. Izukawa, T., Kidd, B.S.L., Moes, C.A.F. *et al.* (1978). Assessment of the cardiovascular system in conjoined thoracopagus twins. *Am. J. Dis. Child.*, **132**, 19
63. Sahn, D.J. (1981). Real-time two-dimensional echocardiography. *J. Pediatr.*, **99**, 175
64. Joffe, H.S., Rose, A., Gersh, B.J. *et al.* (1977). Figure-of-eight circulation in thoracopagus conjoined twins. *Eur. J. Cardiol.*, **6**, 157
65. Marcinski, A., Lopatec, U., Wemenski, K. *et al.* (1978). Angiographic evaluation of conjoined twins. *Pediatr. Radiol.*, **6**, 230
66. Singleton, E.B. (1967). Radiographic studies of thoracopagus twins. In Bergsma, D. (ed.) *Birth Defects Original Article Series: Conjoined Twins*, pp. 89–96. (New York: The National Foundation – March of Dimes)
67. Mulcare, R.J., Bhokakui, P., Potitung, P. *et al.* (1970). The surgical separation of the thoracopagus conjoined twins of Korat, Thailand. *Ann. Surg.*, **172**, 91

68. Bankole, M.A., Oduntan, S.A., Oluwasanini, J.O. *et al.* (1972). The conjoined twins of Warri, Nigeria. *Arch. Surg.*, **104**, 294
69. Towey, R.M., Kisia, A.K.L., Jacobacci, S. *et al.* (1979). Anesthesia for the separation of conjoined twins. *Anaesthesia*, **34**, 187
70. Chao, C.C., Susetio, L., Luu, K.W. *et al.* (1980). Anesthetic management for the successful separation of tripus ischiopagal conjoined male twins. *Can. Anaesth. Soc. J.*, **27**, 565
71. Fournier, L., Goulet, C., Waugh, R. *et al.* (1976). Anesthesia for the separation of conjoined twins. *Can. Anaesth. Soc. J.*, **23**, 425
72. O'Connell, J. (1976). Craniopagus twins: surgical anatomy and embryology and their implications. *J. Neurol. Neurosurg. Psych.*, **39**, 1
73. Pepper, C.K. (1967). Ethical and moral considerations in the separation of conjoined twins. In Bergsma, D. (ed.), *Birth Defects Original Article Series: Conjoined Twins*, pp. 128–34. (New York: The National Foundation – March of Dimes)

Placentation 9

R. Derom, C. Derom and R. Vlietinck

Introduction

In multiple pregnancies, placentation is influenced not only by the number of zygotes but also by the number of blastocysts and, before or after implantation, the division of the inner cell mass. If, in the past, the relationship between the number of the zygotes and their divisions and the gross morphology of the placenta was not always clear, this no longer need be the case. With a minimum of instruction, anyone investigating the placenta of a multiple pregnancy should be able to grasp the link between this structure and the origin of the pregnancy.

Single placentas are generally characteristic of monozygotic (MZ) pregnancies, but can be present in dizygotic (DZ) pregnancies as well. They can be mono- or dichorionic. When they are dichorionic, the single placental mass results from the fusion of two separate placental discs. When two placentas are present, they are almost always dichorionic. Most, but not all, instances of two placentas arise from the DZ twinning process; some also are present in MZ twinning in which division occurs before implantation (Figure 1). Figures 2 and 3 respectively illustrate very early singleton[1] and twin embryos before placentation has been established. In both illustrations, the amnionic membranes are readily visible. The twins shown in Figure 3 are diamnionic and monochorionic.

It is not generally appreciated that twin placentation differs widely by race. Table 1 documents marked differences in the rates of monochorionic and dichorionic placentation in diverse geographic regions inhabited by different ethnic groups. Considering the extent of these differences, any assessment of zygosity based solely on the number of placental discs is of little value. Rather, it is necessary and crucial to consider the number and structure of the membranes as well as the number of placental discs in order to accurately determine zygosity. Whether the placentas are separated or fused may be of crucial importance for fetal growth, as will be shown later in this chapter and is also discussed in Chapter 27.

The principles addressed in the preceding paragraph pertain to triplet and higher order placentation as well. With regard to triplets, a fused placenta is more common, regardless of zygosity, simply because of uterine crowding. Figure 4 shows the mechanisms of MZ, DZ and trizygotic (TZ) triplets with different types of membranes. It is readily apparent that examination of the membranes alone cannot establish zygosity if the placenta is trichorionic. Similarly, if the placenta is dichorionic, the zygosity may be MZ or DZ. Finally, only when the placenta is monochorionic can one truly establish monozygosity, regardless of the number of fetuses. Thus, the principle stated in the preceding paragraph, i.e. that placental examination by itself is insufficient to establish zygosity in all cases, can be extended to the membranes as well. The general rule in triplets is to have a single placenta, and a single placenta can result from MZ, DZ or TZ origins. Table 2 outlines placental structure in triplets and complements data presented in Figure 4.

The relationship between zygosity and placental structure in twins leads to three clinical aphorisms, the last one of which is of paramount importance. As stressed in the preceding comments, one can conclude from a proper examination of the placental membranes (as opposed to

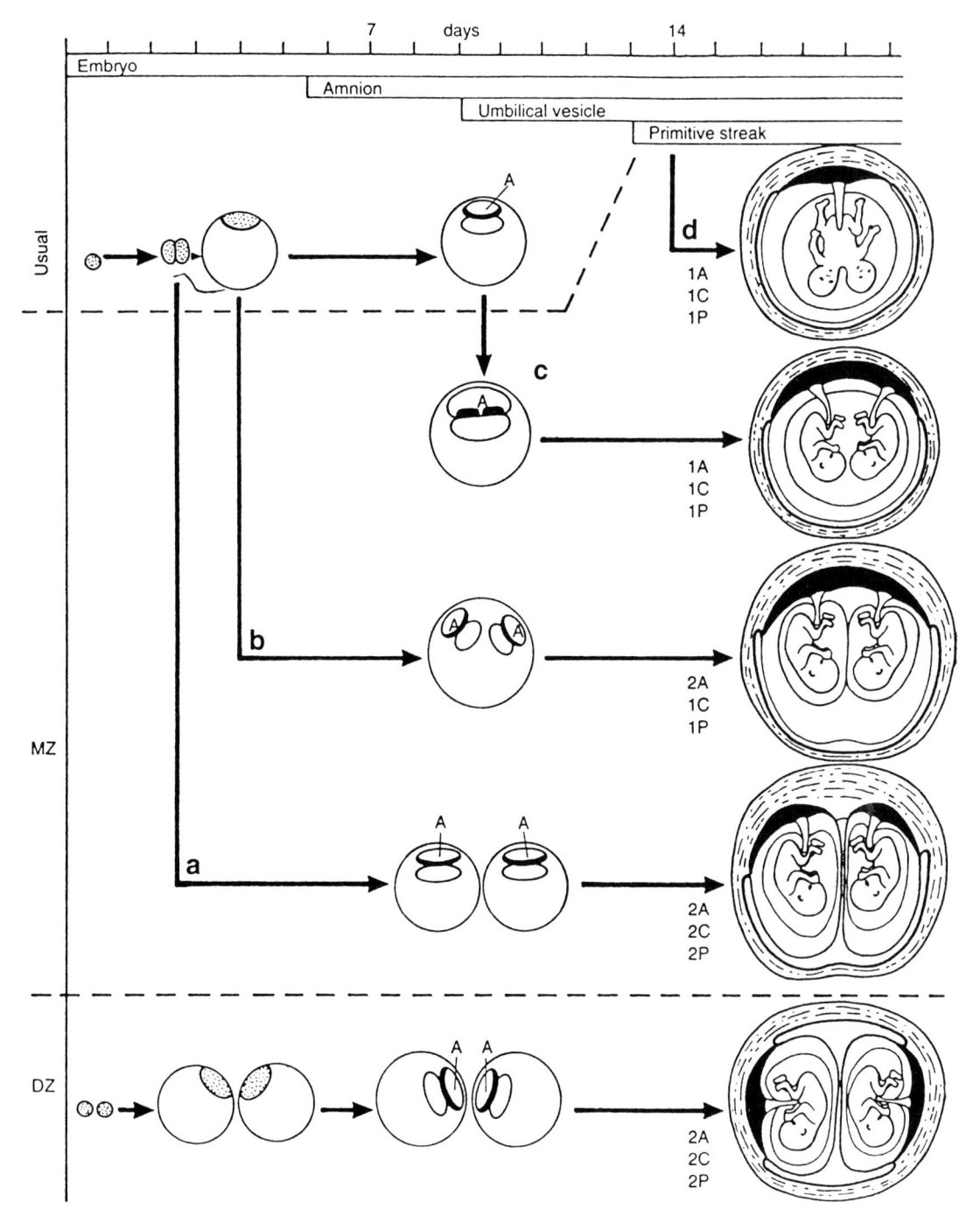

Figure 1 The arrangement of the adnexa (fetal membranes) in twinning. **a–d**, various forms of monozygotic (MZ) twins, **d** being conjoined twins. The uppermost panel shows the usual development, i.e. in singletons, together with an approximate time-scale. A, amnion/amniotic cavity; C, chorion; P, placenta. Reproduced from reference 1, with permission

Placentation

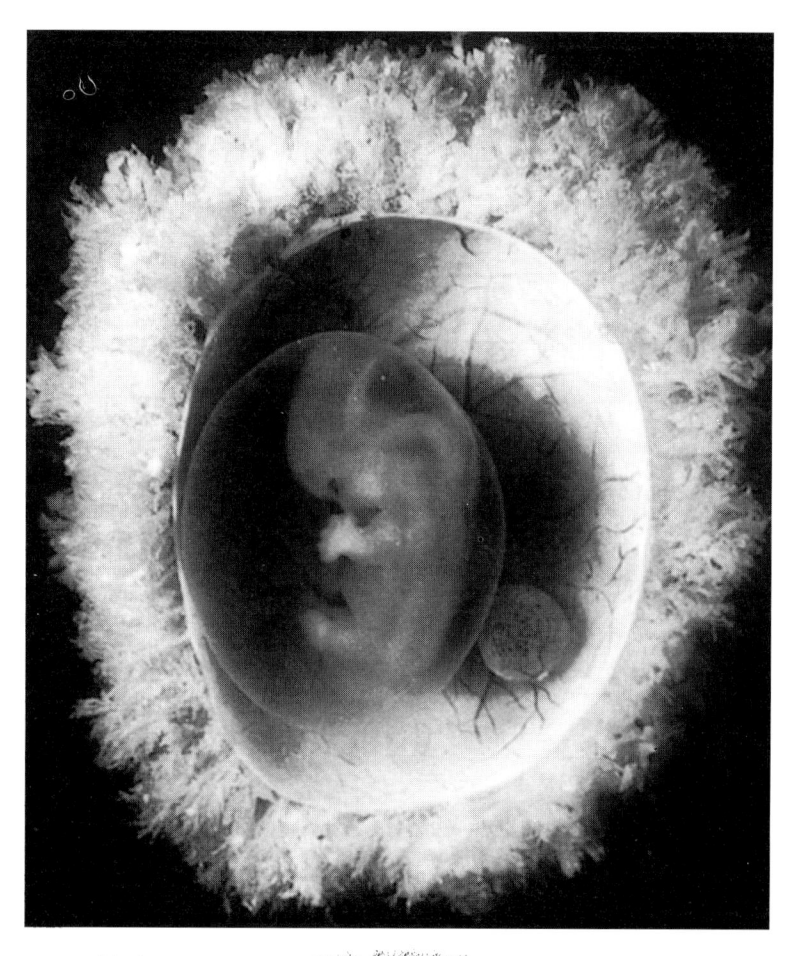

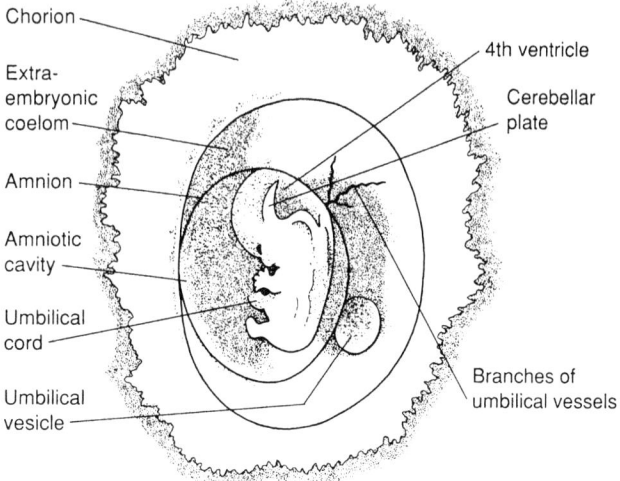

Figure 2 Embryo of 7 weeks surrounded by intact amnion and the bisected leafy mass of the chorion. Villous stems are visible, especially in the left lower quadrant of the chorion frondosum. The future chorion laeve is at the right-hand side of the photograph. Reproduced from reference 1, with permission

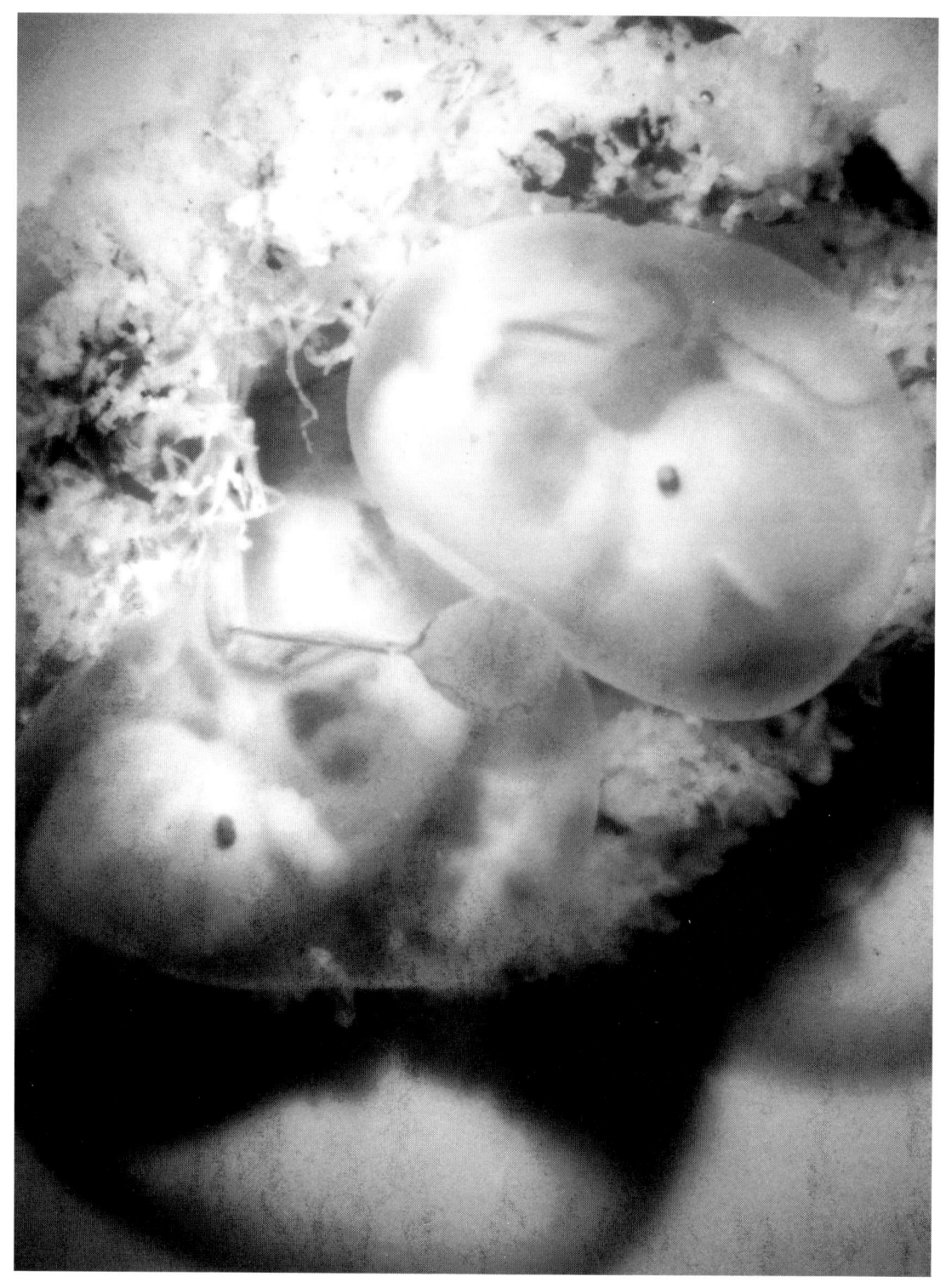

Figure 3 Monochorionic–diamnionic twin embryos. Photograph obtained by Dr John Marlow of Washington, D.C. during treatment of a patient with ectopic pregnancy. Reproduced with permission

Table 1 Geographic distribution of the relative frequency of placental structure of twins

	Monochorionic	Dichorionic		Unknown
		Single and fused	Double or separate	
Ibadan, Nigeria	5.0	51.1	41.2	2.7
Aberdeen, UK	18.7	34.5	41.0	5.6
Oxford, UK	22.5	33.0	42.5	2.0
Birmingham, UK	19.6	80.4		—
East Flanders, Belgium	26.3	37.2	35.3	0.1
Japan	61.8	19.7	18.5	—

	T_1	T_2	T_3
	Monozygotic	Dizygotic	Trizygotic
Number of zygotes	1	2	3
Number of split	2	1	0
Membranes	Trichorionic Dichorionic Monochorionic	Trichorionic Dichorionic	Trichorionic
Genetic markers Sex Blood groups Alkaline phosphatase DNA polymorphisms	1 = 2 = 3	1 ≠ 2 = 3	1 ≠ 2 2 ≠ 3 1 ≠ 3

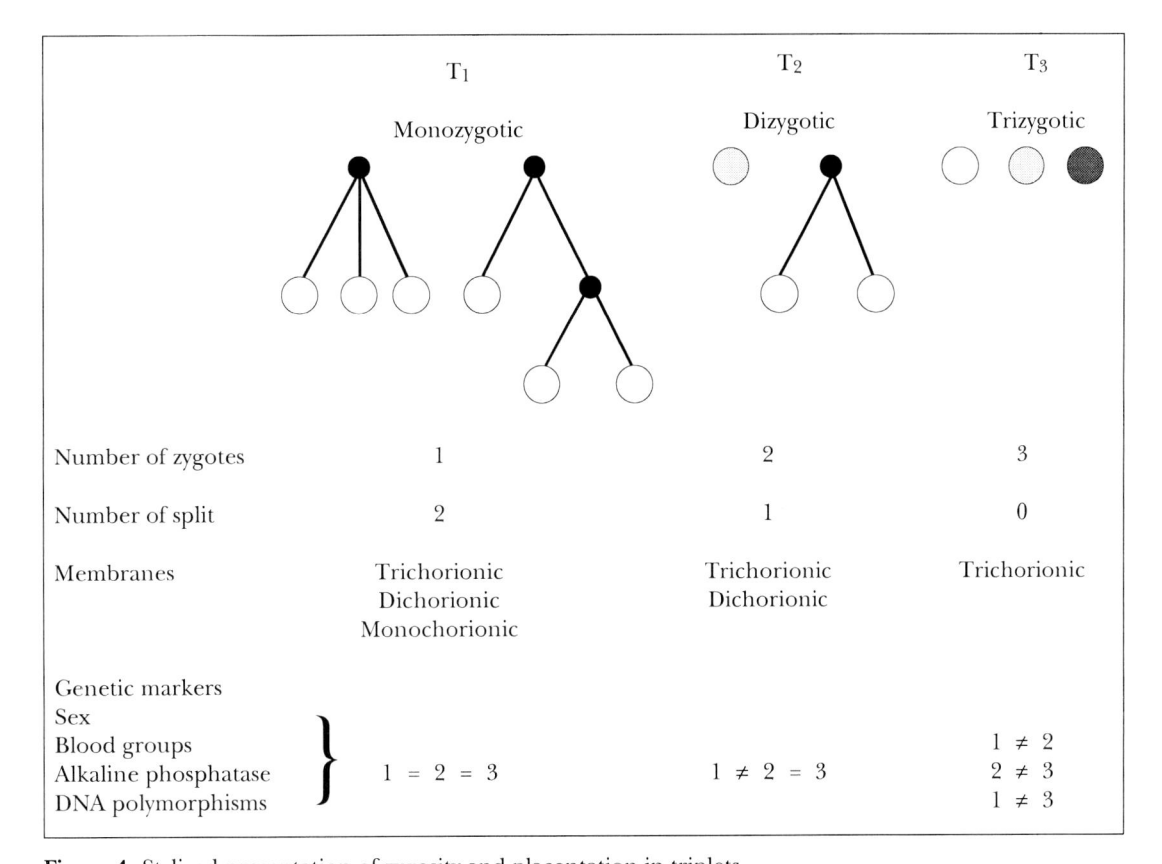

Figure 4 Stylized presentation of zygosity and placentation in triplets

the number of placentas) that a twin pair is monozygotic. The aphorisms are as follows (see Figure 1 for visual confirmation):

(1) Dizygotic twins are dichorionic;
(2) Monozygotic twins are either monochorionic or dichorionic;
(3) A monochorionic placenta is proof of monozygosity.

Only one well-documented exception to this third rule has been published[2], so that, in monochorionic twins, the diagnosis of monozygosity is very close to certainty.

Table 2 Placental structure in triplets

Number of chorionic membranes	Number of amnionic membranes	Denomination
3	3	trichorionic–triamnionic
2	3	dichorionic–triamnionic
	2	dichorionic–diamnionic
1	3	monochorionic–triamnionic
	2	monochorionic–diamnionic
	1	monochorionic–monoamnionic

Table 3 Anastomoses in 39 monochorionic placentae (from reference 5)

Artery-to-artery only	4
Artery-to-artery + artery-to-vein	11****†
Artery-to-artery + vein-to-vein	2†
Vein-to-vein only	0
Artery-to-vein only	2*
Artery-to-vein + vein-to-artery	3**†
Artery-to-vein + vein-to-vein	2
Artery-to-vein + vein-to-vein + artery-to-artery	4**†
Artery-to-vein + vein-to-artery + artery-to-artery	4*
Artery-to-vein + vein-to-artery + artery-to-artery + vein-to-vein	3**
No anastomoses seen	4

*Case of transfusion syndrome; †probable case of transfusion syndrome

The aphorisms for triplets (see Figure 4 for visual confirmation) are as follows:

(1) Trizygotic triplets are trichorionic;
(2) Dizygotic triplets are either di- or trichorionic;
(3) Monozygotic triplets are either tri-, di- or monochorionic;
(4) Dichorionic triplets are either mono- or dizygotic;
(5) Monochorionic triplets are monozygotic.

A unique feature of placentation in multiple pregnancy is the high prevalence of marginal and velamentous insertion of one or more umbilical cords. Among singletons, these variations are found in less than 10%, and less than 2% of cases, respectively, although slightly different rates have been published in various reports[3]. A more complete analysis of velamentous insertion in twins is found later in this chapter along with other data from the East Flanders Prospective Twin Survey. In many, but not all instances, marginal insertions are symmetrical, i.e. present in both twins, all three triplets or all four quadruplets if the placenta is monochorionic[3,4]. Marginal or velamentous insertion of the cord is associated with preterm birth and low birth weight and, if present, should always be noted either in the delivery record, the operation record or the formal report of the pathological examination of the placenta.

Most monochorionic placentas show anastomoses between the arteries and between the veins at the fetal surface. These may be A–A, A–V or V–V. If large enough, A–A and V–V anastomoses are visible to the naked eye (see Chapters 27–29). However, injection techniques are usually required to demonstrate small A–A and V–V anastomoses. Arteriovenous anastomoses can only be demonstrated by special techniques (see p. 122). The complexity and variety of the anastomotic connections in monochorionic twin placentas are shown in Table 3[5] and described more fully in Chapter 27. No clear pattern emerges with regard to the relationships of the type of vascular communications and the occurrence of twin-to-twin transfusion syndrome (TTS), except that it is absent in those cases in which no anastomoses are present, or if they are A–A. As discussed in other chapters in this book, vascular connections in monochorionic placentas may have crucial bearing on birth weight, the nature and severity of TTS, and, in some cases, life and death.

In fused dichorionic twin placentas, the only systematic study of placental vascular anastomoses has been performed by Cameron[6]. This author only found two arterio-arterial anastomoses in a series of some 534 dichorionic placentas. In this instance, the twins were probably monozygotic. In the East Flanders Prospective Twin Survey, we have been unable to demonstrate any vascular communications in a series of 200 dichorionic twins. Undoubtedly, an A–A or V–V anastomosis is a rare event in dichorionic placentation.

The impact of the different types of placental vascular communications is still debated. Clearly, hemodynamic imbalance must result from a one-way twin-to-twin passage of blood. We and others are of the opinion that the superficial A–A and/or V–V anastomoses compensate for exchanges in the deep A–V channels (see Chapters 27–29) and that the TTS mostly or only originates when superficial anastomoses are absent, small or few in number.

The placentation of monochorionic triplets is entirely comparable to that of monochorionic twins, particularly with regard to vascular anastomoses and the presence or absence of a diamnionic dividing membrane. Monochorionic triplets can have one, two or three amnionic membranes. To date, no injection studies have demonstrated the presence of vascular anastomoses in monochorionic triplets. However, it can be assumed that they are present, just as they are in the placentas of monochorionic twins, and in two cases of monochorionic quintuplets[7,8].

Placentation in pregnancies numbering four or more fetuses follows the same pattern as that described for triplets. Theoretically, the placentation of quadruplets can be of 12 types. Tetra-, tri-, di- and monochorionic cases have been described.

Examination of the placenta(s)

In the delivery room, care should be taken to identify the cords according to birth order, and not to damage the placenta as it is being delivered. Labelling the cords of twins, triplets, etc. at the time of birth can be assured by placing one ligature or clamp on the cord of the first baby, two ligatures or clamps on the cord of the second, and so on. Unfortunately, the fetal membranes are easily torn if the maneuvers used to expel the placenta are too energetic: a gentle delivery technique is advisable. In twins, the dichorionic placenta can be identified as such, even when it is damaged, but this is not the case for the monochorionic placenta, in which it is necessary to differentiate the diamnionic from the rare monoamnionic varieties.

Placentation of twins

Besides the protocol used for standard placental examination in singletons, for which we refer the reader to obstetric and pathological textbooks, especially the third edition of *The Human Placenta* by Benirschke and Kaufmann[3], four specific features require attention

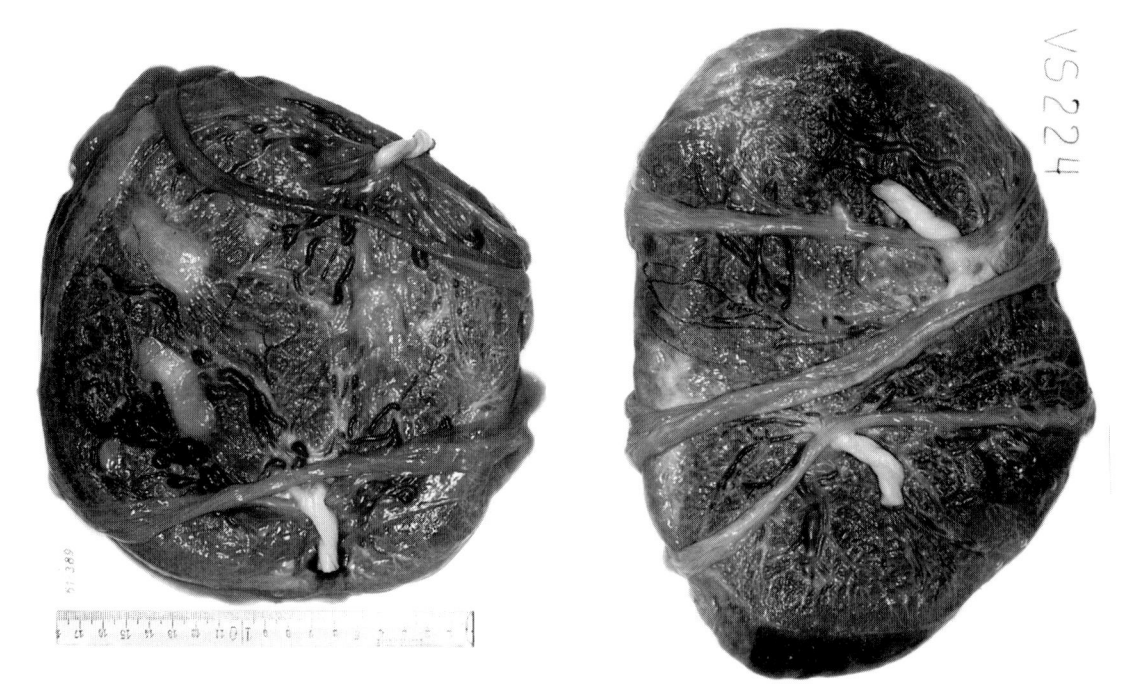

Figure 5 Fused placentas of twins after dissection of the dividing membranes. The left is monochorionic, the right dichorionic

at the time of this examination. All should be noted in the delivery room or operation record. These features include: (1) the structure of the fetal membranes; (2) the unity or division of the placenta; (3) the site of insertion of the umbilical cords; and (4) the nature and the extent of the vascular anastomoses in monochorionic placentas. All are clinically relevant, but of unequal importance. Clinically, the chorion type is most important, followed by the vascular anastomoses in monochorionic placentas, and finally by placental macroscopic structure and site of the insertions of the cords.

Fetal membranes If the twin placentas are separate and not joined by a membranous bridge, the absence of a dividing membrane is indicative of the dichorionic state. If, on the other hand, the placentas are fused or connected by a membranous bridge, the first thing to do is to reconstitute the two embryonic sacs, followed by a search for the dividing membrane. Next, this membrane should be carefully dissected into its constituent appendages by peeling apart the amnionic layer contributed by each twin. In a monochorionic placenta, the two layers of amnion, when separated, are devoid of any chorionic remnants between them. Thus, when the surface of the placenta is reached during the process of peeling apart the two adherent amnions, the amnions will continue to separate from the placenta up to the insertion of the umbilical cords to which they are loosely attached. Once this has been accomplished, the placenta will present a smooth and structureless surface between the two cord insertions (Figure 5). Such a placenta is *mono*chorionic, *di*amnionic. The absence of any septum whatsoever in a well-preserved fetal sac indicates that the placenta is of the rare (1% of all twin placentas) *mono*chorionic–*mono*amnionic type. If the amnionic membranes have been torn or damaged to a significant degree and no septum can be identified, it may be hazardous to conclude that the placenta is monoamnionic. Under these circumstances, it is far better to classify such a specimen as monochorionic with unknown amnionic type.

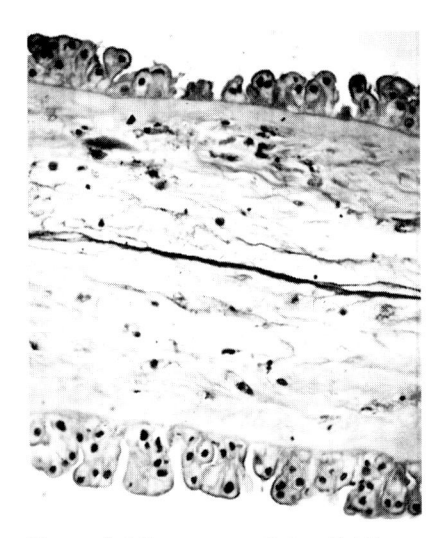

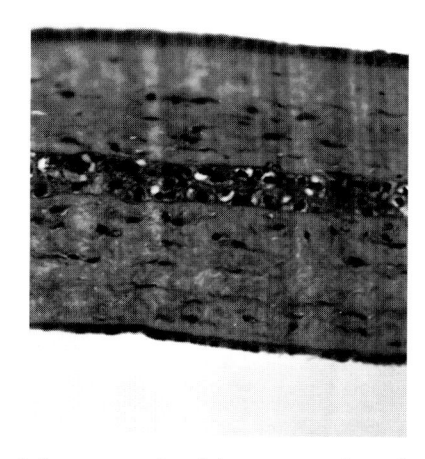

Figure 6 Microscopy of the dividing membranes; left: two amnia; right: two amnia and chorion in between

In the dichorionic placenta, this same dissection reveals a chorionic membrane between the two amnions. This part of the septum is more opaque and is firmly attached to the fetal surface of the placenta. It is constituted of two layers, one from each fetus, and these layers cannot always be separated. Microscopy of the septum confirms the macroscopic findings (Figure 6). Microscopy also has the added advantage of providing permanent evidence of the chorion type. Although microscopic examination is considered of value, it is by no means always necessary, as is the case with opposite sex twins or when the examiner is certain of the macroscopic findings[9].

Although placental examination is not difficult, it requires some degree of expertise and practice. Errors can occur. For example, a dichorionic placenta with a thin septum can erroneously be classified as monochorionic. Because of such inaccuracies, cases of opposite-sex twins with monochorionic placentas have occasionally been reported. At the Chicago Lying-in Hospital, for example, in a Department of Obstetrics and Gynecology with one of the earliest and most prestigious divisions of pathology, two such cases were mentioned in an early paper[10], but subsequently were retracted when it was determined that the placenta had been investigated in Edith Potter's absence[11].

Fusion or separation of the placentas Placentas are fused in half of the cases of dichorionic twins. This is of importance to the clinician for several reasons. First, the cords may not both insert in a central location and predispose the twins to different intrauterine conditions that may affect growth. Second, the fusion may not be located in the center of the placenta, and both halves may have a vastly different functional placental mass from which to derive nutrition, apart from any difference based on the site of the cord insertion. According to Corey *et al.*[12], a comparison of intrapair birth weight variation of monochorionic and dichorionic monozygotic twins revealed significant differences between monochorionic pairs and dichorionic separate pairs and no significant differences between monochorionic pairs and dichorionic fused pairs. These findings suggest that placental proximity may have as important an influence on variation in birth weight as does the presence or absence of vascular anastomoses. The observations of Corey and her co-workers, based on a sizeable but limited number of cases, should be extended in order to reach sex/zygosity/chorion-type subgroups of 100 or more pairs to warrant firm conclusions with regard to the influence of placental proximity. Such a study has been performed in the East Flanders Prospective Twin Survey (see below).

Insertion and vascular anatomy of the umbilical cord The types of insertion of the umbilical cords do not differ from those found in singletons, except for the velamentous insertion which can be located either on the dividing or on the peripheral part of the membranes. Because the single umbilical artery syndrome is more frequent in twins and other multiples[3,13], no examination of the cord is complete without recording the number of umbilical arteries. Histological examination should be performed if one is in doubt about the number of arteries.

Vascular anastomoses Arterioarterial and venovenous anastomoses can be demonstrated by injection of colored or contrast medium into an artery and a vein of one twin and following its path into the vascular system of the other twin (Figures 7 and 8). Whereas superficial communications are readily shown by this method, the demonstration of A–V anastomoses requires the use of radiography after injection of a barium sulphate suspension or, preferably, a solution of an iodine salt, sodium diatrizoate[5] (Figure 9). Using a syringe, we routinely inject the umbilical vessels on one side with a suspension of barium sulphate or a colored fluid. The monograph of Strong and Corney[5] discusses at length the advantages and disadvantages of different injection techniques.

The placentation of triplets and other higher order multiple births

The literature on triplets and higher order multiple births consists to a large part of case reports and small series, most of which fail to discuss placentation. The examination of the placenta(s) from these gestations should proceed along the same lines as indicated for twins. The dividing membranes between each sac should be dissected taking into account the fact that if the placentas are fused, the number of these membranes generally equals the number of fetuses. For example, in a fused trichorionic triplet placenta, dividing membranes are found between triplets 1 and 2, triplets 2 and 3, and triplets 3 and 1, respectively.

The numbers of chorionic and amnionic membranes should always be counted. Table 2 lists the different placental types encountered in triplets. Extension of this table to quadruplets, quintuplets, etc. should follow the same anatomical principles.

Experience of the East Flanders Prospective Twin Survey (EFPTS)

Following the plea of Benirschke[14], and convinced that zygosity determination at birth would be invaluable, not only for the multiples and their families but for medical research, after July 15, 1964 all placentas from twin and higher order multiple births in the Province of East Flanders, Belgium were fully investigated and described[15,16]. Twin and triplet placentas were obtained from participating hospitals and examined according to the guidelines described in this chapter. In addition, blood was collected from the umbilical cords of all infants for determination of blood groups, and samples of placental tissue were deepfrozen for later determination of genetic markers if needed. Alkaline phosphatase was the first marker used, but after 1985 the more exact determination of DNA sequences replaced this[17–19].

Over the years we developed a flow chart for zygosity determination (Figure 10)[16,18]. This chart was of particular value in the population served by physicians practicing in East Flanders. Virtually all multiple births were registered to Caucasian women. In same-sex dichorionic twins or di- and trichorionic triplets with the same blood and placental markers, we calculated the probability of monozygosity[18]. Pairs were classified as monozygotic if the probability was at least 0.95.

Twins

An overview of the placentation and other basic data obtained in East Flanders is presented in Table 4. A total of 3567 twin pairs were available for analysis and these data form the basis of Tables 5–8 (see below). In contrast to most studies performed in the first half of this

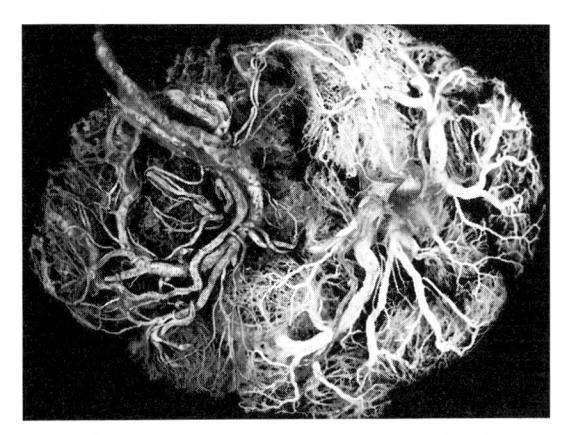

Figure 7 Monochorionic – diamnionic twin placenta that has been injected with colored plastics and then made into a corrosion cast. Many small anastomoses can be seen. Their nature is difficult to delineate. (Reproduced from reference 3, p. 738, with permission)

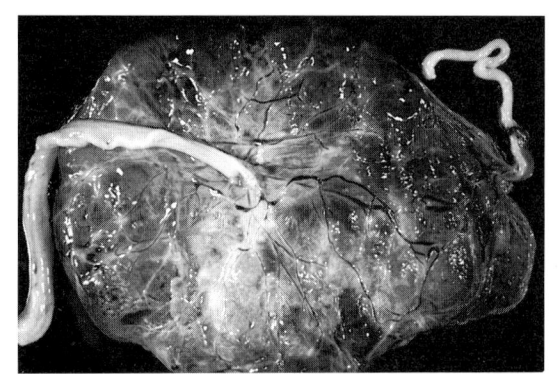

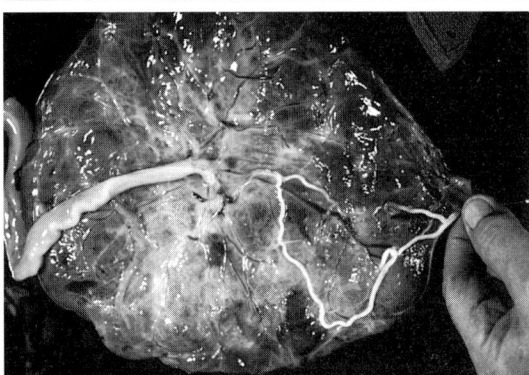

Figure 8 Monochorionic placenta of stillborn twins with hemodynamic imbalance. One larger A–A anastomosis exists. Through this anastomosis, the larger twin, who died last, must have exsanguinated into the plethoric twin. This situation is *not* the transfusion syndrome. (Reproduced from reference 3, p. 773, with permission)

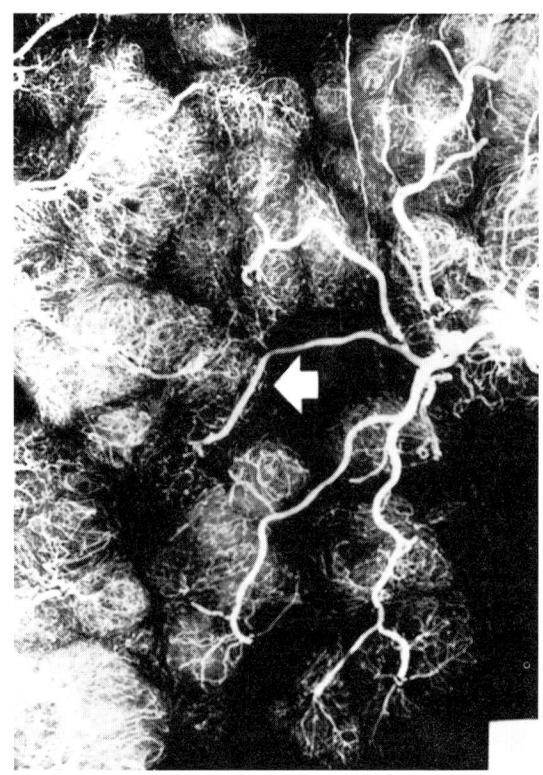

Figure 9 Monochorionic placenta with a shared cotyledon (arrow). Micropaque was injected into the arterial system of the placenta on the right. Only the larger cotyledonary vessels were filled but the contrast material flowed into the vessels of the opposite placenta. (Reproduced from reference 5, with permission)

century in Europe and North America, the proportion of monochorionic twins has increased, at least during the years 1964–79. This period is the last one during which, but for a few exceptions, all twin pregnancies were spontaneously conceived. In contrast, since 1980 increasing numbers of twin pregnancies were related to the use of ovulation-inducing drugs. Because, as a rule, most of these iatrogenic pregnancies were dizygotic and, therefore, dichorionic, the proportion of dichorionic twins has increased.

Structure of the fetal membranes Fetal growth is impaired by monochorionic placentation. The duration of pregnancy being equal, the mean birth weight of twins is highest in dizygotic twins whose placenta is dichorionic, and lowest

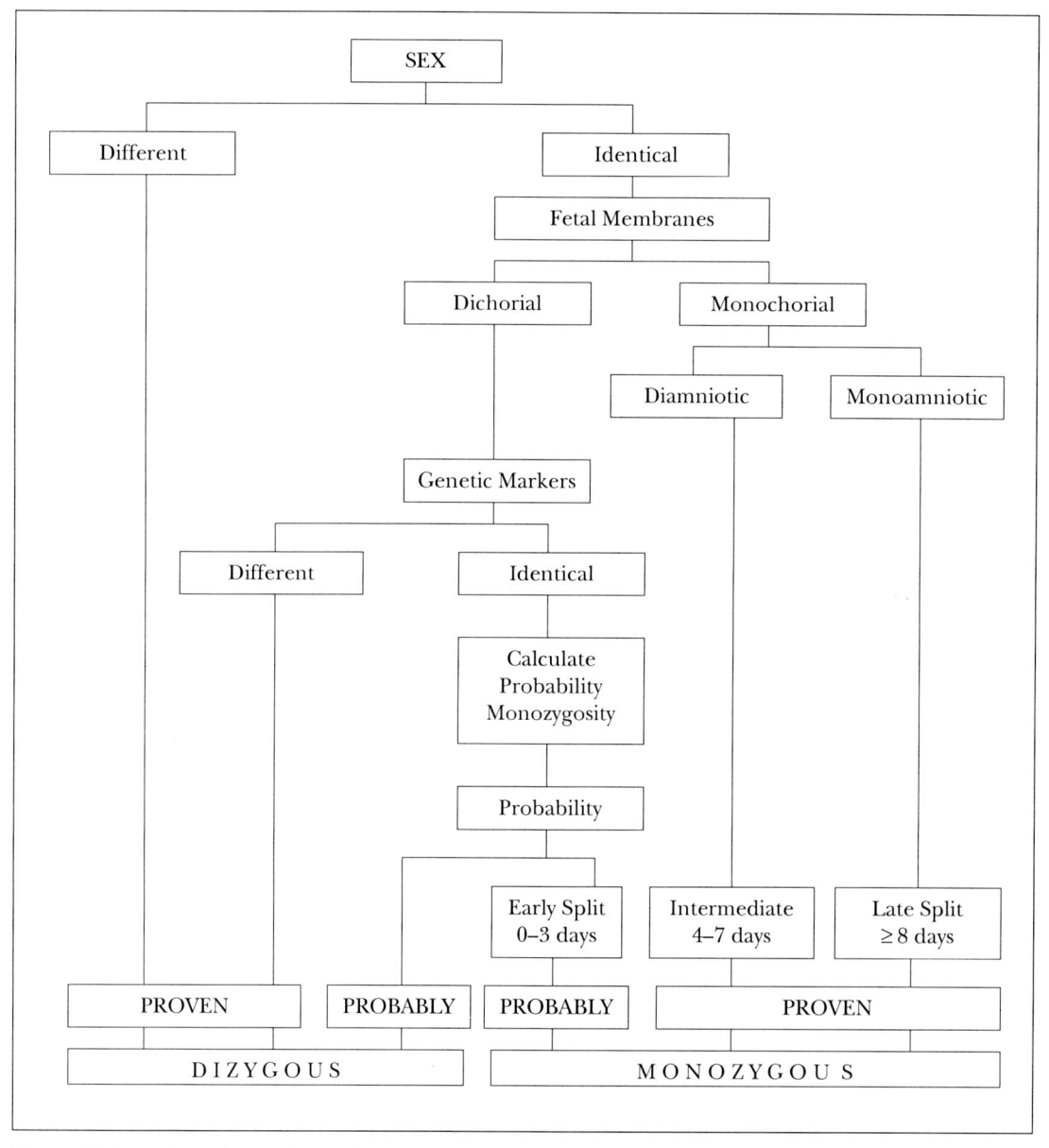

Figure 10 Decision table to determine zygosity and time of splitting. (Reproduced from reference 18, with permission)

in monochorionic twins (Table 5). Note that the birth weight differences are much more influenced by placentation than by zygosity.

Besides the slower intrauterine growth which characterizes monochorionic twinning, one member of the pair may develop intrauterine growth retardation. Tables 6 and 7 compare the weight deficits of monozygotic pairs according to gender and type of placentation. Large deficit, i.e. one of the twins weighs less than 20% of its co-twin, is much more frequent in monochorionic pairs, and more common in females than in males.

Preliminary results on the prevalence of congenital heart disease in monozygotic twins point to a possible association with chorion type[20] (Table 8). Acardia is not included in this series, because this malformation does not

Table 4 East Flanders Prospective Twin Survey. Sex distribution, placentation and perinatal mortality (‰) of twins, 1964–91

Period	Number of pairs and distribution of sex				Placentation				Perinatal mortality[†]			
					Monochorionic		Other		Twin 1		Twin 2	
	MM	MF	FF	Total	DA	MA	(1)	(2)	F	EN	F	EN
1964–79	687	516	647	1850	498	19	1318	15				
					26.9	1.0	71.2	0.8	26.0	36.2	36.2	56.2
1980–91	592	513	613	1718	441	12	1253	12				
					25.6	0.7	73.0	0.7	12.8	18.6	18.0	22.7
Total	1279	1029	1260	3568*	939	31	2571	27				
					26.3	0.9	72.1	0.6	19.6	27.7	27.5	40.0

*Freq. missing = 4; [†]no missing; (1), dichorionic; (2), unknown; DA, diamnionic; MA, monoamnionic; F, fetal; EN, early neonatal

Table 5 Birth weight (g) according to zygosity and chorion type, 1964–91

	MZ twins		DZ twins
	Monochorionic ($n = 987$)	Dichorionic ($n = 373$)	($n = 2136$)
Mean	4576	4838	4976
SD	1178	1240	1066
	$p < 0.001$		

Source: EFPTS

Table 6 Asymmetric growth retardation in male MZ twin pairs, 1964–91 (% weight deficit of smaller twin)

% Weight deficit	Dichorionic ($n = 180$)	Monochorionic ($n = 479$)
0–10	0.64	0.51
11–20	0.24	0.30
>20	0.12	0.19
	$p = 0.02$	

Source: EFPTS

Table 7 Asymmetric growth retardation in female MZ twin pairs, 1964–91 (% weight deficit of smaller twin)

% Weight deficit	Dichorionic ($n = 193$)	Monochorionic ($n = 508$)
0–10	0.61	0.46
11–20	0.33	0.32
>20	0.06	0.22
	$p < 0.001$	

Source: EFPTS

Table 8 Percentage of congenital heart disease according to zygosity and type of placentation, 1963–67. Data from reference 20

Zygosity	Placental structure	No. of infants	No. of cases	Percentage of malformation
DZ	dichorionic	1958	8	0.4
MZ	dichorionic	264	2	0.8
MZ	monochorionic	626	8	1.2

Table 9 EFPTS (1964–1989) Monozygotic twins. Perinatal mortality according to placentation

Placentation	Number of pairs	Perinatal mortality (%)	
		Twin 1	Twin 2
Dichorionic (PMZ ≥ 95%)*	438	14 (3.2%)	26 (5.9%)
Monochorionic–diamnionic	871	65 (7.5%)	84 (9.6%)
Monochorionic–monoamnionic	30	9 (30%)	7 (23%)

*PMZ, probability of monozygosity
Source: EFPTS

Table 10 Sex proportion in monochorionic twin pairs. Data from reference 22

Placentation	Male pairs	Female pairs	Sex proportion
Diamnionic	378	389	0.493
Monoamnionic	6	20	0.231
Total	384	409	0.484

Table 11 MZ dichorionic twins. Birth weight according to fetal sex in fused and separate placentas

	Female pairs			Male pairs		
	Mean	SD	n	Mean	SD	n
Fused	4514	1032	103	4820	1135	91
Separate	5009	1136	91	5090	1119	89

Table 12 Frequencies (%) of marginal and velamentous insertion of the cords according to chorion type (n = 6935*)

Cord insertion	Monochorionic placenta	Dichorionic placenta
Central, paracentral, paramarginal	69	87
Marginal	22	8
Velamentous	9	5

*Total number of cases in the study = 7134

Table 13 Distribution of the frequency (%) of the type of cord insertion according to perinatal outcome (n = 6949*)

Cord insertion	Living and well	Early neonatal death	Stillbirth
Central, paracentral, paramarginal	82.7	81.0	63.1
Marginal and velamentous	17.3	19.0	36.9

*Total number of cases in the study = 7134

occur in dichorionic twins. We acknowledge that the number of cases is small and the difference in rates is not statistically significant. However, we are of the opinion that additional longitudinal investigations may confirm this trend. The single chorionic membrane with its associated twin-to-twin vascular communications represents the major, if not the only, reason why the perinatal mortality rate is so much higher in monozygotic twins. Table 9 presents mortality rates of monozygotic twins as related to the chorion type. The figures for dichorionic twins are comparable to those of their dizygotic counterparts. Monochorionic–diamnionic twins, on the other hand, and especially monochorionic–monoamnionic twins, show markedly elevated mortality rates. Several aspects of the monochorionic placenta account for its deleterious influence on the viability of the fetuses and newborns. Most obvious are the hemodynamic imbalances and the growth retardation described previously. Another factor is the excess of marginal and velamentous cord insertions. Besides these three characteristics of the monochorionic placenta, the monoamnionic variety is associated with two additional hazards: intertwining of the umbilical cords and conjoined twinning.

The sex proportion, i.e. the proportion of male to female twins, is lower in mono- than in dizygotic twins. The figures in the EFPTS are 0.51 to 0.49, respectively. Within the

Table 14 Cord insertion and birth weight (g). Central (c), paracentral (pc) and paramarginal (pm) vs. marginal (m) and velamentous (v)

	Twin no.	Cord insertion	Birth weight
Monochorionic placenta	1	c + pc + pm ($n = 645$)	2395
		m + v ($n = 294$)	2227
	2	c + pc + pm ($n = 649$)	2336
		m + v ($n = 291$)	2154
Dichorionic placenta	1	c + pc + pm ($n = 2198$)	2522
		m + v ($n = 322$)	2364
	2	c + pc + pm ($n = 2181$)	2477
		m + v ($n = 314$)	2294

Table 15 Distribution of chorion type in 92 triplets, from East Flanders Prospective Twin Survey (Derom et al., unpublished data)

	Spontaneous ($n = 31$)	Induced ($n = 61$)
Monochorionic	4	0
Dichorionic	14	4
Trichorionic	13	57

monozygotic group, remarkable changes in this proportion are found with respect to the number of amnionic sacs (Table 10). Whereas the sex proportion in monochorionic–diamnionic twins does not differ from the dichorionic group, it is lowered to 0.23 in monochorionic–monoamnionic twins.

Fusion of the placentas Separate placentas, as might be expected from the writings of Corey et al.[12], should theoretically be more favorable to fetal growth than fused placentas. This is the case in the EFPTS study for monozygotic pairs (Table 11). Here, one witnesses an almost ideal natural experiment in which the location of the placenta is probably the only major variable. The mean weight difference is substantial and amounts to 239 g in male and 524 g in female pairs. Again, as in intrapair differences in birth weight, the female fetus is more sensitive to changes in intrauterine environment. Changes in the same direction are found in dizygotic pairs but they are not statistically significant.

Cord insertions Table 12 presents the prevalence rates of marginal and velamentous insertion of the cords according to the structure of the fetal membranes. Marginal insertion is three times and velamentous insertion somewhat less than two times more frequent in monochorionic placentas. These differences are the same for the first- and the second-born twin.

Insertion of the cord on the periphery of the placenta is deleterious to fetal well-being. Velamentous insertion is two times more frequent in stillbirths and early neonatal deaths than in liveborn twins surviving the early neonatal period (Table 13). The higher prevalence rate of marginal insertion in stillbirths is of borderline significance.

The mean birth weight of twins with marginal or velamentous insertion is 160 to 180 g less than with insertion on the central placental surface, regardless of whether the fetal membranes are mono- or dichorionic (Table 14).

Triplets

Table 15 gives the distribution of the placental structure in a series of 92 triplets registered in the East Flanders Prospective Twin Survey (C. Derom et al. unpublished data). The majority of the spontaneous triplets were dichorionic, whereas all but four induced triplets were trichorionic. The four induced triplets with dichorionic membranes are proof that not all multiple births originating after ovulation induction are polyzygotic[21].

Acknowledgements

Aided by grants No 3.0038.82 of the Fund for Medical Scientific Research (Belgium), No 86/0823 of NATO, and the Association for Scientific Research in Multiple Births (Belgium).

References

1. O'Rahilly, R. and Müller, F. (1992). *Human Embryology and Teratology.* (New York: Wiley-Liss)
2. Bieber, F.R., Nance, W.E., Morton, C.G. *et al.* (1981). Genetic studies of an acardiac monster: evidence of polar body twinning in man. *Science*, **213**, 775
3. Benirschke, K. and Kaufmann, P. (1995). *Pathology of the Human Placenta*, 3rd edn. (New York: Springer-Verlag)
4. Matayoshi, K. and Yoshida, K. (1989). Observation of 11 cases of triplets and their outcome, abstr. p. 92. *Sixth International Congress on Twin Studies*, Rome
5. Strong, S.J. and Corney, G. (1967). *The Placenta in Twin Pregnancy.* (Oxford: Pergamon Press)
6. Cameron, A.H. (1968). The Birmingham twin survey. *Proc. Soc. Med.*, **61**, 229
7. Gibbs, C.E., Boldt, J.W., Dally, J.W. *et al.* (1984). A quintuplet gestation. *Obstet. Gynecol.*, **16**, 464
8. Neubecker, R.D., Blumberg, J.M. and Townsend, F.M. (1962). A human monozygotic quintuplet placenta: report of a specimen. *J. Obstet. Gynaecol. Br. Commonw.*, **69**, 137
9. Nylander, P.P.S. (1970). A simple method for determining monochorionic and dichorionic placentation in twins. *Nig. J. Sci.*, **4**, 239
10. Potter, E.L. and Fuller, H. (1949). Multiple pregnancies at the Chicago Lying-in Hospital 1941–1947. *Am. J. Obstet. Gynecol.*, **58**, 139
11. Potter, E.L. (1963). Twin zygosity and placental form in relation to the outcome of pregnancy. *Am. J. Obstet. Gynecol.*, **87**, 566
12. Corey, L.A., Nance, W.E., Kang, K.W. *et al.* (1979). Effects of type of placentation on birthweight and its variability in monozygotic and dizygotic twins. *Acta Genet. Med. Gemellol.*, **28**, 41
13. Ramos-Arroyo, M.A., Ulbright, T.M., Yu, P.L. *et al.* (1988). Twin: relationship between birth weight, zygosity, placentation, and pathological placental changes. *Acta Genet. Med. Gemellol.*, **37**, 229
14. Benirschke, K. (1961). Accurate recording of twin placentation. A plea to the obstetrician. *Obstet. Gynecol.*, **18**, 334
15. Derom, R., Vlietinck, R.F., Derom, C. *et al.* (1991). Zygosity determination at birth: a plea to the obstetrician. *J. Perin. Med.*, **19**, (Suppl. 1), 234
16. Vlietinck, R., Papiernik, E., Derom, C. *et al.* (1988). The European Multiple Birth Study (EMBS). *Acta Genet. Med. Gemellol.*, **37**, 27
17. Derom, C., Bakker, E., Vlietinck, R. *et al.* (1985). Zygosity determination in newborn twins using DNA variants. *J. Med. Genet.*, **22**, 279
18. Vlietinck, R. (1986). *Determination of the Zygosity of Twins*. Leuven: thesis
19. Derom, C., Vlietinck, R., Derom, R. *et al.* (1991). Genotyping macerated stillborn fetuses. *Am. J. Obstet. Gynecol.*, **164**, 797
20. Cameron, A.H., Edwards, J.H., Derom, R. *et al.* (1983). The value of twin surveys in the study of malformations. *Eur. J. Obstet. Gynecol. Reprod. Biol.*, **14**, 347
21. Derom, C., Vlietinck, R. and Derom, R. *et al.* (1987). Increased monozygotic twinning rate after ovulation induction. *Lancet*, **1**, 1236
22. Derom, C. and Vlietinck, R. (1988). Population-based study on sex proportion in monoamniotic twins. *N. Engl. J. Med.*, **19**, 119

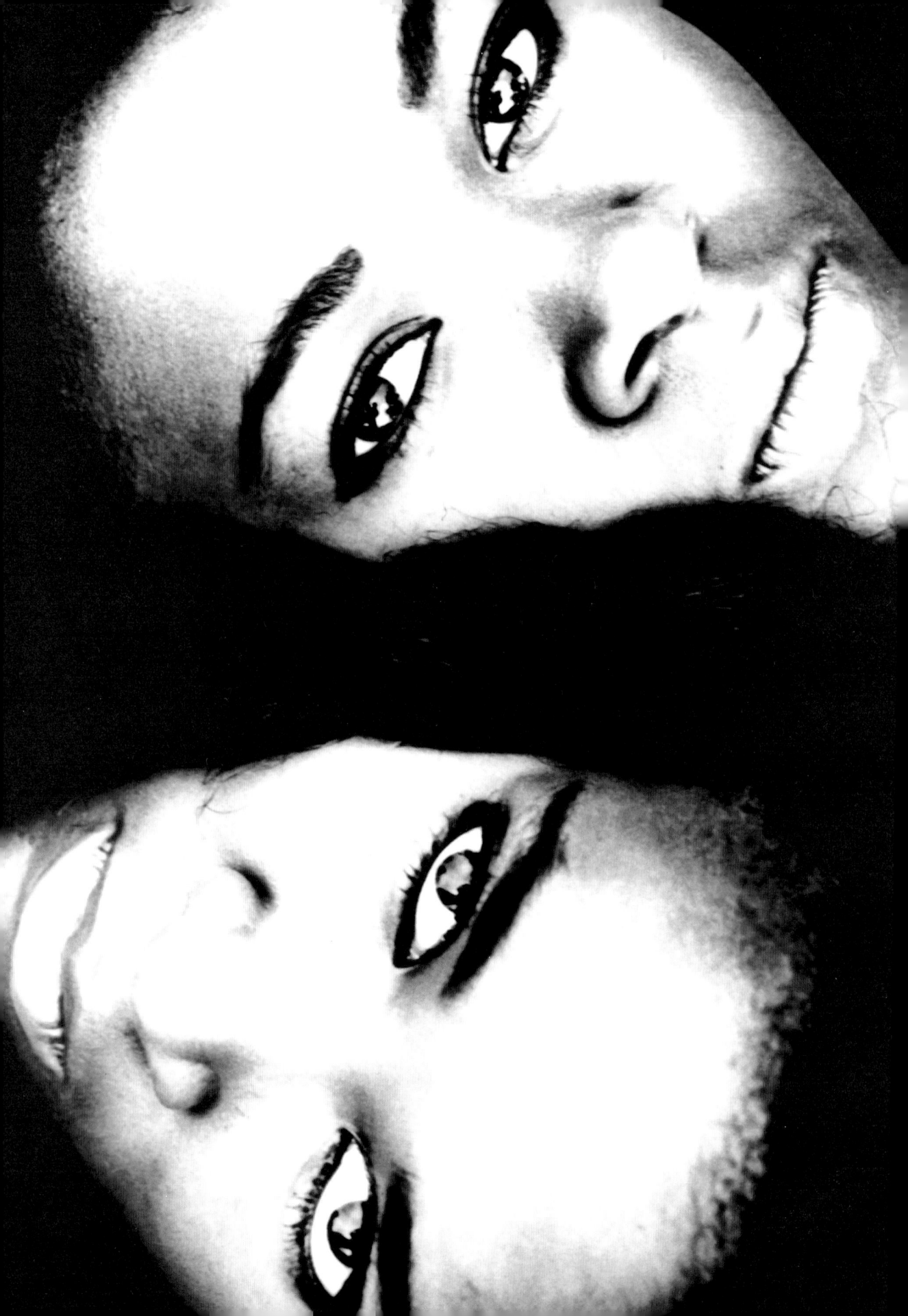

section III
Epidemiology

The Reed Twins

David Teplica, 1990,
Collection of Gary C. Burget, MD, Chicago, Illinois

Demographic trends in twin births: USA 10

S.M. Taffel

Introduction

Since 1917, information on the plurality of births derived from live-birth certificates has been published annually in the United States. Before 1959, the live-birth and fetal death records of sets of multiple births were matched. Beginning with the 1959 data year, however, this matching process was discontinued, and the number and composition of plural sets could no longer be determined. Because of the lack of such information for recent years, tables and discussion in this chapter refer only to the number of live twin births.

At the time this chapter was written, information was available on twin births through the year 1987. Since then, data for the years 1988–92 have become available, and these are presented in Table 1 and Figure 1. However, all of the remaining tables and figures and almost all of the discussion focus on data prior to 1988. The data in the tables and figures in this chapter were, for the most part, specially run and are not reflected in other publications except for reference 1.

Trends in twin birth incidence

Both the number of live twin births and the ratio of twin births per 1000 total live births have risen fairly steadily since the early 1970s (Table 1 and Figure 1). This rise follows a small drop in twin birth ratios from 1950 to the late 1960s. By 1992, there were 23.5 live twin births per 1000 total live births in the United States, an increase of 32% over the twinning ratio of 17.8 in 1971. The 1992 ratio exceeds the highest ratios of the 1950s. A rising proportion of pregnancies resulting in twins since the 1970s has also been noted in England and Wales[2].

The recent rise in twinning incidence reflects both a change in the age distribution of women giving birth (see below) and an increased usage of fertility drugs which greatly increase the incidence of multiple ovulation and the subsequent delivery of multiples (see Chapters 11 and 13).

For all years for which data are available, the twinning ratio for black births exceeded the ratio for white births. In 1992, the ratio of 27.3 for black births was 19% higher than the ratio of 23.0 for white births. This racial differential has narrowed considerably since 1971, however, when the black ratio exceeded the white ratio by 32%. The narrowing of the racial differential is due to the more rapid increase in twinning incidence for white births than for black births (especially among 'older' mothers – see below).

The twin birth ratio for black births has consistently exceeded that for all non-white races combined. This differential has increased in recent years as the proportion of non-white births that are black has declined (from 95% in 1950 to 77% in 1992). The 'non-white' category includes a growing number of Chinese, Japanese, Filipino, other Asian and Pacific Islander, and American Indian births. Twin birth ratios for these groups are substantially lower than the ratio for black births. In 1992 the ratios were 17.8 for American Indian births; 17.2 for Chinese births; 23.1 for Japanese births; 16.3 for Filipino births; 20.7 for Hawaiian births; 16.8 for other Asian and Pacific Islander births.

MULTIPLE PREGNANCY

Table 1 Twin birth ratios by race of child: United States, 1950–92. (Ratios are live births in twin deliveries per 1000 total live births)

	All races			White			All other					
							Total			Black		
Year	Number of twin births	Total births	Ratio	Number of twin births	Total births	Ratio	Number of twin births	Total births	Ratio	Number of twin births	Total births	Ratio
1992	95 372	4 065 014	23.5	72 000	3 131 679	23.0	23 372	933 335	25.0	19 634	719 396	27.3
1991	94 779	4 110 907	23.1	71 593	3 174 030	22.6	23 186	936 877	24.7	19 500	725 163	26.9
1990	93 865	4 158 212	22.6	71 258	3 225 343	22.1	22 607	932 869	24.2	19 000	724 576	26.2
1989	90 118	4 040 958	22.3	68 004	3 131 991	21.7	22 114	908 967	24.3	18 637	709 395	26.3
1988	85 315	3 909 510	21.8	65 136	3 046 162	21.4	20 179	863 348	23.4	17 052	671 976	25.4
1987	81 778	3 809 394	21.5	62 952	2 992 488	21.0	18 826	816 906	23.0	16 042	641 567	25.0
1986	79 485	3 756 547	21.2	61 385	2 970 439	20.7	18 100	786 108	23.0	15 252	621 221	24.6
1985	77 102	3 760 561	20.5	59 420	2 991 373	19.9	17 682	769 188	23.0	15 137	608 193	24.9
1984	72 949	3 669 141	19.9	56 439	2 923 502	19.3	16 510	745 639	22.1	14 111	592 745	23.8
1983	72 287	3 638 933	19.9	55 766	2 904 250	19.2	16 521	734 683	22.5	14 142	586 027	24.1
1982	71 631	3 680 537	19.5	55 229	2 942 054	18.8	16 402	738 483	22.2	14 042	592 641	23.7
1981	70 049	3 629 238	19.3	53 653	2 908 669	18.4	16 396	720 569	22.8	14 340	587 797	24.4
1980	68 339	3 612 258	18.9	52 397	2 898 732	18.1	15 942	713 526	22.3	14 026	589 616	23.8
1979	66 858	3 494 398	19.1	51 372	2 808 420	18.3	15 486	685 978	22.6	13 872	577 855	24.0
1978	64 163	3 333 279	19.2	49 461	2 681 116	18.4	14 702	652 163	22.5	13 116	551 540	23.8
1977	62 880	3 326 632	18.9	48 824	2 691 070	18.1	14 056	635 562	22.1	12 512	544 221	23.0
1976	60 664	3 167 788	19.2	47 521	2 567 614	18.5	13 143	600 174	21.9	11 786	514 479	22.9
1975	59 192	3 144 198	18.8	46 266	2 551 996	18.1	12 926	592 202	21.8	11 674	511 581	22.8
1974	57 836	3 159 958	18.3	45 573	2 575 792	17.7	12 263	584 186	21.0	11 041	507 162	21.8
1973	56 777	3 136 965	18.1	44 452	2 551 030	17.4	12 325	585 935	21.0	11 201	512 597	21.9
1972	59 122	3 258 411	18.1	46 302	2 655 558	17.4	12 820	602 853	21.3	11 670	531 329	22.0
1971	63 298	3 555 970	17.8	49 576	2 919 746	17.0	13 722	636 224	21.6	12 656	564 960	22.4
1970	–	3 731 386	–	–	3 091 264	–	–	640 122	–	–	572 362	–
1969	–	3 600 206	–	–	2 993 614	–	–	606 592	–	–	543 132	–
1968	69 300	3 501 564	19.8	55 464	2 912 224	19.0	13 836	589 340	23.5	–	531 152	–
1967	68 336	3 520 959	19.4	54 123	2 922 502	18.5	14 213	598 457	23.7	–	543 976	–
1966	70 340	3 606 274	19.5	55 430	2 993 230	18.5	14 910	613 044	24.3	–	558 244	–
1965	74 594	3 670 358	20.3	58 436	3 123 860	18.7	16 158	636 498	25.4	–	581 126	–
1964	78 954	4 027 490	19.6	62 076	3 369 160	18.4	16 878	658 330	25.6	–	607 556	–
1963*	80 044	4 098 020	19.5	61 062	3 326 344	18.4	16 356	638 928	25.6	–	580 658	–
1962*	80 180	4 167 362	19.2	61 792	3 394 068	18.2	15 788	641 580	24.6	–	584 610	–
1961	84 926	4 268 326	19.9	67 442	3 600 864	18.7	17 484	667 462	26.2	–	611 072	–
1960	85 440	4 257 850	20.1	68 414	3 600 744	19.0	17 026	657 106	25.9	–	602 264	–
1955	84 394	4 047 295	20.9	69 079	3 458 448	20.0	15 315	588 847	26.0	14 806	558 251	26.5
1954	82 626	4 017 362	20.6	67 705	3 443 630	19.7	14 921	573 732	26.0	14 477	544 288	26.6
1953	81 000	3 902 120	20.8	66 518	3 356 772	19.8	14 482	545 348	26.6	13 998	517 576	27.0
1952	78 457	3 846 986	20.4	65 232	3 322 658	19.6	13 225	524 328	25.2	12 817	497 880	25.7
1951	75 335	3 750 850	20.1	62 772	3 237 072	19.4	12 563	513 778	24.5	12 155	489 282	24.8
1950	73 499	3 554 149	20.7	61 233	3 063 627	20.0	12 266	490 522	25.0	11 794	466 718	25.3

*Figures by race exclude data for residents of New Jersey, which did not report race in this year; –, data not available

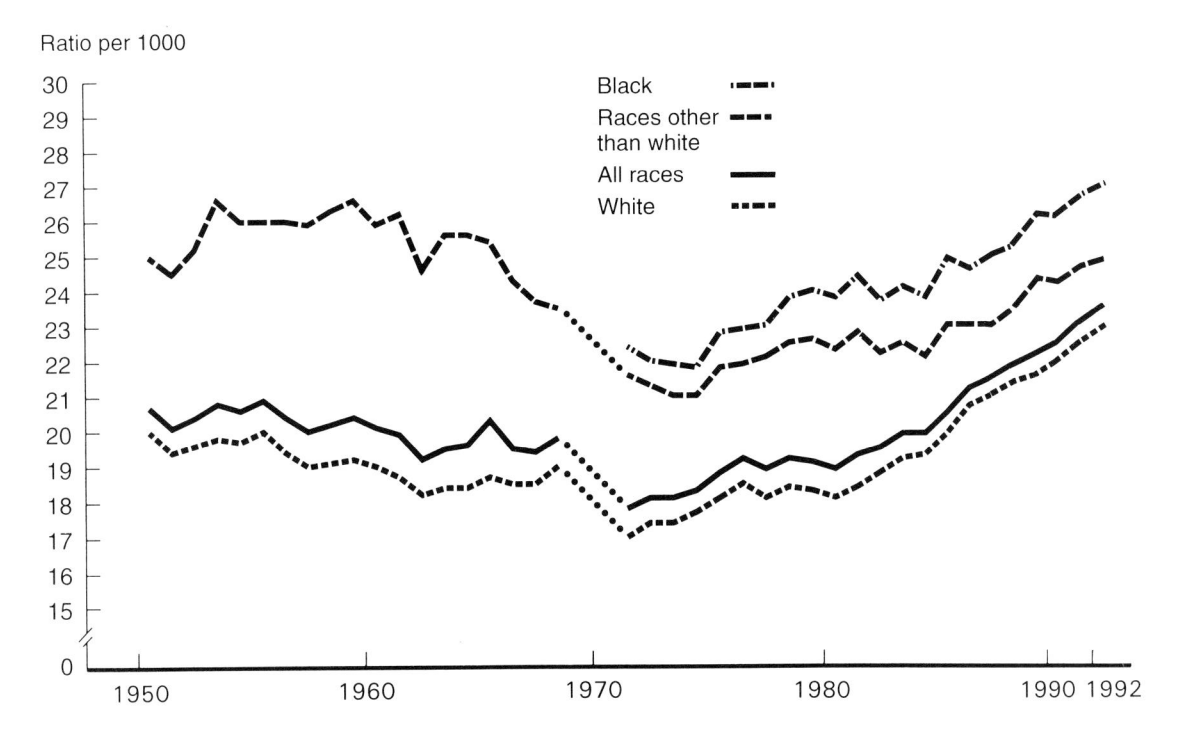

Figure 1 Twin birth ratios by race of child: United States, 1950–92 (ratios are live births in twin deliveries per 1000 total live births) (Source: NCHS, National Vital Statistics System, 1950–92)

Age of mother and live-birth order

The incidence of twinning increases with mother's age up to ages 35–39 years, and then declines (Table 2). This increase, and the subsequent decline evident for both white and black births, has been attributed to the rise in the level of gonadotropin secretion with age, with maximum stimulation of follicles at ages 35–39, and a subsequent decline in ovarian function at older ages[3].

Since the mid-1970s, the proportion of births to women in their thirties has risen steadily. In 1987, 20.0% of all births were to women 30–34 years of age, 75% more than the comparable proportion in 1971 (11.4%). Similarly, in 1987, 6.5% of births were to women 35–39 years of age, up from 4.6% in 1971. This increase in the proportion of older women having children is a major reason for the recent rise in the twinning ratio. If the age distribution of women giving birth in 1987 were exactly the same as in 1971, the twinning ratio

Table 2 Twin birth ratios by age of mother and race of child: United States, 1987. (Ratios are live births in twin deliveries per 1000 total live births in specified group)

	Race of child		
Age of mother	All races*	White	Black
All ages	21.5	21.0	25.0
Under 15 years	10.8	12.0	10.5
15–19 years	14.1	12.9	17.0
20–24 years	18.8	17.6	24.4
25–29 years	22.8	22.2	28.9
30–34 years	25.8	25.7	30.5
35–39 years	27.5	27.5	32.8
40–44 years	20.7	21.6	20.4
45–49 years	24.7	18.3	56.2†

*Includes races other than white and black; †based on less than 10 twin births

Table 3 Observed and adjusted twin birth ratios by race of child: United States, selected years, 1971–87. (Ratios are live births in twin deliveries per 1000 total live births in specified group)

Year	All races*			White			Black		
	Observed	Adjusted†	% Difference‡	Observed	Adjusted†	% Difference‡	Observed	Adjusted†	% Difference‡
1987	21.5	20.2	−6.0	21.0	19.6	−6.7	25.0	23.7	−5.2
1986	21.2	20.0	−5.7	20.7	19.3	−6.8	24.6	23.3	−5.3
1985	20.5	19.5	−4.9	19.9	18.7	−6.0	24.9	23.5	−5.6
1984	19.9	19.0	−4.5	19.3	18.3	−5.2	23.8	22.7	−4.6
1983	19.9	19.1	−4.0	19.2	18.4	−4.2	24.1	23.1	−4.1
1982	19.5	18.8	−3.6	18.8	18.1	−3.7	23.7	22.7	−4.2
1981	19.3	18.8	−2.6	18.4	17.9	−2.7	24.4	23.6	−3.3
1980	18.9	18.5	−2.1	18.1	17.7	−2.2	23.8	23.2	−2.5
1975	18.8	18.8	0.0	18.1	18.1	0.0	22.8	23.1	1.3
1973	18.1	18.1	0.0	17.4	17.4	0.0	21.9	22.2	1.4
1971	17.8	17.8	—	17.0	17.0	—	22.4	22.4	—

*Includes races other than white and black; †adjusted to reflect the age of mother distribution in 1971 of live births in specified racial group; ‡adjusted twin ratio compared with observed twin ratio

Table 4 Twin birth ratios by live-birth order, age of mother and race of child: United States, 1987. (Ratios are live births in twin deliveries per 1000 total live births in specified group)

Age of mother (years) and race of child	Total	Live-birth order				
		1	2	3	4	5 and over
All races*						
All ages	21.5	10.7	22.8	33.0	42.0	46.0
Under 20	14.0	7.2	33.8	51.4	64.3	112.6
20–24	18.8	9.6	21.5	34.1	47.4	68.0
25–29	22.8	12.3	22.0	33.3	43.7	50.3
30–34	25.8	14.8	22.2	32.0	40.9	44.9
35–49	26.7	16.8	23.6	28.2	33.3	36.8
White						
All ages	21.0	10.8	22.5	33.0	41.7	44.6
Under 20	12.9	6.8	33.7	54.9	74.6	154.9
20–24	17.6	9.3	20.9	34.2	48.1	63.5
25–29	22.2	12.3	21.8	33.1	44.0	51.8
30–34	25.7	15.3	22.7	32.3	40.8	44.1
35–49	26.8	17.3	24.2	29.1	33.1	36.1
Black						
All ages	25.0	10.8	26.0	35.4	46.2	55.0
Under 20	16.8	8.5	34.7	48.0	58.7	86.3
20–24	24.4	11.4	24.7	35.2	48.8	77.5
25–29	28.9	13.5	24.9	36.3	46.3	52.0
30–34	30.5	13.4	22.5	32.5	45.6	53.5
35–49	31.4	18.6	23.7	28.2	37.1	44.9

*Includes races other than white and black

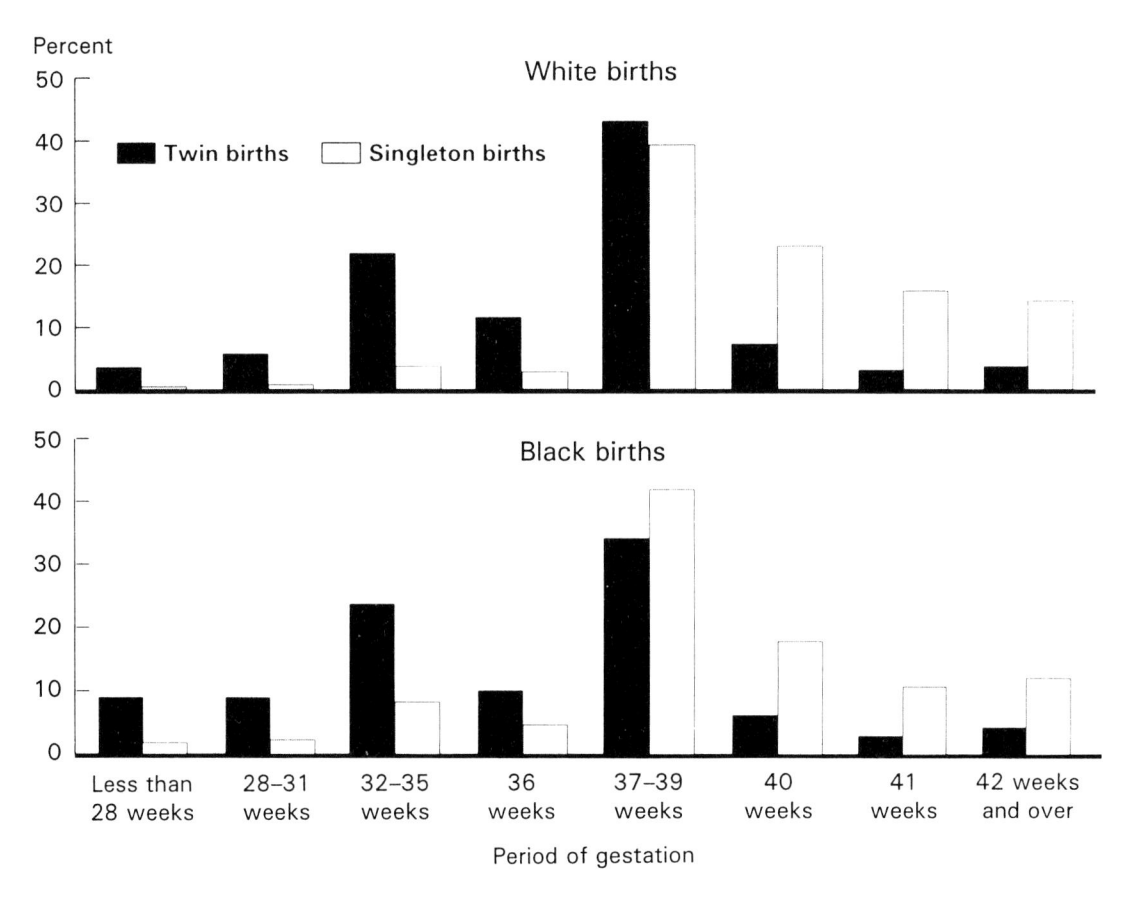

Figure 2 Percentage distribution of twin and singleton live births by period of gestation: United States, 1987. (Source: NCHS, National Vital Statistics System, 1987)

in 1987 would be 6% lower, or 20.2 rather than 21.5 (see Table 3).

An independent effect of parity of equal or greater importance than that of maternal age has been observed in a number of previous studies[4-6]. However, it is not possible to determine the exact influence of parity from data derived from live-birth certificates, because each live-born twin in a twin delivery is assigned a different, adjacent, live-birth order. Thus, if a mother had one previous live-born child, the first born of a set of twins would be assigned live-birth order two, while the second would be assigned live-birth order three. However, despite this shortcoming, it is evident that there is a greatly increased incidence of twinning for high-order compared with low-order births.

As indicated in Table 4, the twinning ratios for 4th or 5th birth orders are about 4 times as high as the ratio for first-order births. These differences are not due to the older ages of women having high-order births. For all maternal ages, and for both white and black births, twinning ratios increase with birth order, and are substantially higher for high than for low birth orders.

Previous studies indicate that the maternal age and birth order effect on twinning incidence is most pronounced for dizygotic twins, with little or no difference for monozygotic twin deliveries[4,5,7].

Sex ratio at birth

There is a distinct difference in the sex ratio at birth (the number of male births per 1000 female births) for twin and singleton live births. In 1987, the sex ratio for singleton live births was 1051, compared with 1013 for twin live

Table 5 Sex ratio of twin and singleton live births by age of mother and race of child: United States, 1987. (Ratios are the number of male births per 1000 female births in specified group)

Age of mother (years)	All races*		White		Black	
	Twin births	Singleton births	Twin births	Singleton births	Twin births	Singleton births
All ages	1013	1051	1008	1055	1027	1028
Under 15	762	1057	920	1105	658	1025
15–19	1038	1053	1016	1060	1082	1037
20–24	1027	1051	1019	1056	1044	1030
25–29	1008	1051	1011	1054	997	1026
30–34	984	1051	980	1055	984	1018
35–39	1046	1048	1027	1049	1082	1014
40–44	1165	1041	1196	1048	1275	1045
45–49	1000†	1089	1000†	1038	667†	1301

*Includes races other than white and black; †based on less than 20 live births

births (Table 5). The ratio is higher for singleton births for all maternal ages except for women 40–44 years old. This same pattern is obvious for white births. For black births, however, there is no consistent pattern by age of mother and the overall sex ratio for black singletons is nearly identical to that of black twin births (1028 compared with 1027).

The sex ratio of both early and late fetal deaths is higher than that of live births[8]. The lower sex ratio for twin than for singleton births implies a higher sex ratio for twin fetal deaths for almost all maternal ages.

Period of gestation and birth weight

The gestational age of a newborn is determined from the first day of the mother's last normal menstrual period and the date of birth. Short gestational periods are far more common for twins than for singletons (Table 6). In 1987, almost five times the proportion of twins to singletons were born preterm (before 37 weeks' gestation) – 44.5% compared with 9.4% (Figure 2).

It has been suggested that the greater risk of preterm delivery for twins is due to uterine over-distension, mechanical stretching of the cervix and decreased uterine blood flow[3]. Preterm birth is the leading cause of neonatal deaths in multiple gestations[9].

Black twin births are more likely to occur preterm than white twin births (52.0% compared with 42.8%). However, the difference in the rate of preterm delivery by plurality is far greater for white than for black births, with nearly six times the proportion of white twins as white singletons born before 37 weeks compared with three times the proportion of black twins as black singletons.

Slightly more than half of twin babies are born at term (37–41 weeks' gestation) compared with about three-quarters of singleton births. There are relatively few twins born post-term (3.8% compared with 13.7% of singletons), and racial differences are minor for post-term deliveries. The average length of gestation for singletons is 39.3 weeks, slightly more than 3 weeks longer than for twins (36.1 weeks). Approximately the same differential is evident for white and black births (Table 6).

Generally speaking, twins weigh less at birth than do singletons. While their lower birth weight is due in part to shorter gestational periods, there are major differences in birth weight for equal periods of gestation (Table 7). More than twice the proportion of twins than singletons born before 37 weeks' gestation weigh less than 2500 g (76.2% compared with

Table 6 Percentage distribution of twin and singleton live births by period of gestation and race of child: United States, 1987

Period of gestation (weeks)	All races*		White		Black	
	Twin births	Singleton births	Twin births	Singleton births	Twin births	Singleton births
Live births[†]	81 778	3 725 477	62 952	2 927 745	16 042	625 265
Total (%)	100.0	100.0	100.0	100.0	100.0	100.0
Less than 28 (%)	4.7	0.7	3.6	0.5	9.0	1.8
28–31 (%)	6.3	1.0	5.7	0.8	9.0	2.3
32–35 (%)	22.3	4.5	21.9	3.7	23.8	8.3
36 (%)	11.3	3.2	11.6	2.8	10.1	4.7
37–39 (%)	41.4	40.0	43.1	39.3	34.3	42.0
40 (%)	7.1	22.1	7.2	23.0	6.3	17.9
41 (%)	3.1	14.8	3.1	15.8	3.0	10.8
42 and over (%)	3.8	13.7	3.7	14.2	4.4	12.2
Less than 37 (%)	44.5	9.4	42.8	7.7	52.0	17.1
Mean (weeks)	36.1	39.3	36.4	39.6	35.2	38.6

*Includes races other than white and black; [†]includes births with period of gestation not stated, which are excluded from the computation of the percent distribution

34.8%). Similarly, more than twice the proportion of premature twins than premature singletons weigh less than 1500 g (20.1% compared with 9.3%). Less than 1% of twins born preterm weigh 3500 g or more, compared with 13.8% of singletons.

For gestations of 40 weeks or longer, the proportion of low birth weight infants (less than 2500 g) declines to 25.9% for twins, but the disparity with singleton birth weight becomes even more evident, with only 1.6% of singletons weighing this little.

The fact that twins have, on the average, far lower birth weights than singletons of matched gestational ages suggests that other factors are responsible for their reduced birth weight. Several explanations have been offered: (1) the overcrowding in the uterus limits the area available for placental growth, leading to placental insufficiency; (2) the inability of the mother to provide adequate nourishment to support optimal growth of two fetuses; and (3) the blood supply to the uterus is not sufficient to support the same rate of growth for a multiple as for a single pregnancy[10]. These factors are discussed in other portions of this book.

Apgar score

The Apgar score is one of a number of parameters used to evaluate the physical condition of an infant at 1 and 5-min after birth. The score is often considered as an indication of whether or not immediate medical attention is required. As indicated in Table 8, almost one-quarter of twins (22.2%) had a 1-min score of less than 7, and a score this low was more common for black twins than for white twins (28.7% compared with 20.5%). A low 1-min score was 2.5 times as frequent for twins as for singletons, regardless of race. Singletons were about 50% more likely than twins to have optimal 1-min scores of 9 or 10 (42.2% compared with 27.7%).

Although 5-min scores are considerably higher than 1-min scores for both twins and singletons, the differential by plurality is still quite marked. A twin is about 4.5 times as likely as a

MULTIPLE PREGNANCY

Table 7 Percentage distribution of twin and singleton live births by birth weight according to period of gestation and race of child: United States, 1987

Period of gestation and birth weight	All races*		White		Black	
	Twin births	Singleton births	Twin births	Singleton births	Twin births	Singleton births
All gestational ages						
Live births†‡	81 778	3 725 477	62 952	2 927 745	16 042	625 265
Total (%)	100.0	100.0	100.0	100.0	100.0	100.0
Less than 1000 g (%)	4.8	0.5	3.9	0.4	8.8	1.3
1000–1499 g (%)	5.1	0.5	4.6	0.4	7.3	1.1
1500–1999 g (%)	12.5	1.0	11.7	0.8	15.8	2.1
2000–2499 g (%)	27.9	3.8	27.2	3.1	29.9	7.0
2500–2999 g (%)	31.4	15.7	32.7	13.8	26.3	23.5
3000–3499 g (%)	15.2	37.1	16.5	36.6	10.2	38.8
3500–3999 g (%)	2.8	30.1	3.1	32.3	1.5	20.9
4000 g or more (%)	0.3	11.2	0.3	12.6	0.2	5.5
Less than 2500 g (%)	50.3	5.9	47.4	4.7	61.8	11.4
Under 37 weeks						
Live births‡	34 740	335 867	25 764	217 758	7 912	102 167
Total (%)	100.0	100.0	100.0	100.0	100.0	100.0
Less than 1000 g (%)	9.8	4.7	8.2	4.0	15.2	6.4
1000–1499 g (%)	10.3	4.6	9.5	4.3	12.7	5.4
1500–1999 g (%)	21.9	8.1	21.5	7.8	23.2	9.1
2000–2499 g (%)	34.2	17.4	35.2	17.2	30.6	18.1
2500–2999 g (%)	19.4	26.8	20.8	26.6	15.0	26.8
3000–3499 g (%)	3.9	24.6	4.3	24.8	2.8	23.6
3500–3999 g (%)	0.4	10.9	0.3	11.8	0.4	8.8
4000 g or more (%)	0.1	2.9	0.1	3.5	0.1	1.8
Less than 2500 g (%)	76.2	34.8	74.5	33.2	81.7	39.0
37–39 weeks						
Live births‡	32 326	1 427 347	25 949	1 104 541	5 213	250 245
Total	100.0	100.0	100.0	100.0	100.0	100.0
Less than 1000 g (%)	0.2	0.0	0.1	0.0	0.4	0.1
1000–1499 g (%)	0.6	0.1	0.5	0.1	1.2	0.1
1500–1999 g (%)	4.7	0.4	4.0	0.3	8.3	0.7
2000–2499 g (%)	23.8	3.5	22.2	3.0	30.2	6.0
2500–2999 g (%)	42.8	19.5	43.5	17.5	39.5	27.3
3000–3499 g (%)	23.7	42.1	25.0	41.9	17.8	42.4
3500–3999 g (%)	3.9	26.8	4.3	28.8	2.4	19.2
4000 g or more (%)	0.3	7.5	0.3	8.3	0.2	4.2
Less than 2500 g (%)	29.3	4.0	26.9	3.4	40.1	6.9

Continued

Table 7 *(Continued)*

	All races*		White		Black	
Period of gestation and birth weight	Twin births	Singleton births	Twin births	Singleton births	Twin births	Singleton births
40 weeks and over						
Live births‡	10 934	1 808 297	8 440	1 490 095	2 084	243 648
Total (%)	100.0	100.0	100.0	100.0	100.0	100.0
Less than 1000 g (%)	0.4	0.0	0.4	0.0	0.6	0.1
1000–1499 g (%)	1.0	0.0	0.8	0.0	1.8	0.1
1500–1999 g (%)	4.3	0.2	3.8	0.1	6.7	0.4
2000–2499 g (%)	20.2	1.4	18.4	1.1	27.7	3.0
2500–2999 g (%)	38.3	10.4	38.0	9.0	39.0	17.9
3000–3499 g (%)	27.5	35.7	29.4	34.4	19.7	41.9
3500–3999 g (%)	7.3	36.5	8.1	38.0	4.2	28.1
4000 g or more (%)	1.0	15.9	1.1	17.3	0.3	8.5
Less than 2500 g (%)	25.9	1.6	23.3	1.3	36.8	3.5

*Includes races other than white and black; †includes births with period of gestation not stated; ‡includes births with birth weight not stated, which are excluded from the computation of the percent distribution

singleton to have a 5-min score of less than 7 (7.1% compared with 1.6%). About seven out of ten twins, compared with about nine out of ten singletons, had high 5-min scores of 9 or 10. Large differentials in 5-min Apgar scores by plurality are evident for both races.

As stated previously, the birth weight of twins is less favorable than that of singletons. About 50% of twins weigh less than 2500 g at birth compared with 6% of singletons. Weight at birth is highly correlated with Apgar scores. At 1 min after birth, low-birth-weight babies are about nine times as likely as those of higher weights to be classified as severely depressed (scores of 0 to 3), and about three times as likely to be classified as moderately depressed (scores of 4 to 6). Differentials by birth weight are even larger for 5-min Apgar scores. This is one of the major reasons for the relatively high proportion of twin births with low 1- and 5-min scores. An additional reason is that a very high proportion of twins are delivered by Cesarean section. In 1986, almost two-thirds of twin deliveries, compared with about one-quarter of singleton deliveries, were by Cesarean section[11]. Apgar scores at 1- and 5-min are both lower for Cesarean than for vaginal deliveries (unpublished data from the 1980 National Natality Survey of the National Center for Health Statistics).

Comment

The health status of twin infants at birth is far more precarious than is the case for singletons. The lower birth weight and higher incidence of preterm delivery for twin births may be associated with other disabilities. A study of congenital anomalies and birth injuries among live births found that the overall incidence of congenital defects was 18% higher among births in plural than in single deliveries, and that for almost all anomalies examined, there was a higher incidence for plural births. Additionally, there was a far greater likelihood of brain, bone, or nerve injury at birth for a multiple than for a single birth[12]. With the continuing growth in the number of twin births in the United States, research into the prevention of preterm delivery and low birth weight for multiple births is of increasing importance.

Beginning with the 1989 data year, a wealth of new information relevant to the demo-

Table 8 Percentage distribution of twin and singleton live births by 1- and 5-min Apgar scores and race of child: total of 46 reporting states and the District of Columbia, 1987

Apgar score	All races*		White		Black	
	Twin births	Singleton births	Twin births	Singleton births	Twin births	Singleton births
1-min score						
Live births†	63 817	2 880 766	48 681	2 251 521	13 481	526 830
Total (%)	100.0	100.0	100.0	100.0	100.0	100.0
0–3 (%)	8.0	2.1	6.9	1.8	12.5	3.6
4–6 (%)	14.2	6.6	13.7	6.4	16.2	7.7
7–8 (%)	50.1	49.0	51.3	49.8	45.3	45.2
9–10 (%)	27.7	42.2	28.1	42.0	26.0	43.5
Less than 7 (%)	22.2	8.8	20.5	8.2	28.7	11.3
5-min score						
Live births†	63 817	2 880 766	48 681	2 251 521	13 481	526 830
Total (%)	100.0	100.0	100.0	100.0	100.0	100.0
0–3 (%)	2.8	0.5	2.3	0.4	4.9	1.0
4–6 (%)	4.3	1.1	3.8	0.9	6.1	1.8
7–8 (%)	20.9	9.5	20.5	9.3	23.0	10.5
9–10 (%)	71.9	89.0	73.5	89.5	66.0	86.7
Less than 7 (%)	7.1	1.6	6.1	1.3	11.0	2.8

*Includes races other than white and black; †includes births with Apgar score not stated which are excluded from the computation of the percentage distribution
Note: Excludes data for California, Delaware, Oklahoma and Texas, which did not report Apgar scores on the birth certificate

graphic and health aspects of multiple births will become available from the revised US Standard Certificate of Live Birth. Included on the new certificate are questions relating to medical risk factors of pregnancy, such as anemia, pregnancy-associated hypertension and eclampsia; and complications of labor and delivery, such as fetal distress and dysfunctional labor. In addition, information will be collected on life style factors – tobacco and alcohol use, and weight gained during pregnancy – as well as method of delivery, and abnormal conditions and congenital anomalies of the newborn[13]. This new information, combined with other socioeconomic and health data available from birth certificates, will provide a clearer and more complete picture of the risks of multiple delivery than is presently obtainable from periodic sample surveys.

Previous versions of the live-birth certificate included open-ended questions on the health of the mother and child, but these were poorly completed. The present revision uses check boxes to obtain such information, and it is believed this will elicit better reporting by providing a more exact description of what information is desired. However, the usefulness of these new items is highly dependent on how carefully birth certificates are completed. It is hoped that recognition by the medical community that the revised birth certificate is a unique source of information on the medical and demographic aspects of birth will stimulate more accurate and complete reporting.

References

1. Taffel, S.M. (1992). Health and demographic characteristics of twin births: United States, 1988. *Vital Health Stat.*, **21**, 1–17
2. Botting, B.J., MacDonald Davies, I. and MacFarlane, A.J. (1987). Recent trends in the incidence of multiple births and associated mortality. *Arch. Dis. Child.*, **62**, 951
3. Danforth, D.N. (1990). *Danforth's Obstetrics and Gynecology*, (6th edn). (Philadelphia: Lippincott)
4. Gittelsohn, A.M. and Milham, S. Jr (1965). Observations on twinning in New York State. *Br. J. Prev. Soc. Med.*, **19**, 8–17
5. Heuser, R.L. (1967). Multiple births: United States, 1964. *Vital Health Stat.*, **21**(14), 1–50
6. Williams, J.W. (1976). *Williams Obstetrics*, (15th edn.) (New York: Appleton-Century-Crofts)
7. Yerushalmy, J. and Sheerar, S.E. (1940). Studies on twins. I. The relation of order of birth and age of parents to the frequency of like-sexed and unlike-sexed twin deliveries. *Hum. Biol.*, **12**, 95–113
8. Querec, L. and Spratley, E. (1978). Characteristics of births, United States, 1973–75. *Vital Health Stat.*, **21**(30), 1–49
9. American College of Obstetricians and Gynecologists (1989). *Multiple Gestation*, ACOG Technical Bulletin No. 131. (Washington: ACOG)
10. Bulmer, M.G. (1970). *The Biology of Twinning in Man.* (Oxford: Clarendon Press)
11. Placek, P.J. and Taffel, S.M. (1988). Recent patterns in Cesarean delivery in the United States. *Obstet. Gynecol. Clin. N. Am.*, **15**, 607–27
12. Taffel, S.M. (1978). Congenital anomalies and birth injuries among live births: United States, 1973–74. *Vital Health Stat.*, **21**(31), 1–58
13. Taffel, S.M., Ventura, S.J. and Gay, G.A. (1989). Revised US Certificate of Birth – new opportunities for research on birth outcome. *Birth*, **16**, 188–93

The epidemiology of multiple births in Europe

11

R. Derom, J. Orlebeke, A. Eriksson and M. Thiery

Secular trends

Twinning rates vary considerably in different parts of the world. In Europe and North America, for example, the twinning rate averaged between 12 and 14 per 1000 maternities during the first seven decades of this century. In contrast, it was only about six per thousand in Japan[1] and about 40 per thousand in Nigeria[2,3] during these same years. Considered over the past three centuries, the secular twinning rate has varied widely in those countries in which records were kept. Prior to 1900, several, albeit unknown, conditions led to considerably higher twinning rates than have been recorded in the twentieth century. In the Scandinavian countries, for example, the frequency of twin births was about 17 per thousand maternities during the second part of the 18th century and even higher (more than 20‰) in areas with a low migration rate, such as the islands in the Baltic sea[4]. The fluctuations in twinning rate over the last 250 years in Sweden are illustrated in Figure 1.

Since 1900, the twinning rate in most European countries has stabilized around 11 to 12 per thousand, presumably because of the disappearance of isolated societies within nations and the concomitant process of industrialization and urbanization[5], but predominantly because of a gradual decline in the mean maternal age and a lower total number of maternities per woman (parity). When twinning rates in different countries and different years are corrected for differences in maternal age and parity, temporal and regional variations in the twinning rate still

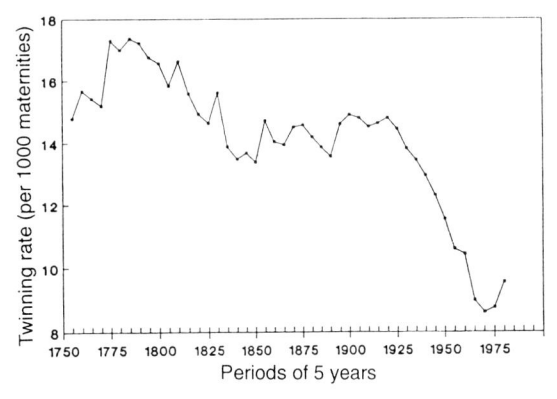

Figure 1 Secular variations in twinning rate in Sweden between 1756 and 1990. Data are averaged per 5-year period

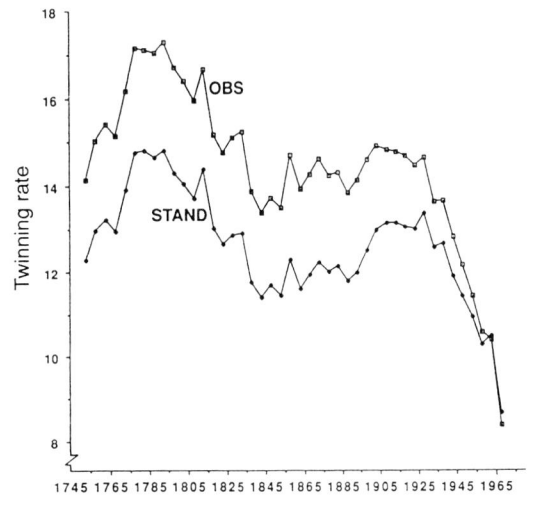

Figure 2 Secular variations in twinning rate in Sweden between 1751 and 1970. The upper curve shows the observed values (corresponding to those in Figure 1); the lower curve represents the same data, corrected for the effect on twinning rate of changes in maternal age

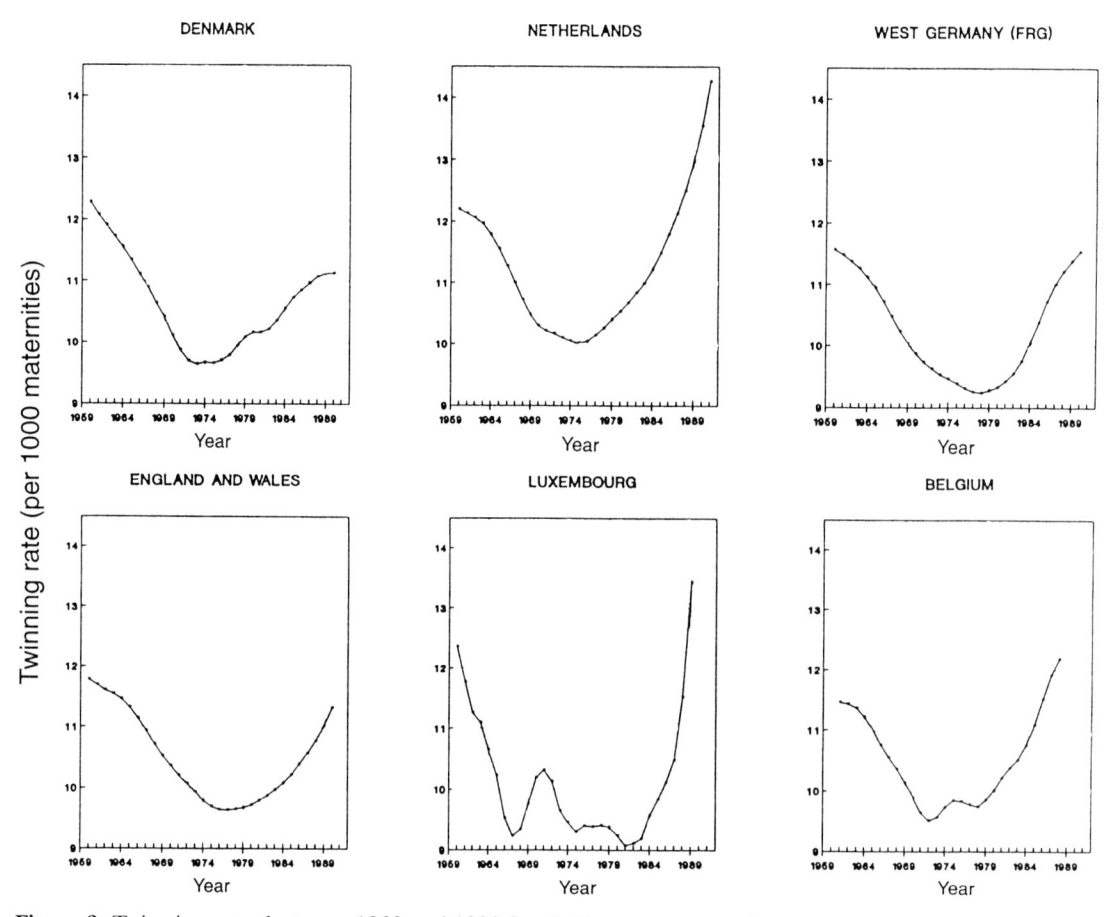

Figure 3 Twinning rates between 1960 and 1990 for six European countries

remain[5–7]. This is amply documented for Sweden during the period between 1870 and 1970[8,9] (Figure 2), a hundred-year period uncontaminated by modern obstetric techniques for the improvement of fertility.

After about 1960, a sudden rapid decline in the twinning rate was observed in most European countries. The nadir of this decline occurred in the middle of the 1970s when twinning rates fell to between 9 and 10 per 1000 maternities. Beyond that point, an equally rapid recovery to the pre-1960 figures – or even higher in recent years – took place. The U-shape of these shifts between 1960 and 1990 as occurred in six representative countries is shown in Figure 3.

The understanding of such a remarkable change in an otherwise rather stable biological phenomenon, presenting itself in nearly the same manner in several countries, is an epidemiological challenge. For the Netherlands (total population of about 15 million people), strong evidence exists that the decline in twinning rate between 1960 and 1975 can be ascribed predominantly to a parallel drop in maternal age at delivery. Several investigators[10,11] have demonstrated that the probability of a dizygotic (DZ) twin pregnancy is twice as great in mothers between 35 and 40 years of age compared to mothers below 25. In the Netherlands, the 1960–1975 fall in the total twinning rate was accompanied by a parallel decline in maternal age at delivery (operationalized as the percentage of deliveries by mothers of 30 years of age and over). These changes are shown in Figure 4.

Figure 4 also shows that the twinning rate increased again after 1975, as did mean maternal

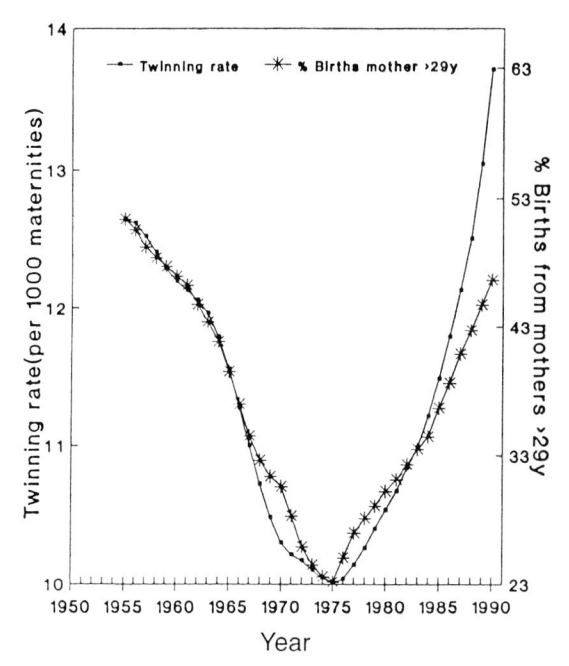

Figure 4 Correspondence in The Netherlands between changes in twinning rate and changes in maternal age (operationalized as percentage of maternities from mothers of 30 years and over). Recent years show a disproportional growth in twinning rate relative to increase in maternal age

age. After about 1984 the increase in the twinning rate became stronger than might be expected from the continuing increase in general maternal age. This 'additional' growth is very likely due to the increasing use of fertility-enhancing substances. The excess number of twin pairs (i.e. more than may be expected from the quantitative relationship between the twinning rate and the proportion of deliveries by mothers of ≥30 years) was about 300 in 1990, or about 10% of all twin pairs born in that year. This number equals the outcome of an independent calculation carried out by Merkus* (personal communication) based on the number of women treated with hormones, in most cases clomiphene citrate (Clomid®).

Stated another way, the left sides of the U-shaped curves in Figures 3 and 4 very likely reflect only the influence of a rapid change in the mean age at which women become pregnant (an interesting societal phenomenon, manifest in most European countries). In contrast, the right sides of the Us are produced by a combination of the increase in maternal age and the application of fertility-improving techniques. The relative contribution of these two factors (from the mid-seventies till now) obviously varies between countries.

Zygosity

It is not presently clear to which degree the epidemiological changes in twin prevalence cited above are related to the occurrence of DZ twins, monozygotic (MZ) twins or both. Figures 3 and 4 present data on all twin maternities. A classic method used frequently to estimate the relative contribution of MZ and DZ twin maternities to the total twinning rate was proposed by Weinberg[12,13] and applied many times since (see Chapter 2 and comments by others). This method assumes that the number of unlike-sexed DZ twin pairs equals that of like-sexed twin pairs. Therefore, twice the number of unlike-sex twin pairs is used as a fair estimate of the total number of DZ twin pairs. Subtracting the latter quantity from the total number of twins yields the number of MZ twins. Applying this method to a year-to-year time series of twin maternities in a given country consistently demonstrates that the changes in total twinning rate can predominantly be ascribed to changes in DZ twinning rate. In contrast, the MZ rate varies much less and hovers around 4 per thousand maternities. Figure 5 gives the results of the application of Weinberg's rule to recent twin prevalence figures in England and Wales and in the Netherlands.

Figure 5 also shows that the MZ twinning rate increased slightly after 1975. This trend has been recorded in several countries[14]. The hypothesis that the use of oral contraceptives is responsible for this phenomenon[15] appears to be untenable, because in several countries the increase in the MZ rate began before the (widespread) use of oral contraceptives, whereas in others it started later. A different

---

* Dr J.M.W.M. Merkus is gynecologist at the Maria Hospital in Tilburg, The Netherlands

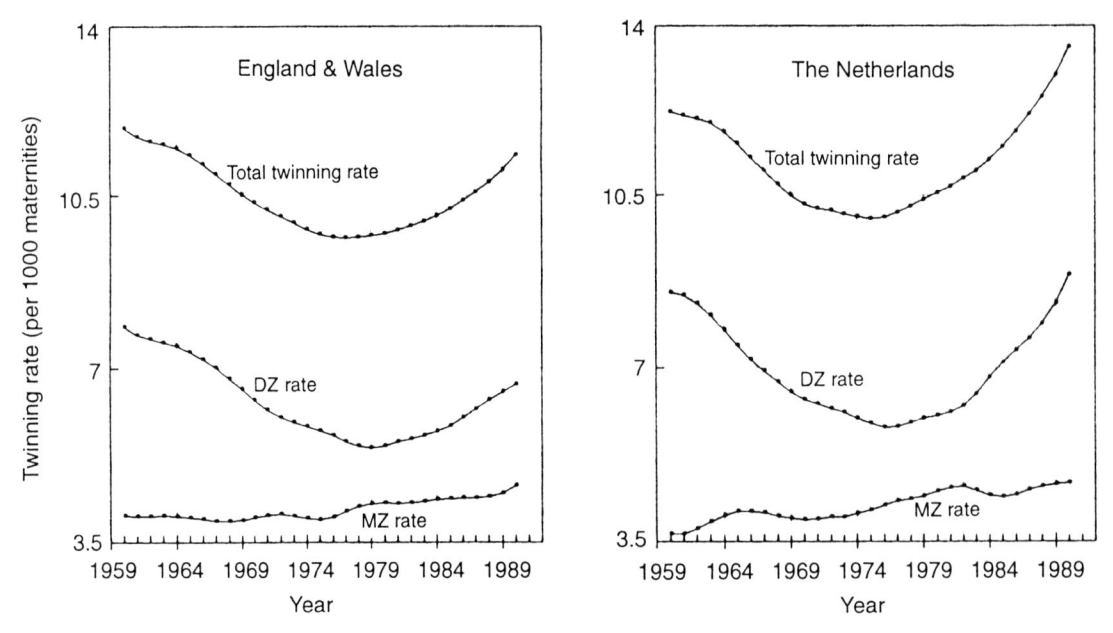

Figure 5 Application of Weinberg's differential rule to twin prevalence figures in England and Wales and in The Netherlands (1959–89)

explanation was proposed by Orlebeke et al.[16], who contend that the rise in the MZ twinning rate is the artificial consequence of another phenomenon, that is, the decrease in twin maternities of unlike sex relative to the number of DZ like-sexed twin maternities. If this latter hypothesis is true, then Weinberg's differential rule loses its basic assumption, that is, the equality of DZ like-sex and DZ unlike-sex prevalence. A relative low number of DZ unlike-sexed twin pairs automatically leads the Weinberg method to overestimation of the MZ rate[16]. Several other authors have also expressed doubt about the DZ like-sex DZ unlike-sex equality assumption[17-20] but still others[21,22] opine that the assumption underlying Weinberg's rule is correct – at least in some countries (see Chapter 2). This discussion is not purely academic, because the Weinberg rule is the major tool available for the study of trends in MZ and DZ twinning rates. A lively debate exists which we will try to summarize in the following paragraphs.

A number of authors[16-20] adhere for several reasons to the hypothesis of a change in the proportion of like/unlike-sex DZ twinning, a change leading to a flaw of the Weinberg rule. First, if one considers the Weinberg-based year-to-year time series of DZ and MZ twinning rates, then a basic prerequisite for the justification of the use of the Weinberg rule is the absence of a correlation between the two series. This is so because the underlying mechanisms of MZ and DZ twinning are unrelated (see Chapter 3). Only if some common external factor would influence the frequency of MZ and DZ twinning or if the assumption about equality of DZ like-sex and DZ unlike-sex frequencies is incorrect could a correlation between the two time series be expected. Orlebeke et al.[16] calculated this correlation for the Netherlands (period 1904–1989), Denmark (1910–1985), Sweden (1961–1985) and Norway (1931–1985). The Pearson correlations for each country were $r = -0.69$; $r = -0.42$; $r = -0.56$ and $r = -0.12$, respectively. A closer look at the data additionally reveals that the MZ twinning rate has increased very slowly from the beginning of the century till the present decade. Stated another way, the increase in 'Weinberg estimated' MZ frequency is not a recent phenomenon (although it has gone up during the last decade), but rather seems to have been present since the beginning of the century. In Germany, for example, the MZ twinning rate was about 3.25 during the second decade of this century, 3.70 during the sixties and about 4.4 during the last few years. A comparable trend is present in the Netherlands: 3.50 around 1915, 3.90 in the sixties and 4.60 during the last few years. In Denmark these figures are 3.67, 4.40 and 4.60, respectively, and for England and Wales 3.38 during the early forties (we did not analyze older data), 3.55 during the sixties and 4.50 in recent years. These arbitrarily selected examples make plausible the concept that a gradual shift in the Weinberg estimations of MZ twinning rate is not a phenomenon of the last one or two decades, but rather one that was present long before the introduction of oral contraceptives and ovulation-inducing drugs, although the latter might be held responsible for the very fast changes in MZ rate during the last decade.

Second, analysis of secular variations in sex combinations of twins in the Åland and the Åboland archipelagos (of Finland) demonstrates that the estimated rate of MZ twin maternities increased consistently during the six 50-year periods between 1650 and 1949[23]. It remains possible that this observation is the result of incompleteness of registration. Mistakes and omissions in the registrations may diminish the proportion of MZ twins because the frequency of stillbirths is higher among MZ than among DZ twins.

The above-mentioned negative correlation between the DZ and MZ time series, combined with the observations of James[20] and others, strongly suggests that the observed MZ twinning rate increase can be ascribed to a gradual shift in the DZ unlike-/DZ like-sex ratio from about unity (or maybe even higher than that) roughly during the first half of this century to less than unity in later years.

Another indication that the number of unlike-sex twin pairs is decreasing comes from the following observation. In all countries from which the total twinning rate is presented in Figure 3, the proportion of unlike-sexed pairs, relative to all twin pairs, is consistently higher (about 31.5%) during the period of a decreasing total twinning rate between about 1965 and 1975 relative to the comparable right part of the curve (about 29%). In other words,

Table 1 Mean proportion (%) of DZ unlike sex twin pairs relative to all twin pairs. Period 1: period of decreasing total twinning rate; period 2: comparable subsequent period of increasing total twinning rate

Country	Period	
	1	2
Belgium	29.9	27.8
Denmark	30.4	28.6
England and Wales	30.4	28.6
Netherlands	30.9	29.4
West Germany	31.0	28.9

when the total twinning rate is the same, then DZ unlike-sex twinning rate declines nevertheless. This trend is summarized in Table 1. It is possible that this observation reflects an increasing MZ rate. Figures from the Dutch Twin Register, however, support the former interpretation. Of 4186 twin pairs in the register (all children below the age of 6), zygosity was assessed by questionnaire filled out by the parents. The parents of 392 twin pairs did not answer the questions (mostly because they were too uncertain). From the remaining 4186 paris, 986 were classified as MZ, 1740 as DZ like sex and 1460 as DZ unlike sex. Application of the Weinberg rule would lead to an estimated number of MZ twins of 1266 (instead of 986) and a number of DZ twins of 2920 (instead of 3200).

The first group of authors[16–20] concluded that there must be some mechanism that has led to a decrease of the number of DZ unlike-sex twin pairs relative to the number of DZ like-sex pairs. The nature of that mechanism is still unclear; it has produced an artificial enhancement in the Weinberg-based estimations of MZ twinning rate during the last 10 to 20 years compared to earlier years. It is possible that the assumption of a constant MZ rate is better for the calculation of zygosity proportions than Weinberg's assumption that DZ unlike- and like-sex numbers are equal.

An opposite view has been put forward by a second group of authors who do not consider the presence of a correlation between the MZ and DZ twinning rates as a reason to invalidate the Weinberg rule. Bulmer[24], writing in 1970, stated: 'It should be observed that m (the MZ rate) and d (the DZ rate) are negatively correlated since the number of unlike-sexed twins occurs in the formulae for both of them but with a different sign. This negative correlation means that m is likely to be an overestimate of the true value when d is an underestimate, and vice versa.' Moreover, in a large population-based registry of multiple births, the East Flanders Prospective Twin Survey (EFPTS)[22], no reason was found to invalidate Weinberg's rule. This survey is characterized by accurate zygosity determinations (see Chapter 9). A total of 2589 twin pairs were investigated, of which 2577 were of known zygosity and placentation. The estimates of Weinberg's rule agreed well with the results of the direct zygosity determination. As pointed out by James[25], in the East Flanders study the area of uncertainty could be reduced in the group in which zygosity diagnosis is most difficult, that is, the group of same-sexed dichorionic pairs. In such pairs monozygosity cannot be diagnosed with certainty. In each pair, according to the number of similar markers, a probability of monozygosity should be computed which should reach at least 0.95 and ideally more than 0.99. In the EFPTS study, about half of the 401 same-sex dichorionic pairs classified as monozygotic had probabilities of monozygosity of less than 0.95. Husby et al.[26], describing a Danish series of 352 consecutive pairs in which direct determination of zygosity was performed, also came to the conclusion that their data were consistent with Weinberg's formulation. James[25] concluded his critical analysis by stating, 'The conclusion of both sets of authors that their data at present are consistent with Weinberg's rule is true but they are also consistent with the hypothesis that the rule is appreciably flawed.'

As suggested by James[25], one way to solve the controversy would be to retest those pairs (or those who survive), especially those with lower probabilities of monozygosity. The uncertain pairs would then be rediagnosed as DZ or reassigned a higher probability of monozygosity. Another way would be to perform population-based studies of placentation. Two-thirds of monozygotic twins are monochorionic. It follows that the number of MZ twins can be calculated by multiplying the number of monochorionic twins by 1.5.

The prevalence of triplets

Compared to the change in twinning rates during the last 15 years (about 30%, produced for the greater part by an increasing maternal age – at least in the Netherlands – and for the rest by use of fertility-enhancing techniques), the increase in triplet deliveries has been much more dramatic. In England and Wales and in West Germany, the triplet rate increased about 170% between 1975 and 1990. In the Netherlands, the increase was more than 300% and in Belgium (figures only available till 1988) still more. Figure 6 depicts the triplet rates between 1971 and 1990 for the countries just mentioned.

Without doubt, ovulation induction and IVF are the principal causes behind this change. Data on the etiology of triplet maternities were collected for 112 triplet sets born between the end of 1986 and the summer of 1991. All sets were part of the Dutch Twin Register. Only 30 sets were spontaneous; 39 were induced and 39 the result of IVF. Four sets were of unknown etiology. Most of the excess triplet sets are trizygotic. The epidemiological counterpart of the Weinberg rule for the estimation of zygosity proportions among triplets was proposed by Allen in 1960[27].

Number of MZ triplets = $L - \frac{1}{2}D - \frac{1}{4}T$

Number of DZ triplets = D = $2(MZ twinning\ \text{rate} \times DZ twinning\ \text{rate})N$

Number of TZ triplets = $T = (U - \frac{1}{2}D)1\frac{1}{3}$

In these formulas, L = number of like-sex triplets, U = number of unlike-sex triplets and N = total number of maternities. Application of the Allen formula to all triplets born in about the same period as the 112 registered triplet sets leads to estimated proportions of 4.5% MZ,

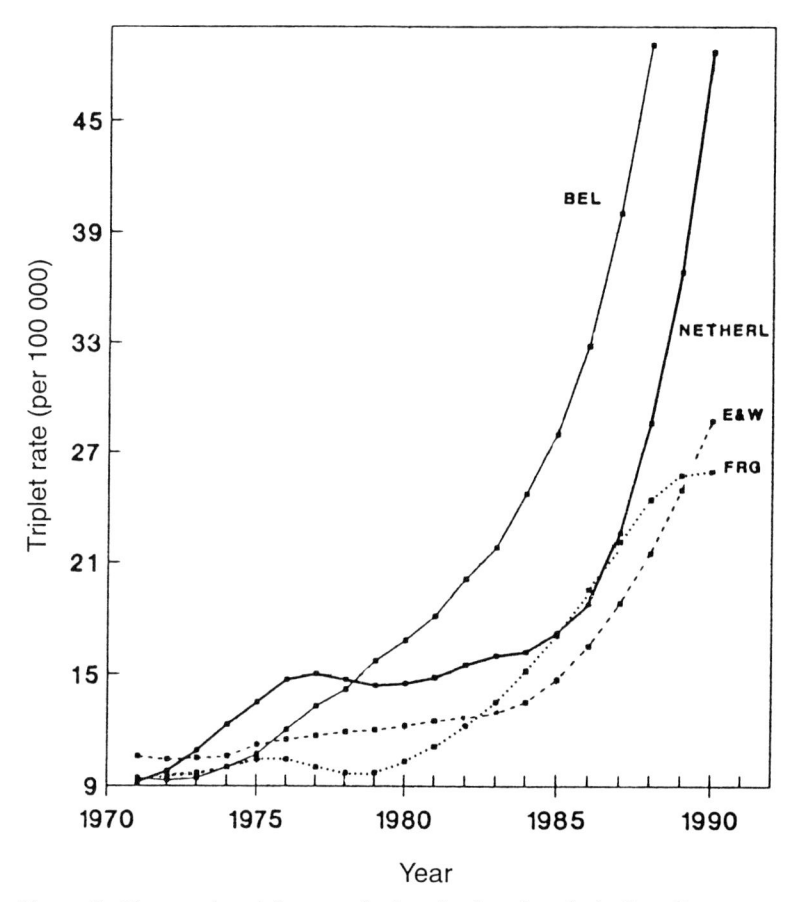

Figure 6 Changes in triplet rate during the last decade in four European countries. Bel, Belgium; Netherl, Netherlands; E & W, England and Wales; FRG, Germany

20.3% DZ and 75.2% TZ. This corresponds rather well with the empirical proportions among the registered 112 triplets: 6.3%, 21.4% and 72.3%, respectively. The Allen method thus seems to be a useful approximation for the estimation of zygosity rates in triplets. If we apply the method to triplet prevalence figures from before 1970 (i.e. when ovulation induction and IVF were still unknown or at least not widely used), zygosity proportions appear to be rather different from those of today, roughly about 20% of all triplets estimated to be MZ, 40% DZ and 40% TZ[28]. In other words, modern obstetric technology has not only increased the triplet rate in general, but has also changed the proportional contribution of zygosity types to the total number of triplets.

Factors determining twinning rates

Twinning rates are influenced by genetic and environmental factors. Some of the latter are undoubtedly related, a circumstance which increases the difficulty of assessing the importance of each factor on its own. Moreover, the actions of genes and environment are interrelated in some instances. Finally, highly significant temporal fluctuations also impact on many of these environmental variables. As a

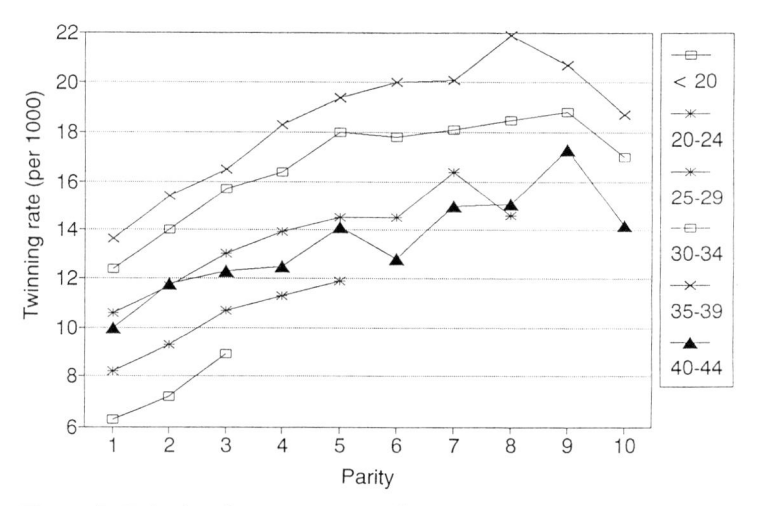

Figure 7 Twinning frequency according to maternal age and parity. England and Wales 1938–48. Drawn from data of Waterhouse[30]

result, great caution is required before assigning a significant role to any of the environmental variables discussed below.

Maternal age

Duncan[29], the famous Scottish obstetrician, was clearly aware of the relationship between maternal age and twinning frequency. In 1865, he stated: 'From the earliest childbearing period till the age of 40 is reached, that is till a period when fecundity has become extraordinarily diminished, the fertility of mothers in twins gradually increases.'

Waterhouse[30] analyzed the total births of England and Wales for the 10-year period, 1938–48 in an attempt to understand how the twinning rate varies with maternal age and parity (Figure 7). Clearly, increased maternal age and increasing parity exert separate and independent positive influences on the twinning rates. However, recent data from the USA[31] do not corroborate the British findings (Figure 8). According to data from Taffel (Chapter 10), only in first US births does the twinning rate increase with maternal age. After live-birth order one, the rates either remain approximately at the same level or are falling. This contrast is of interest and obviously must be explained. To begin with, the respective periods of observation differ by almost 50 years (1938 and 40 years (1948), respectively. During this time, essentially the second half of the 20th century, the entire way of life has changed dramatically. Of all possible changes, the status of women and their reproductive behavior has been modified in ways that could hardly have been conceived in the first part of the century. Much of this change relates to availability of contraception, age at first pregnancy, abortion on demand, smaller family size, infertility treatment and probably other factors as well. Further studies clearly are needed to track the reasons behind this remarkable new phenomenon in the epidemiology of twinning.

Parity

Both the British and American data show the positive influence of parity or live-birth order, respectively, on the twinning rate. There are no directional changes in these trends, as is the case with maternal age, but substantial changes are present in magnitude. Note, for instance, that in the age bracket of 25–29 years, the rates in 1938–48 increased by 37% from parity one to four (Figure 7) but this increase amounted to 129% in 1987 (Figure 8). This almost threefold difference also will require explanation by epidemiologists in the future.

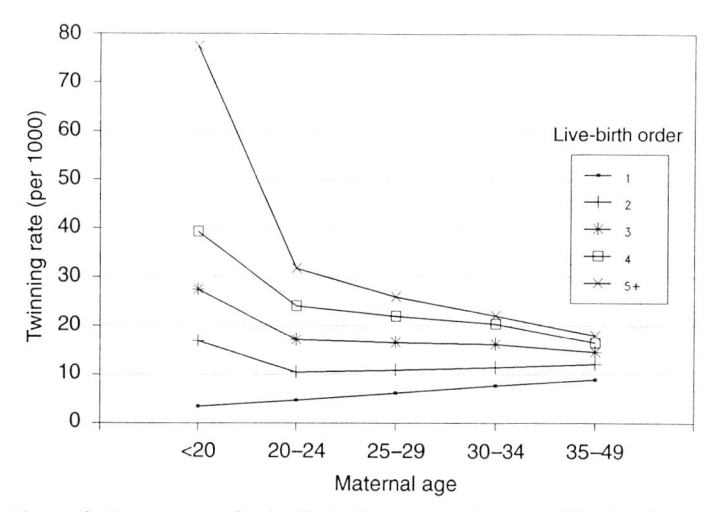

Figure 8 Frequency of twin births by maternal age and live-birth order. US whites, 1987. Drawn from data of Taffel[31]

Height

As long ago as 1877, Tchouriloff[32] suggested that an association was present between height and the rate of twinning in a population. He observed that men rejected for military service because of small stature came from various parts of Europe in which the rate of twinning was known to be low. Studies of the height of mothers of MZ and DZ twins performed in Oxford, England and Aberdeen, Scotland, respectively, support the hypothesis that mothers of DZ twins are taller than those of MZ twins. In reality, the mean difference between the two groups is estimated at 1.03±0.74 cm; mothers of MZ twins resemble mothers of singletons[33].

Geographic variation

The further north, the higher the twinning rate. This relationship, though, is far from close and is limited to DZ twinning. According to James[34], the correlation coefficient between latitude and age-standardized DZ twinning rates in Europe in the late fifties and the early sixties of this century reached a value of +0.68 ($p<0.01$). This trend seems consistent with time, because similar findings had been reported by Davenport[35] in 1930 for the total twinning rate. For US whites, the correlation is +0.54 ($p<0.001$); for US Blacks it is positive (+0.31) but not significant. Bulmer[24] speculated that geographic variations in DZ twinning rates in Europe may have some genetic basis. James[34] observed that there is no reason to suppose that genetic clones in the Old World are duplicated by latitude in the New World. Indeed, the fact that the latitudinal variations in DZ twinning are similar in Europe and the US suggests an environmental rather than genetic cause.

Superimposed on latitude variations are differences between countries and regions. It is not meaningful to report on all or even most national and/or regional figures. Only some examples of differences not fitting the latitude differences will be mentioned. Earlier in this chapter, Finish and Swedish twinning rates were noted to vary between the mainland and islands or groups of islands in which endogamy was important[4,5,23]. Data from France, collected between the years 1858 and 1865, show regional variations ranging from 8.1‰ in the south-west to 11.8‰ in Alsace/Lorraine in the north[36]. In Italy, between 1892 and 1904, not only was there a decrease from north to south, which fits the latitudinal model, but also, a higher frequency of twins was noted in the east as compared with the west, at least in the upper part of the country[37]. Finally, the twinning rate in the Irish Republic is higher than that in the United Kingdom. In 1968, it was 13.6‰ vs. 10.8‰ in Northern Ireland and 10.0‰ in England and Wales, respectively. Only part of the difference is accounted for by the higher age and, to a very small extent, the higher parity of the mothers of the Irish Republic, indicating that the standardized twinning rate is higher in Ireland[38].

Seasonality

Seasonality in the birth rate has been demonstrated in a number of European countries. The peak rate occurs in April–May and the troughs appear in November–December[39]. The question arises whether twinning rates show similar variations. It could even be surmised that during the more fertile months of the year the twinning rate would rise as well. According to James[40], there is good evidence that at least in England and Wales, the incidence of opposite-sexed (and by inference, dizygotic) twin births is seasonal, being about 5% higher in December than in June. Triplet births also show a similar seasonal variation but with double the magnitude. Evidence with regard to seasonal variation in monozygotic twinning rates is equivocal. Richter and co-workers[41] evaluated twinning rates over a period of 250 years (1611–1860) in Görlitz, Germany. The rates were relatively stable in the spring and fall, but varied greatly in the winter and summer. In contrast, analysis of data from the Aberdeen City District (1969–1983) showed little variation in either DZ or MZ twinning by month of last menstrual period[11]. These are but three reports of a voluminous literature which has been critically analyzed by MacGillivray and co-workers[11]. Unfortunately, in many studies clear-cut conclusions cannot be drawn, because of methodological problems, e.g. the use of improper statistical analysis, and the possibility that artifacts in seasonal patterns are caused by the determination of zygosity by the use of an indirect technique such as the Weinberg formula.

According to MacGillivray and co-workers[11] and this is also our view, the seasonal evidence has been inconclusive until the middle of this century. However, circumstances have changed during the last decade or, possibly since the 1970s. Figure 9 shows the seasonal variations in singleton and twin births in the Netherlands from 1987 to 1991. Peaks and troughs for twins are relatively higher and lower than for singletons. Considering the fact that as many as 50% of these pregnancies were planned in Western Europe during these years, one may safely view these variations as resulting from the parents' choice as to the best period of the year to have a baby. Since 1988, the seasonal variations are clearly more pronounced with the twin deliveries.

Genetics

Twins undoubtedly run in families. The mode of inheritance, however, is not clear. Most authors agree that mono- and dizygotic twinning must be considered separately and that the evidence for inheritance is much stronger in the latter. Although only a few studies have examined the heredity of MZ twinning, the strong similarity in their results is remarkable: on the one hand, there is a low increase in the probability of repeat MZ twinning among the relatives of MZ pairs; on the other, there are a small number of case studies of families with more than one pair of MZ twins among the first three degrees of relationship[42]. The best hypothesis seems to be one of monogenic, dominant inheritance with a low penetrance. However, the inheritance seems to be restricted to only a small fraction of the MZ twin families.

Weinberg[12] was the first to investigate the heredity of DZ twinning. He discovered that, in Stuttgart and the areas surrounding Württemberg, Germany, the twinning frequency was increased by almost 54% among mothers of twins, their sisters and daughters, but was not elevated or was even lower among the relatives of fathers of twins. He concluded that the inheritance of DZ twinning is restricted to the female line. A similar study was conducted in the Orkla valley in Norway[43]. Wyshak and White[44] analyzed the offspring of unlike-sexed twin pairs using the archives of the Genealogical Society of the Church of Jesus Christ of Latter Day Saints in Utah, USA. The DZ twinning

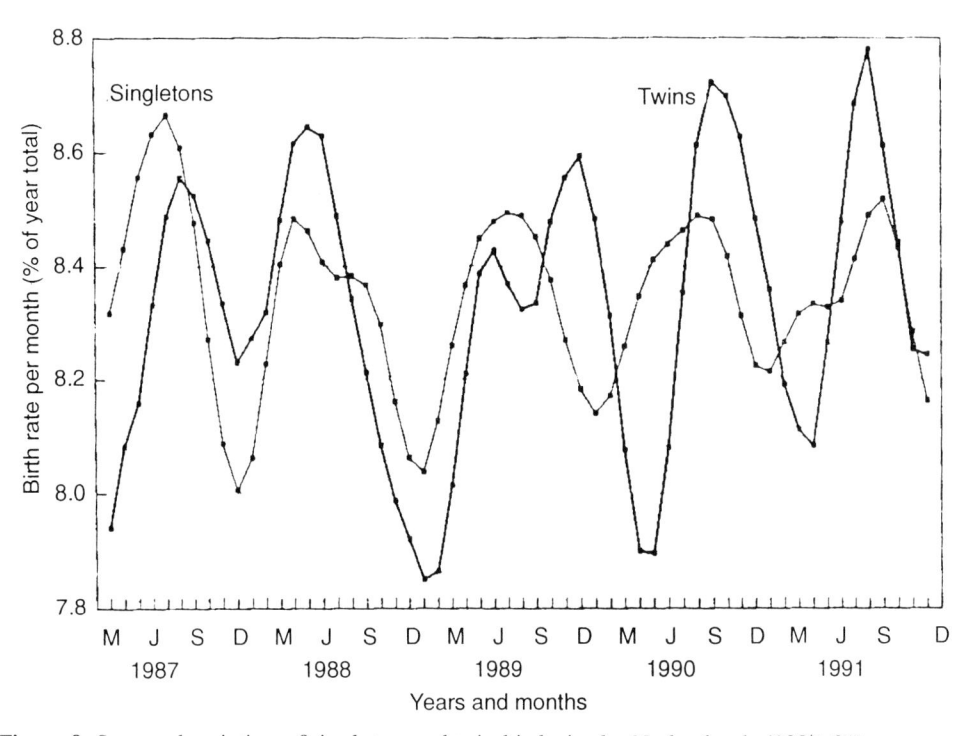

Figure 9 Seasonal variation of singleton and twin births in the Netherlands (1987–91)

frequency computed by the Weinberg method among the offspring of the female twins and their sisters amounted respectively to 14.45 and 16.52 per 1000 maternities compared to 6.86 per 1000 maternities among the offspring of the male co-twins. These findings led Wyshak and White to accept the theory of a maternal autosomal recessive mode of inheritance. Although this point of view is supported by earlier studies[12,43], questions about this type of research remain. Since the hereditary factor interferes with normal ovulation by causing the production of two or more ova, phenotypical proof of the presence of the gene or genes fails on the paternal side. The unobserved transmission in a pedigree through the males may mislead scientists. Indeed, instead of investigating the offspring of the male twin or his male sibs, scanning the offspring of the daughters of the male dizygotic twin and of his male sibs should reveal comparable results. This observation underlines once more the important problem of the sex-limited expression. No doubt rather large samples are needed to detect effects that are diluted 50% by additional segregation.

Eriksson and his co-workers[23,45,46] conducted extensive studies on the secular changes of the DZ twinning rates in Finland and Sweden. These two countries possess the oldest population statistics in the world for a whole nation. In the Åland archipelago in the Northern Baltic Sea, for example, as well as in Sweden, the dizygotic twinning rate has decreased, particularly in the past half century. Until recently, these island populations, particularly the outer parishes, had DZ twinning rates which were significantly higher than on the mainlands of Sweden and Finland. The higher frequencies of multiple maternities in these insular populations may well reflect the effect of inbreeding and endogamy. Indeed, these populations, which have descended from a relatively small group of founding settlers, have a more markedly decreasing trend of twinning, especially DZ twinning, compared to mainland populations. This steep decline in twinning cannot be explained simply by a lower maternal age and parity. The decrease may be partly a consequence of the changes in matrimonial migration patterns, by breaking up of the isolation and by reducing the endogamy. In this case, the high twinning frequencies of previous centuries in these islands are consistent with a recessive mode of inheritance for the dizygotic twinning process.

In the recent analysis of the multiple births by Eriksson et al.[47], high frequencies of multiple maternities were found on the maternal side of families with triplets. The twinning rate among families of mothers with triplets was four times that of normal mothers. According to the senior author of this investigation, a simple genetic model is not sufficient to explain this high frequency. Eriksson's hypothesis is that this higher propensity for twinning, particularly on the maternal side, is caused by multifactorial inheritance.

To conclude, in the majority of instances, the inheritance of DZ twinning possibly results from a recessive character caused by an unknown number of genes. However, recessiveness does not seem to be the only potential mode of inheritance. Indeed, several authors[24,43,48] have already suggested that other modes of inheritance must also be investigated for a dimensionally undefined group of twin mothers. Besides the genetic propensity, environmental factors, such as maternal age, parity and race, increase the individual probability of twin-bearing.

Considering the variety of models which have been suggested up to now and especially the necessity to investigate more fully the hereditary transmission through the female as well as the male line, our group has teamed up with the Genetic Epidemiology Division, Department of Medical Informatics, University of Utah, to conduct a large-scale study of the genetics of twinning on Belgian and Dutch population-based samples. The inheritance of spontaneous dizygotic twinning was investigated in 1422 three-generational pedigrees of mothers of spontaneous dizygotic proband twins. Dizygotic twinning was modelled as a trait of the mother and defined as a dichotomous phenotype. Complex segregation analysis showed that the trait of 'having dizygotic twins' was inherited by an autosomal monogenic dominant model with a gene frequency of 0.035 and a female-specific penetrance of 0.10^{49}.

The same model applies to dizygotic twinning among relatives of induced dizygotic twins, i.e. twins born after artificial induction of ovulation, one of the many modes of treatment of infertility. It seems, therefore, that women over-reacting to the administration of ovulation-inducing drugs are those carrying the twinning gene[50].

Infertility treatment

Recent data pertaining to twin- and triplet-delivery rates in six European nations have been analyzed in the first part of this chapter. Part of the increase has resulted from treatment of infertility. In the East Flanders Prospective Twin Survey (EFPTS) the origin of the pregnancy has been recorded since 1976. From January 1, 1976 to December 31, 1991, a total of 437 multiple births that resulted from artificial induction of ovulation (AIO) were recorded. Only the pregnancies in which one of the children weighed more than 500 g or, if birthweight was unknown, the gestational age was ≥ 22 weeks, have been considered for the present discussion. The zygosities of these pregnancies were compared to the zygosities of spontaneously occurring multiple pregnancies in terms of their relative frequency. All dichorionic monozygotic twins and trichorionic dizygotic triplets born after AIO had a probability of monozygosity and dizygosity, respectively, of at least 0.95.

Figure 10 shows the yearly numbers of spontaneous and induced twin births registered by EFPTS between 1976 and 1992[51]. In 1976, the total number of registered twin births approached 140 per year, whereas by 1991 and 1992 the total numbered more than 200. Figure 10 clearly documents that the increase in the total number of twins is entirely due to the use of fertility-enhancing agents, because the number of spontaneous twin births did not rise appreciably during these years. Between 1976 and 1985 the number of induced twin births increased slowly but substantially, whereas after 1985 it was more dramatic. To be exact, AIO pregnancies accounted for more than one-

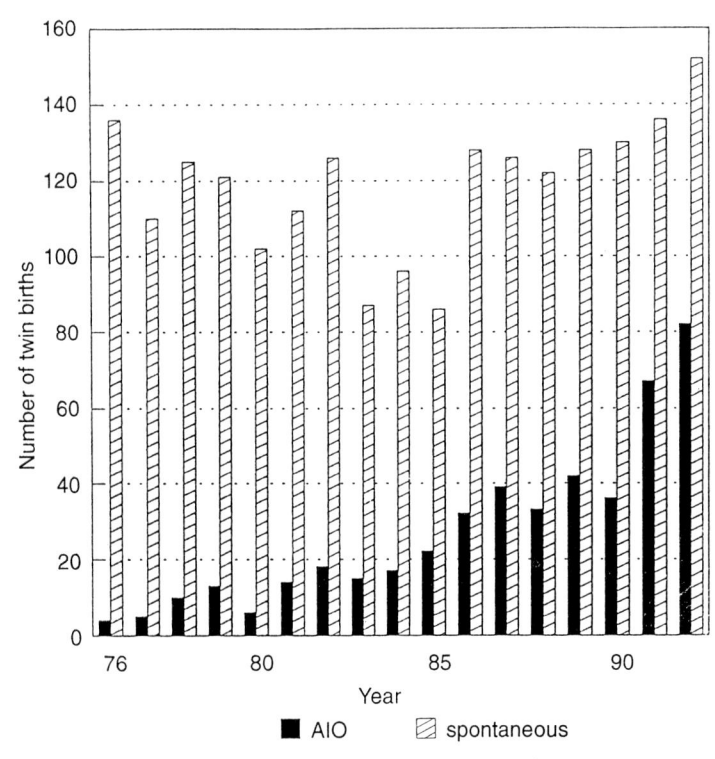

Figure 10 East Flanders Prospective Twin Survey, 1976–1992; yearly numbers of spontaneous and iatrogenic twins. Black bars, artificial induction of ovulation; hatched bars, spontaneous ovulation. (Reproduced from reference 51 with permission)

third of all twin births in 1991 and 1992. The decline in the number of spontaneous twin births during the years 1983, 1984 and 1985 was due to a decrease in the total number of births. Figure 11 extends the analysis by showing the relative frequency of twins and triplets born after AIO between 1976 and 1992. As was the case in the other countries cited above, the increase in the number of triplet births far outweighed the concomitant increase in the number of twin births.

Pooling the data over the years, Table 2 shows that most of the induced multiple gestations in Figures 10 and 11, do not result from the advanced technologies of assisted reproduction such as *in vitro* fertilization and embryo transfer (IVF–ET), gamete intrafallopian transfer (GIFT) and zygote intrafallopian transfer (ZIFT). Rather, they result from the use of fertility-enhancing drugs alone. In 80% of the iatrogenic twin pregnancies and 78% of the iatrogenic triplet pregnancies, AIO was the only treatment. Clomiphene and the sequential use of human menopausal and human chorionic gonadotropin were the regimes most commonly used in the mothers of these multiples. Before 1986, the use of IVF-ET, GIFT and ZIFT was limited in East Flanders. In the last four years, however, the number of pregnancies resulting from these procedures represented more than 35% of all induced twin pregnancies, so that their contribution to the increase in multiple births can no longer be neglected or denied (Figure 11).

In contrast to common expectation, all induced twin and triplet pregnancies were not dizygotic or trizygotic (Table 3). As reported earlier[52], the frequency of zygotic splitting after AIO (1.0%) is higher than observed after spontaneous ovulation (0.45%). There is no significant difference in the rate of zygotic division between the pregnancies which resulted

MULTIPLE PREGNANCY

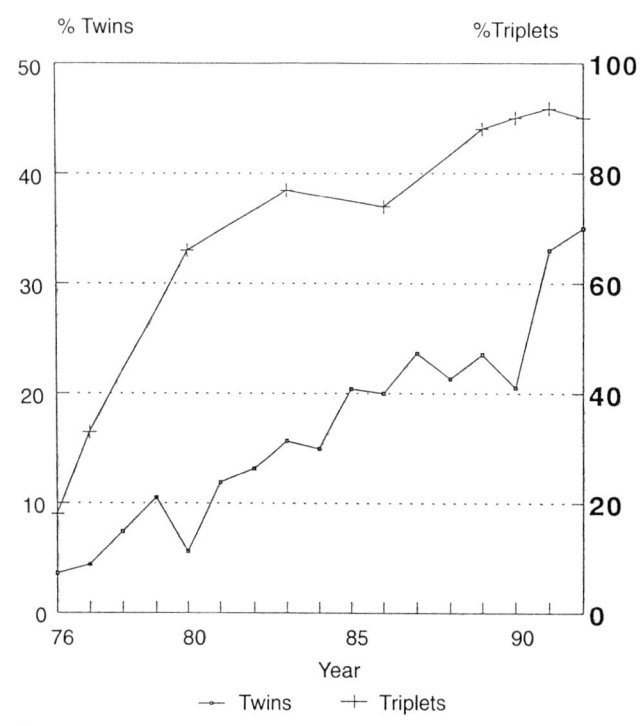

Figure 11 East Flanders Prospective Twin Survey: relative frequency of induced twin and triplet maternities

from AIO only and those which occurred after IVF-ET, GIFT or ZIFT, nor between the pregnancies induced by clomiphene and those induced by gonadotropins.

The increase in the rate of multiple pregnancies represents an important public health problem. If this trend continues, the rates of very preterm births and very-low-birth-weight infants will undoubtedly rise, because the skew of multiple pregnancies with infants whose birth weight is less than 1500 g is dramatic compared to singletons. Because very-low-birth-weight infants have high perinatal mortality and morbidity rates, they represent a high cost to the community in terms of an increased patient load to the neonatal intensive care units and an increased number of lifelong physical and mental handicaps[53–55].

The fact that a number of monozygotic twins are born after AIO and that the frequency of zygotic division after AIO is higher than after naturally occurring ovulation is of fundamental biological importance. It is clear that hormonal induction of ovulation acts not only on the ovary but also on the zygote in as much as it stimulates division. Up to now no conditions were known which could influence the monozygotic twinning rate. Treatment with clomiphene and/or gonadotropins is the first exception.

Sex proportion

The proportion of males in multiple births has been and still is a matter of lively debate. Clearly, there are differences between singleton and multiple births. The question remains, however, as to the explanation for these differences and whether the differences could throw some light on the mechanisms of the human sex proportion at birth.

The proportion of males in the human species decreases with each increase in the number of fetuses per pregnancy. An overview of the sex proportion for 31 million singletons and some ¾ million multiple births in the white population of the United States is shown in Table 4[56].

Table 2 East Flanders Prospective Twin Survey: 1976–1991. Multiple pregnancies after artificial induction of ovulation

	Twins		Triplets	
AIO only	300	(80%)	50	(78%)
IVF–ET, GIFT or ZIFT	73	(20%)	14	(22%)
Total	373		64	

AIO, artificial induction of ovulation; IVF–ET, *in vitro* fertilization and embryo transfer; GIFT–ZIFT, gamete/zygote intrafallopian transfer

Table 3 East Flanders Prospective Twin Survey: 1976–1991. Zygosity of twins and triplets born after artificial induction of ovulation

	Twins	Triplets
Monozygotic (MZ)	25	0
Dizygotic (DZ)	347	7
Trizygotic (TZ)	—	57
Unknown	1	—
Total	373	64

Frequency of zygotic splitting in iatrogenic DZ twinning:

$$\frac{\text{number of DZ triplets}}{2 \times \text{number of (DZ twins + DZ triplets)}} = \frac{7}{2 \times (347 + 7)} = 0.010$$

Twins

In twins, the low sex proportion is for the greater part due to the monozygotic twins (Table 5). In the EFPTS series, the sex proportions of the dizygotic pairs and the singletons did not differ significantly. To our knowledge, no other studies comparing the sex proportion between MZ and DZ twins and singletons have been published. James has studied the sex proportion extensively and has reviewed the literature on monozygotic twins whose sex was ascertained at birth[57–59]. Adding the data from nine studies on Caucasian samples with known placentation, the proportions were as follows: overall 0.499, monochorionic twins 0.492 (in five of the nine reports monoamnionic twins have been omitted) and dichorionic twins 0.571 (only three of the nine authors reported data on these twins). The proportion of 0.499 is lower, but not significantly lower, than that estimated for all Caucasian twins, 0.5047 ± 0.001, by Bulmer[24]. James concludes that there is direct (though admittedly inconclusive) evidence here that MZ twins have a lower sex proportion than DZ twins.

According to our data from East Flanders and data from the literature, it may be concluded that the sex proportion in MZ twins with monochorionic placentas is lowered, albeit to a smaller extent in the diamnionic and a much greater extent in the monoamnionic variety. One can only speculate about the reasons for this remarkable biological phenomenon. Various hypotheses have been put forward. Guerrero[60] and James[61] independently suggest that the sex of a human zygote is influenced by the time of its formation within the menstrual cycle, with more male zygotes being formed on the average both early and very late in the cycle, whereas more female zygotes are formed during the middle of the cycle. Experiments in lower vertebrates such as fish, amphibians and chickens have led to monozygotic twins by retarding the development of the fertilized ova, depriving them of oxygen, or maintaining them at a lower temperature (see Chapter 3). Delayed ovulation seems to induce monozygotic twinning in rabbits[62]. As suggested by James, it seems possible that the delay hypothesized as being associated with the formation of female zygotes runs parallel with the delay associated with the splitting of the ovum. If this is the case, then monozygotic twins could be composed of a higher proportion of females.

One or two per cent of monozygotic pairs of twins share the chorion and the amnion at birth. They represent twinning that occurred after the differentiation of the amnion (about day 7). Incomplete splitting of the embryo gives rise to conjoined twins and could occur even later, after the second week of development. Because of the rarity of conjoined twins, it is as yet unknown whether further subdivision of the monoamnionic twins in unjoined and conjoined pairs will clarify the enigma of their very low sex proportion. As only three conjoined pairs (all of them female) emerged in our relatively large series, only a registry of almost continental scale could provide the amount of data needed to answer

Table 4 Sex proportion (% males) in US white births (1933–48)

Singletons	51.59
Twins	50.85
Triplets	49.54
Quadruplets	46.48

Table 5 Sex proportion (%) in the East Flanders Prospective Twin Survey according to zygosity and placentation (2811 pairs)

Dizygotic	51.8
Monozygotic	
DC	49.3
MC–DA	49.3
MC–MA	23.1
All	48.7

this question. It is well documented that conjoined twins include a high proportion of girls[62] (see Chapter 8).

It is useful to inquire if female embryos are more likely to undergo delayed splitting than male embryos or if embryonal or fetal mortality in the late-splitting group predominantly affects the male embryos. In their series of spontaneously aborted twins, Uchida *et al.*[63] found two male conjoined pairs with normal chromosomes, the result of consecutive abortions in the same mother. Because both conjoined twins and male monoamnionic twins are rare, this single finding could suggest a predominantly male early fetal mortality in monoamnionic twins. With regard to the first question, Burn *et al.*[64] hypothesized that unequal lyonization may represent a cause of late twinning unique to female embryos. If this is true, analysis of the DNA methylation patterns of the X chromosome[65] of monoamnionic twins should throw more light on the question. The sex proportion discussed so far deals with spontaneous twinning, rather than iatrogenic twins. A series of studies have addressed this question, but the results are not in agreement. No large-scale population-based enquiries have been performed. Hence, one can question whether the samples are representative. In the EFPTS, the sex of the iatrogenic and the spontaneous DZ twins do not differ significantly.

Triplets

One finding of the increase in triplet rates (especially TZ) is a decreasing sex ratio. In the population in general about 1000 girls are born per 1045 boys: a sex ratio of 1.045. Among the 336 triplet individuals from the Dutch Twin Register there were 157 boys and 179 girls: a sex ratio of 0.89. The Dutch population triplet sex ratio (i.e. triplets born during about the same period as the sample studied) is 0.87. A closer look at the triplet sets with different etiology reveals that only among the induced triplets does the sex ratio deviate significantly from unity: 50 boys and 67 girls. This supports James' hypothesis[66–68] that hormonal induction of ovulation increases the mother's gonadotropin levels at the time of conception and that this in turn increases the probability of male offspring. In the EFPTS, however, opposite results are found: 47 girls and 66 boys.

Whether the decreasing sex ratio in triplets is unevenly distributed among the three zygosity groups is unknown. Very few population-based studies of zygosity in triplets have been published. In all of these the number of cases is too small to enable one to come to a firm conclusion.

Acknowledgements

Aided by grants no. 3.0038.82 of the Fund for Medical Scientific Research (Belgium), of the Praeventiefonds (The Netherlands), no. 86/0823 of NATO, and of the Association for Scientific Research in Multiple Births (Belgium).

References

1. Imaizumi, Y. and Inouye, E. (1979). Analysis of multiple birth rates in Japan. I. Secular trend, maternal age effect, and geographical variation in twinning rates. *Acta Genet. Med. Gemellol.*, **28**, 107
2. Nylander, P.P.S. (1971). Ethnic differences in twinning rates in Nigeria. *J. Biosoc. Sci.*, **3**, 151
3. Rehan, N. and Tafida, D.S. (1980). Multiple births in Hausa women. *Br. J. Obstet. Gynaecol.*, **87**, 997
4. Eriksson, A.W., Eskola, M.R. and Fellman, J.O. (1976). Retrospective studies on the twinning rate in Scandinavia. *Acta Genet. Med. Gemellol.*, **25**, 29
5. Eriksson, A.W. and Fellman, J.O. (1973). Differences in the twinning trends between Finns and Swedes. *Am. J. Hum. Genet.*, **25**, 141
6. James, W.H. (1982). Second survey of secular trends in twinning rates. *J. Biosoc. Sci.*, **14**, 481
7. Parisi, P. and Caperna, G. (1981). The changing incidence of twinning: one century of Italian statistics. In Gedda, L., Parisi, P. and Nance, W.E. (eds.) *Twin Research 3, Part A, Twin Biology and Multiple Pregnancy*, pp. 35–48. (New York: Alan R. Liss)
8. Fellman, J.O. and Eriksson, A.W. (1987). Statistical models for the twinning rate. *Acta Genet. Med. Gemellol.*, **36**, 297
9. Fellman, J.O. and Eriksson, A.W. (1990). Standardization of the twinning rate. *Hum. Biol.*, **62**, 803
10. Bulmer, M.G. (1976). Is Weinberg's method valid? *Acta Genet. Med. Gemellol.*, **25**, 25
11. MacGillivray, I., Samphier, M. and Little, J. (1988). Factors affecting twinning. In MacGillivray, I., Campbell, D.M. and Thomson, B. (eds.) *Twinning and Twins*, pp. 69–97. (Chichester: Wiley)
12. Weinberg, W. (1901). Beiträge zur Physiologie und Pathologie der Mehrlinggeburten beim Menschen. *Arch. Gesamte Physiol.*, **88**, 346
13. Weinberg, W. (1934). Differenzmethode und Geburtenfolge bei Zwillingen. *Genetica*, **16**, 282
14. Bressers, W.M.A., Eriksson, A.W. and Kostense, P.J. *et al.* (1987). Increasing trend in monozygotic twinning rate. *Acta Genet. Med. Gemellol.*, **36**, 397
15. Emery, A.E.H. (1986). Identical twinning and oral contraception. *Biol. Soc.*, **3**, 23
16. Orlebeke, J.F., Eriksson, A.W., Boomsma, D.I. *et al.* (1991). Changes in the DZ unlike/like sex ratio in The Netherlands. *Acta Genet. Med. Gemellol.*, **40**, 319
17. Renkonen, K.O. (1967). Is Weinberg's rule defective? *Ann. Hum. Genet.*, **30**, 277
18. Nylander, P.P.S. and Corney, G. (1969). Placentation and zygosity of twins in Ibadan, Nigeria. *Ann. Hum. Genet.*, **33**, 31
19. James, W.H. (1971). Excess of like sexed pairs of dizygotic twins. *Nature (London)*, **232**, 277
20. James, W.H. (1979). Is Weinberg's differential rule valid? *Acta Genet. Med. Gemellol.*, **28**, 69
21. Bulmer, M.G. (1959). The effect of parental age, parity and duration of marriage on the twinning rate. *Ann. Hum. Genet.*, **23**, 454
22. Vlietinck, R., Derom, C., Derom, R. *et al.* (1988). The validity of Weinberg's rule in the East Flanders Prospective Twin Survey (EFPTS). *Acta Genet. Med. Gemellol.*, **37**, 137
23. Eriksson, A.W. (1973). *Human Twinning in and around the Åland Islands*. Helsinki: Societas Scientiarum Fennica (academic dissertation)
24. Bulmer, M.G. (1970). *The Biology of Twinning in Man*. (Oxford: Clarendon Press)
25. James, W.H. (1992). The current status of Weinberg's differential rule. *Acta Genet. Med. Gemellol.*, **41**, 33
26. Husby, H., Holm, N.V., Gernow, A. *et al.* (1991). Zygosity, placental membranes and Weinberg's rule in a Danish consecutive twin series. *Acta Genet. Med. Gemellol.*, **40**, 147
27. Allen, G. (1960). A differential method for estimation of type frequencies in triplets and quadruplets. *Am. J. Hum. Genet.*, **12**, 210
28. Allen, G. (1988). Frequency of triplets and triplet zygosity types among US births, 1964. *Acta Genet. Med. Gemellol.*, **37**, 299
29. Duncan, J.M. (1886). *Fecundity, Fertility, Sterility and Allied Topics*. (Edinburgh: A & C Black)
30. Waterhouse, J.A. (1950). Twinning in twin pedigrees. *Br. J. Soc. Med.*, **4**, 197
31. Taffel, S.M. (1995). Demographic trends in twin births: USA. Chapter 10 in this book
32. Tchouriloff, M. (1877). Sur la statistique des naissances gémellaires et leur rapport avec la taille. *Bull. Soc. Anthrop. Paris*, **12**, 440
33. Corney, G., Seedburgh, D., Thompson, B. *et al.* (1979). Maternal height and twinning. *Ann. Hum. Genet.*, **43**, 55

34. James, W.H. (1985). Dizygotic twinning, birth weight and latitude. *Ann. Hum. Biol.*, **5**, 441
35. Davenport, C.B. (1930). Litter size and latitude. *Arch. Rassen. Ges. Biol.*, **24**, 87
36. Puechs, A. (1874). Des accouchements multiples en France et dans les principales contrées de l'Europe. *Ann. Hyg. Publ. II. Sér 41*, p. 197 (cited by Prinzing, reference 37)
37. Prinzing, F. (1907). Die örtlichen Verschiedenheiten der Zwillinghäufigkeit und deren Ursachen. *Z. Geburtsh. Gynäkol.*, **60**, 420
38. Dean, G. and Keane, T. (1972). An investigation of the high twinning rate in the Republic of Ireland. *Br. J. Prev. Soc. Med.*, **26**, 186
39. Huntington, E. (1938). *Season of Birth: Its relation to Human Abilities*. (New York: Wiley)
40. James, W.H. (1980). Seasonality in twin and triplet births. *Ann. Hum. Biol.*, **7**, 163
41. Richter, J., Miura, T., Nakamura, I. *et al.* (1984). Twinning rates and seasonal changes in Görlitz, Germany, from 1611 to 1860. *Acta Genet. Med. Gemellol.*, **33**, 121
42. Sedgwick-Harvey, M.A., Huntley, R.M.C. and Smith, D.W. (1977). Familial monozygotic twinning. *J. Pediatr.*, **90**, 246
43. Bonnevie, K. and Sverdrup, A. (1926). Hereditary disposition to dizygotic twin births in Norwegian peasant families. *J. Genet.*, **16**, 125
44. Wyshak, G. and White, C. (1965). Genealogical study of human twinning. *Am. J. Publ. Health.*, **55**, 1586
45. Eriksson, A.W. (1962). Variations in the human twinning rate. *Acta Genet.*, **12**, 242
46. Eriksson, A.W. and Fellman, G. (1967). Ethnological differences in twinning trends. *Scand. J. Clin. Lab. Invest.*, **19**, (Suppl. 95), 73
47. Eriksson, A.W., Bressers, W.M.A., Kostense, P.J. *et al.* (1988). Twinning rate in Scandinavia, Germany and the Netherlands during years of starvation. *Acta Genet. Med. Gemellol.*, **37**, 277
48. Eriksson, A.W. (1990). Genetic epidemiological aspects on variation in human twinning in Sweden. *VIIth Congress of the European Anthropological Association*
49. Meulemans, W.J., Lewis, C.M., Boomsa, D.I. *et al.* (1995). Genetic modelling of dizygotic twinning among relatives of spontaneous dizygotic twins. *Am. J. Med. Genet.*, submitted
50. Meulemans, W.J., Lewis, C.M., Boomsa, D.I. *et al.* (1994). Segregation analysis of dizygotic twinning in pedigrees of dizygotic proband twins conceived after artificial induction of ovulation. 44th Annual Meeting of the American Society of Human Genetics, Montreal, QE, Canada. *Am. J. Hum. Genet.*, **55** (Suppl.), Abstract 913
51. Derom, C., Derom, R., Vlietinck, R. *et al.* (1993). Iatrogenic multiple pregnancies in East Flanders, Belgium. *Fertil. Steril.*, **60**, 493
52. Derom, C., Derom, R., Vlietinck, R. *et al.* (1987). Increased monozygotic twinning rate after ovulation induction. *Lancet*, **1**, 1236
53. Keith, L., Papiernik, E. and Luke, B. (1991). The cost of multiple pregnancy. *Eur. J. Obstet. Gynecol. Biol. Reprod.*, **36**, 109
54. Luke, B. and Keith, L. (1992). The contribution of singletons, twins and triplets to low birthweight, infant mortality and handicaps in the United States. *J. Reprod. Med.*, **36**, 661
55. Luke, B., Minogue, J. and Witter, F.R. (1993). The role of fetal growth restriction and gestational age on length of hospital stay in twin infants. *Obstet. Gynecol.*, **81**, 949
56. Nichols, J.B. (1952). Statistics of births in the United States. *Am. J. Obstet. Gynecol.*, **64**, 376
57. James, W.H. (1975). Sex ratio in twin births. *Ann. Hum. Biol.*, **2**, 365
58. James, W.H. (1977). The sex proportion of monoamnionic twin pairs. *Ann. Hum. Biol.*, **4**, 143
59. James, W.H. (1980). Sex ratio and placentation in twins. *Ann. Hum. Biol.*, **7**, 273
60. Guerrero, R. (1970). Sex ratio: a statistical association with the type and time of insemination in the menstrual cycle. *Int. J. Fertil.*, **15**, 221
61. James, W.H. (1971). Cycle day of insemination, coitus rate and sex proportion. *Lancet*, **1**, 112
62. Bomsel-Helmrich, O. and Papiernik-Birkhauer, E. (1976). Delayed ovulation and monozygotic twinning. *Acta Genet. Med. Gemellol.*, **25**, 73
63. Uchida, I.A., Freeman, V.C.P., Gedeon, M. *et al.* (1983). Twinning rate in spontaneous abortion. *Am. J. Hum. Genet.*, **35**, 987
64. Burn, J., Povey, S., Boyd, Y. *et al.* (1986). Duchenne muscular dystrophy in one of monozygotic twin girls. *J. Med. Genet.*, **23**, 494
65. Fearon, E.R., Winkelstein, J.A., Civin, C.L. *et al.* (1987). Carrier detection in X-linked agammaglobulinemia by analysis of X-chromosome inactivation. *N. Engl. J. Med.*, **316**, 427
66. James, W.H. (1985). The sex ratio of infants born after hormonal induction of ovulation. *Br. J. Obstet. Gynaecol.*, **92**, 299
67. James, W.H. (1985). Sex ratio, dominance status and maternal hormone levels at the time of conception. *J. Theor. Biol.*, **114**, 505
68. James, W.H. (1986). Hormonal control of sex ratio. *J. Theor. Biol.*, **118**, 427

The role of birth weight, gestational age, race and other infant characteristics in twin intrauterine growth and infant mortality

W.F. Powers, J.L. Kiely and M.G. Fowler

Introduction

The fact that twins are at high risk of multiple adverse outcomes is a recurrent theme throughout this text. In the current literature, demographic characteristics, such as race, gender, birth order, birth weight and gestational age are considered risk factors for unfavorable outcomes, particularly neonatal and infant death[1-4]. Additional characteristics, such as gender pair status (like gender vs. unlike gender) and zygosity, are also deemed risk factors for mortality among twin infants[5]. Unfortunately, the studies that examine infant factors associated with increased mortality among twins during the first year of life provide inconsistent results. For example, some investigators describe higher mortality rates for second born twins[6,7], whereas others do not[8,9]. Similarly, reported differences in mortality rates of like gender vs. unlike gender twins are inconsistent[4,9-10], although almost all studies in which zygosity is known report higher mortality rates for monozygotic twins (particularly monoamniotic twins) compared to dizygotic twins[11].

This chapter uses the US National Natality files[12] to generate intrauterine growth curves for twins and the Linked Birth/Infant Death files[13] to analyze the risk of neonatal and infant death for US black and white twins. Attention will focus upon:

(1) Race-specific intrauterine growth of twins as a function of gestational age;

(2) Comparison of twin and singleton neonatal and infant mortality rates by birth weight and gestational age categories;

(3) Examination of gender difference among twin pairs as a predictor of mortality; and

(4) Definition of a critical duration of pregnancy, which, if not attained, is associated with delivery of twins at very high risk of infant death, as well as the probability of delivery during this critical period.

Before proceeding further, it is necessary to describe specific caveats regarding use of these national data sources. During the years under analysis, the gestational ages recorded on birth certificates were based on the last menstrual period (LMP). In the opinion of some investigators, gestational age estimates based on menstrual dating are frequently erroneous, not necessarily random and offsetting, and potentially systematic and capable of introducing bias[14-16]. Consider, for example, the woman whose best estimate of her LMP is 'the end of October'. If she delivers at a time which would result in an estimate of gestational age of 32 to 34 weeks and the baby is ill, the birth attendant would tend to assign her an LMP which yields a gestational age of 32 weeks. If, on the other hand, she delivers a relatively large and healthy baby, an LMP consistent with 34 weeks is more likely to be assigned. Thus, any prior knowledge of an infant's illness (or early death) might influence the assignment of an LMP, and the apparent relationship between short gestation and neonatal death might be strengthened.

Even though an exclusion algorithm (described below) was used to eliminate infants with implausible birth weight/gestational age combinations, some inaccuracies undoubtedly remain. Because the 1989 revision of the US Standard Birth Certificate not only captures LMP data, but also provides for recording gestational age based on clinical estimates, such as ultrasound, it is anticipated that the accuracy of gestational age as recorded on birth certificates will improve in the future and the potential for bias will diminish.

Despite any present limitations, gestational age information based on LMP is of substantial value. This is primarily because it is consistently available on birth certificates and in antenatal clinical settings. In contrast, birth weight data, although considered far more reliable, is not available until after the infant is born. Moreover, because gestational age is available prospectively and can enter into a variety of clinical decision making processes, outcome analyses based on gestational age are clinically relevant to providers of antepartum care.

The national data sets

The intrauterine growth curves for twins shown in Figure 1 and the race-specific birth weights by gestational age in Table 1 were generated from the twin subset of the 1985–88 National Natality files[12]. All live births to residents of the United States during those years are included. The 1983–85 US Linked Birth/Infant Death files from the National Center for Health Statistics (NCHS)[13] were used for other analyses of infant mortality among twins and singletons. In these files, the 1983 NCHS birth records were linked with infant deaths from the 1983–84 NCHS mortality files, and similar linkages were made for the 1984 and 1985 birth cohorts. These files include birth and death records of US residents that occurred within the US but exclude births and deaths of US residents which took place outside the United States.

Data preparation and analyses

The gestation-specific birth weight curves generated from the Natality files were bimodal at gestational ages under 38 weeks, with an

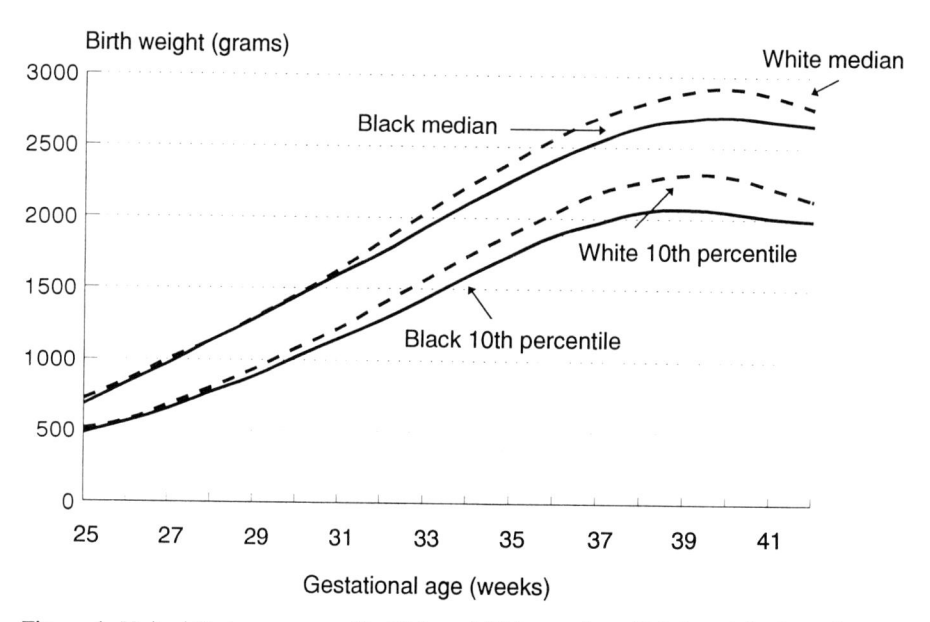

Figure 1 United States race-specific 10th and 50th centiles of birth weight for twins by gestational age (1985–88 data)

Table 1 Centiles of birth weight for US twin infants in 1985–88, by maternal race and gestational age

Gestational age in weeks	Whites			Blacks		
		Birth weight (g)			Birth weight (g)	
	Number	10th centile	50th centile	Number	10th centile	50th centile
25	1052	510	720	529	480	680
26	1216	570	850	636	560	830
27	1493	680	1000	690	650	970
28	1858	800	1130	748	770	1130
29	2279	930	1290	860	880	1280
30	2860	1080	1450	1116	1020	1440
31	4031	1220	1630	1336	1150	1600
32	5555	1390	1830	1749	1280	1750
33	8030	1560	2030	2313	1430	1930
34	12 075	1730	2220	3178	1590	2100
35	18 404	1890	2390	3922	1740	2260
36	25 107	2040	2560	5027	1880	2410
37	31 328	2180	2710	5689	1970	2540
38	33 440	2260	2810	5445	2050	2650
39	26 169	2310	2890	4786	2070	2700
40	15 055	2300	2920	2781	2050	2720
41	6499	2220	2870	1395	2010	2690
42	2979	2130	2780	738	1990	2660

upper, smaller mode generally appearing at about 3000 g. Because this distribution is biologically implausible, the upper mode was smoothed using a method similar to that described by other investigators[17,18]. Normally distributed curves then resulted. The 10th and 50th centiles of birth weight were then calculated for each week of gestation. Blacks and whites were analysed separately because of public health concerns about differences in the respective reproductive outcomes between these groups. Infants of Hispanic ethnicity were not routinely identified as such on birth certificates or in the Linked Birth/Infant Death file for the years in question; hence they were included in either the white or black racial categories. Twins from other racial groups (e.g. Asians and American Indians) were excluded from these analyses because they represent such a small proportion of the entire twin population.

Frequency distributions of live births by race, plurality, gestational age and birth weight were inspected before analyzing gestational age-specific mortality in the 1983–85 Linked Birth/Infant Death files. A small proportion of births with implausible gestational ages was present in each 250-g birth weight category. These were eliminated from subsequent analyses, because they generally represented live births whose birth weights were implausibly high for a given gestational age. The elimination criteria for each week of gestation are presented in Table 2. Infants below 500 g were also eliminated in all subsequent analyses relating birth weight to mortality. Gestational ages of more than 43 weeks were recoded as 43 weeks.

In order to evaluate the relationship of twin pair characteristics to infant mortality, co-twins from the same pregnancy were matched. The variables used for this match included county and state of birth, maternal race, age, county and state of residence, prior live births, month prenatal care began, education and marital status, as well as father's race, age and education. This matching algorithm was not expected to identify 100% of twin pairs[5].

Table 2 Birth weight/gestational age combinations that were excluded from analyses of infant mortality by race and gestational age

For infants of white mothers		For infants of black mothers	
If gestational age was ...	... then the following birth weights were considered implausible	If gestational age was ...	... then the following birth weights were considered implausible
≤21 weeks	≥500 g	≤21 weeks	≥750 g
≤22 weeks	≥750 g	≤22 weeks	≥1000 g
≤23 weeks	≥1000 g	≤23 weeks	≥1250 g
≤24 weeks	≥1250 g	≤24 weeks	≥1500 g
≤25 weeks	≥1500 g	≤25 weeks	≥1750 g
≤26 weeks	≥1750 g	≤26 weeks	≥2000 g
≤27 weeks	≥2000 g	≤27 weeks	≥2250 g
≤28 weeks	≥2250 g	≤29 weeks	≥2500 g
≤30 weeks	≥2500 g	≤30 weeks	≥2750 g
≤31 weeks	≥2750 g	≤31 weeks	≥3000 g
≤32 weeks	≥3000 g	≤32 weeks	≥3250 g
≤33 weeks	≥3250 g	≤33 weeks	≥3500 g
≤34 weeks	≥3500 g	≤34 weeks	≥3750 g
≤35 weeks	≥3750 g		

Final sample size

Data on 199 380 white and 42 938 black twins in the 1985–88 US National Natality files were used to generate Figure 1 and Table 1. After the aforementioned exclusion criteria were applied to the Linked Birth/Infant Death files, a total of 8 720 633 liveborn white singletons, 171 291 white twins, 1 657 757 black singletons and 40 737 black twins remained for the mortality analyses. Of these, 61 853 white singletons, 6730 white twins, 23 628 black singletons, and 2737 black twins died in infancy. Overall infant mortality rates (per 1000) were 7.1 for white singletons, 39.3 for white twins, 14.3 for black singletons and 67.2 for black twins.

Findings

Race-specific intrauterine growth

Figure 1 and Table 1 present the 10th centile and median birth weights for US black and white twins. The median birth weights for twins of both races were very similar until about 31 weeks' gestation. Subsequently, white twins grew at a slightly faster rate than blacks; at term, whites had a median birth weight about 200 g greater than that of black twins. The 10th centiles and medians for US white twins are quite similar to the recently published values for Canadian twins[19].

Birth weight-specific mortality

Birth weight-specific neonatal and infant mortality rates by 250-g categories are presented in Table 3 for white singletons, white twins, black singletons and black twins. The lowest *infant* mortality rates for white singletons are for those infants between 3250 g and 5000 g, for black singletons between 3250 g and 4500 g, and for white and black twins of 3250–3500 g. By race and plurality, black singletons have lower infant mortality rates than white singletons between 500 g and 2500 g, whereas black twins have higher survival rates than white twins for all weight categories below 1750 g (See Figure 2a and b).

Among whites, twins have lower birth weight-specific *infant* mortality rates than singletons between 1000 g and 3000 g, but higher rates above 3000 g. Among blacks, twins have a

Table 3 United States birth weight-specific neonatal and infant mortality rates (per 1000 live births) for black and white singletons and twins (1983–85 data)

Birth weight category (g)	Neonatal mortality rates				Infant mortality rates			
	White singletons	White twins	Black singletons	Black twins	White singletons	White twins	Black singletons	Black twins
500–749	707	806	641	698	755	844	710	770
750–999	356	417	252	277	421	478	343	375
1000–1249	180	162	98	83	222	206	152	136
1250–1499	100	64	53	34	132	91	84	62
1500–1749	65	22	34	14	86	40	57	37
1750–1999	40	10	23	8	57	21	41	26
2000–2249	21	6	12	5	34	13	26	18
2250–2499	11	4	7	3	19	9	16	12
2500–2749	5	3	4	3	11	7	11	12
2750–2999	3	2	2	2	7	4	8	11
3000–3249	2	3	2	3	5	5	6	8
3250–3499	1	2	2	1	3	4	5	4
3500–3749	1	4	2	11	3	6	5	13
3750–3999	1	6	2	14	2	9	4	27
4000–4249	1	25	2	96	3	25	5	96
4250–4499	1	28	2	95	2	28	5	95
4500–4749	2	130	6	375	3	130	8	375
4750–4999	2	182	6	500	3	273	8	500
5000+	9	595	44	533	11	595	53	533
Unknown	190	606	341	512	205	629	364	558

survival advantage over singletons between 1000 g and 2500 g. This pattern of increased mortality for twins of higher birth weight compared to singletons of similar birth weight has been noted previously[2,20]. Similar patterns of lowered *neonatal* mortality rates for twins compared to singletons and blacks compared to whites are displayed in Table 3. Lower neonatal mortality rates are sometimes present over broader birth weight ranges than infant mortality rates. For example, black twins generally have lower neonatal mortality rates than black singletons between 1000 g and 3500 g, whereas lower infant mortality rates are present only between 1000 g and 2500 g. By race and plurality, black singletons have a survival advantage over white singletons between 500 g and 3000 g, and black twins have lower neonatal mortality rates compared to white twins for all birth weight categories less than 3500 g.

These lower *neonatal* mortality rates for black twins and singletons over a broader birth weight range than for *infant* mortality rates could be due to a number of factors. Lower neonatal rates may in part reflect a protective effect among blacks for conditions which result in neonatal death, such as respiratory distress syndrome, or they might reflect increased gestational age of blacks at a given birth weight, which in itself would be protective. In either event, blacks might be more likely to survive those conditions which are common causes of neonatal death. However, this hypothesised protective effect would be less important at the upper birth weight ranges, in which neonatal mortality rates are already quite low. On the other hand, the diminished birth weight range over which blacks have lower *infant* mortality, truncated as it is at the upper end, may be partly explained by the greater susceptibility of blacks compared to

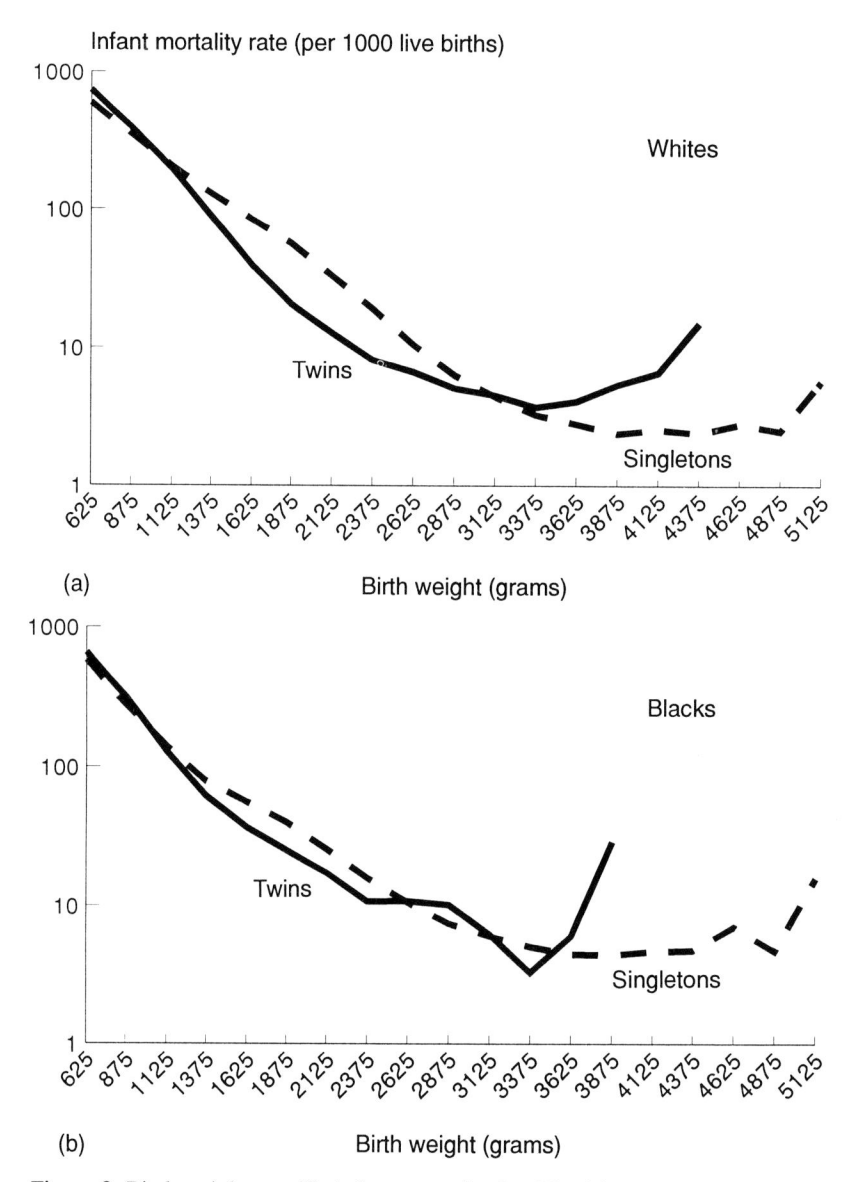

Figure 2 Birth weight-specific infant mortality for US white (a) and black (b) singletons and twins, as calculated from the Linked Birth/Infant Death files for 1983–85

whites for sudden infant death syndrome (SIDS)[21]. The impact of SIDS on *infant* mortality rates in babies of lower birth weight would be masked by their already high rates of *neonatal* death. However, because SIDS generally occurs in the post-neonatal period, it would make a more noticeable contribution to increased *infant* mortality rates among black babies of higher birth weight. The net result would be a narrower range over which black infants have a birth weight-specific survival advantage.

Gestational age-specific mortality

Infant and neonatal mortality rates for white and black singletons and twins by gestational age in weeks are presented in Table 4. The lowest *infant* mortality rate for white singletons was at 40 weeks, for black singletons at 39–40 weeks, for white twins at 39 weeks, and for black twins at 37–38 weeks. Among whites, twins have a survival advantage over singletons between 31 and 36 weeks, whereas black twins have no survival advantage over black singletons at any week of gestation. At gestational ages above 36 weeks, twin infant mortality rates rise dramatically compared to singletons. At 42 weeks the relative risk of infant mortality was 2.8 for white twins and 2.6 for black twins compared to white and black singletons, respectively. The high mortality rates for the implausible birth weight-for-gestational age groups of twins most likely represent gross errors in recorded birth weight or gestation length. Alternatively, some of these may represent true extremes of birth weight at a given length of gestation, reflecting subgroups at particularly high risk for infant mortality. By race and plurality, black singletons born before 36 weeks' gestation are more likely to survive infancy than white singletons of comparable gestational age, whereas only those black twins born before 31 weeks have a survival advantage over white twins (Figure 3).

The patterns for *neonatal* mortality rates by gestational age are similar. Among whites, neonatal mortality rates are lower for twins compared to singletons between 31 and 36 weeks' gestation. However, among blacks, twin neonatal mortality rates are higher than singleton rates at each week of gestation. Comparisons by race and plurality reveal that black singletons have lower neonatal mortality rates than white singletons through 37 weeks' gestation, and black twins have lower neonatal mortality

Table 4 United States gestational age-specific neonatal and infant mortality rates (per 1000 live births) for black and white singletons and twins (1983–85 data)

Gestational age category (weeks)	Neonatal mortality rates				Infant mortality rates			
	White singletons	White twins	Black singletons	Black twins	White singletons	White twins	Black singletons	Black twins
≤23	870	923	793	852	887	930	825	867
24	658	772	509	605	712	794	591	696
25	503	657	349	429	560	706	430	509
26	375	466	260	330	439	522	334	424
27	270	340	170	199	324	401	230	254
28	185	207	117	122	233	252	161	186
29	136	124	72	76	170	162	107	111
30	89	92	57	61	116	121	82	94
31	64	50	32	43	82	76	52	66
32	44	26	21	29	60	39	39	46
33	29	19	14	17	39	27	25	37
34	16	11	9	13	25	19	18	29
35	10	7	6	6	16	14	13	18
36	6	5	5	6	11	10	12	17
37	4	4	3	4	7	8	9	13
38	2	3	2	4	5	8	7	13
39	1	3	2	5	4	7	6	15
40	1	4	2	7	3	8	6	16
41	1	4	3	4	4	8	7	16
42	2	5	3	10	4	12	7	19
43	24	9	3	9	5	17	9	22
Implausible	20	199	30	172	26	205	40	208
Unknown	10	62	20	86	15	76	30	115

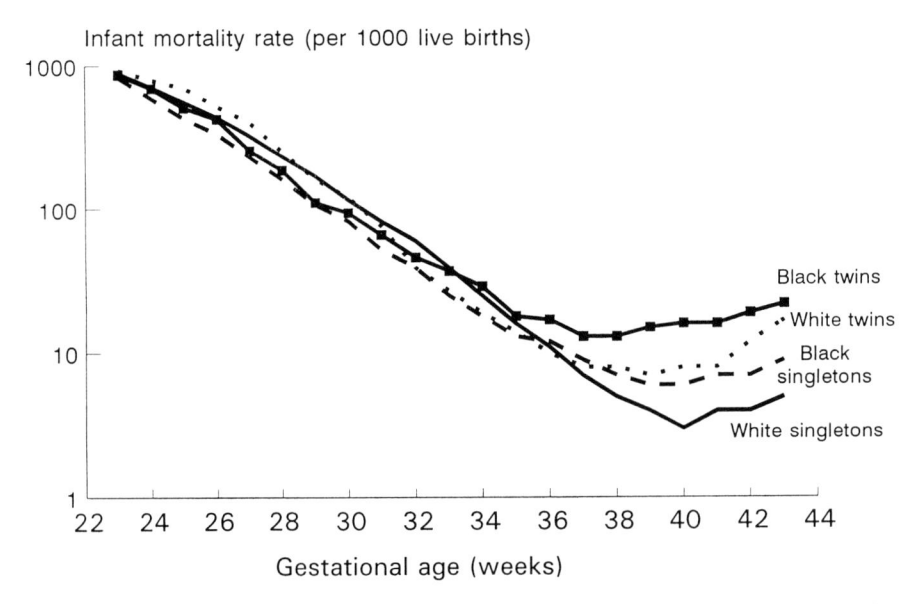

Figure 3 Gestation-specific infant mortality rates for US singletons and twins, as calculated from the US Linked Birth/Infant Death files for 1983–85

rates compared to white twins through 31 weeks' gestation (Table 4).

A number of possible factors might explain the improved survival of white twins over white singletons between 31 and 36 weeks. Twins might be more stressed *in utero*, resulting in increased endogenous steroid production and accelerated pulmonary maturity, and consequently lower rates of and clinically less severe respiratory distress syndrome for a given degree of pre-term birth. A second possibility is that prematurely born singletons are more likely to have a specific precipitating cause for their pre-term birth, such as intrauterine infection or congenital anomalies, whereas pre-term birth in twin pregnancies may be more likely related to uterine constraints imposed by the presence of two *fetuses*, without other specific precipitating causes. The reason or reasons for the lack of survival advantage for black twins compared to black singletons is unclear, unless black singletons are just as likely to be stressed *in utero* and have similar pulmonary maturity as black twins at a given gestational age.

Survival by gender combination of the twin pair

The relationship of gender pair characteristics to twin infant mortality was assessed by comparing unlike-gender pairs to like-gender (male–male and female–female) pairs. The matching criteria previously described resulted in successful matching of 78% of twins. A total of 66 835 white twin pairs and 16 004 black twin pairs were available for analysis. Findings are presented in Table 5 for whites and blacks separately for the cases in which either or both members of a twin pair died. Note that the infant mortality rates are expressed per 1000 *pregnancies*, not per 1000 live births, in order to present the risk of either or both members of the twin pair dying.

Among whites, like-gender pairs, particularly male–male pairs, are at highest risk of infant mortality compared to unlike-gender pairs. White like-gender males have a relative risk (RR) of 2 for both twins dying compared to unlike-gender pairs. Their RR is 1.5 for either twin dying. The risk for white female pairs is intermediate: white female like-gender pairs have 1.6 times the risk of both twins dying but only 1.1 times the risk of either twin dying. In contrast, among blacks, there is much less difference in infant mortality rates by gender pair status. Unlike-gender pairs and female–female gender pairs have equivalent risks of infant death, whereas black males have a 10% increased risk of either twin dying and a 30% increased risk of both twin members dying compared to unlike-gender pairs.

The critical period during which birth of twins is most deleterious

Early definition One of us (WFP) previously reviewed a 1974–77 regional cohort of liveborn twins and noted that 95% of twins who died before hospital discharge were born before completion of 34 weeks' gestation[22]. In contrast, 98% (338/344) of twins born after 34 weeks' gestation survived. Other hospital-based data[23-26] showed similar mortality and survival distributions, namely, rapidly increasing survival rates with gestational age until 34 weeks, and consistently high survival rates thereafter. Most deaths of liveborn twins occurred among infants born before completion of 34 weeks' gestation. These observations led to the definition of a 'critical period' for twin pregnancies which ended at 34 weeks. This critical period was implied to begin at about 26–27 weeks, because this was about the earliest gestational age at which neonatal intensive care was routinely offered to infants born during those study years. Delivery between 26 and 34 weeks was associated with high mortality, and interventions such as the use of prophylactic bed rest or tocolytic agents, designed to decrease mortality in twin pregnancies, would have had to have been applied before or during the critical period to have lowered mortality. Conversely, any intervention beginning or continuing beyond the end of the critical period would have been expected to alter mortality only slightly, because nearly all twins born after 34 weeks survived.

Current definition The NCHS Linked Live Birth/Infant Death file provides a comprehensive basis for redefining the critical period in twin pregnancy (Table 6). Simply put, twins delivering after 32 weeks' gestation have a greater than 95% chance of surviving infancy. Thus, 32 weeks now should mark the end of the critical period.

Moreover, because in at least some institutions, intensive neonatal care is routinely offered to newborns of 24 weeks' gestation, we propose that this lower limit of gestational age now be used to mark the beginning of the critical period, recognizing, of course, that this lower boundary might shift over time and is dependent upon local patterns of care.

Table 5 Gender pair characteristics related to twin infant mortality. 1983–85 US Linked Birth Infant Death cohorts. Infant mortality rates (IMR) per 1000 pregnancies, relative risks (RR) and 95% confidence limits (CL)

	Pregnancies (n)	Both died			Either died		
		IMR	RR	95% CL	IMR	RR	95% CL
Whites							
Unlike gender	17 323	17.0	1.0		47.5	1.0	
Female–female	24 914	26.4	1.6	1.4–1.8	54.0	1.1	1.0–1.2
Male–male	24 598	33.4	2.0	1.7–2.2	69.6	1.5	1.4–1.6
Blacks							
Unlike gender	5811	43.4	1.0		94.8	1.0	
Female–female	5182	43.2	1.0	0.8–1.2	91.1	1.0	0.9–1.1
Male–male	5011	56.3	1.3	1.1–1.6	108.0	1.1	1.0–1.3

Table 6. Twin births and deaths by gestational age as calculated from the 1983–85 US Linked Birth/Infant Death file from the National Center for Health Statistics

Gestational age (weeks)	Neonatal deaths	Post-neonatal deaths	Survived infancy	Total	Percentage infant survival	Cumulative total	Cumulative percentage
≤24	2779	68	424	3271	13.0	3271	1.56
25	807	71	419	1297	32.3	4568	2.18
26	687	102	740	1529	48.4	6097	2.91
27	581	106	1124	1811	62.1	7908	3.77
28	446	111	1664	2221	74.9	10 129	4.83
29	305	98	2224	2627	84.7	12 756	6.09
30	297	99	2925	3321	88.1	16 077	7.67
31	222	111	4066	4399	92.4	20 476	9.77
32	164	83	5787	6034	95.9	26 510	12.65
33	162	90	8172	8424	97.0	34 934	16.67
34	140	119	11 821	12 080	97.9	47 014	22.43
35	116	127	16 611	16 854	98.6	63 868	30.47
36	133	127	21 713	21 973	98.8	85 841	40.96
37	129	137	27 185	27 451	99.0	113 292	54.05
≥38	773	532	94 992	96 297	98.6	209 589	100.00
Total	7741	1981	199 867	209 589	95.4		

Table 6 also shows that about one in eight twin pregnancies resulting in at least one live birth delivers during the critical period. Given today's uncertainty regarding the benefit of prophylactic interventions in twin pregnancy, any practitioner who wishes to use strategies designed to prevent delivery during the redefined critical period might initially feel frustrated. However, the concept of a critical period could still be incorporated into clinical practice and used to delineate a time during which women who experience premature labor or other complications that presage preterm delivery and that warrant hospitalization could preferentially be admitted to hospitals with a Level III Neonatal Intensive Care Unit (NICU) rather than a more convenient or less costly facility lacking an NICU. Of equal importance, reimbursement authorities could be encouraged to develop mechanisms for easy implementation of appropriate patterns of hospitalization. In addition, women carrying twins might be advised early in their pregnancies of the fact that they have at least a one in eight chance of preterm labor and delivery during the critical period. Practitioners must recognise that the critical period as redefined above is characterized solely in terms of infant mortality and that a large proportion of infants born at 33–34 weeks experience substantial morbidity. Thus, the policy of selective hospitalization of women who develop complications threatening early delivery at institutions with a Level III NICU might actually be extended one or two more weeks. After 33–34 weeks, delivery at a more convenient and less expensive hospital may be a reasonable alternative plan.

Because proposed prophylactic interventions for prevention of preterm delivery of twins do not always achieve their goals, it is reasonable to anticipate that research physicians in the future will test additional interventions that might decrease the rate of twin delivery during the critical period. The data in Table 6 will be useful for calculation of sample sizes needed to achieve adequate statistical power in evaluations of these proposed prophylactic interventions.

Summary

The national data on infant mortality presented in this chapter clearly demonstrate that twins have a survival advantage over singletons at certain ranges of both birth weight and gestational age. For birth weight, this advantage is particularly evident between 1000 and 2500 g. Similarly, based on gestational age, white twins have a survival advantage over singletons between 31 and 36 weeks. Despite this, the overall risk of infant death among twins continues to be 4–6 times greater than that of singletons.

The National Linked Birth/Infant Death data also indicate that the optimal duration for twin gestation is 39 weeks for whites (IMR = 7/1000 live births) and 37–38 weeks for blacks (IMR = 13/1000 live births). The optimal birth weight for white twins with respect to infant mortality ranges from 2750 to 3500 g. For blacks, the optimal birth weight range is between 3250 and 3500 g. Note, however, that twins of both races who weigh more than 4000 g are at increased risk for infant mortality.

Clearly, the major cause of increased infant mortality of twins compared to singletons is the much larger proportion of twins born at low birth weight and/or short gestation. Approximately half of white twins are of low birth weight (<2500 g), as are two-thirds of black twins[1]. Over 54% of twins are born before 38 weeks and nearly 13% are born before 33 weeks' gestation. This latter group, born during the critical period characterised by highest infant mortality, are those for whom there is a pressing need to develop and test intervention strategies to prevent preterm delivery.

References

1. Kleinman, J.C., Fowler, M.G. and Kessel, S.S. (1991). Comparison of infant mortality among twins and singletons: United States 1960 and 1983. *Am. J. Epidemiol.*, **133**, 133
2. Ghai, V. and Vidyasagar, D. (1988). Morbidity and mortality factors in twins. An epidemiologic approach. *Clin. Perinatol.*, **15**, 123
3. Grothe, W. and Ruttgers, H. (1985). Twin pregnancies: an 11-year review. *Acta Genet. Med. Gemellol.*, **34**, 49
4. McCarthy, B.J., Sachs, B.P., Layde, P.M., *et al.* (1981). The epidemiology of neonatal deaths in twins. *Am. J. Obstet. Gynecol.*, **141**, 252
5. Fowler, M. G., Kleinman, J.C., Kiely, J.L. *et al.* (1991). Double jeopardy: twin infant mortality in the United States, 1983 and 1984. *Am. J. Obstet. Gynecol.*, **165**, 15
6. Bulmer, M.G. (1970). *The Biology of Twinning in Man*, pp. 47–67. (Oxford: Clarendon)
7. Ellis, R. F., Berger, G.S., Keith, L. *et al.* (1979). The Northwestern University multihospital twin study. II. Mortality of first versus second twins. *Acta Genet. Med. Gemellol.*, **28**, 347
8. Polin, J.I. and Frangipane, W.L. (1986). Current concepts in management of obstetrical problems for pediatricians. II. Modern concepts in the management of multiple gestation. *Pediatr. Clin. N. Am.*, **33**, 649
9. Naeye, R.L., Tafari, N., Judge, D. *et al.* (1978). Twins: causes of perinatal death in 12 United States cities and one African city. *Am. J. Obstet. Gynecol.*, **131**, 267
10. Hoffman, H.J., Bakketeig, L.S. and Stark, C.R. (1978). Twins and perinatal mortality: a comparison between single and twin births in Minnesota and in Norway, 1967–73. In Nance, W.E., Allen, G. and Parisi, P. (eds.). *Twin Research: Biology and Epidemiology*, pp. 133–42. (New York: Alan R. Liss)
11. Lumme, R.H. and Saarikoski, S.V. (1986). Monoamniotic twin pregnancy. *Acta Genet. Med. Gemellol.*, **35**, 99
12. National Center for Health Statistics. (1988). *1985/1986/1987/1988 Detail Natality*, Public Use Data Tape. (Hyattsville, MD: National Center for Health Statistics)
13. National Center for Health Statistics. (1989). *Linked Birth/Infant Death Data Set: 1983/1984/1985 Birth Cohorts*, Public Use Data Tape. (Hyattsville, MD: National Center for Health Statistics)
14. Ahmed, A.G. and Klopper, A. (1986). Estimation of gestational age by last menstrual

period, by ultrasound scan and by SPI concentration: comparison with date of delivery. *Br. J. Obstet. Gynaecol.*, **93**, 122

15. Kramer, M.S., McLean, F.H., Boyd, M.E. *et al.* (1988). The validity of gestational age estimation by menstrual dating in term, preterm, and postterm gestations. *J. Am. Med. Assoc.*, **260**, 3306

16. Treloar, A.E., Behn, B.G. and Cowan, D.W. (1969). Analysis of gestational interval. *Am. J. Obstet. Gynecol.*, **99**, 34

17. Naeye, R.L. and Dixon, J.B. (1978). Distortions in fetal growth standards. *Pediatr. Res.*, **12**, 987

18. David, R.J. (1983). Population-based intrauterine growth curves from computerized birth certificates. *South. Med. J.*, **76**, 1401

19. Arbuckle, T.E. and Sherman, G.J. (1989). An analysis of birth weight by gestational age in Canada. *Can. Med. Assoc. J.*, **140**, 157

20. Kiely, J.L. (1990). The epidemiology of perinatal mortality in multiple births. *Bull. NY Acad. Med.*, **66**, 618

21. Hoffman H.J., Hunter, J.C., Damus, K. *et al.* (1987). Diphtheria–tetanus–pertussis immunization and sudden infant death: results of the National Institute of Child Health and Human Development cooperative epidemiologic study of sudden infant death syndrome risk factors. *Pediatrics*, **79**, 598

22. Powers, W.F. and Miller, T.C. (1979). Bed rest in twin pregnancy: identification of a critical period and its cost implications. *Am. J. Obstet. Gynecol.*, **134**, 23

23. Farooqui, M.O., Grossman, J.H. and Shannon, R.A. (1973). A review of twin pregnancy and perinatal mortality. *Obstet. Gynecol. Surv.* (Suppl.), **28**, 144

24. Ho, S.K. and Wu, P.Y.K. (1975). Perinatal factors and neonatal morbidity in twin pregnancy. *Am. J. Obstet. Gynecol.*, **122**, 979

25. Kauppila, A., Jouppila, M., Koivisto, M. *et al.* (1973). Twin pregnancy. Neonatal morbidity and mortality. *Acta Obstet. Gynecol. Scand.* (Suppl.), **28**, 144

26. Keith, L., Ellis, R., Berger, G.S. *et al.* (1980). The Northwestern University Multihospital Twin Study. I. A description of 588 twin pregnancies and associated pregnancy loss, 1971 to 1975. *Am. J. Obstet. Gynecol.*, **138**, 781

The impact of assisted reproductive technology on the incidence of multiple gestation

13

B.R. Hecht

Introduction

The era of advanced/assisted reproductive technology (ART) began in 1978 with the birth of Louise Brown, a baby conceived 'in vitro' by the late Mr Patrick Steptoe and Dr Robert Edwards[1]. Since then, the subspecialty of reproductive medicine has not only burgeoned but also undergone profound changes. Prominent among these has been the phenomenal growth of ART, as reflected by the number of births in recent years as a result of these procedures. Whereas, in the United States, only 260 infants were born following ART in 1985, this number increased to 5193 births by 1990[2-6] (Table 1). Similar increases have been recorded in other countries as well.

The number of multiple births increased steadily in the United States during the 1980s, partly because of the 'aging' of the female population at the time of reproduction (see Chapter 10), and partly as a consequence of the introduction of assisted reproductive technologies into medical practice. For example, from 1982, following the introduction of *in vitro* fertilization (IVF), through 1988, the last year for which data are available, the number of twin births increased by 18% and triplets or higher order births by 58%, compared to only a 7% increase in total US births[7] (Figure 1). Unfortunately, the relative contributions from the two factors cannot be calculated, because the US Standard Certificate of Live Birth fails to differentiate spontaneous from induced pregnancies.

The American Fertility Society defines 'advanced reproductive technology' procedures as 'those which include the laboratory handling of human oocytes and/or embryos'[8]. For the purpose of examining the overall contribution of current infertility therapies to the rising rate of multiple births, the definition of ART as used in this chapter will also include the use of ovulatory stimulants as well as the handling of male gametes. Although both therapies predate 1978, they have changed significantly as a consequence of the widespread practice of *in vitro* fertilization.

ART has affected the rate of multiple births in two ways. First, the procedures themselves directly impact on the incidence of multiple pregnancy; and second, the number of patients undergoing infertility treatment has increased dramatically. This latter factor undoubtedly has a greater influence on the overall number of multiple births. A discussion

Table 1 US births following ART, 1985–1989

Year	No. births
1985	260
1986	381
1987	1858
1988	3427
1989	4736
1990	5193

Medical Research International and The Society of Assisted Reproductive Technology, The American Fertility Society[2-6]

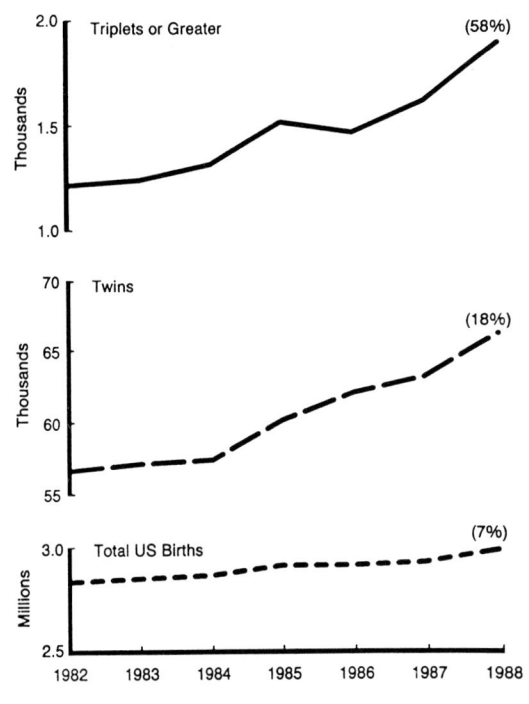

Figure 1 Increase in multiple birth rates

of problems that arise in reviewing the ART literature as it relates to multiple births begins this chapter; this is then followed by examination of the influence of several recent changes in reproductive medicine that have affected the incidence of multifetal pregnancy, including *in vitro* fertilization, gamete intrafallopian transfer (GIFT) and superovulation therapy.

Literature review – methodological problems

It is important to understand the methodological problems associated with a literature review of either ART or multiple birth rates before examining any proposed effect that specific technological advances might exert on the rate of multiple births. Simply stated, for a number of reasons (Table 2), it is not possible to assign specific, cumulative values to the incidence of multiple pregnancy resulting from specific reproductive technologies.

First, the true incidence of multiple pregnancy is underestimated, because vital statistics report live birth rates, not total conceptions.

As a result, early pregnancy wastage invariably leads to under-reporting of multiple pregnancy rates. Moreover, the occurrence of spontaneous reduction ('vanishing sacs'), and the growing practice of partial reduction of multifetal gestations confound the reporting and analysis of the rates of multiple gestations vs. the rate of multiple births.

Second, the interpretation and comparison of 'pregnancy rates' is hampered by non-uniform reporting. This dilemma can be characterized by 'numerator problems' as well as 'denominator problems'[9,10]. Numerator problems occur because of the variable definitions given to 'a pregnancy'. These definitions range from the transient detection of circulating chorionic gonadotropin to the actual delivery of a liveborn infant. Denominator problems also occur, because the data used for the calculation of pregnancy rates may include the total number of patients who begin a fertility treatment cycle or only the number in whom actual transfer of gametes or embryos is performed. Multiple pregnancy rates are also expressed using varying/non-uniform denominators. For the purpose of comparison with the natural incidence, in this chapter iatrogenic multiple pregnancy rates will be expressed as a percentage of ongoing pregnancies or deliveries. For example, a 1991 publication[11] of GIFT procedures reports a pregnancy rate of 96 out of

Table 2 Problems associated with the literature review

Vital statistics record live births, not total pregnancies

Various definitions used for 'pregnancy'

Denominators vary for calculation of 'pregnancy rates'

National information about the extent/outcomes of infertility therapy lacking

Variable/incomplete reporting of outcome statistics (e.g. 'multiple birth' or 'multiple pregnancy')

Evolving treatment protocols within centers and differing protocols between centers

Multiple reports arising from the same data base

399 procedures (24%), and a multiple pregnancy rate of 26 out of 399 procedures (6.5%). However, the multiple pregnancy rate, expressed as a percentage of pregnancies would be 26 out of 96 (27%). The latter method of calculation is clearly more appropriate for comparison to rates of naturally occurring multiples.

Third, any literature analysis is also hampered by a lack of national data regarding the extent and outcomes of infertility therapy. The 1989 revision of the United States Standard Certificate of Live Birth does not include information on prior infertility therapy[12]. Although a standard reporting format with a centralized data base, known as the US IVF Registry, was begun in 1985 by the Society of Assisted Reproductive Technology (SART) in conjunction with the American Fertility Society[2], these data must not be confused with a national registry of all infertility patients. The latter simply does not exist. The more than 150 member clinics of the US IVF registry represent three quarters of all US clinics performing about 90% of the ART procedures nationwide[13], and much of the data presented in the remainder of this chapter derives from their data base.

Finally, a thorough literature review uncovers additional problems associated with the variable reporting of outcomes, such as 'multiple birth' or 'multiple pregnancy', the frequent modifications of technique and protocol within a specific center, the different protocols used at various centers over time, and multiple reports arising from the same data base. All prevent an accurate accumulation of summary statistics.

Specific ART procedures and multiple gestations

In vitro *fertilization embryo transfer*

Of the currently available therapies, *in vitro* fertilization and embryo transfer (IVF–ET) has the longest history and has resulted in the greatest number of published reports. Data from the 1989 IVF Registry report[14] document 2104 IVF–ET births for that year (Table 3). Of these, 32% were multiples (550 twin, 107 triplet and 10 quadruplet pregnancies).

Table 3 IVF outcome: National IVF–ET Registry, 1989

	Number
Embryo transfers	21 870
Clinical pregnancies	5 279 (24%)
Deliveries	4 206 (19%)
Multiple births	667 (32.7%)

Medical Research International and The Society of Assisted Reproductive Technology, The American Fertility Society[14]

In spite of selecting only apparently normal embryos for uterine transfer, IVF–ET pregnancy and birth rates remain low. The initial attempts at IVF–ET were performed in spontaneous (unstimulated) ovulatory cycles with the transfer of a single embryo. Because obtaining an oocyte in a natural (single follicle) cycle was not always possible, and the likelihood of achieving a successful pregnancy was determined to increase with the number of embryos transferred[15], it quickly became standard practice to stimulate the development of multiple ovarian follicles[16]. On occasion, in excess of 20 oocytes can be collected at a single procedure. Without doubt, the simultaneous transfer of multiple embryos initiated the current phenomenon of IVF-related iatrogenic multiple gestations[17]. At present, many physicians in the USA restrict the number of embryos transferred to a maximum of three or four and cryogenically preserve the remainder. (Editor: Others deplore this practice because of the higher likelihood of multiples and restrict this number to two.) However, some clinics still report transferring an average of more than five embryos at a time[5]. Not unexpectedly, multiple births rise in proportion to the number of embryos transferred (Table 4).

The reported rates of multiple gestation from IVF–ET in other national registries are similar to those reported by the US IVF Registry. For example, the Australian *In Vitro* Fertilization Collaborative Group[18] reported the outcome of 244 IVF–ET pregnancies. Twenty-two per cent of ongoing pregnancies were multiples. Of 1092 GIFT

Table 4 IVF outcome by number of embryos transferred

No. embryos transferred	Births/transfer (%)	Multiple births (%)
1	6	0
2	11	3
3	12	21
4	18	17
5	17	31
6	18	50

Medical Research International and The Society of Assisted Reproductive Technology, The American Fertility Society[3]

or IVF–ET pregnancies delivered between 1978 and 1987 in the United Kingdom, 23% were multiples (19% twins and 4% triplets and higher order multiples)[19]. A multinational collaborative study encompassing the years 1979 to 1985 reported detailed data on 1195 IVF–ET births. Of these, 19% were multiples (16.7% twins and 2.6% triplets)[20].

Gamete intrafallopian transfer

Gamete intrafallopian tubal transfer evolved out of IVF–ET technology[21]. GIFT is simpler and utilizes the patient's reproductive physiological functions (including conception *in vivo*) to a greater extent than IVF, but laparoscopy is usually required. The resulting multiple birth rates are similar, however. Of the 848 reported US GIFT births in 1989[5], 34% were multiples. As expected, the multiple birth rate correlates with the number of oocytes simultaneously transferred[22]. Because GIFT is performed in patients with normal tubal patency, there may be an additional risk of multiple pregnancy occurring from naturally ovulated and fertilized oocytes in addition to those collected and mechanically transferred. A sextuplet pregnancy after a transfer of four oocytes probably occurred in this manner[23].

Tubal embryo transfer

Because implantation rates following uterine embryo transfer of apparently viable embryos remain low, many centers presently transfer embryos into the theoretically superior environment of the Fallopian tube in order to take full advantage of the physiological contribution that the tube normally makes to early embryo support[24–32]. This technique is variously referred to as tubal embryo transfer (TET), zygote intrafallopian transfer (ZIFT), or pronuclear stage transfer (PROST), depending on the stage of early pre-embryo development when transfer is performed. Although comparatively small numbers of such transfers were reported in the 1989 Registry[5], 30% of the resulting deliveries were multiple. A retrospective comparison of pregnancy rates between IVF–ET, GIFT and ZIFT showed that the last produced the highest pregnancy rates per transfer[25]. These findings were not supported in a controlled prospective study, however[32]. As noted previously for both IVF–ET and GIFT, the incidence of multiple gestation is strongly associated with the number of embryos per tubal transfer, rising from zero following the transfer of one or two embryos, to 21% multiples with the transfer of three and 57% multiples when four embryos are transferred[30] (Table 5).

As the number of eggs/embryos simultaneously transferred increases, the multiple pregnancy rates rise steeply. In contrast, the overall pregnancy rate is often observed to plateau, despite the increase in eggs/embryos transferred (Tables 4 and 5). This phenomenon occurs with both tubal and uterine embryo transfers. The

Table 5 Tubal embryo transfer outcome by number of embryos transferred

No. embryos transferred	Pregnancies/ transfer (%)	Multiple pregnancies (%)
1	50	0
2	29	0
3	45	21
4	38	57
Total	40	31

Pool *et al.*[30]

'ideal' (maximum) number of eggs/embryos simultaneously transferred at a given center is based on the perceived point at which a balance exists between an 'adequate' pregnancy rate (success) and an 'acceptable' incidence of multiples (risk)[33]. In recent reports, between two and three embryos per tubal transfer procedure have been deemed optimal[25,30,31].

Maternal age, multiple pregnancy and ART

The general trend towards delayed childbearing is intimately related to the increasing number of women in their late 30s and early 40s seeking fertility therapy (see Chapter 10). Under natural circumstances (and also with ART), pregnancy rates decline steadily with increasing female age. Of those who conceive successfully from ART, multiple pregnancy rates also decline with age.

For example, in the 1989 Registry of GIFT pregnancies[5], 44% of women under 30 delivered multiples. This rate declined to 40% for women 30–34 years of age, 25% for women 35–39 and was zero in the 13 pregnancies reported in women over 40. This inverse correlation reached statistical significance in another analysis of 242 GIFT and IVF–ET pregnancies[34], and has been observed in other analyses as well[20,35]. Capitalizing on the apparent decrease in the risk of multiple gestation in women over age 40, while also recognizing the decreased chance of successfully achieving any pregnancy at this age, Craft et al.[22,36] vigorously advocated transfer of all oocytes during GIFT procedures in their older patients. In some cases over 11 oocytes are transferred at a time. Pregnancy rates in the patients over 40 (receiving the high oocyte numbers) were comparable to those in younger women, and the risk of producing multiples was also similar to that seen in the younger patients receiving four or fewer oocytes (18.7 vs. 17.3%).

Risk versus benefit of multiple oocyte/embryo transfer

Ethically, the physician–patient contract is twofold. One element, usually foremost in the mind of the patient, is to achieve a desired goal, e.g. becoming pregnant. The other aspect, probably more strongly regarded by the physician, is the obligation to 'do no harm'. Any morbidity arising from a multiple gestation following the simultaneous transfer of more than one oocyte/embryo clearly represents an iatrogenic complication. Strictly adopting the latter perspective, multiple oocyte/embryo transfers would be contraindicated no matter what the gain in the pregnancy success. However, because virtually all medical interventions entail some risk, assessing the balance between risk and benefit becomes a more realistic approach to examining this physician–patient contract.

The risk to benefit analysis of multiple egg/embryo transfer received early attention in Australia[37]. Strong debate about limiting the number of oocytes/embryos transferred also appeared in the British literature[38]. In 1987, the Voluntary Licensing Authority (VLA) of the United Kingdom imposed voluntary guidelines limiting the number of oocytes/embryos transferred during ART procedures to '3 or exceptionally 4' in response to concern over higher-order multiple births. These recommendations were strongly criticized in the British medical press by Craft et al.[36], in part because they were applied only to ART procedures, which make a minority contribution to the overall incidence of iatrogenic multiples (see below). Craft et al.[36] advocated a flexible code of practice that individualized the number of oocytes or embryos transferred based upon 'the clinician's estimate of risk'. The 1990 Human Fertilization and Embryology Act again codified this protocol. 'No more than three embryos should ever be placed in a woman, though under very special circumstances, such as repeated failures of implantation, occasionally four embryos may be replaced.'[39]. Based on the continuing steep rise in multiple births in Britain and the strain placed on the provision of neonatal services, rigorous enforcement of the Licensing Authority guidelines has been urged[40]. Israeli authors have also called for the development of official policy to reduce multiples[41]. This subject has received less attention in the United States, where no national regulatory body relating to the practice of reproductive medicine yet exists and where free-market forces may encourage an emphasis on achieving maximal pregnancy rates over concern about morbidity arising from multiple gestation.

Factors determining pregnancy/multiple pregnancy

In deciding the optimal/ideal number of oocytes/embryos for transfer, ART teams attempt to achieve a balance between a 'satisfactory' pregnancy rate and an 'acceptable' rate of multiple pregnancy[33]. Many factors contribute to a patient's or clinician's perception of what is 'satisfactory' or 'acceptable', including biological, psychological, ethical and financial considerations. Often, these considerations are not quantifiable and do not fit easily into a risk–benefit analysis. For example, philosophically, is a high-order multiple gestation that fails to result even in a single liveborn baby a 'success'? Should this outcome be considered 'acceptable' from a programmatic standpoint?

Biological factors

The probability that pregnancy (as well as multiple pregnancy) will occur can be reduced to a mathematical formula that includes the following variables: (1) embryo quality; (2) uterine receptivity; and (3) the number of embryos transferred[42]. Unfortunately, the external factors influencing the first two parameters are still poorly understood, and beyond morphology, precise and non-invasive assays for oocyte, embryo or endometrial quality do not currently exist[42–44]. Determinations of metabolic activity (such as lactate excretion of the pre-embryo in culture) may soon permit a more precise identification of the 'healthiest' embryos for transfer[45]. Theoretically, healthier embryos should have a higher probability of survival. A more precise means of selecting only the healthiest embryos would eliminate the current need for multiple embryo transfer in order to achieve a satisfactory pregnancy rate, and the number of multiple pregnancies would then be minimized.

'Transfer efficiency', i.e. the likelihood of pregnancy per embryo transferred, theoretically can be increased either by improving embryo quality or by enhancing uterine receptivity. The practice of embryo cryopreservation[46] has provided additional insight into this biological concept. Prior to the widespread availability of successful embryo cryopreservation, IVF teams were frequently faced with the dilemma of having produced more than four cleaving embryos. At that time, alternatives included either transferring all the embryos to the uterus (and risking high-order multiple pregnancy) or transferring only some embryos and confronting the ethical problems related to disposing of the remainder. The advent of cryopreservation techniques not only helped solve that ethical dilemma, but also helped embryologists examine the hormonal influences on implantation. In cycles in which ovarian hyperstimulation is used to produce multiple follicles for oocyte recovery, the resulting supraphysiological sex steroid levels may have detrimental effects on endometrial synchrony and consequently, decreased uterine receptivity[43,44,47]. Stated another way, the uterine milieu may be *more* receptive to implantation (and the chance of success higher) if an embryo has been collected and cryopreserved in a prior cycle and then transferred into the natural, *unstimulated* endometrium[44,47]. This hypothesis has increased interest in the use of cryopreserved embryos, not only to avoid the problem of multiembryo transfer, but also to increase pregnancy rates. When thawed, 8% of 'cryo' embryo transfers resulted in viable births in 1989, including 23 sets of twins (13%)[5].

Extraordinarily high rates of successful implantation occur in patients with ovarian failure who receive 'donated' oocytes following the administration of carefully controlled quantities of exogenous sex steroids to prepare the uterus for implantation[48]. Because of this, some authors presently contend that the transfer of multiple fresh embryos in stimulated cycles (the current standard practice) be abandoned in favor of routine cryostorage of all embryos and subsequent transfer into an artificially hormone prepared uterus[47]. A controlled comparison of the artificially prepared endometrium vs. the natural endometrium for IVF–ET implantation is currently under way[49]. By increasing transfer efficiency, endometrial manipulations could theoretically allow a reduction in the number of embryos transferred without diminishing the probability of pregnancy per transfer.

Another recent 'innovation' is the return to 'natural cycle' IVF–ET (without ovarian stimulation) and the collection of only a single oocyte per attempt[50,51]. This approach dramatically reduces the cost per cycle by eliminating the use of the expensive medications required to induce ovarian hyperstimulation. Also, the risk of multiple gestation is virtually eliminated by returning to single embryo transfers. Three factors support this approach and may explain the impressive pregnancy rates seen thus far with natural cycle IVF–ET: (1) the use of nature's self-selected 'best' oocyte; (2) the more favorable milieu for implantation; and (3) continuing improvements in embryo culture technique in the laboratory. Widespread adoption of natural cycle IVF–ET could dramatically decrease the risk of multiple pregnancy from IVF–ET. For example, in one report, the combined success of two consecutive 'unstimulated' IVF cycles, each with a single embryo transfer, produced cumulative pregnancy rates and costs similar to a single standard, 'stimulated' IVF cycle, but eliminated the risk of multiple gestation[52].

Social/financial factors

There are many 'pressures' to achieve high pregnancy rates with ART. Primary among these is the fact that for the infertile couple, the birth of one or more babies is the only desired outcome of the enormous emotional and financial sacrifice involved in ART. Unfortunately, the fundamental human urge to procreate frequently is intensified by the frustration and desperation of repeated failure. In many instances, this frustration develops into a focus on success that may overshadow the more theoretical and abstract risks associated with multiple gestation. In addition, there is little doubt that the enormous cost per ART procedure enters into the perception of what is considered a 'satisfactory' pregnancy rate by couples and their physicians. Costs for IVF–ET in the United States currently average over $6000 per attempt. With this level of financial burden, emphasis on achieving a maximal pregnancy rate is also fueled by the desire to achieve a perceived level of cost-effectiveness. If some of the less costly modifications become widely adopted, lower pregnancy rates may be considered 'acceptable', because the cost-effectiveness per procedure may have remained unchanged.

From the 'consumer's' point of view, the quality (and competitive edge) of IVF centers are undoubtedly measured to a large degree by their reported number of pregnancies. With the financial survival of a clinic possibly resting on its 'success rate', as well as the pressures exerted by patients, it is little wonder that clinicians succumb to a success-oriented focus, and multiple pregnancy rates increase as a consequence. Concerns about risks, cost, truth in advertising and the efficacy of modern fertility therapies has led to increased public and governmental scrutiny of providers and pressure for statutory regulations.

Other fertility therapies

No accurate statistics exist to ascertain the proportion of multiples conceived following various fertility therapies. Furthermore, whatever that percentage may actually be at a given time, it does not remain constant. Both the scope of ART practice and the influence on multiples varies as protocols change over time. Although IVF–ET and related technologies produce a large relative excess of iatrogenic multiple gestations, the overall contribution of these procedures to the total number of multiple births is currently small. In contrast, the major cause of multiple births (among women who undergo treatment for infertility) remains *in vivo* conception after the use of ovulatory stimulants. In data compiled from a questionnaire study of patients participating in a multiple pregnancy support group, of 1138 US triplet pregnancies delivered between 1984 and 1989, 38% were conceived spontaneously, 50% following ovulation induction and only 9% following *in vitro* fertilization or GIFT procedures[53]. Similarly, data on 71 quadruplet pregnancies delivered between 1980 and 1989, also obtained by questionnaire, included the following percentages of fertility treatment: 69% ovulation induction; 7% IVF–ET; 18% GIFT and 6% spontaneous[54]. Looking at this problem somewhat differently, of the first 85 patients undergoing multifetal pregnancy reduction reported by Lynch *et al.* in the USA, only 14% and 8% of pregnancies were the product of IVF–ET or GIFT procedures, respectively; the remaining 78% resulted from ovulation induction therapy[55]. The high percentage of multiples arising from ovulation induction reflects the tremendous increase in the use of these agents as well as a major modification in the original philosophy of their use (as described in the next section).

Ovulation induction versus 'superovulation therapy'

Clomiphene citrate and human menopausal gonadotropins (hMG) have been used for many years for the 'induction of ovulation' in women with anovulation, oligo-ovulation or ovulatory dysfunction. The increase in multiple births arising from these therapies is well recognized[56–60]. A review of the literature from 1968 to 1980 summarized over 1000 hMG-induced pregnancies[58]. Multiple pregnancy rates ranged from 16 to 40%, with an average of 25 to 30% multiples. Approximately 75% of the multiples consisted of twins. The magnitude of risk for inducing multiple gestation with hMG therapy varies with the different diagnostic entities being treated[60], as well as the quantity and dosage schedule of the medication (no standard regimen is universally followed). A recent analysis of hMG therapy delivered by pulsatile subcutaneous administration reported a lower rate of multiple gestation as compared with the conventional approach of daily IM injections[61]. The use of these agents has expanded tremendously in recent years, both in IVF–ET and GIFT procedures *per se*, as well as in the practice of 'superovulation therapy'.

With increasing frequency since 1984[62], ovarian stimulants have been administered to *ovulatory* women for the purpose of recruiting multiple follicles/oocytes within a single cycle. This practice clearly increases the number of women exposed to the possibility of iatrogenic multiple pregnancy. Superovulation therapy is also known as 'controlled ovarian hyperstimulation' or by the acronym SOURCE (superovulation, uterine replacement, capacitation, enhancement). Superovulation is often combined with intrauterine insemination of semen that has been washed to separate the sperm from the seminal plasma and further processed by some means of filtration, centrifugation or 'swim-up' technique to yield a highly fertile subpopulation of sperm[62,63].

Superovulation therapy developed from a fortuitous clinical observation. Some patients who received hMG in preparation for an IVF or GIFT cycle attempt had the oocyte aspiration cancelled (due to inadequate follicular stimulation or endogenous luteinizing hormone surge) but became pregnant anyway[64–66]. This observation suggested that multiple follicular recruitment (rather than gamete retrieval or embryo transfer) might be the most critical element contributing to the success of IVF–ET or GIFT in patients with patent Fallopian tubes. Two theories have been offered to explain the improvement in pregnancy rates from this treatment[64]. In women whose ovulatory processes are truly normal, superovulation therapy may enhance fertility by increasing the number of oocytes available per cycle, as well as by increasing the quantity of sperm available for each oocyte. By increasing the numbers of gametes in the reproductive tract, the probability of conception is increased. Alternatively, in women who have subtle (i.e. undiagnosed) ovulatory dysfunction, superovulation therapy may successfully correct such a disorder. The monthly probability of pregnancy (cycle fecundity) following superovulation therapy averages 10–20% per cycle[63,68–70]. With this practice, an increase in the risk of iatrogenic multiple gestation becomes an unavoidable consequence of the intentional increase in available oocytes per cycle. Several large series report multiple pregnancy rates ranging from 7 to 29%[63,68–73]. These reports, however, represent a compilation of data from 'heterogenous groups of patients with dissimilar diagnostic entities, duration of infertility, prior therapy, age and experience of the physician'[68]. Some programs use clomiphene with or without hMG for the same purpose[74].

Several factors distinguish 'superovulation therapy' from the traditional practice of ovulation induction using clomiphene, hMG or both. The foremost difference is that the production of more than one mature follicle was previously a frequent, but inadvertent outcome. With superovulation, it is the intentional goal of therapy. These two fertility treatments are also distinguished by certain subjective elements introduced by the physician. Conventional ovulation induction generally followed a conservative, cautious approach. With superovulation therapy, fewer guidelines exist, and a broader range of 'aggressiveness' is observed, reflected in the quantity of hMG used, the estradiol level achieved and the number of follicles produced, which influences the chance for successful pregnancy[73,75]. Gonadotropin releasing hormone (GnRH) analogs (for example, luprolide acetate) can be added to prevent the spontaneous midcycle luteinizing hormone surge and permit an even greater degree of ovarian stimulation to occur[76].

Traditionally, parameters that are considered predictive for multiple gestation include both the maximum estradiol concentration and the number of large preovulatory follicles observed by ultrasound[77]. However, correlation between the number of apparently mature follicles and the incidence of multifetal gestation is poor[78]. Similarly, peak estradiol levels are poorly predictive of multiple gestation. DeCherney and Laufer[79] reported a quintuplet pregnancy following a peak estradiol level of only 300 pg/ml, a preovulatory estrogen level which is not above normal. Furthermore, in view of the major differences in protocol and in the patients receiving conventional ovulation induction vs. superovulation therapy, the traditional multiple pregnancy risk parameters may no longer be relevant to the current use of hMG therapy[80]. In an analysis of multiple pregnancies from superovulation therapy, neither the patients' clinical characteristics (age, parity, etiology or duration of infertility) nor any features of the stimulation (quantity or duration of hMG therapy, peak estradiol level, number of preovulatory follicles or number of sperm inseminated) correlated with the chance of multiple gestation[80]. Sheldon et al.[72], however, demonstrated a significant correlation between the insemination dose of sperm and the risk of multiple gestation, but a later analysis by Dodson and Haney[68] failed to confirm this observation. In another analysis of almost 800 superovulation cycles by Dickey et al.[73], the number of follicles of ≥ 12 mm correlated with the incidence of multiple gestation. Birth rates rose linearly with the serum estradiol level, but the incidence of multiple gestation was not correlated with the estradiol level. A 29% incidence of multiple birth was observed even when the maximum estradiol level was < 1000 pg/ml, a level ordinarily considered well within safe limits for ovulation induction with gonadotropins.

The risk of multiple pregnancy can be reduced (but not eliminated) by withholding the dose of human chorionic gonadotropin (hCG; used to induce actual ovulation) in the presence of multiple follicles or with excessively high estradiol levels[81]. However, in doing so, pregnancy rates are compromised. Alternatively, in one report, multiple pregnancy rates were reduced substantially when the inseminating dose of sperm was reduced to less than 20 million motile sperm[70].

Freidman[82] reported a case highly illustrative of the inability to predict the occurrence of multiple gestation using current clinical parameters. Sextuplets occurred in a patient with a peak estradiol level of 861 pg/ml and only one follicle fulfilling sonographic criteria for maturity at the time of hCG administration. In this case, 'booster' doses of human chorionic gonadotropin administered following insemination might have caused subsequent release

Table 6 Monozygotic pairs and assisted reproduction

Fixed and universal rate	0.4%
Ovulation induction rate	1.2%*†
IVF–ET rate	~1%*‡

*$p<0.05$ compared to naturally occuring incidence;
† Derom et al.[92]; ‡Edwards et al.[93]

of additional less mature follicles. Septuplets occurred in another patient with only four pre-ovulatory follicles on ultrasound[83], again demonstrating the limitations on predicting or absolutely preventing unanticipated multiple gestations.

Because of the high cost of IVF–ET or GIFT, superovulation therapy has been widely and quickly adopted as a less expensive and non-invasive alternative with perhaps comparable success[63]. The true value of superovulation therapy for the couple with ovulatory infertility has yet to be demonstrated in controlled, prospective studies, however[67,84]. Such a study is essential, because of the known spontaneous pregnancy rate that occurs in some couples, independent of any fertility therapy. If the cost of IVF–ET and other ART procedures can be reduced, the balance may then favor IVF–ET over superovulation therapy for two reasons. First, IVF–ET provides unique, additional information about the normality of the couple's fertilization process; and second, the risk of multiple pregnancy can be controlled (by limiting the number of embryos transferred per cycle). Superovulation and intrauterine insemination could well become obsolete if the cost of IVF–ET becomes more readily attainable for patients, as might be the case for 'natural cycle' IVF. Should this happen, the significant contribution that superovulation therapy is currently making to the number of iatrogenic multiples would be totally eliminated.

Gonadotropin releasing hormone therapy

In contrast to hMG therapy (which overwhelms the endogenous hormonal feedback mechanisms that ordinarily restrain multiple follicular recruitment), the administration of pulsatile GnRH usually allows for appropriate pituitary–ovarian feedback signals, thereby lessening the chance of multiple birth. Recent series of patients treated with GnRH report a 7–10% incidence[85,86] of multiples, usually twins, but occasional reports of higher-order multiples, including quadruplets[87] have appeared. Patient selection and the dose employed affect the likelihood of multiple gestation. There appears to be a significant and consistent association between multiple pregnancy and the *first* cycle of GnRH treatment in patients with hypogonadotropic hypogonadism[85,86,88].

Monozygotic twinning and ART

The observed increase in multiple gestation arising from fertility therapy is ordinarily explained on the basis of fertilization of multiple oocytes, yielding polyzygotic gestations. Unexpectedly, preliminary data presently suggest that the incidence of monozygotic (MZ) splitting, a phenomenon previously thought to be a biological constant, is higher than expected following assisted reproduction[89–93]. Two studies have examined this phenomenon, one following ovulation induction alone[92] and the other dealing with IVF–ET pregnancies[93]. Both investigations demonstrated a significant increase in the number of monozygotic pairs (Table 6).

Theoretically, four factors influence the rate of monozygotic twinning that occurs in conjunction with assisted reproduction. First, as noted by Derom *et al.*[92], ovulation induction alone results in an increased frequency of monozygotic pairs. A 'hardening' of the zona pellucida surrounding the early embryo (from which it 'hatches') is noted in animals after ovulation induction. Derom and co-workers speculated that non-uniform hardening of the zona could lead to herniation of a portion of the blastocyst, ultimately causing formation of two separate embryos surrounded by a dichorionic placenta. The remaining three factors that favor monozygotic splitting relate specifically to the embryo production in the *in vitro* fertilization laboratory: (1) the *in vitro* environment itself may exert detrimental effects on the zona, creating zona defects or non-uniform hardening; (2) routine oocyte and embryo manipulation, such as fine pipetting to remove surrounding granulosa cells, might mechanically cause a bifurcation of the conceptus; and (3) embryo exposure to uterine secretions, possibly including 'lysins', at a sensitive and premature stage of embryo development may also result in embryo splitting[93]. The increased incidence of dichorionic placentation that theoretically would be expected from these early influences on early embryo development has not been observed, however[92].

A certain percentage of implantation failures of IVF–ET embryos may be due to the inability of the embryo to escape ('hatch') from the zona pellucida[92]. 'Assisted hatching' by micromanipulation techniques that either chemically ('zona drilling') or mechanically ('partial zona dissection') create a hole (gap) in the zona pellucida is under intense investigation. The incidence of monozygotic twins is also increased following application of these techniques, especially with partial zona dissection[95]. Biochemical and/or mechanical factors may cause a shearing separation (or loss of intercellular integrity) of the inner cell mass during expulsion of the blastocyst through the artificial zona gap, leading to monozygotic division.

Multifetal pregnancy reduction

In the case of a iatrogenically induced multiple gestation, the ethical considerations of multifetal pregnancy reduction (MPR) are inextricably linked to the ethical conduct of the fertility therapist[96,97]. For induced multiples, it seems appropriate that the physician offer a solution to salvage an otherwise doomed multifetal pregnancy that occurred as a consequence of a lost 'gamble' (of successfully producing a pregnancy, but avoiding a multiple). Recent opinions[98,99] stress the need for infertility spec- ialists to diligently attempt to minimize the risk of inducing multiples and to provide careful, detailed counselling about the risk of complications prior to the initiation of therapy, including an early discussion of MPR. (See Chapters 26 and 27.)

Counselling the infertile couple

Couples joining ART programs are often made aware of the increased risk of multiple pregnancies, but it is unlikely that they fully appreciate the magnitude of physical and psychological harm potentially associated with multiple gestation. The maternal and neonatal morbidity associated with multiple pregnancies has been reviewed in great detail throughout this text[17]. The additional potential for physical and psychological harm from multifetal pregnancy reduction remains to be determined. When couples are being counselled about the risk of multifetal pregnancy arising from fertility therapy, they often initially express the view that a multiple pregnancy would be a welcome 'bonus' outcome of therapy. This attitude probably reflects both ignorance and psychological denial of risk. The counselling process must make clear both the extreme potential for obstetric and perinatal morbidity and also the extraordinary challenges, dilemmas and stresses associated with the parenting of multiples.

The severity of the social and economic strains on the household and the negative psychological reactions of parents of higher-order multiples (ambivalence, shock, shame, feeling cursed and animalistic) have received only limited attention thus far[99,100].

Typically, the costs addressed with infertile couples include only those associated with undergoing a particular procedure in order to achieve a pregnancy. However, in view of the significant risk of multiples, a complete discussion should also include the costs of high-risk pregnancy monitoring, operative delivery, neonatal intensive care and child care. Only when these factors are included is the couple given a complete and realistic appraisal of the financial burden they assume when pursuing aggressive fertility therapy.

Other counselling issues might well include the broader psychosocial consequences unique to couples with *induced* multiples[101]. For example, although more infants delivered after multiple gestations survive as a result of current improvements in neonatal care, severe morbidity and mortality are still common. Guilt or regret over the decision to undergo fertility therapy could result in an exaggerated emotional response if an adverse neonatal outcome does occur. Diminished social support for the parents of iatrogenic multiples also remains a concern. Neglect by friends or relatives might occur as a consequence of a perceived sense that the parents of iatrogenic multiples should be held responsible for the outcome of their fertility therapy. Finally, adequate counselling is imperative to reduce the medical–legal liability of physicians who provide this therapy. The counselling necessary to adequately prepare patients to confront these issues is lengthy, and probably requires special skills. ART programs could undoubtedly enhance the care they deliver when specially trained medical professionals, such as perinatal social workers, are available to offer counselling to infertility patients about the risks of multiple pregnancy, including the practice of multifetal pregnancy reduction.

Concluding considerations

Several fundamental questions remain to be answered regarding the effect of modern reproductive technology on the incidence of multiple pregnancy: (1) What is an acceptable level of pregnancy efficiency per procedure? (2) What incidence of multiple pregnancy is clinically 'acceptable'? (3) Are the risks of iatrogenic multiple pregnancy justified? (4) In what manner, if any, do the problems following multiple birth differ if the multiple pregnancy is spontaneous or induced? (5) How best should couples be counselled regarding the risk–benefit ratio of assisted reproduction? (6) How can the practice of multifetal pregnancy reduction be controlled so that it is used to benefit couples with inadvertent high multiples, but not result in overzealous fertility therapy and in the casual destruction of excess embryos? It may take years before these questions can be satisfactorily answered. In the meantime, we can safely conclude the following:

(1) The incidence of multifetal pregnancy from modern reproductive technology is approximately 25% of births, ranging from a low of 7–9% for clomiphene citrate to a high of 25–40% for hMG and ART.

(2) Recent refinements in clinical practice may greatly reduce the inadvertent production of high-order multiples in the near future.

(3) Ovulation induction (with or without *in vitro* fertilization) may be the first identifiable variable capable of influencing the monozygotic twinning rate.

(4) The risk and benefits of medically assisted reproduction include many complex issues. Proper patient care must include extensive counselling.

References

1. Steptoe, P.C. and Edwards, R.G. (1978). Birth after reimplantation of a human embryo. *Lancet*, **2**, 366
2. Medical Research International, The American Fertility Society Special Interest Group (1988). *In vitro* fertilization/embryo transfer in the United States: 1985 and 1986 results from the National IVF-ET Registry. *Fertil. Steril.*, **49**, 212
3. Medical Research International and the Society of Assisted Reproductive Technology, The American Fertility Society (1989). *In vitro* fertilization/embryo transfer in the United States: 1987 results from the National IVF-ET Registry. *Fertil. Steril.*, **51**, 13
4. Medical Research International and the Society of Assisted Reproductive Technology, The American Fertility Society (1990). *In vitro* fertilization/embryo transfer in the United States: 1988 results from the IVF-ET Registry. *Fertil. Steril.*, **53**, 13
5. Medical Research International and the Society of Assisted Reproductive Technology, The American Fertility Society (1991). 1989 results from the IVF-ET Registry. *Fertil. Steril.*, **55**, 14

6. Medical Research International, Society for Assisted Reproductive Technology (SART), The American Fertility Society (1992). In Vitro Fertilization–Embryo Transfer (IVF–ET) in the United States: 1990 results from the IVF–ET Registry. *Fertil. Steril.*, **57**, 15
7. National Center for Health Statistics: *Vital Statistics of the United States, 1982, 1983, 1984, 1985, 1986, 1987, 1988*, vol I. *Natality*, DHHS publication no. (PHS) 88-1123, Public Health Service. (Washington DC: United States Government Printing Office)
8. American Fertility Society (1990). Revised minimum standards for *in vitro* fertilization, gamete intrafallopian transfer and related procedures. *Fertil. Steril.*, **53**, 255
9. Soules, M.R. (1985). The *in vitro* fertilization pregnancy rate: let's be honest with one another. *Fertil. Steril.*, **43**, 511
10. ACOG Technical Bulletin (1990). *New Reproductive Technologies*, No. 140, **March**
11. Penzias, A.S., Alper, M.M. and Oskowitz, S.P. (1991). Gamete intrafallopian transfer: assessment of the optimal number of oocytes to transfer. *Fertil. Steril.*, **55**, 311
12. Luke, B. and Keith, L.G. (1991). The U.S. Standard Certificate of Live Birth. A critical commentary. *J. Reprod. Med.*, **36**, 587
13. DeCherney, A.H. and Hartz, S.C. (1989). Assisted reproduction: registration vis-à-vis regulation. *Fertil. Steril.*, **51**, 568
14. The American Fertility Society, Society for Assisted Reproductive Technology (1994). Assisted Reproductive Technology in the United States and Canada: 1992 results generated from the American Fertility Society/Society for Assisted Reproductive Technology Registry. *Fertil. Steril.*, **62**, 1121
15. Wood, C., McMaster, R., Rennie, G. *et al.* (1985). Factors influencing pregnancy rates following *in vitro* fertilization and embryo transfer. *Fertil. Steril.*, **43**, 245
16. Quigley, M.M. (1984). The use of ovulation-inducing agents in *in vitro* fertilization. *Clin. Obstet. Gynecol.*, **27**, 983
17. Feldberg, D., Laufer, N., Dicker, D., Goldman, J.A. and DeCherney, A. (1986). Quadruplet pregnancy in IVF. *Eur. J. Obstet. Gynecol. Reprod. Biol.*, **23**, 101
18. Australian *In Vitro* Fertilization Collaborative Group. (1985) High incidence of preterm births and early losses in pregnancy after *in vitro* fertilization. *Br. Med. J.*, **291**, 1160
19. MRC working party on children conceived by *in vitro* fertilization (1990). Births in Great Britain resulting from assisted conception, 1978–87. *Br. Med. J.*, **300**, 1229
20. Cohen, J., Mayaux, M.J. and Guihard-Moscato, M.L. (1988). Pregnancy outcomes after *in vitro* fertilization. *Ann. NY Acad. Sci.*, **541**, 1
21. Asch, R.H., Ellsworth, L.R., Balmaceda, J.P. and Wong, P.C. (1984). Pregnancy after translaparoscopic gamete intrafallopian transfer. *Lancet*, **2**, 1034
22. Craft, I., Al-Shawaf, T., Lewis, P. *et al.* (1988). Analyses of 1071 GIFT procedures – the case for a flexible approach to treatment. *Lancet*, **1**, 1094
23. Batzer, F.R., Gocial, B., Corson, S.L., Weiner, S. and Wapner, R.J. (1988). Multiple pregnancies with gamete intrafallopian transfer (GIFT): complications of a new technique. *J. In Vitro Fert.*, **5**, 35
24. Devroey, L., Braeckmans, P., Smitz, J. *et al.* (1986). Pregnancy after translaparoscopic zygote intrafallopian transfer in a patient with sperm antibodies. *Lancet*, **1**, 1329
25. Yovich, J.L., Yovich, J.M. and Edirisinghe, W.R. (1988). The relative chance of pregnancy following tubal or uterine transfer procedures. *Fertil. Steril.*, **49**, 858
26. Balmaceda, J.P., Gastaldi, C., Remohi, J. *et al.* (1988). Tubal embryo transfer as a treatment for infertility due to male factor. *Fertil. Steril.*, **50**, 476
27. Hamori, M., Stuckensen, J.A., Rumpf, D. *et al.* (1988). Zygote intrafallopian transfer (ZIFT): evaluation of 42 cases. *Fertil. Steril.*, **50**, 519
28. Devroey, P., Staessen, C., Camus, M. *et al.* (1989). Zygote intrafallopian transfer as a successful treatment for unexplained infertility. *Fertil. Steril.*, **52**, 246
29. Scholtes, M.C.W., Roozenburg, B.J., Alberda, A.T. and Zeilmaker, G.H. (1990). Transcervical intrafallopian transfer of zygotes. *Fertil. Steril.*, **54**, 283
30. Pool, T.B. Ellsworth, L.R., Garza, J.R. *et al.* (1990). Zygote intrafallopian transfer as a treatment for nontubal infertility: a 2-year study. *Fertil. Steril.*, **54**, 482
31. Bollen, N., Camus, M., Staessen, C. *et al.* (1991). The incidence of multiple pregnancy after *in vitro* fertilization and embryo transfer, gamete, or zygote intrafallopian transfer. *Fertil. Steril.*, **55**, 314
32. Balmaceda, J.P., Alam, V., Roszjtein, D. *et al.* (1992). Embryo implantation rates in oocyte

donation: a prospective comparison of tubal versus uterine transfers. *Fertil. Steril.*, **57**, 362
33. Bennett, S.J., Parsons, J.M. and Bolton, V.N. (1987). Two-embryo transfer. *Lancet*, **2**, 215
34. Corson, S.L., Dickey, R.P., Gocial, B. *et al.* (1989). Outcome in 242 *in vitro* fertilization embryo replacement or gamete intrafallopian transfer-induced pregnancies. *Fertil. Steril.*, **51**, 644
35. El Khazen, N., Puissant, F., Camus, M., Lejeune, B. and Leroy, F. (1986). A comparison between multiple and single pregnancies obtained by *in vitro* fertilization. *Hum. Reprod.*, **1**, 251
36. Craft, I., Brinsden, P. and Simons, E. (1987). Multiple pregnancy and assisted reproduction. *Lancet*, **2**, 692
37. Kerin, J.F., Quinn, P.J., Kirby, C. *et al.* (1983). Incidence of multiple pregnancy after *in vitro* fertilisation and embryo transfer. *Lancet*, **2**, 537
38. Richards, M. and Price, F. (1987). Licensing work on IVF and related procedures (letter). *Lancet*, **1**, 1373
39. Philipp, E.E. (1993). Impact of the Human Fertilization and Embryology Act (1990) on the practice of reproductive medicine in the United Kingdom. *Fertil. Steril.*, **59**, 285
40. Levene, M.I., Wild, J. and Steer, P. (1992). Higher multiple births and the modern management of infertility in Britain. *Br. J. Obstet. Gynaecol.*, **99**, 607
41. Friedler, S., Mashiach, S. and Laufer, N. (1992). Births in Israel resulting from *in vitro* fertilization/embryo transfer 1982–1989: National Registry of Israel: Association for Fertility Research. *Hum. Reprod.*, **7**, 1159
42. Speirs, A.L., Lopata, A., Gronow, M.J. *et al.* (1983). Analysis of the benefits and risks of multiple embryo transfer. *Fertil. Steril.*, **39**, 468
43. Sharma, V., Whitehead, M., Mason, B. *et al.* (1990). Influence of superovulation on endometrial and embryonic development. *Fertil. Steril.*, **53**, 822
44. Paulson, R.J., Sauer, M.V. and Lobo, R.A. (1990). Embryo implantation after human *in vitro* fertilization: importance of endometrial receptivity. *Fertil. Steril.*, **53**, 870
45. Winston, R.M. (1990). Invited address to the *46th Annual Meeting of the American Fertility Society*, Washington DC, October
46. Trounson, A. and Mohr, L. (1983). Human pregnancy following cryopreservation, thawing and transfer of an eight-cell embryo. *Nature (London)*, **305**, 707
47. Batzofin, J., Tran, C., Tan, T. *et al.* (1991). Is there evidence to support the practice of embryo freezing and halt fresh embryo transfer in stimulated cycles? Abstract P-005, *Abstracts of the 39th Annual Meeting of the Pacific Conference Fertility Society*, Scottsdale, AZ., April, p. A7
48. Navot, D., Laufer, N., Kopolovic, J. *et al.* (1986). Artificially induced endometrial cycles and establishment of pregnancies in the absence of ovaries. *N. Engl. J. Med.*, **314**, 806
49. Bustillo, M., Thorsell, L., Yap, S. *et al.* (1991). Endometrial receptivity after transfer of frozen–thawed human embryos: randomized trial of controlled versus natural cycles. Abstract 161, *Abstracts of the 38th Annual Meeting of the Society for Gynecologic Investigation*, San Antonio, Texas, March, p. 179
50. Garcia, J. (1989). Return to the natural cycle for *in vitro* fertilization (Alleluia! Alleluia!). *J. In Vitro Fert.*, **6**, 67
51. Foulot, M., Ranoax, C., Dubuisson, J.B. *et al.* (1989). *In vitro* fertilization without ovarian stimulation: a simplified protocol applied in 80 cycles. *Fertil. Steril.*, **52**, 617
52. Paulson, R.J., Sauer, M.V., Frances, M.M. *et al.* (1992). *In vitro* fertilization in unstimulated cycles: the University of South California experience. *Fertil. Steril.*, **57**, 290
53. Elster, A.D., Bleyl, J.A. and Craven, T.E. (1991). Birth weight standards for triplets under modern obstetric care in the United States, 1984–1989. *Obstet. Gynecol.*, **77**, 387
54. Collins, M.S. and Bleyl, J.A. (1990). Seventy-one quadruplet pregnancies: management and outcome. *Am. J. Obstet. Gynecol.*, **162**, 1384
55. Lynch, L., Berkowitz, R.L., Chitkara, A. and Alvarez, M. (1990). First-trimester transabdominal multifetal pregnancy reduction: a report of 85 cases. *Obstet. Gynecol.*, **75**, 735
56. Lamont, J.A. (1982). Twin pregnancies following induction of ovulation. A literature review. *Acta Genet. Med. Gemellol.*, **31**, 247
57. Diamond, M.P. and Wentz, A.C. (1986). Ovulation induction with human menopausal gonadotropins. *Obstet. Gynecol. Surv.*, **41**, 480
58. Schenker, J.G., Yarkoni, S. and Granat, M. (1981). Multiple pregnancies following induction of ovulation. *Fertil. Steril.*, **35**, 105
59. Scialli, A.R. (1986). The reproductive toxicity of ovulation induction. *Fertil. Steril.*, **45**, 315
60. Oelsner, G., Serr, D.M., Mashiach, Blankstein, J., Snyder, M. and Lunnenfeld, B. (1978). The

study of induction of ovulation with menotropins: analysis of results of 1897 treatment cycles. *Fertil. Steril.*, **30**, 538

61. Nakamura, Y., Yoshimura, Y., Yamada, H. *et al.* (1989). Clinical experience in the induction of ovulation and pregnancy with pulsatile subcutaneous administration of human menopausal gonadotropin: a low incidence of multiple pregnancy. *Fertil. Steril.*, **51**, 423

62. Sher, G., Knutzen, V.K., Stratton, C.J., Montakhab, M.M. and Allenson, S.G. (1984). *In vitro* sperm capacitation and transcervical intrauterine insemination for the treatment of refractory infertility: phase I. *Fertil. Steril.*, **41**, 260

63. Dodson, W.C., Whitesides, D.B., Hughes, C.L., Easley, H.A. and Haney, A.F. (1987). Superovulation with intrauterine insemination in the treatment of infertility: a possible alternative to gamete intrafallopian transfer and *in vitro* fertilization. *Fertil. Steril.*, **48**, 441

64. Haney, A.F., Hughes, C.L., Whitesides, D.B. and Dodson, W.C. (1987). Treatment-independent, treatment-associated and pregnancies after additional therapy in a program of *in vitro* fertilization and embryo transfer. *Fertil. Steril.*, **47**, 634

65. Curole, D.N., Dickey, R.P., Taylor, S.N. *et al.* (1989). Pregnancies in cancelled gamete intrafallopian transfer cycles. *Fertil. Steril.*, **51**, 363

66. Welner, S., DeCherney, A.H. and Polan, M.L. (1988). Human menopausal gonadotropins: a justifiable therapy in ovulatory women with long-standing idiopathic infertility. *Am. J. Obstet. Gynecol.*, **158**, 111

67. Collins, J.A. (1990). Superovulation in the treatment of unexplained infertility. *Sem. Reprod. Endocr.*, **8**, 165

68. Dodson, W.C. and Haney, A.F. (1991). Controlled ovarian hyperstimulation and intrauterine insemination for treatment of infertility. *Fertil. Steril.*, **55**, 457

69. Chaffkin, L.M., Nulsen, J.C., Luciano, A.A. and Metzger, D.A. (1991). A comparative analysis of the cycle fecundity rates associated with combined human menopausal gonadotropin (hMG) and intrauterine insemination (IUI) versus either hMG or IUI alone. *Fertil. Steril.*, **55**, 252

70. Corsan, G.M., Shelden, R.M. and Kemmann, E. (1989). Multiple gestation with intrauterine insemination and menotropin therapy (letter). *Am. J. Obstet. Gynecol.*, **161**, 1751

71. Remohi, J., Gastaldi, C., Patrizio, P., Gerli, S., Asch, R.H. and Balmaceda, J.P. (1989). Intrauterine insemination and controlled ovarian hyperstimulation in cycles before GIFT. *Hum. Reprod.*, **4**, 918

72. Sheldon, R., Kemmann, E., Bohrer, M. and Pasquale, S. (1988). Multiple gestation is associated with the use of high sperm numbers in the intrauterine insemination specimen in women undergoing gonadotropin stimulation. *Fertil. Steril.*, **49**, 607

73. Dickey, R.P., Olar, T.T., Taylor, S.N. *et al.* (1991). Relationship of follicle number, serum estradiol, and other factors to birth rate and multiparity in human menopausal gonadotropin-induced intrauterine insemination cycles. *Fertil. Steril.*, **56**, 89

74. Dickey, R.P., Olar, T.T., Taylor, S.N., Carole, D.N. and Rye, P.H. (1992). Relationship of follicle number and other factors to fecundability and multiple pregnancy in clomiphene citrate-induced intrauterine insemination cycles. *Fertil. Steril.*, **57**, 613

75. Martinez, A.R., Bernardus, R.E., Voorhorst, F.J. *et al.* (1991). Pregnancy rates after timed intercourse or intrauterine insemination after human menopausal gonadotropin stimulation of normal ovulatory cycles: a controlled study. *Fertil. Steril.*, **55**, 258

76. Frydman, R., Parneix, I., Belaisch-Allart, J. *et al.* (1988). LHRH agonists in IVF: different methods of utilization and comparison with previous ovulation stimulation treatments. *Hum. Reprod.*, **3**, 559

77. Seibel, M.M., McArdle, C.R., Thompson, I.E. *et al.* (1981). The role of ultrasound in ovulation induction: critical appraisal. *Fertil. Steril.*, **36**, 573

78. Stone, S.C., Schimberni, M., Schuster, P.A. *et al.* (1987). Incidence of multiple gestations in the presence of two or more mature follicles in the conception cycle. *Fertil. Steril.*, **48**, 503

79. DeCherney, A.H. and Laufer, N. (1984). The monitoring of ovulation induction using ultrasound and estrogen. *Clin. Obstet. Gynecol.*, **27**, 993

80. Dodson, W.C., Hughes, C.C. and Haney, A.F. (1988). Multiple pregnancies conceived with intrauterine insemination during superovulation: an evaluation of clinical characteristics and monitored parameters of conception cycles. *Am. J. Obstet. Gynecol.* **159**, 382

81. Lipitz, S., Ben-Rafael, Z., Bider, J. *et al.* (1991). Quintuplet pregnancy and third degree ovarian

hyperstimulation despite withholding human chorionic gonadotrophin. *Hum. Reprod.*, **6**, 1478
82. Friedman, A.J. (1990). Sextuplet pregnancy after human menopausal gonadotropin superovulation and intrauterine insemination. *J. Reprod. Med.*, **35**, 113
83. Fedorkow, D.M., Corenblum, B., Pattinson, M.A. and Taylor, P.J. (1988). Septuplet gestation following the use of human menopausal gonadotropin despite intensive monitoring. *Fertil. Steril.*, **49**, 364
84. Wallach, E. (1991). Gonadotropin treatment for the ovulatory patient – the pros and cons of empiric therapy for infertility. *Fertil. Steril.*, **55**, 478
85. Blunt, S.M. and Butt, W.R. (1988). Pulsatile GnRH therapy for the induction of ovulation in hypogonadotropic hypogonadism. *Acta Endocrinol. (Copenh.)*, **288**, 58
86. Homburg, R., Eshel, A., Armar, N.A. *et al.* (1989). One hundred pregnancies after treatment with pulsatile luteinizing hormone releasing hormone to induce ovulation. *Br. Med. J.*, **298**, 809
87. Heineman, M.J., Bouckaert, P.X.J.M. and Schellekens, L.A. (1984). A quadruplet pregnancy following ovulation induction with pulsatile luteinizing hormone-releasing hormone. *Fertil. Steril.*, **42**, 300
88. Braat, D.D.M., Boghelman, D., Coelingh-Bennink, H.J.T. *et al.* (1985). The outcome of pregnancies established in GnRH induced cycles with special reference to the multiple pregnancies in five Dutch centres. In Coelingh-Bennink, H.J.T., Dogerom, A.A., Lappohn, R.E. *et al.* (eds.) *Pulsatile GnRH*, pp. 207–13. (Haarlem, The Netherlands: Ferring)
89. Mettler, L., Riedel, H.H., Grillo, M. *et al.* (1984). Schwangerschaft und geburt monozygoter weiblicher zwillinge nach *in-vitro*-fertilisation und transfer embryo (IVF-ET). *Geburtsch. Frauenheilk.*, **44**, 670
90. Yovich, J.L., Stanger, J.D., Grauang, A. *et al.* (1984). Monozygotic twins from *in vitro* fertilization. *Fertil. Steril.*, **41**, 833
91. Camus, M., Puissant, F., Degueldre, M. *et al.* (1985). Quadruple IVF pregnancy after replacement of three embryos. *4th World Conference on In-vitro Fertilization.* Melbourne, Abstract No. 215A
92. Derom, C., Vlietinck, R., Derom, R. *et al.* (1987). Increased monozygotic twinning rate after ovulation induction. *Lancet*, **2**, 1236
93. Edwards, R.G., Mettler, L. and Walters, D.E. (1986). Identical twins and *in vitro* fertilization. *J. In Vitro Fert.*, **3**, 114
94. Cohen, J., Alikani, M., Trowbridge, J. and Rosenwaks, Z. (1992). Implantation enhancement of selective assisted hatching using zona drilling of human embryos with poor prognosis. *Hum. Reprod.*, **7**, 685
95. Cohen, J. (1991). Assisted hatching of human embryos. *J. In Vitro Fertil. Embryo Transfer*, **8**, 179
96. Weiner, J. (1988). Selective first-trimester termination in octuplet and quadruplet pregnancies: clinical and ethical issues (letter). *Obstet. Gynecol.*, **72**, 871
97. ACOG committee opinion (1991). *Multifetal Pregnancy Reduction and Selective Fetal Termination*, no. 94, April
98. Zaner, R.M., Boehm, F.M. and Hill, G.A. (1990). Selective termination in multiple pregnancies: ethical considerations. *Fertil. Steril.*, **54**, 203
99. Goshen-Gottstein, E.R. (1980). The mothering of twins, triplets and quadruplets. *Psychiatry*, **43**, 189
100. Robin, M., Bydlowski, M., Cahen, F. and Josse, D. (1991). Maternal reactions to the birth of triplets. *Acta Genet. Med. Gemellol.*, **40**, 41
101. Price, F.V. (1988). The risk of high multiparity with IVF-ET. *Birth*, **15**, 157

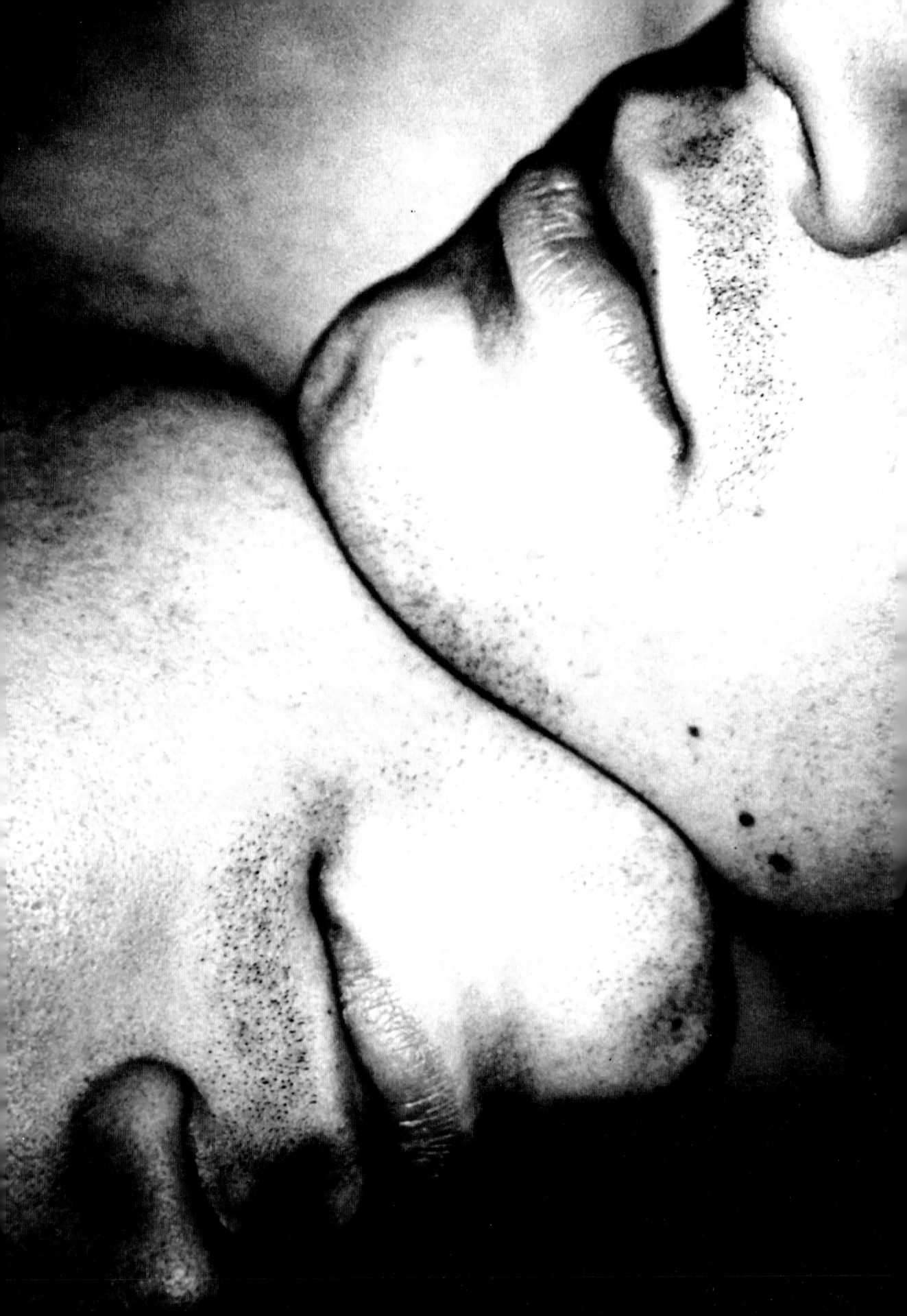

section IV
Diagnosis and General Considerations

The Dworkin Twins

David Teplica, 1990,
The Smart Museum, University of Chicago

Ultrasound scanning techniques

R. Bessis

Introduction

The prognosis of twin pregnancies has improved dramatically since the introduction of ultrasound into clinical practice. Indeed, ultrasound is the only technique that can enhance the clinical examination by monitoring each fetus at times when the apparent well-being of one of them masks the distress of the other. In the last few years, it has become common to refer to the fetus as a patient. In doing so, however, the classic concept of a mother–infant dyad has been restructured, so that each is seen as having a certain amount of independence, albeit within a more encompassing form of dependence. Multifetal pregnancies extend this concept even further, because the fetuses are individuals not only with respect to their mother, but also with respect to each other. The medical impact of these conceptual and, at times, real changes has been enormous. At the same time, the psychological impact for parents is probably of equal magnitude, although data to support this contention are scant. (See Section IX.)

Diagnosis

The major contribution of ultrasound clearly is its ability to obtain a simple and instantaneous confirmation of a clinical suspicion of multifetal pregnancy without risk to the mother or her fetuses. Some departments report that 95% of all twin births are correctly diagnosed prior to delivery[1]. In the last few years, the prenatal diagnosis rate at Hôpital Antoine Béclère in Clamart, France is 100%.

In clinical practice, any size–date discrepancy prior to a presumed gestational age of 18 weeks is sufficient reason for requesting an ultrasound scan[2]. It is important to remember, however, that if scans are not ordered as a routine part of early prenatal care, cases may not always be typical, and clinical perceptions can be adversely affected by a number of factors. The most obvious is an error in the presumed gestational age based on menstrual dates alone. Thus, any doubt concerning gestational age is a valid reason for requesting an ultrasound scan, which can rapidly correct any misperceptions or misdiagnoses.

Principle

Regardless of the clinical context or the reason for ordering a scan, all fetal ultrasound examinations should include a search for multifetal pregnancies. The diagnosis of a twin pregnancy is based on the simultaneous visualization, on the same ultrasound section, of the corresponding body parts of two fetuses. Some years ago, this definition was mainly restricted to fetal heads, which were the only parts that were easy to identify at that time (Figure 1). Currently, however, diagnosis is generally performed during the first trimester, and embryo visualization is more common (Figure 2). Attempts should be made to identify the two embryos on the same initial exploratory examination. Once a twin gestation has been identified, the examination should continue in a logical fashion in order to avoid underestimating a higher-order pregnancy.

Causes of error

Ultrasound diagnosis of multiple pregnancy is theoretically error-free. At 5 weeks of amenorrhea (3 weeks post-fertilization), multiple sacs

MULTIPLE PREGNANCY

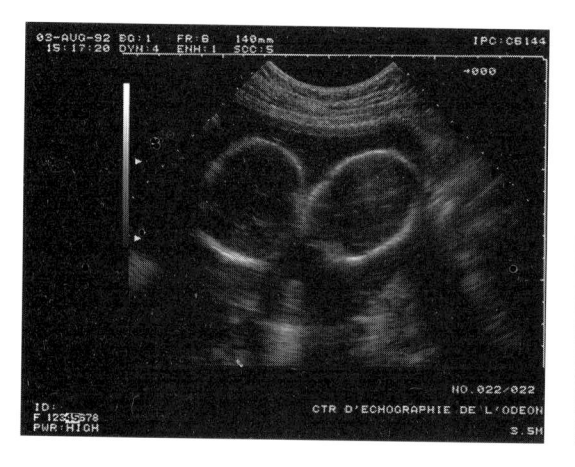

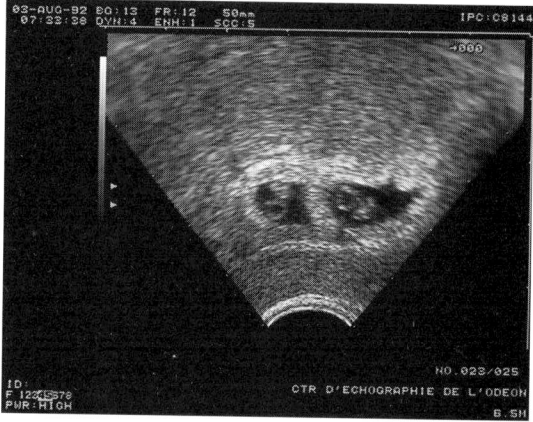

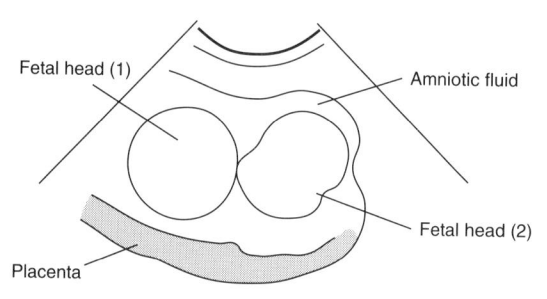

Figure 1 Two fetal heads visible on the same scan (20 weeks)

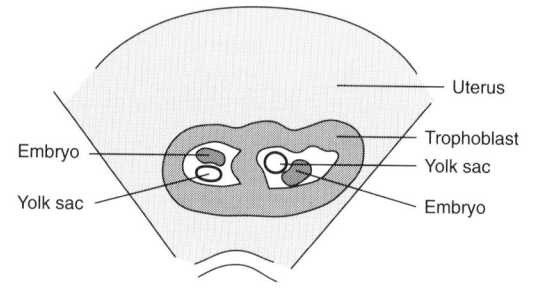

Figure 2 Dichorionic twin pregnancy (6 weeks)

are clearly identifiable. At week 7 (and in some cases earlier, depending on equipment and operator skill) each embryo can be recognized, if only by its pulsatile cardiac activity (which eliminates any suspicion of artifact). In practice, after week 7 of amenorrhea, a firm diagnosis of the number of embryos can be made.

Although errors can arise from haste or inexperience, in fact, few errors are made. The most damaging is a mistaken diagnosis of singleton pregnancy, because this delays the initiation of intensive prenatal care that is required for a multifetal pregnancy. Missing a third or fourth fetus on the initial scan is a far less serious error, because repeat scans are commonly ordered and correct for this error.

Errors related to gestational age

Before 6 weeks, the diagnosis of a monochorial twin pregnancy is not always accurate. Moreover, if the scan is carried out under hurried conditions, a twin pregnancy may be reported and a triplet gestation missed. Additionally, in the very first weeks of pregnancy, it may be difficult to determine whether a gestational sac is present or, more importantly, to be sure that the mass observed in the uterine cavity is actually a gestational sac. Further, the presence of a free extra-ovarian space may make the practitioner hesitate to make a diagnosis, because no embryo is visible. Thus the diagnosis of multifetal gestation should be made with caution before 6 weeks of amenorrhea using a classic abdominal ultrasound scan or 5 weeks of amenorrhea using a vaginal transducer. Given these considerations, the practitioner needs to adopt a middle-of-the-road policy between useless provocation of anxiety and refusal to make a crucial diagnosis. The use of a vaginal transducer cannot always resolve the issue, because the rigidity of the section sweeps may hinder the simultaneous visualization of both sacs as a function of the distance between them and their location within the uterine cavity.

Errors related to type of pregnancy

The relative infrequency of monoamniotic pregnancies leads to confusions between number of embryos and number of visible sacs (Figure 3). For this reason, all scans should be methodological and exhaustive in their approach, regardless of the reason for the scan or the apparent impressions derived from the initial sweeps (Figure 3).

Errors related to technique

If a scan is performed before 7 weeks of amenorrhea, diagnosis is more complicated than one might expect. An abdominal scan is capable of demonstrating two sacs separated by a given distance, and the diagnosis of dichorial pregnancies is relatively straightforward. In contrast, however, some practitioners may miss the thin membrane separating the amniotic and the extra-amniotic spaces. Although vaginal scans more easily identify embryos and the membranes separating them, they lack multi-directional orientation and may miss a dichorial pregnancy because the sacs are too far apart.

Practitioner errors

The accuracy of ultrasound examinations clearly is operator-dependent. The errors described above are basically errors of inexperienced operators, or result from lack of proper equipment or adequate vigilance.

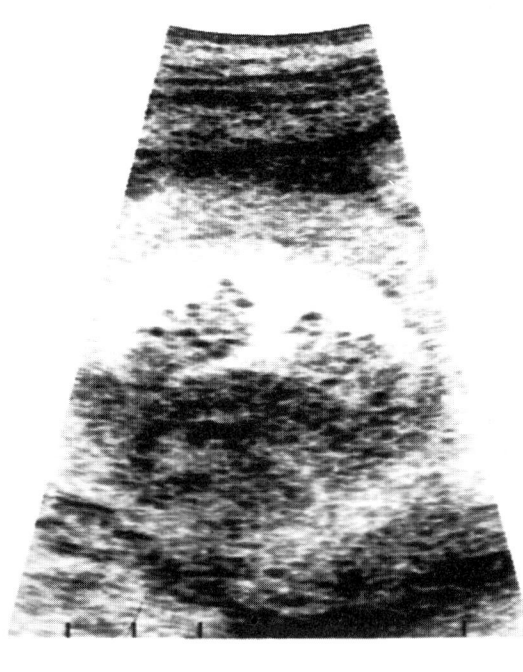

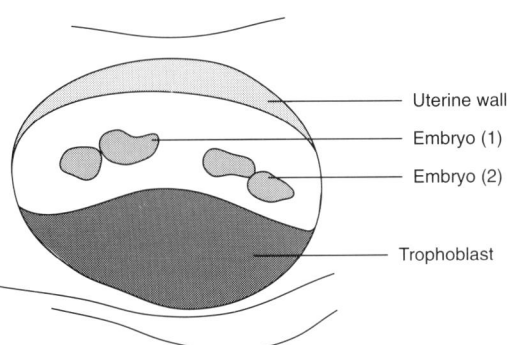

Figure 3 Monoamniotic twin pregnancy (8 weeks)

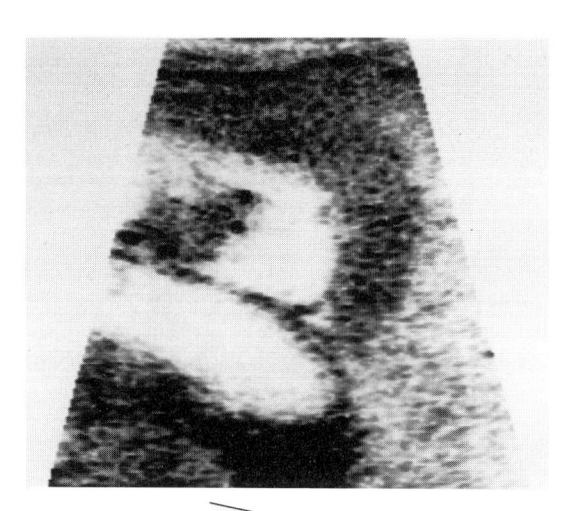

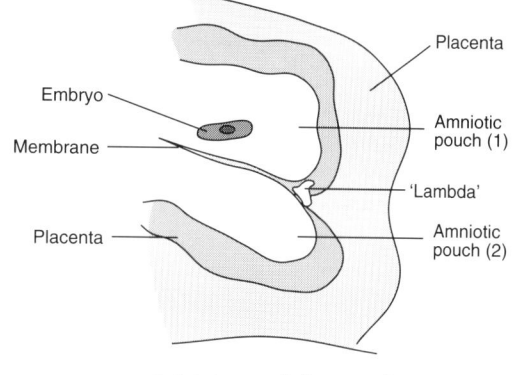

Figure 4 'Lambda' shape of the membrane

Chorionicity

The presence of a webbed, lambda-shaped structure at the end of the inter-ovular membrane at its point of attachment to the placenta is a pathognomonic indication of the dichorial (or multichorial) nature of the pregnancy[3]. This structure is particularly visible between 8 and 15 weeks of amenorrhea, and its presence or absence should be mentioned in any clinical report (Figure 4). In the event of future questions, this information may be crucial but impossible to visualize at a later date. Obviously, however, there is no need to look for the lambda structure if the diagnosis has been established early and if the examination demonstrates two separate sacs, each of which has its own trophoblastic crown.

The thickness of the inter-twin membrane, which some observers consider as an indication of chorionicity[4], may not be a totally reliable measurement, because what is being measured is a wave whose thickness is at least as dependent on the technical conditions as it is on the actual thickness of the structure being examined (Figure 5).

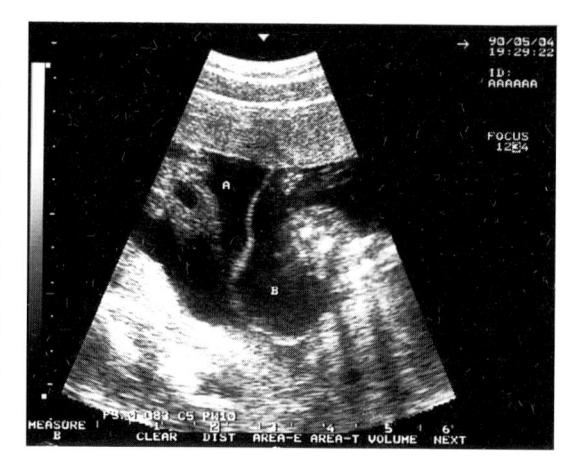

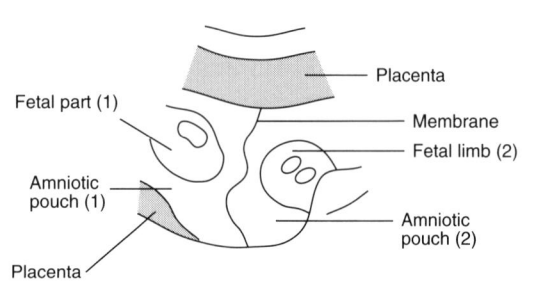

Figure 5 Inter-ovular membrane in a monochorionic pregnancy

Early assessment of prognosis

A hierarchy of risks is often drawn up within the category of multiple pregnancies. The number of fetuses is an important feature of such a schema, as is the existence of mono- or dichorial placentation. During the first trimester, ultrasound scans can provide clearcut, reliable and firm data relating to each of these concerns.

The tabulation of the number of sacs and embryos presents no specific difficulties. Within a given gestational sac, an inter-amniotic membrane may be missed on the first examination and more rarely on the second as well. Relative absence of amniotic fluid in one sac may make the practitioner hesitate, which is one of the major values of a thorough early examination before any pathological syndromes set in. Long before diagnosis of gender, which may or may not confirm the monozygotic or dizygotic nature of pregnancy, observation of the membranes can identify type of placentation. In contrast, gender identification may not be able to do this. In practice, by the end of the first trimester, ultrasound examinations can indicate the nature of pregnancy (twin or higher order), the type of placentation and the gestational age (see Chapter 9).

Vanishing embryos

After the diagnosis of twin pregnancy is established, one of the sacs may cease to develop and undergo resorption without necessarily leaving histopathological stigmata[5]. The possibility of this occurrence was discussed as early as 1945 by Vershuer in Stockel's *Text of Obstetrics*. The earliest ultrasound studies on this topic[6] confirmed the existence of this phenomenon and suggested that it took place in nearly 70% of all twin pregnancies examined before 9 weeks[7]. Clinically, bleeding or

mate the rate of resorption. The Landy cohort[8] is probably the closest to a correct incidence. In this study, 1000 pregnancies were examined systematically by ultrasound during the first trimester. The rate of twin or multiple pregnancies was 3.29% and vanishing sacs were observed for one-fifth (21.5%) of these pregnancies, irrespective of whether the pregnancy was the result of infertility treatment or was spontaneous. Most writers agree that spontaneous resorption following an early cessation of development does not increase the risk to the remaining fetus. Indeed, this phenomenon is now considered to be a physiological incident rather than a pathological accident (see Chapters 4 and 6).

Rejecting diagnoses

Multiple pregnancy must always be suspected when fundal height is disproportionate to presumed gestational age[2] (see above). The possibility of excluding this diagnosis is one of the most important advantages provided by ultrasound, because, once it is excluded, the search for other etiologies of the size–date discrepancy can begin. For example, requesting an ultrasound scan for a suspected twin pregnancy can confirm the presence of macrosomia, polyhydramnios, fetal malformation, non-diagnosed fibroma or, more simply, a major error in the presumed gestational age, once the fact that twin pregnancy is not present has been ascertained.

Biometrics

Clinical examination alone only provides a global overview of twin development and, as noted previously, the well-being of one twin may mask the distress of the other. In contrast, ultrasound scans make it possible to monitor the development of each individual fetus as a separate entity, as would be done for a singleton pregnancy.

Principles

In order to capitalize on recent advances in the field of ultrasound as they relate to twins, it

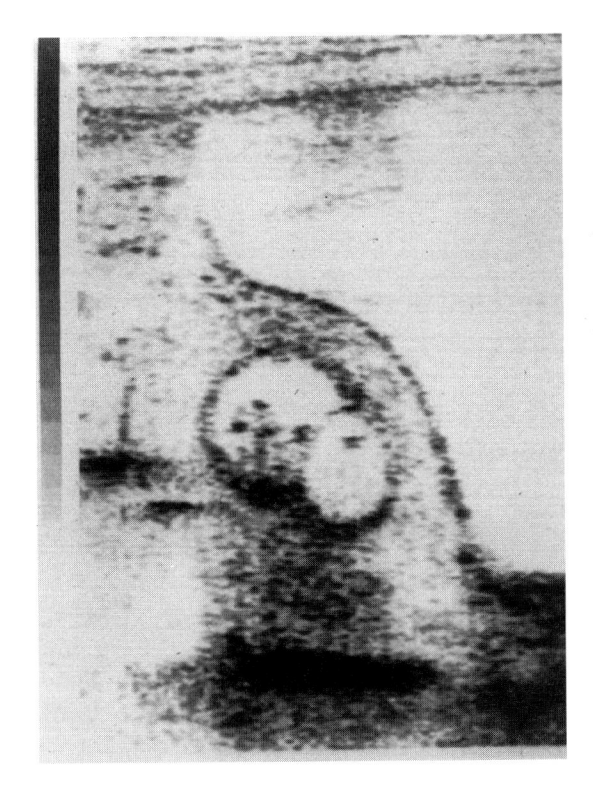

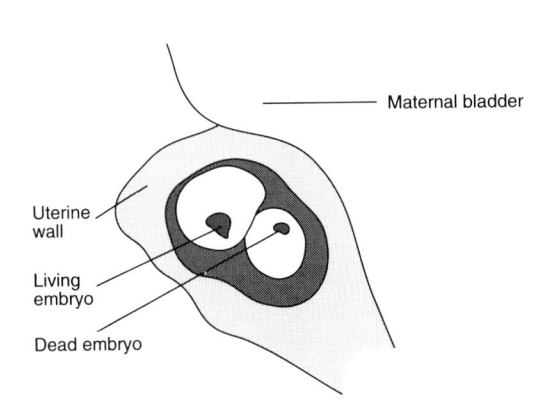

Figure 6 Early embryonic death before vanishing

expulsion of ovular debris were occasionally reported by patients whose remaining singletons then progressed without difficulty until term. More frequently, however, the vanishing sac was not accompanied by any observable signs and could only be documented through repeated ultrasound examinations (Figure 6).

More than likely, biases linked to technical inadequacies led early investigators to overesti-

is necessary to avoid the following common errors:

(1) Assuming it is normal for a fetus to have less than normal measurements simply because it is a twin. Although it is true that twins are particularly susceptible to growth retardation, this is a pathological rather than a physiological situation.

(2) Using one of the fetuses, generally the more developed, as a yardstick for the other(s). One fetus may legitimately develop differently (but normally) from its twin. In addition, one fetus may exhibit a normal biometric record and appear macrosomic compared to its fellow twin. Finally, the twin pair can constitute a growth-retarded or macrosomic pair.

(3) Assuming that any marked disparity in biometric parameters is the sign of a twin–twin transfusion syndrome. This diagnosis should be made based on a combination of clinical, anatomical and hematological criteria: birth weight difference of > 20%, hemoglobin differences of > 5 g/dl, etc. The condition is estimated to occur in one-third or less of monochorionic placentas. (Ed: We cannot agree more strongly. In a recent analysis of more than 200 twin pairs (> 28 weeks, liveborn and non-anomalous from mothers without diabetes, toxemia or other disease) delivered at the Johns Hopkins Medical Institutions between 1979 and 1989, some degree of discordance was common not only in birth weight but also in other parameters measured on ultrasound examination. At present, the literature does not provide a clearcut standard for the definition of 'discordance', and differences in intrauterine growth may not truly be indicative of twin–twin transfusion syndrome.)

Reference curves

Twin pregnancy is generally a rejection criterion when establishing reference samples for biometric curves. It is tempting to reverse this line of reasoning and suggest that this specific population should be monitored with its own curves, as I argued at one time[1]. However, I no longer maintain this position, because fetal growth retardation is a physiological phenomenon. My experience, and that of others[9] shows that weight – and hence biometric curves – are highly dependent on antenatal management conditions. Early diagnosis by ultrasound makes it possible to set a goal of giving twins as good a prognosis as singletons. With respect to ultrasound biometric data, which characterize fetal growth dynamics more fully than merely calculating weight in grams, it is perfectly valid to use the curves established for singletons to monitor twin development *in utero*. The classic skew of the curves for biparietal diameter is mainly due to cases of dolichocephalic fetuses in non-cephalic presentations, a situation that is frequent in twins. The standard curves for abdominal biometrics[10] or femur length[11] can be totally juxtaposed. Under these circumstances, standard reference curves for singleton pregnancies should be used.

Practice

Although much stress has been placed on the value of recent advances in morphological diagnosis, it is equally clear that biometrics is the cornerstone of the contribution of ultrasound to obstetrics practice. It is thus especially important that each ultrasound examination be conducted with a maximum of care, because the findings can only rarely be confirmed by clinical examination which, in any case, is general in its nature. Unfortunately, technical conditions are often less than optimal, and difficulties increase with gestational age. The closer one gets to the time during which growth retardation could take place and an obstetric decision may have to be made, the less reliable is the method. The following factors should be taken into account:

(1) *Scheduling examinations* Normally, ultrasound scans are performed every 4 weeks after diagnosis is made, and the pace of

these examinations increases gradually to once a week by 35 weeks. At this time, examinations are rarely exhaustive and it may be necessary to repeat them in order to confirm specific findings or obtain the missing information.

(2) *Planning examinations* Examinations of twin (or higher order) pregnancies should be performed by well-equipped, well-trained, reliable specialists.

(3) *Integrating the data into a medical procedure* Any doubt that relates to major therapeutic decisions is a clear reason for a repeat ultrasound scan.

Doppler

The Doppler sonographic technique is a major step forward in prenatal management. A variety of sites lend themselves to these examinations, but data obtained on umbilical and cerebral arteries are most valuable in obstetrics decision-making.

Doppler measurement Only the most frequently used techniques will be discussed. All are based on a velocity index score which makes it possible to bypass poorly assessable anatomic sites such as the approach angle of the vessel by the ultrasonic beam or the caliber of the vessel itself[12]. Currently, most writers make Doppler 'samples' on the umbilical artery and measure an index that associates maximum systolic circulatory velocity (S) and residual velocity at the end of diastole (D) (Figure 7).

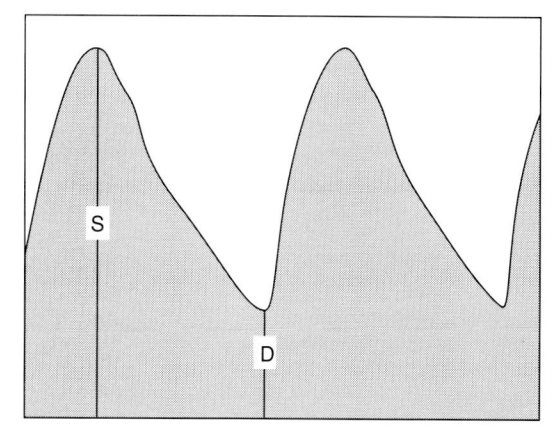

Figure 7 Usual landmarks used for measurement of Doppler indexes

Although other factors, such as volume of the systolic ejection or the cardiac rate, may also play a role, Doppler indices are generally considered to be representative of vascular resistance[12].

Whatever the index used, the pattern is identical: there is a gradual drop in resistance, and a corresponding drop in the index as weeks pass (Figure 8)[13,14].

Difficulties related to twin pregnancies In the case of twin pregnancies, ultrasound scans are more complex, lengthier, and more demanding. With respect to the velocity of flow in the umbilical cord, these difficulties are multiplied by the fact that the target has an extremely low

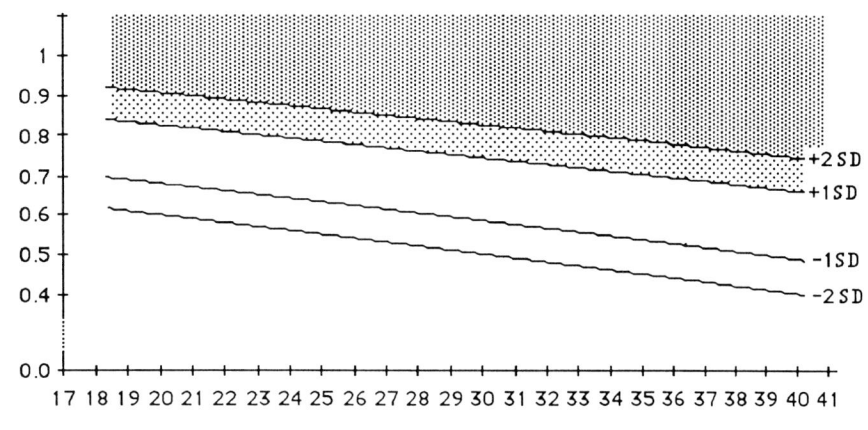

Figure 8 Pourcelot index (umbilical artery) reference curve

Table 1 Predictive values (%) for singletons of the umbilical Doppler index, obtained at the Antoine Béclère Hospital, Clamart, France

	Positive predictive value	Negative predictive value	Sensitivity	Specificity
Index > 1 SD	12	95	45	78
Index > 2 SD	34	89	23	93

volume, is mobile, and is far from the fetal body. It is thus useful to extrapolate the (virtual) fetal positions from the uterine wall on the first scan. Above all, certain artifacts can arise from the inclusion of vessels belonging to both fetuses in the same Doppler measurement. If the heart rates are close, the operator has no way of detecting such a measurement error. It is thus essential to use equipment that permits visualization of the Doppler target; the pulse Doppler which permits precise selection of the volume of measure is by far best suited for this purpose. Often, and in violation of the precept of obtaining velocity measurements near the placenta, the measurement volume should be obtained at the fetal end of the cord to avoid assignment errors.

Reference curves We were able to superimpose the mean observed measurements for singleton pregnancies on 248 twins born at the Antoine Béclère Hospital in Clamart, France between January 1, 1985 and June 30, 1987 (Table 1). Because the standard deviations did not differ significantly, I believe that the curves established for singleton pregnancies are entirely appropriate for the monitoring of twin pregnancies. Being able to use Doppler velocities under the same conditions and with the same reliability as exist for singleton pregnancies represents a major advance in the monitoring of twin pregnancies. If appropriate equipment is used, and a few simple rules are followed, obtaining a Doppler velocity measurement is as elementary as obtaining a biparietal or abdominal diameter measurement. As term approaches, however, biometry is more difficult and less specific, especially if carried out by different technicians. In contrast, a pulse Doppler measurement is only marginally influenced by fetal position or intertwining of the cords in the case of the monoamniotic–monochorionic placenta.

Influence of mode of placentation Monochorial implantations, which have the worst prognosis, probably derive this from the fact that they often have higher Doppler index values than dichorial implantations and that the discordance between values obtained the same day for twins is three times as high (Figure 9)[15].

Placenta

The identification, localization and structural analysis of the placenta present no particular difficulties. At times, however, it is obvious that a given portion of the placental mass is attached to one fetus rather than to the other. Unfortunately, this observation does not always prove that placentation is mono- or dichorionic[5]. The frequency of abnormal insertions of the umbilical cord and their possible effects on the nature of delivery are valid reasons for their careful scrutiny during the final ultrasound examinations (see Chapter 9).

The Grannum classification[16] is often used to characterize placental development in twins.

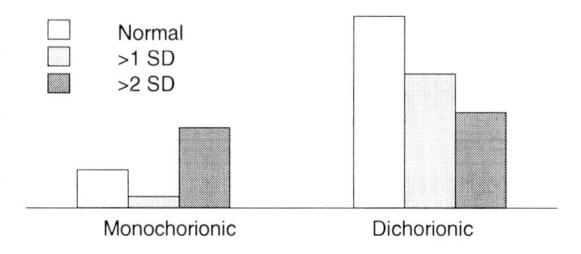

Figure 9 Pathological data are more frequent in monochorionic pregnancies

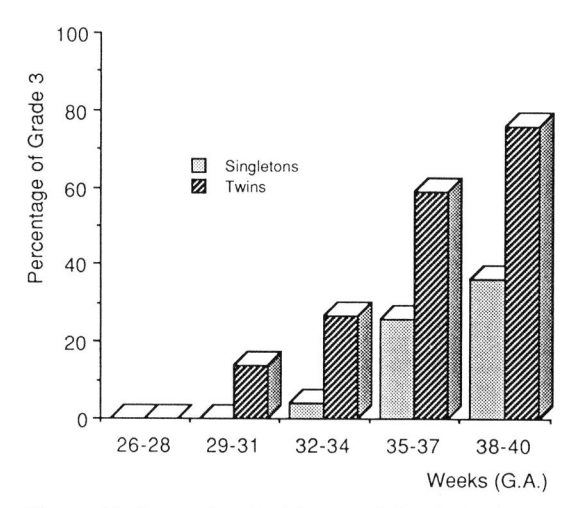

Figure 10 Increasing incidence of Grade 3 placental maturity and gestational age (from reference 18)

Fetal morphology

The study of fetal morphology is now an integral part of routine ultrasound surveillance of all pregnancies (see Chapter 17). In cases of singleton pregnancies, we normally perform a routine scan directed at detection of abnormal fetal morphology at 20 weeks. In twin pregnancies, a repeat morphological scan should be scheduled at a later date as well, because of the particular risks linked to this type of pregnancy. The investigation should be exhaustive, and particular attention should be paid to screening for intracerebral images suggestive of porencephaly and the total autonomy of fetal movement. Some fetal parts tend to be more affected than others[19]: the backbone, the heart, the kidneys, the tracheoesophageal tract, the limbs, and the different components of the VACTERL group (V = vertebra, A = anal, C = cardiac, TE = tracheoesophageal, R = renal, L = limb) (Figure 11).

Most frequently, advanced placental maturity (compared to singleton pregnancies of the same gestational age) is observed (grade 3) (Figure 10). Advanced placental maturity can parallel earlier lung maturity in twins[17], but it can also be observed in cases of growth retardation as a sign of placental alteration. The current state of the art in ultrasound techniques makes it hazardous to draw a direct connection between placental grade and the risk of hyalin membrane disease[18].

Prevention

The early diagnosis of a twin pregnancy makes it possible to set up an appropriate plan for prenatal care. Data from the Antoine Béclère Hospital[20] show that the best prognosis is associated

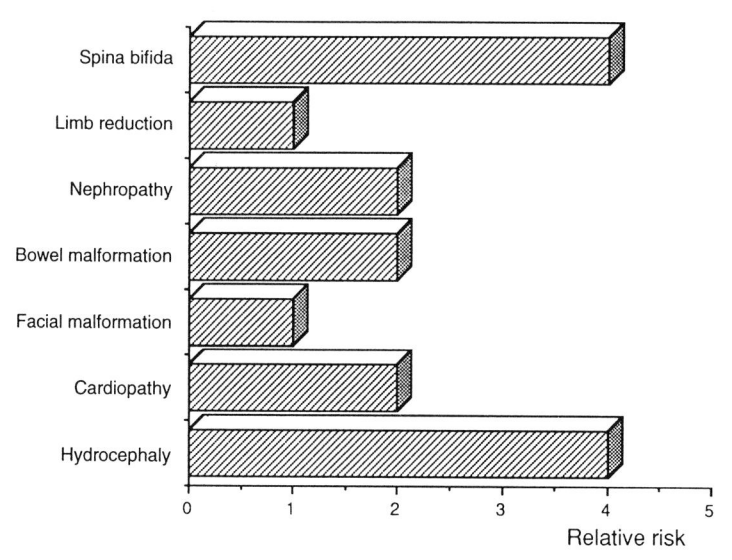

Figure 11 Fetal malformations in twin (actual frequency vs. expected frequency (Källen)

with the earliest onset of intensive management, and the use of preventive interventions[21]. As a function of the time of diagnosis, i.e. in the first trimester or later, the incidence of severe prematurity increased from 8 to 20%, and the number of births at term declined from 74 to 39%. Various other chapters of this book discuss the relationship between early diagnosis and prognosis (see Chapter 15).

References

1. Wenstrom, K.D. and Gall, S.A. (1988). Incidence, morbidity and diagnosis of twin gestations. *Clin. Perinatol.*, **15**, 1
2. Leroy, B., Lefort, F. and Jeny, R. (1984). Uterine height and umbilical perimeter curves in twin pregnancies. *Acta Genet. Med. Gemellol.*, **48**, 405
3. Bessis, R. and Papiernik, E. (1981). Echographic imagery of amniotic membranes in twin pregnancies. In Gedda, L., Parisi, P. and Nance, W.E. (eds.) *Twin Research No. 3, Twin Biology and Multiple Pregnancy*, pp. 183–7. (New York: Alan R. Liss)
4. Barss, V., Benacerraf, B.R. and Frigoletto, F.D. (1985). Ultrasonic determination of chorion type in twin gestation. *Obstet. Gynecol.*, **66**, 779
5. Leroy, B. and Bessis, R. (1980). *Echographie en Obstétrique*, pp. 96–7. (Paris: Masson)
6. Barrat, J. and Leroy, B. (1977). De la résorbtion ovulaire au cours des grossesses multiples. Dépistage échographique. In *Actualités Gynécologiques*. (Paris: Masson)
7. Schneider, L., Bessis, R., Simonnet, T. *et al.* (1979). The frequency of ovular resorbtion during the first trimester of twin pregnancy. *Acta Genet. Med. Gemellol.*, **29**, 271
8. Landy, H.J., Weiner, S., Corson, S.L. *et al.* (1986). The 'vanishing twin': ultrasonic assessment of fetal disappearance in the first trimester. *Am. J. Obstet. Gynecol.*, **155**, 14
9. Gilstrap, L.C., Hankins, G.D., Collins, T. *et al.* (1986). Serial biparietal diameter and femur length measurements in twin gestations. *Am. J. Perinatol.*, **3**, 183
10. Schneider, L., Bessis, R., Tabaste, J.L. *et al.* (1979). Foetal twin ultrasound biometry. *Acta Genet. Med. Gemellol.*, **28**, 299
11. Haines, C.J., Langlois, S.L. and Jones, W.R. (1986). Ultrasonic measurement of fetal femoral length in singleton and twin pregnancies. *Am. J. Obstet. Gynecol.*, **155**, 838
12. Pourcelot, L. (1974). Applications cliniques de l'examen doppler transcutané: vélocimétrie ultrasonore doppler. *Séminaire INSERM*, **34**, 213
13. Arbeille, P., Asquier, E., Mocxhon, E. *et al.* (1983). Nouvelle technique dans la surveillance de la grossesse: l'étude de la circulation foetale et placentaire par les ultrasons. *J. Gynecol. Biol. Reprod.*, **12**, 851
14. Stuart, B., Drumm, J. and Fitzgerald, D.E. (1980). Fetal velocity waveforms in normal pregnancy. *Br. J. Obstet. Gynaecol.*, **87**, 780
15. Bessis, R. (1991). In Papiernik, E. (ed.) *Les Grossesses Multiples*, pp. 105–20. (Paris: Doin)
16. Grannum P.A.T., Berkowitz, R.L. and Hobbins, J.C. (1979). The ultrasonic changes in the maturing placenta and their relation to fetal pulmonic maturity. *Am. J. Obstet. Gynecol.*, **133**, 915
17. Leveno, K.J., Quirk, J.G., Whalley, P.J. *et al.* (1984). Fetal lung maturation in twin gestation. *Am. J. Obstet. Gynecol.*, **148**, 405
18. Ohel, G., Granat, M., Zeevi, D. *et al.* (1987). Advanced ultrasonic placental maturation in twin pregnancies. *Am. J. Obstet. Gynecol.*, **156**, 76
19. Källen, B. (1986). Congenital malformation in twins: a population study. *Acta Genet. Med. Gemellol.*, **35**, 167
20. Bessis, R. (1987). Nombre, sexe et présentation du foetus. Collège National des Gynécologues et Obstétriciens Français, pp. 131–48. (Paris: Vigot)
21. Bessis, R. (1987). Interruption sélective de grossesse. *Horm. Reprod. Metab.*, **4**, 85

Population ultrasound: the Swedish experience

H. Rydhström and L. Grennert

Introduction

Prior to the introduction of ultrasound in Sweden in 1964[1], fewer than 50% of all twins were diagnosed prior to delivery[2]. Perinatal mortality rate was close to 10%, even in the early 1970s (Figure 1). This high rate was the major reason for instituting the first Swedish ultrasound screening program in 1973. Initially this program was proposed for all pregnant women designated to deliver at the University Hospital of Malmö in southern Sweden. The aim of this policy was to detect twins early enough in pregnancy so that measures to prevent preterm delivery could be instituted, primarily in the context of routine antenatal hospital care[3].

This chapter discusses the development of obstetric ultrasound throughout Sweden during the past two decades. Figures are given for the present detection rate of twins, along with a discussion of why some twins are not diagnosed until delivery. The formal organization of training and education in ultrasonography for Swedish specialists in obstetrics is then briefly described[4]. The last part of this chapter deals with the effects of early detection of a twin pregnancy on its prognosis.

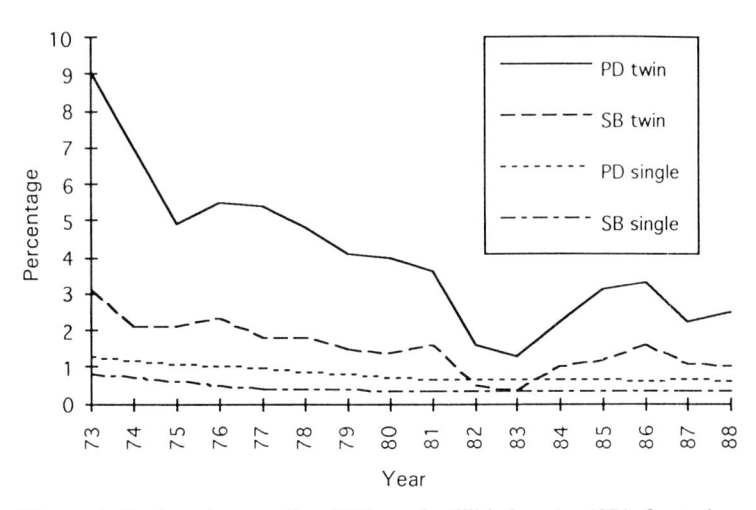

Figure 1 Perinatal mortality (PD) and stillbirth rate (SB) for twins (top lines) and singletons (bottom lines) born in Sweden between 1973 and 1988. Twins have a 4–5-fold greater perinatal mortality than singletons. No single explanation is easily available for the significant rise in PD and SB for twins seen between 1984 and 1986

Development of obstetric ultrasound in Sweden (1970–90)

The first population-based screening program was introduced in the Malmö unit in 1973[3]. The information given in this and the following section is based on three questionnaires distributed in 1983, 1988 and 1990. Only the results from the 1988 investigation have been published[4]. The initial program was intended primarily to detect twin pregnancies. Ten years after introduction (1983), however, similar programs were in place in about 65–70% of all Swedish hospitals (Figure 2), and 67% of all pregnant women received at least one ultrasound examination during their pregnancy. Sweden has 57 delivery units with obstetricians in charge, accounting for >97% of all deliveries. In 1989 the number of deliveries in Sweden was 115 500. By which time 89% of all hospitals had a population-based ultrasound screening program for pregnant women. Only one relatively small antenatal unit had no provisions for a screening program (650 deliveries each year), and five units had partial screening programs which were variably applied to 25–85% of pregnant women. Two of these latter units extended their screening programs to include all pregnant women in 1991. In summary, in the calendar year 1990, more than 97% of the pregnant population in Sweden received a screening ultrasound examination.

Although the obstetrician is responsible for the screening (and its interpretation), midwives perform most of the routine scans. In only one out of 57 hospitals is the X-ray department solely responsible for the screening examination, and in six units the obstetrics and radiology departments collaborate in this endeavor.

The screening of pregnant women is performed at weeks 16–18 of gestation in 90% of all units; a minority (10%) of units adheres to weeks 10–12. The purported benefits of a screening program early in the second trimester are listed in Table 1. Whereas detection of twins was the main reason for introducing ultrasound screening in the early 1970s, we now believe that the most important benefit is a correct assessment of gestational age, because the accuracy of this assessment declines later in pregnancy.

During 1988 and 1989, a total of 2732 twin gestations were delivered in Sweden (unpublished observation). Of these, 30 pairs were not detected until delivery, and the rate of antenatal detection of twins was 98.9%. Eight of the undetected cases had received screening, either from an inexperienced ultrasonographer (in six instances), or before gestational

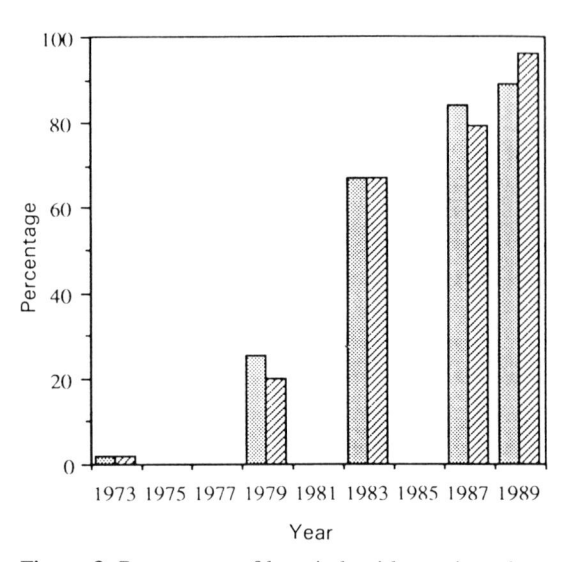

Figure 2 Percentage of hospitals with routine ultrasound screening of all pregnant women between 1973 and 1989 (shaded columns); and percentage of pregnant women participating in the screening program (hatched columns)

Table 1 Benefits of a screening program embracing all pregnant women early in the second trimester (16–18 weeks)

A reliable estimation of gestational age

Detection of twins

Identification of fundal placenta (excluding placenta previa)

Detection of major malformations necessitating abortion (for example, acrania)

Better bonding between mother and fetus/newborn

Table 2 The practical training and theoretical education in diagnostic ultrasonography for Swedish obstetricians

I	*Basic course*	
	Target group	Residents and specialists in obstetrics without any previous formal knowledge or training in ultrasonography
	Aim	To give basic theoretical and practical knowledge
	Course length	5 days
II	*Advanced course*	
	Target group	Residents and specialists who have previously taken the basic course and wish for further experience in practical obstetric ultrasonography
	Aim	To equip staff with necessary knowledge for performing independent diagnostic ultrasound investigations
	Course length	A theoretical 5-day part, 60 participants per course. A practical 3-day part, giving individual training at one of 10 ultrasound units approved for practical training
III	*Special course*	
	Target group	Obtetricians responsible for the ultrasonic unit in each of 57 obstetrical departments throughout Sweden
	Aim	To give a deeper knowledge in a very clearly delimited area within ultrasonography (e.g. fetal echocardiography)

week 12 (in two instances). The remaining 22 women did not receive ultrasound screening, and their twins were detected either in the third trimester or at delivery. Of these women, 14 were not offered screening, two registered for antenatal care very late, and six declined to participate. Three triplet pregnancies were wrongly considered twins. The diagnosis was false positive in one case. In this instance, a twin pregnancy was detected in gestational week 17. The patient and her 'twins' were further evaluated with ultrasonography later in pregnancy, but the mother ultimately delivered a singleton at term. No evidence of a 'vanishing twin' was present, either on ultrasound or upon examination of the placenta. Obviously, the twin diagnosis was incorrect from the beginning.

Our continuing experience with ultrasound screening for virtually all (>99%) pregnant women in the second trimester undoubtedly will be further analyzed in the future. A major factor in our success to date has been the quality of the ultrasound screening.

Training and education in ultrasonography

The Swedish Society of Obstetrics and Gynecology (SFOG) began organizing courses in ultrasonography for specialists in 1981. Prior to that time, courses were given privately. In 1990, a training program was adopted to standardize education throughout the country[4]. This education is not compulsory, in that anyone is able to buy his/her own ultrasound equipment and perform screening without training. However, it is unlikely that many pregnant women choose to obtain care from such inexperienced doctors or midwives.

The program comprises three levels of training to achieve three levels of proficiency (Table 2). The basic course (Level I) provides training and theoretical education for persons not necessarily having had any previous experience with ultrasound. Level II provides training leading to an ability to perform diagnostic ultrasound investigations without supervision. Instruction at Level III is restricted to those individuals who by necessity require insight into a clearly defined area, such as cardiac malformations, or umbilical cord blood sampling.

The recommendations of the SFOG regarding the organization of obstetric ultrasound practice are as follows. First, the unit should work in close collaboration with the department of obstetrics and gynecology. (This dictum includes those units located in private practices outside the hospital. Private obstetricians are offered the same education as those who work in hospitals of municipalities or counties.) Second, the medical and organizational responsibility for the unit should be in the hands of a specialist in obstetrics and gynecology who has passed Levels I and II, and who has several years of practical experience in diagnostic ultrasonography. Third, doctors or midwives who perform obstetric ultrasound independently should have successfully taken Level II instruction and have at least 200 hours of practical experience with a tutor. And finally, evaluation of fetal malformations should be restricted to centers with documented experience. In this regard, Swedish units that conduct less than 500 scans annually are encouraged to send their pregnant women to larger units for screening.

The effect on prognosis of detecting a twin pregnancy before delivery

It is appropriate to ask what benefits can realistically be expected of an early diagnosis of twin pregnancy (Table 3). Traditionally, twins are described as having a perinatal mortality 4–5-

Table 3 Suggested benefits of early diagnosis of twins on short-term and long-term fetal outcome

A reliable estimation of gestational age

A greater awareness of impending complications

The mother induced to be more careful during pregnancy

Expectant mothers given the opportunity to take paid leave of absence from work

Monitoring of twin 2 during labor and delivery

An extremely low rate of entanglement, even when the twins are in breech-vertex presentation

fold higher than singletons. However, when the confounding effect of gestational duration was eliminated, Swedish twins actually had the same – or even lower – perinatal mortality than singletons (Figure 3), at least until the 37th week[5]. This statement applies for Sweden, a country in which the population is homogeneous, medical care is accessible to all and a high level of education (≥ 11 years) for most mothers is virtually universal. This similarity in prognosis until the 37th week for twins and singletons suggests that the major goal following an early twin diagnosis should be prevention of preterm labor and delivery.

In the early 1970s, the diagnosis of twin gestation at the Malmö unit (gestational weeks 16–17) often led to immediate hospitalization; this was continued until gestational weeks 35–36. It was claimed that such treatment was effective in reducing the perinatal mortality to the same level as for singletons[6]. However, larger retrospective studies that included the material of Persson et al.[6] and compared fetal outcome in two neighboring but separate university hospitals (Lund and Malmö) failed to confirm the efficacy of routine hospital care for either the mother or her twins[7]. Therefore, the hospitalization for the Malmö twin pregnant women was abandoned in 1982. Moreover, a prospective randomized study conducted in Australia, and published in 1990, concluded that routine hospital care to prevent preterm labor and delivery was not beneficial because of a significantly higher readmission rate for reasons such as discomfort, hypertension and preterm labor[8]. Indeed, routine hospital admission tended to impair fetal outcome.

After 1985, all women with multiple gestation in Sweden have been entitled to a leave of absence from work from the 24th week onwards, and their salaries are paid at a level of 90%. A prerequisite for this benefit is an early diagnosis of twins. A retrospective study of 78 women who delivered in 1981 and who took advantage of this benefit compared a variety of outcomes with those of 78 controls who did not take work leave. No differences in gestational duration, birth weight, or perinatal mortality were found[9]. This study is small, however, and did not consider all of the social and anthropometric factors that impact on these dependent variables. Clearly more and larger prospective studies investigating this question are needed (see Chapter 33 for French data on this question).

A problem facing all investigators attempting to study the prognostic effects of early diagnosis of twin pregnancy is that a prospective, randomized study, with adequate numbers of twin pregnancies, cannot realistically be performed without the cooperation of several units. In the absence of large numbers and several cooperating centers, data from a single center may not be sufficient to show differences. In one study from Finland, for example, 9310 women took part in a controlled trial of one-stage ultrasound screening in pregnancy[10]. In all, 36 twin pregnancies were found in the screening group and 38 in the control group. No difference was found in the number of pregnancies associated with perinatal mortality (2 vs. 3). In another randomized trial on the effects of ultrasound screening in a total population of pregnant women, about 5000 women had to be included in order to reach valid conclusions[11]. In all, ultrasound screening early in the second trimester detected 24 twin pregnancies. In contrast, 16 of the 20 unscreened women with twin pregnancies were diagnosed later in pregnancy or only at delivery.

Obviously, even the numbers of women included in these trials are insufficient to evaluate the effects (positive or negative) of a screening program, given the low incidence of naturally occurring multiples and the fact that perhaps 20% of twins will undergo spontaneous reduction prior to the initial evaluation.

In order to assess the effects of a screening program on twin prognosis more accurately, we must turn to retrospective studies. As noted above, between 1973 and 1985, the perinatal mortality rate for twins in Sweden declined from 9–10% to 3–4% (Figure 1). Concomitantly, the ultrasound screening program was extended throughout the country. Whereas 1–2% of all pregnant women were screened in 1973, this number rose to 67% in 1983. To evaluate whether a cause–effect correlation existed between an early twin diagnosis and perinatal mortality, we studied all 862 twins with a birth weight of < 1500 g, born in Sweden between 1973 and 1983, regardless of whether the twins were born alive or dead[12].

It was possible to identify the week of detection (by using valid information in the original medical records) in over 90% of all these pregnancies. Surviving twins had a median week of detection about 1.5 weeks earlier than dead

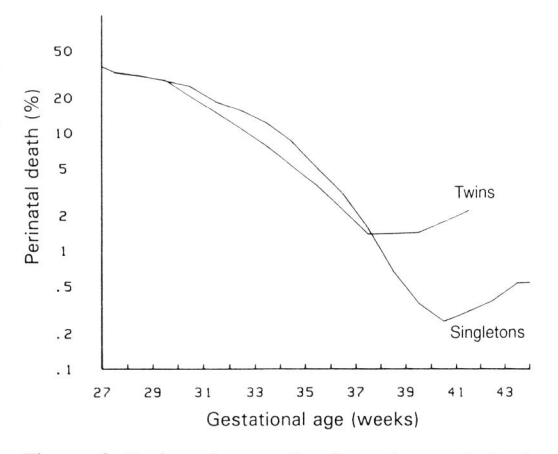

Figure 3 Perinatal mortality for twins and singletons in Sweden between 1973 and 1985 according to gestational age. When the confounding effect of gestational age was eliminated, twins had similar perinatal mortality to singletons up to gestational weeks 37–38. Logarithmic scale

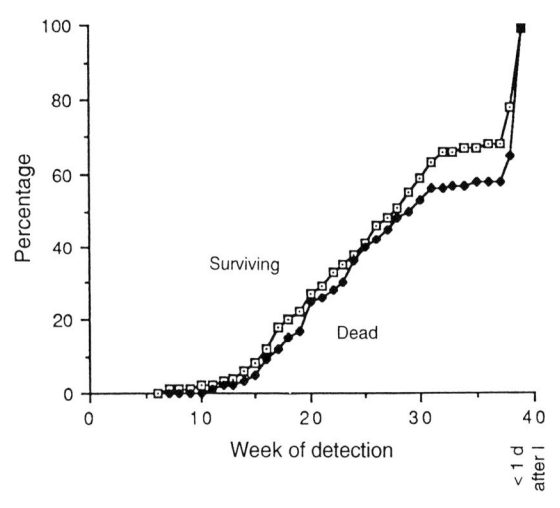

Figure 4 Cumulative distribution of week of detection for twins (surviving and dead) with a birthweight of < 1500 g and born in Sweden between 1973 and 1983. <1 d signifies the percentage of twins detected within 1 day before birth. After I signifies the percentage of twins detected after the birth of twin I

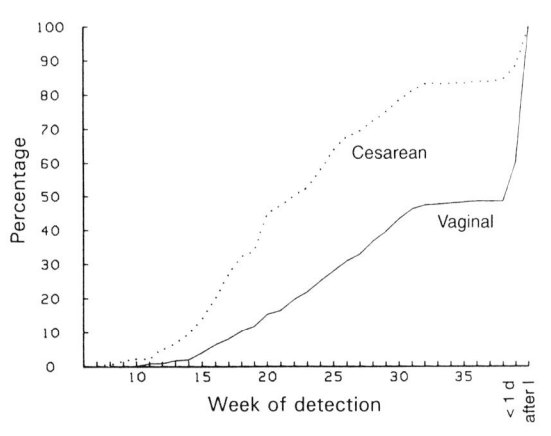

Figure 5 Cumulative week of detection for twins born vaginally and abdominally; identical study population as seen in Figure 4. <1 d signifies detection less than 1 day before birth[12]. In a considerable number of cases, presence of twins was not detected until after the birth of twin I (After I). (Illustration courtesy of the C.V. Mosby Co.)

twins (Figure 4). For the surviving twins, 34% were detected *less than* 24 h before birth (including twins diagnosed after birth of twin 1) compared with 45% for the dead twins ($\chi^2 = 6.1$, $p<0.05$).

Although the material in Figure 4 is population-based, some caution is required when interpreting the results. First, it is possible that some patients who had an early diagnosis benefited from this knowledge in some manner that led to birth weights of >1500 g, and, consequently, exclusion from the study population. Second, the study design could not exclude a confounding effect of higher social class in the women with surviving twins, because higher social class *per se* might have led to an increased rate of ultrasound examination early in pregnancy and thus a better prognosis for the twins, based on considerations other than an early diagnosis. Third, the perinatal mortality for twins was generally higher in the first part of the study period, when ultrasound was less common. This may have led to a later diagnosis for these twins. Fourth, a larger proportion of surviving twins was born during the latter part of the study. At this time, ultrasound was more commonly used, and an earlier diagnosis was more likely. Thus, if the confounding effect of year of birth is taken into consideration, the difference in week of detection between dead and surviving twins is in fact even less than is seen in Figure 4.

We evaluated the effects of Cesarean section on prognosis (Figure 5) in a separate study of the same patient population. We found an appreciable difference in the week of detection between abdominal (median week of detection 22) and vaginal births (median week of detection <1 day before delivery). However, the confounding effect of year of birth was not eliminated, because most of the Cesarean deliveries occurred during the second part of the study. This observation suggests that the difference between the groups is less than is seen in Figure 5.

A similar study was performed for twins with a birth weight between 1500 and 2499 g[13]. A dramatic decrease in perinatal mortality was observed. During the first 4 years (1973–76), 73 twins died, followed by 25 in the next 4 years, and six in the last 3 years (1981–83). For each pregnancy in which one or both twins were

Table 4 Cumulative distribution of week of detection: (A) for twins dead during birth or neonatally ($\mu = 91$), (B) for twins surviving the neonatal period ($\mu = 182$), and (C) for all twins with a handicap (cerebral palsy and/or mental retardation) at 8 years of age or older ($\mu = 99$)

Detection time	A* (%)	B* (%)	C† (%)	χ^2 A–B
<19 weeks	10.1	7.7	5.8	ns
20–29 weeks	28.6	27.5	27.2	ns
30–39 weeks	51.6	52.2	43.7	ns
< 1 day before birth	65.9	66.5	52.4	ns
After birth of twin 1	94.5	94.0	81.6	ns
Total	100.0	100.0	100.0	

*Birthweight 1500–2499 g, birth between 1973 and 1983; †birthweight < 2500 g, birth between 1973 and 1980

dead during birth or died neonatally (< 29 days after delivery), two control twin pregnancies were selected at random. The controls had a similar year of delivery (± 1 year) and a similar birth weight (± 100 g), but no other matching criteria were used. No significant difference was found between cases and controls in terms of gestational week at the time of detection (Table 4). However, cases had a somewhat shorter gestational duration (data shown in the original paper). Because of this, we re-examined the material and calculated the number of weeks between detection and delivery. The median value was 4 weeks, for both cases and controls. The results (disappointingly) seem to indicate that for this group of heavier twins, no obvious difference existed in the week of detection between pregnancies with one or both twins dead and pregnancies in which both twins survived the neonatal period.

Notwithstanding the considerations cited above, after the birth of the first twin, ultrasound monitoring is required to determine the lie of the second twin. It might also be argued that ultrasound should be used during delivery of twin 1 to facilitate the external version of twin 2, or to keep it in a longitudinal position before the birth of twin 1. In addition, electronic fetal monitoring of both twins is a prerequisite of good intrapartum care. However, the *sine qua non* for both interventions is a twin diagnosis before delivery.

A study of all second twins born in Sweden during a 13-year period from 1973 to 1985 determined that, after 1979, no correlation was present between perinatal mortality and the inter-delivery interval[14]. In an unknown but substantial number of deliveries, ultrasound was used for intrapartum monitoring. In contrast, during the period 1973–78, a longer inter-delivery interval was correlated with a greater perinatal mortality for twin 2, and rarely with ultrasound monitoring. We strongly believe (admittedly without any scientific proof) that a significant part of this improved prognosis was due to the increased rate of detection of twins before birth. (Editor: Unpublished data from Northwestern University support prolonged (>30 min) delivery intervals up to 300 min *if* the fetal monitoring strip is reassuring and *if* ultrasound is available in the delivery room to document that the fetus is not in an unsuspected transverse or unstable lie.)

Entanglement during delivery is a rare, but extremely serious complication. According to Nissen[15], the sequence of events leading to entanglement can be catastrophic and tax the ingenuity of even the most resourceful obstetrician. In Sweden the rate of twin entanglement in breech-vertex presentation decreased from one in 74 deliveries between 1961 and 1966 to one in 189 deliveries between 1981 and 1987[16]. The major reason for this decrease, we believe, is the increasing rate of twins detected prenatally, which led to improved monitoring during birth. If entanglement occurs and is recognized early, because of the presence of ultrasound in the delivery room, a rapid Cesarean section allows delivery of both fetuses and reduces the likelihood of extensive trauma or demise to either twin.

Late prognosis

Of all 4719 twins born in Sweden during 1973–1980 with a birth weight between 500 and 2499 g, it was possible to identify 115 twins from 99 pregnancies in which one or both twins were considered handicapped at 8 years of age or later in life[17]. The handicapped twins represent 8.4% of all surviving twins with a birth weight of <1500 g, and 1.9% of all surviving twins with a birth weight of 1500–2499 g born during these years. Unfortunately, the study design precluded quantitation of the degree of cerebral palsy or mental retardation in these individuals. For 19 pregnancies, no information was available regarding week of detection; for the remainder the distribution of week of detection is given in Table 4. For handicapped twins, no major difference appeared to exist when a comparison was made with twins surviving the perinatal period (no control group is available with twins 8 years old, without cerebral palsy and/or mental retardation). Again, it must be emphasized that if this study had been restricted to one single hospital, only one or two mothers with handicapped twins would have been found on the average. It is for this reason that, to our knowledge, no previous study has evaluated the correlation between an early diagnosis of the twin condition and handicap later in life.

Conclusion

To sum up, the perinatal mortality rate for twins in Sweden has decreased concomitantly with an increasing rate of detection of twins. The screening of all pregnant women in Sweden has led to a prenatal detection rate of >98.9% of all twins. We believe that the number of undetected twins will be reduced to a very few select instances in the near future as a result of better training and education of medical care givers.

The improved prognosis seen for twins during the two last decades is explained by several factors. Although it has not been possible to show that an early twin diagnosis *per se* influences perinatal mortality or morbidity for twins of <2500 g, it is our opinion that an early diagnosis is important, nonetheless. It goes without saying that prenatal detection of twins is a prerequisite for monitoring of both twins intrapartum. The lower rate of entanglement during the last decade is undoubtedly an effect of the increased rate of twin detection before delivery. Moreover, an early diagnosis means that the parents can make preparations to care for two babies instead of one, and the bonding between parents and newborns can be facilitated.

We believe it to be important to introduce the screening program in other countries where the greater part of maternity care is in private hands. Compared to ultrasonography, no other single diagnostic modality will achieve the same degree of success in detecting twins during the second trimester.

References

1. Sundén, B. (1964). On the diagnostic value of ultrasound in obstetrics and gynaecology. *Acta Obstet. Gynecol. Scand.*, **43** (Suppl.), 191
2. Grennert, L., Persson, P.H., Gennser, G. and Kullander, S. (1976). Ultrasound and human-placental-lactogen screening for early detection of twin pregnancies. *Lancet*, **1**, 4
3. Grennert, L., Persson, P.-H. and Gennser, G. (1978). Benefits of ultrasound screening of a pregnant population. *Acta Obstet. Gynecol. Scand.*, **78**, 5

4. Jörgensen, C. and Buchhave, P. (1989). The extension of diagnostic ultrasound requires proper training and education. (in Swedish), *Läkartidningen*, **86**, 4605
5. Hoffman, H.J. and Bakketeig, L.S. (1984). Risk factors associated with the occurence of preterm birth. *Clin Obstet. Gynecol.*, **27**, 539
6. Persson, P.H., Grennert, L., Gennser, G. and Kullander, S. (1979). On improved outcome of twin pregnancies. *Acta Obstet. Gynecol. Scand.*, **58**, 3
7. Rydhström, H., Nordensköld, F., Grennert, L. *et al.* (1987). Routine hospital care does not improve prognosis in twin gestation. *Acta Obstet. Gynecol. Scand.*, **66**, 361
8. MacLennan, A.H., Green, R.C., O'Shea, R. *et al.* (1990). Routine hospital admission in twin pregnancy between 26 and 30 weeks' gestation. *Lancet*, **335**, 267
9. Rydhström, H. (1988). Twin pregnancy and the effects of prophylactic leave of absence on pregnancy duration and birthweight. *Acta Obstet. Gynecol. Scand.*, **67**, 81
10. Saari-Kemppainen, A., Karjalainen, O., Ylöstalo, P. and Heinonen, O.P. (1990). Ultrasound screening and perinatal mortality: controlled trial of systematic one-stage screening in pregnancy. *Lancet*, **1**, 387
11. Waldenström, U., Axelsson, O., Nilsson, S. *et al.* (1988). Effects of routine one-stage ultrasound screening in pregnancy: a randomised controlled trial. *Lancet*, **2**, 585
12. Rydhström, H. (1990). Prognosis for twins with a birthweight less than 1500 g: the impact of Cesarean section in relation to fetal presentation. *Am. J. Obstet. Gynecol.*, **163**, 528
13. Rydhström, H. and Ingemarsson, I. (1991). A case–control study on the effects of Cesarean birth on intrapartum and neonatal mortality for twins weighing 1500–2499 g. *Br. J. Obstet. Gynaecol.*, **98**, 249
14. Rydhström, H. and Ingemarsson, I. (1990). Interval between birth of the first and the second twin and its impact on second twin mortality. *J. Perinat. Med.*, **18**, 449
15. Nissen, E.D. (1958). Twins: collision, impaction, and interlocking. *Obstet. Gynecol.*, **5**, 514
16. Rydhström, H. and Cullberg, G. (1990). Pregnancies with growth-retarded twins in breech-vertex presentation at increased risk of entanglement during delivery. *J. Perinat. Med.*, **18**, 45
17. Rydhström, H. (1990). Factors influencing twin perinatal mortality. *Thesis*, Lund, Bloms Tryckeri

Pregnancy dating and evaluation by ultrasonography

R.E. Sabbagha

Introduction

Ultrasound is a non-invasive imaging method for diagnosis of multiple pregnancy and for the longitudinal evaluation of fetal growth and well-being. Ultrasound is not performed routinely on all pregnant women in the United States. As a result, the diagnosis of multiple gestation is inconsistent, particularly during the first trimester. In some large cities where ultrasound is widely available and routinely used, ascertainment is virtually complete, and delivery-room diagnosis a phenomenon of the past. In other areas, however, where ultrasound is unavailable, considered an unwarranted intervention or a non-reimbursable luxury of modern practice, multiple pregnancies still may not be diagnosed prior to delivery. At present, accurate national statistics documenting the extent to which ultrasound is used in the United States are unavailable. (See Chapter 15 for comparison.)

Assuming that ultrasound is not part of the routine prenatal evaluation, the major indications for ordering this test include: (1) poor obstetric history; (2) history of a birth defect; (3) family history of multiple pregnancy; (4) questionable dates; (5) conception by assisted reproductive technology; (6) maternal diabetes mellitus; (7) uterine fundal measurement either smaller or larger than expected for dates; (8) vaginal bleeding in the first or early second trimester; (9) abnormal amniotic fluid alpha-fetoprotein level; and finally (10) abnormal fetal karyotype.

The ultrasound evaluation of a multiple gestation should follow the guidelines of a standard obstetric ultrasound examination, as suggested by the American Institute of Ultrasound in Medicine (AIUM)[1]. In such an examination, the basic areas of investigation should include: (1) duration of pregnancy; (2) evaluation of fetal number, thickness of membranes and placentation; (3) evaluation of individual fetal growth and estimation of fetal weight and percentile ranking; (4) assessment of fetal well-being by biophysical profile and Doppler velocimetry, as indicated; and (5) surveillance of fetal anatomy, including specific views that screen for abnormalities of all systems. The data obtained should then be presented in a concise and complete manner. An example of such a report is shown in Figure 1. A detailed discussion of the areas examined in a standard study follows in the next section.

Pregnancy dating

The use of vaginal (as opposed to abdominal) ultrasound enhances the diagnosis of early gestation. Goldstein *et al.*[2] and Warren *et al.*[3] have pinpointed the exact interval during which the three components of the early embryonic complex first appear. These intervals are: (1) 4 weeks from last menstrual period (LMP) (gestational sac); (2) 5 weeks from LMP (yolk sac); and (3) 6 weeks from LMP (fetal pole). Goldstein *et al.*[2] further defined specific markers of normal embryonic growth as follows: (1) the mean gestational sac diameter is >20 mm during the interval of 6–7 menstrual weeks and is associated with positive fetal heart motion; and (2) the mean gestational sac diameter is >30 mm during the

NM Northwestern Memorial Hospital – Prentice Pavilion	
Standard Ultrasound Obstetrical Examination	

LMP: 7/21/91 Wks by LMP: 42- EDD by LMP: 4/26/92	**Key Fetal Findings**
CURRENT FETAL DATA	Reason for Scan: **Postdates**
(cm) wks %ile (cm) Growth at 35+wks	
CRL: N/A HC/AC : 1.2 >Normal BPD: 8.9 35+ 25-75 FL/BPD : .8 Normal HC-p: 32.4 36 75-90 AC/FL : 4.0 Abnorm AC-p: 28.2 31- <2.5 BPD/OFD: .8 Normal FL: 7.1 36- >95 HC (calc): 32.6 >90 AC (calc): 28.0 <2.5	FINAL ASSIGNED DATES : **35+** Wks EDD: **6/10/92** Date Assignment Based on: Late BPD (+/- 21 days) FETAL HEART BEAT : **PRESENT** FETAL POSITION : **CEPHALIC** NUMBER OF FETUSES : **1** PLACENTAL POSITION : **ANTERIOR**
Placental Grade: 3	ESTIMATED FETAL WEIGHT : **2144** Formula: R.Sabbagha et al BRENNER'S WEIGHT %ILE : **25-50**

Biophysical Profile FBM: 2   FM: 2   FT: 0
                           AVF: 0   NST:
	FETAL GROWTH PATTERN : **At Risk for IUGR**
	                          Abnormal Ponderal Index

Amniotic Fluid Study RUQ: 1.1 RLQ: 0 AFV LUQ: 0 LLQ: 0 Index: 1.1	AMNIOTIC FLUID : **OLIGOHYDRAMNIOS** BIOPHYISICAL PROFILE : **4**
Doppler Study Not Indicated	DOPPLER VELOCIMETRY : **N/A**

PREVIOUS FETAL FINDINGS						
Date	Wks	HC%ile	AC%ile	Growth Pattern	EFW	Wt %ile	AFV

Fetal Anatomy

Cereberal Ventricles	: **Normal**	Stomach Left	: **Normal**
Cerebellum	: **Poor Visualization**	Kidney	: **Normal**
LSP	: **Normal**	Bladder	: **Normal**
Binocular Distance	: **5.6 cm 10-90%ile**	Heart 4CH View	: **Normal**
Nuchal Occip. Thickness	: **Visualization not Possible**	Fetal Other	: **N/A**
Maternal Pelvis	: **Normal**		

Figure 1 In the left upper corner of the report is a display of the data collected. The key fetal findings represent a synthesis of the information that gives the health-care provider a quick glance at all the findings. The method used in assigning dates follows the guidelines discussed in the text and is explained in smaller print under 'final assigned dates'. The middle section displays the growth parameters in the previous two examinations. The section on fetal anatomy displays the areas examined. The responses include one of the following choices: previously normal, normal, suspect, abnormal and poorly visualized

interval of 8–9 menstrual weeks and is associated with embryonic movement.

In a subsequent report, Goldstein[4] demonstrated that conventional crown–rump length (CRL) measurements are only possible when fetal size is 18–20 mm. Prior to this, it is more accurate to use a generic term such as 'early embryonic size' (EES). This is because the relationship of the fetal head and trunk in the early embryo is straight (Figure 2), and extreme flexion of the neck area only develops later. The sequence of anatomic changes is as follows: (1) the embryonic structure at 3–4 mm (6 weeks from LMP) is fairly straight, and measurement of its size is actually its greatest length (Figure 2, left panel); (2) the embryo from 7.2 to 11 mm (7+ to 8– weeks from LMP) shows extreme flexion at the neck. Thus, its greatest length is from neck to rump rather than from crown to rump (Figure 2, right panel); (3) the embryo from 20 to 50 mm (9– to 12+ weeks from LMP) loses the flexion at

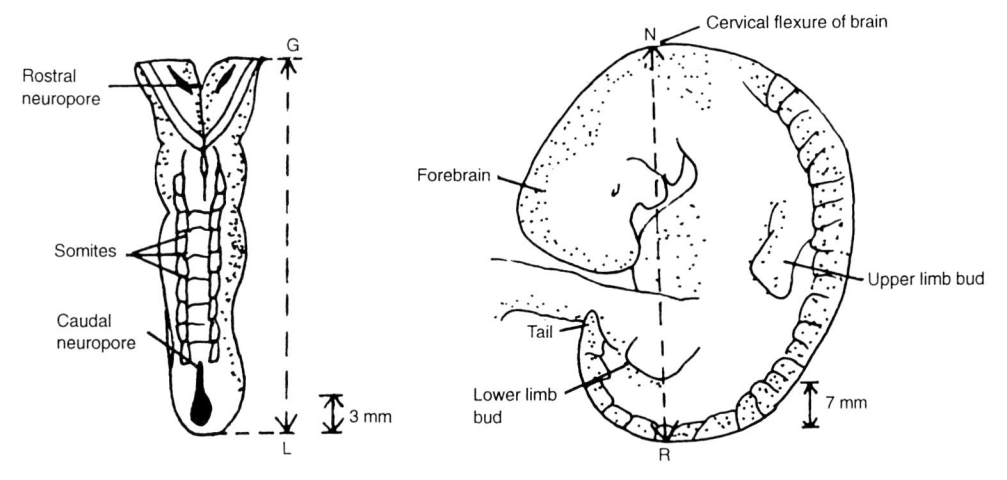

Figure 2 Note the linear fetal pole in an early pregnancy prior to 7 weeks. The fetus at 7–8 weeks' gestation shows extreme flexion at the neck. Thus, terminology in both situations should be early embryonic size (EES). From reference 4, with permission

the neck. As a result, its greatest length is the CRL measurement.

Dating in a multiple pregnancy is accomplished by using ultrasound data derived from singletons. A wide variety of fetal dimensions can be used to estimate dates, including the orbital distance[5] cheek-to-cheek diameter[6], foot length[7], cerebellar diameter[8] and fetal iliac bone measurements[9]. However, because of ease of measurement, the following parameters are used most commonly: CRL, biparietal diameter (BPD), femur length (FL), head circumference (HC) and abdominal circumference (AC). When a discrepancy is noted between fetal measurements in twins, ultrasound dating should be based on the data obtained from the larger twin, because decreased growth in the smaller twin is more likely to underestimate menstrual dates.

CRL and menstrual dates

The fetal CRL is generally considered an accurate means for estimating dates in the first trimester of pregnancy with a ±2 SD variation of 3–5 days. Recently, however, MacGregor et al.[10] determined that the original data relating CRL and dates underestimated the length of pregnancy by an average of 3 days. Data in the cohort described by MacGregor et al.[10] were derived from women with known ovulation dates. Daya[11] also examined the correlation between CRL and dates in very early pregnancy, using data derived from women who underwent in vitro fertilization (IVF). Embryos were transferred into the uterus 2 days after oocyte retrieval and, at that time, the pregnancy was assigned a gestational age of 14 days[11].

The validity of Daya's approach was tested by the almost identical relationship between the normal hCG curve and that derived from IVF pregnancies. The advantage of an IVF model over menstrual dates and possibly ovulation dates is based on several considerations, including: (1) normal ovulation may occur within a range of −4 to +6 days or −6 to +4 days from midcycle, when the LH surge is measured or follicular growth is monitored, respectively; (2) in spontaneous cycles, ovulation can occur from 2 h to 4 days after the follicle reaches the size of 18 mm; and (3) when hCG is administered, ovulation occurs within an interval that extends up to 30 h. Daya's study used polynomial regression analysis to identify the model that provided the best fit for the CRL data[11]. The quadratic model was selected and it showed that CRL growth is curvilinear rather than linear, as previously believed. The 95% confidence interval in pregnancy dates for CRL measurements was 2–3 days prior to 11 weeks and 2–5 days after that interval. Daya[11] also showed that CRL values derived

MULTIPLE PREGNANCY

Table 1 Mean menstrual gestational age in weeks and days relative to fetal early embryonic size (EES) and crown–rump length (CRL) in the first trimester of pregnancy

CRL (mm)	Week +days	CRL (mm)	Week +days
2	6+1	42	11+1
3	6+2	43	11+1
4	6+3	44	11+2
5	6+5	45	11+3
6	6+5	46	11+3
7	6+6	47	11+4
8	7+0	48	11+5
9	7+1	49	11+5
10	7+2	50	11+6
11	7+3	51	12+0
12	7+4	52	12+0
13	7+5	53	12+1
14	7+6	54	12+1
15	8+0	55	12+2
16	8+1	56	12+3
17	8+2	57	12+3
18	8+3	58	12+4
19	8+4	59	12+4
20	8+6	60	12+4
21	9+0	61	12+5
22	9+1	62	12+5
23	9+1	63	12+5
24	9+2	64	12+6
25	9+3	65	12+6
26	9+4	66	12+6
27	9+4	67	12+6
28	9+5	68	12+6
29	9+6	69	13+0
30	9+6	70	13+0
31	10+0	71	13+0
32	10+1	72	13+0
33	10+2	73	13+1
34	10+2	74	13+1
35	10+3	75	13+2
36	10+3	76	13+2
37	10+4	77	13+2
38	10+5	78	13+2
39	10+6	79	13+2
40	10+6	80	13+2
41	11+0		

Adapted from references 10 and 11

from pregnant women with known menstrual dates underestimated as well as overestimated gestational age in the early and late parts of the first trimester of pregnancy, respectively. Further, he noted that CRL values obtained from women with known dates of ovulation also overestimated dates, particularly with CRL of <40 mm. However, the IVF and ovulation CRL data were almost identical in the range of 20–60 mm. This observation lends credence to the study of MacGregor et al.[10], because CRL measurements under 10 mm and above 66 mm were uncommon. A chart combining IVF and ovulation data is shown in Table 1.

BPD/HC/FL evaluation and menstrual dates

From 14 to 26 weeks' gestation, BPD and FL can be used to estimate pregnancy dates. The variation (±2 SD) in the BPD estimate of dates is ±7–11 days. The range for FL is controversial, however, extending from ±11 days to ±18 days[12,13]. Part of the discrepancy may be related to use of sector vs. linear scanners; the latter have poor lateral resolution, which may distort true FL. The error in FL measurements may be reduced if the bone is measured in the longitudinal rather than the horizontal plane.

Recently, Hadlock et al.[14] demonstrated that BPD, FL and HC measurements are quite accurate at 14–26 weeks' gestation and approach the CRL accuracy obtained prior to the 12th week of pregnancy. Additionally, Sabbagha et al.[15] demonstrated that when BPD measuring methodology is standardized, BPD percentile scales are similar in Caucasians and in Black Americans. As a result, the same BPD scale can be used universally. The charts relating BPD, FL, HC and AC to menstrual age are shown in Tables 2 and 3.

Choice of measurements

In every pregnancy the sonographer must choose which measurement(s) to use for estimation of dates. This choice should be based on the ultrasound measurements, the patient's history and the clinical findings. The following guidelines are helpful.

First, the FL should be used if a cephalic abnormality is present, as in hydrocephaly or microcephaly, or when there is side-to-side flattening of the fetal head, a condition known as dolichocephaly. The latter condition is more likely to occur in the presence of fetal crowding, as is the case in multiple pregnancy. By the same token, BPD or HC should be used when the femur is abnormally short, as is the case for most fetuses with skeletal dysplasia. Second, when menstrual dates fall within a week of the estimate defined by CRL, BPD or FL, the role of ultrasound should be to confirm menstrual dates. Third, when gestational age estimates derived from all ultrasonic parameters are close (within a week of each other), but differ from menstrual dates by more than a week, it is acceptable to average the dates derived from all measured parameters, but only if the pregnancy is normal. In other words, averaging dates is justifiable in the absence of growth retardation or growth acceleration. Fourth, when the gestational age estimates of the various parameters are different from each other, averaging dilutes the correct predictor. For example, in asymmetric intrauterine growth retardation (IUGR), the HC should be used to assign dates, because cephalic size in this condition remains normal or near normal, whereas the AC and BPD are likely to be small. Specifically, the AC and BPD are small because of malnutrition and dolichocephaly, respectively. The FL is variable in asymmetric IUGR. Further, in macrosomic fetuses, the AC is expected to be larger than any other parameter and should not be used for pregnancy dating. Finally, in multiple pregnancy, the BPD can be small because of IUGR, oligohydramnios or dolichocephaly. In such pregnancies, the cephalic index or ratio of BPD to occipitofrontal diameter should be obtained. A ratio of <74% implies dolichocephaly. Alternatively, the HC can be measured.

Specific evaluations

Determination of zygosity and placentation

It is crucial to remember that monozygotic (MZ) and dizygotic (DZ) twins both may result in dichorionic/diamniotic (DC/DA) placentation

Table 2 Mean gestational age in weeks relative to fetal BPD, FL, HC and AC in the first two trimesters of pregnancy

Week BPD	Length (cm)	Week FL	Week HC	Perimeter (cm)	Week AC
	0.94				
	1.0	13–			
	1.1	13			
	1.2	13+			
	1.3	14–			
	1.4	14–			
	1.5	14+			
	1.6	15–			
	1.7	15–			
	1.8	15+			
	1.9	16–			
	2.0	16	16	13	17
	2.1	16+	16+	13.5	17+
	2.2	17–	17–	13.8	18
	2.3	17	17	14.5	18+
	2.4	17+	17+	15	19
	2.5	18–	18–	15.5	20–
13+	2.6	18	18	16	21–
14–	2.7	18+	18+	16.5	21
14	2.8	19–	19	17	22–
14+	2.9	19	19+	17.5	22
14+	3.0	19+	—	—	—
15–	3.1	20–	20	18	23–
15	3.2	20	20+	18.5	23–
15+	3.3	20+	—	—	—
15+	3.4	21–	21	19	23
16–	3.5	21+	21+	19.5	24–
16	3.6	22–	—	—	—
16+	3.7	22	22	20	25–
17–	3.8	22+	22+	20.5	25
17	3.9	23–	—	—	—
17+	4.0	23+	—	—	—
18–	4.1	24–	23	21	25+
18	4.2	24–	23+	21.5	26–
18+	4.3	24	24	22	26–
19–	4.4	25–	24+	22.5	26
19	4.5	25	25	23	27+
19+	4.6	25+	26→	24	28
20–	4.7	26–			
20	4.8	26+			
20+	4.9	27–			

Continued

Table 2 (continued)

Week BPD	Length (cm)	Week FL	Week HC	Perimeter (cm)	Week AC
21–	5.0	27	27→	26	28+
21	5.1	27+			
21+	5.2				
22–	5.3				
22–	5.4				
22	5.5				
22+	5.6				
23–	5.7				
23	5.8				
23+	5.9				
24–	6.0				
24	6.1				
24+	6.2				
25–	6.3				
25	6.4				
25+	6.5				
26–	6.6				
26	6.7				
26+	6.8				

BPD, biparietal diameter; FL, femur length; HC, head circumference; AC, abdominal circumference; + or –, plus or minus 1–3 days
Adapted from references 13, 15 and 89, and Tamura, R.K. *et al.*, work in progress

and that the placentas can either be fused or separate (Figures 3 and 4). In addition, the MZ twinning process also can result in monochorionic/diamniotic (MC/DA) and monochorionic/monoamniotic (MC/MA) placentation (Figure 4) (see Chapter 9). The finding of separate placentas on ultrasound readily establishes the presence of DC/DA twinning. However, because a fused placenta may also occur in DC/DA, MC/DA or MC/MA twins, determination of membrane thickness becomes crucial for defining chorionicity (Figure 5)[16]. For example, in 69 twin gestations reported by D'Alton and Dudley[17], counting three or more layers of dividing membranes achieved a 98.5% positive predictive value of dichorionic placentation. Unfortunately, different layers are not always clearly resolved on ultrasound images. Barss *et al.*[18] were able to correctly determine chorionicity in 33 of 34 twin pregnancies. They noted, however, that in MC gestations the amnion may be thin and 'invisible' during the first trimester. In such cases, vaginal ultrasound should be used to enhance visualization of the membranes and/or another scan should be obtained in the second trimester of pregnancy (see Chapter 14).

In DZ twins, the ultrasonographer may either visualize two separate placentas or a single (fused) placenta with thick membranes. Fetal sex may either be the same or different. Similarly, in MZ DC/DA twins, either two placentas or a single fused placenta with thick membranes is possible. However, both twins will have the same sex. The management and outcome of twin pregnancies are clearly related to chorionicity. The best outcome is noted in DC/DA twins, regardless of whether the origin is MZ or DZ.

Table 3 Mean (M) and variability (V) of menstrual dates in weeks relative to fetal BPD, FL, HC and AC in the third trimester of pregnancy

Week/BPD V	Week/BPD M	Length (cm)	Week/FL M	Week/FL V	Week/HC V	Week/HC M	Perimeter (cm)	Week/AC M	Week/AC V
		5.2	28–	3	2	28	26	29–	3
		5.3	28+	3	3	28+	26.5	29–	3
		5.4	29–	3	3	29	27	29	3
		5.5	29+	3	3	30	28	31–	3
		5.6	30–	3	3	31	28.5	33–	3
		5.7	30–	3	3	32–	29	33–	3
		5.8	30+	3	3	32	29.5	33–	3
		5.9	31–	3	3	33	30	34–	3
		6.0	31+	3	3	34	31	35–	3
		6.1	32–	3	3	35	32	35–	3
		6.2	32	3	3	36	32.5	35–	3
		6.3	32+	3	2.5	37	33	35	2+
		6.4	33–	3	2+	38	33	35	2+
		6.5	33+	3	2+	39	33	35	2+
		6.6	34–	3	2+	40	34	36–	2+
		6.7	34+	3			35	37–	2+
		6.8	35–	3			35.5	37	2+
2	27–	6.9	35	3			36	38	2+
2	27	7.0	36–	3			36.5	39	2+
2	27+	7.1	36–	3			37	40	2+
3	28–	7.2	36+	3			38	41	2+
3	28	7.3	37–	3					
3	28+	7.4	37+	3					
3	29–	7.5	38–	3					
3	29	7.6	38+	3					
3	29+	7.7	39–	3					
3	30	7.8	39+	3					
3	30+	7.9	40–	3					
3	31	8.0							
3	31+	8.1							
3	32	8.2							
3	32+	8.3							
3	33–	8.4							
3	33	8.5							
3	33+	8.6							
3	34	8.7							
3	35–	8.8							
3	35+	8.9							
3	36	9.0							
3	36+	9.1							
3	37–	9.2							
3	38–	9.3							
3	39	9.4							
3	40	9.5							

BPD, biparietal diameter; FL, femur length; HC, head circumference; AC, abdominal circumference
Adapted from references 13, 15 and 89, and Tamura, R.K. *et al.*, work in progress

Pregnancy dating and evaluation

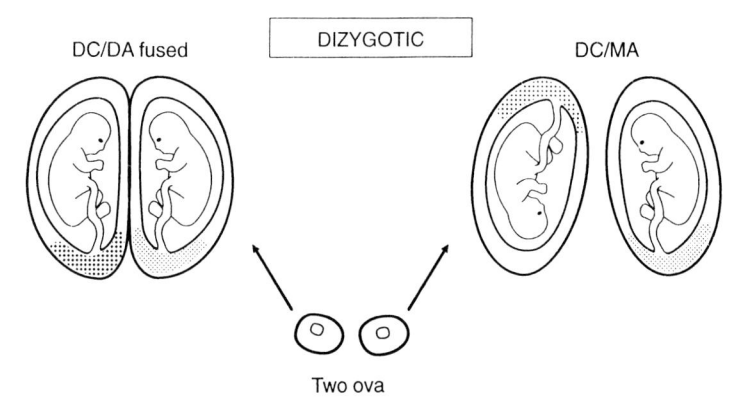

Figure 3 Note that in DZ twinning the result is DC/DA chorionicity, whereby the placentas may either be separate or fused. The membranes between both fetuses represent two amnions and two chorion layers. The total membrane width exceeds 2 mm. From reference 90, with permission

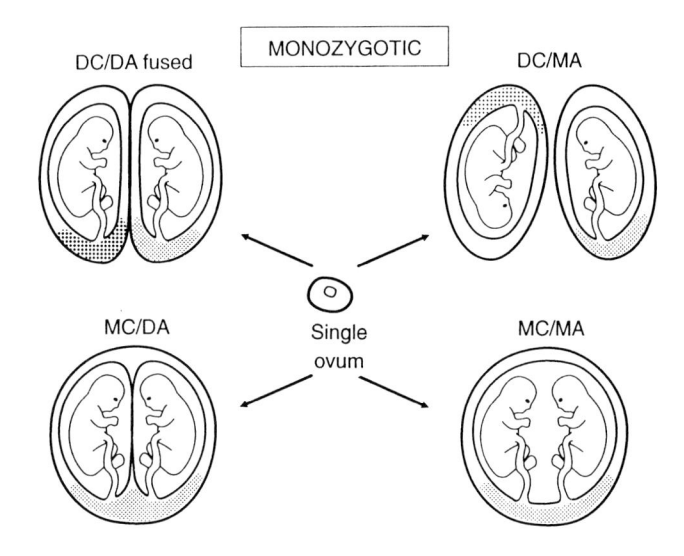

Figure 4 Note that in MZ twinning the chorionicity and amnionicity are variable, as follows: (a) DC/DA chorionicity, with separate or fused placentas; (b) MC/DA placentation with a fused placenta and thin membranes (< 2 mm); and (c) MC/MA placentation with a fused placenta and no membrane between both fetuses. In the last category there is an increased chance of conjoined twinning. In approximately 70% of cases the twins are joined at the thorax (thoracopagus), abdomen (omphalopagus), or a combination of the two. Conjoined twinning can also occur at the head (craniopagus), buttocks (ischiopagus) and cephalothoracopagus. From reference 90, with permission (see Chapter 8)

MZ MC/DA twins

These pregnancies (single placenta, thin membrane and same sex) are associated with a higher rate of growth discordance (≥20% in body weight)[18]. Further, vascular communications may occur and result in twin–twin transfusion syndrome (TTS) and the 'stuck' twin phenomenon (see below). Complications may also occur in the surviving twin if one twin dies (see Chapter 30). Importantly, in this type of twinning, amniotic fluid should be obtained from each sac for evaluating the karyotype of each fetus. The reason for this is that dysjunction or mutation may occur in one twin after the ovum splits[19] (see Chapter 7).

MC/MA twins: diagnosis/management

Although this type of twinning occurs in only 0.1–2.3% of all twin pregnancies, it carries a 50% risk of perinatal mortality. Antenatal diagnosis is essential, because it may lead to altered and aggressive pregnancy management, including possible elective Cesarean section by 34 weeks' gestation to prevent cord accidents[20]. This approach, however, remains controversial[21] (see Chapter 39).

Diagnosis can be made by ultrasound when no membrane is seen intersecting the placenta between the insertion sites of both umbilical cords (Figure 6). In some cases, color Doppler ultrasound has been successfully used to identify the site of placental cord insertions, thus enhancing visualization of the membranes in the surrounding area. Entanglement of the umbilical cords denotes MC/MA twins. Cordocentesis and Doppler studies may show differences in hemoglobin concentration and umbilical velocimetry, respectively (see below).

On occasion, prenatal diagnosis of MA twinning is made when contrast agent is present in the gastrointestinal tract of each fetus following instillation of methylglucamine by single puncture amniocentesis[22]. The importance of establishing this diagnosis relates to the fact that the likelihood of cord entanglement, premature delivery, intrauterine fetal death and lower birth weight is also increased[20]. Additionally, there is a greater chance for antenatal necrosis of the white matter in the brain of one twin; this occurs when the pregnancy is complicated by polyhydramnios, IUFD of the co-twin, hydrops and placental vascular connections, particularly in the presence of a venous anastomosis[23]. Finally, in MC/MA twins there is an increased likelihood of conjoined twinning, and twin reversed arterial perfusion sequence (TRAP; acardiac twin)[20,24].

MC/MA twins: TRAP sequence

When the arterial pressure in one twin exceeds that of the other, blood flow is reversed in the recipient, resulting in the perfusion of deoxygenated blood into the umbilical arteries and, in turn, the iliac arteries and lower body[24]. Thus, varying degrees of upper body reduction anomalies occur, including acardia. Antenatal diagnosis of this condition is possible because cardiac structures and other reduction anomalies can be identified using Doppler ultrasound. Doppler sonography has also been used to demonstrate direct vascular anastomosis between the two fetal circulations[25]. The outcome in such pregnancies is poor, and 100% and 50% mortality of the acardiac and 'pump' twin have been recorded, respectively. Ash *et al.* have successfully controlled polyhydramnios in the 'pump' twin by the administration of indomethacin, a known inhibitor of fetal renal function[24]. In this manner, progression of polyhydramnios is controlled and normal amniotic fluid volume restored. These authors believe that the benefits of administering indomethacin prior to 34 weeks' gestation may exceed the potential side effects of the drug, including temporary constriction of the ductus arteriosus[24]. No permanent loss in renal function was observed in their series. Other methods to improve survival of the 'pump' twin have been tried, including hysterotomy to remove the acardiac twin or occlusion of the anomalous twin's cord. However, these latter methods are currently considered to be unproven and of an investigational nature (see Chapters 7 and 29).

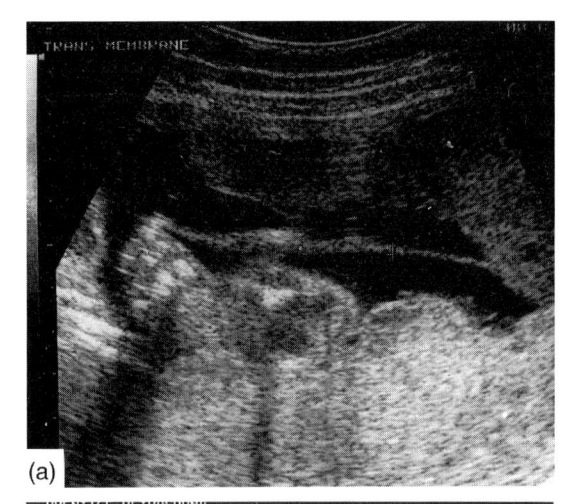

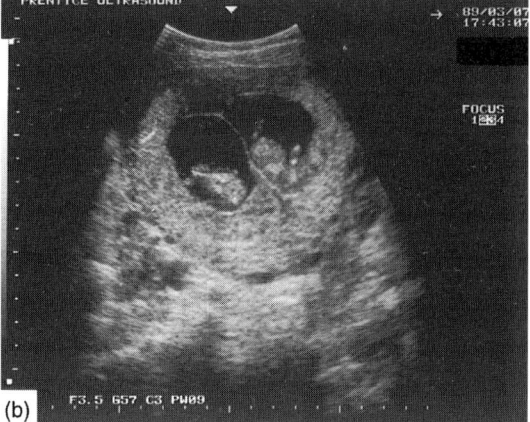

Figure 5 (a) Note the thick membrane (> 2 mm) between the calipers, in DC/DA placentation. (b) A thin membrane is visualized between both twins in MC/DA placentation

TTS and 'stuck' twin phenomenon

The TTS is diagnosed postnatally when fetuses have discordant growth and/or hemoglobin concentrations at delivery. This constellation of findings has a relatively good prognosis[20]. In contrast is the grave prognosis noted in TTS associated with the onset of acute polyhydramnios in one sac and oligohydramnios in the other[20]. These latter findings are more frequently noted in MC/DA twins and usually occur in the early part of the second trimester of pregnancy. In such cases, the donor sac loses its amniotic fluid and the fetus becomes anemic and 'stuck' in a cocoon-like structure formed by its adherent

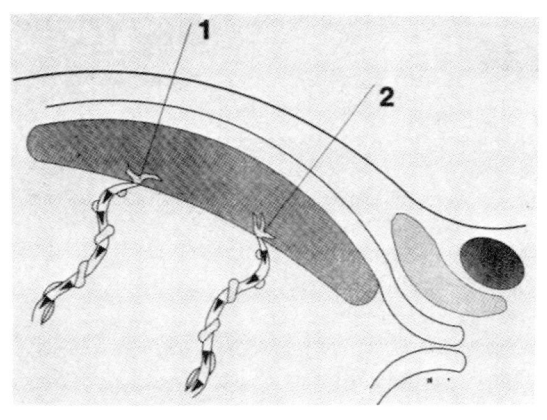

Figure 6 Ultrasonic search for a thin membrane is best performed in the area between the placental insertion of both umbilical cords (1 and 2). From reference 91, with permission

amnion (Figure 7)[20]. In contrast, the recipient twin becomes hydropic[20]. Treatment options include elective termination of pregnancy, selective pregnancy reduction and laser ablation of vascular anastomoses[20,26].

Importantly, however, amniotic fluid volume can be restored to normal in both sacs by aggressive serial amniocenteses. In one study, amniocentesis was performed at a rate of 1–10 procedures per patient, and 225–5000 ml of amniotic fluid was withdrawn each time[20]. With this approach, Elliott et al.[20] reduced perinatal mortality from almost 100% to 21%, without incurring any infectious morbidity or placental abruption. In another report, procedural complications were noted in two of 11 survivors (18%) and these included brain infarction and renal tubular necrosis[27].

Vanishing twin phenomenon

A particularly interesting aspect of the early evaluation of multiple gestation is the 'vanishing twin' phenomenon. Landy et al.[28] reviewed the first trimester ultrasound reports of 1000 pregnancies and reported the incidence of twins confirmed by fetal heart motion to be 3.29%. In 21.2% of these pregnancies, one twin was resorbed or spontaneously aborted; stated another way, it 'vanished'. In 20% of these pregnancies, vaginal bleeding was present although the outcome was not otherwise

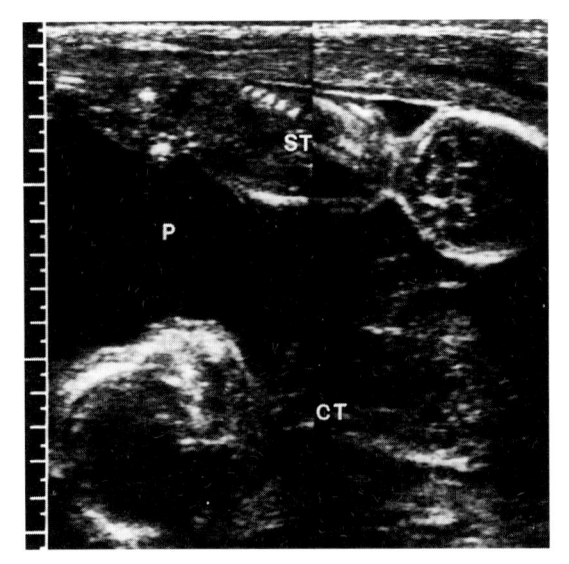

Figure 7 Note the severe oligohydramnios and small size of the stuck twin (ST). The ST is adherent to its amnion, which cannot be visualized in the scan. The co-twin (CT) is larger in size and its sac shows polyhydramnios (P). From reference 27, with permission

more complicated. Based on a critical difference in size of the gestational sac, fetal pole or fetal heart rate, it may be possible at some future time to determine which twin is likely to 'vanish'. This statement is based on the findings of May and Sturtevant, who evaluated 50 early pregnancies (4.5–7.3 weeks' gestation) and found that of the 11 embryos that miscarried, six had initial heart rates below 85 beats per minute; by comparison, all of those that continued to viability exceeded this rate ($p < 0.0001$)[29] (see Chapters 4 and 6).

Assessment of fetal growth

Growth in twins

Some years ago, it was deemed desirable to construct special charts for twin growth. Two recent studies, however, clearly show that the differences in the incremental growth of BPD, HC and FL in normal twins and singletons are not statistically significant[30,31]. As a result, the construction of special charts for these parameters is not warranted. (See comments in Chapter 14.) Notwithstanding, Socol et al. have previously shown that in uncomplicated twin pregnancies a significant decrease of the BPD is noted during the third trimester of pregnancy[32]. Although this decrease is probably the result of dolichocephaly, it emphasizes the need to use HC rather than BPD for determining cephalic size, either to date the pregnancy or to estimate fetal weight. Although Socol et al. also showed that the AC decreased in size after 34 weeks' gestation in twins, this decrease was minimal, reaching only 1 cm at 37 weeks[32]. Indeed, the AC is the most reliable parameter for assessing normality or discordancy of growth in multiple pregnancy. According to Brown et al., in twins an AC difference of ≥ 20 mm is usually associated with a significant growth discordancy[33].

With regard to twin weights, Leroy et al. observed that the 50th weight percentile in twins crossed the 10th weight percentile in singletons at approximately the 37+ weeks of pregnancy (Figure 8)[34]. Similar types of differences occur in triplets as well (Figure 9)[35].

Estimating fetal weight

At this time, the best estimates of fetal weight are derived from a mathematical formula that incorporates HC, AC and FL. Although a general formula was proposed by Hadlock et al.[36] in 1975, formulas targeted to (1) gestational age and (2) fetal size[36] reduce the cumulative absolute 2 SD considerably from 15.6% (Hadlock et al.[36]) to 12.2% (Sabbagha et al.[37]). These formulas are shown in Table 4.

The smaller variation noted with targeted formulas may be related to the fact that the proportional contributions of the HC and AC are in a state of dynamic flux, one that is dependent both on gestational age and the presence of normal vs. altered growth. The following examples illustrate the dynamic state of the HC/AC ratio:

(1) Prior to the 36th pregnancy week, the HC/AC ratio is > 1.0.

(2) Following the 36th pregnancy week, the HC/AC ratio is < 1.0.

Pregnancy dating and evaluation

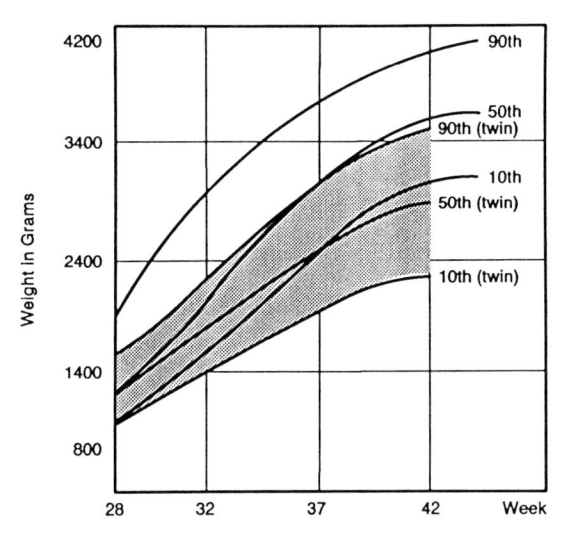

Figure 8 Note that in twin pregnancy the 50th weight percentile crosses the 10th weight percentile of singletons at 37+ weeks. From reference 34, with permission

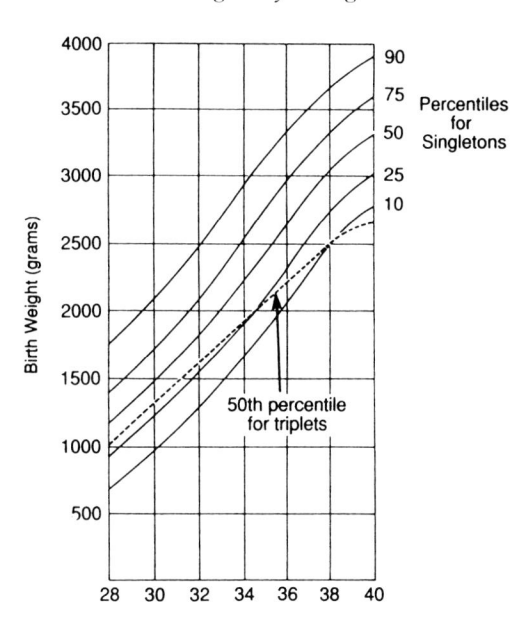

Figure 9 Note that in triplet pregnancy the 50th weight percentile crosses the 10th weight percentile of singletons at 35 weeks. From reference 35, with permission

Table 4 Formulas used in the prospective evaluation of 381 pregnancies

Groups	Formulas
Large for gestational age (LGA)	$5426.9 - (94.98 \times SUM)^* + (0.54262 \times SUM^2)$ ($r = 0.93$, $r^2 = 0.87$)
Appropriate for gestational age (AGA)	$-55.3 - (16.35 \times SUM) + (0.25838 \times SUM^2)$ ($r = 0.97$, $r^2 = 0.94$)
Small for gestational age (SGA)	$1849.4 - (47.13 \times SUM) + (0.37721 \times SUM^2)$ ($r = 0.96$, $r^2 = 0.92$)

LGA, Fetuses with AC ≥90th percentile; AGA, fetuses with AC >5% and <90%; SGA, fetuses with AC ≤5th percentile, for dates. EFW, Estimated fetal weight; AC, abdominal circumference; HC, head circumference; FL, femur length.
*SUM = GA (weeks) + (2 AC) (cm) + HC (cm) + FL (cm).
(From reference 37)

(3) In asymmetric IUGR, the HC/AC ratio is increased, even at term, when the ratio is normally < 1.0.

(4) In symmetric IUGR, the HC/AC ratio is not altered.

(5) In macrosomia, the HC/AC ratio is < 1.0 even before term.

In formulas targeted for the large, appropriate and small-for-gestational-age fetuses, the AC is doubly weighted, because it is the most sensitive parameter for estimating fetal weight. The AC is also used to determine which of the three formulas to use. For example, when the AC is ≥90th percentiles, the formula for the large fetus is used. On the other hand, when

MULTIPLE PREGNANCY

Table 5 Estimates of fetal weight derived from formulas targeted to SGA, AGA and LGA fetuses

Formula 1† Use when abdominal perimeter ≥ 90% Large-for-gestational age group (LGA)			Formula 2† Use when abdominal perimeter >5% <90% Appropriate-for-gestational age group (AGA)			Formula 3† Use when abdominal perimeter ≤ 5% Small-for-gestational age group (SGA)		
SUM*	EFW	Diff	SUM*	EFW	Diff	SUM*	EFW	Diff
102	1385		88	506		81	507	
103	1401	16	89	536	30	82	521	14
104	1418	17	90	566	30	83	536	15
105	1437	19	91	596	30	84	552	16
106	1456	19	92	627	31	85	569	17
107	1477	21	93	659	32	86	586	17
108	1498	21	94	690	31	87	604	18
109	1521	23	95	723	33	88	623	19
110	1545	24	96	756	33	89	643	20
111	1570	25	97	789	33	90	663	20
112	1596	26	98	824	35	91	684	21
113	1623	27	99	858	34	92	706	22
114	1651	28	100	893	35	93	729	23
115	1681	30	101	929	36	94	752	23
116	1711	30	102	965	36	95	776	24
117	1742	31	103	1001	36	96	801	25
118	1775	33	104	1039	38	97	827	26
119	1809	34	105	1076	37	98	853	26
120	1843	34	106	1114	38	99	881	28
121	1879	36	107	1153	39	100	909	28
122	1916	37	108	1192	39	101	937	28
123	1954	38	109	1232	40	102	967	30
124	1993	39	110	1272	40	103	997	30
125	2033	40	111	1313	41	104	1028	31
126	2074	41	112	1354	41	105	1060	32
127	2117	43	113	1396	42	106	1092	32
128	2160	43	114	1438	42	107	1125	33
129	2205	45	115	1481	43	108	1159	34
130	2250	45	116	1524	43	109	1194	35
131	2297	47	117	1568	44	110	1229	35
132	2345	48	118	1613	45	111	1266	37
133	2393	48	119	1658	46	112	1303	37
134	2443	50	120	1703	45	113	1340	37
135	2494	51	121	1749	46	114	1379	39
136	2546	52	122	1795	46	115	1418	39
137	2599	53	123	1842	47	116	1458	40
138	2654	55	124	1890	48	117	1499	41
139	2709	55	125	1938	48	118	1540	41
140	2765	56	126	1986	48	119	1583	43
141	2823	58	127	2035	49	120	1626	43
142	2882	59	128	2085	50	121	1670	44
143	2941	59	129	2135	50	122	1714	44
144	3002	61	130	2185	50	123	1759	45

Continued

Table 5 *(Continued)*

Formula 1[†] Use when abdominal perimeter ≥90% Large-for-gestational-age group (LGA)			Formula 2[†] Use when abdominal perimeter >5% <90% Appropriate-for-gestational-age group (AGA)			Formula 3[†] Use when abdominal perimeter ≤5% Small-for-gestational-age group (SGA)		
SUM*	EFW	Diff	SUM*	EFW	Diff	SUM*	EFW	Diff
145	3064	62	131	2236	51	124	1805	46
146	3127	63	132	2288	52	125	1852	47
147	3191	64	133	2340	52	126	1900	48
148	3256	65	134	2393	53	127	1948	48
149	3322	66	135	2446	53	128	1997	49
150	3389	67	136	2500	54	129	2047	50
151	3458	69	137	2554	54	130	2097	51
152	3527	69	138	2608	54	131	2149	52
153	3598	71	139	2664	56	132	2201	52
154	3669	64	140	2719	55	133	2254	53
155	3742	73	141	2776	57	134	2307	53
156	3816	74	142	2832	56	135	2362	55
157	3891	75	143	2890	58	136	2417	55
158	3966	75	144	2948	58	137	2473	56
159	4044	78	145	3006	58	138	2529	56
160	4122	78	146	3065	59	139	2587	58
161	4201	79	147	3124	59	140	2645	58
162	4281	80	148	3184	60	141	2704	49
163	4363	82	149	3244	60	142	2763	59
164	4445	82	150	3305	62	143	2824	61
165	4529	84	151	3367	62	144	2885	61
166	4613	84	152	3429	62	145	2947	62
167	4699	86	153	3491	62	146	3009	62
168	4786	87	154	3554	63	147	3073	64
169	4874	88	155	3617	63	148	3137	64
170	4963	89	156	3681	64	149	3202	65
171	5053	90	157	3746	65	150	3267	65
172	5144	91	158	3811	65			
173	5236	92	159	3877	66			
174	5329	93						
175	5424	95						
176	5519	95						
177	5616	97						
178	5713	97						
179	5812	99						
180	5912	100						
181	6013	101						

*SUM, sum of fetal parameters constituting independent variables: GA (weeks or weeks plus fractions thereof, e.g. 22.7 weeks) + HC (cm) + 2 AC (cm) + FL (cm)
[†]The equations used to generate the EFW in each subgroup are listed in Table 4
Note: If sum of parameters falls between two numbers, e.g. 82.5, the estimated fetal weight may be extrapolated from the difference (Diff)) between the upper and lower numbers (i.e. 521 and 636). Additionally, the accuracy of the assigned gestational age should be within ± 2 weeks.
Adapted from reference 37

the AC is > 5th and < 90th percentiles, respectively, the formula for the average-sized fetus is used (Table 5). Finally, when the AC is ≤ 5th percentile, the formula for the IUGR fetus is used (Table 5).

In a study of macrosomia reported by Blickstein and Weissman, it was observed that only 3.1% of twins exceeded 3600 g, with the three largest newborns weighing between 4060 g and 4115 g[38]. Because of this, only the formulas for the average and small sized fetuses are used in multiple pregnancy. In another twin study, ultrasound estimates of fetal weight in twins had a higher sensitivity than umbilical Doppler velocimetry in the prediction of intrauterine growth retardation[39]. In still another study, Divon et al. showed that Doppler velocimetry complements ultrasound estimates of fetal weight in the diagnosis of discordant growth (Table 6)[40].

Assessment of fetal well-being

Biophysical profile score (BPS)

The BPS is based on the evaluation of five biophysical functions within an interval of 30 min. These are: (1) amniotic fluid volume (AFV); (2) the non-stress test (NST); (3) fetal breathing movements (FBM); (4) fetal body motion (FM); and (5) fetal tone (FT). A BPS of 2 is assigned for each normal variable and a score of 0 when the biophysical function is lost (see Chapter 23).

Amniotic fluid volume (AFV) The positive predictive value of oligohydramnios in the diagnosis of IUGR is approximately 40%[41]. The sensitivity, however, is quite poor (16%)[41]. Nonetheless, the presence of oligohydramnios remains a useful clinical tool for the evaluation of high-risk pregnancies. For example, fetuses with oligohydramnios and an estimated weight of < 10th percentile are likely to have high morbidity, particularly in post-term pregnancies[42]. In contrast, it is estimated that 25% of fetuses with polyhydramnios have congenital anomalies.

Phelan and co-workers introduced the concept of the amniotic fluid index (AFI) for evaluation of AFV[43]. Specifically, they divided the pregnant uterus into four quadrants by two imaginary lines, one running vertically across the linea nigra and the other transversely across the umbilicus. The vertical diameter of the largest pocket in each of the four quadrants was determined and the sum defined as the AFI. An AFI of ≤ 5 cm was used to define oligohydramnios, because it was associated with poor perinatal outcome[44]. Conversely, an AFI of ≥ 24 was used to define polyhydramnios because of the significant association with congenital anomalies.

Unfortunately, in twin gestations it is impossible to divide the pregnant uterus into four quadrants for each of two fetuses. Thus, the ultrasonographer must use the largest pocket of amniotic fluid in each sac to decide whether the volume is normal or abnormal. Although there is some controversy as to the exact measurement that should be used, it is generally agreed that oligohydramnios is diagnosed when the largest pocket of fluid in a particular pregnancy sac is < 2 cm[45–47]. By comparison, polyhydramnios is diagnosed when the largest pocket of amniotic fluid in a particular pregnancy sac is ≥ 8 cm[45].

NST A normal or reactive NST is defined as one that shows at least two fetal heart rate (FHR) accelerations, each equal to 15 beats per minute (BPM), during a 20-min examination[48]. Additionally, the baseline FHR should fall between 120 and 160 BPM and no decelerations should be noted. The presence of decelerations, particularly with oligohydramnios, may be associated with poor outcome. For example, in prolonged pregnancy the presence of oligohydramnios or an umbilical cord diameter of < 1.6 cm was associated with significant 'cord compression FHR patterns' and increased peripartum morbidity[49].

The predictive value of an abnormal NST is low, however; it ranges from 3 to 29%. The reason is partly related to the normal periodicity intervals that characterize biophysical functions. In other words, lack of motion during the 20-min window may be an indication that the fetus is in a sleep cycle rather than in a

Table 6 Sensitivity, specificity and positive and negative predictive values for single and combinations of test results

	Sensitivity (%)	Specificity (%)	Positive predictive value (%)	Negative predictive value (%)
ΔS/D > 15%	66	64	55	75
ΔEFW > 15%	47	81	56	74
ΔBPD > 6 mm	30	88	50	75
ΔAC > 20 mm	53	77	53	77
ΔFL > 5 mm	28	92	63	72
Either ΔS/D >15% or ΔEFW >15%	78	87	73	90

Adapted from reference 40

Table 7 Comparison of standard diagnostic tests in prediction of adverse perinatal outcome (prevalence: 27.7%)

	MCA	UA	Cerebral-umbilical ratio
Sensitivity	24.0	64.0	68.0
Specificity	100.0	90.7	98.4
Positive predicitve value	100.0	72.7	94.4
Negative predictive value	77.3	86.7	88.8
Accuracy	78.8	83.3	90.0

MCA, middle cerebral artery; UA, umbilical artery
Data are presented as percentages; from reference 76

state of flaccidity caused by hypoxia. Under these circumstances, the finding of an abnormal NST often causes the physician to order one or more complementary tests to determine whether the fetus may be in jeopardy.

Fetal body movement/fetal movement/fetal tone (FBM/FM/FT) FBM is considered normal when it is noted at least once during a 30-min interval of real-time evaluation of the fetus and when breathing activity continues for 30 s. During the same 30-min interval, at least three fetal body movements should be observed. Fetal tone is best assessed by visualization of the hands opening and closing. The presence of all three biophysical functions is reassuring. However, absence of one or other function may result from normal periodicity rather than hypoxia (see Chapter 24).

Fetal acoustic stimulation (FAS)
To reduce testing time, as well as the number of false positive NSTs, many clinicians use the FAS test to awaken the fetus and bring on a state of reactivity[50,51]. The mechanism for reactivity, and in turn the tachycardiac response, may be independent of the function of higher cortical centers[52,53].

In the FAS test, an artificial larynx is used to produce an acoustic vibratory stimulus lasting 2–5 s. A 3-s sound stimulus, however, appears to be adequate for awakening the fetus[54]. Strong application of the artificial larynx over the abdomen results in greater transmission of sound than does mild application[55]. The average sound intensity produced at 1 m is 82 dB, and the frequency of the emitted sound is 80 Hz with harmonics in the range 20–9000 Hz[50].

To assess the intensity of sound on the fetus, Nyman et al. placed a sterile hydrophone in the uterus of 16 women in labor with ruptured membranes[56]. The hydrophone was placed in close proximity to the fetal head. The mean recorded sound pressure level after FAS with an artificial larynx was 115 dB. The highest level was 119 dB. By comparison, background noise was 63.5–80.5 dB. Such high sound levels cause cochlear damage in adult animals[57]. However, it is possible that before reaching the cochlea of the fetus, the sound levels are reduced by the surrounding amniotic fluid as well as the fluid in the middle ear[57]. In support of this hypothesis, Ohel et al. and Arulkumaran et al. found no evidence of hearing loss in children exposed to FAS in utero[58,59].

According to Sherer et al., 57% of FHR accelerations in twins coincide, that is, occur within 15 s of each other. This is thought to result from the first twin's spontaneous movement evoking a tactile response and movement of the second twin[60]. Sherer et al. also showed that when FAS was applied to nine sets of twins, vigorous simultaneous movements of both twins occurred, an observation suggesting that different mechanisms may be responsible for spontaneous vs. evoked fetal movements in twins[61] (see Chapter 24).

BPS and acid–base status

Vintzileos et al. evaluated 124 women within 6 h of elective Cesarean section and found a clear association between BPS and fetal acid–base status; the sensitivity, specificity, and positive and negative predictive values were 90%, 96%, 82% and 98%, respectively[62]. These authors theorized that the nervous system centers that controlled individual biophysical components malfunctioned at varying degrees of acidemia. Abnormalities appeared in (1) FHR reactivity at a pH of < 7.2; (2) FBM at a pH of < 7.2; and (3) FM and FT at a pH of < 7.1. In contrast, Sassoon and colleagues suggested that the regulation of FHR and FBM in the acidemic fetus during labor may differ from the regulation of these activities before labor ensues[63]. In a blinded prospective evaluation of 95 pregnant women in labor, these investigators observed no relationship between BPS and neonatal acid–base status[63]. The last BPS taken prior to delivery failed to identify 50% of fetuses who were acidemic at delivery. Although significant decreases in FHR and FBM were recorded as labor progressed, the presence of these two biophysical functions was not reliable in ruling out acidemia.

Weighted biophysical profile

The relative importance of the five biophysical functions in predicting poor outcome was studied by Manning et al.[64]. The distribution of score combinations within fetal subgroups was not equal, and the positive predictive accuracy was not constant across all possible combinations of the biophysical components and varied by composition of the components. Specifically, these authors showed that:

(1) For a BPS of 6, the possibility of fetal distress or death when the NST and FT were abnormal was significantly higher than with a BPS of 6 attributed to absent FT and FBM. Similar significant variations in outcome appeared with different combinations yielding a BPS of 4. Thus, for fetuses with a BPS of 4 and normal NST and AFV, repeat testing rather than intervention may be appropriate.

(2) A reactive NST in the presence of absent FHR, FBM, FT and oligohydramnios was still associated with a 17-fold increase in perinatal death.

(3) For any abnormal end-point outcome, the relative weighting was highest for the non-reactive NST and least for absent FBM. Thus, the NST, AFV and FBM emerged as the most powerful variables for all end-points.

The interdependence of various components of the score still remains unclear. For example, although a reactive NST implies fetal movement, examples of a reactive NST with abnormal FM were noted by Manning et al.[64]. Further, although a BPS of 4 in which the NST was reactive and AFV was normal had a positive predictive accuracy similar to a score of 6, the risk of adverse outcome was still increased[64]. Thus, the concept proposed by Clark *et al.*, i.e. that antepartum testing should be reduced to NST and AFV determinations[65], cannot be supported.

Recently, a weighted BPS was proposed by Petrikovsky and Baker[66]. They retrospectively assigned the following weighted scores in 600 high-risk pregnancies: 4 for normal AFV (AFI of 10–20 cm); 3 for reactive NST; 2 for FBM (at least one 30-s episode in 30 min); 1 for FBM (at least three episodes in 30 min); 0 for FT. Unfavorable outcome was judged by abnormal FHR patterns in labor, 5-min Apgar score of < 7, IUGR with birth weight of < 5th percentile for age, abnormal cord pH of < 7.2, and admission to intensive neonatal care nursery. With a weighted BPS of 6, perinatal outcome was normal in 95% of fetuses. With a traditional BPS of 4, 12% of fetuses had an unfavorable outcome; in contrast, with a weighted BPS of 4, 48% had an unfavorable outcome. Similarly, with a traditional BPS of 2, 78% of fetuses had an unfavorable outcome[66], whereas with a weighted BPS of 2, 88% now had an unfavorable outcome. These data suggest that an unfavorable outcome[66] correlates in a more consistent fashion with the weighted score.

Doppler assessments

Doppler examinations have recently been added to the group of examinations used to assess fetal well-being. Doppler studies are used to assess blood velocity in a number of vessels, including umbilical, middle cerebral, renal and uterine arteries. These arteries reflect resistance in the placental bed, fetal cerebrum, kidneys and maternal vasculature. The recent introduction of color coding enhances the ultrasonographer's the ability to identify the middle cerebral and uterine arteries.

The recognition of abnormal Doppler velocimetry is beneficial in the determination of fetal-risk status, false-positive electronic FHS tests, IUGR and TTS. Three methods are used to assess Doppler velocimetry:

(1) Systolic/diastolic (S/D) ratio, measuring:

$$\frac{\text{peak arterial velocity}}{\text{end-diastolic velocity}}$$

(2) The resistance index (RI) or Pourcelot's index, measuring:

$$\frac{\text{peak arterial velocity} - \text{end-diastolic velocity}}{\text{end-diastolic velocity}}$$

(3) The pulsatility index (PI), measuring:

$$\frac{\text{peak arterial velocity} - \text{end-diastolic velocity}}{\text{mean velocity}}$$

Maulik *et al.* showed that of the various Doppler indices the RI is the best predictor of perinatal compromise[67]. However, the position of the RI measurement along the umbilical cord affects the result[68]. Measurements near the placental insertion tend to be lower than those near the fetal insertion by approximately 28%. The longer the cord, the greater the expected variation in RI values. Thus, the position of the measurement is an important factor for the pathophysiological interpretation of the RI, and should be known when comparing data from different studies. In normal twin pregnancies, the relationship between the S/D ratios of the umbilical arteries and gestational age is similar to that in normal singleton pregnancies[69] (see Chapters 14 and 23).

Doppler and fetal outcome

Giles *et al.* evaluated the relationship between routine use of S/D ratios in twin pregnancies and perinatal outcome[70]. They obtained S/D ratios in two groups of women with twin gestations. In the first 100 women, the S/D ratios were not communicated to the physician. In the second 172 women, the S/D ratios were obtained at 28–32 weeks' gestation and the results were forwarded to the health-care providers, in order to allow discriminatory prescription of bed rest and close fetal surveillance. The corrected perinatal mortality in the second group was reduced to 8.9 per 1000 from 42.1 per 1000. Similarly, Gaziano *et al.* also showed that abnormal Doppler velocimetry correlated highly with poor outcome[71]. Specifically, twin fetuses with abnormal Doppler findings were born 3–4 weeks earlier and exhibited a greater number of stillbirths and structural anomalies, or were either recipients or donors in the TTS.

Doppler and electronic testing

Pattinson et al. studied 369 high-risk pregnancies and showed that a high umbilical artery RI identified those fetuses with abnormal NST[72]; the sensitivity was 93.1% and the normal predictive value was 99.8%. However, the positive predictive value was very poor. Falsely increased RIs occurred in 293 of 320 normal NSTs[72].

According to Arduini et al., in fetal cerebral arteries a nadir of vasodilatation is reached 2 weeks before the onset of antepartum FHR decelerations[73]. By comparison, significant changes in umbilical velocimetry occur close to the onset of abnormal FHR patterns.

Small-for-gestational age (SGA) fetuses with normal S/D ratio are at significantly lower risk than those with abnormal ratios[74]. It is possible that the S/D ratio might discriminate late decelerations that constitute a false positive test; in the study of Brar et al., there was no difference in the incidence of adverse perinatal outcome in the late deceleration group with normal S/D ratios compared with controls[75].

Doppler and IUGR

Gramellini et al. evaluated 45 IUGR fetuses and 45 normal controls by umbilical and cerebral Doppler velocimetry. These authors showed that in the last 10 weeks of pregnancy the cerebral/umbilical ratio was constant, with a normal cutoff level equal to 1.08[76]. Thus, a value of >1.08 was normal and <1.08 was abnormal. They also showed that the ratio was a better predictor of IUGR and adverse perinatal outcome than either the middle cerebral or umbilical pulsatility indexes alone (Table 7). Mari and Deter demonstrated that the IUGR fetus with a normal middle cerebral artery PI is at lower risk than the fetus with abnormal PI values[77], and Vyas et al. investigated the middle cerebral artery in 81 SGA fetuses by color-coded Doppler[78]. These authors also obtained blood by cordocentesis in all fetuses and measured blood gases. A significant quadratic relation was found between fetal hypoxemia and the degree of reduction in middle cerebral artery PIs. The maximum reduction in PIs was noted when the fetal pO_2 was 2–4 SD below the normal mean for gestation[78].

Absent end-diastolic velocity (AEDV)

A number of authors agree that AEDV as well as reverse end-diastolic velocity in the umbilical arteries is associated with poor perinatal outcome[79,80]. Fetuses with AEDV have a higher incidence of IUGR, admission to intensive-care units, low Apgar scores, congenital anomalies including lethal malformations, aneuploidy and are more likely to have come from mothers with pregnancy-induced hypertension and Cesarean section for fetal distress. Wenstrom et al. noted that the etiology of AEDV is variable and in some cases it cannot be determined[81]. Thus, in any evaluation of a fetus with AEDV, a knowledge of fetal karyotype and anatomy, gestational age, maternal status, and fetal status as determined by tests other than Doppler, is required to optimize outcome. Interestingly, Henretty et al. reported a case complicated by pregnancy-induced hypertension in which the end diastolic velocity reappeared after treatment[82]. Sengupta et al. also showed that a subset of patients with abnormal Doppler velocimetry improved on bed rest and had a better perinatal outcome compared to other patients in whom the abnormal S/D ratios persisted[83].

Doppler and TTS

The use of Doppler in the diagnosis of TTS is controversial. Saldana et al. showed that in twins a difference in the S/D ratio of <0.4 was highly predictive (91%) of concordant fetal growth[84]. However, there was only a 42% predictive value for discordancy with an S/D ratio difference of ≥0.4. Yamada et al. also demonstrated that between 24 and 31 weeks' gestation, six out of seven pregnancies complicated by TTS had a PI of >0.5; this level was significantly greater than the PI in four discordant and 21 concordant twins[85]. Pretorius et al. studied eight twin pairs suspected of TTS because of disparity in size, separate umbilical cords, single placenta and hydrops of one fetus[86]. The authors observed that the differences in the S/D ratios was >0.4 in all eight cases. However, they could not use Doppler velocimetry to differentiate the donor twin from the recipient or even provide prognostic data regarding outcome[86].

In contrast, Giles et al. studied 11 pregnancies with TTS; these were identified on the basis of like sex, monochorionic placentation, and hemoglobin differences of >5.0 g/l at delivery. They showed that the umbilical artery S/D ratios were concordant even in the presence of discordant fetal size[87]. Interestingly, Fusi et al. suggested that acute TTS, rather than disseminated intravascular coagulation, might be the mechanism for brain-damaged survivors after intrauterine death of an MC twin[88].

References

1. Editorial (1986). Antepartum obstetrical ultrasound examination guidelines. *J. Ultrasound Med.*, **5**, 241
2. Goldstein, I., Zimmer, E.A., Tamir, A. et al. (1991). Evaluation of normal gestational sac growth: appearance of embryonic heart beat and embryo body movements using the transvaginal technique. *Obstet. Gynecol.*, **77**, 885
3. Warren, W.B., Timor-Trisch, I., Peisner, D.B. et al. (1989). Dating the early pregnancy by sequential appearance of embryonic structures. *Am. J. Obstet. Gynecol.*, **161**, 747
4. Goldstein, S.R. (1991). Embryonic ultrasonographic measurements: crown–rump length revisited. *Am. J. Obstet. Gynecol.*, **165**, 497
5. Jeanty, P., Cantraine, F., Cousaert, E. et al. (1984). The binocular distance: a new way to estimate fetal age. *J. Ultrasound Med.*, **3**, 241
6. Abramowicz, J.S., Sherer, D.M., Bar-Tov, E. et al. (1991). The cheek-to-cheek diameter in the ultrasonographic assessment of fetal growth. *Am. J. Obstet. Gynecol.*, **165**, 846
7. Mercer, B.M., Sklar, S., Shariatmadar, A. et al. (1987). Fetal foot length as a predictor of gestational age. *Am. J. Obstet. Gynecol.*, **156**, 350
8. Lee, W., Barton, S., Comstock, C.H. et al. (1991). Transverse cerebellar diameter: a useful predictor of gestational age for fetuses with asymmetric growth retardation. *Am. J. Obstet. Gynecol.*, **165**, 1044
9. Apuzzio, J.J., Adhate, A., Ganesh, V. et al. (1992). Prenatal ultrasonographic fetal iliac bone measurement correlation with gestational age. *J. Reprod. Med.*, **37**, 348
10. MacGregor, S.N., Tamura, R.K., Sabbagha, R.E. et al. (1987). Underestimation of gestational age by conventional crown–rump length dating curves. *Obstet. Gynecol.*, **70**, 344
11. Daya, S. (1993). Accuracy of gestational age estimation using fetal crown–rump length measurements. *Am. J. Obstet. Gynecol.*, **168**,, 903
12. Hadlock, F.P., Harrist, R.B., Deter, R.L. et al. (1983). A prospective evaluation of fetal femur length as a predictor of gestational age. *J. Ultrasound Med.*, **2**, 111
13. Jeanty, P., Rodesch, F., Delbeke, D. et al. (1984). Estimation of gestational age from measurements of fetal long bones. *J. Ultrasound Med.*, **3**, 75
14. Hadlock, F.P., Harrist, R.B., Martinez-Poyer, J. et al. (1991). How accurate is second trimester fetal dating. *J. Ultrasound Med.*, **10**, 557
15. Sabbagha, R.E. and Hughey, M. (1978). Standardization of sonar cephalometry and gestational age. *Obstet. Gynecol.*, **52**, 402
16. Townsend, R.R., Simpson, G.F. and Filly, R.A. (1988). Membrane thickness in ultrasound prediction of chorionicity of twin gestations. *J. Ultrasound Med.*, **7**, 326
17. D'Alton, M.E. and Dudley, D.K. (1989). The ultrasonographic prediction of chorionicity in twin gestation. *Am. J. Obstet. Gynecol.*, **160**, 557
18. Barss, V.A., Benacerraf, B.R. and Frigoletto, D. (1985). Ultrasonographic determination of chorion type in twin gestation. *Obstet. Gynecol.*, **66**, 779
19. Watson, W.J., Katz, V.L., Albright, S.G. et al. (1990). Monozygotic twins discordant for partial trisomy 1. *Obstet. Gynecol.*, **76**, 949

20. Elliott, J.P., Urig, M.A. and Clewell, W.H. (1991). Aggressive therapeutic amniocentesis for treatment of twin–twin transfusion syndrome. *Obstet. Gynecol.*, **77**, 537
21. Tessen, J.A. and Zlatnik, F.J. (1991). Monoamniotic twins: a retrospective controlled study. *Obstet. Gynecol.*, **77**, 832
22. Finberg H.J. and Clewell, W.H. (1991). Definitive prenatal diagnosis of monoamniotic twins. Swallowed amniotic contrast agent detected in both twins on sonographically selected CT images. *J. Ultrasound Med.*, **10**, 513
23. Bejar R., Vigliocco G., Gramajo, H. *et al.* (1990). Antenatal origin of neurologic damage in newborn infants II. Multiple gestations. *Am. J. Obstet. Gynecol.*, **162**, 1230
24. Ash, K., Harman, C.R. and Gritter, H. (1990). TRAP sequence – successful outcome with indomethacin treatment. *Obstet. Gynecol.*, **76**, 960
25. Pretorius, D.H., Leopold, G.R., Moore, T.R. *et al.* (1988). Acardiac twin. Report of Doppler sonography. *J. Ultrasound Med.*, **7**, 413
26. De Lia, J.E., Cruikshank, D.P. and Keye, W.R., Jr (1990). Fetoscopic neodymium:YAG laser occlusion of placental vessels in severe twin–twin transfusion syndrome. *Obstet. Gynecol.*, **75**, 1046
27. Mahoney, B.S., Petty, C.N., Nyberg, D.A. *et al.* (1990). The 'stuck twin' phenomenon: ultrasonographic findings, pregnancy outcome, and management with serial amniocenteses. *Am. J. Obstet. Gynecol.*, **163**, 151
28. Landy, H.J., Weiner, S., Corson S.L. *et al.* (1986). The 'vanishing twin': ultrasonographic assessment of fetal disappearance in the first trimester. *Am. J. Obstet. Gynecol.*, **155**, 14
29. May, D.A. and Sturtevant, N.V. (1991). Embryonal heart rate as a predictor of pregnancy outcome: a prospective analysis. *J. Ultrasound Med.*, **10**, 593
30. Reece, A.E., Yarkoni, S., Abdalla, M. *et al.* (1991). A prospective longitudinal study of growth in twin gestations compared with growth in singleton pregnancies I. The fetal head. *J. Ultrasound Med.*, **19**, 439
31. Reece, A.E., Yarkoni, S., Abdalla, M. *et al.* (1991). A prospective longitudinal study of growth in twin gestations compared with growth in singleton pregnancies II. The fetal limbs. *J. Ultrasound Med.*, **10**, 445
32. Socol, M.L., Tamura, R.K., Sabbagha, R.E. *et al.* (1984). Diminished biparietal diameter and abdominal circumference growth in twins. *Obstet. Gynecol.*, **64**, 235
33. Brown, C.E., Guzick, D.S., Leveno, K.G. *et al.* (1987). Prediction of discordant twins using ultrasound measurement of biparietal diameter and abdominal perimeter. *Obstet. Gynecol.*, **70**, 677
34. Leroy, B., Lefort, F., Neveu, P. *et al.* (1982). Intrauterine growth charts for twin fetuses. *Acta Genet. Med. Gemellol.*, **31**, 199
35. Elster, A.D., Bleyl, J.L. and Craven, T.E. (1991). Birth weight standards for triplets under modern obstetric care in the United States, 1984–1989. *Obstet. Gynecol.*, **77**, 387
36. Hadlock, F.P., Harrist, R.B., Sharman, R.S. *et al.* (1975). Estimation of fetal weight with the use of head, body, and femur measurements – a prospective study. *Am. J. Obstet. Gynecol.*, 151, 333
37. Sabbagha, R.E., Minogue, J., Tamura, R.K. *et al.* (1989). Estimation of birth weight by the use of ultrasound formulas targeted to large, appropriate, and small for gestational age fetuses. *Am. J. Obstet. Gynecol.*, **160**, 255
38. Blickstein, I. and Weissman, A. (1990). Macrosomic twinning: a study of growth-promoted twins. *Obstet. Gynecol.*, **76**, 822
39. Scorza, W.E., Nardi, D., Vintzileos, A.M. *et al.* (1991). The relationship between umbilical artery Doppler velocimetry and fetal biometry. *Am. J. Obstet. Gynecol.*, **165**, 1013
40. Divon, M.Y., Girz, B.A., Sklar, A. *et al.* (1989). Discordant twins: a prospective study of the diagnostic value of real time ultrasonography combined with umbilical artery velocimetry. *Am. J. Obstet. Gynecol.*, **161**, 757
41. Philipson, E.H., Sokol, R.J. and Williams, T. (1983). Oligohydramnios: clinical associations and predictive value for intrauterine growth retardation. *Am. J. Obstet. Gynecol.*, **6**, 271
42. Phelan, J.P., Platt, L.D., Yeh, S.Y. *et al.* (1985). The role of ultrasound assessment of amniotic fluid volume in the management of the postdate pregnancy. *Am. J. Obstet. Gynecol.*, **151**, 304
43. Phelan, J.P., Ahn, M.O., Smith, C.V. *et al.* (1987). Amniotic fluid index measurements during pregnancy. *J. Reprod. Med.*, **32**, 601
44. Rutherford, S.E., Phelan, J.P., Smith, C.V. *et al.* (1987). The four quadrant assessment of amniotic fluid volume: an adjunct to antepartum fetal heart rate testing. *Obstet. Gynecol.*, **70**, 353
45. Chamberlain, P.F., Manning, F.A., Morrison, I. *et al.* (1984). Ultrasound evaluation of am-

niotic fluid volume. *Am. J. Obstet. Gynecol.*, **150**, 245

46. Crowley, P., O'Herlihy, C. and Boylan, P. (1984). The value of ultrasound measurement of amniotic fluid volume in the management of prolonged pregnancies. *Br. J. Obstet. Gynaecol.*, **91**, 444
47. Bottoms, S.F., Welch, R.A., Zador, I.E. *et al.* (1986). Limitations of using maximum vertical pocket and other sonographic evaluations of amniotic fluid volume to predict fetal growth: technical or physiologic. *Am. J. Obstet. Gynecol.*, **155**, 154
48. Lavery, P.J. (1982). Nonstress fetal heart rate testing. *Clin. Obstet. Gynecol.*, **25**, 689
49. Silver, R.K., Dooley, S.L., Tamura, R.K. *et al.* (1987). Umbilical cord size and amniotic fluid volume in prolonged pregnancy. *Am. J. Obstet. Gynecol.*, **157**, 716
50. Smith, C.V., Phelan, J.P., Paul, R.H. *et al.* (1985). Fetal acoustic stimulation testing: a retrospective experience with the fetal acoustic stimulation test. *Am. J. Obstet. Gynecol.*, **153**, 567
51. Smith, C.V., Phelan, J.P., Platt, L.D. *et al.* (1986). Fetal acoustic stimulation testing II. A randomized clinical comparison with the nonstress test. *Am. J. Obstet. Gynecol.*, **155**, 131
52. Devoe, L.D., Murray, C., Faircloth, D. *et al.* (1990). Vibroacoustic stimulation and fetal behavioral state in normal term human pregnancy. *Am. J. Obstet. Gynecol.*, **163**, 1156
53. Kisilevsky, B.S., Muir, D.W. and Low, J.A. (1989). Human fetal responses to sound as a function of stimulus intensity. *Obstet. Gynecol.*, **73**, 971
54. Pietrantoni, M., Angel, J.L., Parsons, M.T. *et al.* (1991). Human fetal response to vibroacoustic stimulation as a function of stimulus duration. *Obstet. Gynecol.*, **78**, 807
55. Graham, E.M., Peters, A.J.M., Abrams, R.M. *et al.* (1991). Intraabdominal sound levels during vibroacoustic stimulation. *Am. J. Obstet. Gynecol.*, **164**, 1140
56. Nyman, M., Arulkumaran, S., Hsu, T.S. *et al.* (1991). Vibroacoustic stimulation and intrauterine sound pressure levels. *Obstet. Gynecol.*, **78**, 803
57. Bohne, B. and Clark, W. (1982). Growth of hearing loss and cochlear lesion with increasing duration of noise exposure. In Hamernik, R.P., Henderson, D. and Salvi, R. (eds.) *New Perspectives on Noise-induced Hearing Loss.* (New York: Raven Press)
58. Ohel, G., Horowitz, E., Linder, N. *et al.* (1987). Neonatal auditory acuity following *in utero* vibratory acoustic stimulation. *Am. J. Obstet. Gynecol.*, **157**, 440
59. Arulkumaran, S., Skurr, B., Tong, H. *et al.* (1991). No evidence of hearing loss due to fetal acoustic stimulation test. *Obstet. Gynecol.*, **78**, 283
60. Sherer, D.M., Nawrocki, M.N., Peco, N.E. *et al.* (1990). The occurrence of simultaneous fetal heart accelerations in twins during nonstress testing. *Obstet. Gynecol.*, **76**, 817
61. Sherer, D.M., Abramowicz, J.S., D'Amico, M.L. *et al.* (1991). Fetal vibratory acoustic stimulation in twin gestations with simultaneous fetal heart rate monitoring. *Am. J. Obstet. Gynecol.*, **164**, 1104
62. Vintzeleos, A.M., Gaffney, S.E., Salinger, L.M. *et al.* (1987). The relationship between fetal biophysical profile and cord pH in patients undergoing Cesarean section before the onset of labor. *Obstet. Gynecol.*, **70**, 196
63. Sassoon, D., Castro, L.C., Davis, J.L. *et al.* (1990). The biophysical profile in labor. *Obstet. Gynecol.*, **76**, 360
64. Manning, F.A., Morrison, I., Harman, C.R. *et al.* (1990). The abnormal fetal biophysical profile score V. Predictive accuracy according to score composition. *Am. J. Obstet. Gynecol.*, **162**, 918
65. Clark, S.L., Sabey, P. and Jolly, K.. (1989). Nonstress testing with acoustic stimulation and amniotic fluid volume assessment: 5973 tests without unexpected fetal death. *Am. J. Obstet. Gynecol.*, **160**, 694
66. Petrikovsky, B.M. and Baker, D.A. (1991). A new proposal for a fetal biophysical scoring system. *Am. J. Gynecol. Health*, **2**, 15
67. Maulik, D., Yarlagadda, P., Youngblood, J.P. *et al.* (1991). Comparative efficacy of umbilical arterial indices for predicting adverse perinatal outcome. *Am. J. Obstet. Gynecol.*, **164**, 1434
68. Vieyres, P., Durand, A., Patat, F. *et al.* (1991). Influence of the measurement location on the resistance index in the umbilical arteries: a hemodynamic approach. *J. Ultrasound Med.*, **10**, 671
69. Gerson, A., Johnson, A., Wallace, D. *et al.* (1998). Umbilical arterial systolic/diastolic values in normal twin gestation. *Obstet. Gynecol.*, **72**, 205
70. Giles, W.B., Trudinger, B., Cook, C. *et al.* (1988). Umbilical artery velocity waveforms

and twin pregnancy outcome. *Obstet. Gynecol.*, **72**, 894

71. Gaziano, E., Knox, E.G., Wager, G.P. *et al.* (1988). The predictability of the small for-gestational-age infant by real-time ultrasound-derived measurements combined with pulsed Doppler umbilical artery velocimetry. *Am. J. Obstet. Gynecol.*, **158**, 1431
72. Pattinson, R., Dawes, G., Jennings, J. *et al.* (1991). Umbilical artery resistance index as a screening test for fetal well-being I: prospective revealed evaluation. *Obstet. Gynecol.*, **78**, 353
73. Arduini, D., Rizzo, G. and Romanini, C. (1992). Changes of pulsatility index of fetal vessels preceding the onset of late decelerations in growth retarded fetuses. *Obstet. Gynecol.*, **79**, 605
74. Rochelson, B.L., Schulman, H., Fleischer, A. *et al.* (1987). The clinical significance of Doppler umbilical artery velocimetry in the small for gestational age fetus. *Am. J. Obstet. Gynecol.*, **156**, 1223
75. Brar, H.S., Platt, L.D. and Paul, R.H. (1989). Fetal umbilical blood flow velocity waveforms using Doppler ultrasonography in patients with late decelerations. *Obstet. Gynecol.*, **73**, 363
76. Gramellini, D., Folli, M.C., Raboni, S. *et al.* (1992). Cerebral–umbilical Doppler ratio as a predictor of adverse perinatal outcome. *Obstet. Gynecol.*, **79**, 416
77. Mari, G. and Deter, R.L. (1992). Middle cerebral artery flow velocity waveforms in normal and small-for-gestational-age fetuses. *Am. J. Obstet. Gynecol.*, **166**, 1262
78. Vyas, S., Nicolaides, K.H., Bower, S. *et al.* (1990). Middle cerebral artery velocity waveforms in fetal hypoxaemia. *Br. J. Obstet. Gynaecol.*, **97**, 707
79. Rochelson, B., Schulman, H., Farmakides, G. *et al.* (1987). The significance of absent end-diastolic velocity in umbilical artery velocity waveforms. *Am. J. Obstet. Gynecol.*, **156**, 1213
80. Brar, H.S. and Platt, L.D. (1988). Reverse end-diastolic flow velocity on umbilical artery velocimetry in high-risk pregnancies: an ominous finding with adverse pregnancy outcome. *Am. J. Obstet. Gynecol.*, **159**, 559
81. Wenstrom, K.D., Weiner, C.P. and Williamson, R.A. (1991). Diverse maternal and fetal pathology associated with absent end-diastolic flow in the umbilical artery of high risk fetuses. *Obstet. Gynecol.*, **77**, 374
82. Henretty, K.P., Whittle, M.J. and Rubin, P.C. (1988). Reappearance of end-diastolic velocity in a pregnancy complicated by severe pregnancy-induced hypertension. *Am. J. Obstet. Gynecol.*, **158**, 1123
83. Sengupta, S., Harrigan, J.T., Rosenberg, J.C. *et al.* (1991). Perinatal outcome following improvement of abnormal umbilical artery velocimetry. *Obstet. Gynecol.*, **78**, 1062
84. Saldana, L.R., Eads, M.C. and Schaefer, T.R. (1987). Umbilical blood waveforms in fetal surveillance of twins. *Am. J. Obstet. Gynecol.*, **157**, 712
85. Yamada, A., Kasugal, M., Ohno, Y. *et al.* (1991). Antenatal diagnosis of twin–twin transfusion syndrome by Doppler ultrasound. *Obstet. Gynecol.*, **78**, 1058
86. Pretorius, D.H., Manchester, D., Barkin, S. *et al.* (1988). Doppler ultrasound of twin transfusion syndrome. *J. Ultrasound Med.*, **7**, 117
87. Giles, W.B., Trudinger, B.J., Cook, C.M. *et al.* (1990). Doppler umbilical artery studies in the twin–twin transfusion syndrome. *Obstet. Gynecol.*, **76**, 1097
88. Fusi, L., McParland, P., Fisk, N. *et al.* (1991). Acute twin–twin transfusion: a possible mechanism for brain-damaged survivors after intrauterine death of a monochorionic twin. *Obstet. Gynecol.*, **78**, 517
89. Tamura, R.K. and Sabbagha, R.E. (1980). Percentile ranks of sonar fetal abdominal circumference. *Am. J. Obstet. Gynecol.*, **138**, 475
90. Sabbagha, R.E. (ed.) (1993). *Ultrasound Applied to Obstetrics and Gynecology*, 3rd edn., Chapter 36. (Philadelphia: J.B. Lippincott)
91. Shah, D.M. (1989). Diagnosis of trisomy 18 in monozygotic twins by cordocentesis. *Am. J. Obstet. Gynecol.*, **16**, 214

Diagnosis of fetal congenital anomalies by ultrasonography

17

R.E. Sabbagha

Introduction

Ultrasonography is currently the principal method for detection of fetal congenital anomalies. The recent development of high resolution machines equipped with curvilinear and multifocal transducers has further enhanced the utility of this modality. Despite this, ultrasonography is still dependent on the skill of the sonographer in targeting and obtaining detailed fetal anatomic views of normal or abnormal structures.

The term used to describe the detailed ultrasound study required for the diagnosis of congenital anomalies is targeted imaging for fetal anomalies (TIFFA)[1]. Just as in singleton pregnancies, TIFFA studies in twin gestations are based on one of the following indications:

(1) Low level of maternal serum alpha-fetoprotein (MSAFP) or amniotic fluid alpha-fetoprotein AFAFP);
(2) Abnormalities of amniotic fluid volume – polyhydramnios or oligohydramnios;
(3) History of a previous defect;
(4) Maternal diabetes mellitus;
(5) Intrauterine growth retardation (IUGR);
(6) Breech presentation at term;
(7) Suspicion of an anomaly on a standard obstetric study;
(8) Exposure to a teratogenic agent; and
(9) Abnormal Doppler velocimetry in the form of absent end-diastolic velocity (AEDV).

At least 37 specific views and measurements of the fetus are targeted and photographed in a TIFFA study (Figure 1). For good record keeping, a comment should be made for each of these views indicating whether the image appears to be normal, abnormal, or is simply poorly visualized (Figure 1). This latter situation occurs in women with a large body habitus or when fetal position or movement make it impossible to image the area in question.

In twins, a TIFFA study requires 1.5–2 h for completion and documentation, or approximately double the time allotted for a singleton pregnancy. The finding of any abnormality further extends the time of the examination.

Anomalies of the central nervous system (CNS)

The frequency of central nervous system anomalies is approximately 2:1000 newborns, but varies according to geographic area and race. The recurrence risk is approximately 1–2%. The major CNS anomalies that can be detected by ultrasonograph include:

(1) Anencephaly/exencephaly;
(2) Microcephaly;
(3) Meningocele and encephalocele;
(4) Hydrocephalus;
(5) Choroid plexus cysts;
(6) Other intracranial abnormalities;

Detailed Study of Fetal Anatomy

CENTRAL NERVOUS SYSTEM		CARDIO-PULMONARY		G.U. & G.I.	
Cranium	:Normal	4 Chamber View	:Normal	Diaphragm	:Normal
Lateral Ventricles	:Normal	Short Axis	:Normal	Stomach (left)	:Normal
Third Ventricle	:Normal	Long Axis	:Normal	Bowel Pattern	:Normal
Thalami	:Normal	Great Vessel View	:Normal	ABD Wall/Cord Inst	:Normal
Posterior Fossa	:Normal	Aortic Arch	:Poor Visualization	Kidneys	:Suspect
Spine – Neck	:Normal	Pericardial Area	:Normal	Bladder	:Normal
Spine – Thoracic	:Normal	Pulmonary Area	:Normal	Ureters	:Suspect
Spine – Lumbosacral	:Normal			Genitalia	:Normal

EXTERNAL BODY DEFECTS		SPECIFIC FETAL MEASUREMENTS		OTHER AREAS	
Skeletal dysplasia	:None Noted	V/H Ratio	:19.3%	# Cord Vessesls: 3	
Cystic Hygroma	:None Noted	Cerebellum	:3.3 cm 25–50%ile	Maternal Pelvis: Vis. Prev.: No	
Hydrops	:None Noted	Binocular Distance	:4.7 cm 10–90%ile		
Tumors	:None Noted	Nuchal Occip. Thickness	:Vis. Prev.: Normal	PREGNANCY HISTORY	
Face	:None Noted	Thoracic circumference	:N/A	G: 1 P: 0 A:	
		Right Kidney Circumference	:N/A	Amnio	:
		Left Kidney Circumference	:N/A	CVS	:

COMMENTS: OF THE ANOMALIES THAT MAY BE VISUALIZED, THE FOLLOWING IS/ARE NOTED:
Bilateral pelviectasis is still seen (L = 3.5 mm, R = 6 mm). The amniotic fluid index = 22.4 cm which is consistent with a high normal level.
The previously noted anterior myoma-like echo remains unchanged.

Figure 1 Computer generated form describing the anatomic views and the fetal measurements obtained in a detailed targeted scan. Note that bilateral pelviectasis or pyelectasis is observed and reported

(7) Agenesis of the corpus callosum;

(8) Abnormalities of the posterior fossa; and

(9) Spina bifida.

Anencephalus/exencephalus/iniencephalus

In anencephalus the cerebral hemispheres and overlying skull and scalp are absent. This diagnosis can now be made by 12 weeks' gestation, particularly if a high-frequency vaginal ultrasound probe is used[2]. In women who have previously delivered an infant with anencephalus, screening for the abnormality may begin in the first trimester of pregnancy.

In exencephalus (acrania), the cranial bones are absent, but a large amount of disorganized brain tissue is seen overlying the surface of the head. This diagnosis can be made as early as the late part of the first trimester of pregnancy[3].

In iniencephaly, the skull defect occurs in the area of the occiput (inien). The fetal head is dorsiflexed and the spine is deformed and short. A number of other anomalies complicate this condition, including cyclopia, facial cleft, arthrogryposis and clubfoot[4].

Microcephalus

The distinctive features of microcephalus include: (1) head circumference (HC) $\leq 3\,SD$ below the mean for dates[5,6]; and (2) reduction in the size of the frontal aspect of the fetal head. Thus, sonographic measurement of the frontal lobe (frontal horn size + distance to inner aspect of skull) may be a helpful tool in the diagnosis of microcephalus. The normal frontal lobe measurement in the pregnancy interval of 17–20 weeks is 1.6–1.7 cm $(2\,SD = \pm 0.2\,cm)$[7].

When a positive family history of microcephalus is present, serial ultrasonic studies beginning as early as 16 weeks' gestation showing an HC around the 50th rather than the 5–10th percentile ranks are reassuring.

Table 1 Ultrasonic characteristics and differential diagnosis of fetal cranial and craniocervical masses with no apparent defect in the neural tube

Differential diagnosis	Ultrasonic characteristics of mass			
	Outer margin	Size and shape	Concomitant motion with fetal head	Other possible findings
Meningocele	thin*	variable	yes	bone defect
Fetal edema	thick	uniform, semicircular, simulates contour of fetal head and neck	yes	ascites
Intrauterine fetal death	thick	uniform, semicircular	—	collapse of sutures
Cystic hygroma	thick†	uniform, circular or near circular; sometimes bilateral with multiple septations circular or oblong	yes	pleural or cardiac effusion, or both
Teratoma		variable	yes	clumps of echogenic material

*<3 mm; †thickness of margin (3–5 mm) may not be apparent until 18 to 20 week's gestation. From reference 8, with permission

The etiology of microcephalus is variable, including: (1) syndromes, such as those of Meckel–Gruber, Roberts, Seckel and Bloom; (2) chromosomal abnormalities, such as trisomy 13 and 18 and Del (4p), (13q), (18 p); and (3) exposure to environmental agents, such as alcohol, aminopterin, hydantoin, infections such as rubella and conditions such as maternal phenylketonuria. The differential diagnosis includes severe intrauterine growth retardation.

Meningocele/encephalocele

In cranial or spinal meningocele, the meninges protrude through a bony defect in the skull. Occipital meningoceles are the most common form of the defect. In encephaloceles brain tissue is present within the meningocele. The differential diagnosis of cranial meningocele is that of cranial and craniocervical masses, including cystic hygroma, fetal edema, intrauterine fetal death, and teratoma (Table 1)[8].

Hydrocephalus

The flow of cerebrospinal fluid (CSF) progresses as follows: lateral ventricles → foramen of Monro → 3rd ventricle → aqueduct of Sylvius → 4th ventricle → foramina Luschka and Magendie → cisterns.

In aqueductal stenosis, the 3rd ventricle (situated proximally) is enlarged, a finding that is detectable by ultrasonography. The etiology of aqueductal stenosis includes: (1) recessive inheritance; (2) X-linked inheritance; and (3) infection with cytomegalovirus or toxoplasmosis. Calcification may also be noted by ultrasound in fetuses with hydrocephalus secondary to infection[8].

Atretic foramina Luschka and Magendie may occur in the Dandy–Walker malformation, but in such cases the clue to the diagnosis would be the posterior fossa cyst (Figure 2).

Abnormalities of the subarachnoid space as in the Arnold–Chiari II syndrome also result in hydrocephalus; however, this condition is associated with spina bifida, an abnormal cerebellum (see banana sign), dilatation of all

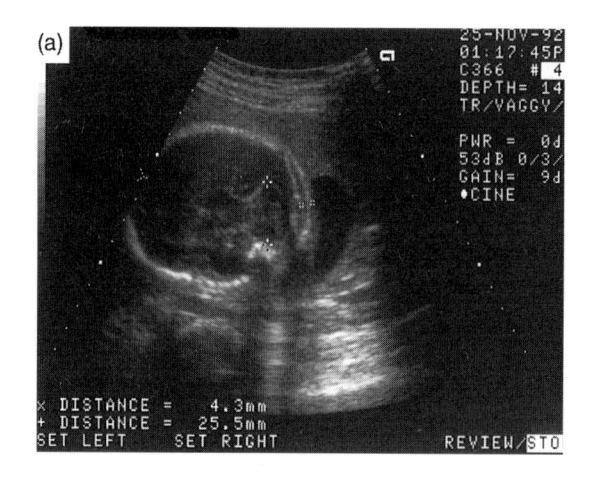

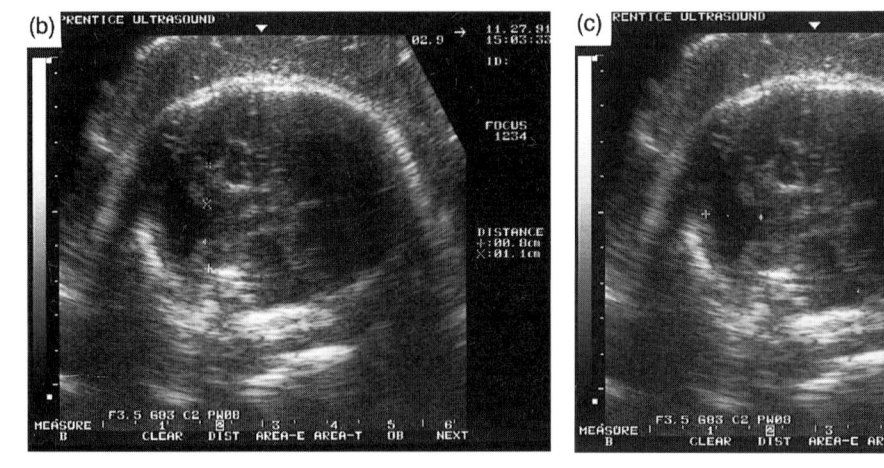

Figure 2 (a) Scan of fetal head, showing the normal appearance of the cerebellar bodies (+ signs). Note how the cerebellar bodies are well apposed. The thin dark area to the right of the cerebellar bodies is the cisterna magna, which appears normal (< 10 mm). The nuchal occipital fold is measured in this plane (rectangular signs) and is normal or < 6 mm. (b) Scan of fetus with Dandy–Walker malformation, showing hypoplastic cerebellar bodies (× and + signs) that are widely separated by the posterior fossa cyst. Arachnoid cysts are not known to separate the cerebellar bodies. (c) Same fetus as in (b), showing abnormal dilatation of the area of the cisterna magna. This dilatation is attributed to absence of the cerebellar vermis and protrusion of the 4th ventricle into the area of the cisterna magna. See text for differential diagnosis of enlarged posterior fossa

ventricles, and forward scalloping of the brain (lemon sign) (see spina bifida). Other causes of abnormalities of the subarachnoid space include cerebral infection[9], achondroplasia and Hurler syndrome.

Hydrocephalus occurs as an isolated finding in approximately 15% of such cases. Thus, in the majority of affected fetuses a variety of other conditions are associated with hydrocephalus. These may involve the skeletal, cardiac, renal and central nervous systems. Fetal karyotype is also abnormal in approximately 25% of cases. Other specific associated conditions include: (1) Apert and Roberts syndromes; (2) osteogenesis imperfecta; (3) thanatophoric dwarfism; (4) trisomy 13, 18, 21; (5) triploidy; (6) aneurysm of the vein of Galen[10]; and (7) papilloma of the choroid plexus – the last resulting in overproduction of CSF.

Diagnosis of fetal anomalies by ultrasonography

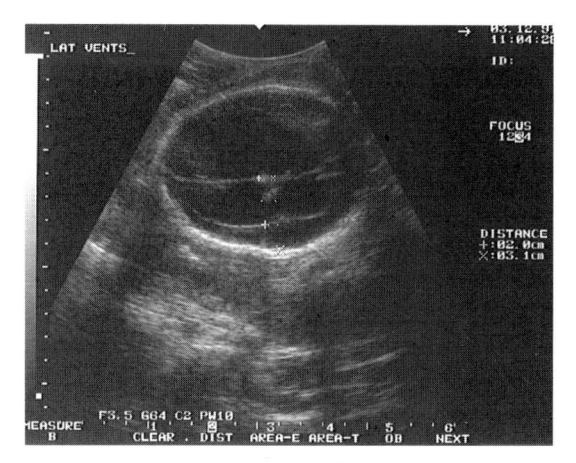

Figure 3 Scan of fetus with hydrocephalus. Note dilatation of the distal ventricle and a small compressed choroid plexus just beneath the midline echo. The size of the ventricle is measured between the + signs. The hemispheric size is measured from the midline echo to the inner aspect of the skull echo-complex (× signs). The ventricular:hemispheric ratio in this case was 66% and was abnormal, indicating ventriculomegaly (see text)

Hydrocephalic fetuses should not be delivered prior to the fetus having attained pulmonary maturity, because correlation between compression of the cerebral cortex and degree of mental retardation is poor. On the other hand, the size of the fetal head should dictate the route of delivery, i.e. vaginal or abdominal. In fetuses with a favorable prognosis, vaginal delivery may not be advisable when: (1) the HC at term is ≥ 90th percentile; or (2) a spina bifida is present (see spina bifida). In contrast, when hydrocephalus is associated with conditions incompatible with life, such as renal agenesis, thanatophoric dwarfism or trisomy 18, then cephalocentesis (a potentially lethal procedure) may be used to facilitate delivery.

In contrast to ventriculomegaly, hydrocephalus is frequently progressive, and compression of the choroid plexus may be noted. The ventricular/hemispheric ratio is used to assess progression of hydrocephalus (Figure 3)[11]. The size of the atrium of the lateral ventricle can also be used to diagnose hydrocephalus (Figure 4)[12,13].

Choroid plexus cyst

The discovery of small cystic areas within the choroid plexus during the second trimester of pregnancy (Figure 5) has become a cause for concern. The reason is related to the 1–2% association between choroid plexus cysts and chromosomal abnormalities[14]. Although these cysts occur in only 1:1000 pregnancies, affected women should be offered amniocentesis for fetal karyotype, because trisomy 18 and 21 have both been reported with this condition[15–18]. The karyotype of affected fetuses who reach the 24th week of pregnancy may be mapped using

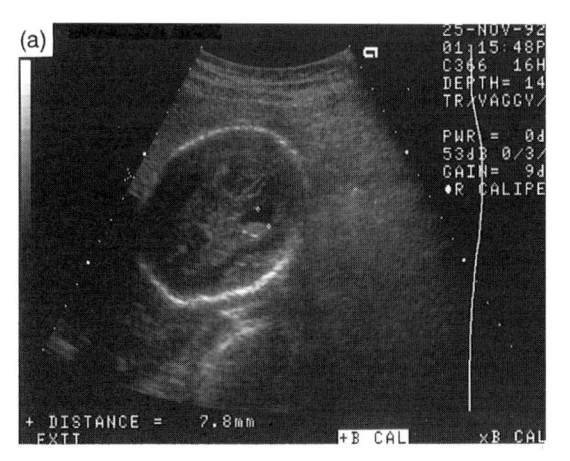

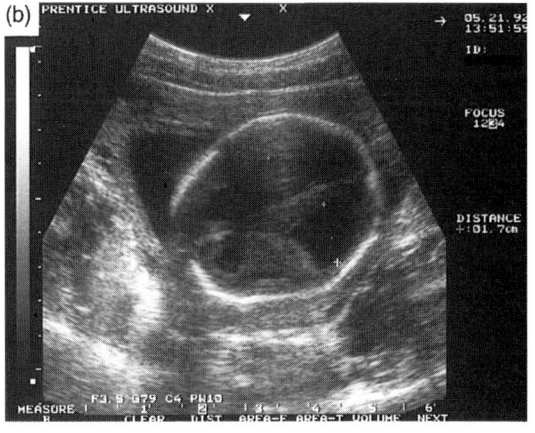

Figure 4 (a) Scan of fetal head, showing normal lateral ventricles at the level of the ventricular atrium (+ signs), adjacent to the choroid plexus. The atrium measured 7.8 mm and was normal. (b) Scan of fetus with hydrocephalus. Note marked dilatation of the ventricular atrium (+ signs). The atrium was more dilated than the remaining ventricle, an abnormality also consistent with agenesis of the corpus callosum

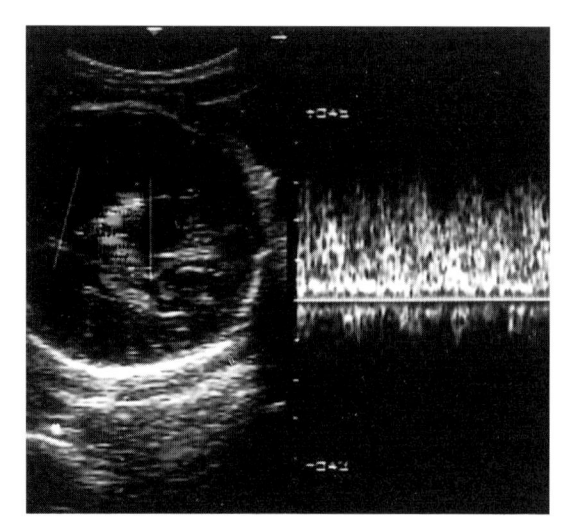

Figure 5 Scan of fetal head with a central cystic area that could not be differentiated from an arachnoid cyst or a porencephalic cyst. However, its location near the cerebral ventricle and the fact that blood vessels were noted to traverse the mass (red and blue coded vessels) led to the diagnosis of dilated vein of Galen

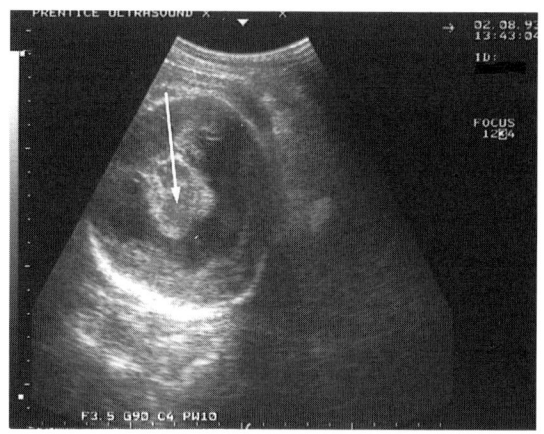

Figure 6 Cerebral scan in a fetus with trisomy 13 and holoprosencephaly. Note that the base of the brain (arrow) is surrounded by a single ventricle (dark area). The adjacent cerebral tissue is disorganized and thinned out

placental biopsy or percutaneous umbilical blood sampling (PUBS).

The risk for chromosomal abnormalities decreases if the cysts are either < 1 cm in size or decrease in size with serial scanning. However, recently this possibility has been challenged in two publications[15–17]. When a choroid plexus cyst is associated with other anomalies, the likelihood of a chromosomal abnormality increases[14].

However, recent data indicate that risk of aneuploidy is 1:25 even with isolated choroid plexus cyst[19].

Other cranial abnormalities

A number of relatively rare cranial abnormalities may be differentiated from hydrocephalus. The first is the alobar form of holoprosencephaly, a condition where the cerebral hemispheres fail to separate, resulting in a single ventricle (Figure 6). Hypotelorism is characteristic of the abnormality and can be diagnosed by a short orbital distance. Other varieties of holoprosencephaly include the semilobar and lobar forms both representing a slightly greater degree of brain development. Fetal karyotype is abnormal in 50% of fetuses with holoprosencephaly and trisomy 13 is the most frequent abnormality.

The second rare cranial abnormality is hydranencephaly in which the cerebral hemispheres are completely atrophic and thus not visualized. This condition results from early bilateral vascular thrombosis of the carotid arteries. The cerebellum, midbrain and basal ganglia are seen in the lower aspect of the cranium surrounded by a fluid interface.

The third is porencephaly, a localized condition of brain atrophy secondary to vascular accident. Differentiation from arachnoid cyst may be difficult.

The fourth is aneurysm of the vein of Galen[10]. The two veins of Galen drain the choroid plexuses of the lateral and 3rd ventricles. Subsequently they unite into a single vein – the great vein of Galen. This joins the straight sinus at the junction of the falx cerebri and tentorium.

Dilatation of the vein of Galen results from an arteriovenous malformation in which one or more arterioles feed the vein of Galen and distend it. The distension may result in hydrocephalus and the condition may lead to high output cardiac failure. The dilated vein of Galen resembles a porencephalic or arachnoid cyst. However, the diagnosis can be readily made by color Doppler velocimetry (Figure 5).

The fifth is an arachnoid cyst. Such cysts can be of variable size and location and should be considered in the differential diagnosis of any of the above conditions.

Agenesis of the corpus callosum (ACC)

The corpus callosum is a bundle of fibers interconnecting the cortical hemispheres. The corpus callosum forms the roof of the cavum septi pellucidi and the third ventricle. It develops first rostrally and then caudally, completely forming by approximately 18–20 weeks' gestation[20,21]. Diagnosis prior to this gestational interval is not possible. Moreover, in most cases, the diagnosis remains indirect, because a coronal cut of the fetal head is difficult to obtain. Secondary abnormalities that can be visualized in a transverse plane of a fetus include:

(1) Dilated ventricular atrium, an abnormality that may be the first clue of complete or partial ACC (Figure 4)[22]. Frequently, a disproportionate increase in the size of the occipital horns is also noted[22].

(2) Lateral displacement of the bodies of the lateral ventricle, particularly the frontal horns. This results in marked approximation of the walls of the frontal horns and, in conjunction with the dilated atria, produces a 'teardrop' ultrasonic image[23].

(3) Enlargement and upward displacement of the 3rd ventricle. In this situation, the 3rd and lateral ventricles are seen in the same plane. A similar image is produced in some fetuses with Dandy–Walker malformation, but in such cases the posterior fossa abnormality leads to the correct diagnosis (Figure 2).

Interestingly, the enlargement of the 3rd ventricle in fetuses with ACC is variable, and if excessive results in the appearance of a midline interhemispheric cyst. The differential diagnosis of such a cyst would include arachnoid cyst and malformation of the vein of Galen (see below).

In partial ACC, the posterocaudal portion of the corpus callosum is absent. Embryologically, this is the last segment of the corpus callosum to develop. In such cases the cephalad displacement of the 3rd ventricle is not so evident and there is less displacement of the frontal horns of the lateral ventricles[22]. Instead, the atrium and posterior horns of the lateral ventricle are dilated (Figure 4).

Although some children with ACC may be normal, as many as 85% have additional CNS anomalies and up to 62% have extra-CNS malformations. Frequently, a seizure disorder or developmental delay brings attention to ACC as the etiologic factor[23].

The posterior fossa The posterior fossa houses the cerebellum and the cisterna magna (Figure 2). It is best imaged by angling the transducer 30° in relation to the axial plane. Normally, the cisterna magna measures 1–10 mm. Abnormal enlargement of the cisternal magna is seen in cases of trisomy 18, Dandy–Walker malformation, arachnoid cysts, and possibly in pregnant women infected with the human immunodeficiency virus[24–26]. These three entities can be differentiated by careful attention to detail, as illustrated in Figure 2[24–26].

Spina bifida

Spina bifida is visualized ultrasonographically as a splaying of the posterior ossification centers of the spine. The size of the defect may vary from tiny to one involving many segments of the spine (myeloschisis).

Occasionally, small spina bifidas located in the lumbosacral area are visualized by imaging the spine in a sagittal plane. In contrast, careful cross-sectional imaging is more likely to delineate a small lumbosacral spina bifida in the interval of 18–22 weeks' gestation (Figure 7). An Arnold–Chiari type II malformation exists in almost all cases of spina bifida. As a result, forward scalloping of the frontal aspect of the fetal head (lemon sign) and a banana shaped abnormal cerebellum (banana sign) are present (Figure 8). These signs should alert the sonographer to the possibility of a spina

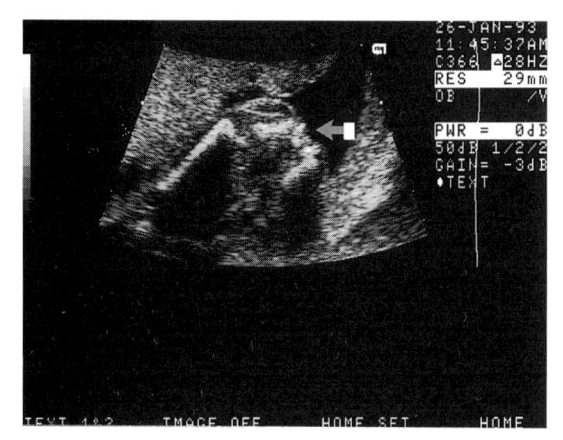

Figure 7 Cross sectional scan of sacrum at approximately 18 weeks' gestation. Note the U-shaped open spina bifida (arrow)

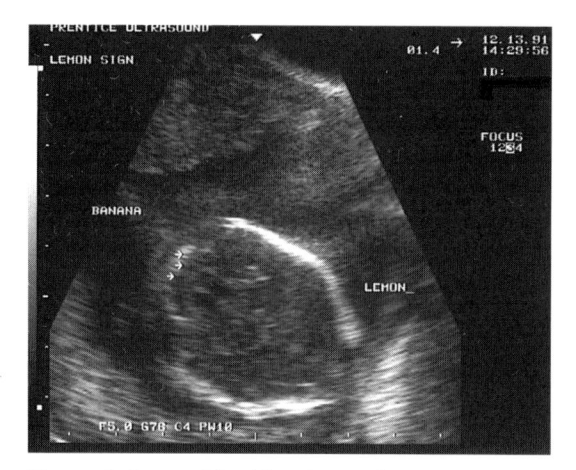

Figure 8 Scan of fetal head, showing angulation of the frontal bones (lemon sign) and a banana-shaped cerebellum (arrows). These findings are predictive of an associated spina bifida

bifida and lead to careful cross-sectional evaluation of the fetal spine[27].

The mode of delivery of the fetus with spina bifida remains controversial, because no controlled prospective studies address this subject. As a result, Cesarean section is still favored by many obstetricians, as no data exist to suggest that vaginal delivery does not adversely influence outcome. In fact, a recent retrospective study by Luthy *et al.* showed that the mean motor functional level of infants delivered by Cesarean section was at the 4th lumbar vertebra, whereas the mean functional level in those delivered vaginally was at the 2nd lumbar vertebra[28]. From a clinical point of view, this two-segment difference may translate into whether or not a child can walk[29].

Congenital heart disease (CHD)

The frequency of CHD is approximately 8:1000 newborns. However, epidemiological reviews which exclude patent ductus arteriosus suggest a lower prevalence of 3.7:1000 newborns[30,31]. The recurrence risk is 8–10%.

The etiology of CHD remains uncertain in 75% of cases. It is related to familial, chromosomal or environmental causes in the remaining 25% of affected newborns. Despite advances in diagnosis, as well as medical and surgical therapies, data from two recent studies suggest that the overall survival rate of fetuses with CHD is poor, ranging from 17 to 24%[32,33].

In evaluating the fetal heart, the sonographer should maintain the format of at least four cardiac images in mind. These include: (1) the four-chamber view (Figure 9); (2) the parasagittal view (Figure 10); (3) the short axis view (Figure 11); and (4) the great vessel view (Figure 12). In addition, the 'crisscross' of the pulmonary artery and aorta should be evaluated, because this view is essential for the possible diagnosis of transposition of the great arteries (Figure 13). An image of the aortic arch should also be obtained (Figure 14).

Importantly, the four-chamber view in and of itself may fail to demonstrate CHD in approximately 39–63% of cases[34,35], and multiple cardiac views remain crucial for the detection of cardiac lesions. The data reported by Copel *et al.* suggesting a 92% sensitivity of the four-chamber view in detecting cardiac abnormalities may have resulted from the nature of their patient population, namely referrals of patients whose fetuses were found to have abnormal four-chamber views on 'standard ultrasound' studies[36].

Sharland and Allan obtained the dimensions of the ventricles in the four-chamber projection at the end of diastole when the atrioventricular valves are closed[37]. They also

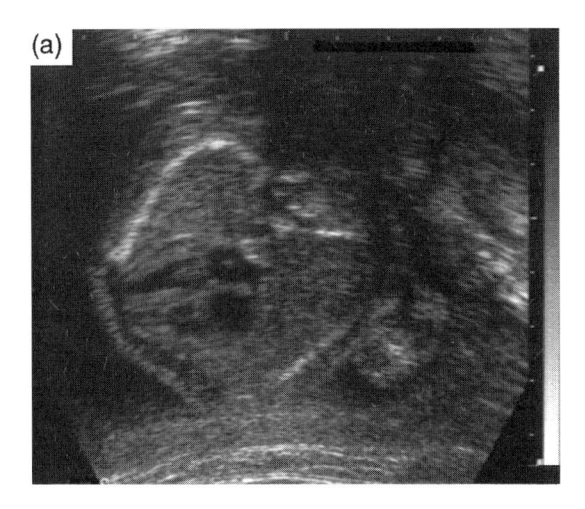

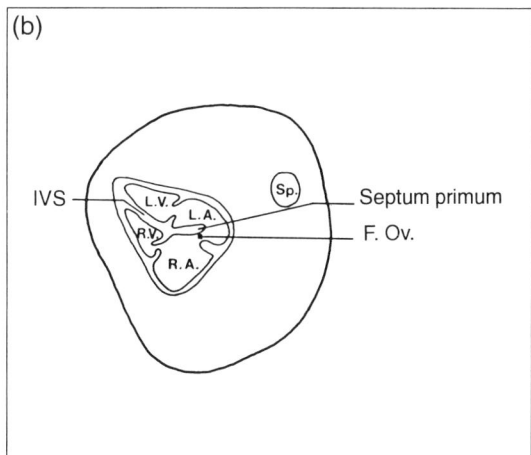

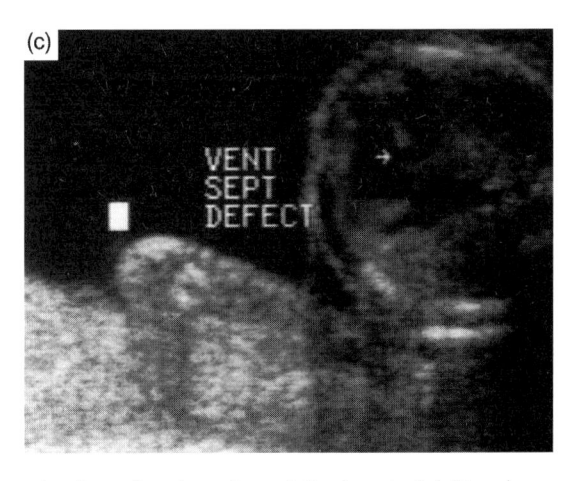

Diagnosis of fetal anomalies by ultrasonography

Figure 9 (a) Scan showing the four-chamber view of the heart. (b) Drawing corresponding to (a). Note equality in the size of the ventricles and atria. The interventricular septum is intact. The left ventricle is closer to the fetal spine. The atrioventricular valves are normally inserted. The moderator band (echogenic area at the base of the right ventricle) is clearly seen. (c) Scan of fetal heart showing a large ventricular septal defect (arrow)

measured: (1) the mitral and tricuspid valve rings during diastole when the valves are open; and (2) the internal diameters of the aorta and pulmonary artery during diastole in the parasagittal and short axis planes, respectively. Their data showed that in early pregnancy the right and left ventricular measurement are equal. The outflow tracts are also near equal in size (Figures 12 and 13). In later pregnancy, however, the right-sided structures appear slightly larger than the left.

Comstock *et al.* showed that the pulmonary to aortic (PA:AO) ratio is independent of gestational age with a mean value of 1.09 (2 SD = 0.75–1.43) (Figures 12 and 13)[38].

A list of the cardiovascular malformations according to relative frequency is shown in Table 2. A discussion of the congenital heart lesions which may be diagnosed by a detailed study of all cardiac views follows.

Interventricular septum (IVS)

An IVS defect is the most frequent structural abnormality of the heart (Figure 9). The defect can either be isolated or associated with a

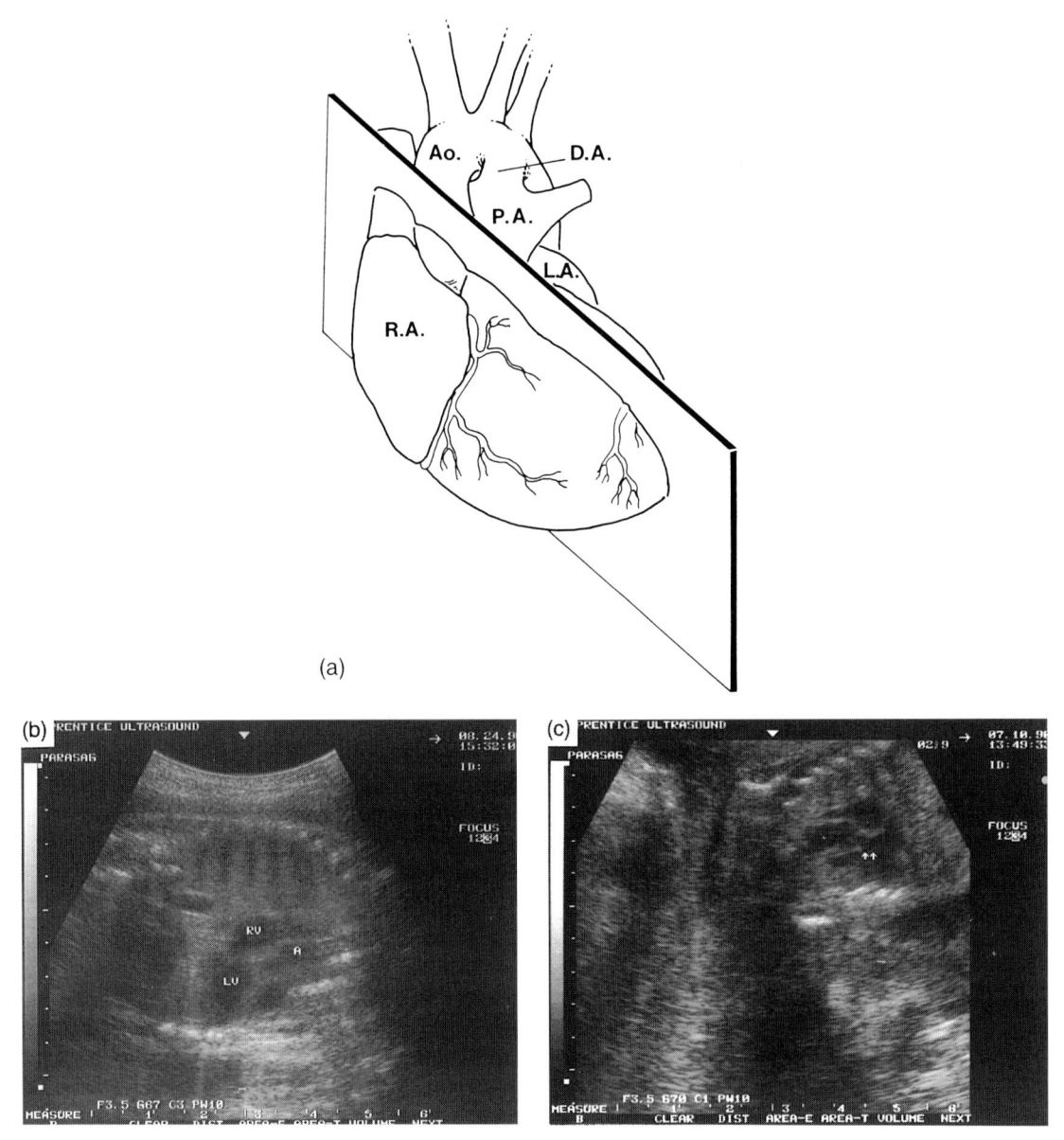

Figure 10 (a) Drawing to illustrate the plane used to obtain a parasagittal view of the heart. (b) Parasagittal view of the fetal heart, showing left ventricular outflow tract from left ventricle (LV) to aorta (A). Note the intact membranous portion of the interventricular septum at the base of the right ventricle (RV). (c) Parasagittal scan of fetus with tetralogy of Fallot. Note the enlarged over-riding aorta and membranous septal defect (arrows). The defect was not apparent on the four-chamber view. See text

variety of abnormalities, including: transposition of great arteries (TGA), tetralogy of Fallot, cushion defect, double outlet right ventricle, aneuploidies, renal anomalies and tracheoesophageal fistula.

Importantly, IVS defects are commonly located in the membranous part of the IVS, subaortically. Thus, small membranous IVS defects may not be visualized in the apical four-chamber view, because the plane of the scan is

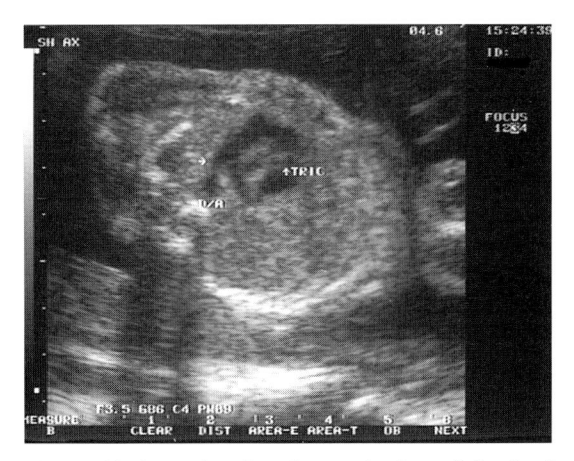

Diagnosis of fetal anomalies by ultrasonography

Figure 11 Scan showing short-axis view of the fetal heart. Note tricuspid valve on right side of circular aorta. To the left of the aorta is seen the ductus arteriosus (arrow and D/A) and the right branch of the pulmonary artery as it courses beneath the aorta

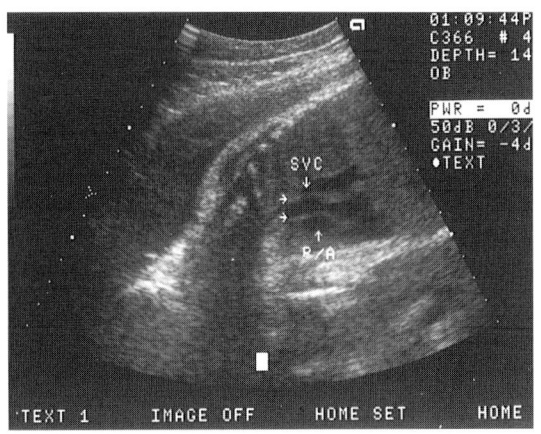

Figure 12 Scan showing the great vessel view. The superior vena cava (SVC) is shown by the top arrow. It overlies the aorta (double arrows) and the pulmonary artery (P/A). Note that the pulmonary and aortic dimensions are equal. See text for pulmonary/aortic ratio

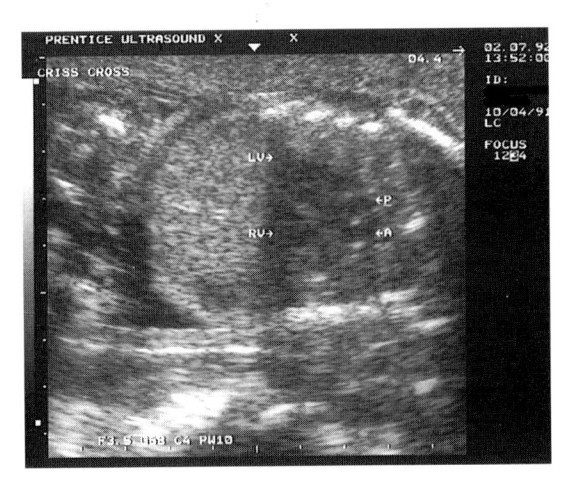

Figure 13 Scan to show the crossing of the great arteries ruling out transposition. The left ventricle (LV) leads to the aorta (A) and the right ventricle (RV) leads to the pulmonary artery (P). Again, the pulmonary (P) and aortic arteries (A) appear equal in size

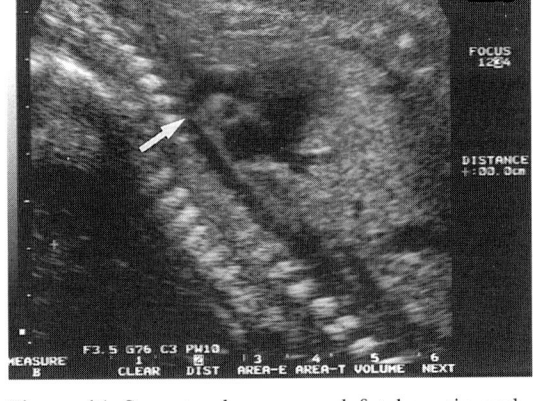

Figure 14 Scan to show normal fetal aortic arch. There is a normal degree of minimal constriction at the area of the ductal insertion (isthmus). See text

along the anterior aspect of the IVS. Such membranous IVS defects are best visualized in a parasagittal slice of the fetal heart showing the aortic outflow tract (Figure 10).

Infants with IVS defect are usually asymptomatic at birth, because the pressure in both ventricles is similar. For the same reason, color Doppler frequently fails to show any jet stream either way. In contrast, a left to right shunt occurs in the neonate because of increased systemic pressure and decreased pulmonary pressure. Interestingly, 25% and 65% of small membranous and muscular IVS defects close by 5 years of age[39].

Table 2 Congenital heart abnormalities possibly diagnosable by ultrasound. List shows relative frequency of the abnormality

Interventricular septal defect	(14%)
D-transposition of the great arteries	(13%)
Complex cardiac defect	(10%)*
Left ventricular hypoplasia	(9%)
Coarctation of the aorta	(9%)
Tetralogy of Fallot	(8%)
Right ventricular hypoplasia	(7%)
Pulmonary stenosis	(3%)
Endocardial cushion defect	(3%)
Cardiomyopathy	(2%)
Total anomalous pulmonary venous return	(2%)
Truncus arteriosus	(2%)
Aortic stenosis	(1%)
Ebstein anomaly	(<1%)
Arteriovenous malformation	(<0.5%)

Arrhythmia, cardiac tumors, idiopathic infantile arterial calcification, increased right ventricular dimensions in the post-term fetus, and patent ductus arteriosus are excluded, bringing the total to <100%.

*Group with complex cardiac defects including relative frequency are single ventricle (4%), dextrocardia (3%), asplenia/polysplenia (1.5%), double outlet right ventricle (1%), and L-transposition of great arteries (0.5%) Adapted from Rowe, R.D., Freedom, R.M., Mehirizi, A. and Bloom, K.R. (eds.) (1981). *The Neonate with Congenital Heart Disease*, 2nd edn., p. 106. (Philadelphia: W.B. Saunders)

Right ventricular hypoplasia

This abnormality comprises two entities: (1) hypoplastic right heart + pulmonary atresia with an intact IVS; and (2) hypoplastic right heart + tricuspid atresia + defects of the IVS + atrial septum. In 30% of cases, transposition of the great vessels is also noted[40]. Both conditions can be diagnosed by multiple cardiac views.

Left ventricular hypoplasia

This defects ranks fourth in relative frequency and can be detected on the four-chamber and aortic outflow tract views, because the left ventricle, mitral valve, aortic valve and aorta are underdeveloped. The isthmic portion of the aortic arch can also be small, because diminished left ventricular output results in decreased blood flow through the aortic isthmus, thus restricting its growth and size[41]. Approximately 40% of such fetuses will have associated extracardiac or karyotype abnormalities[42].

From a pathophysiological point of view, the right ventricle supplies all the blood to the systemic circulation via the ductus arteriosus. As a result, neonatal survival is ductus-dependent. Prenatal diagnosis allows for immediate administration of prostaglandin E_1 infusion to maintain ductal flow and prevent hypoxia with ensuing acidosis and death.

Prenatal counselling is quite important. Ethical issues include: (1) respect for parental autonomy; (2) promotion of the infant's welfare; and (3) fairness in distributing scarce medical resources such as cardiac transplants[43], which may result in survival rates of 70%[44].

Coarctation of the aorta

Coarctation is most frequently seen in the juxtaductal portion of the aortic arch. Unfortunately, in the term fetus the diameter of the aortic isthmus is normally smaller than that of the aorta, thus making the prenatal diagnosis of coarctation difficult (Figure 14). In the normal neonate, ductal closure is followed by isthmic enlargement unless extensive smooth muscle proliferation and coarctation are present.

Another condition resulting in coarctation is the *in utero* underdevelopment of the left outflow tract. Decreased flow through the aorta results in hypoplasia. Coarctation has also been reported in fetuses in which the left ventricle is only slightly smaller than the right[41]. Importantly, fetal karyotype should be assessed in suspected cases because there is an association with trisomy 9 and Turner syndrome. Interventricular septal defect, subaortic obstruction, atrial septal defect, malposition of great arteries and mitral valve abnormalities occur with coarctation of the aorta and should be carefully looked for during the ultrasound study.

Tetralogy of Fallot

This condition is characterized by four abnormalities of varying severity: subaortic (membranous) IVS defect, over-riding aorta, varying degrees of underdevelopment in the subpulmonary conus, and right ventricular enlargement. In mild cases the membranous IVS defect may not be seen, even in the parasagittal plane, and the condition may be totally missed by a scan at 18–20 weeks' gestation (Figure 10). In more severe cases, the aortic root is dilated and its large size relative to that of the pulmonary artery is a marker for tetralogy of Fallot (Figure 10)[45]. The development of extracorporeal circulation has led to correction of the primary anatomic defects with a survival rate of 85%.

Transposition of the great arteries (TGA)

Two types of transposition have been reported. In *l*-transposition, the moderator band is seen on the left side of the heart (transposed right ventricle) (Figure 9). The condition is asymptomatic, unless associations such as IVS defect or Ebstein-like tricuspid valve co-exist.

In *d*-transposition, the right ventricle gives rise to the aorta and the left ventricle to the pulmonary artery. The normal crossing of the great vessels is lost (Figure 13). In most cases the aorta is anterior and to the right of the pulmonary artery. Pulmonary stenosis is likely to occur, regardless of whether the IVS is intact or not. Abnormalities of the mitral or tricuspid valves, with varying degrees of right or left ventricular under-development, occur.

Truncus arteriosus

This condition is characterized by the presence of a single arterial vessel arising from the base of the heart and giving rise to the systemic, pulmonary and coronary vessels. It is usually associated with an IVS defect. In truncus arteriosus, a single arterial vessel over-rides the ventricular septum, a finding similar to that of tetralogy of Fallot with pulmonary atresia. However, the two conditions differ in that with truncus arteriosus the pulmonary artery originates from the truncus. An increased number of leaflets (2–6) is also noted in the latter, but the vessel usually remains incompetent, leading to right ventricular overload after birth. Most infants die of congestive heart failure in the first year of life. However, the use of a conduit connecting the right ventricle to the pulmonary artery prior to 6 months of age has improved the survival rate to approximately 88%[46].

Double outlet right ventricle (DORV)

In this condition, an IVS defect is present and both arterial trunks emerge completely from the right ventricle. In over 95% of fetuses, blood flows normally from the right atrium to the right ventricle and from the left atrium to the left ventricle. Associated anomalies include situs inversus, dextrocardia, pulmonary stenosis, coarctation of the aorta, atrial septal defects, total anomalous pulmonary venous connections, asplenia/polysplenia, aneuploidy, cleft lip/palate and tracheoesophageal fistula. Both hemodynamics and surgical treatment are influenced by the associated lesions.

Atrioventricular septal defects (ASDs)

The incomplete variety of ASD is characterized by an ostium primum defect. The atrioventricular valves are normally inserted on an intact IVS, but the left atrioventricular valve has three leaflets.

The complete form is characterized by absence of the septum primum as well as the upper part of the interventricular septum. Thus, the defect is large and the atrioventricular valves are abnormally attached to the small ventricular septum by chordae tendinea or by anomalous papillary muscles. The septum secundum can also be absent, resulting in a common atrium.

This condition may be associated with malposition of the heart, tetralogy of Fallot, double outlet right ventricle, transposition of the great arteries, pulmonary stenosis, coarctation of the aorta and asplenia and polysplenia syndromes, the last frequently associated with total anomalous pulmonary venous return (TAPVR). Distortion of the conduction tissue also leads to atrioventricular block and marked bradycardia. Berger and associates reported 91% long-term survival following intracardiac repair[47].

Cardiosplenic syndromes

Asplenia syndrome (situs ambiguous) In this condition, the spleen is absent (most cases), the liver is centrally located, the gut is malrotated, the stomach lies on either side of the abdomen and bilateral superior vena cava is present. The sonographer should look for the location of the inferior vena cava and aorta on the left and right aspects of the spine. In asplenia the vessels are abnormally located on the same side (right or left side).

TAPVR is also seen in almost all such fetuses and the condition may also be associated with IVS defect, single ventricle, transposition of great arteries and pulmonary stenosis.

Polysplenia syndrome (presence of two or more spleens) In this condition, the stomach may be located on the right side and the gut malrotated. A midline aorta, bilateral superior vena cava and an absent or interrupted inferior vena cava (with blood drained by an azygous vein) may also be present. Other associations include TAPVR (in 70% of fetuses), dextrocardia, atrial septal defect, IVS defect, transposition of great arteries and double outlet right ventricle.

Total anomalous pulmonary venous return

In TAPVR the pulmonary veins drain into the right atrium rather than into the left atrium. In the first form (supracardiac drainage), the anomalous pulmonary veins follow the tract of the left innominate vein and the persistent left superior vena cava.

In the second form (infradiaphragmatic drainage) the pulmonary venous channel is directed to the liver, inferior vena cava or portal vein. The diagnosis of this condition is difficult in the fetus but attention to it derives from the presence of asplenia or polysplenia. Color Doppler mapping may help to identify the anomalous channel[47].

Ebstein anomaly

This condition is characterized by downward displacement of the septal insertion of the tricuspid valve. The right ventricle is thus divided into two compartments: a superior atrialized portion and an inferior chamber. Pulmonary blood flow is reduced, because part of the right ventricle (the atrialized portion) is relaxed during systole. Further, the tricuspid valve is usually incompetent and the main and branch pulmonary arteries are small. The right atrium becomes very large and congestive heart failure develops. Ebstein anomaly may also be associated with other cardiac anomalies, including ASD, IVS defect, tetralogy of Fallot, coarctation of the aorta and transposition of the great arteries.

In the neonate with severe hypoxia, pulmonary blood flow can be increased by a prostaglandin E infusion. However, in the absence of tricuspid regurgitation, the condition may be asymptomatic.

Other cardiac abnormalities

These include single ventricle, cardiac myopathy, endocardial fibroelastosis, cardiac tumors, ectopia cordis, ventricular aneurysm, enlargement of the heart secondary to arteriovenous malformation (Klippel–Trenaunay–Weber syndrome), idiopathic infantile arterial calcification, right ventricular enlargement in the compromised post-term fetus and arrhythmia.

The thickness of the cardiac chambers, including the IVS, should be carefully evaluated to rule out cardiomyopathy. The etiology of this condition is variable and includes: (1) hypertrophic myopathy in infants of diabetic mothers (IDMs); (2) myocarditis from virtually all known bacteria and viruses, including TORCH organisms and resulting in enlarged fetal heart on ultrasound; and (3) idiopathic obstructive myopathy, a condition characterized by massive hypertrophy of both ventricles and the IVS[48]. Approximately one-third of these cases are familial and approximately 25% show outflow obstruction[48]. It is difficult to distinguish this condition from hypertrophic cardiomyopathy in IDMs. However, unlike as is the case with infants of IDMs, there is a progressive increase in the septal dimension and the prognosis is guarded. Finally, one must consider endocardial fibroelastosis, a cardiomyopathy characterized by diffuse endocardial thickening. The foramen ovale is closed in approximately 50% of such cases. In most infants, obstruction to left ventricular flow and congestive heart failure are present.

The differential diagnosis of cardiomyopathy includes cardiac tumors, such as rhabdomyoma, myxoma, lipoma, teratoma, angioma, hamartoma and papilloma[50]. The most common tumor is rhabdomyoma, a condition associated with tuberous sclerosis in about 50% of affected fetuses[51]. The disorder is associated with mental deficiency and an intractable seizure disorder. Inheritance is by an autosomal dominant trait. Linkage studies with restriction fragment length polymorphism (RFPL) have located the mutant gene on chromosome 9.

Pericardial tumors generally cause cardiac compression. On the other hand, an intracardiac growth may result in inflow or outflow tract obstruction and arrhythmia. Non-immune hydrops may result from altered cardiac dynamics[52].

Ventricular aneurysm has been diagnosed *in utero* with color Doppler ultrasound[53]. In idiopathic infantile arterial calcification (IIAC), a rare and usually fatal disorder, diffuse calcification is noted in soft tissue and arteries[54].

In the post-term fetus, Horenstein and associates recently showed that M-mode measurements of the right ventricular inner dimensions (RVID), left ventricular inner dimensions (LVID), and RVID/LVID ratio were 1.7–4 times better than the non-stress test in predicting abnormal intrapartum heart patterns in post-term pregnancies[55].

A discussion of arrhythmia is beyond the scope of this chapter, and the treatment of arrhythmia remains one of the most specialized aspects of cardiology. It is noteworthy, however, that tachycardia refractory to maternally administered medication can be reverted by direct fetal therapy[56]. This is particularly applicable to hydropic fetuses with suboptimal placental absorptive function.

Table 3 Ultrasonically recognizable abnormalities of the pulmonary system and the gastrointestinal (GI) tract

Esophageal atresia
Pulmonary cystic adenomatoid malformation
Pulmonary hypoplasia
Diaphragmatic hernia
GI obstructive lesions (duodenal, jejunal, ileal atresia)
Other obstructive GI lesions
Hyperechogenic bowel
Ventral wall defects

Abnormalities of the chest and gastrointestinal (GI) tract

A list of the ultrasonographically recognizable abnormalities in the chest and GI tract is shown in Table 3.

Esophageal atresia

This is a very rare anomaly (1:25 000 births), and its antenatal diagnosis is difficult because, in 90% of such cases, the stomach remains ultrasonically visible, as a result of a communication between the esophagus, trachea and stomach. This communication allows a normal flow of amniotic fluid to the stomach. A dilated proximal esophagus, an absence of the normal stomach echo and polyhydramnios are present in the 10% of fetuses who lack this conduit to the stomach[57].

Pulmonary cystic adenomatoid malformation

This abnormality is characterized by the conglomeration of multiple cystic areas within the lung tissue. The resulting mass can result in a

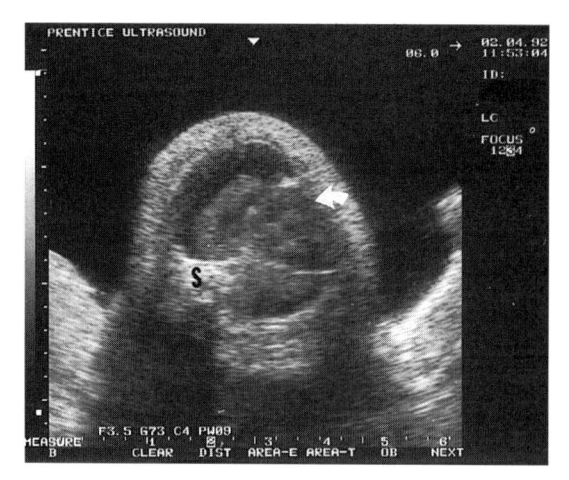

Figure 15 Cross-sectional scan of fetal chest, showing spine (S) and heart (arrow). The lungs are seen adjacent to the heart and markedly compressed by hydrothorax

shift of the mediastinum to the right or left. Three types have been described[49]. In type I, the cysts are large (≥2 cm) but the prognosis is good, following resection of that portion of the lung. In type II, the cysts are < 1 cm in size, and the condition is associated with other anomalies of the renal or GI tract. In type III malformation, the lesion is large, more echogenic and carries a worse prognosis. The differential diagnosis includes pulmonary sequestration and some forms of diaphragmatic hernia[58].

Pulmonary hypoplasia

Poor development of the lungs leading to pulmonary hypoplasia is associated with a high mortality rate. In this condition, neonatal lung weight at autopsy is ≤2 SD of the normal mean weight[59]. Pulmonary hypoplasia can occur as a primary condition. However, it more commonly is associated with oligohydramnios or follows compression of the lungs.

Oligohydramnios can result from severe obstructive uropathies, severe IUGR, and prolonged rupture of membranes. By comparison, pulmonary compression results from a myriad of causes, including hydrothorax (Figure 15), pulmonary tumor (cystic adenomatoid malformation), chest mass (teratoma, anterior thoracic meningocele), diaphragmatic hernia, and

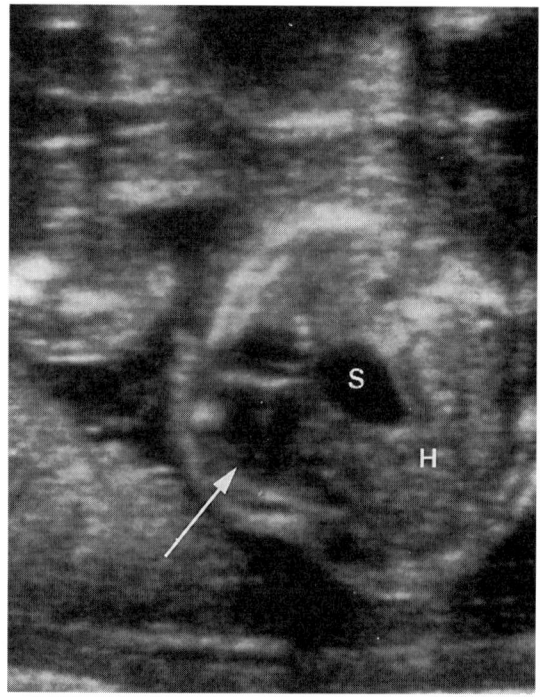

Figure 16 Cross-sectional scan of fetal chest, showing large left-sided diaphragmatic hernia (H) adjacent to the fetal stomach (S). Note how the heart is markedly displaced to the right side of the chest

elevation of the diaphragm in the presence of severe ascites or obstructive uropathy.

Although lung tissue may be visualized adjacent to the heart if high-resolution equipment is used, most studies dealing with pulmonary hypoplasia have focused on reduced chest size as a predictor of pulmonary hypoplasia[60]. The chest circumference/abdominal circumference ratio has been used to diagnose pulmonary hypoplasia; this ratio is constant throughout gestation and equals 0.89±0.12 (2 SD). Values of ≤0.77 are consistent with pulmonary hypoplasia[60]. In cases in which the fetal abdomen is altered in size, as is the case with obstructive uropathies and diaphragmatic hernia, the chest circumference/femur length ratio may be used. The 5th percentile values for this ratio equal 4.0 and 3.4 from 18–24 and 25–40 weeks' gestation, respectively[61].

The highest sensitivity (85%) and positive predictive value (83%) for the diagnosis of pulmonary hypoplasia was reported by Vintzileos et al.[62]. These investigators traced the chest circumference at the midpoint of the chest wall. Their calculations were based on: (chest area − heart area) × 100/chest area. This ratio is independent of gestational age and is abnormal at or below 62 (5th percentile).

Diaphragmatic hernia

In this condition, some of the abdominal contents are displaced into the chest as a result of congenital defects in the diaphragm (Figure 16). The most common defect (1 : 3000 births) is that involving the foramen of Bochdalek, situated in the posterolateral aspect of the diaphragm[63]. Usually, these hernias include fetal stomach and bowel, but part of the liver and pancreas can also be displaced into the chest. The condition may be associated with trisomy 13, 18 and 21.

In utero corrective surgery by 30 weeks' gestation has been successful in some isolated cases of diaphragmatic hernia in which the liver and pancreas are not displaced into the chest[64]. However, the success rate of *in utero* surgery has not been proven to be superior to treatment of affected neonates with the use of extracorporeal oxygen membrane oxygenation[65].

A rarer type of diaphragmatic hernia is anteromedial in location, traversing the foramen of Morgagni. In this condition, the prognosis is poor, because of associated anomalies, including hydrocephalus, cardiac anomalies and trisomies[63].

Eventration or thinning of the diaphragm may result in displacement of visceral contents into the chest. However, this condition is not an actual diaphragmatic hernia and differentiation from the latter may be difficult.

GI obstructive lesions

Duodenal atresia results from failure of recanalization of the upper GI tract in the interval of 8 weeks' gestation. In this condition the stomach and proximal part of the duodenum (double bubble sign) appear sonographically dilated, particularly after the 20th week of pregnancy, an interval when the quantity of swallowed amniotic fluid exceeds the resorptive capacity of the gut[66]. The condition may be associated not only with anomalies involving the gastrointestinal, cardiac and renal systems but also with trisomy 21.

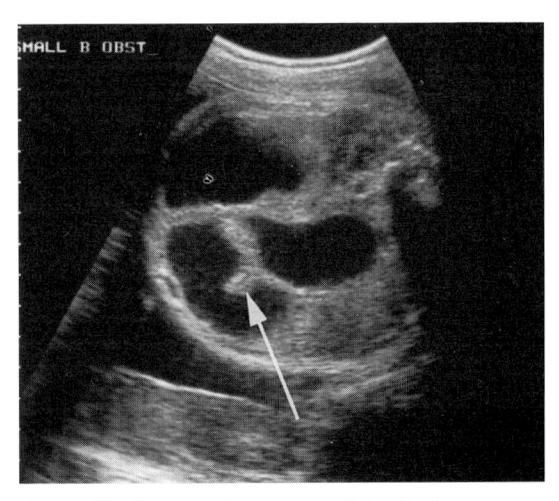

Figure 17 Cross-sectional scan of the fetal abdomen in a case of jejunal atresia. Note the markedly dilated small bowel loops characterized by valvular flaps

In contrast, obstruction at the level of the jejunum and ileum is caused by *in utero* vascular accidents resulting in avascular necrosis of small bowel segments. The dilated bowel loops, situated proximal to the atretic segments, are characterized by the presence of valvular flaps projecting into the lumen (Figure 17).

Other obstructive GI lesions such as malrotation of the bowel, volvulus, intussusception and Hirschprung's disease (congenital intestinal aganglionosis) produce some abnormal dilatation of the bowel. However, neither the onset nor the pattern of this bowel dilatation is specific enough to allow for a precise antenatal diagnosis using ultrasonography.

Hyperechogenic bowel

The presence of hyperechogenic bowel has recently assumed significance, because of the association with cystic fibrosis and trisomies[67]. Although the outcome in some of these fetuses may be normal[68], when this finding is present

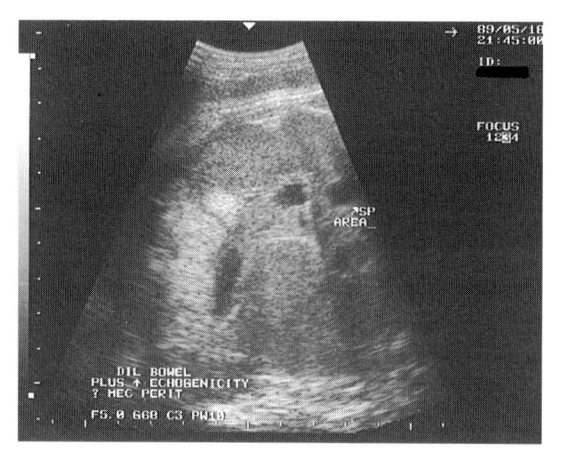

Figure 18 Cross-sectional scan of the fetal abdomen in a case of meconium peritonitis. Note the large area of increased echogenicity adjacent to dilated bowel, left side of scan. The area of the spine is seen on the right side of the image (SP area) See text for differential diagnosis

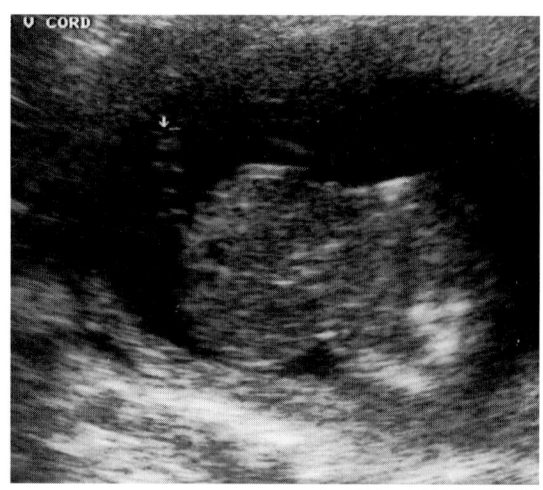

Figure 19 Cross-sectional scan of the fetal abdominal area showing a large omphalocele. Note the umbilical cord (arrow) and its insertion into the apex of the omphalocele. This image is diagnostic of omphalocele

couples should be counselled regarding antenatal testing for fetal karyotype and cystic fibrosis.

Hyperechogenic bowel may also result from a small perforation of a dilated segment of bowel, one which usually induces an inflammatory response followed by adhesions and calcium deposition in the area. This entity is known as meconium peritonitis (Figure 18). Differentiation from hyperechogenic bowel without perforation may be possible in some cases.

Ventral wall defects

Omphalocele and gastroschisis occur at a rate of approximately 1:2500 births. Their ultrasonographic appearance is different. In omphalocele, the umbilical cord is inserted at the apex of the herniated bowel (Figure 19). In contrast, in gastroschisis the umbilical cord inserts into the fetal abdomen to the left of a small 2–5 cm abdominal defect, which is believed to result from abnormal involution of the right umbilical vein.

Approximately 50% of fetuses with omphalocele are either chromosomally abnormal, particularly if the fetal liver is not part of the hernia[69,70], or have other anomalies involving the cardiac, skeletal, renal, or central nervous systems. In particular, the Beckwith–Weidman syndrome of organomegaly and hypoglycemia has been described with omphalocele.

Interestingly, the fetal bowel is normally located outside the abdomen in the first trimester of pregnancy, an observation described as physiological herniation. This phenomenon can be visualized using transvaginal sonography[71,72]. To avoid errors, the diagnosis of omphalocele should not be made prior to the 14th week of pregnancy.

In the presence of a ventral wall defect, the mode of delivery (vaginal vs. Cesarean section) remains controversial[73,74]. However, vaginal delivery is preferable when the hernia is small and the liver is not herniated.

Urinary tract abnormalities

The frequency of urinary tract abnormalities is approximately 7:1000 newborns, and the recurrence risk is 8–10%. The thought process regarding the etiology of urinary tract abnormalities should extend beyond the apparent site of the lesion. For example, dilatation of the ureteropelvic junction (UPJ) may result

Table 4 Ultrasonically recognizable urinary tract abnormalities

Bladder dilatation
Urethral obstruction
Prune-belly syndrome
Persistence of cloaca
Megacystis–microcolon–intestinal hypoperistalsis syndrome

Megaureter
Urethral obstruction
Prune-belly syndrome
Persistence of cloaca
Non-obstructive, non-reflux megaureter
Ureterovesical junction (UVJ) obstruction
Ureterovesical junction (UVJ) reflux
Ureterocele

Pyelectasis
Ureterovesical junction (UVJ) reflux
Chromosomal abnormality

Ureteropelvic (UPJ) dilatation and hydronephrosis
Urethral obstruction
Persistence of cloaca
Prune-belly syndrome
Ureterovesical junction (UVJ) obstruction
Ureterovesical junction (UVJ) reflux
UPJ dysfunction

Renal anomalies
Renal agenesis
Unilateral empty renal fossa (crossed fused ectopic kidney, pelvic kidney)
Infantile polycystic kidney disease (IPKD)
Adult polycystic kidney disease (APKD)
Multicystic dysplastic kidney
Other conditions, including horseshoe kidney, ectopic ureter, adrenal cysts, congenital mesoblastic nephroma and Wilms' tumor

Adapted from reference 90, with permission

not only from obstruction at that level but also from increased intraluminal pressure secondary to a lower abnormality, one involving the ureters, ureterovesical junction (UVJ), or posterior urethral valve (PUV).

A list of ultrasonically recognized urinary abnormities is shown in Table 4. This list is arranged to show lesions of the lower urinary tract first and then progresses to renal abnormalities. A discussion of urinary tract abnormalities follows.

A posterior urethral valve (PUV) is a major etiological factor for markedly dilated fetal bladders (Figure 20). The condition is usually associated with convoluted large ureters and hydronephrosis. The fetal abdomen may also be quite distended and the diaphragm elevated, a condition which, together with oligohydramnios, prevents appropriate pulmonary development and leads to pulmonary hypoplasia.

The affected fetus may benefit from open fetal surgery or use of a catheter to drain the contents of the urinary bladder into the abdominal cavity[75,76]. To prevent pulmonary hypoplasia, however, fetal surgery or single or multiple drainage procedures must be performed early in the second trimester of pregnancy. Thus,

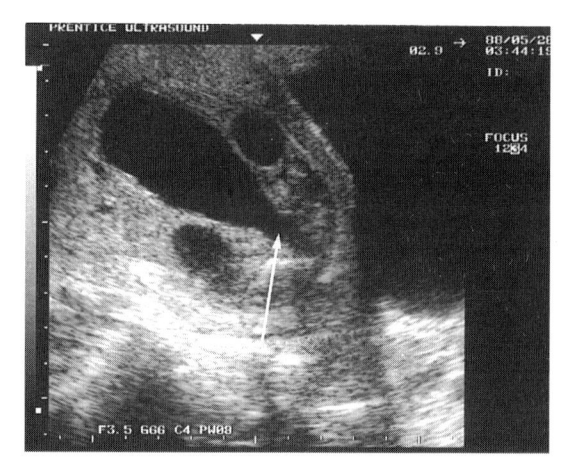

Figure 20 Scan of fetus with posterior urethral valve (PUV). Note dilated bladder (center) surrounded by dilated ureters (dark circles on each side of bladder). The proximal urethra (arrow) is dilated and diagnostic of PUV

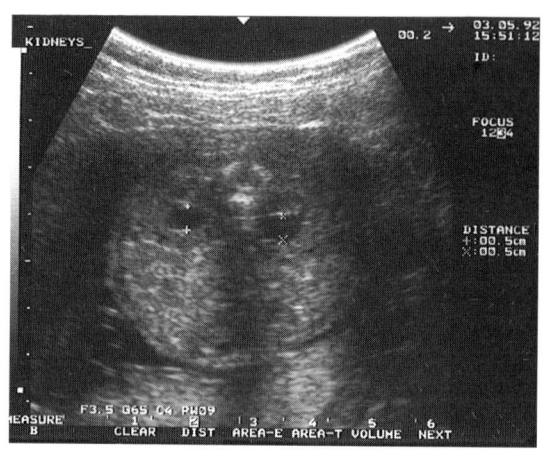

Figure 21 Cross-sectional scan of the fetal abdomen at the level of the kidneys. Note bilateral dilatation of the renal pelvis or pyelectasis (+ and × signs). Each pelvis measures 5 mm in the anteroposterior plane. See text for significance of pyelectasis

early diagnosis is mandatory in these fetuses. Unfortunately, early diagnosis is at present based on chance, because obstetric ultrasound examinations are not yet routinely performed.

The indications for fetal surgery include: (1) early diagnosis prior to 20 weeks' gestation; (2) a fetal urine sample showing concentrations of sodium of <100 mg/dl, chloride <90 mg/dl, and osmolality of 210 mosm/dl – all indirectly pointing to the ability of the kidneys to function in conserving salt; and (3) progressive oligohydramnios.

Prune-belly syndrome (dilated urinary bladder, lax abdominal wall, and undescended testicles – cryptorchidism) is frequently noted in fetuses with severe PUV[77]. However, it is also believed that prune-belly syndrome may result from a primary mesoderm defect in the abdominal wall and urinary tract muscles[77].

Importantly, the urethral obstruction in most cases with PUV is incomplete and allows for some fetal urination and maintenance of near normal amniotic fluid volume. The bladder diameters in the incomplete form fall in the 3–4 cm range and the ureteral dilatation, with or without a UPJ dilatation, is minimal to moderate.

A rare etiology of bladder dilatation is the megacystis–microcolon–hypoperistalsis syndrome. This syndrome is characterized by a large, unobstructed and thick walled bladder in conjunction with dilatation of the small bowel and polyhydramnios[78–81]. The abnormalities may not always be apparent prior to 24 weeks' gestation. The prognosis is poor.

Dilatation of the ureteropelvic junction (UPJ) occurs secondary to abnormal recanalization of the upper part of the ureter or absence of the longitudinal muscle fibers in the area. The UPJ is surrounded by both circular and longitudinal muscle fibers. Absence of the latter component interferes with the UPJ function of propelling boluses of urine forward, resulting in dilatation of the UPJ[82]. Dilatation of the UPJ may also occur secondary to obstruction or reflux at the ureterovesical junction (Figure 21).

In UPJ dilatation, males are affected more frequently than females, the ratio being 5:1. The condition occurs more frequently on the left side, but can be unilateral in 70% of cases. Importantly, however, UPJ dilatation may be associated with other anomalies involving the fetal cardiac, gastrointestinal and central nervous systems.

Pyelectasis or dilatation of the renal pelvis may occur secondary to any abnormality of the urinary tract below that level. Severity is

Diagnosis of fetal anomalies by ultrasonography

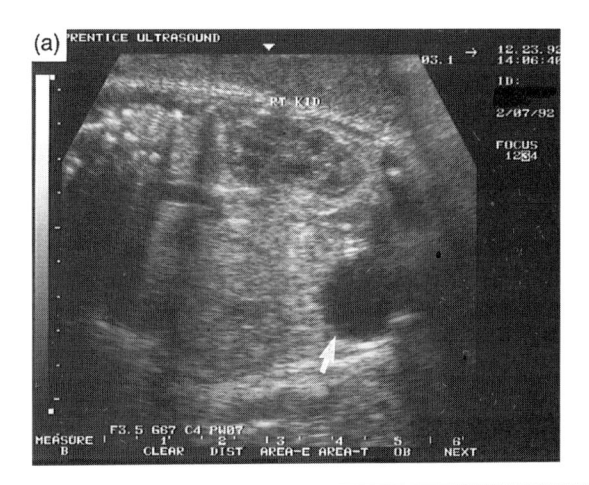

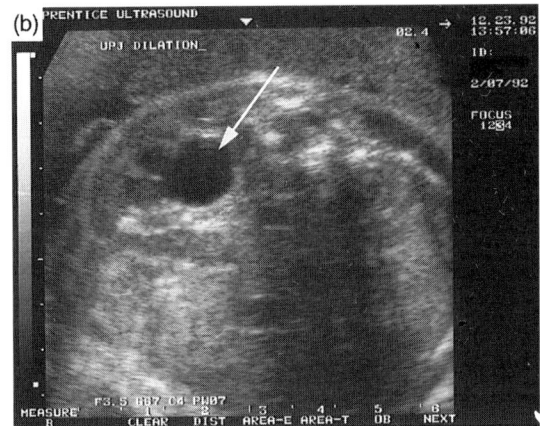

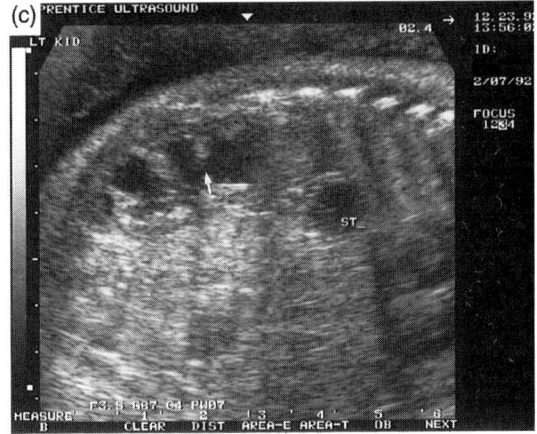

Figure 22 (a) Oblique scan of fetal abdomen, showing normal right kidney (RT KID). A normal bladder is also seen (arrow). (b) Oblique scan of the left ureteropelvic junction (UPJ) of same fetus. Note UPJ dilatation (arrow). (c) Oblique scan of left hydronephrotic kidney of same fetus. Note communication between the dilated calyces typical of hydronephrosis. In this fetus, dilatation of the left UPJ and the left hydronephrosis resulted from reflux at the ureterovesical junction

gauged by the size of the anteroposterior diameter of the renal pelvis. Mild pyelectasis (A–P diameter ≤5 mm) may be associated with normal outcome[83]. An A–P diameter of ≥4 mm or ≥7 mm before and after 33 weeks' gestation, respectively, warrants postnatal follow up[84]. Recent data[85] suggest that the positive predictive value for pathological hydronephrosis or need for corrective surgery is as shown in Table 5.

Of importance is the fact that approximately 3.3% of fetuses with pyelectasis in the range of 3–5 mm have an associated chromosomal abnormality, including Down's syndrome[86]. Interestingly, although 25% of fetuses with Down's syndrome have pyelectasis, only 2.8% of fetuses with normal karyotype have a dilated renal pelvis[86].

Dilatation of the renal calyceal system, or hydronephrosis, results from various abnormalities below that level (Table 4 and Figure 22). It is differentiated from multicystic dysplastic disease by the ultrasonic visualization of radially placed calyces communicating with each other or with the renal pelvis (Figure 22). In addition, renal cortical tissue is also seen (Figure 22).

Ultrasonographic diagnosis of hydronephrosis, pyelectasis, or UPJ dilatation is of

Table 5 Positive predictive value (%) for pathological hydronephrosis or need for corrective surgery

Pelvic diameter (mm)	Gestational age (weeks)		
	<24	24–33	>33
4–6	14	45	29
7–9	78	54	73
≥10	100	92	90

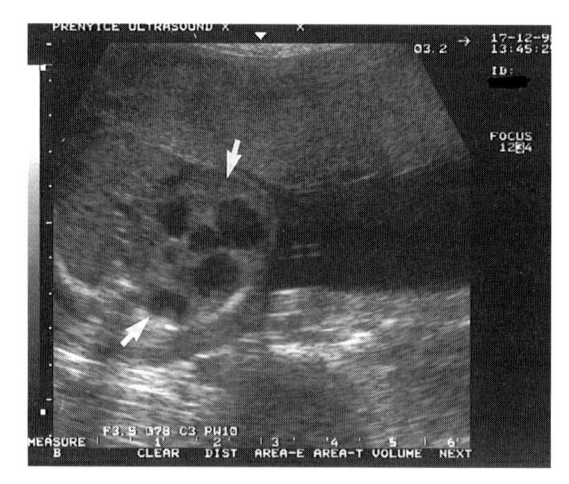

Figure 23 Cross-sectional scan of the fetal abdomen at the level of the kidneys. Note large multicystic right kidney (arrows). The cysts are of varying size and do not communicate with each other. Compare with hydronephrosis in Figure 21

importance, because it leads to careful postnatal evaluation and early treatment of affected infants prior to irreversible compromise of the kidneys.

Renal agenesis

This condition is often an isolated finding, occurring with a frequency of 1:4000 births. On the other hand, it may also occur secondary to a chromosomal or genetic disorder (recessive or dominant mode of inheritance). Further, it may be part of the VATER association (vertebral defects, anal atresia, tracheoesophageal fistula, and radial and renal dysplasia). The risk of recurrence is 3%[87]. Renal agenesis is usually bilateral, but unilateral empty renal fossa has been reported[88]. The outcome of fetuses with renal agenesis is poor, because of pulmonary hypoplasia secondary to severe oligohydramnios.

Ultrasound diagnosis is difficult and the sensitivity is low, approximating 50%[89]. The difficulty is related to the presence of oligohydramnios and enlarged adrenal glands that fill the renal spaces, projecting an image similar to that of the kidneys[89]. Recently, the diagnosis of renal agenesis has been enhanced by the use of color Doppler velocimetry, a method that may help determine the absence of renal vessels[90].

The differential diagnosis includes severely growth-retarded fetuses who also have oligohydramnios secondary to low urine output. In such fetuses, urine production remains low, even following maternal administration of furosemide (40 mg IV).

Infantile polycystic kidney disease (IPKD)

This condition is transmitted as an autosomal recessive disease. Characteristically, the kidneys show a multicystic appearance and are enlarged. The ratio of kidney circumference to abdominal circumference exceeds the normal range of 0.3[91].

Renal enlargement in IPKD may not always occur prior to 24 weeks' gestation[92]. Several subtypes of IPKD exist and these vary in onset and severity. In contrast, adult polycystic kidney disease (APKD) is rarely detected *in utero*, although the diagnosis has been made prenatally in pregnant women with a positive family history[93].

Multicystic, dysplastic kidneys

This condition occurs sporadically at a rate of 1:10 000 births. It is unilateral in 75% of cases. The male:female ratio is 2:1. Etiology is either secondary to a chromosome/gene disorder resulting in poor induction of nephron formation or early obstructive uropathy. If the 'insult' occurs early in embryogenesis, nephron formation is compromised, resulting in a very small kidney which may weigh as little as 1 g and exhibit small cysts microscopically. This abnormality is classified as Potter type II B

Diagnosis of fetal anomalies by ultrasonography

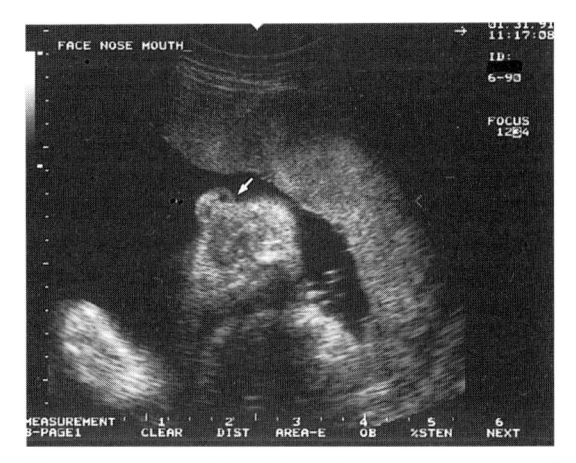

Figure 24 Scan of fetal face, showing lower part of the nose and the nostrils (arrow). Note the normal formation of the lips clearly ruling out cleft lip

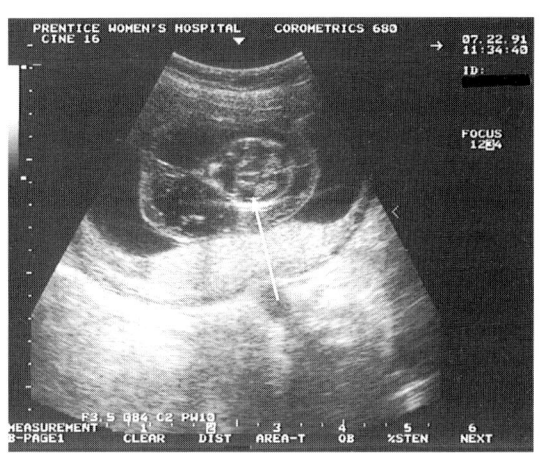

Figure 25 Cross-sectional scan of the fetal neck (arrow). Note bilateral large masses surrounding the fetal neck consistent with cystic hygromas

dysplastic kidney[94]. If, on the other hand, the insult occurs at 9–13 menstrual weeks, the kidney assumes a large multicystic appearance (Figure 23). Unlike hydronephrosis, the cystic areas do not communicate with each other (Figures 22 and 23).

Some externally visible body defects

A number of anomalies occur in this category, including cleft lip/palate, cystic hygroma, non-immune fetal hydrops, sacrococcygeal teratoma and skeletal abnormalities.

The fetal face and the nose and lower lips can easily be outlined to rule out cleft lip and cleft lip/palate (Figure 24). The former is genetically and probably etiologically different from cleft lip/palate and is more likely to occur in females (female:male ratio = 2:1). Importantly, cleft lip and cleft lip/palate may be components of other genetic or chromosomal abnormalities.

Cystic hygroma

This abnormality is rare, occurring in 1:6000 pregnancies. It results from poor development of the communication channels between the jugular veins and the cervical lymph sacs. It is referred to as the jugular lymphatic obstruction sequence.

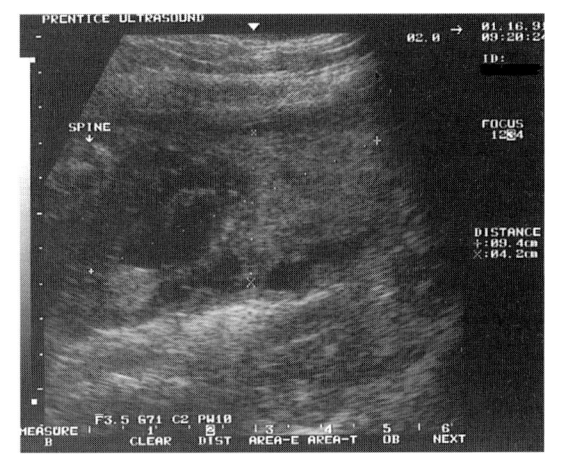

Figure 26 Scan of very large predominantly echogenic sacrococcygeal teratoma (+ and X signs). The mass is attached to the lower end of the fetal spine (arrow on left)

Cystic hygromas vary in size, depending on the degree to which lymph can be drained into the jugular veins (Figure 25). Interestingly, in a few cases the nuchal mass has been noted to regress, implying the occurrence of delayed but otherwise normal development of communication channels between the lymph sacs and the venous system[95]. In severe cases, massive fetal hydrops develops, resulting in intrauterine fetal death during the second trimester of pregnancy. Although a recessive mode of inheritance is implicated, the anomaly is usually

Table 6 Etiologic factors leading to non-immune fetal hydrops

Infection with TORCH organisms*
Fetal–maternal hemorrhage
Fetal cerebral hemorrhage
Twin-to-twin transfusion syndrome
Inherited metabolic diseases (Gaucher or Tay-Sachs disease)
Alpha thalassemia
Cardiac arrhythmia
Structural defects of the heart
Other abnormalities, including cystic hygroma, hydrothorax, chylothorax, cystic adenomatoid malformation of the lung, teratoma, bladder perforation resulting from posterior urethral valve

*Toxoplasmosis, other, rubella, cytomegalovirus, and herpes virus

a sporadic event. Nonetheless, 75% of cases have an associated chromosomal abnormality, including 45,XX (two-thirds of cases), and trisomies 21, 18, 13 and 47,XY.

Non-immune fetal hydrops

This term describes massive fetal edema with accumulation of fluid in some or in all serous cavities. Although chromosomal abnormalities are noted in 15% of cases, non-immune fetal hydrops can occur secondary to many etiologies (listed in Table 6).

Sacrococcygeal teratoma

This tumor appears as a predominantly echogenic mass attached to the sacrococcygeal area (Figure 26). It is rare (1 : 40 000 births). Size is variable; in approximately 10% of cases the tumor is ≥ 10 cm at term and requires delivery by Cesarean section[96]. Although it is usually considered a benign lesion, sacrococcygeal teratoma has the potential of becoming malignant. Thus, excision should be performed prior to 2 months of age and the operation often incorporates the coccyx.

Skeletal abnormalities

These are a heterogeneous group of abnormalities characterized by variability in the mode of inheritance, recurrence risk, gene penetrance, and type of limb shortening[97]. Some are lethal, including achondrogenesis, thanatophoric dwarfism, chondrodysplasia (recessive form), congenital lethal hypophosphatasia, short rib polydactyly, campomelic dysplasia and osteogenesis imperfecta (type II).

It is beyond the scope of this chapter to detail the ultrasonographic findings in each possible skeletal abnormality. However, the sonographer should be able to place the defect into a general category based on:

(1) The specific segment of long bone shortened, that is, whether rhisomelia, mesomelia or acromelia exists;

(2) The presence of facial abnormalities;

(3) Hypoplasia of the radius;

(4) The appearance of a small or barrel-shaped chest;

(5) Demineralization of bone; and

(6) Other features indicative, for example, of sirenomelia sequence (caudal regression syndrome), lobster claw deformity, arthrogryposis, or craniocytostosis (premature closure of the cranial sutures) (see Chapter 7).

Table 7 groups different forms of skeletal dysplasias according to the presenting ultrasound feature.

Table 7 Abnormal ultrasonographic features in various skeletal dysplasias

Abnormal ultrasonographic feature	Skeletal dysplasias
Amniotic fluid volume/ polyhydramnios	Robert syndrome, VATERS association
Acromelia	Ellis-van Creveld dysplasia Poland sequence, acrodysostosis
Bowing of long bones Tibia Femur	Campomelic dysplasia, metaphyseal chondrodysplasia, split hand syndrome
Cardiac abnormalities	thanatophoric dysplasia, chondroectodermal dysplasia, short rib polydactyly, campomelic dwarfism, Robert syndrome
Cleft lip/palate	all facial skeletal dysplasias, diastrophic dwarfism, chondroectodermal dysplasia, short rib polydactyly, campomelic dwarfism,
Contractures:	femoral hypoplasia-unusual facies syndrome, popliteal web syndrome, sirenomelia sequence, arthrogryposis
Demineralization/poor calcification of bone mainly noted in spine mainly noted in skull mainly noted in long bones with fractures	achondrogenesis hypophophatasia osteogenesis imperfecta
Femoral hypoplasia	femoral hypoplasia-unusual facies syndrome ectrodactyly–ectodermal–dysplasia–clefting syndrome
Fetal motion absence	arthrogryposis
Finger abnormalities/ triphalangeal thumb	ectrodactyly–ectodermal–dysplasia–clefting syndrome
Head shape abnormalities brachycephaly dolichocephaly hydrocephaly	craniosynostosis, acrodysostosis, achondroplasia, (heterozygous form) craniosynostosis, trilobed or clover leaf skull thanatophoric dwarfism, osteogenesis imperfecta
Hydropic appearance	achondrogenesis, short rib polydactyly, (Saldino–Noonan type)
Hypertelorism	cleidocranial cleidostosis, acrodysostosis, VATERS association
Intrauterine growth retardation	Robert syndrome, VATERS association
Kyphoscoliosis	metatropic dysplasia
Limbs/lower fusion	caudal regression syndrome

Continued

Table 7 *Continued*

Abnormal ultrasound feature	Skeletal dysplasias
Long bones/↑thickness	diastrophic dysplasia
Macrocephaly	achondroplasia, campomelic dysplasia
Mesomelia	Neivergelt or Langer dysplasia
Micromelia (severe)	Robert syndrome, type II osteogenesis imperfecta, achondrogenesis
Microcephalus	Robert syndrome, thanatophoric dwarfism, De Lange syndrome, chondrodysplasia punctata
Protuberant abdomen	achondrogenesis, thanatophoric dwarfism, short rib polydactyly (Majewski type)
Radial bone hypoplasia	Miller syndrome, TAR syndrome, Aase syndrome, VATERS association, acromelia
Renal disease	short rib polydactyly, campomelic dwarfism, asphyxiating thoracic dysplasia (Jeune type), short rib polydactyly
Thorax/↓ size	thanatophoric dwarfism, achondrogenesis, metatrophic dwarfism, asphyxiating thoracic dysplasia, (Jeune type), short rib polydactyly, campomelic dysplasia, cleidocranial dysostosis, metatropic dwarfism
Umbilical cord Single umbilical artery	VATERS association

Adapted from reference 98, with permission

References

1. Sabbagha, R.E., Sheikh, Z., Tamura, R.K. *et al.* (1985). Predictive value, sensitivity, and specificity of ultrasonic targeted imaging for fetal anomalies in gravid women at high risk for birth defects. *Am. J. Obstet. Gynecol.*, **152**, 822
2. Rottem, S., Bronstein, M. and Thaler-Brandes, J.M. (1989). First trimester transvaginal sonographic diagnosis of fetal anomalies. *Lancet*, **1**, 444
3. Kennedy, K.A., Flick, K.J. and Thurmond, A.S. (1990). First trimester diagnosis of exencephaly. *Am. J. Obstet. Gynecol.*, **162**, 461
4. Meizner, I., Levi, A., Katz, M. and Maor, E. (1992). Iniencephaly. A case report. *J. Reprod. Med.*, **37**, 885
5. Chervenak, F.A., Rosenberg, J., Brightman, R.C., Chitkara, U. and Jeanty, P. (1987). A prospective study of the accuracy of ultrasound in predicting fetal microcephaly. *Obstet. Gynecol.*, **69**, 908
6. Chervenak, F.A., Jeanty, P., Cantraine, F. *et al.* (1984). The diagnosis of fetal microcephaly. *Am. J. Obstet. Gynecol.*, **149**, 512
7. Goldstein, I., Reece, A., Pilu, G. *et al.* (1988). Sonographic assessment of the fetal frontal lobe: a potential tool for prenatal diagnosis of microcephaly. *Am. J. Obstet. Gynecol.*, **158**, 1057
8. Sabbagha, R.E., Tamura, R.K. and DalCompo, S. (1980). Fetal cranial and craniocervical masses: ultrasound characteristics and differential diagnosis. *Am. J. Obstet. Gynecol.*, **138**, 511
9. Ghidini, A., Sirtori, M. and Vergani, P. (1989). Fetal intracranial calcifications. *Am. J. Obstet. Gynecol.*, **160**, 8622

10. Jeanty, P., Kepple, D., Roussis, P. and Shah, D. (1990). *In utero* detection of cardiac failure from aneurysm of the vein of Galen. *Am. J. Obstet. Gynecol.*, **163**, 50
11. Pretorius, D.H., Drose, L.A. and Manco-Johnson, M.L. (1986). Fetal lateral ventricular ratio determination during the second trimester. *J. Ultrasound Med.*, **5**, 121
12. Pilu, G., Reece, A., Goldstein, I., Hobbins, J.C. and Bovicelli, L. (1989). Sonographic evaluation of the normal developmental anatomy of the fetal cerebral ventricles: the atria. *Obstet. Gynecol.*, **73**, 2505
13. Cordoza, J.D., Goldstein, R.B. and Filly, R.A. (1988). Exclusion of fetal ventriculomegaly with a single measurement of the width of the lateral ventricular atrium. *Radiology*, **169**, 711
14. Chitkara, U., Cogswell, C., Norton, K., Wilkins, I.A., Mehalek, K. and Berkowitz, R.L. (1988). Choroid plexus cysts in the fetus: a benign anatomic variant or pathologic entity? Report of 41 cases and review of the literature. *Obstet. Gynecol.*, **72**, 185
15. Gabrielli, S., Reece, A.E., Pilu, G., Perolo, A., Rizzo, N., Bovicelli, L. and Hobbins, J.C. (1989). The clinical significance of prenatally diagnosed choroid plexus cysts. *Am. J. Obstet. Gynecol.*, **160**, 1207
16. Rotmensch, S., Luo, J.S., Nores, J.A. *et al.* (1992). Bilateral choroid plexus cysts in trisomy 21. *Am. J. Obstet. Gynecol.*, **166**, 591
17. Platt, L.D., Carlson, D.E., Medearis. A.L. *et al.* (1991). Fetal choroid plexus cysts in the second trimester of pregnancy: a cause for concern. *Am. J. Obstet. Gynecol.*, **164**, 1652
18. Benacerraf, B.R., Harlow, B. and Frigoletto, F. (1990). Are choroid plexus cysts an indication for second-trimester amniocentesis? *Am. J. Obstet. Gynecol.*, **162**, 1001
19. Kupfermink, M.J., Tamura, R.K., Sabbagha, R.E. *et al.* (1994). Isolated choroid plexus cyst(s): an indication for amniocentesis. *Am. J. Obstet. Gynecol.*, **171**, 1068
20. Lemire, R.J., Loeser, J.D., Leech, R.W. *et al.* (1975). *Normal and Abnormal Development of the Human Nervous System*, pp. 260–77. (New York: Harper & Row)
21. Bertino, R.E., Nyberg, D.A., Cyr, D.R. and Mack, L.A. (1988). Prenatal diagnosis of agenesis of the corpus callosum. *J. Ultrasound Med.*, **7**, 251
22. Lockwood, C.J., Ghidini, A., Aggarawal, R. and Hobbins, J.C. (1988). Antenatal diagnosis of partial agenesis of the corpus callosum: a benign cause of ventriculomegaly. *Am. J. Obstet. Gynecol.*, **159**, 184
23. Comstock, C. (1992). Agenesis of the corpus callosum in the fetus: diagnosis and significance. *Female Patient*, **17**, 40
24. Sabbagha, R.E. (1990). Targeted imaging for fetal anomalies: clues to reaching a correct diagnosis. *Obstet. Gynecol. Rep.*, **2**, 142
25. Byrd, S.E. and Thomas, N.P. (1988). Common congenital brain anomalies. *Radiol. Clin. N. Am.*, **26**, 755
26. Thurmond, A.S., Nelson, D.W., Lowensohn, R.I. *et al.* (1989). Enlarged cisterna magna in trisomy 18, prenatal ultrasonographic diagnosis. *Am. J. Obstet. Gynecol.*, **161**, 83
27. Van den Hof, M.C., Nicolaides, K.H. and Campbell, S. (1990). Evaluation of the lemon and banana signs in one hundred thirty fetuses with open spina bifida. *Am. J. Obstet. Gynecol.*, **162**, 322-37
28. Luthy, D.A., Wardinsky, T., Shurtleff, D.B. *et al.* (1991). Cesarean section before the onset of labor and subsequent motor function in infants with meningomyelocele diagnosed antenatally. *N. Engl. J. Med.*, **162**, 624
29. Hobbins, J.C. (1991). Diagnosis and management of neural tube defects today. *N. Engl. J. Med.*, **324**, 690
30. Boughman, J.A., Berg, K.A., Astemborski, J.A. *et al.* (1987). Familial risks of congenital heart disease in a population based epidemiologic study. *Am. J. Med. Genet.*, **26**, 839
31. Ferencz, C., Rubin, J.D., McCarter, R.J. *et al.* (1985). Congenital heart disease: prevalence at livebirth. The Baltimore–Washington Infant Study. *Am. J. Epidemiol.*, **121**, 31
32. Ferrazi, E., Fesslova, V., Bellotti, M., Agostoni, G., Pardi, G. and Makowski, E.L. (1989). Prenatal diagnosis of and management of congenital heart disease. *J. Reprod. Med.*, **34**, 207
33. Crawford, D.C., Chita, S.K. and Allan, L.D. (1988). Prenatal detection of congenital heart disease: factors affecting obstetric management and survival. *Am. J. Obstet. Gynecol.*, **159**, 352
34. Wigton, T.R., Sabbagha, R.E., Tamura, R.K. *et al.* (1993). Sonographic diagnosis of congenital heart disease: comparison between the 4-chamber view and multiple cardiac views. *Obstet. Gynecol.*, **82**, 219
35. Bromley, B., Estroff, J.A., Sanders, S.P. *et al.* (1992). Fetal echocardiography: accuracy and

limitations in a population at high risk for heart defects. *Am. J. Obstet. Gynecol.*, **166**, 1473
36. Copel, J.A., Pilu, G., Green, J. *et al.* (1987). Fetal echocardiographic screening for congenital heart disease: the importance of the four-chamber view. *Am. J. Obstet. Gynecol.*, **157**, 648
37. Sharland, G.K. and Allan, L.D. (1992). Normal fetal cardiac measurements by cross sectional echocardiography. *Ultrasound Obstet. Gynecol.*, **2**, 175
38. Comstock, C.H., Riggs, T., Lee, W. *et al.* (1991). Pulmonary-to-aorta diameter ratio in the normal and abnormal fetal heart. *Am. J. Obstet. Gynecol.*, **165**, 1038
39. Alpert, B.S., Mellitus, E.D. and Rowe, R.D. (1973). Spontaneous closure of small ventricular septal defects. Probability rates in the first five years of life. *Am J. Dis. Child.*, **125**, 194
40. Vlad, P. (1989). Tricuspid atresia. In Keith, J.D., Rowe, R.D. and Vlad, P. (eds.) *Heart Disease in Infants Children and Adolescents*, 4th edn., p. 348. (Baltimore: Williams and Wilkins)
41. Benacerraf, B.R., Saltzman, D.H. and Sanders, S.P. (1989). Sonographic signs suggesting the prenatal diagnosis of coarctation of the aorta. *J. Ultrasound Med.*, **8**, 65
42. Blake, D.M., Copel, J.A. and Kleinman, C.S. (1991). Hypoplastic left heart syndrome: prenatal diagnosis, clinical profile, and management. *Am. J. Obstet. Gynecol.*, **165**, 529
43. Veille, J.C., Mahowald, M.B. and Sivakoff, M. (1989). Ethical dilemmas in fetal echocardiography. *Obstet. Gynecol.*, **73**, 710
44. Baily, L.L. and Gundry, S.R. (1990). Hypoplastic left heart syndrome. *Pediatr. Clin. N. Am.*, **37**, 137
45. DeVore, G.R., Siassi, B. and Platt, L.D. (1988). Fetal echocardiography VIII. Aortic root dilation – a marker for tetralogy of Fallot. *Am. J. Obstet. Gynecol.*, **159**, 129
46. Ebert, P.A., Turley, K. and Stranger, P. *et al.* (1984). Surgical treatment of truncus arteriosus in the first 6 months of life. *Ann. Surg.*, **200**, 451
47. Berger, T.J., Blackstone, E.H., Kirklin, J.W. *et al.* (1979). Survival and probability of cure without and with operation in complete atrioventricular canal. *Ann. Thorac. Surg.*, **27**, 104
48. Spray, T.L., Maron, A.G., Morrow, A.G. *et al.* (1978). Clinical pathologic conference. Discussion on hypertrophic cardiomyopathy. *Am. Heart J.*, **95**, 511
49. Stocker, J.T., Modewell, J.E. and Grake, R.M. (1977). Congenital cystic adenomatoid malformation: classification and morphologic spectrum. *Hum. Pathol.*, **8**, 155
50. Green, W.K., Bors-Koefoed, R., Pollack, P. *et al.* (1991). Antepartum diagnosis and management of multiple cardiac tumors. *J. Ultrasound Med.*, **10**, 697
51. Cassidy, S. (1984). Tuberous sclerosis in children: diagnosis and course. *Comprehens. Ther.*, **101**, 43
52. Veille, J.C. and Sivakoff, M. (1988). Fetal echocardiographic signs of congenital endocardial fibroelastosis. *Obstet. Gynecol.*, **72**, 219
53. Jacobsen, R.I., Meyer, R.A., Miodovnik, M. *et al.* (1991). Prenatal diagnosis of fetal left ventricular aneurysm: a case report and review. *Obstet. Gynecol.*, **78**, 525
54. DiSessa, T.G., Emerson, D.S., Felker, R.E. *et al.* (1990). Anomalous systemic and pulmonary venous pathways diagnosed *in utero* by ultrasound. *J. Ultrasound Med.*, **9**, 311
55. Horenstein, J., DeVore, G.R., Platt, L.D. *et al.* (1991). The use of fetal echocardiography for predicting intrapartum fetal heart rate patterns in the post-term fetus. *Ultrasound Obstet. Gynecol.*, **1**, 395
56. Hansmann, M., Gembruch, U., Bald, M. *et al.* (1991). Transplacental and direct treatment of the fetus – a report of 60 cases. *Ultrasound Obstet. Gynecol.*, **1**, 162
57. Farrant, P. (1988). The antenatal diagnosis of oesophageal atresia by ultrasound. *Br. J. Radiol.*, **53**, 1202
58. Mariona, F., McAlpin, G., Zador, I., Philippart, A. and Jafri, S.Z.H. (1986). Sonographic detection of fetal extrathoracic pulmonary sequestration. *J. Ultrasound Med.*, **5**, 283
59. Thibeault, D.W., Beatty, E.C., Hall, R.T. *et al.* (1985). Neonatal pulmonary hypoplasia with premature rupture of membranes and oligohydramnios. *J. Pediatr.*, **107**, 273
60. Chitkara, U., Rosenburg, J., Chervenak, F.A. *et al.* (1987). Prenatal sonographic assessment of the fetal thorax: normal values. *Am. J. Obstet. Gynecol.*, **156**, 1069
61. Fong, K., Ohlsson, A. and Zaber, A. (1988). Fetal thoracic circumference: a prospective cross sectional study with real time ultrasound. *Am. J. Obstet. Gynecol.*, **158**, 1154
62. Vintzileos, A.M., Campbell, W.A., Rodis, J.F. *et al.* (1989). Comparison of six different ultra-

sonographic methods for predicting lethal fetal pulmonary hypoplasia. *Am. J. Obstet. Gynecol.*, **161**, 606

63. Sabbagha, E.R. and Comstock, C.H. (1993). Abnormalities of the gastrointestinal system. In Sabbagha, R.E. (ed.) *Ultrasound Applied to Obstetrics and Gynecology*, 3rd edn., (Philadelphia: J.B. Lippincott)

64. Harrison, M.R., Adzick, N.S., Longaker, M.I. *et al.* (1990). Successful repair of a fetal diaphragmatic hernia after removal of herniated viscera from the left thorax. *N. Engl. J. Med.*, **322**, 1582

65. Wenstrom, K.D., Weiner, C.P. and Hanson, J.W. (1991). A five-year statewide experience with congenital diaphragmatic hernia. *Am. J. Obstet. Gynecol.*, **165**, 838

66. Nelson, L.H., Clark, C.E., Fishburne, J.I. *et al.* (1982). Value of serial sonography in the *in utero* detection of duodenal atresia. *Obstet. Gynecol.*, **59**, 657

67. Paulson, E.K. and Hertzberg, B.S. (1991). Hyperechoic meconium in the third trimester fetus: an uncommon normal variant. *J. Ultrasound Med.*, **10**, 677

68. Pretorius, D., Budorick, N., Cahill, T. *et al.* (1992). Mid-trimester echogenic bowel and chromosomal abnormalities. SPO abstract 20. *Am. J. Obstet. Gynecol.*, **166**, 283

69. Benacerraf, B.R., Saltzman, D.H., Esteroff, J.A. and Frigoletto, F.D. (1990). Abnormal karyotype of fetuses with omphalocele: prediction based on omphalocele contents. *Obstet. Gynecol.*, **75**, 317

70. Nyberg, D.A.S., Fitzsimmons, J., Mack, L.A., Hughes M Pretorius, D.H., Hickok, D. and Shepard, T.H. (1989). Chromosomal abnormalities in fetuses with omphalocele: significance of omphalocele contents. *J. Ultrasound Med.*, **8**, 299

71. Green, J.J. and Hobbins, J.C. (1988). Abdominal ultrasound examination of the first trimester fetus. *Am. J. Obstet. Gynecol.*, **159**, 165

72. Gray, D.L., Martin, C.M. and Crane, J.P. (1989). Differential diagnosis of first trimester ventral wall defect. *J. Ultrasound Med.*, **8**, 255

73. Kirk, P.E. and Wah, R.M. (1983). Obstetric management of the fetus with omphalocele or gastroschisis: a review and report of 112 cases. *Am. J. Obstet. Gynecol.*, **146**, 512

74. Sipes, S.L., Weiner, C.P., Sipes II, D.R., Grant, S.S. and Williamson, R.A. (1990). Gastroschisis and omphalocele: does either antenatal diagnosis or route of delivery make a difference in perinatal outcome? *Obstet. Gynecol.*, **76**, 19557

75. Evans, M.I., Sacks, A.J., Johnson, P.M. *et al.* (1991). Sequential invasive assessment of fetal renal function and the intrauterine treatment of fetal obstructive uropathies. *Obstet. Gynecol.*, **77**, 545

76. Estes, J.M., Adzick, N.S. and Harrison, M.R. (1993). Antenatal open surgery for the abnormal fetus. In Sabbagha, R.E. (ed.) *Ultrasound Applied to Obstetrics and Gynecology*, 3rd edn. (Philadelphia, J.B. Lippincott)

77. Garris, J., Kangarloo, H., Sarti, D. *et al.* (1980). The ultrasound spectrum of prune-belly syndrome. *J. Clin. Ultrasound*, **8**, 117

78. Berdon, W.E., Baker, D.H., Blanc, W.A. *et al.* (1976). Megacystis–microcolon–intestinal hypoperistalsis syndrome: a new cause of intestinal obstruction in the new born. Report of radiologic findings in 5 newborn girls. *Am. J. Radiol.*, **126**, 957

79. Vintzileos, A.M., Eisenfeld, L.I., Herson, V.C. *et al.* (1986). Megacystis–microcolon–hyperistalsis syndrome – prenatal sonographic findings and review of the literature. *Am. J. Perinatol.*, **3**, 297

80. Penman, D.G. and Lilford, R.J. (1989). The megacysitis–microcolon–intestinal hypoperistalsis syndrome: a fatal recessive condition. *J. Med. Genet.*, **26**, 66

81. Young, I.D., Mckeever, P.A., Brown, L.A. *et al.* (1989). Prenatal diagnosis of the megacystis–microcolon–intestinal hypoperistalsis syndrome. *J. Med. Genet.*, **26**, 403

82. Antonakopoulos, G.N., Fuggle, W.J., Newman, J. *et al.* (1985). Idiopathic hydronephrosis. *Arch. Path. Lab. Med.*, **109**, 1097

83. Hoddick, W.K., Kogan, B.A., Jeffry, R.B. *et al.* (1985). Minimal fetal renal pyelectasis. *J. Ultrasound Med.*, **4**, 85

84. Corteville, J.E., Gray, D.L. and Crane, J.P. (1991). Congenital hydronephrosis: correlation of fetal ultrasonographic findings with infant outcome. *Am. J. Obstet. Gynecol.*, **165**, 384

85. Wickstrom, E.A., Maizels, M., Sabbagha, R.E. *et al.* (1994). Prenatal detection of dilation of the fetal urinary tract: analysis of prognostic factors for postnatal outcome. Personal communication

86. Benacerraf, B.R., Mandell, J., Estroff, J.A. *et al.* (1990). Fetal pyelectasis: a possible association with Down syndrome. *Obstet. Gynecol.*, **76**, 5855

87. Carter, C.O. (1984). The genetics of urinary tract malformations. *J. Genet. Hum.*, **32**, 23

88. Jeanty, P., Romero, R., Kepple, D. *et al.* (1990). Prenatal diagnosis in unilateral empty renal fossa. *J. Ultrasound Med.*, **9**, 651
89. Romero, R., Cullen, M., Grannum, P. *et al.* (1985). Antenatal diagnosis of renal anomalies with ultrasound. III. Bilateral renal agenesis. *Am. J. Obstet. Gynecol.*, **151**, 38
90. Sabbagha, R.E. (1993). Renal abnormalities. In Sabbagha, R.E. (ed.) *Ultrasound Applied to Obstetrics and Gynecology*, 3rd edn. (Philadelphia, J.B. Lippincott)
91. Grannum, P., Bracken, M., Silverman, R. and Hobbins, J.C. (1980). Assessment of fetal kidney size in normal gestation by comparison of ratio of kidney circumference to abdominal circumference. *Am. J. Obstet. Gynecol.*, **136**, 249
92. Simpson, J.L., Sabbagha, R.E., Elias, S. *et al.* (1982). Failure to detect polycystic kidneys *in utero* by second trimester ultrasonography. *Hum. Genet.*, **60**, 295
93. Pretorius, D.H., Lee, E., Manco-Johnson, M.L. *et al.* (1987). Diagnosis of autosomal dominant kidney disease *in utero* in the young infant. *J. Ultrasound Med.*, **6**, 249
94. Potter, E.L. (1972). *Type II Cystic Kidney: Early Ampullary Inhibition in Normal and Abnormal Development of the Kidney*, p. 154. (Chicago: Year Book Publishers)
95. Macken, M.B., Granmyre, E.B. and Vincer, M.J. (1989). Regression of nuchal cystic hygroma *in utero*. *J. Ultrasound Med.*, **8**, 101
96. Salerno, A.P. (1985). Fetal sacrococcygeal teratoma. *Perspect. Probl. Obstet. Gynecol.*, **1**, 3
97. Smith, D.W. (1976). *Recognizable Patterns of Human Malformation.* (Philadelphia: W.B. Saunders)
98. Sabbagha, R.E., Toig, R.M. and Sheikh, Z. (1993). Skeletal abnormalities. In Sabbagha, R.E. (ed.) *Ultrasound Applied to Obstetrics and Gynecology*, 3rd edn. (Philadelphia: J.B. Lippincott)

Maternal adaptation to multifetal pregnancy

18

S.N. MacGregor and R.K. Silver

Introduction

Maternal adaptation to pregnancy is initiated by the production of protein and steroid hormones by the fetus and the placenta. These changes begin shortly after conception and continue throughout gestation. The scope of these adaptations are particularly profound, considering the relatively short span of pregnancy in humans. Whereas an understanding of most physiological adaptations to singleton pregnancies has increased in recent years, the unique physiological circumstances of multifetal gestation are as yet not thoroughly understood. In this chapter, we review available data regarding the adaptation of the major maternal organ systems to multifetal pregnancy.

Cardiovascular system

Plasma volume

The maternal plasma volume begins to increase during the first trimester, expands most rapidly during the second trimester, rises at a much slower rate during the third trimester and finally plateaus during the last weeks prior to delivery. The degree of plasma volume expansion varies considerably from patient to patient. In singleton pregnancies, the plasma volume near term is approximately 45% above non-pregnant levels[1,2]. However, in one study comparing singleton and twin pregnancies with a dye technique (Figures 1 and 2), plasma volume nearly doubled in twin pregnancies compared to non-pregnant levels, and was greater in multiparous compared to primiparous patients[3].

It is probable that the increased rates of aldosterone and mineralocorticosteroid secretions are important in the plasma volume expansion that accompanies pregnancy. Not only do the maternal adrenal glands secrete increased amounts of aldosterone[4], but the maternal serum levels of renin and angiotensin II substrate also increase, especially during the latter half of pregnancy. These last two hormones in all probability account for the markedly elevated secretion of aldosterone[5]. In addition, the maternal levels of deoxycorticosterone increase markedly as a result of the peripheral 20-hydroxylation of progesterone in maternal tissues[6,7]. It has been suggested that the increased secretion of aldosterone affords protection against the natriuretic affects of progesterone and atrial natriuretic peptides which are also increased during pregnancy[8,9].

Blood pressure and regional blood flow

In pregnant women, arterial blood pressure is markedly affected by changes in posture. Typically, arterial blood pressure is lowest in the lateral recumbent position, intermediate in the supine position, and highest when the woman is sitting. In contrast, diastolic blood pressures are lower in pregnant compared to non-pregnant women. Diastolic blood pressures generally are lowest during mid-pregnancy and increase slightly during the latter stages[10]. The systolic blood pressure decreases, although to a lesser degree than diastolic blood pressure. As is the case with diastolic pressures, systolic

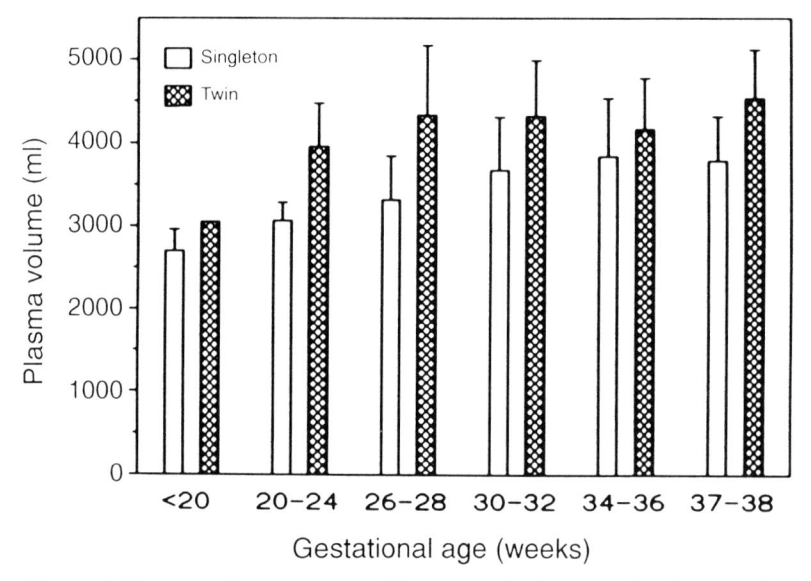

Figure 1 Plasma volume compared between singleton and twin gestations among primigravid women (adapted from reference 3)

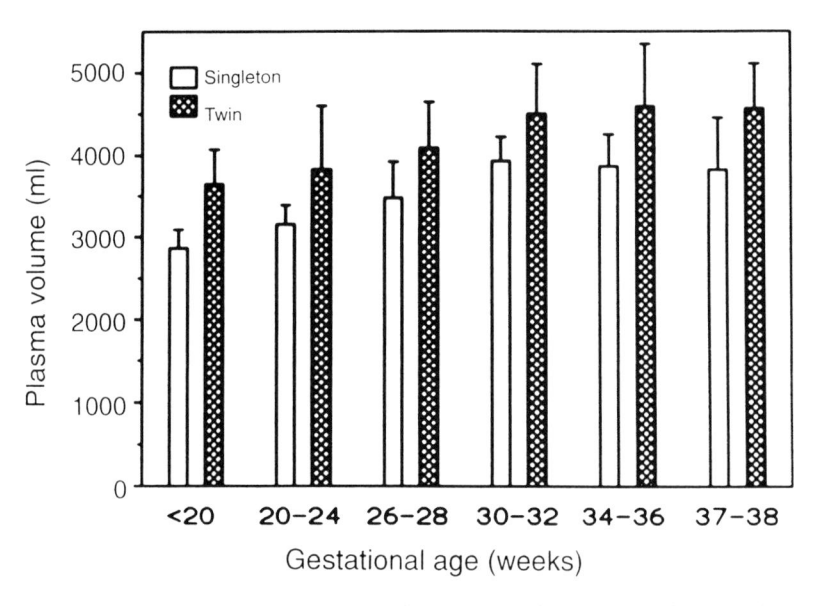

Figure 2 Plasma volume compared between singleton and twin gestations among multigravid women (adapted from reference 3)

blood pressure increases slightly during the latter portion of pregnancy.

It is surprising that blood pressures normally decrease during pregnancy, despite considerable increase in the formation of aldosterone, deoxycorticosterone and angiotensin II. Pressor responsiveness to angiotensin II and the renin–angiotensin–aldosterone system is markedly altered in pregnant women compared to non-pregnant women[11,12]. This blunted pressor response to angiotensin II is not observed in women destined to develop pre-eclampsia. It is likely that the refractoriness to angiotensin II is mediated, in part, by prostaglandin related substances (produced by the vascular endothelium), in addition to the influence of progesterone[13,14].

Campbell and Campbell found that the reduction in diastolic blood pressure in mid-pregnancy (compared to non-pregnant levels) was greater in twin than singleton pregnancies[15]. Similar observations were not made for systolic blood pressure, however. This study additionally demonstrated that twin pregnancies exhibited a greater increase in diastolic pressure near term compared to singleton pregnancies. Despite lower diastolic pressures in mid-pregnancy, pre-eclampsia occurs with greater frequency in twin compared to singleton pregnancies for reasons that are presently unclear[15,16].

Placental perfusion by maternal blood is dependent upon blood flow to the uterus through the uterine and ovarian arteries. Adequate placental perfusion of the intervillous space is essential for growth and metabolism of the fetus(es) and placenta(s). During pregnancy, uteroplacental blood flow increases progressively. The average uteroplacental blood flow in singleton pregnancies is approximately 500 ml/min in the late third trimester[17,18] but this value is certainly higher in twin gestations. Among individual patients, the intervillous and myometrial blood flow varies appreciably[19]. In addition, appreciable changes in intervillous and myometrial blood flow are induced by changes in body position[20]. In the third trimester, the large pregnant uterus compresses the venous system and impedes the return of blood from the lower half of the body. The retarded blood flow and increased lower extremity venous pressure both contribute to the development of dependent edema and varicose veins in the legs and vulva, as well as hemorrhoids. Venous distention secondary to uterine compression of the inferior vena cava is understandably greater in women with twin compared to singleton gestations and complications related to venous stasis are more common.

Compression of the venous system by the large pregnant uterus also reduces cardiac filling and, therefore, cardiac output. Venous compression by the uterus is greatest in the supine position and may be associated with significant arterial hypotension, occasionally referred to as the 'supine hypotensive syndrome'[21]. (Editor: Recently, it has also been shown that standing for prolonged periods of time creates essentially the same problem.) In the supine position, the enlarged uterus may compress the aorta sufficiently to reduce perfusion pressure in arteries located below the level of compression[22]. Measurements of the blood pressure in the brachial artery may not provide a reliable estimate of pressure in the uterine artery. Compression of the aorta by the uterus, especially in multiple gestations, increases the likelihood of reduced uterine arterial pressure and increases the risk of reduced uteroplacental blood flow following regional anesthesia.

Uterine contractions, either spontaneous or induced, cause a decrease in uteroplacental blood flow that is directly proportional to the intensity of the contraction[23]. Doppler velocimetry of the uterine artery, correlating these Doppler waveforms with intrauterine pressure readings, shows an almost linear correlation between pressure and decreased velocity[24]. It is likely that similar findings are observed in multiple gestations.

Cardiac function

The maternal heart is displaced to the left and upward as the diaphragm is progressively elevated during pregnancy. As a result, the cardiac silhouette appears increased in size on X-ray. Normal pregnancy induces no characteristic changes in the electrocardiogram other than a slight left axis deviation as a result of the altered position of the maternal heart. Cardiac size does not appear to be increased in twin pregnancies compared to singleton pregnancies. Thus, the susceptibility to cardiac arrhythmias is probably similar for both singleton and twin gestations.

Left ventricular wall mass and end-diastolic dimensions all increase during pregnancy, as does heart rate, calculated stroke volume and cardiac output[25]. In singleton pregnancies, there is little change in the inatropic state of the myocardium, and changes in stroke volume are directly proportional to the increase in end-diastolic volume.

In twin pregnancies, end-diastolic ventricular dimensions are comparable to those in singleton pregnancies. However, cardiac output is greater during twin than during singleton pregnancy. The increase in cardiac output in twin pregnancies results from greater increase in maternal heart rate and stroke volume. Increased stroke volume results from an increased inatropic effect as measured by increased fractional shortening of the ventricular diameters[26–28]. Not all studies support these observations in twin pregnancies, however. Campbell *et al.* suggested that neither stroke volume nor cardiac output are significantly different between twin and singleton pregnancies[29]. The increased maternal heart rate and contractility during twin gestations suggest that cardiovascular reserve is reduced. This possibility should be considered when recommending changes in maternal activity levels or when multiple gestation coexists with maternal cardiovascular conditions. In addition, cardiac output in response to physical activity is greatest late in pregnancy. During the first stage of labor, maternal cardiac output increases moderately, with appreciably greater increases in cardiac output occurring with vigorous expulsive efforts during the second stage of labor. During labor, a condition of reduced cardiovascular reserve, in combination with the reduced colloid osmotic pressure, may act synergistically to increase susceptibility to fluid overload, congestive heart failure and pulmonary edema, especially during the intrapartum and early postpartum periods.

Hematological profile

The total iron requirement for a normal singleton pregnancy equals about 1 g. This includes 300 mg actively transferred to the fetus and placenta, 200 mg representing obligatory losses, and the 500 mg of iron required for the increase in maternal red cell volume[30]. Transfer of iron to the fetus and placenta, as well as obligatory losses, occur even if the mother is iron-deficient. Iron absorption from the gastrointestinal tract is moderately increased[31]. The plasma iron-binding capacity or transferring level increases, probably as a result of increased levels of maternal estrogen[32]. Although these physiological changes are intended to help meet the increased iron requirements of normal pregnancy, many women require iron supplementation during the second half of pregnancy. Indeed, without supplemental iron therapy, bone marrow iron stores often decrease.

Folate requirements also increase during pregnancy. Megaloblastic anemia, characterized by the presence of macrocytosis with hypersegmentation of neutrophils, may occur secondary to folate deficiency. Whereas megaloblastic anemia is uncommon, reduced red cell folate levels and megaloblastic changes in the bone marrow are not uncommon during pregnancy[33]. The frequency of megaloblastic changes in the bone marrow is significantly reduced in singleton pregnancies by the addition of daily supplementation of 100 μg of folate[33].

Hall *et al.* evaluated peripheral blood and performed bone marrow aspiration in twin pregnancies[34]. Because iron deficiency anemia and megaloblastic anemia secondary to folate deficiency were uncommon, this study concluded that it was not necessary to prescribe prophylactic iron or folate to women with twin gestations in the absence of significant anemia. However, in this study bone marrow aspirates in twin pregnancies show deficient iron stores (40%) and megaloblastic changes (30%). In our opinion, the increased requirements for iron and folate in twin gestations, combined with the frequent observation of iron and folate deficiencies in the bone marrow of women with twin pregnancies, suggest that iron and folate supplementation during the second half of pregnancy in twin gestations are prudent.

Total red cell volume increases markedly in twin compared to singleton pregnancy[27,35] (Table 1). Despite the increase in red cell mass in both singleton and twin pregnancies, hemoglobin concentration decreases during pregnancy. The reduction in hemoglobin concentration is dilutional; plasma volume increases to a greater degree than total red cell volume.

Table 1 Total red cell volume in twin and singleton pregnancy

Gestational age (weeks)	Singleton red cell volume (ml)	Twin red cell volume (ml)
Primigravidae		
30	1732 ± 328	1944 ± 297
34	1694 ± 323	2037 ± 312
38	1797 ± 352	2272 ± 122
Multigravidae		
30	1612 ± 281	1897 ± 359
34	1710 ± 283	2097 ± 465
38	1677 ± 291	2042 ± 395

Adapted from reference 35

Maternal platelet counts also decrease moderately during pregnancy[36]. Although this decrease is also likely to be dilutional, it may be a consequence of increased platelet consumption. In contrast, many of the levels of blood coagulation factors are increased. Plasma fibrinogen increases approximately 50%, with a range of 300–600 mg/dl in later pregnancy. Other clotting factors which are increased include factor II, factor VII, factor VIII, factor IX and factor X. In contrast, factors XI and XIII are usually somewhat decreased[37].

The level of maternal plasminogen (profibrinolysin) in the plasma increases during pregnancy and results from elevated estrogen levels. However, plasmin or fibrinolytic activity is prolonged compared with that of the non-pregnant patient. It has been suggested that the placenta is responsible for the reduced fibrinolytic activity[38]. It is likely that these quantitative and functional changes in coagulation are similar in both singleton and twin gestations.

Pulmonary system

The level of the diaphragm rises during pregnancy. The subcostal angle widens and the thoracic circumference increases; however, these increases are insufficient to prevent reductions in the residual lung volume secondary to the elevated diaphragm[39]. In twin pregnancies, it is likely that the level of the diaphragm rises higher than the normal 4 cm observed in singleton pregnancy, resulting in further reduction in the pulmonary residual volume. Because diaphragmatic excursion is greater during pregnancy compared to the non-pregnant state, the tidal volume increases. It has been suggested that tidal volume increases to a greater degree in twin gestations compared to singleton gestations[40].

Oxygen consumption increases, primarily due to fetal and placental oxygen consumption. It must be assumed that oxygen consumption would be further increased in twin pregnancies, as the result of increased fetal and placental mass. However, the amount of oxygen delivered by increased tidal volume exceeds the oxygen need imposed by the pregnancy. In addition, cardiac output increases, as does the total oxygen-carrying capacity (resulting from increased maternal red cell mass). Therefore, maternal arteriovenous oxygen difference is decreased during pregnancy.

Ventilatory volume and minute oxygen uptake increase as pregnancy progresses. In contrast, the respiratory rate, maximum breathing capacity and vital capacity are changed little. As mentioned above, residual volume, as well as functional residual capacity, are decreased as a consequence of elevation of the diaphragm. Table 2 summarizes the resting pulmonary function parameters during pregnancy[41].

Table 2 Resting pulmonary function tests in pregnancy

Function	Non-pregnant	Pregnant	% Change
Respiratory rate	15	16	—
Tidal volume (ml)	487	678	+39
Minute ventilation (ml)	7270	10 340	+42
Vital capacity	3260	3310	—
Maximum breathing capacity (predicted; %)	102	97	—
Inspiratory capacity (ml)	2625	2745	—
Residual volume (ml)	965	770	−20

Adapted from reference 41

The increased respiratory effort results in a reduction of pCO_2 during pregnancy. This hyperventilatory state appears to be hormonally mediated, primarily by increased progesterone levels. Progesterone increases respiratory drive, an action that is probably centrally mediated through a direct stimulatory effect on the medullary respiratory center[42]. In twin pregnancies, the effect of increased progesterone levels on pulmonary function is unknown; however, it seems likely that these increased levels could lead to further stimulation of the respiratory center.

Urinary system

Anatomic changes

The maternal kidneys increase slightly in size during pregnancy[43]. This increase may, in part, result from increased cardiac output, and the concomitant augmentation in blood flow to the kidneys. The enlarging uterus compresses the ureters as they enter the pelvis. The degree of this compression increases with advancing gestational age. Typically, ureteral dilatation is more marked on the right side[44]. Increased intraureteral tone above the level of the pelvic compression may be associated with mild hydronephrosis[45]. An additional mechanism causing hydronephrosis and hydroureter is the effect of progesterone, dilating the smooth muscle of the renal collecting system[46]. The observation of hydronephrosis and hydroureter in a donor kidney after transplantation to the iliac fossae supports such a hormonal mechanism. Both obstruction of the ureters by enlargement of the uterus and relaxation of the renal collecting system as a result of increased progesterone levels are exaggerated during twin pregnancy. It has been suggested that dilatation of the urinary collecting system and urine stasis increase the risk of upper urinary tract infection[47]. The presumed greater extent of dilatation of the collecting system in twin gestations may likewise be associated with a higher risk of urinary tract infections; however, such an increased risk of infection in twin gestations has not been confirmed[48].

The urinary bladder trigone becomes elevated and its posterior margin thickened as the uterus enlarges and the surrounding pelvic tissues undergo hyperplasia. By the end of pregnancy, there is a marked deepening and widening of the bladder trigone, and the bladder pressure doubles[49]. To compensate for reduced bladder capacity and to preserve continence, both urethral length and maximal urethral pressure increase with advancing gestation. At the end of pregnancy, the pressure of the presenting fetal part impairs drainage of blood and lymph from the base of the bladder. This process often results in edema and an increased susceptibility to infection. Following vaginal delivery, the urethral pressure and length are reduced, potentially contributing to the pathogenesis of urinary stress incontinence[50]. It is likely that the changes in the urinary bladder are similar for both singleton and twin gestations.

Modifications in renal function

The glomerular filtration rate (GFR) and renal plasma flow begin to increase early in pregnancy with the highest rates of increase in the first and early second trimester. The GFR increases nearly 50% above non-pregnant levels by 20 weeks' gestation; the rate of increase slows markedly, with no more than an additional 10% increase during the remainder of pregnancy[51,52]. Renal plasma flow increases to approximately 35% above non-pregnant levels, reaching a maximum in the second trimester and decreasing slightly near term. As is the case with cardiac output, renal plasma flow varies late in pregnancy with changes in posture. Cardiac output is increased in twin pregnancies compared to singleton pregnancies and these changes may influence renal function. It has been suggested that GFR and renal plasma flow are greater in twin compared to singleton pregnancy[40]. The greater enlargement of the uterus associated with twin pregnancy could conceivably enhance changes in GFR and renal plasma flow observed with changes in posture.

The filtered sodium load is increased during pregnancy, as is the tubular reabsorption of sodium. The management of sodium by the kidney is intricately involved in the fluid balance during pregnancy. Numerous factors promote sodium excretion (e.g. increased GFR, increased progesterone levels, increased antidiuretic hormone and decreased systemic vascular resistance), whereas additional factors tend to decrease sodium excretion (e.g. increased levels of aldosterone, cortisol, placental lactogen, estrogen and prolactin). In addition, the supine position may decrease sodium excretion by more than 50%. The plasma sodium concentration decreases only slightly in pregnancy, primarily as a result of water retention and a slight excess of solute. The mechanisms for these changes are unclear, but the nature of these changes are probably quite similar in singleton and multiple gestation.

Gastrointestinal system

Anatomic and functional changes

The stomach and intestines are increasingly displaced by the enlarging uterus as the pregnancy progresses. The significance of positional changes in the viscera is that physical findings in certain disease states may be altered. The appendix, for example, is displaced upward and lateral as the uterus enlarges, potentially confusing the diagnosis of acute appendicitis. In addition to displacement, the motility and tone of the gastrointestinal tract are reduced, gastric emptying is delayed and intestinal transit time is prolonged. The decreased tone and motility result from increased progesterone levels. Delayed gastric emptying, especially during labor, increases the likelihood of aspiration during general anesthesia. Pyrosis or heartburn is common, resulting from reflux of acid secretions into the lower esophagus. Delayed gastric emptying, altered position of the stomach, and reduced esophageal sphincter tone predispose to gastroesophageal reflux. Hemorrhoids are also common. Apart from a congenital predisposition, the cause of hemorrhoids probably relates to elevated venous pressure resulting from vessel compression by the enlarged uterus, as well as constipation from reduced gastrointestinal tone and motility with delayed intestinal transit time. It is likely that the frequency of these complications is greater in twin compared to singleton pregnancies, since progesterone levels are increased in twin pregnancies.

Hepatic and biliary function

The liver undergoes no morphological changes during pregnancy. However, functional changes occur. In particular, plasma albumin concentrations decrease, and serum globulin concentration increases slightly[53]. These changes result in a decrease in the albumin to globulin ratio, similar to that observed in certain liver diseases. Alkaline phosphatase activity doubles, primarily as a result of increased production by the placenta, in addition to a lesser contribution by the liver itself[54]. Plasma cholinesterase activity is reduced, and leucine amniopeptase activity is markedly elevated during pregnancy compared to non-pregnant values[54,55]. The significance of these changes is unknown. However, reduced plasma cholinesterase activity may be significant in women abusing cocaine, because levels of this drug may be maintained at higher concentrations for prolonged periods of time as a result of decreased metabolism[54].

The biliary tract also demonstrates delayed emptying during pregnancy. The gall bladder may be distended and somewhat hypotonic, with thickened biliary secretions[56]. Decreased gall bladder motility and thickening of the biliary secretions predispose to cholelithiasis. The differences in liver and biliary function between singleton and multiple pregnancy have not been elucidated.

Summary

Maternal adaptation to multifetal pregnancy results in profound physiological changes within a short period of time. In general, the maternal response to multifetal pregnancy is similar to that of singleton pregnancy; however, the magnitude of the respective changes is often exaggerated. These exaggerated physiological responses are of enormous potential clinical significance in the management of multifetal pregnancy.

References

1. Pritchard, J.A. (1965). Changes in the blood volume during pregnancy and delivery. *Anesthesiology*, **26**, 393
2. Ueland, K. (1976). Maternal cardiovascular dynamics: VII. Intrapartum blood volume changes. *Am. J. Obstet. Gynecol.*, **126**, 671
3. MacGillivray, I. and Campbell, D.M. (1977). Maternal physiological responses and birthweight in singleton and twin pregnancies by parity. *Eur. J. Obstet. Gynecol. Reprod. Biol.*, **7**, 17
4. Watanbe, M., Meeker, C.I., Gray, M.J. *et al.* (1963). Secretion rate of aldosterone in normal pregnancy. *J. Clin. Invest.*, **42**, 1619
5. Geelhoed, G.W. and Vander, A.J. (1968). Plasma renin activities during pregnancy and parturition. *J. Clin. Endocrinol.*, **28**, 412
6. Nolten, W.E., Lindheimer, M.D., Oparil, S. and Ehrlich, E.N. (1978). Desoxycorticosterone in pregnancy: I. Sequential studies of the secretory patterns of desoxycorticosterone, aldosterone and cortisol. *Am. J. Obstet. Gynecol.*, **132**, 414
7. Winkel, C.A., Parker, C.R. Jr, Milewich, L., Simpson, E.R., Gant, N.F. and MacDonald, P.C. (1980). The conversion of plasma progesterone to desoxycorticosterone (DOC) in men, nonpregnant and pregnant women, and adrenalectomized subjects: evidence for steroid 21-hydroxylase activity in non-adrenal tissues. *J. Clin. Invest.*, **66**, 803
8. Landau, R.L. and Lugibihl, K. (1961). The catabolic and natriuretic effects of progesterone in man. *Rec. Prog. Horm. Res.*, **17**, 249
9. Sagnella, G.A., Markandu, N.D., Shore, A.C. and MacGregor, G.A. (1985). Effects of changes in dietary sodium intake and saline infusion on immunoreactive atrial natriuretic peptide in human plasma. *Lancet*, **1**, 1208
10. Wilson, M., Morganti, A.A., Zervoudakis, J. *et al.* (1980). Blood pressure, the renin–aldosterone system and sex steroids throughout normal pregnancy. *Am. J. Med.*, **68**, 97
11. Gant, N.F., Daley, G.L., Chand, S., Whalley, P.J. and MacDonald, P.C. (1974). The nature of pressor responsiveness to angiotensin II in human pregnancy. *Obstet. Gynecol.*, **43**, 854
12. Chesley, L.C. (1978). Renin, angiotensin, and aldosterone in pregnancy. In Chesley, L.C. (ed.) *Hypertensive Disorders in Pregnancy*, p. 236. (New York: Appleton-Century-Crofts)
13. Broughton-Pipkin, F. and Meirelles, R.S. (1982). Prostaglandin E2 attenuates the pressor response to angiotensin II in pregnant subjects but not in nonpregnant subjects. *Am. J. Obstet. Gynecol.*, **142**, 168
14. Everett, R.B., Worley, R.J., MacDonald, P.C. and Gant, N.F. (1978). Modification of vascular responsiveness to angiotensin II in pregnant women by intravenously infused 5α-dihydroprogesterone. *Am. J. Obstet. Gynecol.*, **131**, 352
15. Campbell, A.J. and Campbell, D.M. (1985). Arterial blood pressure – the pattern of change in twin pregnancies. *Acta Genet. Med. Gemellol.*, **34**, 217
16. MacGillivray, I. (1988). Some observations on the incidence of pre-eclampsia. *J. Obstet. Gynaecol. Br. Emp.*, **65**, 536
17. Blechner, J.N., Stenger, V.G. and Prystowsky, H. (1975). Blood flow to the human uterus during maternal metabolic acidosis. *Am. J. Obstet. Gynecol.*, **121**, 789
18. Metcalfe, J., Romney, S.L., Ramsey, L.H., Reid, D.E. and Burwell, C.S. (1955). Estimation of uterine blood flow in normal human pregnancy at term. *J. Clin. Invest.*, **34**, 1632
19. Rekonen, A., Luotola, H., Pitkanen, M., Kuikka, J. and Pyorala, M. (1976). Measurement of intervillous and myometrial blood flow by an intravenous Xe method. *Br. J. Obstet. Gynaecol.*, **83**, 723
20. Kauppila, A., Koskinen, M., Puolakka, J., Tuimala, R. and Kuikka, J. (1980). Decreased intervillous and unchanged myometrial blood flow spinal recumbency. *Obstet. Gynecol.*, **55**, 203
21. Howard, B.K., Goodson, J.H. and Mengert, W.F. (1953). Supine hypotensive syndrome in late pregnancy. *Obstet. Gynecol.*, **1**, 371
22. Bieniarz, J., Branda, L.A., Mqueda, E., Morozovsky, J. and Caldeyro-Barcia, R. (1968). Aortocaval compression by the uterus in late

pregnancy: III. Unreliability of the sphygmomanometric method in estimating uterine artery pressure. *Am. J. Obstet. Gynecol.*, **102**, 1106
23. Assali, N.S., Dilts, P.V., Pentl, A.A., Kirschbaum, T.H. and Gross, S.J. (1968). Physiology of the placenta. In Assali, N.S. (ed.) *Biology of Gestation*, vol. I. *The Maternal Organism.* (New York: Academic Press)
24. Janbu, T. and Nesheim, B.-I. (1987). Uterine artery blood velocities during contraction in pregnancy and labour related to intrauterine pressure. *Br. J. Obstet. Gynaecol.*, **94**, 1150
25. Katz, R., Karliner, J.S. and Resnik, R. (1978). Effects of a natural volume overload state (pregnancy) on left ventricular performance in normal human subjects. *Circulation*, **58**, 434
26. Veille, J.C., Morton, M.J. and Burry, K.J. (1985). Maternal cardiovascular adaptations to twin pregnancy. *Am. J. Obstet. Gynecol.*, **153**, 261
27. Rovinsky, J.J. and Jaffin, H. (1966). Cardiovascular hemodynamics in pregnancy. II. Cardiac output and left ventricular work in multiple pregnancy. *Am. J. Obstet. Gynecol.*, **95**, 781
28. Rovinsky, J.J. and Jaffin, H. (1966). Cardiovascular hemodynamics in pregnancy. III. Cardiac rate, stroke volume, total peripheral resistance, and central blood volume in multiple pregnancy. Synthesis results. *Am. J. Obstet. Gynecol.*, **95**, 787
29. Campbell, D.M., Haites, N., MacLennan, F. and Rawles, J. (1985). Cardiac output in twin pregnancy. *Acta Genet. Med. Gemellol.*, **34**, 225
30. Widdowson, E.M. and Sprag, C.M. (1951). Chemical development *in utero*. *Arch. Dis. Child.*, **26**, 205
31. Hahn, P.F., Carothers, E.L., Darby, W.J., Martin, M., Sheppard, C.W., Cannor, R.O., Beam, A.S., Densen, P.M., Peterson, J.C. and McClellan, G.S. (1951). Iron metabolism in human pregnancy as studied with the radioactive isotope FE. *Am. J. Obstet. Gynecol.*, **61**, 477
32. Sturgeon, P. (1959). Studies of iron requirements in infants: III. Influence of supplemental iron during normal pregnancy on mother and infant: A. The mother. *Br. J. Haematol.*, **5**, 31
33. Chanarin, I., Rothman, D., Ward, A. and Perry, J. (1968). Folate status and requirement in pregnancy. *Br. Med. J.*, **2**, 390
34. Hall, M.H., Campbell, D.M. and Davidson, R.J. (1979). Anaemia in twin pregnancy. *Acta Genet. Med. Gemellol.*, **28**, 279
35. MacGillivray, I., Campbell, D.M. and Duffus, G.M. (1971). Maternal metabolic response to twin pregnancy in primigravidae. *Br. J. Obstet. Gynaecol.*, **78**, 530
36. Pitkin, R.M. and Witte, D.L. (1980). Platelet and leukocyte counts in pregnancy. *J. Am. Med. Assoc.*, **242**, 2696
37. Coopland, A., Alkjaersig, N. and Fletcher, A.P. (1969). Reduction in plasma factor XIII (fibrin stabilization factor) concentration during pregnancy. *J. Lab. Clin. Med.*, **73**, 144
38. Astedt, B. (1972). Significance of placenta in depression of fibrinolytic activity during pregnancy. *J. Obstet. Gynaecol. Br. Commonw.*, **79**, 205
39. Mobius, W.V. (1961). Abrung und Schwangerschaft. *Munchener Med. Woschr.*, **103**, 1389
40. MacGillivray, I. (1975). Physiologic changes in twin pregnancy. In MacGillivray, I., Nylander, P.P.S. and Corney, G. (eds.) *Human Multiple Reproduction*, p. 107. (London: W.B. Saunders)
41. Cugell, D.W., Frank, N.R., Gaensler, E.A. and Badger, T.L. (1953). Pulmonary function in pregnancy. I. Serial observations in normal women. *J. TB*, **67**, 568–97
42. Sutton, F.D., Zwillich, C.W., Creagh, E., Pierson, D.J. and Wiel, J.V. (1975). Progesterone for outpatient treatment of Pickwickian Syndrome. *Ann. Intern. Med.*, **83**, 476
43. Bailey, R.R. and Rolleston, G.L. (1971). Kidney length and ureteric dilatation in the puerperium. *J. Obstet. Gynaecol. Br. Commonw.*, **78**, 55
44. Peake, S.L., Roxburgh, H.B. and Langlois, S.L.P. (1983). Ultrasonic assessment of hydronephrosis of pregnancy. *Radiology*, **146**, 167
45. Rubi, R.A. and Sala, N.L. (1968). Ureteral function in pregnant women: III. Effect of different positions and of fetal delivery upon ureteral tonus. *Am. J. Obstet. Gynecol.*, **101**, 230
46. Van Wagenen, G. and Jenkins, R.H. (1939). An experimental examination of factors causing ureteral dilatation of pregnancy. *J. Urol.*, **42**, 1010
47. Cunningham, F.G. (1987). Urinary tract infections complicating pregnancy. *Clin. Obstet. Gynaecol. (Ballières)*, **1**, 891
48. Guttmacker, A.F. (1939). An analysis of 573 cases of twin pregnancy. *Am. J. Obstet. Gynecol.*, **38**, 277
49. Iosif, S., Ingemarsson, I. and Ulmsten, U. (1980). Urodynamic studies in normal pregnancy and the puerperium. *Am. J. Obstet. Gynecol.*, **137**, 696

50. Van Wagenen, G. and Jenkins, R.H. (1939). An experimental examination of factors causing ureteral dilatation of pregnancy. *J. Urol.*, **42**, 1010
51. Chesley, L.C. (1963). Renal function during pregnancy. In Carey, H.M. (ed.) *Modern Trends in Human Reproductive Physiology*. (London: Butterworth)
52. Dunlop, W. (1981). Serial changes in renal haemodynamics during normal pregnancy. *Br. J. Obstet. Gynaecol.*, **88**, 1
53. Mendenhall, H.W. (1970). Serum protein concentrations in pregnancy. 1. Concentrations in maternal serum. *Am. J. Obstet. Gynecol.*, **106**, 388
54. Song, C.S. and Kappas, A. (1968). The influence of estrogens, progestins and pregnancy on the liver. *Vitam. Horm.*, **26**, 147
55. Kamban, J.R., Perry, S.M., Entman, S. and Smith, B.E. (1988). Effect of magnesium on plasma cholinesterase activity. *Am. J. Obstet. Gynecol.*, **159**, 309
56. Potter, M.G. (1936). Observations of the gall bladder and bile during pregnancy at term. *J. Am. Med. Assoc.*, **106**, 1070

Maternal clinical and biochemical changes

A.M. Peaceman

Introduction

The presence of more than one fetus alters numerous aspects of prenatal care. Twin gestations are at increased risk of preterm delivery, as well as fetal growth abnormalities, intrauterine demise, congenital anomalies and delivery complications, but intervention strategies aimed at decreasing these risks can be applied only if the presence of more than one fetus is known and appreciated.

The early diagnosis of multifetal gestation

The diagnosis of multifetal gestation was imprecise at best prior to the widespread use of antepartum ultrasound examinations. More than one fetus could be suspected if the uterine size appeared to be abnormally large for gestational age; however, such discrepancies could also be explained by an inaccurate assessment of gestational age, or the presence of excess amniotic fluid, fetal macrosomia, or a fetal anomaly. Accordingly, the discovery of a second fetus after the delivery of the first was not unusual. In 1955, Kurtz *et al.*[1] reported on 500 consecutive cases of twin gestation. Only 52.2% (261 sets) were diagnosed prior to entry into the delivery room. Isolated reports from the same era claimed higher rates of predelivery detection[2], but early diagnosis in the second trimester, when intervention strategies might have begun, was much less frequent as a rule. The experience at Northwestern University reported in 1980 was similar to that of Kurtz *et al.*, even though it was 20 years later and ultrasound was available, if not performed routinely. In almost half of the cases, the diagnosis of multiple gestation was made in the third trimester; in one-quarter of the cases, the diagnosis was made only after labor had begun or after the first twin had been delivered[3].

Efforts toward prenatal confirmation of the diagnosis of multifetal gestation began with radiological examinations, because radiographs could demonstrate more than one fetal skeleton, as well as their orientation. However, radiographs were often incorrect, as a second fetus could be missed if the study was performed prior to sufficient mineralization of the fetal skeleton (approximately 20 weeks' gestation). Other causes of missing the identification of a second twin on radiographic examinations included maternal obesity with inadequate tissue penetration, fetal movement during exposure, hydramnios, and inappropriately small fields of examination[4]. Radiographs for fetal position still have an occasional place in the intrapartum management of twin gestations, however, ultrasound examinations have all but replaced them as a means of diagnosis, not only because of their greater accuracy at all gestational ages but also because of safety concerns.

Another method of documenting twin gestation involves auscultation of fetal heart rates with baselines differing by more than 10 beats per minute. Such a finding can be confirmed by phonocardiography. As with radiological examination, however, this technique is only helpful if the diagnosis is already suspected clinically. Not infrequently, this method is associated with false positive (auscultation of the same fetus twice) and false negative (failing to appreciate a different rate for the second fetus) results. A variety of investigations have used biochemical parameters as screening tools for the detection of multifetal pregnancies, including hormone levels known to be elevated in multiple gestation. Although these methods have demonstrated reasonable sensitivity and specificity, they are not currently applied widely.

Today, the percentage of multiple gestations detected prior to labor varies directly with the degree to which ultrasound examinations are used. In centers where the majority of patients receive at least one obstetric sonogram, undiagnosed twins at the time of delivery are an unusual occurrence[5]. Even in situations where universal real-time ultrasound screening is routine, in the second trimester, a failure to diagnose a multiple gestation will occasionally occur, due to technical difficulties in the sonographic examination, or the patient not obtaining timely prenatal care[6].

Despite its usefulness, universal ultrasound examination is currently not advocated in the United States for all patients[7]. Indeed, in many clinical settings this diagnostic modality is not available or is under-used. For these patients, the antenatal detection of multiple gestations and selection of patients for confirmatory studies depends upon clinical findings. In this chapter, we review clinical signs related to the diagnosis of multiple gestations, as well as the alterations in biochemical parameters associated with twinning.

Clinical parameters of multiple gestation

The most commonly noted physical finding associated with multiple gestation is a discrepancy between uterine size and the purported age of gestation. This circumstance is predicated upon the correct assessment of gestational age; when gestational age is overestimated, a twin pregnancy may not appear inappropriately large. As measured from the top of the symphysis, the height of the uterine fundus in centimeters will approximate the weeks of gestation in normally growing singleton pregnancies from 18 to 34 weeks[8]. When the fundal height measurement (in centimeters) exceeds the gestational age in weeks by more than two, the uterus may be overly enlarged. Other than multiple gestation, additional causes of a large uterine measurement include hydramnios, fetal macrosomia, fetal malformations, uterine myomas and ovarian masses. Ultrasound examination is the best means by which to differentiate these conditions.

Differences in opinion exist as to when in gestation it is first discernable that the uterus is enlarged. Some clinicians argue that the increased intrauterine volume associated with multiple gestations can cause the uterus to feel enlarged on pelvic bimanual examination by 8 weeks' gestation. Others argue that uterine enlargement in the first trimester is primarily due to muscular growth under hormonal influences, and that the presence of more than one fetus cannot be discerned by physical examination until early in the second trimester. Little published data exist to support either point of view. If accurate gestational age is known, and the patient obtains early prenatal care, examination will most likely demonstrate accelerated uterine growth in a majority of cases by 14 weeks' gestation, with pregnancies of higher order than twins being larger than expected for dates even earlier.

Certain other data from a patient's history and physical examination might also suggest an increased chance of carrying more than one fetus. Although a family history of twinning is often sought during the patient's initial interview, a positive history generally affects one's chances of having multiples very little. The effects of family history, age and parity are only discernable on the rate of dizygotic twinning, and the relative risk is roughly 1.1. Of much greater import is a history of the use of one of a number of procedures commonly characterized as assisted reproductive technology to overcome infertility (see Chapter 13). The use of agents to promote ovulation or the placement of multiple fertilized ova in the upper genital tract both increase the chances of multiple gestation if pregnancy is achieved. Indeed, use of these techniques is the primary factor responsible for the increases in the numbers of higher order multiple gestations observed in many countries over the past decade.

Another important clinical finding associated with the presence of a multiple gestation is polyhydramnios. Most patients with excess amniotic fluid will already be undergoing ultrasound examination for inappropriately large fundal height, and this physical finding alone will detect very few additional cases. Unexplained anemia early in the second trimester has also been linked with multiple gestation. Even in patients with normal iron stores, the dilutional effect of increased plasma volume over the increase in red blood cell mass associated with twins can result in a marked anemia with normal red blood cell indices. Such an anemia generally appears in the second trimester, when plasma volume is significantly increased compared to levels seen in singleton pregnancies of the same gestational age. The dilutional effect is maximal early in the third trimester. The vast majority of anemic patients, however, have only one fetus, and this physical finding leads to a diagnosis of twins in very few instances.

Biochemical parameters of multiple gestation

Beginning in the first trimester, the placenta manufactures steroid and protein hormones that enter the maternal circulation in measurable amounts. With the evolution of accurate assays for these hormones over the past 25 years, repetitive analyses reveal patterns of production characteristic of normal pregnancies. Deviations from expected values are useful in identifying abnormal pregnancies. Expected values of specific hormones are significantly elevated in multiple gestations, either as a result of increased placental mass for those hormones synthesized by trophoblastic cells, or because of increased total amount of fetal tissue for those hormones produced by the fetus. For hormone levels to be clinically useful, however, expected values require adjustment for multiple gestations. Indeed, differences in certain hormone levels between singleton and multiple gestations have been used as screening tests to detect the presence of more than one fetus.

The remainder of this chapter will concern hormone levels, their usefulness in detecting the presence of multiple gestations, and their clinical utility in managing these pregnancies.

Human chorionic gonadotropin

Human chorionic gonadotropin (hCG) is a glycoprotein produced by the syncytiotrophoblast cells of the placenta. By sensitive assay, this hormone can be detected in maternal serum around the time of implantation. The level of hCG in maternal serum rises exponentially during the first 2 months of pregnancy, doubling every 1.4 to 2 days in normal gestations. In singleton pregnancies, the hCG levels rise exponentially until 10–12 weeks of gestation, and then fall precipitously. Recognition of these propensities has led to a number of clinical uses for monitoring hCG levels serially. These include early pregnancy detection, assessment of viability, and detection of extrauterine implantation. In addition, monitoring serial levels of hCG is useful in the evaluation of progress during therapy for gestational trophoblastic disease.

In general, hCG levels in twin gestation are higher than those found in singleton pregnancies at similar gestational ages (Figure 1). Jovanovic et al.[9] screened 590 women in the first trimester, and identified nine patients with significantly elevated hCG levels, all of whom were later determined by pelvic ultrasound to have twin gestations. In this study, the hCG levels in twin pregnancies from 4 to 10 weeks' gestation were 3–10 times higher than corresponding levels in singleton pregnancies. On the basis of this high predictive value of a single elevated hCG, these authors suggested that this test might serve as an early screening test for twins. O'Keane et al.[10] evaluated hCG levels from twin, triplet and quadruplet pregnancies, and found increasing levels with pregnancy order. They also noted that the successful pregnancy reduction of a quintuplet pregnancy to twins was followed by a five-fold

MULTIPLE PREGNANCY

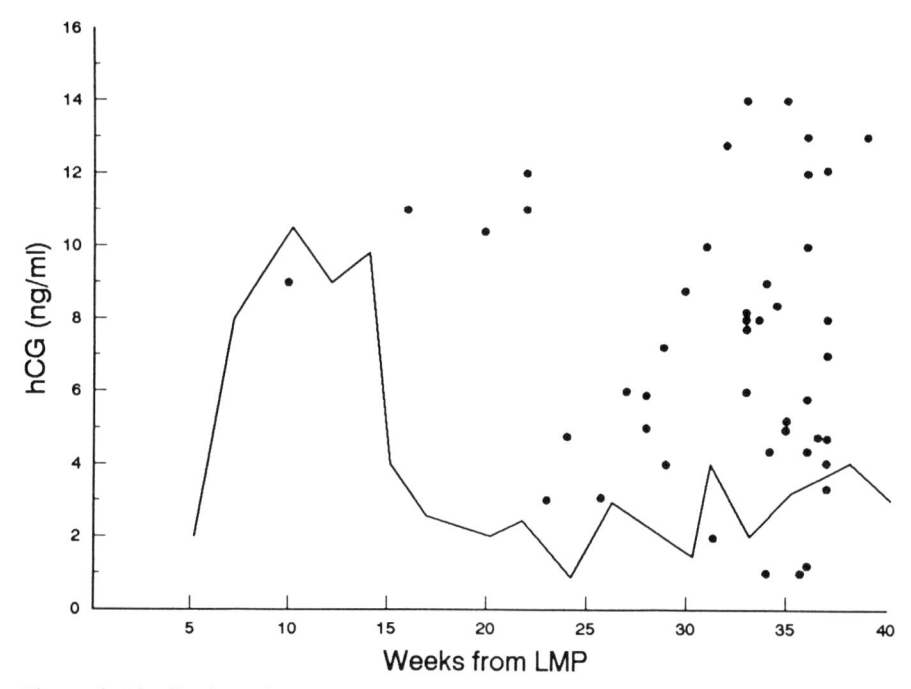

Figure 1 Distribution of maternal serum hCG levels in 12 twin pregnancies with normal fetal outcome. The solid line represents mean serum levels in singleton pregnancies. Adapted from reference 11

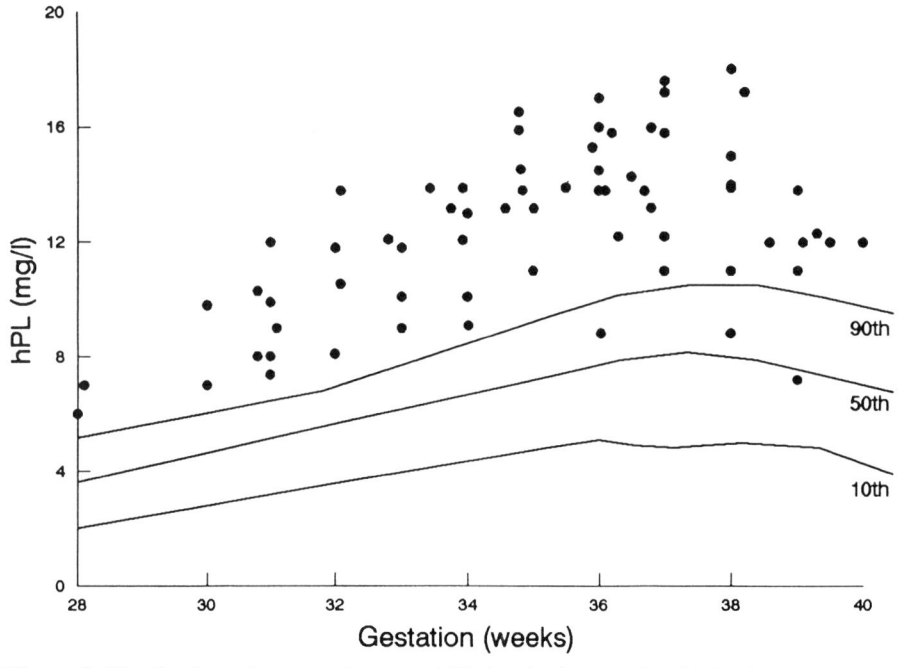

Figure 2 Distribution of maternal serum hPL levels during the third trimester in 17 twin pregnancies with normal fetal outcome. The solid lines represent the 10th, 50th and 90th centiles for singleton pregnancies. Adapted from reference 21

reduction in the hCG level over a 4-week period. Reuter et al.[11] found hCG levels elevated above the range expected for singleton pregnancies in 45 of 52 (86%) samples taken in 12 twin gestations after the first trimester.

Unfortunately, not all studies have been able to demonstrate consistent differences between hCG levels in singleton and twin gestations. For example, Harrison et al.[12] followed a single patient with a normal twin pregnancy with twice weekly β-hCG levels, and found the level to be elevated over the mean for singletons only from weeks 10–14, and even then the difference was not greater than one standard deviation above the mean. Thiery et al.[13] found hCG levels more than two standard deviations above the mean for singleton pregnancies in only five of nine women (56%) tested at least twice in the first trimester. Crosignani et al.[14] demonstrated elevated hCG levels after 12 weeks' gestation in less than half of 22 women carrying twins. Because many studies have demonstrated significant overlap of hCG levels between singleton and twin pregnancies[12–14], the value of hCG as a screening test for multiple gestation is problematic. (Editor: The hCG level is generally not used in practice to arrive at diagnosis.)

Human placental lactogen

Human placental lactogen (hPL) is a polypeptide hormone synthesized and secreted by the syncytiotrophoblast cells of the placenta. Maternal levels of hPL can be detected soon after conception but, unlike hCG, these levels continue to rise steadily until the end of pregnancy. Although levels of hPL are directly proportional to placental mass, they do not correlate as well with birth weight[13,15]. Historically, hPL levels were used to monitor fetal well-being, as falling levels occasionally were present in association with a deteriorating fetal condition. This method of fetal assessment has presently been supplanted by electronic fetal heart rate monitoring and evaluation of other biophysical parameters, because these tests are associated with improved sensitivity and specificity.

As with hCG, maternal serum levels of hPL also tend to be elevated in twin gestations compared with levels obtained from singleton pregnancies at similar gestational ages[13,16]. Elevations in hPL levels are detectable as early as 9 weeks' gestation[17], and are maintained throughout pregnancy. The distribution of hPL values for twin pregnancies in relation to the distribution for singleton gestations is displayed in Figure 2.

Mägiste et al.[18] first suggested using maternal serum hPL levels as a screening test for twin gestation. With a cutoff value of 5.0 μg/ml at 29 to 30 weeks' gestation, 13.4% of the population tested was found to have an elevated hPL level. Twin gestation was confirmed in 13.6% of those patients with an elevated level. In this study, the use of hPL as a screening test yielded a sensitivity of 100% with a specificity of 88%. Spellacy et al.[19] also determined that elevated hPL levels at 30 and 36 weeks were of value in screening for twin gestation, but with cutoff values of 8.0 and 9.0 μg/ml, respectively. Using these critical values, however, only 32% of twin pregnancies were recognized at 30 weeks' gestation, and 56% at 36 weeks' gestation. Grennert et al.[20] did not use a specific gestational age or an absolute value for screening, but found 37 of 39 twin pregnancies between 24 and 30 weeks' gestation to have maternal hPL values greater than one standard deviation above the mean for singleton pregnancies, giving a sensitivity of 95%, with 84% specificity.

Although the investigators cited above generally found maternal hPL levels of value in detecting the presence of more than one fetus, absolute cutoff values have not yet been established, and appropriate cutoff values may indeed vary among different populations. More importantly, use of hPL as a screening tool has not been tested prior to the third trimester, when efforts at diagnosis may prove to be of the greatest clinical value.

Estrogens and progesterone

Three estrogens are produced by the fetoplacental unit – estrone (E_1), estradiol (E_2) and estriol (E_3). All are produced by the placenta from fetal precursors, and subsequently cross to the maternal circulation. Normal ranges for these estrogens have been calculated for singleton gestations, and the levels of all three rise throughout gestation. In uncomplicated singleton pregnancies, urinary excretion of estriol increases with gestational age, and this property is the basis for its utility in fetal surveillance. In contrast, investigations of maternal estrogen levels in multiple gestations yield mixed results[16,21–26]. Some authors have shown that maternal serum estrogen levels in the third trimester of twin pregnancies appear to be significantly elevated over singleton levels[16,21–24]; however, others have been unable to demonstrate such a difference[25,26]. Because of these differences and the large inter-patient variations, estrogens have not proven useful for detection of multiple gestation and have been replaced by the assessment of fetal biophysical parameters as the preferred method of surveillance in multifetal pregnancies.

Changes in progesterone levels in twin gestations have not been studied as extensively as have those of estrogens. Progesterone levels in multiple gestations appear to be significantly elevated over those in singleton pregnancies; once again, however, the wide inter-patient variations have precluded assigning clinical usefulness to these assessments.

Alpha-fetoprotein

Alpha-fetoprotein (AFP) is a protein hormone found in significant quantities in the maternal serum during pregnancy. It differs from the hormones previously discussed in that it is produced by the fetal liver rather than the placenta. AFP is a plasma protein during fetal life, and is normally found in the amniotic fluid as well. Like the other fetal hormones of a proteinaceous nature, maternal levels increase with gestational age, as a result of increasing fetal production and transplacental transfer.

During the 1970s, preliminary work in the United Kingdom associated elevated levels of maternal serum alpha-fetoprotein (MSAFP) with open fetal neural tube defects (ONTDs)[27].

Concomitantly, investigations of normal singleton pregnancies revealed relatively small variations from median values in the early second trimester. As a result of these observations, it was proposed that testing maternal serum for levels of AFP at 15–20 weeks' gestation could serve as a valuable screening tool for detection of ONTDs[28]. The basis for this suggestion lay in the fact that exudation of large amounts of fetal plasma occurs through open defects in the body wall and that the levels of AFP in the amniotic fluid rise, as a result. Because the excess amniotic AFP is transferred to the maternal circulation, it can be detected by screening. Even today, with the advances in imaging technology, MSAFP testing appears to be more sensitive, more available, and less costly than ultrasound examination as a screening tool for neural tube defects in the first half of pregnancy.

Screening protocols using AFP for detection of open neural tube defects often use relatively low cutoff values to improve their sensitivity. However, more than 90% of ONTDs will be detected using 2.5 multiples of the median (MoM) for gestational age as the critical value[29]. With this cutoff value, however, approximately 5% of mothers have an elevated level, of which only one in 25 have a fetus with a neural tube defect[29]. Factors which can explain approximately half of AFP elevations include underestimated gestational age, multiple gestation, fetal death, early pregnancy bleeding, congenital nephrosis, and other defects in the fetal skin that allow plasma transudation into the amniotic cavity (e.g. abdominal wall defects)[29–31]. The relative contributions of a number of these factors are listed in Table 1.

Table 1 Ultrasound findings (%) in patients with elevated MSAFP. From references 29 and 30

Underestimated gestational age	21
Multiple gestation	13
Fetal death	7
Open neural tube defects	5
Oligohydramnios	2
Other anomalies	1
No explanations	51

Table 2 Distribution of MSAFP levels in twin pregnancies. From references 32 and 33

MoM*	n	%
< 2	76	26.9
2–2.5	69	24.4
2.5–3	51	18.0
3–4	53	18.7
> 4	34	12.0
Total	283	100

*Multiples of the median for singleton gestation

Ultrasound examination detects the majority of these conditions, and is the logical next step after the MSAFP level is found to be elevated.

If ultrasound fails to provide an explanation, as is the case in approximately 2% of all patients screened, amniocentesis for amniotic fluid levels of alpha-fetoprotein and acetylcholinesterase (AChE) will detect almost all neural tube defects not previously found. In those pregnancies with elevated MSAFP and normal amniotic fluid alpha-fetoprotein (AFAFP), poor pregnancy outcomes are more common, with increased rates of preterm birth, fetal growth retardation, pre-eclampsia, and perinatal death compared to the general population[29]. A possible explanation for this association may be that these pregnancies have intrinsic placental abnormalities which lead to pregnancy complications and, in addition, allow more fetal AFP to cross into the maternal circulation.

MSAFP levels are significantly elevated in multiple gestations compared to singleton pregnancies, and these differences continue to be present throughout the second and third trimesters[32]. The median value of MSAFP levels in twin gestations from 14–20 weeks is 2.5 times the median curve for singleton gestations[33,34]. Table 2 details the distribution of MSAFP values in twin pregnancies in the early second trimester; almost three-fourths of twin pregnancies have levels greater than two multiples of the singleton median. From 10–20% of elevated MSAFP levels are explained by the presence of more than one fetus[33]. As a result, MSAFP screening programs contribute significantly to the early detection of multiple gestations, especially in populations that do not receive routine early ultrasound examinations. Detection rates vary with the level used as a critical value.

Although most twins will be identified by this test, the percentage of patients who would normally have been diagnosed on clinical grounds is not clear. In the population studied by Johnson et al., MSAFP screening was responsible for the detection of 40.5% of the twin gestations[33]. Clearly, the true value of MSAFP screening for detection of multiple gestations varies among different clinical settings, depending on the frequency of early routine ultrasound examination, prenatal care prior to 20 weeks' gestational age, and utilization of genetic amniocentesis (see Chapters 7, 15 and 22).

Once it is recognized that multiple gestation is present, the practitioner is faced with the question of how to use elevated levels of MSAFP in the search for ONTDs in one or both fetuses. As with MSAFP screening in singleton gestations, a cutoff level must be chosen for further diagnostic testing. Cuckle et al.[35] identified 46 twin pregnancies with open neural tube defects who had had MSAFP screening. If a critical value of 3.0 multiples of the singleton median was chosen, only 13% of affected pregnancies would have been missed, but almost 20% of all twin pregnancies would have screened positive and needed further evaluation. If the critical value of 5.0 MoM was used, only 3.3% of the twin population would have screened positive, but 40% of the ONTDs would have been missed, most of which were spina bifida. All of these patients presumably would have had ultrasound examinations for the detection of twin gestation, but how many of these ONTDs would have been detected during this initial sonography is not known.

Follow up with amniocentesis of both sacs can be performed, but results can be misleading, because both AFP and AChE can cross the amniotic membranes. Numerous investigators have found twin gestations discordant for ONTDs where AFP and AChE are elevated in both sacs[36]. The degree to which these proteins cross between sacs is dependent on how much is present in the sac of the affected twin, and also whether the twins are monochorionic or dichorionic. Because of these considerations, twin pregnancies with MSAFP levels above the chosen critical value should all have careful ultrasound examinations of the cranium and spine (see Chapter 17). If no defect is identified, amniocentesis of both sacs can be helpful in assuring normal AFAFP levels. If, however, an abnormality is identified by sonography in one or both twins, amniocentesis may not be helpful. In multiple pregnancies beyond two, and in twin pregnancies remaining after selective reduction, MSAFP screening has not yet been tested sufficiently to be clinically useful.

As noted above, an increased rate of complications is observed in singleton pregnancies found to have elevated MSAFP levels without ONTD. This appears to be true for twin pregnancies as well. Wald et al.[37] first recognized the negative correlation between MSAFP levels in twin gestations and combined birth weight. This finding has been confirmed by other investigators[33,34]. Furthermore, significantly elevated MSAFP levels (more than four multiples of the singleton median) have been associated with increasing rates of premature delivery, birth weight discordance, and fetal and neonatal death. MSAFP levels of >5 MoM are rarely associated with term delivery of normal twins. Thus, whereas MSAFP screening may be of relatively little benefit in the diagnosis of twins, it can be useful to assess perinatal risk.

In 1984, Merkatz et al.[38] first noted the association between low MSAFP levels and chromosomal abnormalities. Since then, MSAFP levels have been used in calculating age-related risks of chromosomal aberrations. Maternal serum levels of hCG and estriol have been added to testing protocols to increase sensitivity. To date, however, MSAFP testing has not been investigated as a screening test for chromosomal abnormalities in twin gestations.

Summary

Significant progress has been made over the past two decades in increasing the percentage of multiple gestations diagnosed early in pregnancy. This progress is due primarily to the widespread availability and use of ultrasound. As a result, it is very unusual to discover an unexpected second fetus in the delivery room. Although numerous physical or biochemical parameters may be helpful in selecting patients for further study with ultrasound, some multiple gestations will still be missed, unless programs involving universal ultrasound screening are incorporated into routine obstetric care. Biochemical parameters initially showed promise in increasing the detection of twin gestations, but have not proven to be of sufficient sensitivity to justify their use in screening for twins. Elevated levels of MSAFP, however, still have important clinical utility in screening for open neural tube defects, and may contribute to the identification of multiple gestations in some populations.

References

1. Kurtz, G.R., Keating, W.J. and Loftus, J.B. (1955). Twin pregnancy and delivery: analysis of 500 twin pregnancies. *Obstet. Gynecol.*, **6**, 370
2. Powers, W.F. (1973). Twin pregnancy: complications and treatment. *Obstet. Gynecol.*, **42**, 795
3. Keith, L., Ellis, R., Berger, G.S. *et al.* (1980). The Northwestern University multihospital twin study – a description of 588 twin pregnancies and associated pregnancy loss, 1971 to 1975. *Am. J. Obstet. Gynecol.*, **138**, 781
4. Cunningham F.G., MacDonald, P.C. and Gant, N.F. (eds.) (1989). Multifetal pregnancy. *Williams Obstetrics*, 18th edn., p. 637. (Norwalk: Appleton and Lange)
5. Chervenak, F.A., Youcha, S., Johnson, R.E. *et al.* (1984). Twin gestation: antenatal diagnosis and perinatal outcome in 385 consecutive pregnancies. *J. Reprod. Med.*, **29**, 727
6. Persson, P.H. and Kullander, S. (1983). Long-term experience of general ultrasound

screening in pregnancy. *Am. J. Obstet. Gynecol.*, **146**, 942
7. ACOG (1988). *Ultrasound in Pregnancy*. American College of Obstetricians and Gynecologists Technical Bulletin #116, May
8. Quaranta, P., Currell, R., Redman, C.W.G. *et al.* (1981). Prediction of small-for-dates infants by measurement of symphysial-fundal-height. *Br. J. Obstet. Gynaecol.*, **88**, 115
9. Jovanovic, L., Landesman, R. and Saxena, B.B. (1977). Screening for twin pregnancy. *Science*, **198**, 738
10. O'Keane, J.A., Yuen, B.H., Farquharson, D.F. *et al.* (1988). Endocrine response to selective embryocide in a gonadotropin-induced quintuplet pregnancy. *Am. J. Obstet. Gynecol.*, **155**, 364
11. Reuter, A.M., Gaspard, U.J., Deville, J.L. *et al.* (1980). Serum concentrations of human chorionic gonadotrophin and its alpha and beta subunits during normal singleton and twin pregnancies. *Clin. Endocrinol.*, **13**, 305
12. Harrison, R.F., O'Moore, R.R. and McSweeney, J. (1980). Maternal plasma β-hCG in early human pregnancy. *Br. J. Obstet. Gynaecol.*, **87**, 705
13. Thiery, M., Dhont, M. and Vandekerckhove, D. (1976). Serum hCG and hPL in twin pregnancies. *Acta Obstet. Gynecol. Scand.*, **56**, 495
14. Crosignani, P.G., Trojsi, L., Attanasio, A.E.M. *et al.* (1974). Value of hCG and hCS measurement in clinical practice. *Obstet. Gynecol.*, **44**, 673
15. Sciarra, J.J., Sherwood, L.M., Varma, A.A. *et al.* (1968). Human placental lactogen (HPL) and placental weight. *Am. J. Obstet. Gynecol.*, **101**, 413
16. Trapp, M., Kato, K., Bohnet H.-G. *et al.* (1986). Human placental lactogen and unconjugated estriol concentrations in twin pregnancy: monitoring of fetal development in intrauterine growth retardation and single intrauterine fetal death. *Am. J. Obstet. Gynecol.*, **155**, 1027
17. Harrison, R.F. and Biswas, S. (1980). Maternal plasma, human placental lactogen, α-fetoprotein, prolactin and growth hormone in early pregnancy. *Int. J. Gynecol. Obstet.*, **17**, 471
18. Mägiste, M., von Schenk, H., Sjöberg, N.-O. *et al.* (1976). Screening for detecting twin pregnancy. *Am. J. Obstet. Gynecol.*, **126**, 697
19. Spellacy, W.N., Buhi, W.C. and Birk, S.A. (1978). Human placental lactogen levels in multiple pregnancies. *Obstet. Gynecol.*, **52**, 210
20. Grennert, L., Persson, P.-H., Gennser, G. *et al.* (1976). Ultrasound and human-placental-lactogen screening for early detection of twin pregnancies. *Lancet*, **1**, 4
21. Westergaard, J.G., Teisner, B., Hau, J. *et al.* (1985). Placental protein and hormone measurements in twin pregnancy. *Br. J. Obstet. Gynaecol.*, **92**, 72
22. MacGillivray, I., Campbell, D. and Duffus, G.M. (1971). Maternal metabolic response to twin pregnancy in primigravidae. *J. Obstet. Gynaecol. Br. Commonw.*, **78**, 530
23. Duff, G.B. and Brown, J.B. (1974). Urinary oestriol excretion in twin pregnancies. *J. Obstet. Gynaecol. Br. Commonw.*, **81**, 695
24. Dawood, M.Y. and Ratnam, S.S. (1974). Serial estimation of serum unconjugated estradiol-17β in high-risk pregnancies. *Obstet. Gynecol.*, **44**, 200
25. Khoo, S.K. and Mackay, E.V. (1970). Urinary oestriol excretion in multiple pregnancy. *Med. J. Austral.*, **1**, 896
26. Batra, S., Sjöberg, N.O. and Åberg, A. (1978). Human placental lactogen, estradiol-17β, and progesterone levels in the third trimester and their respective values for detecting twin pregnancy. *Am. J. Obstet. Gynecol.*, **131**, 69
27. Brock, D.J.H., Bolton, A.E. and Monaghan, J.M. (1977). Prenatal diagnosis of anencephaly through maternal serum alpha-fetoprotein measurements. *Lancet*, **2**, 923
28. Wald, N.J., Cuckle, H. and Brock, D.J. (1977). UK collaborative study on alpha-fetoprotein in relation to neural tube defects: maternal serum alpha-fetoprotein measurements in antenatal screening for anencephaly and spina bifida in early pregnancy. *Lancet*, **1**, 1323
29. Milunsky, A., Jick, S.S., Bruell, C.L. *et al.* (1989). Predictive values, relative risks, and overall benefits of high and low maternal serum α-fetoprotein screening in singleton pregnancies: new epidemiologic data. *Am. J. Obstet. Gynecol.*, **161**, 291
30. Burton, B.K., Sowers, S.G. and Nelson, L.H. (1983). Maternal serum α-fetoprotein screening in North Carolina: experience with more than twelve thousand pregnancies. *Am. J. Obstet. Gynecol.*, **146**, 439
31. Haddow, J.E., Kloza, E.M., Smith, D.E. *et al.* (1983). Data from an alpha-fetoprotein pilot screening program in Maine. *Obstet. Gynecol.*, **62**, 556
32. Ishiguro, T. (1975). Serum α-fetoprotein in hydatidiform mole, choriocarcinoma, and twin pregnancy. *Am. J. Obstet. Gynecol.*, **121**, 539

33. Johnson, J.M., Harman, C.R., Evans, J.A. *et al.* (1990). Maternal serum α-fetoprotein in twin pregnancy. *Am. J. Obstet. Gynecol.*, **162**, 1020
34. Redford, D.H.A. and Whitfield, C.R. (1985). Maternal serum α-fetoprotein in twin pregnancies uncomplicated by neural tube defect. *Am. J. Obstet. Gynecol.*, **152**, 550
35. Cuckle, H., Wald, N., Stevenson, J.D. *et al.* (1990). Maternal serum alpha-fetoprotein screening for open neural tube defects in twin pregnancies. *Prenat. Diagn.*, **10**, 71
36. Johnson, V.P., Vidgoff, J., Wilson, N. *et al.* (1989). Alpha-fetoprotein and acetylcholinesterase in twins discordant for neural tube defect. *Prenat. Diagn.*, **9**, 831
37. Wald, N.J., Cuckle, H., Stirrat, G.M. *et al.* (1978). Maternal serum alpha-fetoprotein and birth weight in twin pregnancies. *Br. J. Obstet. Gynaecol.*, **85**, 582
38. Merkatz, I.R., Nitowsky, H.M., Macri, J.N. *et al.* (1984). An association between low maternal serum α-fetoprotein and fetal chromosomal abnormalities. *Am. J. Obstet. Gynecol.*, **148**, 886

Psychophysiological adaptation to multiple pregnancy

E. Noble

Introduction

The adjustment to multiple pregnancy varies with each woman and depends on many factors, including the amount and nature of the support provided by her partner and family, marital and economic status, age and number of prior children, fertility history and her general state of health. Also of importance are past or present acquaintances with other families of multiples, and the events surrounding the woman's birth and upbringing.

Becoming a mother is an endless growth process during which the woman confronts her limits and learns to stretch beyond them. Being pregnant with multiples poses many more challenges than does a singleton gestation. Table 1 depicts the two extremes of potential reactions. Because ambivalence is common in pregnancy, most women fluctuate between positive and negative reactions, especially when a multiple gestation is involved. It is particularly important for health-care providers to recognize real or perceived negative reactions on the part of either parent and to deal with them by providing information, counselling and support. Many of the emotional issues that arise during a multiple pregnancy are of unconscious origin and, on occasion, hypnotherapy can be helpful. Additional support can be derived from the networks, clubs and newsletters of the various multiple birth associations (see Resources, in the Appendix).

The earlier the satisfactory acceptance and adjustment to the concept of a multiple pregnancy, as well as the physical experiences associated with it, the more likely that adequate psychological adaptation and bonding will occur.

Acceptance

Acceptance is the first step in the process of psychological adaptation. To a large extent, acceptance depends on how, when and where the diagnosis is disclosed. Although many mothers suspect that they are carrying twins, confirmation of their intuition often represents a major transition. Indeed, the news may be accompanied by feelings of excitement and wonder, or powerlessness, regret, fear of the future or complete devastation. This is especially true for women who have conceived after the use of assisted reproductive technologies or ovulation-inducing treatments and who had, in their 'heart of hearts', only wanted one child. Some of these expectant mothers may have been inadequately warned of the possibility of multiples, others may not have been forewarned at all, and still others may have chosen to ignore the warnings in the belief that it could only happen to other couples. In this regard, the sudden swing from infertility to abundance can be an enormous shock. In such circumstances, Cheek and Le Cron[1], have aptly noted that patients with idiopathic infertility often were neither biologically nor emotionally ready to conceive. This observation is of particular relevance today, when previously infertile women comprise a growing number of mothers of multiples, some of whom may be faced with the additional dilemma posed by the real or perceived need for selective reduction (see Chapters 25 and 26).

The diagnosis of multiple pregnancy should be disclosed by the midwife or doctor with the utmost sensitivity, in an open-ended session. To say the least, joking over the ultrasound

Table 1 Reactions to pregnancy

Negative	Positive
Suspected twin pregnancy insensitively disclosed by technician or doctor	Suspected twin pregnancy, confirmed with sensitivity and support
News experienced as a shock	News received as a wonderful surprise or dream come true
Unplanned pregnancy; unwilling to bear multiples	Planned pregnancy/conscious conception, optimistic about outcome of fertility treatments
Perceives large abdomen as 'too fat'	Enjoys blossoming of her body
Feels like a sow, like she's having a litter	Grateful for abundance – 'two babies for the price of one'
Resents size, appearance, social comments	Welcomes questions about large belly, due date
Anxious about high-risk pregnancy and going to term	Strongly motivated to learn how to achieve term pregnancy and to meet parents of multiples
Irritated by bodily changes and discomforts of pregnancy	Views adaptation of body with sense of wonder and appreciation
Unaware of differences between babies; just feels kicks	Begins prenatal bonding with babies as unit and individually
Fears labor, sees Cesarean as an easy way out	Looks forward to labor, finds providers to support natural birth
Rejects idea of breast feeding	Joyfully anticipates breast feeding
Feels overwhelmed by the thought of having and caring for two or more babies	Sets up support systems for birth and postpartum

machine is an inappropriate form of disclosure. *Immediate* contact with other parents of multiples should be arranged to avoid feelings of isolation or despondency. In addition, the newly informed woman (or couple) should not leave the doctor's office without appropriate phone numbers (of mothers of multiples, the local or national Mothers of Twins Club, or Twin Services, and ideally, some literature such as *Twins* magazine, *Double Talk*, or books about twins and other reading and resource lists). In order not to waste time, the health-care professional should have these documents at hand.

Adjustment can be more complicated if there are other children in the family. Not infrequently, the impending arrival of multiples may stress resources that already are at their limits. Multipara often become pregnant 'to have an even number of children' or to try for a girl or boy. When multiples are diagnosed such plans are upset, and health-care providers should not be surprised if the woman's reaction is less than enthusiastic at hearing the news.

Without doubt, two or more babies represent a huge burden on space, time, income and life style. The totality of these burdens and the changes that accompany them place families of multiples at increased risk of postpartum depression, drug and alcohol abuse, child abuse and divorce. Child abuse can be physical, verbal or emotional, or can simply result from neglect. In half the families studied by Groothuis *et al.*[2], only the elder or younger sibling, not either of the twins, was abused.

Because individuals who were abused as children tend to repeat this behavior, it is important to ask questions about past childhood abuse as part of the general prenatal historical survey. Evans[3] found that if a woman had experienced sexual abuse by a care-taker prior to the age of 18, she was twice as likely to deliver before 34 weeks of gestation, and two and a half times more likely to have a newborn with a medical problem, regardless of the number of previous pregnancies, education, race, use of alcohol or cigarettes, or history of additional physical abuse in childhood. Considering that sexual abuse presently is estimated to occur in 60% of girls[4], this topic should be part of every prenatal interview, not only for those of mothers of multiples.

The reproductive history of the expectant mother and that of her own mother (which has been a major influence during the expectant mother's formative years) is significant, as is the history and psychosocial experiences of twinning in the extended family. Positive or negative attitudes of other family members impact on family adjustment, whether they reflect feelings of pride or pity, or whether the expectant mother is treated like a queen or an invalid.

In order to foster the process of acceptance, it is useful to help all newly-informed patients to arrange a personal meeting with other mothers of multiples, both during pregnancy and well into the postpartum period. These encounters help to reassure apprehensive women that a huge belly is normal and that with exercise it will return to its former size in due time. Fatigue, and the great increase in body size and weight, conspire against feelings of sensuality and sexuality for many women. To assist the mother in accepting the temporary nature of the stressful situation, care-providers should recommend patience, as well as a sense of humor, and emphasize that the pregnancy lasts only nine months.

Education and supportive measures

It is important that the mother be informed and feel empowered to cope with the many changes that await her. Most important to her personal health and well-being is optimal nutrition and adequate rest (at least twice daily for a minimum of a half-hour). Both help to reduce fatigue and combat depression in addition to facilitating carrying the multiples to term.

Ongoing support, financial as well as emotional, is helpful to prepare parents adequately for the physical and social stress of multiples. Material needs must be accurately assessed and prioritized. A larger car, house, and more income often are deemed necessary, just at the moment when the mother is asked to quit work. However, as Zazzo[5] has so correctly noted, it is 'indecent' to recommend a larger house, for example, if no financial means are available. Thus, housing and child care subsidies, food supplements, extended leave from work, postpartum home care and homemaker services for teens and single parents should be sought as soon as possible from community resources, in order to reassure anxious mothers that they will be able to cope. Many patients deeply appreciate help from a social service agency at this time.

Frequently, financial burdens mean that the father has to seek extra work and has even less time to help at home. In the nuclear family, the father's assistance is of primary importance to the mother's perception of being able to cope. Maternity-care providers must encourage the partner to attend as many prenatal visits as possible, as well as the birth.

Regardless of the partner's willingness or ability to assist the mother, it is important that help from family and neighbors be solicited and organized well in advance for the postpartum months. Invariably, families are reluctant to ask for help from outsiders and struggle to cope alone. Regardless, health-care providers often know individuals who would be glad to be of assistance. As one mother of twins said, 'Never deprive anyone of the chance to do a good deed!'

It is crucial that the woman has confidence in her obstetrician and that he/she has the requisite skills to handle multiples, particularly breech delivery. Couples expecting twins and higher order multiples should visit a neonatal intensive-care nursery and take Cesarean preparation classes, so that they are well-informed if a need for either arises. They may actually prefer to deliver in a level III hospital so that a transfer will not be required if the newborns should need intensive care.

Ideally, the need to 'be prepared for the worst' should not discourage, but rather encourage a woman to take the appropriate prenatal steps to minimize the likelihood of an adverse outcome. This she can clearly do by making nutrition, rest, appropriate exercise (strengthening rather than contraction-producing) and self-education her top priorities. A strong commitment to optimal health during pregnancy may diminish problems later on.

Because half of the mothers of twins *do* reach their due date, all women should be encouraged to think positively about carrying to term, even when they have triplets. In my opinion, intense preoccupation and worries about risks and complications conveyed by the physician may become self-fulfilling prophesies and lead to preterm labor, the need for anesthesia or Cesarean section. In the case of multiples, the term 'special needs' is always preferable to 'high risk'.

Concerns which health-care providers might view as 'trivial' should never be dismissed – deeper issues may lie beneath. Often, a patient is simply testing the environment to see if she feels safe and supported so that she may speak about a larger problem. Bland reassurance, however well-intentioned, can be interpreted as a put-down. Rather, health-care professionals should listen actively, and encourage the patient to elaborate verbally, to explore presently occurring bodily sensations and to recall any prior similar experiences and outcomes. An open-ended dialogue which allows the patient to use her inner resources for creative solutions is ideal.

Finally, the value of the informal network should never be underestimated. By this I mean those experts (parents) who have personally experienced the multiple-birth process. Couples expecting multiples should have the opportunity to share their fears, expectations and experiences with other couples in prenatal and postpartum support groups. Expectant parents of multiples can learn invaluable lessons from real parents of multiples. Additionally, some clinics and hospitals offer special classes for parents of multiples (see Chapters 50 and 52). Whether or not these exist, anxious mothers and fathers should have the opportunity to talk with an experienced psychologist or social worker who has counselled other parents-to-be with anxiety so that concerns about bearing multiples can be recognized and dealt with.

Prenatal bonding

The increasingly routine use of prenatal screening means that more parents know the sex, placentation and perhaps the zygosity of their infants before birth. This information can be used to enhance bonding with each twin as an individual with both babies as a dyad.

Piontelli[6] studied twins with ultrasound and confirmed that they interact in myriad ways and are clearly capable of expressing their separate identity and responding in different ways to their respective positions in the uterus. She pointed out that myths, legends and popular beliefs about twins attribute a 'much more lively and adult life' to them than to singletons, who continue to be seen to some extent as 'more passive, amorphous and little differentiated creatures, as if the fact of sharing the nine months of the pregnancy gave twins some kind of special attributes'.

Psychological adaptation and prenatal bonding develop simultaneously. After the mother has adapted to her diagnosis, she must begin to accept her babies as unborn *persons*. In the beginning, it is often easier for mothers to bond with the unit. Only later does differentiation of specific members occur. In the case of twins, the risk of polarization is always present in which one twin is viewed as active and the other passive, large or small, extrovert or introvert, etc. Such differences may indeed exist or may result from parental projection or need to find distinguishing characteristics for each infant. Often mothers of triplets are especially tempted to separate their babies into a 'pair and a spare' or may occasionally state that they are carrying twins and a single baby, in order to make the situation seem unusual. Mothers and fathers often can 'visualize' their babies by remaining open to their dreams and to images, hunches, and other dimensions of human intuition. At the same time, actual photographs of the infants can be obtained with ultrasonography, either still or real-time (see Chapters 14, 16 and 24).

Parents must realize that each fetus is aware from a very early age and is sensitive to sound, touch and emotional states. Because the experience of twinship *in utero* is generally one of a struggle for space, the process of sharing should be explained to the twins prenatally in the form of maternal verbal reassurance. When one baby is felt kicking, it is necessary to reassure the other that s/he is safe. Kicking, as distinct from turning and stretching, may be a sign of distress and related to tense uterine walls. Many babies must assume a 'malpresentation' because the uterus is too tense for them to change position. In multiple pregnancy, the natural desire to change position is complicated by the presence of an additional fetus.

Tension of the uterine musculature is not under conscious control, but reduced muscle tone can be induced through techniques of imagery, mediation and haptonomy. Haptonomy[7], which is well known in Europe (especially France), involves the use of touch to actually change the tension in the muscle spindles of the gamma nervous system. (This approach is of great value for obstetricians who perform external version.)

It is important for the parents to encourage activity in the 'quieter' twin by touching, talking and singing, and haptonomic preparation. It is useful to encourage the mother to let her uterus 'soften' on exhalation to allow more room for the babies. I suggest that the mother envisage a relaxed uterus that will allow each baby to stretch and turn comfortably. I also recommend that parents place their hands on the uterus as they reassure their babies inside that there is enough room, enough oxygen, enough nutrients and enough love and attention.

Concepts of up, down, right, left, back and front, and body parts can also be introduced to the babies when mothers, fathers and indeed siblings, talk and use their hands to communicate with each baby. Family members should state their names each time they speak to the fetuses. A statement such as, 'This is your brother, Joe', links the touch, voice and family relationship in an instant.

The psychological adjustment of each baby and the parents is enhanced if the individuality of each twin can be affirmed. To facilitate this, the midwife or doctor can draw each baby's position on the skin with a felt-tipped pen at every prenatal visit. Referring to each by name and gender (if it is known), also helps the babies with their ego boundaries. As psychiatrists Bernabei and Levi[8] point out, 'more than other people, twins must in each moment live with the problem and the question of identity of the "I" and of the "you" and their continuing relation' (see Chapter 1). At no time is this situation more pronounced than during prenatal development and the effects of this interaction last a lifetime.

Our general understanding of the memories of birth and the prenatal period is hampered by the almost universal belief that we do not have such memories. Chamberlain proposes that memory is innate rather than developmental, noting that after 70 years of intensive research, our understanding of memory storage and retrieval is still incomplete. However, the growing body of evidence regarding memories of intrauterine experiences is impressive (see Chapter 24). Anecdotes dealing with early twin experiences that were recalled with various regression therapies are described in my books *Having Twins*[9] and *Primal Connections*[10].

Journal writing

Encourage parents to keep a journal. This helps them express both negative and positive feelings toward the pregnancy and to bond with the twins as a unit and as individuals. It also creates a wonderful record of the multiple's prenatal existence. These early writings have additional importance, because often there is little time to maintain the journal after the delivery. As Leonardo da Vinci noted: 'the child grows daily more when in the body of its mother than when it is outside'. This fact of life should not be overlooked or forgotten.

Psychological support at the time of complications

Allopathic medical professionals often treat symptoms without exploring the cause; therefore, the psychological dimensions of specific complications may be overlooked. Every symptom has an underlying emotion that should be considered, especially in pregnancy. Mothers of twins who develop contractions of preterm labor or high blood pressure can often resolve these complications if encouraged to talk frankly about what is going on in their lives. If this is not possible, hypnosis may be tried.

According to David Cheek, an obstetrician of 35 years' experience, preterm labor is caused by unconcious fears[11-13]. These fears become reinforced by dreams of losing a baby/ies that lead to increased sensitivity to the normal Braxton–Hicks contractions. As the contractions become more painful, the fear becomes conscious. Ideomotor questioning techniques under hypnosis can easily locate the fears and help the mother to resolve them. With his last 250 patients, Cheek avoided preterm deliveries by encouraging women (who had presented with contractions) to call him – even during the night (half of his patients would wake from their sleep with contractions). He conducted the hypnosis over the telephone (D. Cheek, personal communication to author). Cheek has now retired from clinical work and is further studying the therapeutic value of ideomotor questioning. He will provide consultation by phone if the obstetrician makes the call and gives him a definitive diagnosis of preterm labor (cervical changes) for the purpose of his statistical research. However, from a preventive aspect, he prefers to contact the women when they first experience preterm contractions. In view of the benign nature of this therapy (and the failure of tocolytics in many cases), it is certainly worthy of the most serious consideration. Because Dr Cheek is gathering data for a research project, he does not charge for his services in this regard. Other practitioners offering telephone hypnosis for resolving preterm labor are listed in the Appendix.

In view of the success of hypnosis in the treatment of preterm labor and hypertension by Cheek[11-13] and Peterson[14], this modality should be considered as a low-risk alternative.

Bed rest

Although I advocate resting twice daily for at least a half-hour, total confinement in bed can create a paradoxical situation. On the one hand, the mother may believe that she is helping her babies achieve maturity; on the other, she may feel guilty that she needs to rest because her 'body is failing her'. Additional guilt may develop if the mother feels that she is neglecting her house, her other children and/or her job. Full bed rest should be avoided if possible and used only as a temporary last resort if other means do not resolve the problem.

Whenever a mother's activities are restricted, regular telephone and personal contact is essential. In Freeman's[15] symposium on home monitoring of contractions, one group found that daily contact with the medical staff was very important, especially if the medical staff initiated it. A reduction in the incidence of preterm labor was observed even when the monitor strips were not interpreted and the phone calls were the primary intervention.

The mother's confidence and well-being will be greatly improved by physical therapeutic to provide appropriate exercise. Such activity ameliorates the physical problems as well as the mental depression that is frequently associated with prolonged confinement. In this regard, the anxiety, tension, excitement and insomnia that may result from the use of tocolytic drugs can also be relieved by the use of a bath or pool. Water facilitates movement as well as relaxation, and provides resistance for gentle strengthening exercise. Even if the mother requires transport by wheelchair, the benefits of immersion to reduce swelling, diminish uterine contractions and improve morale are certainly worth the effort.

Mothers of multiples are often well aware of the potential problems associated with pregnancy and birth, having heard plenty of 'glad it is you and not me' comments and disaster stories. Comments that may seem relatively benign to a health professional, such as 'your cervix is a little soft' or 'you're not very tall to be carrying twins', often cause significant anxiety and stress. At an unconscious level, often during sleep, a woman may perceive her Braxton–Hicks contractions as painful. According to Cheek and Le Cron[1], the mother then becomes more tense and anxious and a vicious cycle sets up that indeed may culminate in preterm labor.

The birth and after

Vaginal delivery

Natural childbirth, without medication/anesthesia, and breast feeding are important psychologically for the mother to feel that her body has functioned normally despite the additional challenge of multiples.

Cesarean delivery

Unfortunately, operative delivery has become more common for twins and is virtually assured for quadruplets and many triplets. (Editor: This is true at least in the United States. Professor Derom of Belgium and his group in East Flanders, as well as their colleagues in The Netherlands, are firm proponents of vaginal delivery.) This circumstance is not always considered in the best interests of all, as Chervenak points out in Chapter 36. Because the postpartum demands related to the care of two or more babies are so rigorous, surgery should be avoided if possible. If, however, the mother has to undergo Cesarean delivery, it is particularly important for her to breast feed in order to experience the special intimacy of nursing her children and to support her self-esteem. This intimacy is especially important for mothers of multiples, who sometimes feel that they do not give each baby 'enough' closeness.

Just as Cesarean babies need additional cuddling, body contact and massage (lacking the experience of contractions at vaginal delivery), Cesarean mothers need extra care, too. Physical rehabilitation to restore normal muscle strength and to prevent backache and injury also returns a sense of mastery over one's own body. Physical therapy by trained therapists should commence in the recovery room.

Unless the infants require special attention or admission to the intensive-care nursery, it is important that the mother hold them as soon as possible after delivery. In this way, she can physically experience the reality of two or more babies. Hospital staff can help by assisting the mother with simultaneous breast feeding, positioning for cuddling, etc.

During the hospital stay, twins should share the same crib if at all possible. That this practice is virtually unheard of indicates the poor appreciation of the emotional needs of newborn multiples both by society and by the medical profession. When the babies require intensive care, this argument is even more persuasive. Failure to thrive can occur from lack of touch and human contact in early life. By the same token, a sick multiple, separated both from his or her sibling, as well as from his or her mother, suffers even greater stress and anxiety.

Breast feeding

Doctors and nurses often discourage breast feeding in the case of twins and particularly higher-order multiples. *This is a grave disservice to parents as well as the babies.* The physiological and emotional advantages of nursing must be emphasized, and these benefits are even more valuable in cases of prematurity and illness (see Chapter 41). Moreover, the financial cost and labor associated with bottle feeding should not be minimized. While breast feeding is often difficult for single, working or poor mothers, as well as mothers with other children, bottle feeding is *not* the solution. Instead, more financial support, home help and encouragement by maternity-care providers is required to ensure successful breast feeding for *at least* 5–6 months.

Postpartum adjustment

Postpartum adjustment depends to a great extent on the quantity and quality of preparation and planning that the couple were able to institute in the prenatal period. 'Twin shock' can overwhelm the best-prepared mother as she copes with marathon feedings, lack of sleep and crying babies, all of which are particularly exhausting if she must return to work.

Difficulty in distinguishing identical twins or preferring one over the other often leads to feelings of guilt, because new mothers have not as yet worked through a series of changing attachments. This is particularly true in the radical change with regard to her partner. The new mother and her partner are now parents first, and spouses and lovers second.

The antepartum 'Supermom' image should be tossed aside. Both parents can make the adjustment with twins easier by co-sleeping and co-bathing, to ensure that they do not 'lose touch' with each other and at the same time to feel that their twins are enjoying extra contact. The family bed and bath save time and extra equipment, and mean more rest for everyone. For reassurance about sexual opportunities, smothering and other unfounded anxieties about this age-old custom, the reader should consult Thevenin's *The Family Bed*[16].

Dealing with older sibling(s)

The older sibling(s) often represents a major source of stress. Regressive behavior such as bed wetting, nail biting and increased incidence of minor accidents is not uncommon with the arrival of any younger sibling. Twins, of course, are not just siblings but celebrities. This possibility must be dealt with from the outset by making extra efforts to ensure that the older child(ren) feels affirmed of his/her/their worth and value to the family unit. Not to do so may engender hostility, indifference and, in some instances, aggressive feelings toward the twins. Ideally, each sibling should have supervised time with each twin separately. Sensitive friends and families will offer special gifts and invitations to the siblings, as well as the twins.

Infant hospitalization

Any situation which separates the multiples is very taxing for both mother and child(ren). If one baby is struggling to survive, it is difficult for the mother to bond with the healthy baby while attempting to 'do enough' for the one who is ill. It is important that the healthy multiple(s) and sibling(s) – no matter how young – visit and have close contact with the baby who is ill. Otherwise, the healthy child(ren) will be disturbed by this absence, which further increases maternal stress. Infant twins are highly distressed by separation, although they may be too sick to show it.

Coping with fetal loss

Many more twins exist in the shadowy world of prenatal ultrasound (some estimates are as high as 70%) than are born (see Chapters 4–6). Although a vanishing twin is a benign medical event, it may be a turbulent emotional experience. At any stage of the pregnancy, women need to grieve after their loss, *particularly in the case of multiples where the couple must continue to bond with the surviving baby/ies*. Every possible memento should be saved; scans, autopsy report, lock of hair and, if possible, photographs of the twins *together*, in any condition. The parents should hold the dead baby/ies as often and as long as they wish, without pressure from the staff to look after the living baby/ies.

The mother should never be told that she is lucky to have another living baby, or that God didn't mean for her to handle extra baby/ies, or that it is just as well, because something was wrong. A loss is a loss and should be treated as such[17]. Because loss among multiples occurs more frequently than with singletons, maternity-care providers need to develop bereavement skills; these are outlined in the Appendices of *Having Twins*[9]. Allowing the parents to grieve fully after a loss actually facilitates the processes of letting go and bonding with the survivor(s). Memories of traumatic events, which later become unconscious, may adversely affect the health and development of the surviving multiple(s) if the death is not openly discussed during the formative years.

It is important to remember that mothers always think of their offspring in the original number. As for the survivor, he/she is still a twin (triplet etc.) regardless of what society says. Respecting this reality is essential for family dynamics as well as for the survivors themselves, so that each one knows if s/he was once a twin, triplet, etc. Unfortunately, society almost invariably accentuates the loss by statements such as 'What a cute baby', not recognizing that the baby once had a twin or that the twins once had one or more siblings. (Editor: This process continues into adulthood when the survivor still speaks of his or her 'twin', despite the loss having occurred years earlier. Singletons cannot easily deal with this, but the Editors ask their forebearance.)

In summary, multiple pregnancy has the potential to be an exciting and fulfilling time or an anxious struggle beset with complications. Earlier diagnosis with sensitive disclosure, indepth interviews, education and counselling, plus utilization of the available support networks can help to facilitate the psychological adaptation to multiple pregnancy.

References

1. Cheek, D. and Le Cron, L. (1993). *Clinical Hypnotherapy*. (Needham, MA: Allyn and Bacon)
2. Groothuis, J.R. (1982). Increased child abuse in families with twins. *Pediatrics*, **70**, 769
3. Evans, A. (1989). Address at *Pre- and Perinatal Psychology Association of North America, Fourth Congress*, Amherst, MA, August
4. DeMause, L. (1991). The universality of incest. *J. Psychohistory*, **19**, 123
5. Zazzo, R. (1989). In Lebatard, C. (ed.) *Une aventure tridimensionelle. Naissances Multiples*, 26 juin
6. Piontelli, A. (1989). A study on twins before and after birth. *Int. Rev. Psycho-Anal.*, **16**, 413
7. Veldman, F. (1989). *Haptonomie: Science de L'Affectivité*. (Paris: Presses Universitaires de France)
8. Bernabei, P. and Levi, G. (1976). Psychopathologic problems in twins during childhood. *Acta Genet. Med. Gemellol.*, **25**, 381
9. Noble, E. (1991). *Having Twins*. (Boston: Houghton Mifflin)
10. Noble, E. (1993). *Primal Connections*. (New York: Simon and Schuster)
11. Rossi, E.L. and Cheek, D.B. (1988). *Mind–body Therapy: Methods of Idiodynamic Healing in Hypnosis*. (New York: Norton)
12. Cheek, D.B. (1969). The significance of dreams in initiating premature labor. *Am. J. Clin. Hypnosis*, **12**, 5
13. Cheek, D.B. (1965). Some newer understanding of dreams in relation to threatened abortion and premature labor. *Pac. Med. Surg.*, **73**, 379
14. Peterson, G. (1987). Prenatal bonding, prenatal communicating and the prevention of prematurity. *Pre- Peri-nat. Psychol.*, **2**, 87
15. Freeman, R.K. (1988). Symposium: Home monitoring of uterine contractions. *Contemp. OB/GYN*, **32**, 173
16. Thevenin, T. (1987). *The Family Bed*, revised edn. (New Jersey: Avery)
17. Bryan, E. (1986). The death of a newborn twin: how can support for parents be improved? *Acta Genet. Med. Gemellol.*, **5**, 115

Maternal characteristics and prenatal nutrition

B. Luke

Introduction

The incidence and type of twinning worldwide vary by a number of maternal characteristics, including age and race. Whereas monozygotic (MZ) twinning rates are remarkably constant at about 3–4 per 1000 live births, the dizygotic (DZ) twinning rate varies between racial groups and with maternal age. Within racial groups, DZ twinning is at least partially related to a maternal recessive trait[1]. An estimated 11–27% of Caucasian women may be twin prone, much more than the proportion who actually bear twins[1].

In the United States, the multiple birth ratio (MBR) (the number of multiple births/1000 total live births), an indicator of the overall rate of twinning, differs considerably between ethnic and racial groups. It ranges from a high of 25.8 for blacks and 24.9 for Alaskan natives, 19.6 for whites, 18.8 for American Indians, to 17.0 for Japanese, 15.3 for Hawaiian, 13.2 for Filipino, and 11.2 for Chinese[2,3].

Increases in MBR parallel increasing maternal age, and are differentially higher for blacks compared to whites. For example, the MBR for women aged 30–34 is more than twice that of women under the age 20 years.

Physical characteristics

No particular maternal physical characteristics are associated with MZ twinning, but women who conceive DZ twins are different from women who conceive singletons or MZ twins, being older, of higher parity, taller and heavier. The proportion of twin births to women aged 35 and older in the United States has more than doubled between 1982 and 1992. Several studies have reported that twinning rates are higher among overweight and obese women[4–6]. The increased twinning rate among this group of women may be due to the accompanying greater age and parity, however.

Maternal height is positively correlated with the rate of twinning[7], and therefore may partially explain the mechanism by which zygosity influences birth weight. In addition, mothers of DZ twins are taller than mothers of MZ twins and mothers of singletons[8], but the heights of mothers of MZ twins and singletons do not differ.

Menstrual and hormonal differences

The physical differences noted above may reflect underlying hormonal differences between women who conceive twins and those who conceive singletons. For example, in a study of reproductive and menstrual characteristics, mothers of multiples had an earlier age at menarche and shorter menstrual cycles than mothers of singletons[6]. Mothers of like-sexed twins experienced an earlier menopause compared to mothers of singletons[9]. The earlier the twin birth, the shorter the menstrual life thereafter[9]. Women who have twins have a higher level of follicle stimulating hormone (FSH) compared to women who have singletons. Mothers of DZ twins have an earlier age of menarche and a lower frequency of menstrual irregularities compared to mothers of singletons[10]. Obese women have elevated levels of circulating estrogens, and presumably this circumstance is associated with higher levels of FSH[11]. FSH levels increase with age[12] and may account in part for the effect of maternal age on DZ twinning rates[8]. The increased height among mothers of DZ twins may also reflect an additional manifestation of anterior pituitary activity, namely growth hormone secretion.

Physiologic changes and adaptations to multiple gestation

Endocrine and metabolism

Adaptation to multiple pregnancy is in many ways an exaggerated version of the maternal response to a singleton pregnancy. The trigger to the physiologic response is hormonal, with increased production of both steroid and protein hormones from the fetoplacental unit during multiple pregnancy, primarily due to an increase in placental mass. Urinary and plasma estriol levels increase in twin pregnancies to more than double the singleton mean by term[13]. Progesterone is also increased during twin pregnancies above that observed in singleton pregnancies[14]. Other hormones that increase above singleton pregnancy levels include human placental lactogen (hPL) and Schwangerschafts protein (SP_1)[15,16]. α-Fetoprotein levels are indicative of fetal abnormalities in singleton pregnancies. There is a difference in the production of α-fetoprotein levels in MZ vs. DZ twin pregnancies, which may be related to differences in placentation[17].

The hormonal changes in multiple pregnancy also result in alterations in metabolism. Women with twin pregnancies have significantly lower blood glucose and insulin levels[18,19]. Despite these differences, women with twin pregnancies do not have an increased frequency of gestational diabetes[20].

Uterine changes

At the beginning of the second trimester, the total intrauterine volume in twin pregnancy is similar to that of a singleton pregnancy; by 18 weeks' gestation, however, the uterus of a twin pregnancy is twice as large as that of a singleton pregnancy[21]. By 25 weeks' gestation, the uterus of a twin gestation is equivalent to a singleton uterus at term. By term, the uterus of a singleton pregnancy has a total intrauterine volume of about 5000 ml, compared to nearly 10 000 ml in a twin pregnancy[21].

Weight gain

Twin gestations A major physiologic response to pregnancy is gestational weight gain. Generally, the weight gain with multiple pregnancy is greater and of a different pattern than in singleton pregnancies. MacGillivray and Campbell[4] reported that weight gain in the first trimester was much higher among mothers with twins compared to mothers of singletons and greater than expected. Campbell et al.[22] also reported that women with twin pregnancies tended to gain more weight and in a different pattern than women with singleton pregnancies. In a study of 378 primiparas who delivered twins between 1950 and 1969, Campbell and her group found the mean total weight gain for women with twins to be 14.6 kg (32.1 lb) compared to 11.1 kg (24.4 lb) for singletons. These authors noted that the maximum rate of gain in twin pregnancies occurs during the early and late weeks of gestation compared to mid-gestation for singletons.

Konwinski et al.[23] had previously reported that, among twin gestations, the rate of preterm delivery was higher among women with pregravid weights less than 136 lb and who had inadequate gestational weight gain: less than 6 kg (13.2 lb) by 28 weeks, or less than 8 kg (17.6 lb) by 36 weeks.

In a study of weight gain in twin pregnancies, Pederson et al.[24] reported that optimum pregnancy outcome (≥37 weeks' gestation, both infants ≥2500 g, each infant with Apgar scores ≥7) was associated with weight gains of 20 kg (44 lb) vs. 16.8 kg (37 lb) for women with less-than-optimum outcomes. These investigators also found that the weight gain patterns of both groups were parallel until 30 weeks' gestation, at which time weight gain slowed in the less-than-optimum group.

Brown and Schloesser[5] investigated the relationships between pregravid weight, gestational weight gain, and outcome in 922 twin births delivered at term using linked birth and death certificates in Kansas between 1980 and 1986. These investigators found a positive linear relationship between gestational weight gain and infant birth weights in women who were underweight or normal weight before conception, but not for those who were overweight or obese. They also found that the proportion of low birth weight infants declined as pregravid weight increased. The mean gestational weight gain of underweight women who were delivered of twin infants at term with birth weights in the range of the lowest perinatal mortality (3001–3500 g)[25] was 44.2 lb; for normal pregravid weight women, the corresponding figure was 40.9 lb.

A recent study by Luke et al.[26] examined the association between maternal pregravid weight, weight gain to selected weeks of gestation, and average birth weight as the mean of the twin pair and as a ratio derived by dividing the average birth weight by the 50th percentile weight for gestation. This study reported that, regardless of maternal pregravid weight, twin birth weight >2500 g was associated with higher maternal weight gains at 24 weeks' gestation, higher rate of gain and total gain, shorter newborn length of hospital stay, and higher birth weight ratios (Table 1). Among preterm births, women who gave birth to twins with birth weights >2500 g had higher early (before 24 weeks' gestation) and late (after 24 weeks' gestation) rates of gain, longer length of gestation, higher mean birth weights and birth weight ratios, and shorter length of stay compared to their preterm low birth weight counterparts (Table 2). Among term pregnancies, women who gave birth to twins with birth weights >2500 g had significantly higher early rate of gain and total gain, and their infants had higher birth weights, birth weight ratios, and shorter length of stay compared to their term low birth weight counterparts (Table 2). Total weight gain of 40–45 lb and a rate of gain of 1.25 lb/week were significantly associated with higher twin birth weights and better intrauterine growth for gestational age.

In a follow-up study by Luke et al.[27], ten models were formulated using multiple regression and multiple logistic regression, including absolute birth weight (sum of twin pair, smaller of twin pair), larger of twin pair, birth weight ratio (observed twin birth weight divided by expected singleton birth weight for that gestational age, for average of twin pair, smaller of twin pair, and larger of twin pair), birth weight ≤10th percentile for smaller and larger of twin pair. The last two models characterized the ideal twin pregnancy as (model I): birth weight of the smaller of the twin pair >10th percentile for gestational age and length of stay ≤8 days for each twin; and (model II): same as model I but also including gestation of 35–38 weeks. In the models of birth weight, gestations of 28–36 weeks and 39–41 weeks, black race, ≥15% discordancy, and smoking were all significant negative factors. The pattern of early low weight gain (≤0.85 lb/week before 24 weeks) and late low weight gain (<1.0 lb/week after 24 weeks) was negatively associated with all eight models of intrauterine growth. *Based on these studies, the recommended rate of gain for twin gestations is 24 lb by 24 weeks, and a rate of gain of 1.25 lb/week thereafter.*

Triplet and higher-order gestations

There are much less data and currently no recommendations on maternal weight gain in triplet and higher-order gestations. When weight gain data have been reported, it has usually been on case reports or small series, and frequently did not consider the factors of maternal pregravid weight or parity, nor the pattern of gain. For example, Seoud et al.[28] reported on 15 triplet and four quadruplet pregnancies that resulted from *in vitro* fertilization. In the triplet gestations, maternal weight gain averaged 50.6 lb in 31.8 weeks. In the quadruplet gestations, maternal weight gain averaged 68.2 lb in 31 weeks. In their review of 71 quadruplet pregnancies, Collins and Bleyl[29] reported an average maternal weight gain of

Table 1 Comparison of perinatal outcomes by maternal body mass index categories by average of twin birth weights <2500 g vs. ≥2500 g. Adapted from reference 26

Pregravid weight for height and birth weight categories	n	Gain			Length of gestation (weeks)	Birth weight (g)	Length of stay (days)	Birth weight ratio
		Rate of gain (lb/week)		Total (lb)				
		Early	Late					
All weights								
<2500 g	105	0.90	1.09	33.1	34.6	1989	16.2	0.885
≥2500 g	58	0.94	1.44	42.5	37.8	2865	5.9	0.959
p value		NS	<0.001	<0.001	<0.001	<0.001	<0.001	0.03
Underweight								
<2500 g	26	0.85	1.09	32.5	34.8	1948	16.9	0.816
≥2500 g	14	0.96	1.45	43.6	38.3	2918	6.9	0.944
p value		NS	0.03	0.008	<0.001	<0.001	0.005	0.002
Normal weight								
<2500 g	63	0.87	1.12	32.4	34.4	1983	16.3	0.905
≥2500 g	36	0.94	1.43	41.9	37.5	2836	5.5	0.972
p value		NS	0.01	0.001	<0.001	<0.001	<0.001	NS
Overweight								
<2500 g	16	1.13	0.92	36.7	34.8	2076	14.4	0.922
≥2500 g	8	0.93	1.51	43.5	38.1	2903	5.7	0.927
p value		NS	0.02	NS	0.01	<0.001	0.01	NS

NS is not significant at the 0.05 level (two-tailed)

Table 2 Comparison of perinatal outcomes by term vs. preterm and by average of twin birth weights <2500 g vs. ≥2500 g. Adapted from reference 26

Pregravid weight for height and birth weight categories	n	Gain			Length of gestation (weeks)	Birth weight (g)	Length of stay (days)	Birth weight ratio
		Rate of gain (lb/week)		Total (lb)				
		Early	Late					
Preterm*	90	0.93	1.13	33.2	33.6	2024	16.3	0.973
Term[†]	73	0.90	1.31	40.5	38.4	2641	7.8	0.836
p value		NS	0.03	0.001	<0.001	<0.001	<0.001	<0.001
Preterm								
<2500 g	78	0.92	1.10	32.2	33.3	1921	18.1	0.948
≥2500 g	12	1.03	1.35	39.6	35.1	2693	4.5	1.135
p value		NS	NS	NS	0.01	<0.001	<0.001	0.01
Term								
<2500 g	27	0.87	1.05	35.7	38.2	2184	10.6	0.704
≥2500 g	46	0.92	1.47	43.3	38.5	2910	6.2	0.913
p value		NS	<0.001	0.02	NS	<0.001	<0.001	<0.001
≥2500 g								
Preterm	12	1.03	1.35	39.6	35.1	2693	4.5	1.135
Term	46	0.92	1.47	43.3	38.5	2910	6.2	0.913
p value		NS	NS	NS	<0.001	0.01	0.03	<0.001

NS is not significant at the 0.05 level (two-tailed); *preterm is defined as <37 completed weeks of gestation; [†]term is defined as ≥37 completed weeks of gestation

45.8 lb in 31.4 weeks. A recent analysis of data from 1138 surveys of mothers of triplets indicated an average maternal weight gain of 45.1 lb in 33.8 weeks[30]. Based on these reports, *it seems reasonable to recommend weight gain of 36 lb by 24 weeks, and a rate of gain of 1.25 lb/week thereafter for triplet gestations.*

Cardiovascular and hematologic changes

Other adaptations made to a greater degree in twin compared to singleton pregnancies include cardiovascular and hematologic changes (see Chapter 19). Some of the earliest adaptations in pregnant women are cardiovascular changes. Total peripheral resistance is lowered even further in a twin pregnancy because of the greater production of progesterone and prostaglandins, resulting in vasodilatation and a lowering of diastolic blood pressure.

Other related changes include the plasma volume and constituents of the blood. From about 20 weeks onwards, the plasma volume in twin gestations is approximately 20% greater than in singleton gestations[13]. Total red cell volume also increases above singleton levels in twin pregnancy by about 25%[13]. This is indicative of a markedly increased oxygen-carrying capacity required for the oxygen transfer for two fetuses. The increase in red cell volume is not as great as that of the plasma, resulting in a more exaggerated hemodilution. The hemoglobin concentration for women with twins averages 10 g/dl from 20 weeks' gestation onwards[31]. During pregnancy, hematologic values change substantially. For women with adequate iron stores, hemoglobin and hematocrit values begin to decline during the first trimester, reach a nadir by the end of the second trimester, and gradually rise again during the third trimester[32–35]. However, because of the concomitant changes in hemoglobin and hematocrit during pregnancy, iron deficiency anemia ideally should be characterized according to the specific stage of gestation. Table 3 gives the mean hemoglobin values by week of gestation, as well as cut-off values of hemoglobin and hematocrit defining anemia as suggested by the Centers for Disease Control.

Table 3 Pregnancy month-specific hemoglobin and hematocrit cut-offs. Adapted from CDC criteria for anemia in children and childbearing-aged women. *MMWR*, **38**, 400–4, 1989

Gestation (weeks)	Mean hemoglobin (g/dl)	5th percentile hemoglobin (g/dl)	5th percentile hematocrit (%)
12	12.2	11.0	33.0
16	11.8	10.6	32.0
20	11.6	10.5	32.0
24	11.6	10.5	32.0
28	11.8	10.7	32.0
32	12.1	11.0	33.0
36	12.5	11.4	34.0
40	12.9	11.9	36.0

The principal goals of therapy for the treatment of iron deficiency anemia are the correction of the iron deficit and replenishment of the iron stores. The absorption of iron supplements is influenced by the solubility of the compound, dosage, timing of administration (with or between meals), concurrent medications (alone or as part of a vitamin–mineral supplement), and the extent of physiologic iron stores. The therapeutic dosage of iron supplements should be evaluated in terms of the amount of iron in the compound, the equivalent in elemental iron, and the presence of additional ingredients that could potentially reduce iron absorption. Hydrated ferrous sulfate contains 20% iron by weight, and therefore 60 mg of elemental iron in a 300 mg tablet[36]. Ferrous gluconate contains 12% iron by weight, and ferrous fumarate contains 32% iron by weight, and therefore a 300 mg tablet would contain, respectively, 36 mg and 96 mg of elemental iron. The highest availability of therapeutic iron is from ferrous sulfate and such organic complexes or chelates of iron as the ascorbate, fumarate and citrate complexes; reduced metallic iron is intermediate. Iron phosphates, carbonates, or EDTA complexes exhibit poor bioavailability. The absorption of iron is greater when the supplement contains only an iron salt than when the iron is part of a vitamin–mineral compound[37]. Calcium

Table 4 Heme-rich dietary sources of iron. Calculated from US Department of Agriculture, Human Nutrition Information Service. Home and Garden Bulletin No. 72: *Nutritive Value of Foods*. Washington, DC: US Government Printing Office, 1985

Food and method of preparation	Iron content (mg)	
	Per 100 g	Per 100 kcal
Pork sausage (Braunschweiger)	9.3	2.6
Chicken liver (cooked)	8.5	5.7
Oysters (breaded, fried)	6.7	3.3
Oysters (raw)	6.5	9.8
Beef liver (fried)	6.2	2.9
Clams (canned)	4.1	4.1
Sirloin steak (lean, broiled)	3.3	1.6
Sardines (canned)	3.1	1.5
Duck (roasted)	2.7	1.3
Turkey (dark meat, roasted)	2.4	1.3
Lamb chops (lean, broiled)	2.0	0.9
Shrimp (canned)	1.6	1.4
Ocean perch (breaded, fried)	1.4	0.6
Turkey (light meat, roasted)	1.3	0.8
Fried chicken	1.3	0.5
Ham (lean roasted)	1.1	0.6
Roasted chicken	1.0	0.6
Veal cutlet (broiled)	0.9	0.4
Canadian bacon (fried)	0.9	0.5
Tuna (solid white, canned)	0.7	0.4

carbonate, citrate and phosphate all have been shown to inhibit iron absorption[37,38], as do magnesium[37] and zinc[39–41].

The Institute of Medicine's 1990 report on nutrition during pregnancy[42] recommended the routine use of 30 mg of ferrous iron per day beginning at about the 12th week of gestation. For these reasons, the iron supplement should include a type of iron which has a high bioavailability (ferrous sulfate or fumarate), is free from additional ingredients which would lower the absorption of iron (such as calcium, magnesium, or zinc), and, if part of a multivitamin, does not contain excessive levels of additional vitamins or minerals.

Multiple gestation imposes a special demand for iron which may not be adequately met in women with low or absent iron stores. An early and thorough hematologic evaluation is important to establish the extent of iron stores at the onset of pregnancy and to prescribe appropriate therapy. Of the oral medications, ferrous sulfate has the highest bioavailability. Animal sources of iron are the best absorbed dietary sources of this mineral because of their content of heme iron (Table 4). Because iron deficiency anemia during pregnancy is associated with an increased risk of morbidity and mortality for both the mother and her unborn children, assessment of iron status and provision of appropriate therapy are important considerations of optimal prenatal care.

The Institute of Medicine[42] recommends the following clinical regimen to prevent iron deficiency during pregnancy:

(1) The routine use of 30 mg ferrous iron per day beginning at about 12 weeks' gestation, in conjunction with a well-balanced

diet that contains enhancers of iron absorption (ascorbic acid, meats).

(2) The supplemental iron should be taken between meals with liquids other than milk, tea, or coffee.

(3) Hemoglobin and hematocrit should be routinely determined at the first prenatal visit in order to detect pre-existing anemia. Hemoglobin levels below 11 g/dl during the first or third trimesters or below 10.5 g/dl during the second trimester are characteristic of anemia. When accompanied by a serum ferritin concentration <12 μg/dl, iron deficiency anemia can be diagnosed with certainty and required treatment with 60–120 mg/day of ferrous iron prescribed. When the hemoglobin concentration becomes normal for the stage of gestation, the iron dose can be decreased to 30 mg/day.

Dietary recommendations

At present there are no specific dietary recommendations for women pregnant with twins, triplets, or higher-order multiples. *The most current guidelines on gestational weight gain from the National Academy of Sciences[42] suggest a range of gain of 25–35 lb for a singleton gestation, depending on the mother's pregravid weight. Current research suggests optimal weight gain for twin gestations to be 24 lb by 24 weeks' gestation, and 1.25 lb/week thereafter; for triplet and higher-order multiple gestations, weight gain should be about 36 lb by 24 weeks' gestation, and 1.25 lb/week thereafter.*

Good maternal nutrition is central to achieving optimal fetal growth and development, and to maintaining maternal health and well-being. Through the Recommended Dietary Allowances (RDAs), the National Academy of Sciences recommends levels of essential nutrients to meet the additional nutrient

Table 5 Summary of RDAs for women aged 25 and older, pregnant with singletons vs. twins. Adapted from the pregnancy RDAs in National Academy of Sciences: *Recommended Dietary Allowances*, 10th edition, Washington, DC: National Academy Press, 1989

Nutrient	Singleton pregnant	Twin/triplet pregnant	Dietary sources
Folic acid	400 μg	800 μg	leafy vegetables, liver
Vitamin D	10 μg	15 μg	fortified dairy products
Iron	30 mg	50 mg	meats, eggs, grains
Calcium	1200 mg	1800 mg	dairy products
Phosphorus	1200 mg	1800 mg	meats
Pyroxidine	2.2 mg	4.0 mg	meats, liver, grains
Thiamine	1.5 mg	3.0 mg	enriched grains, pork
Zinc	15 mg	30 mg	meats, seafood, eggs
Riboflavin	1.6 mg	3.0 mg	meats, liver, grains
Protein	60 mg	120 mg	meats, fish, poultry, dairy
Iodine	175 μg	300 μg	iodized salt, seafood
Vitamin C	70 mg	150 mg	citrus fruits, tomatoes
Energy	2500 kcal	3000 kcal	protein, fat, carbohydrate
Magnesium	320 mg	450 mg	seafood, legumes, grains
Niacin	17 mg	25 mg	meats, nuts, legumes
Vitamin B_{12}	2.2 μg	3.0 μg	animal proteins
Vitamin A	800 μg	1000 μg	dark green, yellow, or orange fruits and vegetables, liver

demands of a singleton pregnancy. At present, there are no guidelines for women pregnant with a twin, triplet, or higher-order pregnancy. In the absence of such guidelines and in view of the established need for substantially higher weight gains, it seems reasonable to propose a 50–100% increase in the RDAs for singleton pregnancy for women pregnant with multiples. Table 5 outlines a modified RDA for women pregnant with multiples.

References

1. Wyshak, G. and White, C. (1965). Genealogical study of human twinning. *Am. J. Public Hlth.*, **55**, 1586–93
2. Taffel, S.M. (1987). Characteristics of American Indian and Alaska Native births, United States, 1984. *Monthly Vital Statistics Report*, Vol. 36, No. 3, Supplement, June 19
3. Taffel, S.M. (1984). Characteristics of Asian births: United States, 1980. *Monthly Vital Statistics Report*, Vol. 32, No. 10, Supplement, February 10
4. MacGillivray, I. and Campbell, D.M. (1978). The physical characteristics and adaptations of women with twin pregnancies. In Allen, G., Nance, W.E. and Parisi, P. (eds.) *Twin Research: Clinical Studies*, pp. 81–6. (New York: Alan R. Liss)
5. Brown, J.E. and Schloesser, P.T. (1990). Prepregnancy weight status, prenatal weight gain, and the outcome of term twin gestations. *Am. J. Obstet. Gynecol.*, **162**, 182–6
6. Wyshak, G. (1981). Reproductive and menstrual characteristics of mothers of multiple births and mothers of singletons only: a discriminant analysis. In Gedda, L., Parisi, P. and Nance, W.E. (eds.) *Twin Research 3: Twin Biology and Multiple Pregnancy*, pp. 95–105. (New York: Alan R. Liss)
7. Campbell, D.M., Campbell, A.J. and MacGillivray, I. (1974). Maternal characteristics of women having twin pregnancies. *J. Biosoc. Sci.*, **6**, 463–70
8. Corney, G. Seedburgh, D., Thompson, B., Campbell, D.M., MacGillivray, I. and Timlin, D. (1981). Multiple and singleton pregnancy: differences between mothers as well as offspring. In Gedda, L., Parisi, P. and Nance, W.E. (eds.) *Twin Research 3: Twin Biology and Multiple Pregnancy*, pp. 107–14. (New York: Alan R. Liss)
9. Philippe, P. (1988). The end of reproductive life in mothers of twins: epidemiologic analysis of a large data base. *Acta Genet. Med. Gemellol.*, **37**, 249–62
10. Bonnelykke, B. (1989). Menstrual characteristics of mothers of twins. *J. Biosoc. Sci.*, **21**, 329–34
11. Siiteri, P.K., Schwartz, B. and MacDonald, P.C. (1974). Oestrogen receptors and the oestrone hypothesis in relation to endometrial and breast cancer. *Gynecol. Oncol.*, **2**, 228
12. Reyes, F.I., Winter, J.S.D. and Faiman, C. (1977). Pituitary–ovarian relationships preceding the menopause. *Am. J. Obstet. Gynecol.*, **129**, 557–64
13. Campbell, D.M. (1988). Physiological changes and adaptation. In MacGillivray, I., Campbell, D.M. and Thompson, B. (eds.) *Twinning and Twins*, pp. 99–109. (New York: John Wiley)
14. Tambyraja, R.L. and Ratnam, S.S. (1981). Plasma steroid changes in twin pregnancy. In Gedda, L., Parisi, P. and Nance, W.E. (eds.) *Twin Research 3: Twin Biology and Multiple Pregnancy*, pp. 189–95. (New York: Alan R. Liss)
15. Grennert, L., Gennser, G., Persson, P., Kullander, S. and Thorell, J. (1976). Ultrasound and human placental-lactogen screening for early detection of twin pregnancies. *Lancet*, **1**, 4–6
16. Jandial, V., Horne, C.H.W., Glover, R.G., Nisbet, A.D., Campbell, D.M. and MacGillivray, I. (1979). The value of measurement of pregnancy-specific proteins in twin pregnancies. *Acta Genet. Med. Gemellol.*, **28**, 319–25
17. Thom, H., Buckland, C.M., Campbell, A.G.M., Thompson, B. and Farr, V. (1984). Maternal serum alpha-fetoprotein in monozygotic and dizygotic twin pregnancy. *Prenatal Diagn.*, **4**, 341–6
18. Spellacy, W.N., Buhi, W.C. and Birk, S.A. (1980). Carbohydrate metabolism in women with a twin pregnancy. *Obstet. Gynecol.*, **55**, 688–91
19. Campbell, D.M. and MacGillivray, I. (1979). Glucose tolerance in twin pregnancy. *Acta Genet. Med. Gemellol.*, **28**, 283–7
20. Kohl, S.G. and Casey, G. (1975). Twin gestation. *Mt. Sinai J. Med. NY*, **43**, 523

21. Redford, D.H.A. (1982). Uterine growth in twin pregnancy by measurement of total intrauterine volume. *Acta Genet. Med. Gemellol.*, **31**, 145–8
22. Campbell, D.M., MacGillivray, I. and Tuttle, S. (1982). Maternal nutrition in twin pregnancy. *Acta Genet. Med. Gemellol.*, **31**, 221–7
23. Konwinski, T., Gerard, C., Hult, A.M. and Papiernik-Berhauer, E. (1974). Maternal pregestational weight and multiple pregnancy duration. *Acta Genet. Med. Gemellol.*, **22**, 44–7
24. Pederson, A.L., Worthington-Roberts, B. and Hickok, D.E. (1989). Weight gain patterns during twin gestation. *J. Am. Dietet. Assoc.*, **89**, 642–6
25. Williams, R.L., Creasy, R.K., Cunningham, G.C., Hawes, W.E., Norris, F.D. and Tashiro, M. (1982). Fetal growth and perinatal viability in California. *Obstet. Gynecol.*, **59**, 624–32
26. Luke, B., Minogue, J., Abbey, H., Keith, L., Witter, F.R., Feng, T.I. and Johnson, T.R.B. (1992). The association between maternal weight gain and the birthweight of twins. *J. Matern. Fetal Med.*, **1**, 267–76
27. Luke, B., Minogue, J., Witter, F.R., Keith, L.G. and Johnson, T.R.B. (1993). The ideal twin pregnancy: patterns of weight gain, discordancy, and length of gestation. *Am. J. Obstet. Gynecol.*, **169**, 588–97
28. Seoud, M.A.F., Toner, J.P., Kruithoff, C. and Muasher, S.J. (1992). Outcome of twin, triplet and quadruplet *in vitro* fertilization pregnancies: the Norfolk experience. *Fertil. Steril.*, **57**, 825–34
29. Collins, M.S. and Bleyl, J.L. (1990). Seventy-one quadruplet pregnancies: management and outcome. *Am. J. Obstet. Gynecol.*, **162**, 1384–92
30. Elster, A.D., Bleyl, J.L. and Craven, T.E. (1991). Birth weight standards for triplets under modern obstetric care in the United States, 1984–89. *Obstet. Gynecol.*, **77**, 387–93
31. Hall, M.H., Campbell, D.M. and Davidson, R.J.L. (1979). Anaemia in twin pregnancy. *Acta Genet. Med. Gemellol.*, **28**, 279–82
32. Svanberg, B., Arvidsson, B., Norrby, A., Rybo, G. and Solvell, L. (1975). Absorption of supplemental iron during pregnancy: a longitudinal study with repeated bone-marrow studies and absorption measurements. *Acta Obstet. Gynecol. Scand.* (Suppl.), **48**, 87–108
33. Sjostedt, J.E., Manner, P., Nummi, S. and Ekenved, G. (1977). Oral iron prophylaxis during pregnancy: a comparative study on different dosage regimens. *Acta Obstet. Gynecol. Scand.* (Suppl.), **60**, 3–9
34. Puolakka, J., Janne, O., Pakarinen, A., Jarvinen, A. and Vihko, R. (1980). Serum ferritin as a measure of iron stores during and after normal pregnancy with and without iron supplements. *Acta Obstet. Gynecol. Scand.* (Suppl.), **95**, 43–51
35. Taylor, D.J., Mallen, C., McDougall, N. and Lind, T. (1982). Effect of iron supplementation on serum ferritin levels during and after pregnancy. *Br. J. Obstet. Gynaecol.*, **89**, 1011–17
36. Scott, D.E. and Pritchard, J.A. (1974). Anemia in pregnancy. *Clin. Perinatol.*, **1**, 491–502
37. Seligman, P.A., Caskey, J.H., Frazier, J.L., Zucker, R.M., Podell, E.R. and Allen, R.H. (1983). Measurements of iron absorption from prenatal multivitamin–mineral supplements. *Obstet. Gynecol.*, **61**, 356–62
38. Babior, B.M., Peters, W.A., Briden, P.M. and Cetrulo, C.L. (1985). Pregnant women's absorption of iron from prenatal supplements. *J. Reprod. Med.*, **30**, 355–7
39. Crofton, R.W., Gvozdanovic, D., Gvozdanovic, S., Khinn, C.C., Brunt, P.W., Mowat, N.A.G. and Agget, P.J. (1989). Inorganic zinc and the intestinal absorption of ferrous iron. *Am. J. Clin. Nutr.*, **50**, 141–4
40. Sandstrom, B., Davidson, L., Cederblad, A. and Lonnerdal, B. (1985). Oral iron, dietary ligands and zinc absorption. *J. Nutr.*, **115**, 411–14
41. Solomons, N.W. (1986). Competitive interaction of iron and zinc in the diet: consequences for human nutrition. *J. Nutr.*, **116**, 927–35
42. National Academy of Sciences (1990). *Nutrition During Pregnancy*. (Washington DC: National Academy Press)

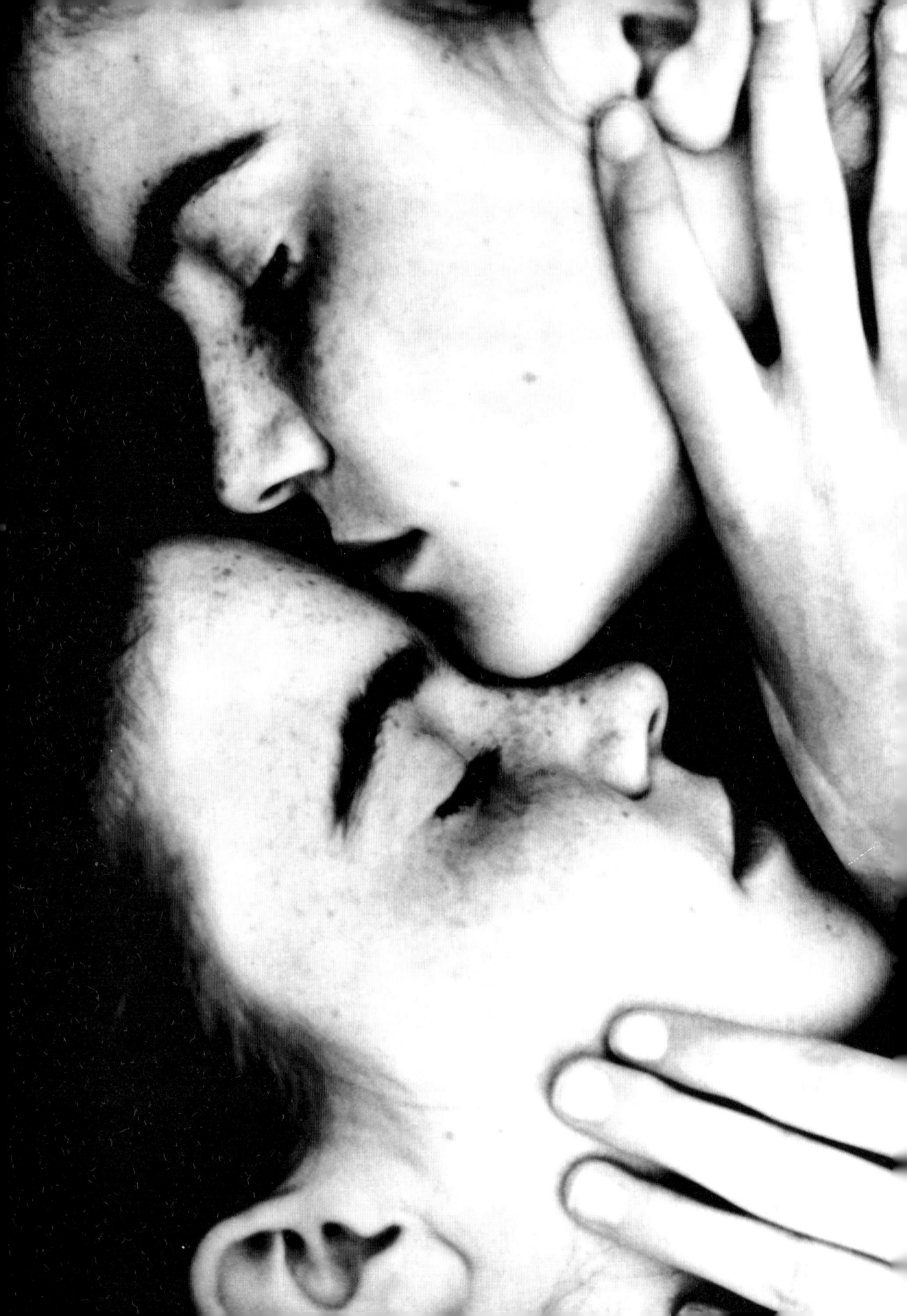

section V
Assessment and Management of Fetal Well-being

The Schell Twins

David Teplica, 1990,
Palmer Museum of Art, University Park, Pennsylvania

Prenatal genetic diagnosis: amniocentesis and chorionic villus sampling

E. Pergament

Introduction

Prenatal diagnosis is considered a standard of care for women at significant risk of having a child with a genetic disorder. For the past quarter of a century, women of advanced maternal age (35–37 years and older), women with a previous chromosomally abnormal conception, and known carriers of single gene mutations have routinely been offered second-trimester amniocentesis. During the past 5 years, however, first-trimester chorionic villus sampling (CVS) has been available as an alternative approach to the fetal diagnosis of genetic disorders.

When amniocentesis was first introduced into clinical practice, the major concerns surrounding its use were the obstetric risk to the mother and her fetus and the accuracy of the genetic analyses. These concerns were adequately resolved over the years. More recently, multicenter, national studies have determined that the safety and accuracy of first-trimester transcervical and transabdominal CVS compares favorably with the safety and accuracy of midtrimester amniocentesis (L. Jackson *et al.*, submitted for publication). Currently, transabdominal CVS is being applied in the second as well as the third trimester, particularly in cases in which the fetus has been judged at risk for a chromosomal aberration or in which a structural anomaly has been detected by ultrasound examination[1]. Unfortunately, most studies on the safety and the accuracy of prenatal genetic diagnosis have been based on singleton pregnancies[2,3] and only a limited number of reports discuss the issues as they relate to amniocentesis or CVS performed in multifetal pregnancy. (Editor: The term 'multifetal pregnancies' as used in this chapter refers to twins, triplets or higher order gestations.)

Prenatal diagnosis in multifetal pregnancy may differ in several ways compared to singleton gestations.

First, the obstetric risks following amniocentesis or CVS are likely to be qualitatively as well as quantitatively higher. Second, the rate of diagnostic error is likely to be increased, because the errors resulting from maternal cell contamination must be added to those of possible fetal–fetal cell contamination. Third, when only one fetus of a multifetal pregnancy is determined to be genetically abnormal, the prospective parents may experience additional medical and psychological problems.

Finally and more importantly, most obstetricians performing amniocentesis have considerably less experience with genetic diagnostic procedures performed on multifetal pregnancies than on singleton pregnancies. Despite this, because of the accepted safety of amniocentesis with singleton pregnancies, amniocentesis has also been accepted as safe and efficacious for genetic diagnosis in twin and triplet pregnancies. At present, experience with CVS for genetic diagnosis in multifetal pregnancy is far less well-documented than is the case for amniocentesis.

This chapter evaluates the effectiveness of both amniocentesis and CVS in the diagnosis of genetic disorders, focusing in particular on the incidence and types of obstetric risks associated with each procedure and the accuracy of the genetic analyses. Although published data pertain mainly to twins, the term multifetal will be used, because a growing number of reports discuss these analyses in triplet and quadruplet pregnancies.

Indications for prenatal diagnosis

The indications for prenatal genetic diagnosis in multiple gestations are essentially the same as in singleton pregnancies. These include advanced maternal age, a previous conceptus with a chromosomal abnormality, a parent with a structural chromosome rearrangement and the presence of genes associated with inborn errors of metabolism, e.g. Tay–Sachs disease, sickle cell disease or thalassemia, in both parents. On occasion, prenatal genetic diagnosis is also provided because of 'parental anxiety'. When such procedures are deemed necessary, it is important to explain in detail the risks and benefits of such an undertaking in the genetic counselling that precedes the intervention.

Two potential indications require specific comment. The first relates to reports that twin gestations are associated with a higher incidence of chromosome aneuploidy[4,5]. These reports raise the question of whether amniocentesis or CVS should routinely be recommended in all multifetal pregnancies. Data presented in this chapter address this question.

The second relates to the interpretation of the results of maternal serum alpha-fetoprotein (MSAFP) screening. This test is now offered routinely to all pregnant women between the 16th and 18th week of gestation. One of the common explanations for an 'abnormally elevated' MSAFP concentration is a multiple gestation. A twin pregnancy, for example, on the average exhibits an MSAFP concentration twice that of a singleton pregnancy[6,7]. Under these circumstances, higher levels of MSAFP are not unexpected and, in fact, represent a major source in the initial detection of a multifetal gestation. Approximately 40% of twin pregnancies are associated with MSAFP levels of more than a 2.5 multiple of the median (MoM) at 16 weeks' gestation[7]. Unfortunately, although the presence of twins or triplets may explain the elevation in MSAFP, the possibility of an open neural tube defect in one or more fetuses is not precluded. Despite the fact that each fetus in a multifetal gestation can be evaluated by ultrasound for the presence of any congenital anomalies, in twin pregnancies where the MSAFP level exceeds 5 MoM, amniocentesis should be performed and the amniotic fluid AFP in each amniotic sac analyzed separately, regardless of the ultrasound findings[8].

Thorough genetic counselling by a board-certified clinical geneticist and/or genetic counsellor is essential prior to performing *any* obstetric procedure for fetal diagnosis. As a result of the recent increasing commercialization of prenatal diagnostic services in the United States, in which cytogenetic laboratories have become private enterprises and amniocentesis is performed outside the hospital, the stage has been set for compromise in accurate and informative genetic counselling with parents of multiples being treated virtually the same as those with a singleton pregnancy. This is a highly questionable practice, because prenatal diagnostic procedures with multiples require a level of expertise most frequently found only at major medical centers and hospitals.

Amniocentesis

All prenatal diagnostic procedures must be preceded by a detailed ultrasound evaluation by an ultrasonographer knowledgeable in fetal development. Each fetus must be carefully examined for the presence of congenital anomalies, gestational age, and the location of placenta and extra-embryonic membranes. These data should be recorded on video film as well as in the patient's medical chart. It may be appropriate for the entire evaluation to be confirmed by a second, experienced ultrasonographer and/or reviewed by the obstetrician prior to performing any invasive procedure.

For amniocentesis performed in the second trimester, the abdominal site is cleansed appropriately and sterile technique maintained throughout the procedure. A 20- or 22-gauge needle is introduced transabdominally under continuous ultrasound visualization. After removal of a sufficient quantity of amniotic fluid, usually 15–20 ml or 3–5 ml of Indigo Carmine dye is injected into this sac, in order to assure that aspiration of amniotic fluid from the second (or next) sac is not merely a repetition of the first.

Because instances of bacterially contaminated dye samples have been reported, the following precautions are advised. Prior to the use of a dye lot, one vial should be opened and the fluid cultured to determine sterility; for further security, following the use of a specific vial of dye, a sample should be cultured to assure sterility before the vial is discarded. Finally, if ultrasound examination fails to identify the individual membranes separating each fetus, the second needle insertion should be performed near the small parts of the remaining fetus(es).

CVS

A detailed transabdominal ultrasound evaluation is required prior to undertaking CVS. Those parameters to be determined include: (1) viability of each fetus; (2) crown–rump length of each fetus; (3) number and location of each placenta; and (4) location and thickness of dividing membrane(s) (see Chapter 16). Pregnancies with two (or three) distinct placental implantation sites demarcated by a thick, dividing membrane can usually be sampled individually without difficulty. In pregnancies with an identifiable but thin membrane and only one distinguishable placental site, sampling in the area nearest the insertion of the cord is advised. In instances in which no separating membrane is observed and the sites of umbilical cord insertion cannot be identified, either opposite ends of the fused chorions are sampled or only a single sample of chorionic villus is taken. These two last situations may require diagnostic confirmation by a follow-up midtrimester amniocentesis. Despite the potential need for follow up, CVS can be performed in these cases, in order to detect a chromosomal aberration in one or more fetuses and thereby make possible a choice of either a selective or elective termination during the first trimester. As many as 5–7% of patients with multifetal pregnancy who undergo first-trimester CVS may require a follow-up midtrimester amniocentesis in order to confirm that both chorions were sampled or to further evaluate the clinical significance of chromosomal mosaicism (R.J. Wapner et al., submitted for publication). This number is considerably higher than the number of follow-up amniocenteses required (0.8%) of singleton pregnancies undergoing CVS[3].

Careful ultrasound examination usually determines how the chorion of each fetus will be sampled, i.e. transcervically or transabdominally. Between 1983 and 1987, CVS was almost exclusively performed transcervically; subsequently, the transabdominal approach was added. Obstetric aspects of each method are highlighted later in this section.

A major concern in undertaking prenatal diagnostic studies is obtaining a sample of tissue that accurately represents the genotype of each fetus. In contrast to amniocentesis, in which dye can be injected into one of the amniotic cavities, no similar technique is available with CVS to minimize the problems of maternal cell contamination or twin–twin contamination. In the case of fused or joined placentas, CVS may be at a distinct disadvantage compared with amniocentesis. The following steps are suggested.

(1) Each implantation site and its borders should be meticulously demarcated by ultrasound evaluation;

(2) The catheter or needle should be placed in close proximity to the site of insertion of each umbilical cord prior to sampling; and

(3) Identical twins should be identified by the presence and thickness of the dividing chorionic membrane.

In performing transcervical CVS, the patient is placed in the lithotomy position, the vaginal vault thoroughly cleansed with antiseptic solution (e.g. Betadine®) and the excess removed. Under ultrasound guidance, the catheter is introduced through the cervix and into the longest axis of the chorion frondosum. The stylet is removed and a syringe filled with collecting media (e.g. Puck's or Hank's basic salt solution) containing heparin and antibiotics (penicillin and streptomycin) is attached to the catheter. As the catheter is slowly retracted through the chorion frondosum, negative pressure (10–15 ml) is applied to the syringe and then released. The application of negative pressure, then release, is repeated three or four times. For technical reasons, at certain times it may be possible to sample only in a limited area of the chorion. In either circumstance, as the catheter is removed from the chorion frondosum, negative pressure must be applied and then constantly maintained during passage through the cervical canal. The contents of the syringe are then placed in a petri dish and observed either visually or with a dissecting microscope. The morphology of the villous tissue is easily distinguishable from that of maternal decidua. In most circumstances, no more than two samplings are attempted, each time with a fresh, sterile catheter. Generally, the villi are first prepared for short-term tissue culture, which allows for a chromosomal analysis, the determination of enzyme activity in cases of inborn errors of metabolism, or analysis of gene mutations by means of recombinant DNA technology. Alternatively, these analyses can be performed by direct processing of the villi, without the need for tissue culture.

Transabdominal CVS is performed in a manner similar to amniocentesis. A careful ultrasound evaluation is critical, not only to outline the location of the placenta but also to document that no bowel is obstructing the proposed sampling path. Under ultrasound guidance, a sterile 20-gauge needle of sufficient length (commonly, a spinal needle) is introduced transabdominally through the uterine wall and into the longest possible axis of the chorion frondosum. After removal of the stylet and the addition of a 20-ml syringe containing collecting media with heparin and antibiotics (see above), the needle is moved back and forth four to five times through the chorion while a series of negative pressures are applied to the syringe. The number of aspirations should not exceed four or five, in order to minimize the potential for fetal loss. As the needle is removed, constant negative pressure should be maintained. Minor alterations to the single needle technique of transabdominal CVS have been described, including the use of a double-needle[9] and the use of a handle on the syringe to generate sufficient negative pressure during aspiration of the villi[10,11].

Each of the two approaches (transcervical and transabdominal) have advantages and disadvantages. The 'learning curve' for transcervical CVS appears to involve several hundred patients for most operators[12] and, save for the introduction of transabdominal CVS, would probably have required an even greater patient experience. Technically, transcervical CVS may be more difficult to perform than transabdominal CVS. Despite the presence of an inner aluminum stylet, the placement of the catheter into the chorion frondosum is occasionally impeded by the natural shape and form of the cervical canal and the uterus. Because transabdominal CVS is technically similar to midtrimester amniocentesis, it has gained quicker acceptance and application than its transcervical counterpart. Not only is the approach with transabdominal CVS more direct, but the needle is not subjected to forces that alter its course to the chorion. At the same time, the amount of tissue obtained with transabdominal CVS is characteristically smaller than that obtained by the transcervical route. In instances where a large sample is necessary, e.g. to establish sufficient cultures to monitor for an inborn error of metabolism, this difference may influence the choice of sampling method.

Obstetric outcome following amniocentesis

Since 1980, nine series reporting midtrimester amniocentesis performed on multifetal pregnancies have been published[13–21]. These reports analyzed multifetal pregnancies for obstetric outcomes following amniocentesis. Of these, 648 were twin pregnancies and 12 were triplet pregnancies (Table 1). Of a total

Table 1 Obstetric results following amniocentesis in multiple gestations, according to nine sources, given by reference number

	13	14	15	16	17	18	19	20	21
Total number of gestation	26	47			70	53		339	
Number identified at amniocentesis	25	29	13	31	68	52	83	316	58
Pregnancies undergoing amniocentesis	20	29	13	31	62	48	83	316	58
Fetuses sampled	39	55	24	65	111	94	160	629	116
Success (%)	98	95	92	100	90	98	96	100	100
Elective terminations	—	4	—	4	—	—	2	6	2
Lost to follow up	—	—	—	—	—	—	—	8	2
Selective reduction	—	—	—	—	—	—	—	7	—
Delivery cohort after successful amniocentesis	39	51	24	61	111	94	158	607	112
Pregnancy loss through 28 weeks									
Number	0	9	2	5	6	1	2	24	7
% loss	0	17.6	8.3	8.2	5.4	1.1	1.2	4.0	6.1
Intrauterine fetal demise	1	1	0	0	9	5	6	6	5
Neonatal death	0	0	0	3	5	2	3	2	0
Perinatal mortality rate/1000	26	24	0	54	133	75	58	14	48
Total fetal loss									
Number	1	10	2	8	20	8	11	32	12
% of delivery cohort	2.6	19.6	8.3	13.1	18.0	8.5	7.0	5.3	10.7

of 1320 fetuses that underwent amniocentesis, 1293 or 98% were successfully sampled. This rate is only slightly less than the success rate for singleton pregnancies (99.5%)[3]. The fetal loss rate before 28 weeks ranged between zero and 17.6% but averaged 5.0% for the nine studies (Table 1). This average exceeds more than fivefold the loss rate of singleton pregnancies (0.6–1%) having amniocentesis under similar conditions[3,20]. The perinatal mortality included 33 intrauterine fetal demises and 15 neonatal deaths, resulting in an overall perinatal mortality rate for the nine studies of 40.6/1000. This rate also considerably exceeds the perinatal mortality rate in singleton pregnancies of 7.9/1000 in the multicenter study reported by Rhoads et al.[3] or of 12.1/1000 in the single-center study of Anderson et al.[20]. The total fetal loss rate was 8.3% (104 fetuses) for the nine studies in a delivery cohort of 1257. This rate likewise exceeds the total fetal loss rate for singleton pregnancies of 1.8 and 1.9%, respectively, as reported in two recent studies[3,20].

The incidence of complications varied considerably (Table 1). Some investigators found that amniocentesis conferred a small additional risk when performed in twin pregnancies[13,18,19]; others concluded that there is an increased risk above that present in singleton pregnancies in terms of spontaneous abortion and stillbirth rates[14,17,20]. Palle et al.[14] concluded that in twin pregnancies amniocentesis on both sacs required multiple needle insertions and this technical necessity was directly responsible for a significantly increased risk of spontaneous abortion. Of twin pregnancies, 17% spontaneously aborted following amniocentesis, vs. only 6% of women with undetected twin pregnancies and 3% of singleton pregnancies undergoing amniocentesis[14]. The number of punctures per sac and obstetric risk were related: a 22% loss for twin pregnancies with at least two punctures in one or more sacs, 15% with one puncture in each sac, and 6% where only one sac was punctured, because the twin pregnancy was undetected[14]. Whereas the study by Anderson et al.[20] also demonstrated

Table 2 Chromosomal aberrations detected in multiple gestations following amniocentesis, according to nine sources, given by reference number

	13	14	15	16	17	18	19	20	21
Total population									
Twins	20	29	13	28	62	48	83	307	58
Triplets	—	—	—	3	—	—	—	9	—
Chromosomes									
Normal	39	52	24	62	111	94	160	619	114
Abnormal	—	3	—	3	—	—	—	10*	2
XXY		2							
trisomy 21		1		3					
marker									2

* Types of chromosome aberrations not defined

that the spontaneous abortion rate in multiple gestations (3.57%) exceeded the control singleton loss rate (0.6%), their data did not support the conclusions of Palle *et al.*[14], because more than 90% of their procedures required only one needle entry per sac. In six of the nine studies listed in Table 1[14–17,20,21], the fetal loss rate through 28 weeks appeared significantly to exceed that of singleton pregnancies undergoing amniocentesis at similar gestational ages[22,23]. Unfortunately, no comparable data exist on the spontaneous loss rate from 16 to 28 weeks in multifetal pregnancies. The overall perinatal mortality rate in the nine studies, 40.6/1000 births, does not appear to be different from twin pregnancies not undergoing amniocentesis, however[24].

Genetic outcome following amniocentesis

For each patient, the clinician must be concerned with the critical question of how many times each sac is actually sampled, as opposed to one (or more) amniotic sac being inadvertently sampled twice. The introduction of dye to 'mark' the first sac prior to sampling the second (or third, etc.) has virtually eliminated the failure to recognize and correct for this potential problem. An equally if not more important question is whether twin (or triplet) pregnancies are associated with an increased occurrence of chromosomal anomalies, in either one or more of the fetuses. Table 2 lists the number of chromosomal anomalies detected in each of the nine studies listed in Table 1. Of the 332 pregnancies in which ascertainment of whether one or both twins were chromosomally normal was undertaken, a total of five were detected in which a chromosome aberration was present. The risk of a karyotypic anomaly per multiple gestation was therefore 1.5%. Of the 1293 fetuses, a total of 18 were chromosomally abnormal, and the risk of a karyotypic anomaly in a fetus from a multifetal pregnancy was therefore 1.4%. Given that the indication for amniocentesis was primarily advanced maternal age in the cited studies, the risk of a chromosome abnormality in either a pregnancy or a fetus was remarkably low in these reports and not dissimilar to the risk for a singleton pregnancy undergoing amniocentesis for the same indication. One can reasonably conclude that multiple gestations are not associated with an obvious increased risk of chromosomal anomalies, at least based on their evaluation at the time of midtrimester amniocentesis.

Obstetric outcome following CVS

CVS offers numerous advantages over midtrimester amniocentesis, several of which are particularly significant for multiple gestations.

Of special interest is the fact that CVS can be performed earlier than amniocentesis, routinely between 9 and 12 weeks of gestation. Since transcervical and transabdominal approaches to CVS are available, obtaining villus tissue from each chorion may be technically easy and safe. Results of chromosomal and genetic analyses can usually be obtained much more rapidly than with amniotic fluid cells, either in hours by direct preparation of the cytotrophoblast layer or in 3–7 days by tissue culture of the villus' mesenchymal core. Elective termination is generally considered safer and easier in the first trimester than in the second. In the case of a multifetal pregnancy with discordant genetic results, the opportunity for selective termination in the first trimester offers enormous clinical and psychological benefits compared to second-trimester procedures. Finally, the issue of privacy is of great concern. CVS can be performed when there are no physical signs of pregnancy, and any decision to continue a pregnancy or to selectively terminate an affected fetus can be made in private before the pregnancy has become apparent.

When a twin pregnancy is first detected in a woman considering CVS, the prospective parents must be counselled concerning the following points: first, midtrimester amniocentesis on each gestational sac is an alternative to CVS; second, it is possible that twin–twin contamination of chorionic villi will occur, i.e. one chorion being sampled twice whereas the other is not sampled at all; third, genetic results may be discordant; fourth, the parents must face an increased risk of pregnancy loss after genetic testing of a multiple gestation. This last concern is primarily based on the generally poor obstetric outcome in twin pregnancies undergoing midtrimester amniocentesis, combined with the limited experience with CVS in the case of multiple gestations, mostly twins.

Table 3 summarizes the obstetric outcomes from five centers experienced in performing CVS in multiple gestations, mostly twins. The success rate for obtaining villus tissue was higher than 99%; the one unsuccessful sampling represented an operator's second attempt at CVS. A single sampling was performed in 19 cases (9.4%) because it was not possible to delineate separate placentas nor to assure that individual sites of implantation were sampled at the time of CVS. When demarcation of the placental borders was possible in twin pregnancies, the number of procedures required to obtain an adequate sample approached the ideal number (two) at all centers (Table 3).

Fourteen of the 202 pregnancies, or 7.0%, experienced the loss of one or more fetuses (Table 3): five (2.5%) prior to 20 weeks' gestation; four (2.0%) between 20 and 28 weeks' gestation; and five (2.5%) after 28 weeks' gestation. In six of these pregnancies, the loss involved both fetuses, including a documented set with the twin–twin transfusion syndrome. Of the 409 fetuses undergoing CVS, a total of 20 losses occurred, or 4.9%. Among these losses were included fetuses with chromosomal aberrations, one 47,XY,+21 that died spontaneously at 12 weeks' gestation and two mosaics (45,X/46,XY and 46,XX/46,XXr11) (Table 4). When only chromosomally normal pregnancies are considered, the overall loss rate becomes 3.7%, which is considerably less than that of amniocentesis.

Genetic outcome

Since CVS is usually performed at 9–11 weeks' gestation, the incidence of fetal chromosomal abnormalities is expected to be significantly higher than in women having amniocentesis. In the five centers cited in Table 3, a karyotypic abnormality was present in ten (5%) of the 202 pregnancies and involved a total of 14 (3.4%) of the 409 fetuses. Excluding the one high-risk pregnancy in a set of twins with partial trisomy (case 4, Table 4), the corrected incidence of chromosomal abnormalities in the CVS population is 2.9%, a rate that is twofold greater than that diagnosed at the time of amniocentesis, 1.4% (Table 2).

These comparisons seem reasonable, however, in view of the fact that advanced maternal age is the major indication for fetal diagnosis, regardless whether CVS or amniocentesis is chosen. Thus, approximately half

Table 3 Pregnancy outcome in multiple gestations following CVS, in five centers

	Center									
	1		2		3		4		5	
	Pregnancy	Fetus	Pregnancy	Fetus	Pregnancy	Fetus	Pregnancy	Fetus	Pregnancy	Fetus
Patients	46	93	54	108	13	26	15	31	74	151
Failed procedures	0	0	0	0	1	2	0	0	0	0
Therapeutic abortion	1	1	3	4	0	0	1	1	3	5
Elective abortion	1	2	0	0	0	0	0	0	0	0
Spontaneous abortion (SAB)										
<20 weeks	0	0	1	2	1	1*	1	2	2	3†
20–28 weeks	0	0	0	0	1	2‡	0	0	3	4
Perinatal loss										
>28 weeks	2**	2	0	0	1	1	0	0	2	3
SAB <28 weeks (%)	0		1.9		12.5		6.7		4.8	
Total loss (%)		2.2		1.9		16.7		6.7		6.8

Center 1: Michael Reese/Illinois Masonic Hospitals, Chicago, IL; Center 2: Genetics & IVF Institute, Fairfax, VA; Center 3: Baylor College of Medicine, Houston, TX; Center 4: Northwestern School of Medicine, Chicago, IL; Center 5: Thomas Jefferson Medical College, Philadelphia, PA
*Anticipated loss as no yolk sac present at time of procedure; †included one trisomy 21 fetus with spontaneous demise at 12 weeks; ‡elevated serum alpha-fetoprotein and documented twin–twin transfusion syndrome; **included one monozygotic male twin in triplet pregnancy and one intrauterine fetal demise at term

of the chromosomally abnormal multifetal conceptions appear to be spontaneously lost between 9 and 16 weeks' gestation. If indeed half of the viable multiple conceptions with chromosome anomalies spontaneously abort sometime before the midtrimester, a comparison of the safety of the two procedures becomes a primary issue.

As diagnostic problems with CVS have been sufficiently described in singleton pregnancies, along with the steps necessary for their resolution, their occurrence is not unexpected in multiple gestations. For example, chromosomal mosaicism may be confined to the direct preparation of the cytotrophoblast layer of the chorion but is unlikely to be clinically significant if the villus tissue culture is chromosomally normal. In one set of twins, trisomy 13 mosaicism (46,XX/47,XX+13) was present in the direct preparation only (Table 4); amniocentesis showed a normal chromosomal complement. The pregnancy continued and a normal female was delivered at term. Alternatively, in case 9 (Table 4), in which monochorionic twins were suspected on the basis of ultrasound, the direct preparation was chromosomally normal (46,XY), whereas tissue culture revealed a 45,X/46,XY mosaic. These cases reaffirm an earlier conclusion: although chromosomal analysis of the cytotrophoblast layer and of the mesenchymal core of the villi are both extremely accurate, the latter has consistently been the most reliable measure of the fetal karyotype[25]. To date, false-negative results with CVS have not been reported with multiple gestation, i.e. a normal CVS cytogenetic analysis followed by the birth of a newborn with a chromosomal abnormality. Concern about such an occurrence is warranted in multiple gestations, because in addition to maternal cell contamination, the possibility of twin–twin cell contamination also exists. In the series reported by Pergament et al.[26], the overall frequency of cell contamination in multiple gestation was 6.2% and included two cases where contamination was complete and individual fetal karyotypes

Table 4 Chromosomal aberrations in multiple gestations undergoing CVS*

	Case	Twin A	Twin B	Outcome
Center 1	1	46,XX	45,X/46,XXr	selective termination
Center 2	2	46,XX	46,XY/47,XXY	selective termination
	3	47,XXY	47,XXY	elective termination
	4	46,XY+10p	46,XY+10p	elective termination
Center 3	—	—	—	—
Center 4	5	46,XX	47,XX+13	selective termination
Center 5	6	47,XY+21	46,XX	selective termination
	7	47,XY+21	46,XX	twin A: SAB, 12 weeks
	8	45,X/46,XY	45,X	spontaneous abortion
	9	45,X/46,XY	45,X/46,XY	twin A: selective termination twin B: IUFD
	10	46,XX/46,XX r(11)	46,XX	twin A: neonatal demise

*Centers cited in Table 3

were never determined. In the series evaluated by Wapner et al.[21], there was one case (of 101) in which contamination of one twin sample from villi from the co-twin led to an incorrect sex prediction. These cases of undetected maternal or twin–twin cell contamination pose a serious potential problem, that is, the failure to identify the presence of a potential chromosomal abnormality in one or both twins. Maternal decidua as a source of contamination can be avoided by performing chromosomal analyses on direct preparations of chorionic villi, because only cells from the cytotrophoblast layer exhibit mitotic activity suitable for karyotyping. Direct preparations, however, do not eliminate diagnostic problems generated by twin–twin cell contamination in cases involving cytogenetic studies, inborn errors of metabolism or DNA analysis.

Based on a limited number of cases in newborns, Lubs and Ruddle[4] suggested that the risk of a cytogenetic abnormality was increased in multiple compared to singleton pregnancies. More recent reports do not support this observation. The 1.4% of karyotypic abnormalities detected in multifetal pregnancies after midtrimester amniocentesis (18 out of 1293 fetuses, Table 2) is comparable to that found in singleton pregnancies[20,25]. For patients with advanced maternal age undergoing CVS, the frequency of clinically significant cytogenetic abnormalities in fetuses of multiple gestation is 2.4%[26]. This rate is similar to that of patients with singleton pregnancies undergoing CVS[25].

Because chromosomally discordant results must be anticipated, it is critical that an accurate delineation of the fetal and placental relationships be determined prior to CVS, if selective termination is contemplated. At the time of selective termination, a standard practice is to confirm the original diagnosis in both fetal and chorionic tissues.

Comparison of amniocentesis and CVS

Preliminary evidence suggests that fetal diagnosis performed in the first trimester by means of CVS may be less of a risk in terms of obstetrical outcome than second-trimester amniocentesis. In a prospective comparison between these two procedures, Wapner et al.[21] compared 58 women who underwent amniocentesis and 101 women who chose CVS. The total fetal loss rate following amniocentesis was 10.7%, with a loss rate to 20 weeks' gestation of 6.3%; in contrast, the loss rates for CVS were 6.8 and 3.2%, respectively. The spontaneous abortion rate after CVS performed in four centers[26] was compared to that of seven studies of amniocentesis in twin pregnancies conducted during the past 10 years[13-19]. Fetal losses following amniocentesis prior to 20 weeks' gestation averaged (weighted mean) 3.6%; for the CVS population it was 1.9%, indicating that in prenatal diagnosis involving multiple gestations, CVS compared favorably to amniocentesis in terms of immediate post-procedural losses. After 20 weeks' gestation, however, fetal losses were 9.5% (weighted mean) for the seven amniocentesis studies of twin gestations and only 1.6% for the patients who underwent CVS. The results of these two studies[21,26], suggest that CVS may actually be a safer obstetric procedure than amniocentesis in the prenatal diagnosis of genetic disorders in twins. If the obstetric outcome should prove to be more favourable with CVS, this would differ from that of singleton pregnancies, wherein amniocentesis is still considered to carry a slightly lower risk than CVS[3]. Notwithstanding this advantage, CVS in twins is associated with a higher risk of maternal and twin–twin cell contamination than amniocentesis. Cell contamination occurring in long-term tissue cultures was not a significant diagnostic problem in the series described by Pergament *et al.*[26]: in the cases where a mixture of XX and XY cells occurred, no patients were referred for follow-up amniocentesis and there were no incorrect sex predictions or cytogenetic diagnostic errors in the liveborn. Nevertheless, in the series evaluated by Wapner *et al.*[21], one case of complete twin–twin cell contamination occurred in which one twin was sampled twice; in the series reported by Pergament *et al.*[26] two such cases were present. In sum, failure to correctly sample a fetus using CVS occurs about 1.3% of the time. This rate is approximately six times higher than that of amniocentesis. Such a possibility emphasizes that care must be taken to assure that individual sites are sampled.

Early amniocentesis and late CVS

After first-trimester CVS was described, other alternatives to midtrimester amniocentesis have also been considered, e.g. amniocentesis prior to 15–16 weeks' gestation[27] and transabdominal CVS in the second and third trimesters[1]. To date, these approaches have been applied almost exclusively to singleton pregnancies, are experimental in nature and, despite claims to the contrary, cannot be considered as 'standard of care' until their safety and efficacy has been established in randomized trials.

Transabdominal CVS performed after the first trimester is unlikely to incur any additional risks over amniocentesis, but this conjecture remains to be demonstrated in a randomized study. A major advantage of transabdominal CVS in the second or third trimesters is that the genetic analysis can be completed within 24–48 h, whereas similar studies with amniotic fluid cells would probably required 2–4 weeks. This time difference could be clinically important in the management of patients who initially present themselves late in the second trimester. Transabdominal CVS may also have a direct impact on obstetric management in which structural anomalies are diagnosed by ultrasound in one of the fetuses. On the other hand, with early amniocentesis, there remains significant concern that removal of amniotic fluid prior to 15 weeks' gestation may be associated with skeletal deformations and respiratory compromise (Fairweather, personal communication, 1983). A randomized trial comparing early amniocentesis with transabdominal CVS is required in singleton pregnancies before it may be appropriate to use for multiple gestations.

Future prospects

Two new approaches to fetal genetic diagnosis are the subject of considerable clinical investigation. One approach attempts to isolate, then analyze for genetic disorders, those fetal blood cells circulating in the maternal peripheral blood[28]. The advantage of such an approach is obvious: the obstetric risks of CVS and amniocentesis would be circumvented by a blood sample drawn from the patient's arm at the appropriate time in pregnancy. However, the possibility of an unrecognized multifetal pregnancy represents a major confounding factor.

Simply stated, if such techniques were to be developed, their application would require not only separation of the fetal from the maternal cells, but also separation of the cells from each fetus. Although the possibility of performing genetic analysis on fetal cells obtained from a sample of maternal blood is inherently attractive, its role in those pregnancies involving multifetal gestations may be limited because of this requirement.

A second approach that may prove of value is preimplantation genetic diagnosis, that is the testing of an embryo for a genetic mutation and replacing (transferring) only those embryos shown to be unaffected[29]. This approach involves applying the conventional techniques of *in vitro* fertilization (IVF), biopsying and analyzing one or more embryonic or extra-embryonic cell(s) from each embryo, and then transferring 1–4 unaffected embryos in each cycle. The use of drugs to enhance fertility and techniques that increase the risk of multiple gestations, e.g. IVF and preimplantation diagnosis, both require that all aspects of prenatal diagnosis receive careful attention and monitoring[29].

Summary

In multiple gestations, the prenatal diagnosis of genetic disorders is safe and effective when performed by either first-trimester CVS or midtrimester amniocentesis. Preliminary studies suggest that although CVS may entail a slightly lower risk of procedure failure and of fetal loss than amniocentesis, it also carries a higher risk of maternal cell and twin–twin cell contamination. Issues related to the obstetric safety of different techniques, efficacy of sampling at different times in pregnancy and accuracy of genetic analysis have not as yet been completely resolved in the case of multiple gestations. Additional studies are required to clarify these important questions, if women with multiple gestations are to receive the highest standard of care possible.

References

1. Holzgreve, W., Miny, P. and Schloo, R. (1990). 'Late CVS' international registry compilation of data from 24 centres. *Prenat. Diagn.*, **10**, 159
2. Tabor, A., Madsen, M. Obel. E. *et al.* (1986). Randomized controlled trial of genetic amniocentesis in 4606 low risk women. *Lancet*, **1**, 1287
3. Rhoads, G.G., Jackscon, L.G., Schlesselman, S.E. *et al.* (1989). The safety and efficacy of chorionic villus sampling for early prenatal diagnosis of cytogenetic abnormalities. *N. Engl. J. Med.*, **320**, 609
4. Lubs, H.A. and Ruddle, F. (1970). Chromosomal abnormalities in the human population: estimation of rates based on New Haven newborn study. *Science*, **169**, 495
5. Milunsky, A. (1979). Prenatal diagnosis of chromosomal disorders. In Milunsky, A. (ed.). *Genetic Disorders and the Fetus: Diagnosis, Prevention and Treatment*, p.123. (New York: Plenum Press)
6. Wald, N.J., Barker, S. and Peto, R. *et al.* (1975). Maternal serum alpha-fetoprotein in multiple pregnancy. *Br. Med. J.*, **1**, 651
7. Gardner, S., Burton, B. and Johnson, A.M. (1981). Maternal serum alpha-fetoprotein screening: a report of the Forsyth County Project. *Am. J. Obstet. Gynecol.*, **140**, 250
8. Ghosh, A., Woo, J.S.K., Rawlinson, H.A. and Ferguson-Smith, M.A. (1982). Prognostic significance of raised serum alpha fetoprotein levels in twin pregnancies. *Br. J. Obstet. Gynaecol.*, **89**, 817
9. Smidt-Jensen, S. and Hahnemann, H. (1984). Transabdominal fine needle biopsy from chorionic villi in the first trimester. *Prenat. Diagn.*, **4**, 163
10. Brambati, B., Oldrini, A. and Ianzani, A. (1987). Transabdominal chorionic villus sampling: a freehand ultrasound-guided technique. *Am. J. Obstet. Gynecol.*, **157**, 134
11. Elias, S., Simpson, J.L., Shulman, L.P. *et al.* (1989). Transabdominal chorionic villus sampling for first trimester prenatal diagnosis. *Am. J. Obstet. Gynecol.*, **160**, 879

12. Report of a WHO Consultation on First Trimester Diagnosis (1986). Risk Evaluation in CVS. *Prenat. Diagn.*, **6**, 451
13. Elias, S., Gerbie, A.B., Simpson, J.L., *et al.* (1980). Genetic amniocentesis in twin gestations. *Am. J. Obstet. Gynecol.*, **138**, 169
14. Palle, C., Andersen, J.W., Tabor, A. *et al.* (1983). Increased risk of abortion after genetic amniocentesis in twin pregnancies. *Prenat. Diagn.*, **3**, 83
15. Bovicelli, L., Michelacci, L., Rizzo, N. *et al.* (1983). Genetic amniocentesis in twin pregnancy. *Prenat. Diagn.*, **3**, 101
16. Filkins, K., Russo, J., Brown, T. *et al.* (1984). Genetic amniocentesis in multiple gestations. *Prenat. Diagn.*, **4**, 223
17. Librach, C.L., Doran, T.A., Benzie, R.J. *et al.* (1984). Genetic amniocentesis in seventy twin pregnancies. *Am. J. Obstet. Gynecol.*, **148**, 585
18. Tabsh, K.M.A., Crandall, B., Lebherz, T.B. *et al.* (1985). Genetic amniocentesis in twin pregnancy. *Obstet. Gynecol.*, **65**, 843
19. Pijpers, L., Jahoda, M.G.J., Vosters, R.P.L. *et al.* (1988). Genetic amniocentesis in twin pregnancies. *Br. J. Obstet. Gynaecol.*, **95**, 323
20. Anderson, R.L., Goldberg, J.D. and Golbus, M.S. (1991). Prenatal diagnosis in multiple gestation: 20 years' experience with amniocentesis. *Prenat. Diagn.*, **11**, 263
21. Wapner, R.J., Johnson, A., Davis, G., Urban, A., Morgan, P. and Jackson, L. (1993). Prenatal diagnosis in twin gestations: a comparison between second-trimester amniocentesis and first-trimester chorion villous sampling. *Obstet. Gynecol.*, **82**, 49–56
22. NICHD Study Group (1976). Midtrimester amniocentesis for prenatal diagnosis. *J. Am. Med. Assoc.*, **236**, 1471
23. Simpson, N.E., Dallaire, L., Miller, J.R. *et al.* (1976). Prenatal diagnosis of genetic disease in Canada: report of a collaborative study. *Can. Med. Assoc. J.*, **115**, 739
24. Ho, S.K. and Wu, J.K. (1975). Perinatal factors and neonatal morbidity in twin pregnancy. *Am. J. Obstet. Gynecol.*, **122**, 979
25. Ledbetter, D.H., Martin, A.O., Verlinsky, Y. *et al.* (1990). Cytogenetic results of chorionic villus sampling: high success rate and diagnostic accuracy in the U.S. Collaborative study. *Am. J. Obstet. Gynecol.*, **162**, 495
26. Pergament, E., Schulman, J.D., Copeland, K. *et al.* (1992). The risk and efficacy of chorionic villus sampling in multiple gestations. *Prenat. Diagn.*, **12**, 377–84
27. Hanson, F.W., Zorn, E.M., Tennant, F.R. *et al.* (1987). Amniocentesis before 15 weeks' gestation: outcome, risks and technical problems. *Am. J. Obstet. Gynecol.*, **156**, 1564
28. Bianchi, D.W., Flint, A.F., Pizzimenti, M.F. *et al.* (1990). Isolation of fetal DNA from nucleated erythrocytes in maternal blood. *Proc. Nat. Acad. Sci. USA*, **84**, 3279
29. Pergament, E. (1991). Preimplantation diagnosis: a patient perspective. *Prenat. Diagn.*, **11**, 493

Biophysical assessment

J.A. Lopez-Zeno

Introduction

The increased perinatal mortality and morbidity associated with twin gestations requires specific antenatal surveillance measures. The principal source of morbidity for the gravida with twins is prematurity. The second source of morbidity is intrauterine growth retardation (IUGR), manifested in the form of a delivery weight of <10th percentile for gestational age or discordant growth between the twins.

The definition and prognosis of intrauterine growth discrepancy varies among different authors from 15–25% of estimated fetal weight[1]. The etiology of growth discrepancy is not clear in all instances. In some it may result from monochorionic placentation (as documented by the twin–twin transfusion syndrome); in others, it may represent unequal competition for nutrients in dichorionic placentation; in still others, it may result from differences in genetic potential, as would be the case with dizygotic twins or trizygotic triplets.

It is important to understand that not all twin gestations share the same types or degrees of morbidity and/or risk for mortality. In a healthy gravida undergoing an uncomplicated gestation, the greatest predictor for the development of fetal compromise is chorionicity. With real-time ultrasound, a diagnosis of dichorionic placentation can be made indirectly by documentation of different fetal sex, separate placentas, amniotic sac membrane thickness of ≥2 mm, or the presence of three or four layers in the membranes[2,3]. Such information can assist the clinician in determining when to start antenatal surveillance. Monoamniotic (monochorionic) gestations are at the highest risk for morbidity and mortality[4]. The lowest level of risk for IUGR is associated with diamniotic–dichorionic gestations, whereas diamniotic–monochorionic gestations are associated with an intermediate risk.

Serial ultrasound is of great help for the diagnosis of fetal growth abnormalities in diamniotic–dichorionic and diamniotic–monochorionic gestations. If found, they indicate a need for antenatal surveillance using the non-stress test (NST) every week. In contrast, a diamniotic–dichorionic twin gestation with no growth abnormality and no other complication does not require antenatal surveillance prior to 34 weeks. Indeed, one group of authors have expressed an opinion that this type of twin gestation may not even need routine antenatal surveillance in the form of NST[5]. However, this opinion seems not to have many proponents.

Several options for antenatal surveillance should be included in the antenatal plan of care for twin gestations. These include the NST, the contraction stress test (CST), the biophysical profile (BPP) and Doppler umbilical velocimetry studies. Normal antenatal surveillance tests are associated with a decreased perinatal mortality. It is necessary to remember, however, that even with a negative or normal antenatal surveillance test, perinatal deaths still occur and infants still suffer morbid events. This fact should be clearly communicated with the patient and her partner prior to the onset of antenatal surveillance.

Non-stress test

The NST test involves the use of continuous electronic fetal monitoring for the documentation of fetal heart rate accelerations associated with fetal movements. The test is classified as reactive or non-reactive. A reactive test is the one that demonstrates two accelerations of the fetal heart rate, of at least 15 beats per minute, for at least 15 s in 20 min. According to one group of authors[6] some degree of variation exists in the number of accelerations and the total examination time required for the diagnosis of reactivity. A non-reactive test should not be considered as an indication for immediate delivery. More than 50% of all the non-reactive NST examinations are false-positive tests due to being obtained during a fetal sleep cycle[7]. Unless some additional abnormal signs are present, such as the presence of late or variable decelerations, the examination cycle should be extended to a total of 90 min, after which an alternate surveillance method should be used to confirm the diagnosis of fetal compromise and the consideration of an intervention. The discussions of CST, BPP and Doppler later in this chapter will look at the possibility of using these methods for that purpose.

Although a voluminous literature has been published on the use of the NST, only six of these articles relate to twins[8–13]. Some of the initial articles on the use of the NST for the surveillance of singletons were performed in a blinded manner, in which the results of the test were not made available to the clinician caring for the particular patient. From these blinded studies, it was possible to estimate the level of perinatal mortality associated with normal and abnormal tests. In contrast, none of the studies performed on twins was blinded to the clinician. This problem is further compounded by the fact that the investigations on twins generally comprised small series, thus making it difficult to establish reliable estimates of perinatal mortality.

Bailey et al.[8] followed 50 twin gestations with weekly NSTs starting at 32 weeks. There were no perinatal deaths in 96 reactive tests. Of five non-reactive, non-stress tests (NR-NST), there were two intrauterine and two neonatal deaths.

Devoe and Huguette[9] studied 24 twin pregnancies in which the incidence of non-reactive, non-stress tests (NR-NST) was 23%. The two intrauterine demises of this study were in the NR-NST group. In addition, the group with NR-NST had double the incidence of intrauterine growth retardation (IUGR).

Blake et al.[10] evaluated 94 multiple gestations with NST. A total of 25 fetuses had a NR-NST. All patients who had a NR-NST were immediately followed by a CST. Based on this relatively small number, a perinatal mortality was calculated, of 12/1000 for a reactive NST vs. 80/1000 for NR-NST. In addition, general morbidity was increased in the NR-NST group, including IUGR (see discussion below).

Lenstrup[11] evaluated 27 twin gestations, of which four were complicated by abnormal NST, all of which were small for gestational age (SGA) neonates. No mortality was recorded in this study.

Knuppel et al.[12] utilized a historical cohort design to show the significant decrease in mortality associated with the routine use of a NST in twin pregnancies. Of the 90 twins managed in the prospective arm of this study, there was no mortality. In contrast, six intrauterine fetal demises (IUFD) occurred in the historical arm in which control patients did not receive antenatal surveillance with the NST.

Patkos et al.[13] reported on 90 sets of twins. Their study documented the higher incidence of NR-NST (31.1%) in fetuses between 26 and 31 weeks compared with fetuses between 32 and 36 weeks (12.1%) and those at term (6.2%). This observation suggests that there is a normal progression toward reactive NST in twins with advancing maturation. A similar progression occurs in singletons. This study serves to emphasize the point that in a preterm twin pregnancy, it is of even greater importance that an abnormal NST be followed by a confirmatory alternative antenatal surveillance test before intervention is considered.

Clinicians or their designees performing NSTs on twins should be aware of the possibility of inadvertently monitoring or performing the test twice on the same twin. The use of simultaneous monitors and/or ultrasound localization of the fetus can obviate this technical

Contraction stress test

The CST involves the use of spontaneous or induced contractions to evaluate signs of uteroplacental insufficiency. A test is considered negative (or normal) if three contractions are present in 10 min, and no late decelerations of the fetal heart rates are evident. Positive tests are those in which persistent late decelerations of the fetal heart rate are observed. The presence of intermittent decelerations classifies the test as equivocal, with further surveillance being required. A positive test may be considered as an indication for delivery. In twin gestations, the use of a CST could theoretically trigger premature labor or, if the pregnancy were complicated by polyhydramnios, a placental abruption. Only two investigations have evaluated twins with this test[10,12].

Blake et al.[10] followed their NR-NSTs with CST. A total of 61% of the CSTs were positive. This finding was considered as an indication for delivery. The fetuses with a negative CST after a NR-NST were managed conservatively, but the frequency of antenatal testing performed on this subgroup was not specified. Knuppel et al.[12] also used CST after a NR-NST, and also considered a positive CST as an indication for delivery. Despite the theoretical possibility of complications mentioned above, neither of these reports mentions any complications arising from the use of this test.

Biophysical profile

The BPP involves the use of the NST as well as real-time ultrasound for the documentation of fetal movement, tone, breathing activity and amniotic fluid volume determination. According to Manning et al.[14], the presence or absence of each one of these parameters is given a score of 2 or 0, respectively. An alternative scoring system developed by Vintzileos et al.[15] uses a score of 1 for an intermediate result, and adds a sixth parameter, namely placental grading. Using this latter scoring system, Lodeiro et al.[16] reported using BPP on 49 twin gestations. A total of 64 fetuses had a reactive NST (R-NST), and all of them had a BPP score of ≥ 8. Of these 64 fetuses, only two died after birth because of the complications of prematurity. Of the 34 fetuses with a NR-NST, 28 had a BPP ≥ 8, and all had good outcomes. Only six fetuses had a BPP of < 8, and even though none died, all had signs of fetal compromise at birth. This study provides strong support to the concept that the BPP tests may serve as a reasonable confirmation of fetal compromise after a NR-NST. In addition, this test may be easier to perform, and has less potential risks than the CST.

Doppler

The use of the physical principle of the Doppler wave shift has led to rapid interest in its use as a means for antenatal surveillance. The bulk of the data published to date evaluates flow of blood through the umbilical cord of the fetus. With the waveform obtained from the Doppler shift, a value is assigned to the flow present during systole and diastole (see Chapter 14). Several indices and ratios can be calculated from these two values, including the S/D ratio, and the resistance and pulsatility indices. Most studies have evaluated the S/D ratio and its role in the diagnosis and management of IUGR. Some pregnancies complicated by placental insufficiency have an increased resistance to blood flow through the umbilical cord, which can be detected and followed with Doppler flow studies. Obviously, twin pregnancies are at a higher risk than singleton gestations for development of growth-related abnormalities. This fact has led several investigators to evaluate the use of the Doppler for the diagnosis or detection of growth retardation in twins[17–25].

In the case of twins, any clinician who wishes to evaluate fetal well-being with Doppler should use a pulsed (duplex) wave. This technology permits direct visualization of the umbilical cord at the same time that the Doppler is obtained. Unless the examiner uses real-time ultrasound to identify the location of the cord before performing a continuous wave Doppler examination, the examination essentially will be blinded. Even if an ultrasound evaluation is performed initially, the possibility of movement of one or both twins is always present, and it is conceivable that the examination is being performed twice on the same cord. Only the use of pulsed wave for the detection of growth abnormalities carries a sensitivity and specificity that could approach that of real-time ultrasound in the diagnosis of IUGR. Before considering the routine use of Doppler for this purpose in twins, additional confirmatory studies on the pulsed wave technique are needed.

If a twin gestation is found to have IUGR by ultrasound, the use of umbilical cord Doppler evaluation may have value in antenatal surveillance. A worsening Doppler evaluation may suggest a worsening of the IUGR. Signs of deterioration include an abnormal S/D ratio, the absence of umbilical blood flow during diastole, or even the reverse of flow during diastole. In order to ascertain if the S/D ratio is abnormal, its value is plotted against gestational age using published tables[23]. These tables are essentially similar for singletons and twins. Singleton data suggest a potential role for serial umbilical Doppler examinations. The ideal frequency of performing this examination is unclear from the literature. Further data in this regard are needed both in twin and in singleton gestations.

One other possible use for Doppler is in the diagnosis of the twin–twin transfusion syndrome. In the syndrome, one of the fetuses is growth retarded and anemic, whereas the other is hydropic and plethoric. This difference is secondary to a shunting of blood through vessel-to-vessel anastomoses associated with monochorionic placentation. As a result of an abnormal hemodynamic state, either an elevated umbilical S/D ratio is seen on the smaller twin (due to increase in resistance), or a wide difference in the S/D ratio is present between the two fetuses due to the abnormalities in flow. Reports of umbilical artery Doppler in the twin–twin transfusion syndrome are conflicting, ranging from normal to elevated[16,17]. Because of this lack of consensus, the predictive value of a negative or normal report is limited, but close attention should be paid to grossly abnormal ones.

Recommendations

Twin gestations require increased antenatal surveillance compared to singleton gestations. The intensity of such surveillance depends not only on the existence of maternal medical or obstetric complications, but also on chorionicity as determined antenatally by ultrasound. The following broad recommendations are offered, and the clinician must consider alternative protocols depending on different risk status.

Monoamniotic–monochorionic

Start NST at 28 weeks, twice weekly. Consider intervention if a repetitive cord compression pattern develops during a NST. A reactive NST deceleration may not be sensitive nor predictive of a cord accident. No adequate alternate surveillance method is available to predict a cord accident.

Monochorionic–diamniotic

Start NST at 30–32 weeks, and repeat NST every week until delivery. If IUGR is diagnosed, then move to twice weekly NST and weekly umbilical Doppler studies.

Dichorionic

Start NST at 34 weeks, and repeat NST every week. Possibly start NST earlier, if IUGR is diagnosed or if there are any other obstetric or medical complications. If IUGR is diagnosed, then move to twice weekly NST, and weekly umbilical Doppler studies.

For any of the above

NR-NST Follow up immediately with a BPP. If BPP is reassuring, repeat the NST in 4–7 days, depending on the level of risk of the pregnancy. If BPP is non-reassuring, consideration should be given to delivery, if possible by the vaginal route.

Abnormal umbilical cord Doppler study May require assessment in conjunction with all the other antenatal surveillance tests. An elevated S/D ratio may raise concerns of IUGR. If no diastolic flow is present, a careful review of the clinical condition is indicated. Reversal of umbilical blood flow during diastole in a fetus with IUGR may be ominous. The use of Doppler as a routine screening test or first-line antenatal surveillance test is not warranted at present, and use of this test should be limited to pregnancies with anomalies of fetal growth diagnosed by serial ultrasound determinations.

References

1. Blickstein, I. (1990). The twin–twin transfusion syndrome. *Obstet. Gynecol.*, **76**, 714
2. D'Alton, M.E. and Dudley, D.K. (1989). The ultrasonographic prediction of chorionicity in twin gestation. *Am. J. Obstet. Gynecol.*, **160**, 557
3. Winn, H.N., Gabrielli, S., Reece, E.A. *et al.* (1989). Ultrasonographic criteria for the prenatal diagnosis of placental chorionicity in twin gestations. *Am. J. Obstet. Gynecol.*, **161**, 1540
4. Carr, S.R., Aronson, M.P. and Coustan, D.R. (1990). Survival rates of monoamniotic twins do not decrease after 30 weeks' gestation. *Am. J. Obstet. Gynecol.*, **163**, 719
5. MacLennan, A.H. (1989). Clinical characteristics and management. In Creasy, R.K. and Resnik, R. (eds.) *Maternal–Fetal Medicine: Principles and Practice*, 2nd edn., pp. 580–91. (Philadelphia: W.B. Saunders)
6. Devoe, L.D., Castillo, R.A. and Sherline, D.M. (1985). The nonstress test as a diagnostic test: a critical reappraisal. *Am. J. Obstet. Gynecol.*, **152**, 1047
7. Brown, R. and Patrick, J. (1981). The nonstress test: how long is enough? *Am. J. Obstet. Gynecol.*, **141**, 646
8. Bailey, D., Flynn, A.M., Kelly, J. *et al.* (1980). Antepartum fetal heart rate monitoring in multiple pregnancy. *Br. J. Obstet. Gynaecol.*, **87**, 561
9. Devoe, L.D. and Huguette, A. (1981). Simultaneous nonstress fetal heart rate testing in twin pregnancy. *Obstet. Gynecol.*, **58**, 450
10. Blake, G.D., Knuppel, R.A., Ingardia, C.J. *et al.* (1984). Evaluation of nonstress fetal heart rate testing in multiple gestations. *Obstet. Gynecol.*, **63**, 528
11. Lenstrup, C. (1984). Predictive value of antepartum non-stress test in multiple pregnancies. *Acta Obstet. Gynecol. Scand.*, **63**, 597
12. Knuppel, R.A., Rattan, P.K., Scerbo, J.C. *et al.* (1985). Intrauterine fetal death in twins after 32 weeks of gestation. *Obstet. Gynecol.*, **65**, 172
13. Patkos, P., Boucher, M., Broussard, P.M. *et al.* (1986). Factors influencing nonstress test results in multiple gestations. *Am. J. Obstet. Gynecol.*, **154**, 1107
14. Manning, F.A., Platt, L.D. and Sipos, L. (1980). Antepartum fetal evaluation: development of a fetal biophysical profile. *Am. J. Obstet. Gynecol.*, **136**, 787
15. Vintzileos, A.M., Campbell, W.A., Ingardia, C.J. *et al.* (1983). The fetal biophysical profile and its predictive value. *Obstet. Gynecol.*, **62**, 271
16. Lodeiro, J.G., Vintzileos, A.M., Feinstein, S.J. *et al.* (1986). Fetal biophysical profile in twin gestations. *Obstet. Gynecol.*, **67**, 824
17. Giles, W.B., Trudinger, B.J. and Cook, C.M. (1985). Fetal umbilical artery flow velocity–time waveforms in twin pregnancies. *Br. J. Obstet. Gynaecol.*, **92**, 490
18. Farmakides, G., Schulman, H., Saldana, L.R. *et al.* (1985). Surveillance of twin pregnancy with umbilical arterial velocimetry. *Am. J. Obstet. Gynecol.*, **153**, 789
19. Saldana, L.R., Eads, M.C. and Schaefer, T.R. (1987). Umbilical blood waveforms in fetal surveillance of twins. *Am. J. Obstet. Gynecol.*, **157**, 712
20. Giles, W.B., Trudinger, B.J., Cook, C.M. *et al.* (1988). Umbilical artery flow velocity waveforms and twin pregnancy outcome. *Obstet. Gynecol.*, **72**, 894

21. Nimrod, C., Davies, D., Harder, J. et al. (1987). Doppler ultrasound prediction of fetal outcome in twin pregnancies. *Am. J. Obstet. Gynecol.*, **156**, 402
22. Gerson, A.G., Wallace, D.M., Bridgens, N.K. et al. (1987). Duplex Doppler ultrasound in the evaluation of growth in twin pregnancies. *Obstet. Gynecol.*, **70**, 419
23. Gerson, A., Johnson, A., Wallace, D. et al. (1988). Umbilical arterial systolic/diastolic values in normal twin gestation. *Obstet. Gynecol.*, **72**, 205
24. Divon, M.Y., Girz, B.A., Sklar, A. et al. (1989). Discordant twins – a prospective study of the diagnostic value of real-time ultrasonography combined with umbilical artery velocimetry. *Am. J. Obstet. Gynecol.*, **161**, 757
25. Hastie, S.J., Danskin, F., Neilson, J.P. et al. (1989). Prediction of the small for gestational age twin fetus by Doppler umbilical artery waveform analysis. *Obstet. Gynecol.*, **74**, 730

Intrauterine behavior

24

B. Arabin, U. Gembruch and J. van Eyck

Introduction

For a long time, delivery was regarded as the 'start in life'. Indeed, prior to birth, fetal activity was generally assessed only via the mother's perceptions, and it was not possible to describe fetal behavior until the development of real-time ultrasound. Subsequently, real-time ultrasound has been used to record fetal behavior in the first trimester of pregnancy[1], and, in the second trimester fetal heart rate (FHR) monitoring was additionally applied[2]. By including fetal eye movements (FEM) during the last weeks of pregnancy as an additional aspect of fetal behavior, Nijhuis et al.[3] established definitions of fetal behavior during the last gestational weeks based on an earlier classification of neonatal behavior described by Prechtl[4]. In this manner, it became obvious that delivery only marks a transition from the prenatal to the postnatal environment.

To date, interest in the scientific investigation of human fetal developmental behavior, including perception, sensation, emotional and neuromotor development and expression, is relatively scant. Figure 1 is a schematic representation of various factors that potentially affect fetal behavior. Until publication of our first study[5], fetal behavior in human multiple pregnancies had not been described. Regardless, such pregnancies are ideal for the simultaneous evaluation of fetuses of the same gestational age who share the same 'environment' but may differ in zygosity, gender, placentation, position, hemodynamics, morphological malformation or exposure to teratogenic substances. Moreover, multiple pregnancies facilitate the investigation of any 'interfetal influences' that are present over and above the relationship between the mother and her unborn children.

This chapter describes the first attempts to evaluate fetal behavior in multiple gestations and suggests possible clinical and scientific applications of these findings.

Methods for detection of intrauterine behavior

Ultrasound observations

The investigation of fetal behavior utilizes data from numerous disciplines and integrates them into a cohesive whole. The following sections describe various techniques and discuss their application to the overall evaluation of fetal intrauterine behavior.

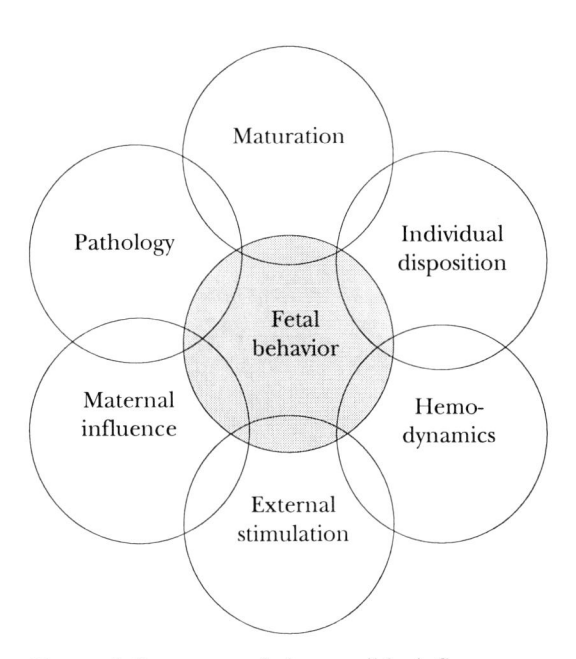

Figure 1 Spectrum of the possible influences on fetal behavior

Spontaneous fetal movement in early singleton pregnancy has been studied for years with ultrasound[6]. Early documentation of fetal behavior is best accomplished using real-time ultrasound to describe fetal somatic movement, respiratory activity, heart motion and complex specific movement patterns and in twins first contacts with each other. Up to around 12 weeks we prefer transvaginal ultrasound for documenting first twin behavior.

In advanced pregnancy, ultrasound is absolutely necessary for the simultaneous documentation of specific fetal movements, breathing movements and fetal eye movements.

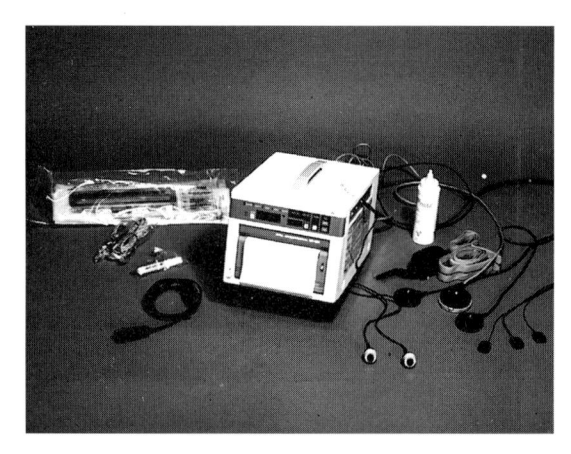

Figure 2 Example of equipment for FHR and FM registration of multiples (actocardiograph MT 430)

Zygosity determination

Examination of placentation and gender is sufficient to establish zygosity in around 50% of cases. However, zygosity is unclear in cases with same-sex, dichorionic placentation and the same blood group phenotypes (see Chapter 9). DNA-fingerprinting of each twin's leukocytes or tissue of the placenta or the umbilical cord provides the most accurate means for the determination of zygosity in the postnatal period (see Chapter 47)[7]. Placental investigation was performed for all cases of behavioral investigation described in the sections that follow, and DNA-fingerprinting was used for final diagnosis of zygosity.

Documentation of fetal movements and fetal heart rate

Although the fetal activity of twins has been documented and compared in several studies[8–10], important methodological differences exist between these investigations. These differences relate to whether fetal movements (FM) were recorded by real-time ultrasound, the mother's perception or by electromagnetic devices.

Up to now, the FHR of twins has been recorded antenatally by use of separate cardiotocographs, either consecutively or simultaneously. Use of this technology, however, does not always allow identification of each individual twin or determine whether one twin has been studied twice. In contrast, *the simultaneous recording of both FHR patterns on one tracing permits clear identification of individual FHRs and fetal behavior.* Portable equipment is presently available for simultaneous recordings of both FHR and FM in twins (Actocardiograph MT 430 Toitu, Japan). This machine was originally designed for singleton pregnancies, and the prototype MT 320 and technical details have been described[11,12].

The actocardiograph MT 430 permits FHR and FM of each twin fetus to be simultaneously documented by using separate transducers with a frequency of 1.1 MHz and an intensity of $<1.1\,mW/cm^2$. The device captures the signals of FHR and FM with one external Doppler transducer for each twin (Figure 2). These signals are then simultaneously recorded on separate channels. The FHR is documented according to the autocorrelation principle at a range of 50–240 beats per minute (bpm). FM are simultaneously documented in an analog manner by 'spikes'. The density of the spikes reflects the frequency of the FM, whereas the height of the spikes reflects the velocity. Additional information (e.g. FM perceived by the mother or FEM observed by the examiner) is documented by a double push-button system. Since all information is recorded simultaneously on one tracing, both FHR and FM patterns can be interpreted accurately and compared with each other or to additional information provided by the mother or the examiner.

Documentation of fetal behavior using the Doppler device requires a high sensitivity and specificity for the recognition of FM compared to ultrasound studies of singleton pregnancies[12–14]. At the same time, it requires less staff and is reproducible. Maeda *et al.* have developed computer-generated three-dimensional histograms[15] for more specific analysis of FM, e.g. fetal breathing movements, hiccups, etc.

In our own studies, we determine the presentation and size of the twin by ultrasound at the beginning of each session, and document the distance between the two transducers on the mother's abdomen. If the distance is small, superimpositions must be considered, although it is easy to recognize this phenomenon by simultaneous documentation. We use simultaneous ultrasound observations if the FM pattern cannot be interpreted by the actocardiograph alone. Interferences with Doppler signals of the actocardiograph must be considered if the ultrasound transducers are located close to the transducers of the actocardiograph. This phenomenon is dependent on the frequencies and qualities of the ultrasound transducers.

The additional use of real-time transducers is obligatory for the observation of the FEM during the last weeks of pregnancy[3], though this may cause interferences with twin FHR tracings to a degree that the interpretation may be impaired. Technical developments that may facilitate future documentation of fetal behavior include special computer programs applied to the Hewlett Packard system (Arduini, personal communication), but this technology has not yet been developed for multiple gestations.

External stimulation

Fetal reactions to external stimuli can also be tested by acoustic, vibroacoustic, light or tactile stimulations. Fetal reactions towards maternal intestinal sounds, which are presumed to function as intrinsic acoustic stimulation, can be studied by auscultation of the maternal abdomen. Various kinds of sound are used as sources of external acoustic stimulation.

The external tactile stimulation afforded by palpating or feeling the baby through the maternal abdomen is hard to quantify as a stimulus in multiple pregnancy. Even so, this type of activity should be considered, because babies are capable of reacting to all kinds of external touching of the mothers' abdomen. In order to compare the rate of incidental reactions to the stimulus when the instrument (e.g. flashlight or larynx-vibrator) in our investigations is attached to the maternal abdomen, sham stimuli are conducted (e.g. touching the maternal abdomen with the instrument)[16].

A larynx-vibrator is the usual instrument for testing reactions towards vibroacoustic stimulation[17]. In multiple pregnancies, it can be applied to the mother's abdomen between the heads of twins or even triplets. The position of the vibroacoustic stimulator does thus not affect the fetal response[18], making it attractive for twin research. Flashlights are applied to the head of each twin for testing fetal reactions towards light stimulation. The effect of the stimulus depends on the position of the fetal eyes with regard to the light beam. Although this can be determined by ultrasound, it is difficult to quantitate.

Reactions to tactile stimulation of the other twin can be examined by real-time ultrasound.

Definition of behavioral states

The description of fetal behavior during the first 20 weeks of gestation in singletons is up to now based on real-time observations of fetal movement patterns according to the descriptions of de Vries *et al.*[1]. Despite the fact that respiratory activity, hiccups, isolated arm and leg movements or yawning can be demonstrated in early pregnancy, these movements are not yet organized in a coordinated fashion. In addition to the criteria of de Vries, we define movement patterns like 'twisting' (which is a lateral bowing of the body) and jumping from the uterine wall. In twins, it is essential to compare their first activities and their activity cycles and, last but not least, to observe their first contacts. This is possible from 8 to 12 weeks by transvaginal and until around 20

MULTIPLE PREGNANCY

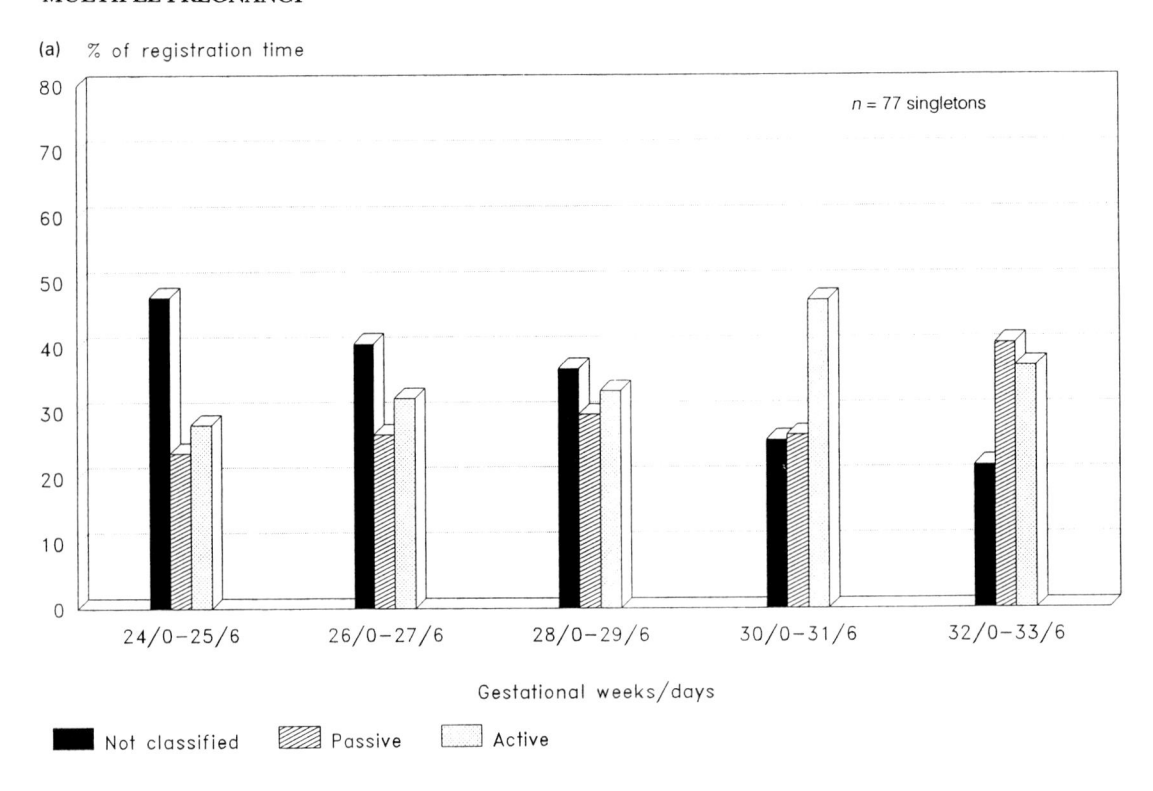

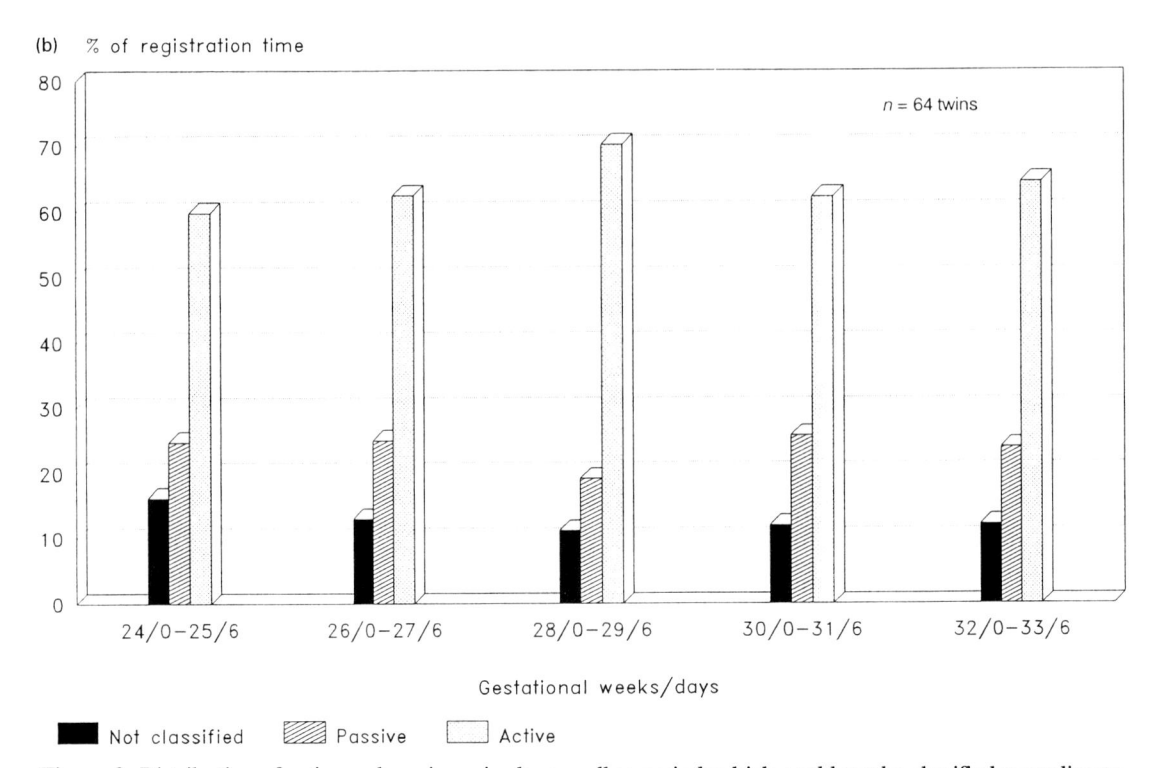

(a) % of registration time

(b) % of registration time

Figure 3 Distribution of active and passive episodes as well as periods which could not be classified according to standardized criteria[19] in singletons (a) and twins (b)

Intrauterine behavior

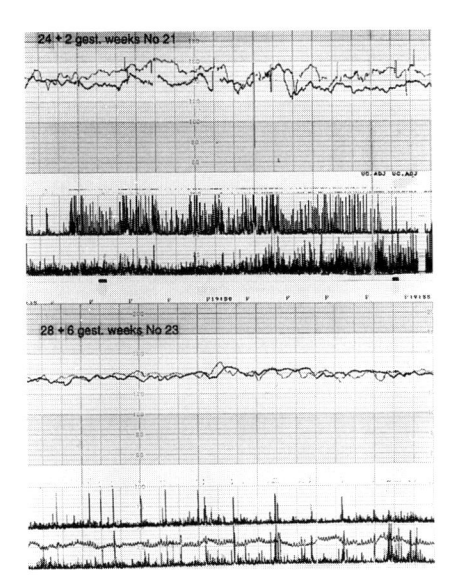

Figure 4 Development of spontaneous fetal behavior in a twin pregnancy of 24 (top) and 28 (bottom) completed gestational weeks. In the upper tracing, no cyclic differences or even similar reactions of twins can be differentiated. In the lower tracing, the simultaneous movements are observed

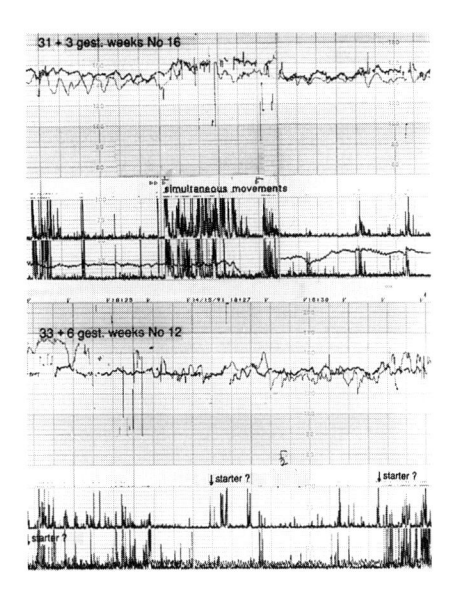

Figure 5 Development of spontaneous fetal behavior in a twin pregnancy of 31 (top) and 33 (bottom) completed gestational weeks. In the upper tracing, simultaneous clusters of FM combined with FHR accelerations of both twins can be observed. In the lower tracing, one fetus seems to 'start' moving, followed by the other. Ultrasound observations may substantiate the patterns of the actocardiograph and help to differentiate between primary and induced activity

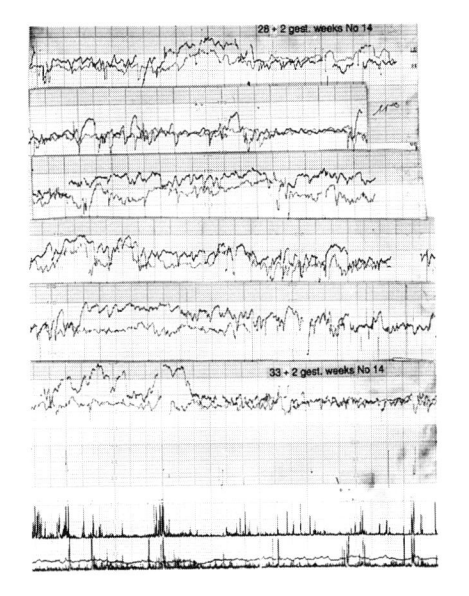

Figure 6 Comparison of spontaneous behavior in a twin pregnancy from 28 to 33 completed gestational weeks (longitudinal course of weekly settings). Twin 1 (dark tracing) always demonstrates a higher baseline and more pronounced accelerations. These characteristics become more obvious in advanced pregnancies but are observed continuously throughout pregnancy

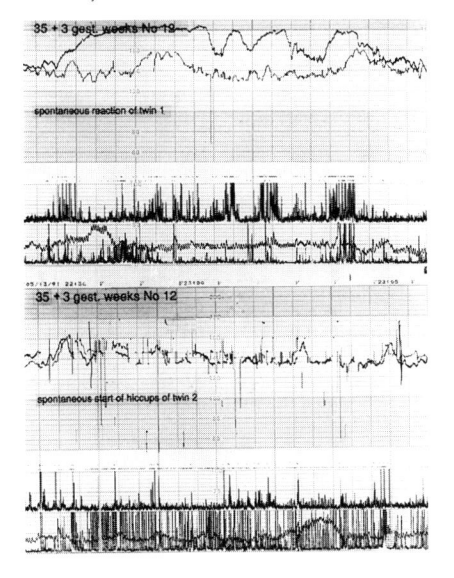

Figure 7 Comparison of spontaneous behavior in a twin pregnancy at 35 completed gestational weeks. In the upper tracing, one twin demonstrates sudden tachycardia. In the lower tracing, the other develops hiccups

Table 1 First inter-twin contacts and reactions in mono- and dichorionic twin pairs, retrospectively analyzed from video tapes of weekly ultrasound observations from 8 weeks' gestation onwards

	First inter-twin contacts and reactions (postmenstrual days)	
Kind of contact	Monochorionic twins ($n=2$)	Dichorionic twins ($n=8$)
First touch	66	75
First reaction towards touch	72	79
First gentle head contact	72	79
First gentle body contact	72	79
First gentle leg contact	72	79
First gentle arm contact	73	79
First violent leg contact (kicking)	79	88
First violent body contact	80	85
First violent arm contact (boxing)	80	94
First violent head contact	92	85
First 'embracing'	86	107
First 'kiss'	92	107

weeks by transabdominal ultrasound. Table 1 summarizes the criteria of first contacts that we have so far analyzed.

From about 24 weeks of gestation onwards, fetal behavior can be classified by analysis of FHR and FM patterns: both active and passive periods can be differentiated[19]. Our own analysis of 77 singleton pregnancies studied at regular intervals after 24 completed weeks showed characteristic active and passive periods, with a mean value of 5 min of passive and 6 min of active behavior, respectively. These durations increased to 12- and 14-min intervals, respectively, after 32 completed weeks, and the percentage of intervals which could not be classified as either active or passive decreased from 49 to 24% (Figure 3a). Breathing movements are common in both active and passive periods. (In twins, we observe a significantly higher rate of active in comparison to passive periods, while periods without classification were short (Figure 3b). This phenomenon may be explained by frequent 'inter-twin stimulations', while one twin induces either passive or active reactions of the co-twin.)

Only a small percentage of twin pregnancies we evaluated could be studied after 36 gestational weeks, because gestation length expectedly was less than 40 weeks for many of the pregnancies. If the pregnancy is not foreshortened during the last week, study of FEM should be considered for the classification of fetal behavior into four categories: 1F, 2F, 3F and 4F[3,20]. Should this be the case, the effort for recording and documentation, particularly in multiples will increase dramatically and has not yet been performed systematically in twins.

Specific aspects of fetal behavior

One of the most fantastic issues in twin research is the early observation of the first attempts of inter-human contacts. This is best visualized either by video tapes or in numerous still pictures. In this section we concentrate on the documentation of twin behavior after 24 weeks. To give some impression of the development of inter-twin contacts and reaction, we have summarized the most evident criteria of first occurence in mono- and dichorionic twins in Table 1.

The effect of maturation

From 24 gestational weeks onwards, the FHR as well as the FM patterns of twins can easily be

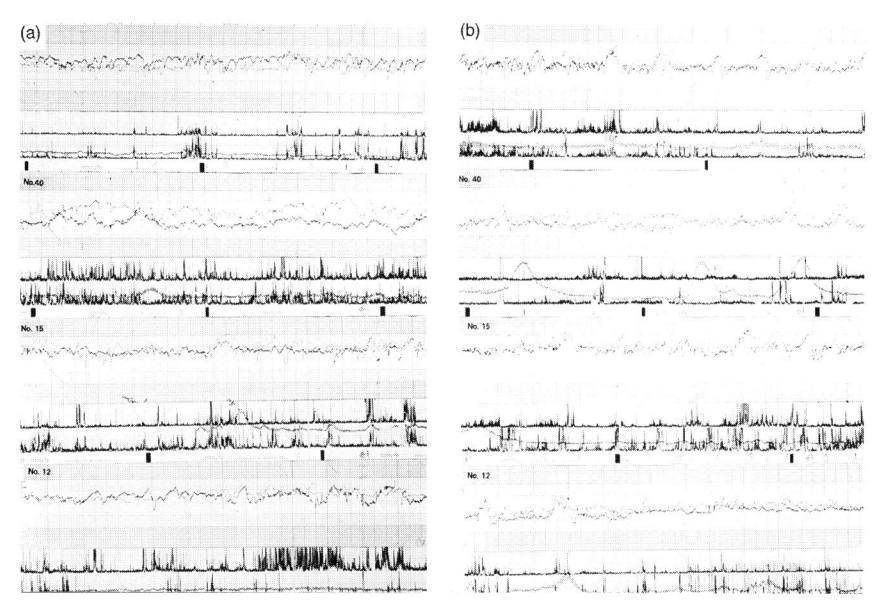

Figure 8 Longitudinal FHR and FM tracings of twin pregnancies at 28 (a) and 36 (b) completed weeks

differentiated by the actocardiograph. Before 30 gestational weeks, however, it is difficult to decide whether simultaneous common behavioral patterns exist in both twins (Figure 4, top), because cycles of defined activity are still short. We rarely observe common FHR accelerations of both twins in combination with FM.

In 'passive' periods, singular common spikes of FM occur without FHR accelerations, reflecting singular common movements (Figure 4, bottom). After 30 or even 32 gestational weeks, it is easier to differentiate the occurrence of common FM or FHR changes of both twins, due to the increasing coordination of FM and FHR (Figure 5). In active periods, we can easily recognize common spikes in combination with FHR accelerations and common clusters, i.e. the occurrence of a multitude of spikes reflecting several FMs of rapid sequences combined with a common increase of FHR, (Figure 5, top). If the movements of one fetus obviously start earlier than those of the other, it remains unclear whether the second twin's FM are induced by those of the first (Figure 5, bottom) or just an expression of his or her own primary activity.

Individual differences

FM and FHR patterns of twins may be compared either in single tracings or longitudinally. In single tracings, we can see whether and to what degree the behavior of both twins shows similar or different reactions. In a longitudinal analysis, on the other hand, we can determine whether the differences in behavioral patterns of one twin, compared to the other, are just occasional or reproducible throughout pregnancy.

It is possible to differentiate between concordant and discordant behavioral patterns in either type of evaluation. For example, if both twins occasionally 'behave' in a concordant manner in a single tracing, i.e. they both show similar FHR and FM patterns at the same time, this activity can be characterized as 'occasionally concordant spontaneous behavior' (Figure 5, top). On the other hand, if one fetus always reacts in the same manner relative to the other twin, e.g. with a higher baseline or with more pronounced accelerations, this activity can be characterized as 'continuously concordant spontaneous behavior'.

Figure 6 is an example in which the first twin always has a higher heart rate (dark line) than the second (light line). This characteristic, like others, is independent of fetal sex or the presence or absence of pathology. In this case, both fetuses were male, with a weight difference of <200 g, a dichorionic (DC) placenta and a normal pregnancy course.

The same definitions hold for discordant behavior. Each fetus may demonstrate a behavior which seems to be independent of the other. This activity is characterized as 'occasionally discordant spontaneous behavior' and is depicted in Figure 7. Here the first twin reacts spontaneously with an increase of the FHR without any obvious reason, and the second twin spontaneously starts to hiccup 10 min later. Again, these differences were independent of sex (both were female) or any obvious pathology. Discordant behavior patterns occur throughout pregnancy. In these instances, both fetuses continuously demonstrate a discrepancy compared to the preceding tracing. This activity is called 'continuously discordant spontaneous behavior'.

We developed a score to consider various degrees of differences in FHR and FM patterns (Table 2). The score ranges from 0 to 10 points. Low scores represent fewer similarities in the pattern of FHR and FM. The score is computed by using 3-min windows for a tracing of at least 30 min.

Scores were calculated for each week in a series of 32 normal twin pregnancies studied longitudinally from the 26th to the 36th gestational week. In general, we observed a slight increase of differences with advanced gestation and a lowering of the mean score from 7.1 points at 26 weeks to 6.1 at 36 weeks. Figure 8(a) and (b) demonstrates longitudinal FHR and FM tracings of twin pregnancies at 28 (a) 36 (b) completed gestational weeks. Although an increase of accelerations is seen, mainly in combination with FM and contractions, the differences between both twin tracings remain fairly stable.

Up to now, we have not been able to discern significant differences in the spontaneous behavior of both twins in the following groups: (1) MC–DA pregnancies ($n=7$, mean score 6.7), (2)

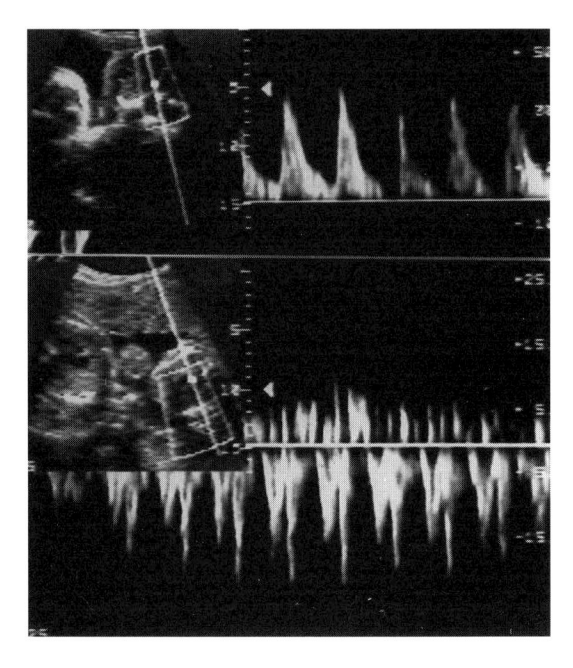

Figure 9 Blood flow velocity waveforms of the foramen ovale and the corresponding middle cerebral artery in a twin pregnancy

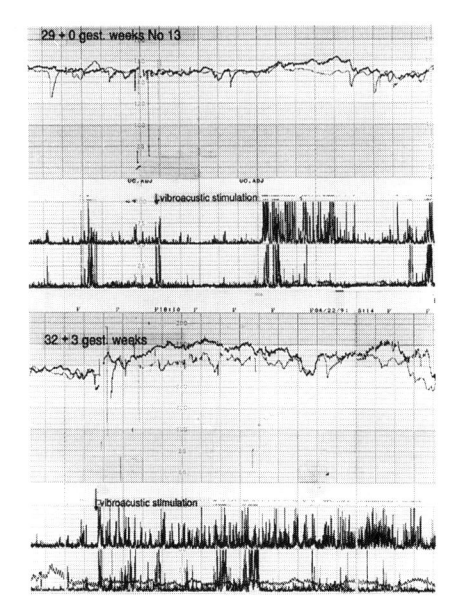

Figure 10 Reactions of twins towards vibroacoustic stimulation at 29 and 32 completed gestational weeks. In the upper tracing, only a short reaction of both FM, and in the lower tracing, a lasting reaction of FHR and FM patterns of both twins are observed

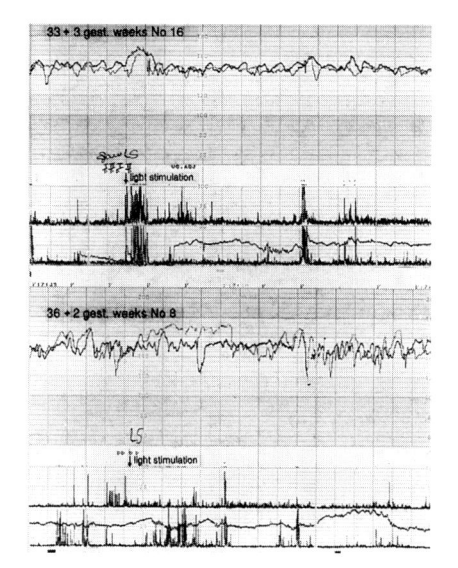

Figure 11 Reaction of twins towards separate light stimulation at 33 and 36 completed weeks. In the upper tracing, a short increase is seen in the FHR and FM of both twins, and in the lower tracing, a lasting reaction of FHR (lighter line) and FM of twin 2 is observed

DC pregnancies with different sex ($n = 18$, mean score 6.5) or the same sex ($n = 17$, mean score 6.2), all of whom had a normal pregnancy course.

Hemodynamic considerations

In early singleton pregnancies, the embryonic heart rate has been investigated by transvaginal ultrasound[21,22]. Meanwhile, we have also studied the development of heart rate and Doppler flow patterns of the umbilical artery in twin pregnancies from 8 weeks onwards. There was a decrease in heart rate from 170 beats/min at 9 weeks to 144 beats/min at 16 weeks, and a decrease in the pulsatility index from 3.2 to 1.5, respectively. Inter-twin differences may be due to differences in the implantation process or even activity.

Later in pregnancy, fetal blood flow velocity waveforms of the aorta and cerebral arteries change with the activity state[23]. As such, the waveforms represent an additional parameter of fetal behavior. Supposedly this holds true also for multiples.

After 36 gestational weeks, the end-diastolic blood flow velocities of the internal carotid artery and the fetal aorta, as well as of the foramen ovale, change significantly between states 1F and 2F. Blood flow velocity waveforms of the foramen ovale and cerebral arteries are linked to each other (Figure 9), because in state 2F more oxygenated blood is directed to the brain. Therefore, although analysis of fetal behavior is of clinical value in the interpretation of fetal hemodynamics in singleton pregnancies[24–26], this remains to be shown in multiple pregnancies.

Data relating to venous flow in the ductus venosus or inferior vena cava are now established in twins and might even change with behavioral states (Hofstaeffer, personal communication).

External stimuli

In general, the stimuli experienced by the fetus may differ to some extent from the stimuli presented from outside, primarily because the maternal abdomen alters the quality of the stimulus. Moreover, fetal perception depends on the fetal stage of development and the corresponding sensory abilities. Under these circumstances, it is not surprising that the results from investigations of various researchers differ. Twin studies represent an ideal tool for clarifying whether reactions are incidental or systematic.

Fetal reactions towards sound and the development of hearing are the most commonly studied of all fetal sensory capabilities. Reactions occur as early as from 26 weeks onwards[27,28]. A large variety of stimuli have been used. Responsiveness has been shown to sounds ranging from 83 to 5000 Hz[29,30]. Sources of sound may arise from the intra- or extrauterine environment (e.g. maternal heartbeat or borborygmi from the digestive system). Such sounds are called 'internal' or 'external' auditory stimuli, respectively. By inserting a small microphone into the uterine cavity after rupture of the membranes, we were able to demonstrate that external sounds can be heard above the internal background noise.

Table 2 Score for comparison of spontaneous and reactive FHR and FM patterns of twins with a 3-min window (tracing of twin 1/twin 2, for 30 min or for the duration of the reaction)

	0 Points	1 Point	2 Points	3 Points	4 Points
Movements	cluster/no FM	cluster/no FM	cluster/spikes/	cluster/cluster	cluster/cluster
		spikes/no FM	spikes/spikes	spikes/spikes	
			no FM/no FM	no FM/no FM	
Similarity (%)	< 20	20–40	40–60	60–80	80–100
Baseline	> 10 bpm	5–10 bpm	< 5 bpm		
Variability (amplitude of oscillation)	> 10 bpm	5–10 bpm	< 5 bpm		
Accelerations	different in number	different in amplitude > 5 bpm	equal		
Simultaneous	(−)	(+)	(+)		

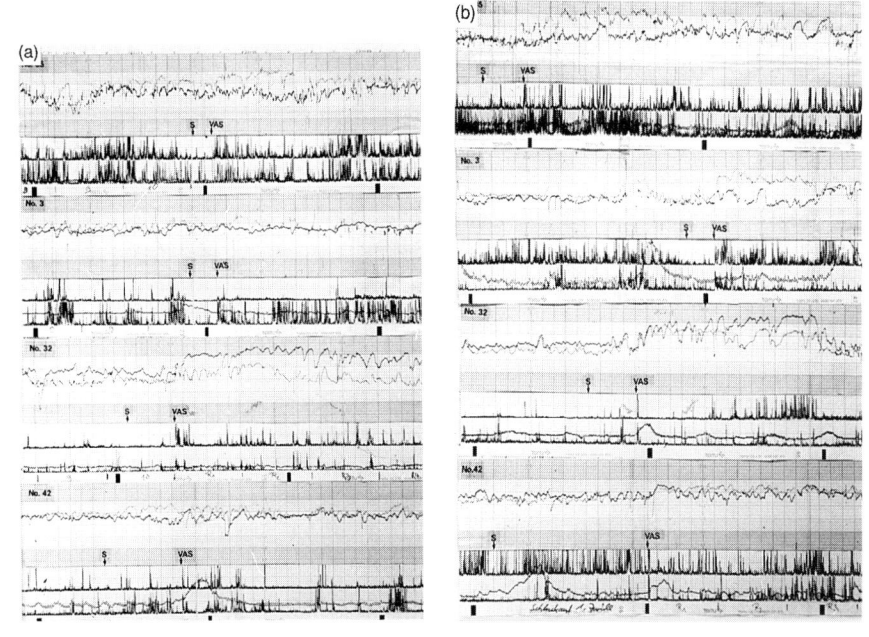

Figure 12 Longitudinal FHR and FM tracings of twins at 28 (a) and 38 (b) completed gestational weeks, all with vibroacoustic stimulation

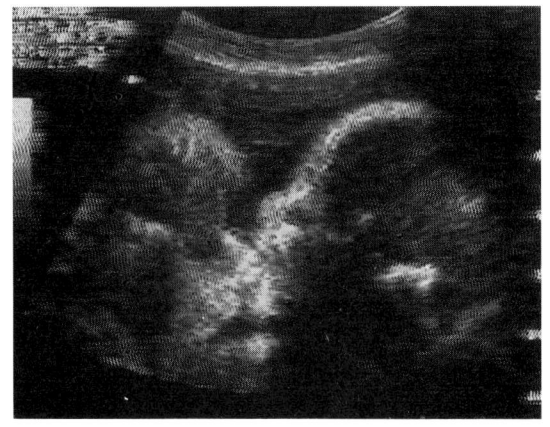

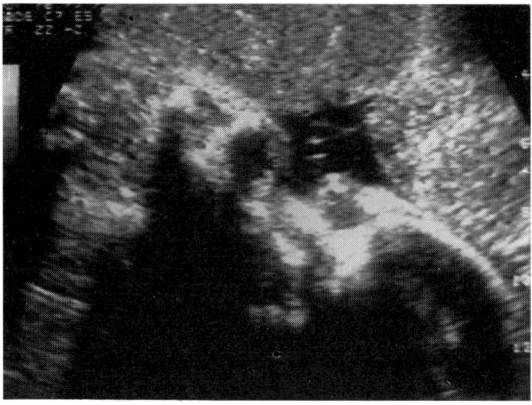

Figure 13 Face contact of two fetuses with the lips (top) and the nose (bottom)

with an increase of FHR and FM were also seen (Figure 10, below). It is important to remember, however, that because of the variable fetal position of the slight reactions such as twinkling of the eyes might be missed, not only by the combination of FHR and FM registration, but also by ultrasound observations.

The fetus may respond to external light from 26 weeks of pregnancy onwards by an increase of FHR or FM[31]. We observed an initial reaction towards light in a twin pregnancy of 26 weeks. Although we tried to provide light stimuli in twin pregnancies by using two flashlights, common reactions of twins are more difficult to quantitate, due to the positions of the fetuses vis-à-vis the light. This might be the reason that common reactions towards light stimulation (Figure 11, top) were rare in early gestation. Nearly all were 'short reactions'. Reactions of longer duration were only observed in four cases of all the light stimulations performed, but never in both twins at the same time (Figure 11, bottom).

We primarily used the above-mentioned score for analyzing differences in fetal reactions towards vibroacoustic or light stimulation (Table 2). This score ranges from 0 points,

Because the common FHR accelerations of twins have been explained by internal stimuli such as borborygmi, we documented bowel sounds of the mother by auscultation throughout our observation periods of 1 h. Surprisingly, we were unable to document correlations between the fetal twin reactions and the maternal bowel sounds as we had expected from reports in the literature. In our opinion, this discrepancy may arise from some type of habituation to these low-frequency sounds.

In contrast, after stimulating the twin fetuses with a standardized external vibroacoustic sound of 2 s duration, similar fetal reactions of both twins were observed in many cases (76%) (Figure 10). The earliest reaction of both twins was documented at 27 weeks. Before 30 weeks, we observed mainly reflex-like FM reactions (Figure 10, top). At more advanced gestational ages, long-lasting reactions

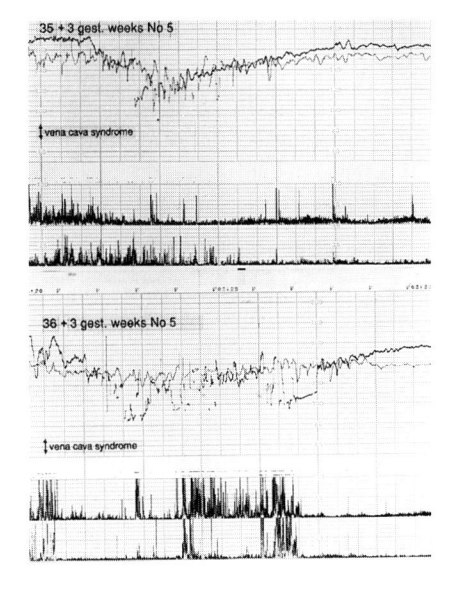

Figure 14 Reaction of FHR and FM towards a decrease of maternal blood pressure at 35 and 36 completed gestational weeks

Table 3 Significant parameters influencing different reactions of corresponding twins. ($n = 390$ twin reactions of 32 pairs to vibroacoustic stimulations/multivariate analysis)

Kind of reaction	Up to 30 weeks	31–33 weeks	33–36 weeks
Short reaction		state/zygosity	presentation
Long reaction > 3 min	state	state/zygosity	state/sex/presentation
Change of state	state	state/sex	state/sex
Score to compare FHR and FM of corresponding twins	presentation	zygosity	sex

which represents the highest differences in fetal reaction, to 10 points, which represents reactive similarity. The score was applied using a 3-min window in reactions of prolonged duration. Tracings of 30 twin pregnancies were analyzed systematically from 26 to 36 completed gestational weeks. In general, the number and degree of FHR and FM reactions increased (Figure 12), although the character of the differences between both twins remained fairly constant. The mean scores changed from 7 points at 26 weeks to 6.2 points at 36 weeks. We have looked at different groups of monochorionic–diamniotic (MC–DA) pregnancies ($n = 7$, mean score 6.5), dichorionic (DC) pregnancies with different sex ($n = 8$, mean score 5.4) or DC pregnancies of either male ($n = 9$, mean score 6.2) or female sex ($n = 11$, mean score 5.9), all of whom had a normal pregnancy course. By multivariate analysis, we could prove that there are significant differences in the kind of reaction in corresponding twins. Twins in the same position, of the same state, sex or zygosity more often demonstrate similar short or lasting reactions than twins where these parameters differ. This is even more pronounced at an advanced gestational age (Table 3).

Fetuses appear to respond reflexively to touch as early as at the end of the 7th week[32]. Initially, the response to touch on the cheek is to move away and only subsequently to move toward the touch. In a singleton pregnancy, the fetus may only touch itself around the facial region, which may be particularly sensitive to tactile stimulation. In twins, on the other hand, the potential for tactile stimulation by the co-twin represents a continuous source of contact which can be characterized as 'interfetal stimulation'.

Figure 13 demonstrates various forms of 'interfetal' communication. It shows that twins not only may touch each other with their legs or hands, but also can initiate face contact or even touch each other with their lips. In real-time ultrasound observations, we see twins approaching each other continuously with their hands or faces. Given this fact, at least some accelerations of FM and also some simultaneous FM of twins may be interpreted as a reaction of one twin following the tactile stimulation of the other. The real cause of similar reactions of both twins might only become clearly differentiated if one fetus begins to demonstrate movements of a 'starter or initiative-taker' type that subsequently induce the other to specific reactions. Unfortunately the state of the art of FHR or FM tracings is still not sufficiently developed to answer this question. More carefully executed real-time observations will be necessary before it is possible to fully describe this type of behavior. (Editor: Dr Rudy Sabbagha has described one twin 'punching' its co-twin, but he did not have the video recorder on at that instant.)

Maternal influences on fetal behavior

Maternal influences of a physical and psychological nature have been described in terms of their relation to fetal behavior. Twins are an

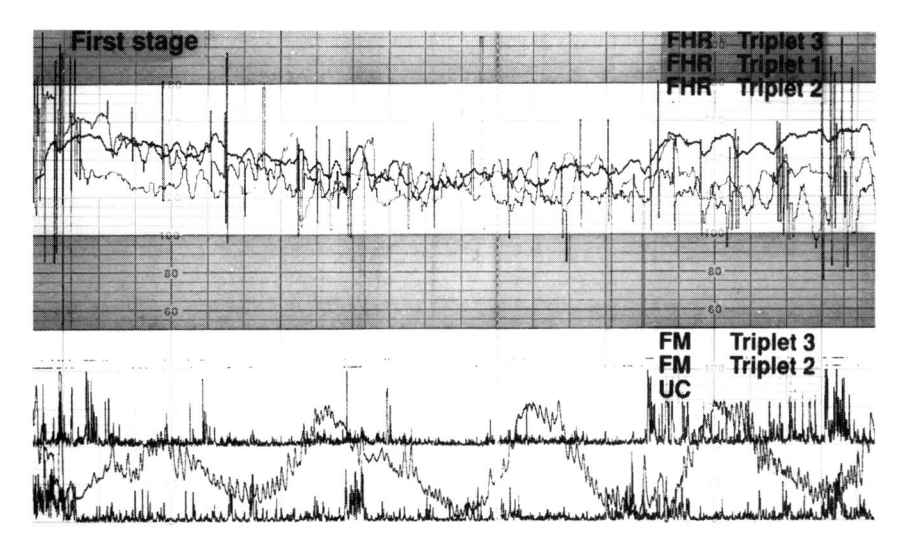

Figure 15 FHR and FM tracing of triplets during delivery

ideal model to examine these concepts. Under physiological conditions, a sudden decrease of maternal blood pressure, as might occur in the aorta–vena-cava syndrome, induces a change of FHR and FM. We observed this repeatedly in one twin pregnancy, even though the mother had been placed in a semi-recumbent position. Both twins reacted with a similar pattern of FM and FHR and even had the same difference of their baseline before and after the FHR decrease (Figure 14). It is obvious that FM stop only after the deceleration.

It has also been suggested that sounds from the maternal intestine may provoke an increase of FHR and FM by stimulating the fetus. In theory, the twin model should reveal systematic reactions in both twins. We accordingly documented maternal bowel sounds throughout our 1-h settings by auscultation but were unable to show any relationship between bowel sounds and FHR acceleration or FM.

A loss of fetal activity cycles was described after adrenectomy in singleton pregnancies – though not yet in twins – suggesting that cortisol has an important influence on cyclic fetal activity[33,34]. The literature concerning maternal prenatal emotional influences is extensive and diverse. Mothers under severe emotional stress may have hyperactive fetuses[35,36]. FHR changes, characterized as tachycardia, change in the beat-to-beat variability or decelerations have been described in mothers who were emotionally upset, subject to psychological stress or highly anxious with high adrenalin levels[37–39]. Unfortunately, fetal behavior was not systematically examined in any of these studies. By performing a careful longitudinal study, Van den Bergh et al.[40] found a positive correlation between permanent, actual maternal anxiety states and fetal and neonatal behavior in singletons.

Severe fetal bradycardia was documented during an air raid in Israel in which patients and health care personnel had to wear gas masks because of the possibility of a poison-gas attack. The bradycardia resolved when the all-clear signal was heard (personal communication to L. Keith by Moishe Hod, 1992). Despite these interesting observations, the changes of fetal behavior described as a higher incidence of state 4F or fetal activity must be interpreted with caution.

Because the twin model is ideal for examining the influence of spontaneous or induced psychological stress, we investigated the influence of induced (positive and negative) maternal emotions on FHR and FM in up to now ten twin pregnancies using the method described by Lang[41] Thus far we have been unable to discern systematic changes of FHR or FM

MULTIPLE PREGNANCY

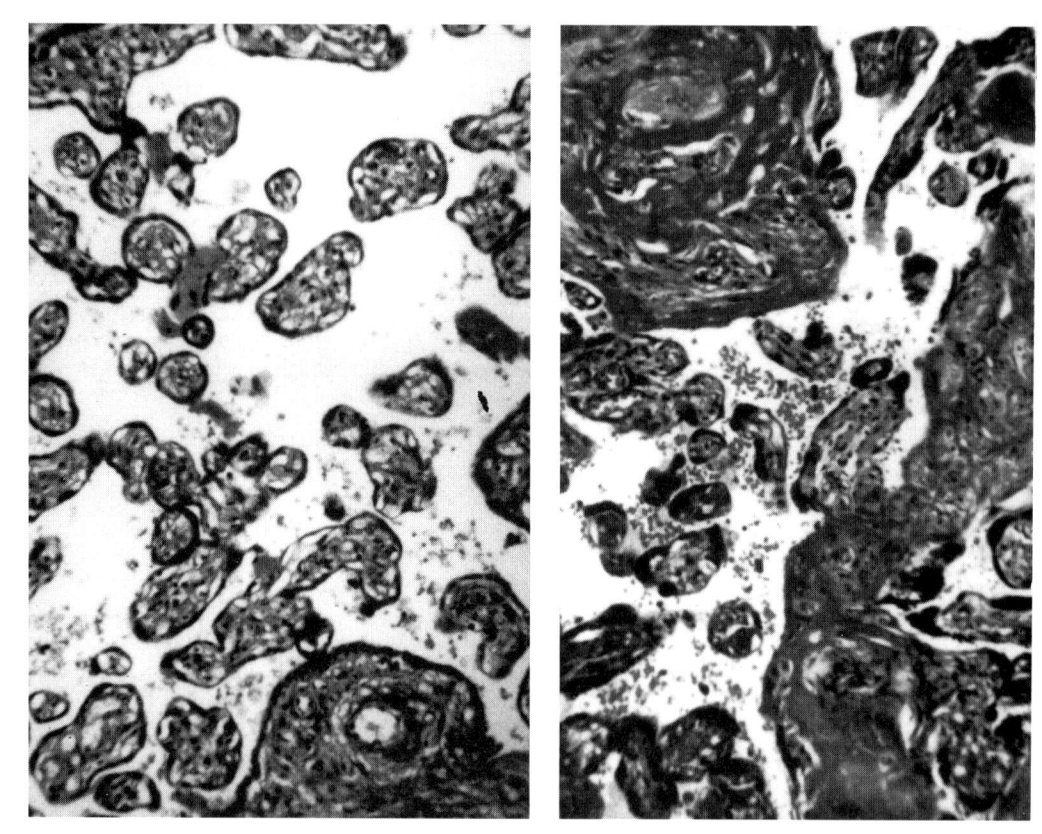

Figure 16 Left: separate dichorial placenta of the first twin (3080 g): placental weight 430 g, surface area 298 cm^2, normal histomorphological pattern. Right: second twin (1440 g): placental weight 200 g, surface area 200 cm^2, perivillous fibrin deposits, villous fibrosis and degenerative patterns of the epithelium

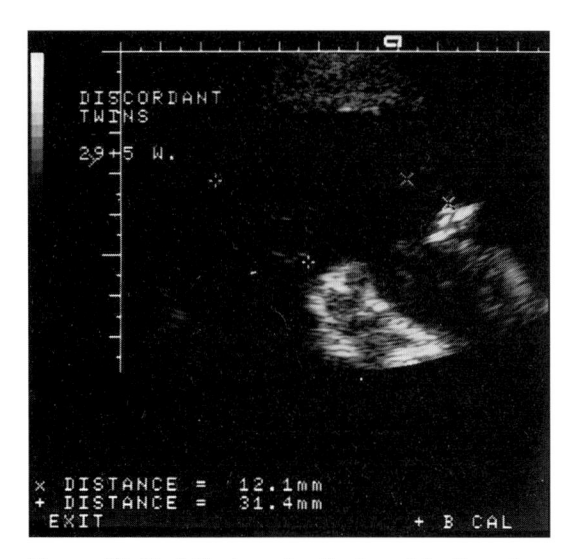

Figure 17 Umbilical cords of twins with discordant growth

patterns. However, this might be due to the fact that the number of our observations was too small, the periods of induced emotions too short or the methods of observation not sufficiently specific.

Fetal behavior during delivery

During delivery, the fetus exhibits behavioral characteristics that resemble late fetal and early neonatal behavior[42]. Fetal movements continue during labor in singleton as well as in twin pregnancies. In singleton pregnancies, FHR accelerations contribute to the effect of rest–activity cycles on the FHR during labor[43]. Most FM during labor are associated with uterine contractions and accounts for FHR accelerations. In a study of singleton pregnancies with continuous FHR recording during labor, Spencer and Johnson[43] demonstrated that

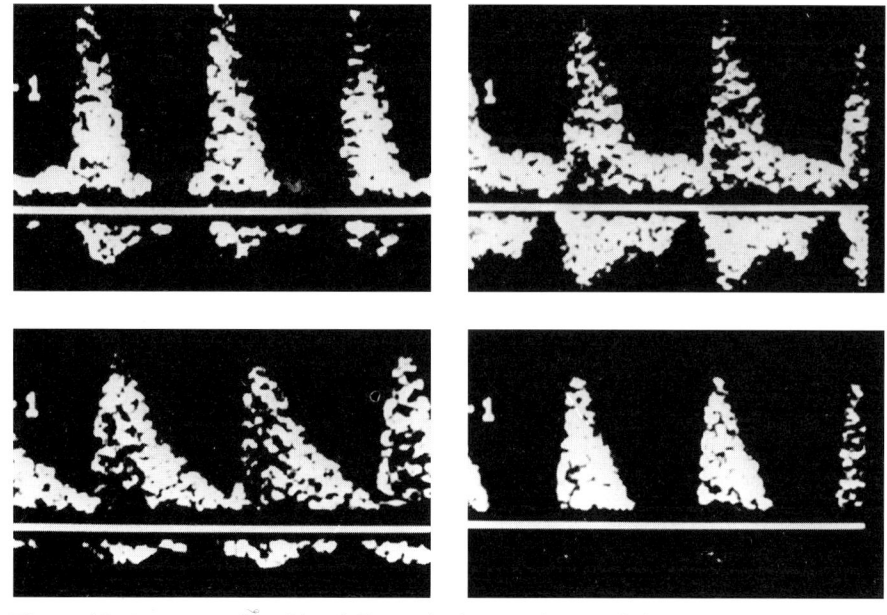

Figure 18 Corresponding blood flow velocity waveforms of the common carotid artery (top) and the fetal descending aorta (bottom), showing redistribution of the fetal circulation in the second twin (right)

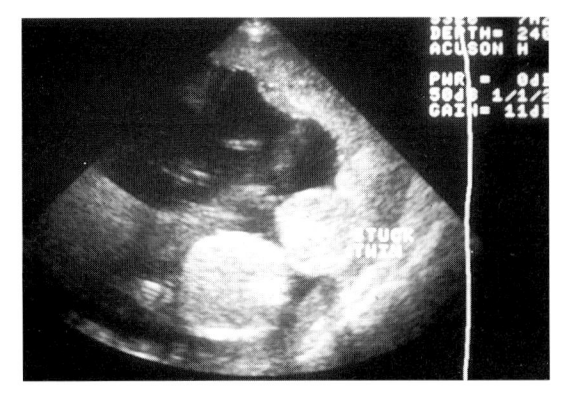

Figure 19 Feto-fetal transfusion syndrome, 28 weeks. One twin has polyhydramnios, the other appears as a 'stuck twin' without any amniotic fluid

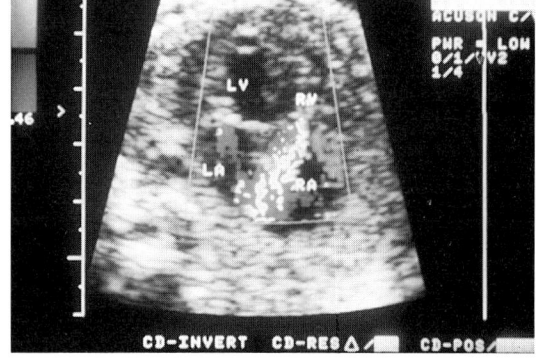

Figure 20 Recipient of the twin pregnancy with feto-fetal transfusion syndrome, demonstrating non-immunological hydrops following insufficiency of the atrio-ventricular valves, and cardiomegaly

fetal behavioral cycles were absent in around 50% of cases with healthy neonates.

FM and FHR recording was performed during labor in twin and triplet pregnancies using the actocardiograph MT 430[44]. Although we could demonstrate that the method provides an ideal tool for antepartum investigation of multiple pregnancies, to date the number of cases examined is too small to develop systematic data on the influence of labor on fetal behavior in twin or triplet pregnancy (Figure 15).

The presence of pathology

Fetal behavioral patterns are a potential tool for fetal surveillance in singleton pregnancies in which there is suspicion either of hypoxia or malformations, combined with neuromotor

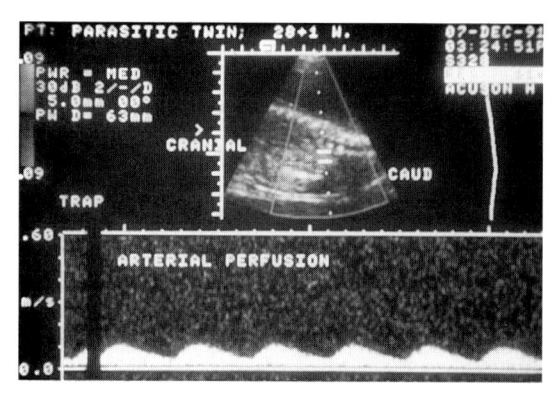

Figure 21 Parasitic twin, 28 weeks. Blood flow through the umbilical and the iliac arteries into the descending aorta can be demonstrated

disorder[45,46]. The comparison of fetal behavior might provide additional hints for the diagnosis of these complications. Preliminary results with multiples are available.

Congenital anomalies in multiple births present a wider range of problems than those in singleton births. Some anomalies are unique to multiple pregnancy (e.g. conjoined twins, acranius/acardius). Several genetic disorders and malformations are increased in multiple pregnancies, including trisomy 21, Klinefelter's or Turner's syndrome, hydrocephalus, neural tube defects, or cardiac defects. Discordant anomalies have been observed in trisomy 18 in MZ twins[47]. Movement patterns of fetuses with chromosomal anomalies differ from those of healthy fetuses[48]. We observed fetal behavior in a triplet pregnancy with trisomy 21 of one triplet. The affected triplet differed from the other two in behavioral patterns. In general simultaneous reactions, such as FM in combination with FHR accelerations, were decreased.

Little is known about the occurrence of functional anomalies, especially those related to the central nervous system (CNS) and their influence on later outcome or psychological impact[49]. Neurological disorders may exist in the absence of gross structural deficits and only become apparent after birth or emerge later in childhood. There is strong evidence that many neurological disorders have prenatal origins and are not related to the management of the delivery. Because fetal behavior is a reflection of fetal neuromotor development, in twins behavioral changes may signal the later diagnosis of conditions that depend on differences in placental nutrition or genetic makeup. Though no systematic data presently exist to support these contentions, it is quite possible that future behavioral studies will be of help in formulating the prognosis for later neuromotor development.

In twin pregnancies with discordant growth, the differences of FM and FHR patterns depend to a certain extent on the differences of placental blood supply to each fetus and thus on differences of placental anatomy (Figure 16). In these situations, multiple pregnancies may be characterized by similar uteroplacental and vastly different fetoplacental blood supply. The differences in umbilical blood flow velocity waveforms might also be due to differences in umbilical vessel diameter (Figure 17). Low pH and pO_2 levels may lead to severe circulatory centralization of the smaller compared to the larger twin (Figure 18). Based on these considerations, we observed differences of FHR and FM patterns that correlated with weight differences and differences of blood flow velocity waveforms[50]. Future systematic investigations should simultaneously consider the placental morphology and Doppler blood flow velocimetry.

The basic pathophysiology is more complex in the twin–twin transfusion syndrome. Our observations in 25 cases revealed compromised FHR patterns and a reduction of FM in both the acceptor and the donor. These changes and mainly the neonatal outcome were dependent on the severity of growth retardation in the donor and the degree of tricuspid valve regurgitation mainly of the acceptor[51].

Characteristic patterns cannot as yet be defined. Although Giles et al.[52] suggested that fetal umbilical blood flow parameters (S/D ratio) were not different in the twin–twin transfusion syndrome, this study did not apply sufficiently specific diagnostic criteria (only monochorionicity and Hb difference of >5 g% were used).

In contrast, we found great differences (>50–200%) of indices of blood flow velocity waveforms in the umbilical arteries of affected twins. Despite this, a fixed increase or decrease of either the donor or the acceptor was not present independent of the degree of cardiac insufficiency (Figure 20) or the Hb difference of the twins.

It is therefore impossible to interpret behavioral changes in the twin–twin transfusion syndrome merely on the basis of umbilical hemodynamics. Only in twins with retrograde arterial perfusion is it easy to interpret the retrograde blood flow in either the umbilical vein or the descending aorta (Figure 21) Even cordocentesis and determination of hemoglobin or hematocrit levels are unreliable to determine the severity of the problem and the prognosis for the fetuses. Given these circumstances, it seems of great importance to have additional tools for determining fetal well-being or the necessity for intervention in the case of twin–twin transfusion. Twin behavior studies might be one of these in the future.

Prognosis and future development

The increasing survival rate of immature twins and other multiples contributes substantially to the group of infants who may be handicapped after delivery[53]. It also encourages us to continue to evaluate antenatal neuromotor behavior in the hopes that these studies might be used to detect or prevent neuromotor disease prenatally.

Multiple pregnancies require intensive monitoring of the fetal condition, particularly during the last months of pregnancy. Recording fetal behavior allows us to investigate intrauterine development in twin and even triplet pregnancies to compare behavioral patterns of fetuses of the same gestational age and 'environment'. The methodology described and definitions used in this chapter should be applied in the future for comparison of twins and higher-order multiples under a variety of intrinsic or extrinsic physiological or pathological conditions. Evidence from animal research[54] and child psychology[55] suggests that placentation and zygosity may have an impact on neonatal and child behavior.

In our opinion, a new field is about to open that not only assists the clinical evaluation of complicated twin pregnancies, but also allows for basic research on the possible impact of late intrauterine neurological development on later life of multiples. More than that, human behavior can be compared by considering 'interfetal communication' in its earliest stages.

Acknowledgements

I thank Professor H.T. Versmold, Benjamin Franklin Univ.-Kinderklinik Berlin-Steglitz, R. Rijlaorsdam, H. Adt and B. Güner for encouragement, advice and practical help.

References

1. De Vries, J.I.P, Visser, G.H.A. and Prechtl, H.R.F. (1982). The emergence of fetal behavior. I Qualitative aspects. *Early Hum. Dev.*, **7**, 301
2. Arduini, D., Rizzo, G., Giolandino, C. *et al.* (1985). The fetal behavioural states. *Prenat. Diagn.*, **5**, 269
3. Nijhuis, J.G., Prechtl, H.F.R., Martin, C.B. Jr *et al.* (1982). Are there behavioural states in the human fetus? *Early Hum. Dev.*, **6**, 177
4. Prechtl, F.R. (1974). The behavioural states of the newborn infant. *Brain Res.*, **5**, 477
5. Arabin, B., van Eyck, J., Wisser, J. *et al.* (1991). Fetales Verhalten bei Mehrlingsgravidtät: Methodische, klinische und wissenschaftliche Aspekte. *Geburtsh. Frauenheilk.*, **51**, 869
6. Reinold, E. (1973). Clinical value of fetal spontaneous movements in early pregnancy. *J. Perinat. Med.*, **1**, 65
7. Jeffrey, A.J., Brookfield, J.F.Y. and Semeonoff, R. (1985). Positive identification of an immigration test case using human DNA fingerprints. *Nature (London)*, **317**, 818
8. Ohel, G.A., Samueloff, A., Navot, D. *et al.* (1985). Fetal heart rate accelerations and fetal

movements in twin pregnancies. *Am. J. Obstet. Gynecol.*, **152**, 686

9. Sadovsky, E., Ohel, G. and Simon, A. (1987). Ultrasonographical evaluation of the incidence of simultaneous and independent movements in twin fetuses. *Gynecol. Obstet. Invest.*, **23**, 5

10. Zimmer, E.Z., Goldstein, I. and Alglay, S. (1988). Simultaneous recording of fetal breathing movements and body movements in twin pregnancy. *J. Perinat. Med.*, **16**, 109

11. Maeda, K. (1984). Studies on new ultrasonic Doppler fetal actograph and continuous recording of fetal movement. *Acta Obstet. Gynaecol.*, **36**, 280

12. Arabin, B., Riedewald, S., Zacharias, C. *et al.* (1988). Quantitative analysis of fetal behavioural patterns. *Gynecol. Obstet. Invest.*, **26**, 211

13. Schwöbel, E., Fallenstein, F., Huch, R. *et al.* (1987). Combined electronic FHR and FM monitor – a preliminary report. *J. Perinat. Med.*, **15**, 179

14. Besinger, R.E. and Johnson, T.R.B. (1985). Doppler recordings of fetal movement: clinical correlation with real-time ultrasound. *Am. J. Obstet. Gynecol.*, **152**, 686

15. Maeda, K., Tatsumura, M., Nakajima, K. *et al.* (1988). The ultrasonic Doppler fetal actocardiogram and its computer processing. *J. Perinat. Med.*, **16**, 327

16. Schmidt, W., Boos, R., Gnirs, J. *et al.* (1985). Fetal behavioral states and sound stimulation. *Early Hum. Dev.*, **12**, 145

17. Gagnon, R., Hunse, C. and Foreman, J. (1989). Human fetal behavioral states after vibratory stimulation. *Am. J. Obstet. Gynecol.*, **161**, 1470

18. Eller, D.P., Robinson, L.J. and Newman, R.B. (1992). Position of the vibroacoustic stimulator does not affect fetal response. *Am. J. Obstet. Gynecol.*, **167**, 1137–9

19. Arduini, D., Rizzo, G., Giorlandino, C. *et al.* (1986). The development of fetal behavioral states: a longitudinal study. *Prenat. Diagn.*, **6**, 117

20. Arabin, B. and Riedewald, S. (1992). An attempt to quantify characteristics of behavioral states. *Am. J. Perinat.*, **9**, 115

21. Schats, R., Jansen, C.A.M. and Wladimiroff, J.W. (1990). Embryonic heart activity: appearance and development in early human pregnancy. *Br. J. Obstet. Gynaecol.*, **97**, 989

22. Wisser, J. and Dirschede, P. (1994). Embryonic heart rate in dated human embryos. *Early Hum. Devel.*, **37**, 107–15

23. Arabin, B. (1990). *Pathophysiological and Clinical Value of Doppler Ultrasound of Uteroplacental and Fetal Vessels.* (Heidelberg, Berlin, New York: Springer-Verlag)

24. van Eyck, J., Wladimiroff, J.W, Noordam, M.J. *et al.* (1985). Blood flow velocity waveform in the fetal descending aorta: its relationship to fetal behavioral states in normal pregnancy. *Early Hum. Dev.*, **12**, 137

25. van Eyck J., Wladimiroff, J.W., van den Wijngard J.A.G.W. *et al.* (1987). Blood flow velocity waveforms in the internal carotid and umbilical artery: its relationship to fetal behavioural states in normal pregnancy at 37–38 weeks. *Br. J. Obstet. Gynaecol.*, **94**, 736

26. van Eyck, J., Stewart, P.A. and Wladimiroff, J.W. (1990). Human fetal foramen ovale flow velocity waveforms relative to behavioral state in normal term pregnancy. *Am. J. Obstet. Gynecol.*, **163**, 1239

27. Hepper, P.G. and Shahidulla, S. (1992). Habituation in normal and Down syndrome fetuses. *Q. J. Exp. Psych.*, **44**, 305

28. Timor-Tritsch, I.E. (1986). The effect of external stimulation on fetal behavior. *Eur. J. Obstet. Reprod. Biol.*, **21**, 321

29. Lecanuet, J.P., Granier-Deferre, C. and Busnel, M.C. (1988). Fetal cardiac and motor response to octave-band noises as a function of central frequency, intensity and heart rate variability. *Early Hum. Dev.*, **18**, 81

30. Madison, L.S., Adubato, S.A, Madison, J.K. *et al.* (1986). Fetal response decrement: true habituation. *Dev. Behav. Pediatr.*, **7**, 14

31. Peleg, D. and Goldman, J.A. (1980). Fetal heart rate acceleration in response to light stimulation as a clinical measure of fetal well being. A preliminary report. *J. Perinat. Med.*, **8**, 38

32. Hooker, D. (1952). *The Prenatal Origin of Behavior.* (Kansas: University of Kansas Press)

33. Arduini, D., Rizzo, E., Parlati, E. *et al.* (1986). Modification of ultradian and circadian rhythms of fetal heart rate and fetal–maternal adrenal gland suppression: a double blind study. *Prenat. Diagn.*, **6**, 409

34. Arduini, D., Rizzo, G., Parlati, E. *et al.* (1987). Loss of circadian rhythms of fetal behavior in a totally adrenalectomized pregnant woman. *Gynecol. Obstet. Invest.*, **23**, 226

35. Ferreira, A.J. (1965). Emotional factors in prenatal environment. *J. Nerv. Ment. Dis.*, **141**, 108
36. Wolkind, S. (1990). Prenatal emotional stress: effects on the foetus. In Wolkind, S. and Zajicek, E. (eds.) *Pregnancy: A Psychological and Social Study*, pp. 177–94. (London: Academic Press)
37. Eskes, T.K.A.B. (1985). Verkloskundige consequenties van niet verwerkte rouw over een perinatal gestorven kind. *Ned. Tijdschr. Geneesk.*, **129**, 433
38. Talbert, D.G, Benson, P. and Dewhurst, J. (1982). Fetal response to maternal anxiety: a factor in antepartum heart rate monitoring. *Br. J. Obstet. Gynaecol.*, **3**, 34
39. Lederman, E., Lederman, R.P., Work, B.A. *et al.* (1981). Maternal psychological and physiological correlates of fetal newborn health status. *Am. J. Obstet. Gynecol.*, **139**, 956
40. van den Bergh, B.R., Mulder, E.J.H., Poelman-Wesjes, G. *et al.* (1989). The effect of (induced) maternal emotions on fetal behavior: a controlled study. *Early Hum. Dev.*, **9**, 9
41. Lang, P. (1979). Emotional imaging: theory and experiment on instructed somatovisceral control. In Kimmel, H.D. (ed.) *Biofeedback and Self-regulation*. (New York: Erlbaum)
42. Griffin, R.L., Caron, F.J. and van Gejn, H.P. (1985). Behavioral states in the human fetus during labor. *Am. J. Obstet. Gynecol.*, **152**, 828
43. Spencer, J.A.D. and Johnson, P. (1986). Fetal heart rate variability changes and fetal behavioural cycles during labour. *Br. J. Obstet. Gynaecol*, **93**, 314
44. van Eyck, J. and Arabin, B. (1992). Actocardiographic monitoring of triplets during vaginal delivery. *Am. J. Obstet. Gynecol.*, **166**, 1293
45. Rizzo, G., Arduini, D, Pennestri, F. *et al.* (1987). Fetal behavior in growth retardation: its relationship to fetal blood flow. *Prenat. Diagn.*, **7**, 229
46. Arduini, D., Rizzo, G., Caforio, L. *et al.* (1987). Development of behavioral states in hydrocephalus fetuses. *Fetal Ther.*, **2**, 135
47. Mulder, A.F.P., van Eyck, J., Groenendaal, F. and Wladimiroff, J.W. (1989). Trisomy 18 in monozygotic twins. A case report. *Hum. Genet.*, **83**, 300
48. Boue, J., Vignal, P., Aubry, J.P. *et al.* (1982). Ultrasound movement patterns of fetuses with chromosome anomalies. *Prenat. Diagn.*, **2**, 61
49. Versmold, H.T. (1990). Outcome von 93 Drillingen, 40 Vierlingen, 15 Funflingen. In Saling, E. and Dudenhausen, J.W. (eds.) *Perinatale Medizin Band XIV*, pp. 28–30 (*Stuttgart: Thieme Verlag*)
50. Arabin, B., Jimenez, E. and Saling, E. (1987). Die Bedeutung von Doppler-Blutflußmessungen bei Geminigravidität. *Z. Geburtsh. Perinat.*, **191**, 99
51. Gembruch, U. and Arabin, B. (1994). Twin to twin transfusion syndrome. In Van Geijn, H.P. and Copray, F.J.A. (eds.) *A Critical Appraisal of Fetal Surveillance*, pp. 169–80. (Amsterdam: Elsevier)
52. Giles, W.B., Trudinger, B.J., Cook, C.M. *et al.* (1990). Doppler umbilical artery studies in the twin–twin transfusion syndrome. *Obstet. Gynecol.*, **76**, 1097
53. Uverbrant, P. (1988). Hemiplegic cerebral palsy. Aetiology and outcome. *Acta Paed. Scand.*, **345**, 5
54. Baunack, E., Falk, U. and Gaertner, K. (1984). Monozygotic vs. dizygotic twin behavior in artificial mouse twins. *Genetics*, **106**, 463
55. Reed, T., William, C., Rose, R. *et al.* (1991). Effect of chorion type on cognitive and personality factors in young monozygotic twins. Proceedings of the 8th International Congress of Human Genetics. *Am. J. Hum. Genet.*, **49**, 174

25 The natural history of grand multifetal pregnancies and the effect of pregnancy reduction

L. Lynch and R.L. Berkowitz

Introduction

The incidence of multifetal pregnancy has increased greatly since the introduction of ovulation-inducing drugs in the early 1960s. Depending upon the medications, the incidence of multiples ranges from a low of 7–9% with clomiphene citrate to a high of 39% with human menopausal gonadotropins[1-3].

In vitro fertilization (IVF) and related techniques also contribute to the rising rate of multiple gestations[4]. Presently, no consensus exists regarding the optimal number of embryos or oocytes to be transferred during IVF, zygote intrafallopian transfer (ZIFT), or gamete intrafallopian transfer (GIFT) procedures. Clearly, the pregnancy rate improves as the number of embryos or oocytes transferred increases, but so does the rate of multiple pregnancies.

The risk of extreme prematurity is directly proportional to the number of fetuses within the uterus. Some premature infants die in the neonatal period, whereas many others survive but develop severe complications and sequelae as a result of their early preterm delivery. Reduction in the number of fetuses has been proposed as a means to improve perinatal outcome in grand multifetal pregnancy.

This chapter reviews the literature on the natural course of pregnancies consisting of three or more fetuses and the effect of multifetal pregnancy reduction procedures on specific outcome variables.

Natural history of grand multifetal pregnancies

The most important complication of pregnancies consisting of three or more fetuses is preterm delivery, with its concomitant increase in perinatal morbidity and mortality. Accurate data about the outcome of grand multifetal pregnancies is limited for several reasons. First, the number of cases reported prior to the use of ovulation induction is limited by the low natural incidence of higher order multifetal pregnancies. Second, the majority of reports only contain information about pregnancies attaining 20 or 24 weeks' gestation and provide little data relating to spontaneous abortion rates. Third, as most published series concern triplets, the natural course of pregnancies consisting of four or more fetuses must often be extrapolated or inferred from secondary data. Finally, most published reports only present perinatal mortality data, with very little attention given to perinatal morbidity or long-term follow up of the survivors. Despite these limitations, some insights into the subject can be gained by reviewing published series.

Table 1 summarizes data from seven series reporting the natural course of triplet gestations[4-10]. The four most recent of these studies are relatively comparable, because they concern deliveries conducted during the past 15 years. In 1988, the Australian *In Vitro* Fertilization Collaborative Group reported their experience

Table 1 Natural course of triplets (series published up to 1990)

Authors	Delivery Years	Delivery No.	Mean age at delivery (weeks)	Delivery (%) < 37 weeks	Delivery (%) < 32 weeks	Delivery (%) < 28 weeks	Perinatal mortality (/1000)
Australian IVF[4]	1979–85	32	—	97	39	3	—
Newman et al.[5]	1985–88	198	34	88	20	7*	50
Lipitz et al.[6]	1975–88	78	33	86	26	10	93
Gonen et al.[7]	1978–88	24	32	100	—	—	69
Itzkowic[8]	1946–76	59	33	83	25	10	273
Syrop and Varner[9]	1946–83	20	33	75	—	15	216
Holcberg et al.[10]	1960–79	31	32	87	35	16	312/33†
Total		442	33	88	29	10	

*Less than 29 weeks; †delivery by vaginal and Cesarean route, respectively

with 1510 pregnancies conceived between 1979 and 1985[4]. Included were 32 sets of triplets that reached at least 20 weeks of gestation. Virtually all (87%) delivered before 37 weeks, 39% before 32 weeks and 3% before 28 weeks. Morbidity and mortality data were not reported separately for the triplets in this series.

In 1989, Newman et al.[5] described 198 sets of triplets delivered in a number of disparate settings between 1985 and 1988. These patients were followed using ambulatory contraction monitoring, and the data in this report were obtained from the records kept by a private monitoring service. The mean gestational age at delivery was 33.6 weeks. Despite intensive prenatal surveillance, 88% of the patients delivered before 37 weeks, 20% before 32 weeks and 6.6% before 28 weeks. The corrected perinatal mortality in this series rate was 50/1000.

Also in 1989, Lipitz et al.[6] reported 78 triplet pregnancies delivered between 1975 and 1988. This report was limited to patients reaching at least 20 weeks' gestation. The mean gestational age at delivery was 33.2 weeks. Eighty-six per cent of women delivered before 37 weeks, 26% before 32 weeks and 10% before 28 weeks. The perinatal and neonatal mortality rates were 93/1000 and 51/1000, respectively. In contrast to other reports, follow-up data for at least 1 year (range 1 to 6 years) were available for 38 of 48 surviving infants with birth weight of <1500 g. Four of the infants (10.5%) had severe neurological handicaps and eight (21%) had mild disabilities, predominantly abnormalities of muscle tone or attention deficit disorders.

Finally, in 1990, Gonen et al.[7] reported the outcome of 24 triplet, five quadruplet and one quintuplet pregnancies. Seventy-nine per cent of the mothers with triplets, all mothers with quadruplets, and the mother of the quintuplets experienced preterm labor. All the deliveries occurred prematurely with 47% occurring before 32 completed weeks of gestation. The perinatal mortality for the triplets was 69.4/1000, and the incidence of respiratory distress syndrome was 41%, bronchopulmonary dysplasia 4%, retinopathy of prematurity 4%, and intraventricular hemorrhage 4%. Follow up of 1–10 years among all survivors documented only one child with moderate delay in gross and fine motor skills as well as social adaptive and language developmental delays.

Although data regarding the natural course of quadruplets are more limited (Table 2), they cover the same time span of the more recent triplet series[7,11–13]. The largest report by Collins and Bleyl[11] consisted of 71 cases. Data were obtained by sending questionnaires to patients registered with a support group for patients with multifetal pregnancies (The Triplet Connection). Despite a less than optimal response rate and the limitations of this

Table 2 Natural course of quadruplets (series published up to 1990)

Authors	Delivery		Gestational age at delivery			
	Years	No.	Mean (weeks)	< 37 weeks (%)	< 32 weeks (%)	< 28 weeks (%)
Collins and Bleyl[11]	1980–89	71	31	97	61	20
Gonen et al.[7]	1978–88	5	30	100	—	—
Lipitz et al.[12]	1975–89	8	31	100	50	25
Vervliet et al.[13]	1985–88	5	31	100	60	20
Total		89	31	98	57	22

type of data collection, these self-reported pregnancy outcomes were not significantly different from smaller single-institution series. Virtually all patients with quadruplets delivered before term, approximately half delivered before 32 weeks and one-fifth delivered before 28 weeks. The perinatal mortality in this series was 67 per 1000.

Lipitz et al.[12] reported long-term follow up of 11 pregnancies consisting of four or more fetuses (eight quadruplets, two quintuplets and one sextuplet). Two women delivered stillborn quadruplets at 25 and 26 weeks, respectively, and one 310-g fetus of a quadruplet pregnancy died. Six of these nine stillborn fetuses weighed less than 500 g. Twenty-nine (74%) of the liveborn infants weighed less than 1500 g and 16 (41%) were small for gestational age. The total fetal loss rate was 23%, and the perinatal mortality rate, excluding stillborn fetuses weighing less than 500 g, was 119 per 1000 births. All but one of the liveborn quadruplets survived. The one that died had trisomy 18. Most of the surviving infants were followed for at least two years. Thirty per cent were found to have neurodevelopmental abnormalities, including 27% of surviving quadruplets.

The multifetal pregnancies described above were also associated with significant maternal risks. Mothers carrying triplets had a 20% incidence of pre-eclampsia, an 11–35% incidence of anemia and a 35% incidence of postpartum hemorrhage[6,9]. In Collins and Bleyl's series of 71 quadruplets, 32% of the women developed pre-eclampsia, 25% became anemic and 21% experienced postpartum hemorrhage[11].

In summary, the rate of preterm delivery in triplets has not changed to a great extent over the past two or three decades; in contrast, perinatal mortality rates have declined markedly, most probably due to improved neonatal care. The average gestational age at delivery for triplets in all published series consistently hovers around 33 weeks. In general, about 85–90% of triplets deliver before 37 weeks, 20–30% before 32 weeks and 5–10% before 28 weeks. Data regarding the natural course of quadruplets are insufficient to develop comparable rates for comparable stages of gestation; however, it appears that almost all experience preterm delivery, half before 32 weeks and one-quarter before 28 weeks.

Fetal reduction procedures

Selective termination was first described in twins who were discordant for congenital anomalies. In 1978, Aberg et al.[14] reported a successful selective termination of a twin with Hurler's syndrome. The authors utilized cardiac puncture to cause the death of the affected twin, and the patient went on to deliver a normal singleton at 33 weeks. In the second report of selective termination resulting in a term delivery of a normal child, hysterotomy was performed to remove the affected fetus at 22 weeks of gestation[15].

Since these initial reports, various methods for selective termination during the second trimester have been utilized in an attempt to refine the technique and to decrease the rate and risk of potential complications. Rodeck[16] published a report on six cases of second-trimester selective twin terminations performed by injecting air into the fetal circulation (to create an embolus) under fetoscopic visualization. Although he was successful in all instances, others subsequently determined that air embolization markedly reduced the ability to visualize the fetal heart ultrasonically. Since the development of percutaneous fetal blood sampling (PUBS), most termination procedures have been performed using percutaneous cardiac or umbilical vein puncture and injection of a cardiotoxic substance, such as potassium chloride[17,18].

The initial report of first-trimester reduction of grand multifetal pregnancies (three or more fetuses) was published in 1986. Dumez and Oury[19] reported 15 transcervical aspirations of multifetal pregnancies reduced to four singletons, ten sets of twins and one set of triplets. At the time their report was written, nine patients had successfully delivered, four pregnancies were ongoing and two women had lost their entire pregnancy. In the same year, Kanhai et al.[20] reported reduction of a quintuplet pregnancy to twins by thoracic puncture under ultrasonic visualization. Their patient delivered healthy twins at term.

Our group published the first series of transabdominal multifetal pregnancy reductions[21,22]. The first three procedures were performed using transcervical aspiration; however, the third patient experienced intractable bleeding secondary to placental separation. We then switched to a transabdominal approach, which we have utilized subsequently. Because of the risk of infection and uteroplacental bleeding with transcervical aspiration, most other centers also prefer transabdominal thoracic puncture.

The New York Mount Sinai experience

As of November 1991, 200 first-trimester multifetal pregnancy reductions had been performed at the Mount Sinai Medical Center in New York[23]. Eighty-eight patients presented with triplets, 89 with quadruplets, 16 with quintuplets, five with sextuplets, one with septuplets and one with nontuplets. All pregnancies resulted from ovulation induction, except one set of spontaneous quadruplets. All of the pregnancies were reduced to twins except for 11. Of these, five were reduced to triplets; in one case the presenting twins were monochorionic and the other four patients requested a reduction from a higher number to triplets. The remaining six pregnancies were reduced to a singleton, because of the presence of significant additional risk factors predisposing to preterm delivery.

Of the first 200 completed pregnancies, 19 (9.5%) were lost completely, and 181 patients have delivered viable infants: 171 twins, three triplets and seven singletons. The mean gestational age at delivery for the entire group was 35.7 weeks. Only 16 patients delivered before 32 weeks.

The only immediate, albeit uncommon, complication following the procedure was a self-limited leakage of amniotic fluid from the sacs of the terminated fetuses in a small number of patients. Our patients were not generally followed with serial coagulation profiles, but no cases of clinically evident disseminated intravascular coagulation (DIC) were apparent. In addition, no cases of intrauterine infections occurred secondary to the procedure.

Of the 19 pregnancies that were lost completely, only one occurred within the 2 weeks following the procedure, and ten occurred more than 8 weeks later. It is unclear why these patients experienced a pregnancy loss so many weeks after the procedure had been performed. Since the background rate of spontaneous second-trimester abortions in twin gestation is not known, the number of procedure-related losses cannot be ascertained.

Our experience suggests that perinatal morbidity and mortality are likely to be improved when pregnancies with four or more fetuses are reduced to smaller numbers. The mean age of delivery in 89 reported quadruplet pregnancies was 31 weeks, and 22% delivered before 28 weeks (Table 2). In our series, the mean age of delivery for women who presented with quadruplets and underwent reduction was 35.4 weeks, and only 4/82 (5%)

delivered before 28 weeks. It is reasonable to assume that this trend would be equally or more obvious with higher numbers of fetuses. However, the advantages of reducing fetal number in triplet pregnancies are not clearcut. As mentioned above, data on the natural history of triplets suggest that mean gestational age at delivery is generally around 33 weeks. More importantly, published series indicate that 20–39% of triplets deliver before 32 weeks, and 3–10% prior to 28 weeks. The outcome in our series is encouraging, in that only four of the patients who initially had triplets delivered before 32 weeks, none delivered earlier than 28 weeks, and all of the neonates were healthy at the time of discharge from the hospital (Table 3). Currently, long-term follow-up data in reported triplet series are insufficient to determine whether first-trimester reduction procedures are truly beneficial.

Technical considerations

In our opinion, the best time to perform first-trimester transabdominal reduction procedures is between the 11th and 12th weeks of gestation. Although it is feasible to carry out the procedure earlier, it is technically more difficult. The reverse is probably the case when the transvaginal approach is utilized, because the uterus rises out of the pelvis as pregnancy progresses. We also prefer to wait until the end of the first trimester, because it allows more time for spontaneous losses to occur. A number of our patients with grand multifetal pregnancies spontaneously lost one or more fetuses after cardiac activity had been demonstrated. We see no advantage in delaying the procedure beyond the 12th week of gestation, however, because if all fetuses are alive and are of appropriate size at that time, spontaneous losses are unlikely in the next few weeks. Moreover, the later in pregnancy the termination is performed, the more probable it is that fetal resorption will be incomplete. This, in turn, may increase the rare chance that maternal disseminated intravascular coagulation will develop.

At the Mount Sinai Medical Center in New York, reduction procedures are performed by transabdominal intrathoracic injection of potassium chloride. Other authors have advocated a transvaginal approach. In 1989, Itskovitz et al.[24] reported two quadruplet pregnancies successfully reduced to twins by transvaginal ultrasonography-guided aspiration of the gestational sacs. This procedure is similar to transvaginal oocyte retrieval, and is generally performed at an earlier gestational age than when the transabdominal approach is used. Also in 1989, Shalev et al.[25] reported 20 reductions of multifetal pregnancies, half performed transvaginally, and half by the transabdominal route. Four (40%) patients who underwent transabdominal procedures lost the entire pregnancy, vs. one (10%) in the transvaginal group. Although these authors proposed that transvaginal fetal reductions may offer better outcomes, larger series clearly are necessary before this position can be substantiated. Presently, it is not clear that one approach is better than the other.

Most of the multiple gestations conceived through ovulation induction are di- or multi-

Table 3 Triplets: comparison between published data and triplet pregnancies that underwent pregnancy reduction at Mt Sinai Hospital, New York, prior to November 1991

	Total	Gestational age at delivery			
		Mean (weeks)	< 37 weeks (%)	< 32 weeks (%)	< 28 weeks (%)
Natural history	442	33	88	29	10
Current series	81	36.1	41	5	none

zygotic. In spite of this, monozygotic pairs do occur. Prior to the contemplated reduction, the membranes separating the sac of each fetus should be carefully evaluated using ultrasound. If a dividing membrane is not seen, or if it is extremely thin, it is reasonable to presume that these fetuses are very likely to be monochorionic. If this situation is encountered, *both* fetuses should be either terminated or left alone, because of the high probability of vascular connections existing between the placentas of monochorionic fetuses. If not, the selective termination of one twin may cause death or severe damage to the co-twin. Although this complication has not been reported in first-trimester reduction procedures, it is well documented after the spontaneous death of one monochorionic twin[26] or second-trimester selective terminations of monochorionic discordant twins[18].

The primary criterion for selecting a fetus for termination by the transabdominal approach is its proximity to the maternal abdominal wall. In our opinion, the fetus in the sac immediately adjacent to the internal os should generally not be terminated. It is possible that devitalization of the membranes in the leading sac may cause their rupture which in turn could set the stage for an ascending uterine infection. Having said this, if one of the fetuses has an obvious abnormality or a significantly smaller crown–rump length than its siblings, that fetus should be selected for termination, even if it is in the lowest sac.

Prenatal care after reduction procedures

Patients who undergo reductions of multifetal pregnancies to twins should be treated as if they had conceived two fetuses, with two exceptions. First, after a reduction procedure the maternal serum alpha-fetoprotein (MSAFP) will always be abnormally elevated, sometimes extremely so[27]. This is due to the presence of the dead fetus(es) and not to fetal or placental disorders. If these patients were not going to have invasive diagnostic studies performed for other indications (such as maternal age), amniocentesis is not indicated solely on the basis of the elevated MSAFP value. However, since these fetuses can also have the type of anomalies that are associated with elevated MSAFP levels, a thorough ultrasound examination must be performed at an appropriate fetal age to rule out morphological abnormalities (see Chapter 9).

Second, because some of our patients experienced pregnancy losses many weeks after the procedure and presented with uterine contractions which they were unable to perceive, we currently recommend outpatient contraction monitoring beginning at approximately 20 weeks' gestation in an attempt to provide earlier awareness of premature labor, intended to prevent these losses.

Conclusion

Grand multifetal pregnancies are at significant risk of preterm delivery. Although perinatal mortality rates have decreased considerably in recent years, preterm delivery rates have not declined in a similar fashion, either for singleton or multiple pregnancies. Our data suggest that first-trimester reduction lessens the incidence of preterm deliveries in all pregnancies with three or more fetuses. It is reasonable to assume that this procedure improves the outcome of quadruplets or pregnancies of higher order. The benefits of reducing triplets to twins are less clear, because the perinatal mortality for these pregnancies is low and sufficient long-term morbidity data are not yet available for meaningful numbers of triplet pregnancies. Nevertheless, we believe that multifetal pregnancy reduction offers a reasonable alternative to couples whose only choices in the past were limited to accepting the risk of extreme prematurity or terminating the entire pregnancy.

References

1. Schenker, J.G., Yarkoni, S. and Granat, M. (1981). Multiple pregnancies following induction of ovulation. *Fertil. Steril.*, **35**, 105
2. Caspi, E., Ronen, J. and Schreyer, P. (1976). The outcome of pregnancy after gonadotrophin therapy. *Br. J. Obstet. Gynaecol.*, **83**, 967
3. Navot, D., Bergh, P.A., Drews, M. et al. (1991). The role of ultrasound in ovulation induction. In Grunfeld, L. (ed.), *Infertility and Reproductive Medicine. Clin. N. Am.*, **2**, 741
4. Australian In Vitro Fertilization Collaborative Group (1988). In-vitro fertilization pregnancies in Australia and New Zealand, 1979–1985. *Med. J. Aust.*, **148**, 429
5. Newman, R.B., Hamer, C. and Clinton Miller, M. (1989). Outpatient triplet management: a contemporary review. *Am. J. Obstet. Gynecol.*, **161**, 547
6. Lipitz, S., Recihman, B., Paret, G. et al. (1989). The improving outcome of triplet pregnancies. *Am. J. Obstet. Gynecol.*, **161**, 1279
7. Gonen, R., Heyman, E., Asztalos, E.V. et al. (1990). The outcome of triplet, quadruplet and quintuplet pregnancies managed in a perinatal unit: obstetric, neonatal and followup data. *Am. J. Obstet. Gynecol.*, **162**, 454
8. Itzkowic, D. (1979). A survey of 59 triplet pregnancies. *Br. J. Obstet. Gynaecol.*, **86**, 22
9. Syrop, C.H. and Varner, M.W. (1985). Triplet gestations: maternal and neonatal implications. *Acta Genet. Med. Gemellol.*, **34**, 81
10. Holcberg, G., Biale, Y., Lewenthal, H. et al. (1982). Outcome of pregnancy in 31 triplet gestations. *Obstet. Gynecol.*, **59**, 472
11. Collins, M.S. and Bleyl, J.A. (1990). Seventy-one quadruplet pregnancies: management and outcome. *Am. J. Obstet. Gynecol.*, **162**, 1384
12. Lipitz, S., Frenkel, Y., Watts, C. et al. (1990). High-order multifetal gestation – management and outcome. *Obstet. Gynecol.*, **65**, 215
13. Vervliet, J., De Cleyn, K.I., Renier, M. et al. (1989). Management and outcome of 21 triplet and quadruplet pregnancies. *Eur. J. Obstet. Gynecol. Biol. Reprod.*, **33**, 61
14. Aberg, A., Miterian, F., Cantz, M. et al. (1978). Cardiac puncture of fetus with Hurler's disease avoiding abortion of unaffected co-twin. *Lancet*, **2**, 990
15. Beck, L., Terinde, R. and Dolff, M. (1980). Zwillingsschwangerschaft mit freier Trisomie 21 eines Kindes: Sectio parva mit Entfernung des Kranken und Spatere gebert des gesunden Kindes. *Geburtsh. Fraunheilkd.*, **40**, 397
16. Rodeck, C. (1984). Fetoscopy in the management of twin pregnancies discordant for a severe abnormality. *Acta Genet. Med. Gemellol.*, **33**, 57
17. Chitkara, U., Berkowitz, R.L., Wilkins, I.A. et al. (1989). Selective midtrimester termination of the anomalous fetus in twin pregnancies. *Obstet. Gynecol.*, **73**, 690
18. Golbus, M.S., Cunningham, N., Goldberg, J.D. et al. (1988). Selective termination of multiple gestations. *Am. J. Med. Genet.*, **31**, 339
19. Dumez, Y. and Oury, J.F. (1986). Method for first trimester selective abortion in multiple pregnancy. *Contr. Gynecol. Obstet.*, **15**, 50
20. Kanhai, H.H.H., van Rijssel, E.J.H.C., Meerman, R.J. et al. (1986). Selective termination in quintuplet pregnancy during first trimester. *Lancet*, **1**, 1447
21. Berkowitz, R.L., Lynch, L., Chitkara, U. et al. (1988). Selective reduction of multifetal pregnancies in the first trimester. *N. Engl. J. Med.*, **318**, 1043
22. Lynch, L., Berkowitz, R.L., Chitkara, U. et al. (1990). First trimester transabdominal multifetal pregnancy reduction: a report of 85 cases. *Obstet. Gynecol.*, **75**, 735
23. Berkowitz, R.L., Lynch, L., Lapinski, R. and Berger, P. (1993). First trimester transabdominal multifetal pregnancy reduction: a report of two hundred completed cases. *Am. J. Obstet. Gynecol.*, **169**, 17
24. Itskovitz, J., Boldes, R., Thaler, I. et al. (1989). Transvaginal ultrasonography-guided aspirations of gestational sacs for selective abortion in multiple pregnancy. *Am. J. Obstet. Gynecol.*, **160**, 215
25. Shalev, J., Frenkel, Y., Goldenberg, M. et al. (1989). Selective reduction in multiple gestations: pregnancy outcome after transvaginal and transabdominal needle-guided procedures. *Fertil. Steril.*, **52**, 416
26. D'Alton, M.E., Newton, E.R. and Cetrulo, C.L. (1984). Intrauterine fetal demise in multiple gestation. *Acta Genet. Med. Gemellol.*, **33**, 43
27. Lynch, L. and Berkowitz, R.L. (1993). Maternal serum α-fetoprotein and coagulation profiles after multifetal pregnancy reduction. *Am. J. Obstet. Gynecol.*, **169**, 987

Multifetal pregnancy reduction and selective second-trimester termination

M.I. Evans, N.B. Isada, P.G. Pryde and J.C. Fletcher

Introduction

In Chapter 25, Drs Lynch and Berkowitz have described the natural history of grand multifetal pregnancy and the effect of fetal reduction on the clinical outcome of multiple pregnancies. Their discussion was based on the initial experience at the Mount Sinai Hospital and Medical Center in New York City. Their group, as well as ours, is among a small number of clinicians throughout the world who have published their experience with the management of iatrogenic multifetal pregnancies. Without doubt, the technique of multifetal pregnancy reduction (MFPR) has reduced the morbidity and mortality associated with quadruplet and higher-order gestations and, arguably, that of triplets[1-6]. This chapter reviews the worldwide experience in MFPR and discusses selective termination for cause in the second trimester, because these procedures are used for different reasons.

Elective multifetal pregnancy reduction

Recently, several groups of investigators pooled their results into a collaborative effort that documents a total of 1074 MFPR procedures[7]. The salient feature of this report is that MFPR can be performed by experienced clinicians in essentially 100% of cases in which the procedure is deemed appropriate. Fetal losses within 1 week occurred in about 3.5% of cases, were 4.5% at 2 weeks, and 6% at 4 weeks, respectively. Overall, the loss rate is 13% by 24 weeks of gestation. However, these rates are comparable with the spontaneous loss rate of twins and higher-order multiple pregnancies, especially among those pregnancies diagnosed early in gestation. In this report, the loss rates were categorized according to the number of fetuses at the start of the procedure and the number that remained after the procedure. Procedures that terminated with two fetuses (twins) had better outcomes than those reduced either to three fetuses (triplets) or singletons (Table 1).

The distribution of patients in the collaborative study who delivered a potentially viable child(ren) is as follows: very premature births (25–28 weeks) were observed in approximately 5.5% of patients; 10% delivered between 29 and 32 weeks, 33% between 33 and 36 weeks, and 50% delivered at at least 37 weeks or more (Figure 1). Further analysis shows that gestational age in this cohort correlates directly with the original 'starting number' of the pregnancy, Stated another way, even if MFPR is performed successfully, it is not without problems. More specifically, preterm delivery is not totally eliminated and the higher the original number of fetuses, the shorter the gestation duration (Table 2). This observation suggests that crowding alone may not be the sole reason that preterm delivery is so common in multiple pregnancies. Despite this, these data argue quite convincingly that, in experienced hands, MFPR is a safe, reliable procedure that reduces the infant mortality rate associated

Table 1 Loss of pregnancy ≤ 24 weeks by finishing number

Finishing number	Starting number				Totals
	2	3	4	5+	
Singletons					
Losses	4	9	4	2	19
Total	37	44	11	3	95
Percentage	10.8	26.5	36.1	66.7	20.0
Twins					
Losses		16	36	24	76
Total		305	313	94	712
Percentage		5.2	11.5	25.5	10.7
Triplets					
Losses			2	7	9
Total			19	19	38
Percentage			10.5	36.8	23.7

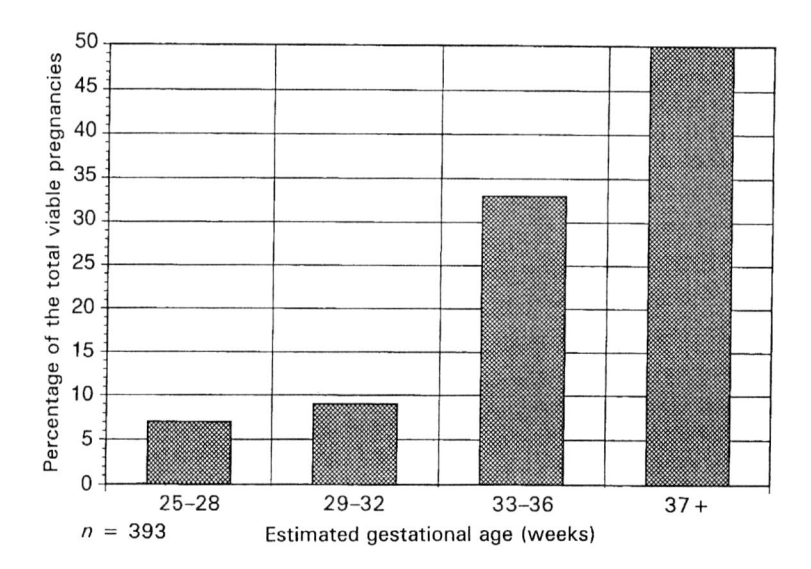

Figure 1 Gestational age at delivery following multifetal pregnancy reduction

with iatrogenic or spontaneous multiple pregnancies.

Ethical considerations of MFPR

Our writings on the subject of fetal reduction have evolved over the past 5 years after we published the first series of such cases[2–4]. At that time, we argued that, principally because of risks to the surviving fetuses, the procedure should never be considered frivolously and should only be performed for medical indications[2]. However, as we began to appreciate the relative safety of the procedure, our thinking evolved to allow greater patient autonomy and choice in the decision-making process. At

Table 2 Gestational age at delivery by starting number

Starting number	Gestational age (weeks)				Mean gestational age (weeks)
	25–28	29–32	33–36	37+	
5+	8	4	18	25	34.7
4	12	19	64	69	35.3
3	7	13	55	84	36.1
2	1	1	3	10	37.3
All	28	37	140	188	35.3

χ^2 = NS

present, considerable differences of opinion exist, based on medical data as well as ethical positions, about the appropriateness of MFPR in different situations. Some physicians, such as Professor Manfred Hansmann of Bonn, Germany (personal communication) propose that there is no justification for ever reducing a pregnancy to less than three fetuses. At the same time, others believe that, because the safety of the procedure is now reasonably known, no restrictions need be placed upon its use. Specifically, some believe that reducing triplets to a singleton is no different from eliminating a single fetus when that is deemed necessary or desirable. However, our collaborative experience shows that, whereas the gestational age at delivery of MFPR singletons is greater than MFPR twins, the loss rate of pregnancies reduced to singletons is greater than twins[6,7]. These data are confounded, unfortunately, by some degree of selection bias. Many of the centers collaborating only perform a reduction to a singleton in patients at high risk with twins who may inherently have had a greater risk for loss. Such a gradual shift of philosophy is based upon increasing comfort with the procedure, and, most importantly, the actuarial data showing that the real risks of MFPR lie in pregnancy loss, not in damaged survivors.

An issue presently being discussed is the reality that twins deliver on average a month prematurely and have a 5% incidence of long-term adverse sequelae compared to a 2–3% chance for a singleton pregnancy. It is, therefore, being argued that such a difference alone might be sufficient to make fetal reduction to a singleton ethically appropriate in selected circumstances. In our opinion, intelligent and well-meaning people can look at the same facts and reach entirely opposite conclusions in a pluralistic society. Thus, we believe that selective termination of a high-order multiple pregnancy to a singleton can be justified on the grounds of a more favorable fetal outcome, particularly if there are mediating circumstances that would make a twin pregnancy difficult for the mother to carry. In contrast, we do not believe that such a decision should be based on convenience or sex preference. We also believe that, in the majority of instances, a reduction of a high-order pregnancy to twins is appropriate, and strongly argue against the routine reduction of twins to singletons. We do not believe that the difference in outcome between twin and singleton pregnancies in this country justifies the utilization of this invasive procedure in an effort to improve the favorable outcome by reduction of uncomplicated twin pregnancies to singletons.

Whereas some individuals do not believe that a damaged survivor is worse than a loss, this concept is held by many practitioners of MFPR, and in our experience, most of our patients. Nevertheless, this difference of opinion reinforces our position that MFPR is a medical procedure that should not be used frivolously. Because we feel deeply about this issue, we argue against those who prescribe aggressive endocrine treatments for ovulation induction and then, when faced with iatrogenic high-order multiples, adopt the philosophy that MFPR is just another aspect of fertility treatment with little thought to the ethical consequences of such an approach[8,9].

Selective termination in the second trimester

Treatment of an 'abnormal' twin

In contrast to the previous discussion of too many, albeit presumably normal, fetuses is the more common problem of a twin pregnancy in which one fetus is abnormal. In the not too distant past the only rational approach involved keeping or terminating both fetuses. However, in 1978, Aberg *et al.* published the first report of a selective termination procedure performed on a fetus affected with Hurler's syndrome. This operation was followed by the delivery of a healthy, unaffected co-twin at term[10]. In 1981, Kerenyi and Chitkara reported selective birth in a twin pregnancy discordant for Down's syndrome[11]. These authors remarked that the mother had threatened to abort both fetuses unless the novel technique of selective termination of the affected fetus was attempted.

During the 1980s several case series appeared, adding substantially to the limited experience. In two of these, Rodeck *et al.* published six cases of selective termination in the second trimester[12,13]. Five of the six cases resulted in the subsequent live birth of a normal twin. In the sixth case, however, the delivery occurred at 29 weeks, and the fetus died at 1 month of age from necrotizing enterocolitis. In 1988, Golbus *et al.* reported on selective termination procedures performed in 22 patients. Nineteen of these operations were performed for a fetal abnormality discovered in a twin pregnancy[14]. Outcomes were satisfactory in all but one of the 17 dichorionic pregnancies. In contrast, four out of the five monochorionic pregnancies were complicated by loss of the normal fetus after the selective termination. Six of 18 pregnancies that continued were complicated by preterm labor and delivery.

Shortly thereafter, Chitkara *et al.* reported on 17 discordant anomalous twin pairs managed by selective termination[15]. Outcomes were excellent in 13 of the cases; the other four were complicated by losses of the normal fetus. We have recently published a collaborative series of 188 cases from nine centers which reveals viable pregnancies in 88% of cases and a distinct correlation between gestational age at both procedure and losses (< 24 weeks) and severe prematurity (25–28 weeks). These data emphasize the desirability of early diagnosis in twin pregnancies[16,17].

The technique of KCl injection

A variety of techniques has been reported in the literature with variable success. The collaborative data show that KCl is the most efficacious technique with the lowest complication rate[15]. Because we have extensively commented on other techniques[16], we will focus on the use of KCl in the paragraphs that follow.

All percutaneous techniques require accurate placement of a needle into the fetal cardiac chambers. In contrast to first-trimester procedures, in which the needle may be placed anywhere within the thoracic cavity with no effect on the success rate, in second-trimester procedures, true intracardiac placement of the needle is critical. We generally prefer a 20-gauge needle positioned carefully above the fetal thorax. Using ultrasound, the needle position is confirmed in both the longitudinal and the transverse planes. The needle is then inserted into either cardiac ventricle with a sharp thrust. Since even minor movements of the needle are sufficient to displace it, some authors suggest having an assistant remove the stylet and attach a 3-ml syringe to the operating needle to confirm fetal blood flow. The combination of ultrasound verification demonstrating intracardiac placement and a low resistance blood return in the operating needle are considered the criteria that guarantee vascular access and the subsequent success of the procedure. A fetal blood sample can then be obtained for determination (or confirmation) of fetal karyotype if indicated. Once the clinician has determined that the needle is accurately and faultlessly placed, a separate and clearly labelled syringe containing 5 ml of potassium chloride (2 mEq/ml solution) is attached to the operating needle and 2 ml of KCl is injected briskly into the fetal heart. A decrease in fetal heart rate occurs almost immediately, with complete cessation typically noted within 1 min. The requisite amount of KCl required to achieve cardiac standstill varies from as little as 1 ml to as much as 6 ml, depending upon fetal age and needle positioning. The needle should not be removed until the operator is absolutely convinced that cardiac activity has ceased. One published report describes re-initiation of fetal cardiac activity several minutes after the intracardiac infusion of an insufficient dose of KCl[18]. We recently have suggested that the KCl can be injected via the umbilical cord[19]. This technique has the added benefit of providing experience in cordocentesis.

Regardless of whether injection of KCl or another technique is used, it is absolutely crucial to make certain that one is injecting the correct fetus. In *multifetal pregnancy reduction*, in which the absolute number of fetuses *per se* is the indication for the procedure, it probably does not matter from a clinical point of view which fetus(es) are affected. In contrast, because a *selective termination* procedure is performed specifically on the basis of a fetal abnormality in one twin, *definitive identification* of the affected fetus becomes absolutely essential. This can be very easy in cases in which the affected twin has obvious structural defects or in which a chromosome abnormality is discovered in one member of a twinship discordant for sex. On the other hand, specific fetal verification becomes much more difficult if the abnormality involves a subtle anatomical defect or chromosomal aneuploidy in twins concordant for sex. Such issues point to the importance of documentation of fetal orientation and position when prenatal diagnostic procedures are first undertaken.

Special concerns

Preterm delivery, even many weeks following an uncomplicated procedure, is a consistent problem in the reported series of second-trimester selective termination procedures. Anecdotally, this observation appears to occur more frequently in second-trimester selective termination procedures than with first-trimester high-order multiple pregnancy reductions. One can speculate that the cause of such events is related to the amount of residual fetal tissue left *in utero* (intuitively, a single 18-week fetus weighs more than several 10-week fetuses added together). In some places where a rigid gestational age limit on abortions for anomalies is not mandated by law, selective termination of an abnormal twin is delayed until 30 weeks, so that iatrogenic extremely early preterm delivery will not occur. What is not known, however, is whether the likelihood of a 25–28-week delivery is greater with twins both of whom are alive or with twins in which one is normal and alive and the other is abnormal and dead.

As changes in medical practice propel first–trimester prenatal diagnosis toward a standard of care for many patients, centers involved either in selective termination or in multifetal pregnancy reduction no doubt will diagnose the presence of fetal anomalies at earlier gestational ages, so that these operations can be undertaken earlier in pregnancy. Such a shift is likely to produce far better outcomes, with decreased incidences of preterm delivery and neonatal morbidity and mortality. Unfortunately, as long as there are patients who do not receive prenatal care in the first trimester or whose ultrasound diagnoses of fetal abnormalities are not made until the late second trimester, the necessity for second-trimester procedures will persist, and the difficulties associated with them will remain.

We are in agreement with Golbus *et al.*[14], that one must use extreme caution when considering a selective termination on monochorionic twins, or in the extremely rare case of shared circulation in non-monochorionic twins. Data from a number of centers suggest that the risks of the normal twin dying are considerably increased under these circumstances, regardless of the technique used to perform the selective termination. Several explanations have been proposed regarding the mechanism of death in the co-twin. One possibility is a twin-to-twin transfusion-like phenomenon in which the healthy twin essentially exsanguinates following the death and decreased vascular resistance in the treated twin. Another potential mechanism involves the evolution of fetal coagulopathy due to the release of tissue thromboplastin and similar procoagulants from the decomposing dead twin into the living twin's circulatory system. Finally, there is evidence to suggest thromboembolic phenomena within the circulatory systems of the co-twins. Anderson *et al.*[20] and Melnik[21] have reported four cases of neurological damage of an embolic nature in surviving monochorionic twins of both naturally dying and selectively terminated fetuses. Clearly, one must proceed with extreme caution before declaring that there are no vascular communications between twin fetuses when considering a selective termination by any technique. It is under such circumstances, if ever, that hysterotomy or one of the proposed cord obstructing or vascular connection ablation procedures might be considered on an investigational basis.

Another concern is that of potential risks to the parturient. The first is that of post-procedural amnionitis resulting in pregnancy loss and potential life-threatening maternal infection. Although amnionitis has been reported after these operations and has been implicated in pregnancy losses, there have been no reported cases of ensuing life-threatening maternal infections. This is not surprising, given the extremely low rate of severe maternal infection after other pregnancy-related, invasive diagnostic and/or therapeutic procedures. An additional theoretical risk to the patient is that of evolving coagulopathy secondary to the phenomenon of the continuation of a pregnancy with a dead second-trimester fetus *in utero* (the 'fetal death syndrome'). Although this complication has not been observed in reported cases of second-trimester selective termination, there are insufficient data upon which to draw a definitive conclusion that it could never occur. In the collaborative project there was none[21]. In a comprehensive review of pregnancies complicated by spontaneous demise of one twin, only three cases of antenatal maternal disseminated intervascular coagulation were noted[22]. Despite this, it is necessary to closely monitor patients for the evolution of coagulopathy. We have recently shown that the umbilical cord of an acardiac fetus can be ligated endoscopically which should allow selective termination while minimizing the vascular risks[23,24].

Ethical considerations of selective termination in the second trimester

To many people, any deliberate termination of a fetus is inherently wrong. When selective termination is compared to multifetal pregnancy reduction, the ethical arguments which have been detailed elsewhere contain many parallels[24]. At the same time, there are important ethical differences between selective termination/multifetal pregnancy reduction and 'voluntary interruption of pregnancy' *per se*. The principal difference is that a woman has a 'voluntary interruption of pregnancy' because she has decided for whatever reason that she does not wish to have the child. In contrast, a woman undergoes elective multifetal pregnancy reduction or selective termination precisely because she *does* wish to have a healthy child in circumstances that make having that child very difficult, if not impossible, either because of the number of fetuses or because a fetal abnormality has been detected in one of the twins or a higher-order group. In the past, the only options were to keep all fetuses and commit oneself to the care of potentially severely handicapped infant(s), or to abort all fetuses and terminate the otherwise healthy, and wanted fetus(es). However, selective termination allows couples in this very serious situation to attempt to have a presumably healthy infant while being spared the emotional and financial trauma that accompanies the birth of a severely handicapped infant. Indeed, the Ethics Committee of the American College of Obstetricians and Gynecologists has endorsed the ethical probity of offering selective termination under such circumstances[25]. In a society that legally permits abortion, there is no ethical justification for attempting to impose legal sanctions against selective termination as has been proposed but not enacted in a number of jurisdictions in the United States.

A potential for abuse certainly exists if sex selection is the indication for the operation. Such instances have been described anecdotally, but the absolute incidence is probably extremely low[26]. In our opinion, sex selection should not be condoned, because it crosses the line between treatment for genetic disease and eugenics. However, beyond the indication of sex selection (or ethically equivalent selection criteria), we believe that selective termination for a significant fetal abnormality is justifiable in a pluralistic society in which abortion can be considered an acceptable option under a variety of circumstances. We also believe that all couples should be allowed to make this difficult choice for themselves based on known clinical facts, and that different personal perceptions of risk and burden cannot be ethically legislated or imposed. Given that a fundamental tenet of genetic counselling is that it be conducted in a non-directive manner, the imposition of one's personal view of what are acceptable versus unacceptable abnormalities is neither ethical nor justifiable.

As with all procedures, as experience increases and the degree of safety becomes more appreciated, the unequivocal indications will likely become more clearly delineated. In concert with our opinion about multifetal pregnancy reduction, we do not believe that selective termination should ever be considered a frivolous procedure performed merely for patient convenience.

References

1. Bronsteen, R.A. and Evans, M.I. (1989). Multiple gestation. In Evans, M.I., Fletcher, J.C., Dixler, A.O. and Schulman, J.D. (eds.) *Fetal Diagnosis and Therapy: Science, Ethics, and the Law*, pp. 242–66. (Philadelphia: Lippincott Harper)
2. Evans, M.I., Fletcher, J.C., Zador, I.E. *et al.* (1988). Selective first trimester termination in octuplet and quadruplet pregnancies: clinical and ethical issues. *Obstet. Gynecol.*, **71**, 289
3. Berkowitz, R.L., Lynch, L., Chitkara, U. *et al.* (1988). Selective reduction of multifetal pregnancies in the first trimester. *N. Engl. J. Med.*, **318**, 1043
4. Evans, M.I., May, M., Drugan, A. *et al.* (1990). Selective termination: clinical experience and residual risks. *Am. J. Obstet. Gynecol.*, **162**, 1568
5. Wapner, R.J., Davis, G.H., Johnson, A. *et al.* (1990). Selective reduction of multifetal pregnancies. *Lancet*, **335**, 90
6. Evans, M.I., Dommergues, M., Wapner, R.J. *et al.* (1993). Efficacy of transabdominal multifetal pregnancy reduction: collaborative experience among the world's largest centers. *Obstet. Gynecol.*, **82**, 61–7
7. Evans, M.I., Dommergues, M., Timor-Tritsch, I. *et al.* (1994). Transabdominal and transcervical multifetal pregnancy reduction: international collaborative experience of more than 1000 cases. *Am. J. Obstet. Gynecol.*, **170**, 902–9
8. Evans, M.I. and Fletcher, J.C. (1992). Multifetal pregnancy reduction and selective termination. In Reece, E.A. (ed.) *High Risk Pregnancy Management Options*, pp. 136–41. (Philadelphia: Lippincott)
9. Ayers, J.W.T., Peterson, E.P., Knight, L. *et al.* (1991). Incorporation of transvaginal embryo reduction with an aggressive IVF/GIFT/ZIFT program to optimize pregnancy outcome. *Fertil. Steril.*, **36** (Suppl.), S173
10. Aberg, A., Miterian, F., Cantz, M. *et al.* (1978). Cardiac puncture of fetus with Hurler's disease avoiding abortion of unaffected co-twin. *Lancet*, **2**, 990
11. Kerenyi, T. and Chitkara, U. (1981). Selective birth in twin pregnancy with discordancy for Down's syndrome. *N. Engl. J. Med.*, **304**, 1525
12. Rodeck, C., Mibashan, R., Abramowitz, J. *et al.* (1982). Selective feticide of the affected twin by fetoscopic air embolization. *Prenat. Diag.*, **2**, 189
13. Rodeck, C. (1984). Fetoscopy in the management of twin pregnancies discordant for a severe abnormality. *Acta Genet. Med. Gemellol.*, **33**, 57

14. Golbus, M.S., Cunningham, N., Goldberg, J.D. et al. (1988). Selective termination of multiple gestations. *Am. J. Med. Genet.*, **31**, 339
15. Chitkara, U., Berkowitz, R.L., Wilkens, I.A. et al. (1989). Selective second-trimester termination of the anomalous fetus in twin pregnancies. *Obstet. Gynecol.*, **73**, 690
16. Evans, M.I., Goldberg, J.D., Dommergues, M. et al. (1994). Efficacy of second trimester selective termination for fetal abnormalities: international collaborative experience among the world's largest centers. *Am. J. Obstet. Gynecol.*, **171**, 90–4
17. Evans, M.I., Pryde, P.G., Johnson, M.P. et al. (1993). Management of multifetal pregnancies discordant for fetal anomalies. In Simpson, J.L. and Elias, S. (eds.) *Essentials of Prenatal Diagnosis,* pp. 331–45.(London: Churchill Livingstone)
18. Still, K., Kolatat, T., Corbett T. et al. (1989). Early third trimester selective feticide of a compromising twin. *Fetal Ther.*, **4**, 83
19. Isada, N.B., Pryde, P.G., Johnson, M.P. et al. (1992). Fetal intracardiac potassium chloride injection to avoid the hopeless resuscitation of an abnormal abortus: I. Clinical issues. *Obstet. Gynecol.*, **80**, 296
20. Anderson, R.L., Golbus, M.S., Curry, C.J.R. et al. (1990). Central nervous system damage and other anomalies in surviving fetus following second trimester antenatal death of co-twin. *Prenat. Diag.*, **10**, 513
21. Melnick, M. (1977). Brain damage in survivor after *in-utero* death of monozygous co-twin. *Lancet*, **2**, 1287
22. Lowery, M.F. and Stafford, J. (1988). Northern Region twin survey. *J. Obstet. Gynecol.*, **8**, 228–34
23. Quintero, R.A., Reich, H., Puder, K.S. et al. (1994). Umbilical cord ligation of an acardiac twin by fetoscopy at 15 weeks of gestation. *N. Engl. J. Med.*, **330**, 469–71
24. Evans, M.I., Fletcher, J.C. and Rodeck, C. (1989). Ethical problems in multiple gestations: selective termination. In Evans, M.I. Fletcher, J.C., Dixler, A.O.and Schulman, J.D. (eds.) *Fetal Diagnosis and Therapy: Science, Ethics, and the Law*, pp. 266–76. (Philadelphia: Lippincott Harper)
25. ACOG Ethics Statement (1990). Multifetal pregnancy reduction and selective fetal termination. The Committee on Ethics, American College of Obstetricians and Gynecologists, November
26. Evans, M.I., Drugan, A., Koppitch, F.C. et al. (1989). Genetic diagnosis in the first trimester: the norm for the 90's. *Am. J. Obstet. Gynecol.*, **160**, 1332

27
The twin–twin transfusion syndrome: vascular anatomy of monochorionic placentas and their clinical outcomes

G.A. Machin and K. Still

Introduction

Spontaneous multiple pregnancies are associated with an 8–10-fold increase in the risk of perinatal mortality and neonatal morbidity compared to singleton pregnancies. Although several factors contribute to these increased risks, the risks themselves are largely, but not entirely, confined to monozygotic (MZ) twins who are monochorionic (MC). Thus, studies of clinical outcomes in twin and higher-order multiple pregnancies depend heavily on an accurate diagnosis of zygosity and also of chorionicity (see Chapter 9).

The relative frequency of twinning by zygosity and chorionicity in North America and Europe, is shown in Table 1 and Figure 1[1–4]. Because these series originated from referral centers, they probably over-represent the frequency of MC twins. In a general Anglo-Saxon-derived population, MZ pairs probably account for 30% of twins; of these, only about two-thirds are MC. The remaining one-third are dichorionic (DC). All dizygotic (DZ) twins are DC. In terms of risk, MC twins (who are all MZ) are at highest risk for complications. Reported mortality rates in spontaneous twins by chorionicity are as shown in Table 2[1,5–9]. Birth weight by chorionicity is shown in Table 3[3].

Table 1 Chorionicity and amnionicity in 2029 twin pairs[1-4]

	n	%
Dichorionic	1515	74.7
Monochorionic/diamniotic	468	23.1
Monochorionic/monoamniotic	46	2.3
Total	2029	100

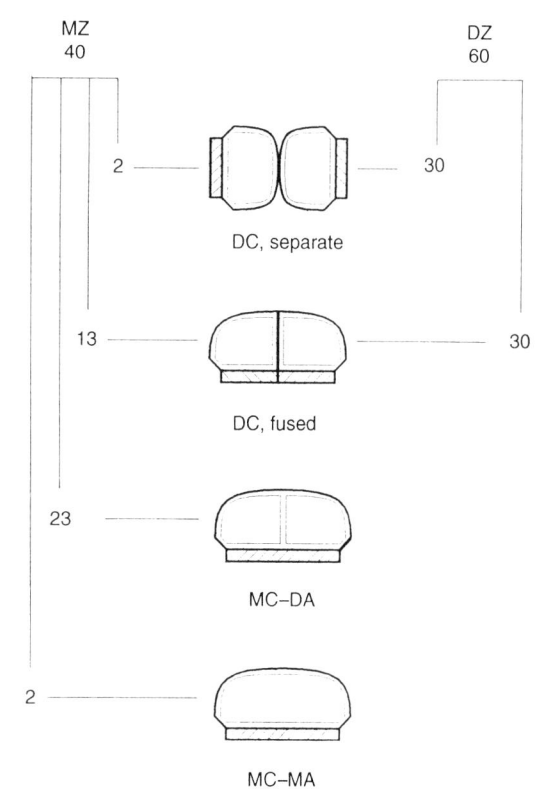

Figure 1 Frequency of zygosity and chorionicity in twins, based on four large series from tertiary centers[1-4]

Table 2 Perinatal mortality (/1000 births) by chorionicity and amnionicity[1,5–9]

Chorion, amnion status	Total twins	Stillborn	Neonatal death	Perinatal death No.	%
DC,DA separate placentas	280	10	29	39	13.9
DC,DA fused placenta	412	11	23	34	8.3
MC,DA	198	15	30	45	22.7
MC,MA	20	4	5	9	45.0
Total	910	40	87	127	14.0

Table 3 Birth weight at delivery by chorionicity (MC, MA twins excluded)[3]

Chorion status	<1500 g No.	%	1501–2500 g No.	%	2501–3000 g No.	%	>3000 g No.	%	Total No.	%
DC,DA separate placentas	36	13	123	45	63	23	52	19	274	100
DC,DA fused placenta	40	10	212	52	105	26	53	13	410	100
MC,DA	42	22	93	49	44	23	11	6	190	100
Total	118	14	428	49	212	24	116	13	874	100

The large differences between outcomes in MC and DC twins are almost entirely related to the fact that the MC placenta is truly a single placenta perfused by two fetuses. The great majority of MC placentas have inter-fetal vascular anastomoses (IFVA) of various kinds (Table 4)[2,10–13]. *It is the particular anatomical arrangement of these vessels that largely determines the poorer outcomes of MC pregnancies, including various forms of twin–twin transfusion syndrome (TTTS).*

This chapter reviews the literature concerning the frequency of types of IFVA and clinical outcomes reported in MC twins. It also presents the results of a detailed study by the authors to correlate IFVA patterns with clinical outcomes in the MC twins at our institution in 1987–92. In particular, we present in detail the vascular anatomy that underlies acute prenatal TTTS.

Vascular anastomoses and perfusion in MC placentas

The details of placental vasculogenesis are not known with certitude in humans. The general pattern is that a peripheral vascular bed is formed in the branching villi. At the same time, the central vascular tree, including the umbilical vessels, is laid down in the embryo. These two systems eventually coalesce, giving rise to a variety of patterns of cord insertion and an equal variety of branching patterns of chorionic vessels. In the MC twin placenta, the chorionic parenchyma is truly single (i.e. not fused), and the connections of the peripheral villous vasculature to the two central fetal umbilical circulations are not precisely patterned. Presumably, the rapidity of the arrival and spread of fetal vessels into the chorionic plate determines two factors:

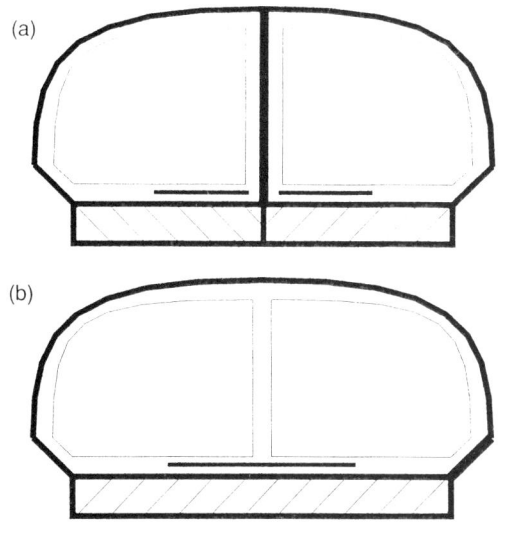

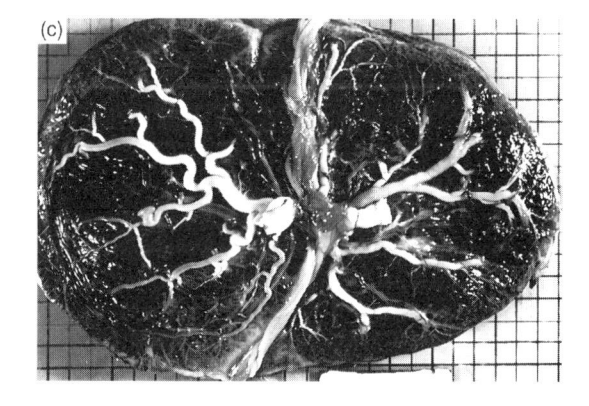

Figure 2 (a) Because of the presence of chorion (broad, solid black) in the septum, inter-fetal anastomoses do not occur in DC placentas. (b) The septum of MC placentas does not contain chorion; therefore, vascular zones are not delimited strictly, and anastomoses are common in MC placentas. (c) Fetal surface of fused DC placenta. By convention, in this and subsequent figures, twin A is on the left unless otherwise specified. The septum is equatorial, and was prenatally documented as DC. Arteries of twin A and vein of twin B were perfused; there were no anastomoses and parenchymal sharing was roughly equal. Gestation was 36 weeks. Twin A female, 1505 g, double outlet right ventricle prenatally diagnosed. Twin B female, 2330 g, normal clinical course. The twins were MZ by DNA restriction fragment length polymorhism (RFLP), but discordant for major congenital cardiovascular anomaly that was unrelated to flow phenomena of MC placenta (compare with case in Figure 7b), that may have accounted for growth discordance

(1) The anastomotic linkages of vessels in the chorionic plates and in the perfusion zones (cotyledons); and

(2) The 'sharing' of the parenchymal mass by the two fetal circulations, in terms of both arterial supplies and venous returns.

The developmental timing of these events, and, therefore, their relative extent, may not be equal for each of the co-twins. It is not presently known whether MZ twin pairs have approximately equal cell populations derived from the inner cell mass. If there should indeed be an unequal allocation of cells into the two fetuses, this process could account for differences in the sizes of vascular perfusion zones in the MC placenta.

The majority of MC twin placentas have IFVA: these are virtually always limited to MC placentas (Figure 2), and are present only very rarely in fused DC placentas (the twins usually being MZ). The frequency and types of IFVAs reported in the literature are analyzed in Table 4[2,10–13]. IFVAs are of three types, and any combination of the three may be seen in any MC placenta. In general, the patterns are simple. Only rarely does one detect multiple and complex IFVAs. The types and patterns of IFVA are illustrated in Figures 3–9. The three types of IFVA are:

(1) Arterio-arterial anastomoses (A–A) in the chorionic plate. These are frequent (Table 4).

(2) Veno-venous anastomoses (V–V) in the chorionic plate. These are rare (Table 4), but may be of considerable clinical significance[14].

(3) Arterio-venous anastomoses (A–V) are not present in the chorionic plate; they represent normal artery–capillary–vein flow in a perfusion zone (e.g. a cotyledon); however, the arterial inflow to the

Table 4 Frequencies of vascular anastomoses in MC placentas

Authors	Cases	A–A present		V–V present		A–V present		Placentas with one or more types of anastomosis	
		No.	%	No.	%	No.	%	No.	%
Benirschke[2]	60	36	60	8	13	29	48	51	85
Strong and Corney[10]	39	31	79	14	36	29	74	35	90
Galea et al.[11]	32	22	71	3	9	2	6	22	69
Arts and Lohman[12]	23	17	74	2	9	15	65	20	87
Sekiya and Hafez[13]	44	33	75	18	41	21	48	—	—
Total	198	139	70	45	23	96	48	128	83*

*Excluding reference 13

cotyledon is supplied by one fetus, while the venous return is to the other twin. *When this is the only anastomotic pattern present, uncompensated TTTS occurs.*

The most common pattern is a combination of A–A and A–V anastomosis (Figure 3a).

In addition to the patterns of IFVA, it is also necessary to consider the extent to which the placental parenchyma is equally or unequally perfused by the two fetal circulations. Because V–V anastomoses are uncommon, the two venous fields are often independent[15]; however, because A–A anastomoses are relatively common, the arterial systems of the two twins may frequently function as one unit. In addition, the extents of venous sharing of the placental parenchyma by the two fetal circulations are more likely to be unequal than are the extents of arterial sharing. Because the area of venous return determines the benefit derived by the fetus from placental perfusion, the twin with the larger venous share may experience better fetal growth than the other twin, quite independently of any considerations of TTTS. These two factors, i.e. the presence and type of IFVA and the degree of unequal venous sharing, should be considered together in the genesis of A–V anastomoses. It is probable that A–V anastomoses represent perfusion zones in which the chorionic arterial trees of the two twins are roughly equal, but the venous zone of the 'recipient' is larger than that of the 'donor' (Figure 3b). This anatomical difference allows the 'recipient' to receive venous blood in a zone that was arterially perfused by the 'donor'.

It is important to remember that the vascular patterns observed in MC placentas after birth do not necessarily accurately reflect the anatomy at all times in prenatal life. Changes in vascular status do occur in MC pregnancy, as reflected in well-documented cases of spontaneous resolution of TTTS[16,17]. (Editor: Emphasis added.) Almost certainly, the development of hydramnios in TTTS modifies the function, and, ultimately, the structure of IFVA.

The twin–twin transfusion syndrome (TTTS)

Acute prenatal TTTS (PreTTTS) is the result of *unidirectional* A–V anastomosis in the absence of superficial A–A or V–V anastomoses. It presents in the second trimester with growth discordance, 'stuck' oligohydramniotic donor and hydramniotic recipient[18–21]. Onset is usually sudden, often with spontaneous premature rupture of membranes (SPROM) and/or premature labor. One or both twins may be hydropic. Fetal mortality is near 100% without active management[22]. Growth discordance is usually present along with differences in cord blood hematocrits.

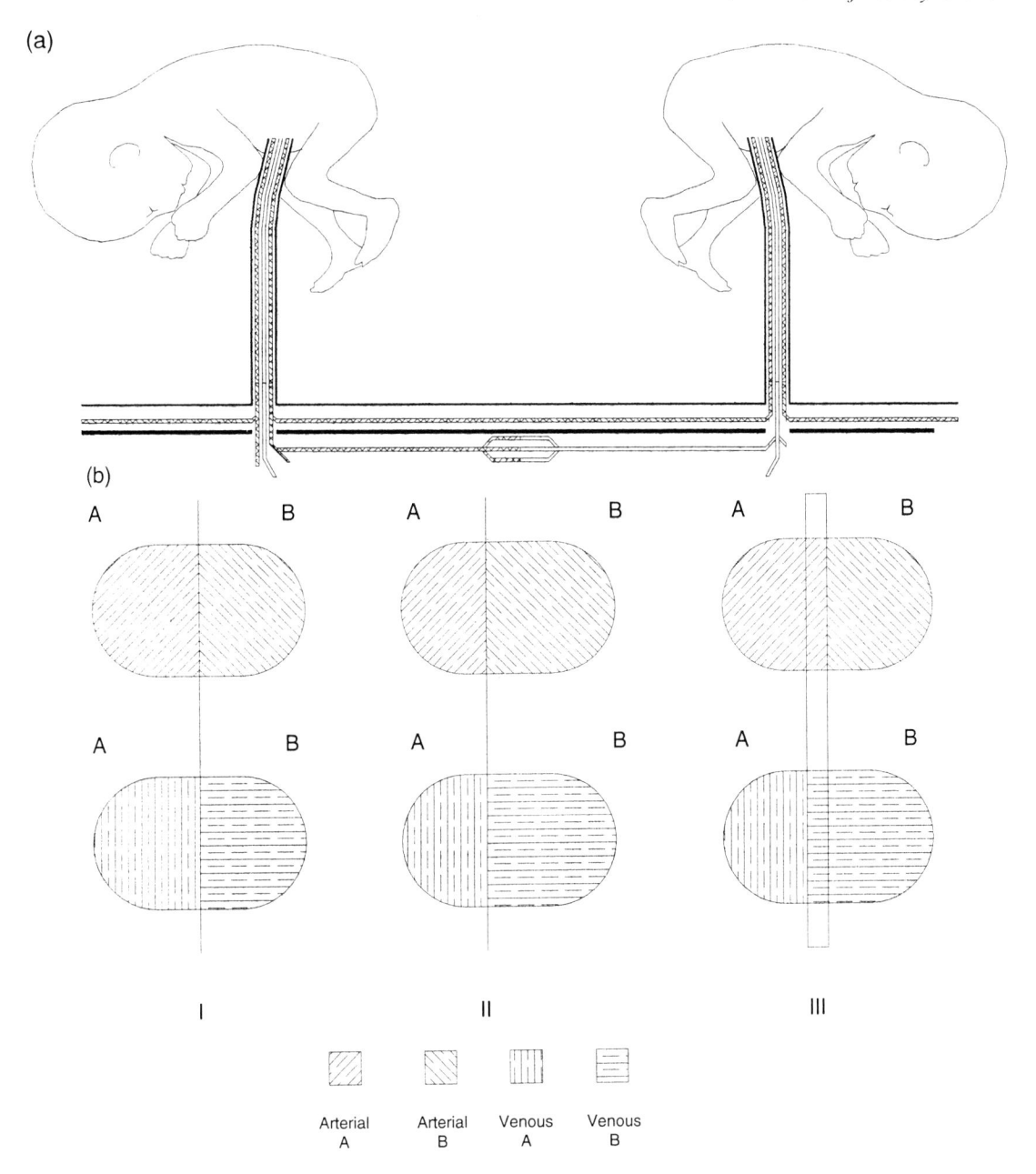

Figure 3 (a) Lateral sketch of MC twins and placenta; umbilical arteries cross-hatched, veins open, chorionic plate bold black. In the most common anastomotic pattern, there is A–A anastomosis superficial to the chorionic plate, with A–V in the chorionic parenchyma. (b) The arterial and venous zones of MC placentas develop separately, and may be equal or unequal in size. Because A–A anastomoses are so common, the arterial zones are usually considered to function as an equilibrated, 'syncytial' network; V–V are uncommon, so the venous zones usually function independently. On the left (I), the arterial zones are equal and correspond with the size of the venous zones. At the center (II), the arterial zones are unequal (A < B) and the venous zones are correspondingly unequal with the same bias as the arteries, i.e. A < B. This pattern may be associated with growth discordance. On the right (III), the arterial zones are equal, but A < B for venous return. An equatorial zone is also present in which the arterial supply is from A (donor), and the venous return is to B (recipient). In the absence of superficial anastomoses, TTTS will result

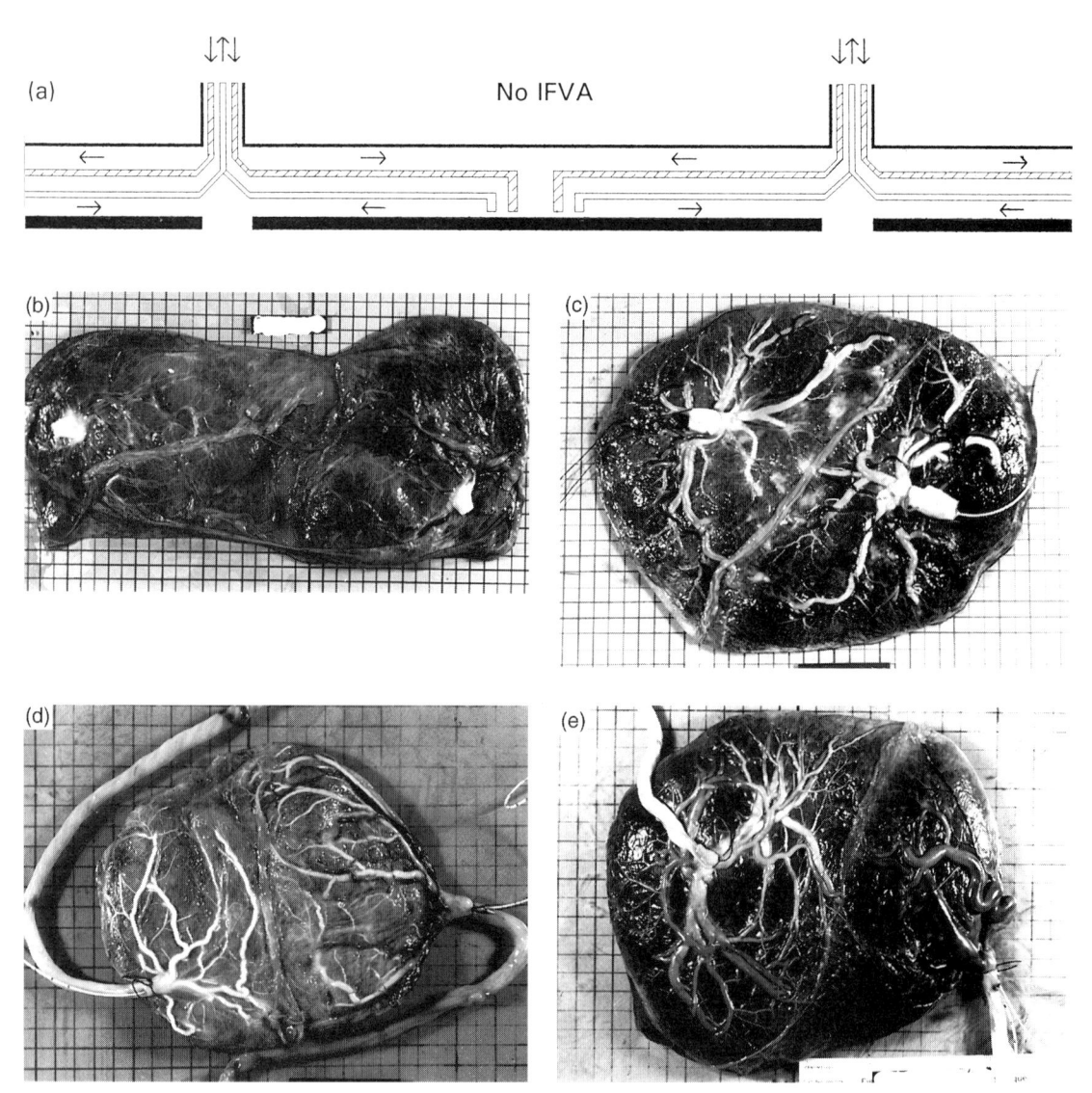

Figure 4 (a) Sketch of lateral view of MC placenta with no anastomoses. (b) This MC placenta had separate parenchymal disks and an MC septum. There were no anastomotic vessels in the chorion laeve between the two disks; the parenchymal sizes are roughly equal. Gestation is 33 weeks. Twin A female, 1750 g; twin B female, 1900 g. No complications. MZ status confirmed by DNA RFLP. (c) MC–DA placenta with no anastomoses, discordance or complications. The veins of both twins were perfused; the septum was left in place; equal parenchymal sharing. Gestation is 33 weeks. Twin A male, 2755 g; twin B male, 2795 g. MZ status confirmed by DNA RFLP. (d) MC–DA placenta with no anastomoses. Cervical incompetence with SPROM at 23 weeks. Chorionamnionitis of sac of twin A. The twins were liveborn, but were not resuscitated. Twin A female, 395 g; twin B female, 300 g. The arteries of twin A and vein of twin B were perfused, showing no anastomoses; parenchymal sharing was equal. Premature delivery and neonatal death of both MC twins caused by cervical incompetence; there was no TTTS. (e) MC–DA placenta with no anastomoses. Parenchymal sharing was unequal, A > B. The parenchyma of twin A showed extensive perivillous fibrin deposition, while the parenchyma of twin B was normal. Gestation was 35 weeks. Twin A female, 1755 g; twin B female, 1725 g. No complications; no growth discordance, and growth of twin A was probably retarded by placental parenchymal intervillous fibrin deposition despite unequal sharing. Venous sharing was *unequal*, but there is no birth weight discordance, so the placenta of twin A was probably less efficient

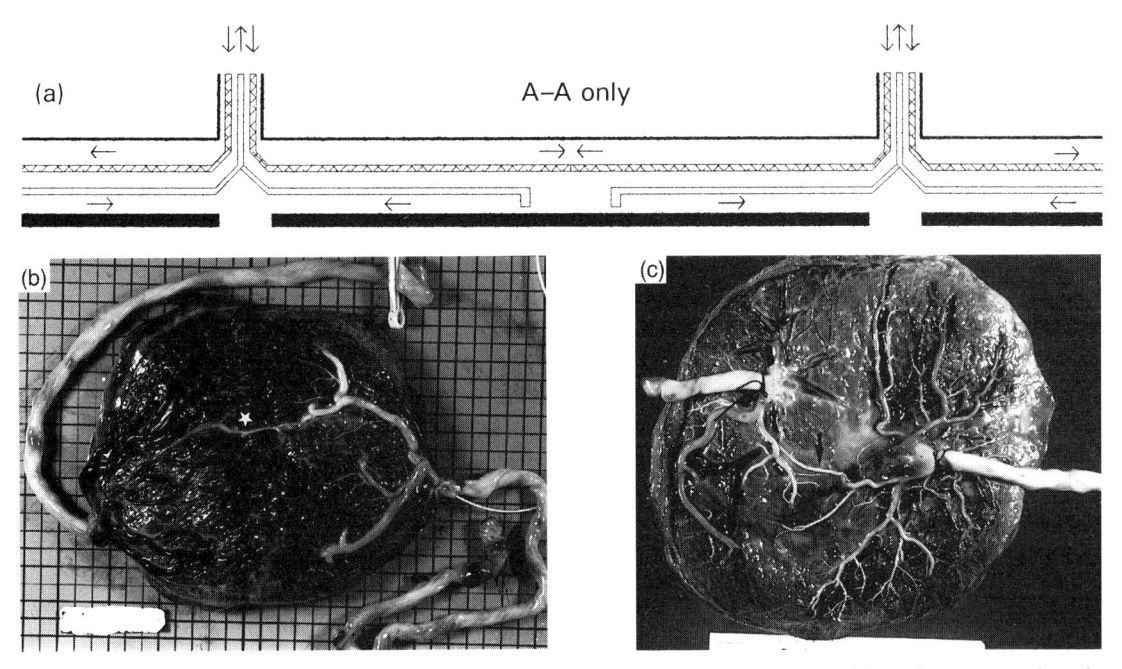

Figure 5 (a) Sketch of lateral view; A–A anastomosis only. (b) MC–DA placenta with A–A anastomosis only (asterisk). Artery of twin B was perfused. Gestation was 39 weeks. Twin A male, 2710 g; twin B male, 2985 g; no complications. (c) MC–DA placenta with A–A anastomosis only (arrow). Arteries of both twins were perfused. Gestation was 40 weeks. Twin A female, 2440 g; twin B female, 2715 g. No complications

The diagnosis of PreTTTS is readily made prenatally if all the criteria described above are present[23–27]. It is also obvious at birth, when low rates of survival are to be expected. At birth, the chronic 'recipient' twin usually has a high hematocrit, whereas the 'donor' is anemic. Classic PreTTTS is not the only consequence of IFVA, however. Three other syndromes are also important:

(1) Twin-reversed arterial perfusion (TRAP), or holoacardius acephalus, results from the presence of large, direct A–A and V–V anastomoses between the two cords (Figure 10)[28–32]. As the cardiac function of the acardiac fetus declines, its circulation is dominated by that of the 'pump' twin. Arterial flow in the acardiac cord is reversed, flowing from the placenta to the acardiac twin (Figure 10)[33–35]. Mortality and morbidity are high in the 'pump' twin[29,36].

(2) Acute perinatal twin transfusion (APeriTTS)[14,18,37] may occur if, after cord clamping of the first-born MC twin, the blood in the placental parenchyma drains back into the second twin during the delivery interval. This can occur in the presence or absence of superficial anastomoses, but is more likely to be severe when V–V anastomoses are present. In the case of PreTTTS, the chronic donor 'stuck' twin is less accessible and is likely to be born second, either by vaginal or Cesarean delivery. In the presence of superimposed acute PeriTTTS, the chronic donor may appear paradoxically plethoric (Figure 9h, i). Treatment of APeriTTTS may be required for donor and recipient.

(3) Complications may arise in the surviving MC twin if the co-twin dies *in utero*, the so-called 'twin-embolization syndrome'. In the event of fetal death of either donor or recipient twin with PreTTTS, the surviving twin is at risk for at least two possible reasons: (*continued on page 377*)

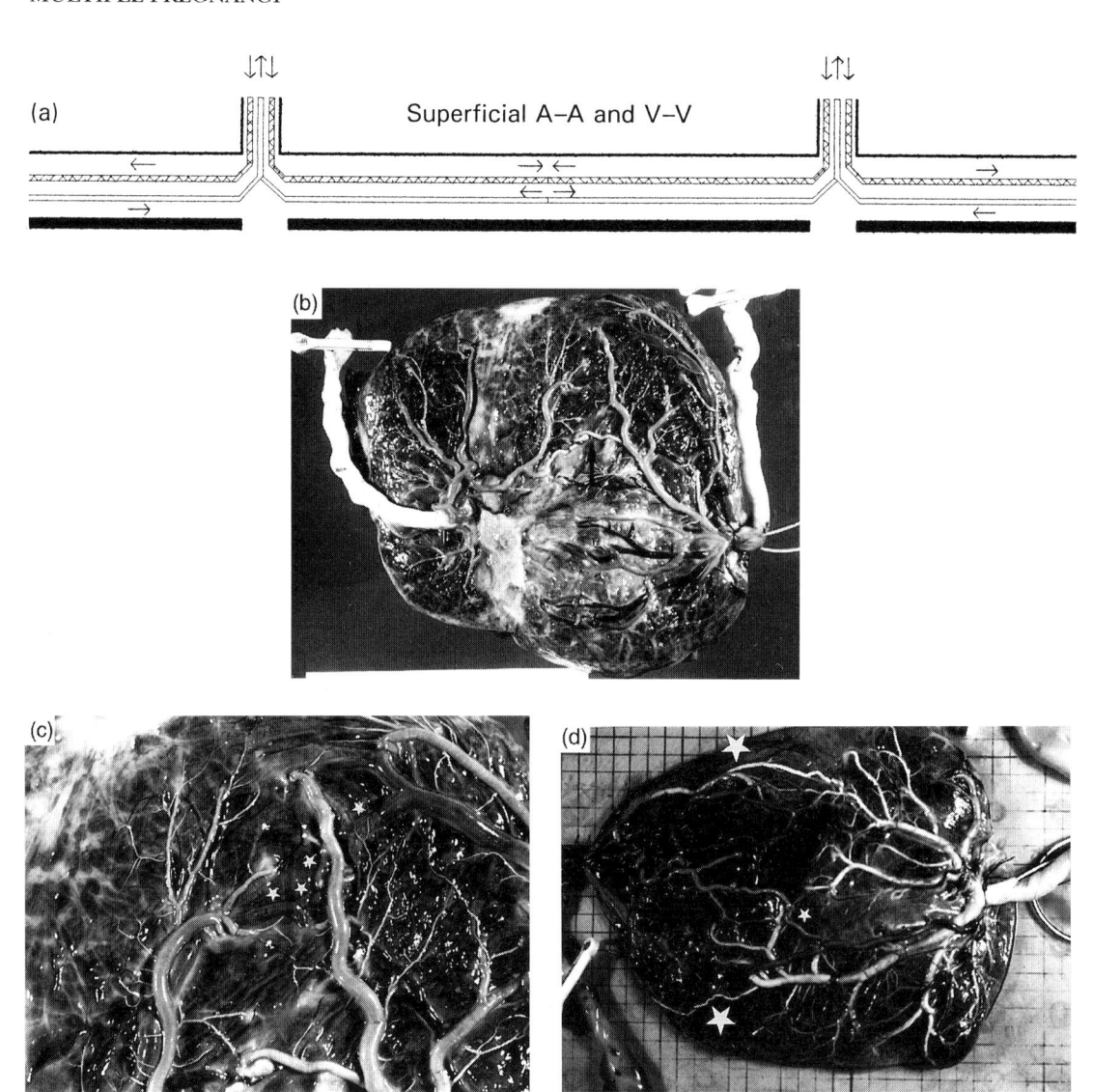

Figure 6 (a) Sketch of lateral view, A–A and V–V anastomoses present. Superficial (superf) anastomoses only. (b) MC–DA placenta with A–A and V–V anastomoses. A–A (large arrow) is at the center. (c) Close-up view of Figure 6b. V–V (asterisks) is beneath large artery. Gestation was 40 weeks. Twin A male, 2880 g; twin B male, 2810 g; no complications. (d) MC–DA placenta with A–A and V–V. Cord A was velamentously inserted and contained little Wharton's jelly; cord B was thick and slightly edematous. Markedly unequal venous sharing was present, B>A. The arteries of twin A and vein of twin B were perfused. One A–A anastomosis was present at the equator (small asterisk), and two V–V (large asterisks) at the margins. No A–V were noted. Gestation was 31 weeks. Twin A male, 970 g; twin B male, 1475 g. No TTTS. Growth discordance was secondary to unequal venous sharing, despite presence of superficial IFVA

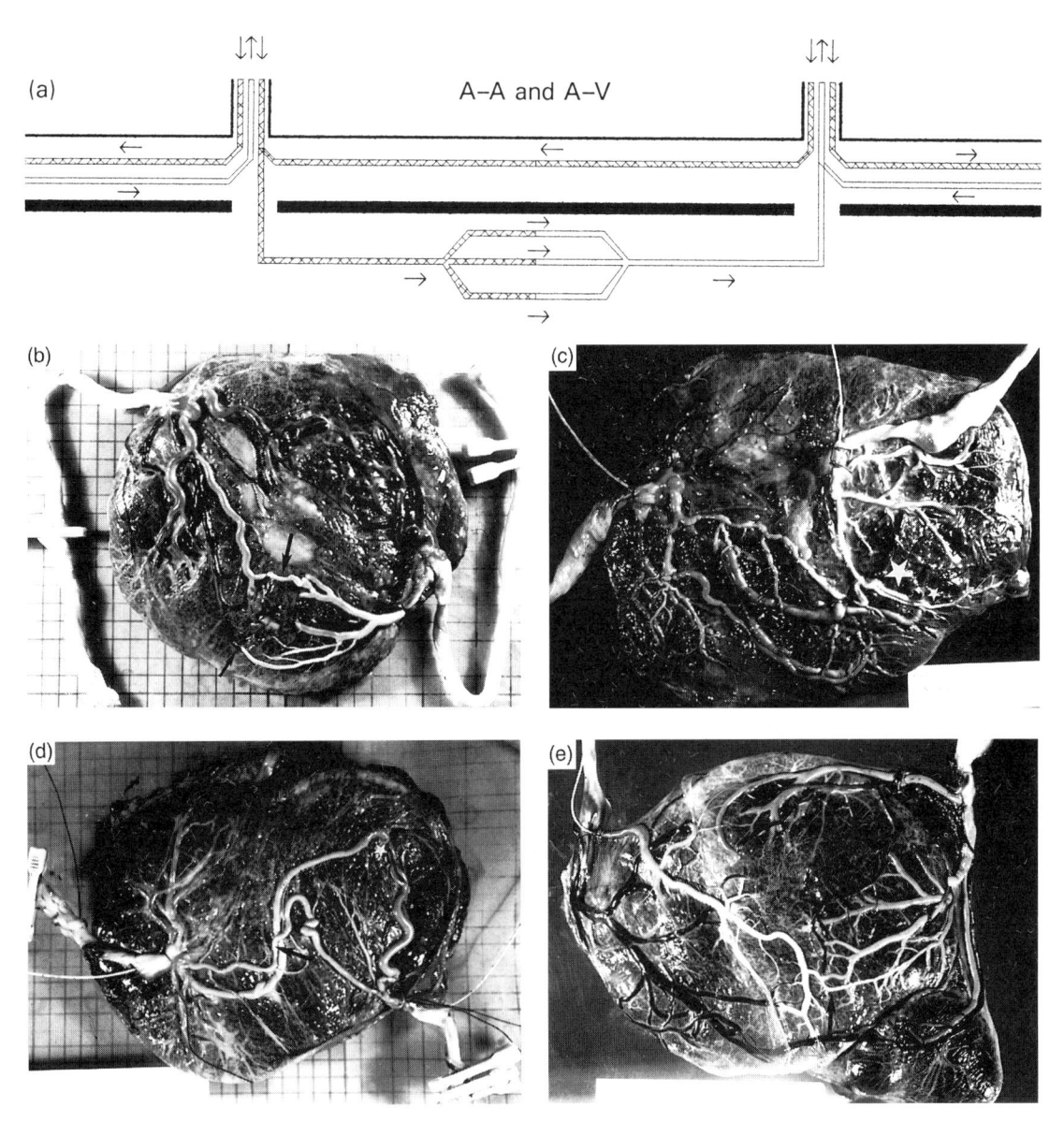

Figure 7 (a) Sketch of lateral view; A–A and A–V anastomoses are present. This is the most common vascular pattern in MC twin placentas. (b) MC–DA placenta with A–A and A–V anastomoses. Cord A was thicker than cord B. One artery of twin B was perfused; a single, central A–A (large arrow) was present along with a zone of A–V perfusion (small arrow), with twin B as the donor. Gestation was 37 weeks. Twin A male, 2850 g; twin B male, 2500 g. Twin A had a hypoplastic aortic arch (possible flow-type congenital heart lesion); twin B was normal. Significant growth discordance was present in the absence of TTTS. Twins were confirmed as MZ by DNA RFLP. (c) MC–DA placenta with A–A and A–V. Twin B had a thin cord. Arteries of both twins were perfused, together with the vein of twin A. Unequal venous sharing was present, A > B. A large venous branch arose to the right and extended inferiorly to cord A (small arrow). An A–A anastomosis (large asterisk) was present along with a zone of A–V (small asterisk) with twin B as donor. Gestation was 40 weeks. Twin A female, 3050 g; twin B female, 2655 g; no complications. Growth discordance was attributable to unequal venous sharing with A–V; no TTTS because an A–A was present. (*Continued overleaf*)

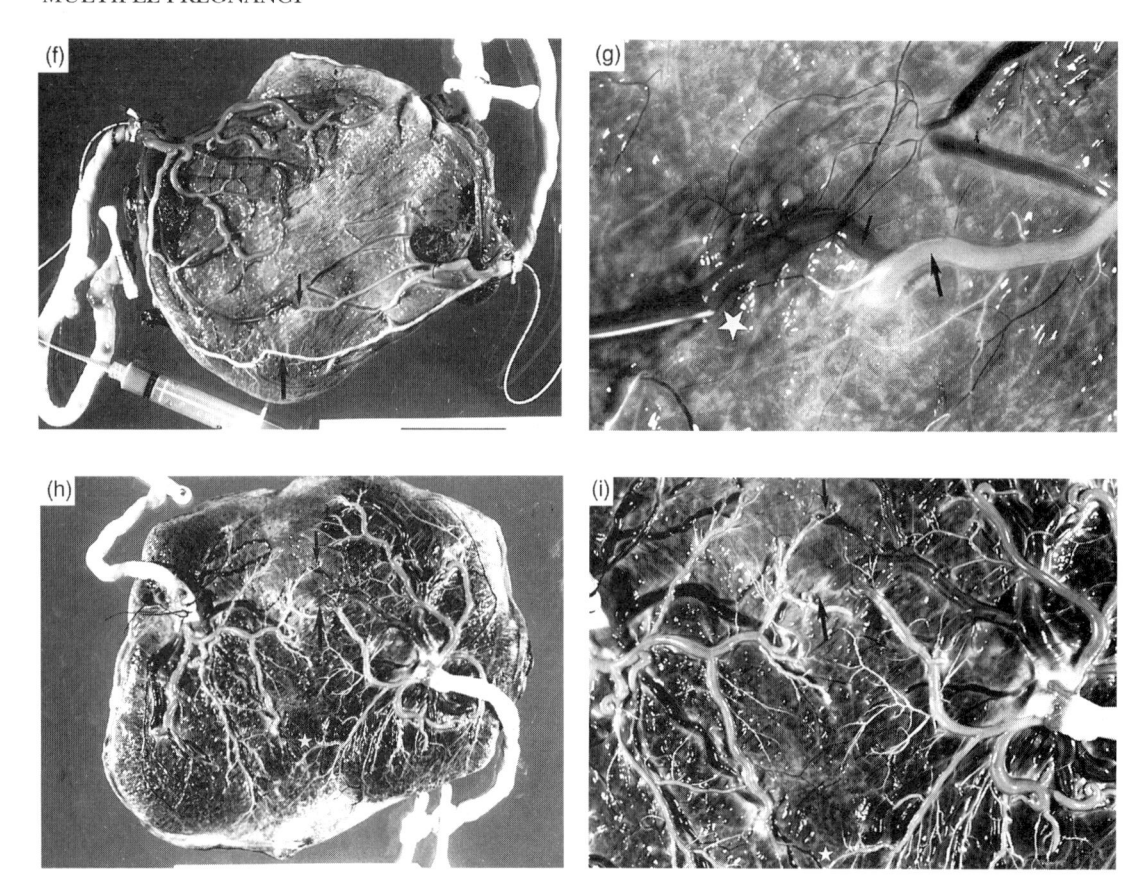

Figure 7 *(continued)* (d) MC–DA placenta with A–A and A–V. An artery of twin B and the vein of twin A were perfused. One equatorial A–A (large arrow) was present; venous sharing was unequal (A>B), with a large venous branch (small arrows) coursing from the arterial perfusion zone of twin B to the cord of twin A. A zone of A–V (asterisk) was supplied by an artery of twin B (donor) and drained by the long venous branch of twin A. A prenatal diagnosis of discordant omphalocele and hydramnios of twin B was made. Gestational age was 35 weeks. Twin A female, 2270 g; twin B female, 1960 g. MZ status was confirmed by DNA RFLP. Despite hydramnios, growth discordance and MC placentation, no TTTS was present; a zone of A–V was compensated by the A–A. (e) MC–DA placenta with A–A and A–V anastomoses. Velamentous insertions of both cords; the cord of twin B thicker than cord of twin A. A succenturiate lobe was present on the lower right. An artery of twin A and the vein of twin B were perfused. A single A–A (large arrow) was noted, along with an A–V arising from the A–A (small arrow), with twin A as the donor. Venous sharing was unequal (B>A). Gestation was 35 weeks. Twin A male, 1905 g; twin B male, 2470 g. No complications; growth discordance was attributable to unequal venous sharing and an A–V, but no TTTS was present because of a compensating A–A. (f) MC–DA placenta with A–A and A–V. Cord A was velamentously inserted. An artery of twin B and the vein of twin A were perfused. An A–A was present at the lower margin (large arrow) along with a zone of A–V (small arrow) with twin B as donor. (g) Close-up view of Figure 7f showing zone of A–V from artery of twin B (large arrow) to vein of twin A (small arrow); note catheter tip (asterisk) in vein of A, close to A–V perfusion zone. Gestation was 35 weeks. Twin A male, 2580 g; twin B male, 2420 g. Although venous sharing was unequal (A>B), growth discordance was not significant. No TTTS because an A–A anastomosis was present. (h) MC–DA placenta with A–A and two, bidirectional A–V anastomoses. An artery of twin A and the vein of twin B were perfused. A single A–A dipped beneath a large vein (large arrow); an A–V (donor A) was present in the upper field (small arrow) along with a second A–V (donor B) in the lower field (asterisk). (i) Close-up view of Figure 7h to show A–A (large arrow) and two A–V anastomoses (small arrow, asterisk), as shown in Figure 7h. Gestation was 39 weeks. Twin A female, 2920 g; twin B female, 2915 g. No complications

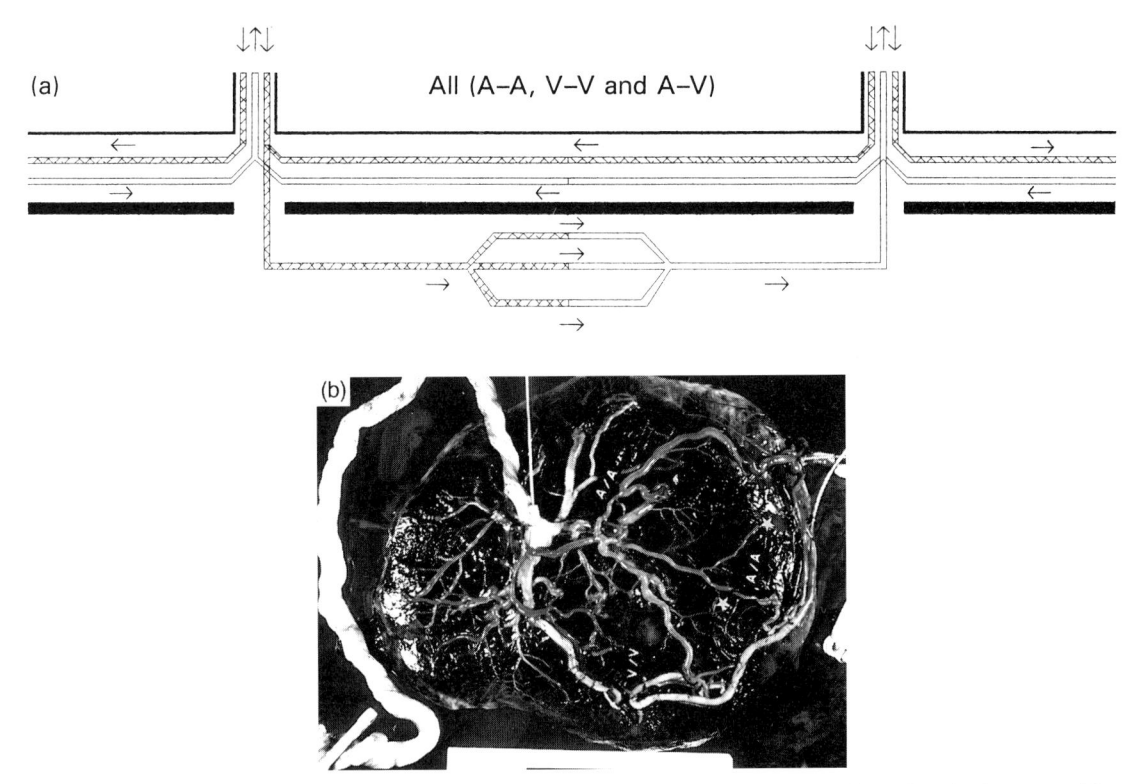

Figure 8 (a) Sketch of lateral view; all three types of anastomosis are present. (b) MC–DA placenta with two A–A, one V–V and several zones of A–V anastomoses. The cord of twin B was velamentously inserted, with single umbilical artery. The cord of twin B was thicker than the cord of twin A. An artery of twin B and the vein of twin A were perfused. Two A–A (labelled) and one V–V (labelled) were present. Venous sharing was unequal (A > B). Sites of A–V (donor B) are shown with asterisks. Gestation was 37 weeks. Twin A female, 3060 g; twin B female, 2100 g. No complications despite growth discordance secondary to unequal venous sharing

(a) The placental parenchyma, no longer perfused by the deceased twin, may act as a pool for blood from the survivor, with hypotension and hypovolemia resulting in visceral shutdown and organ infarction[38,39].

(b) The deceased twin may liberate thromboplastins, which passively return into the survivor via IFVA[40–42].

The result of either of these events may be multi-organ infarction in two main patterns, depending on the fetal age at death. In the second trimester, the surviving twin may develop aplasia cutis congenita and/or multiple bowel atresia[43–47]. In contrast, in the third trimester, visceral infarction usually involves brain, lungs, kidneys and liver[44,48–51].

PreTTTS was originally recognized in newborn MC twins who were growth-discordant and had different hemoglobin concentrations. Because of the complexity of the consequences of MC placentation, there are no simple criteria for the diagnosis of TTTS in the prenatal patient[27]. Growth discordance, which is usually present in PreTTTS, may also be caused by unequal venous sharing without PreTTTS. Hydramnios may result from fetal malformation (e.g. Figure 7d). Major malformation may affect only one twin of an MC pair. Hydrops may be caused by a number of factors other than PreTTTS, including feto-maternal hemorrhage. Anemia may also be caused by hydrops, feto-maternal hemorrhage and PeriTTTS without the need to invoke PreTTTS. Likewise, plethora can be caused by PeriTTTS.

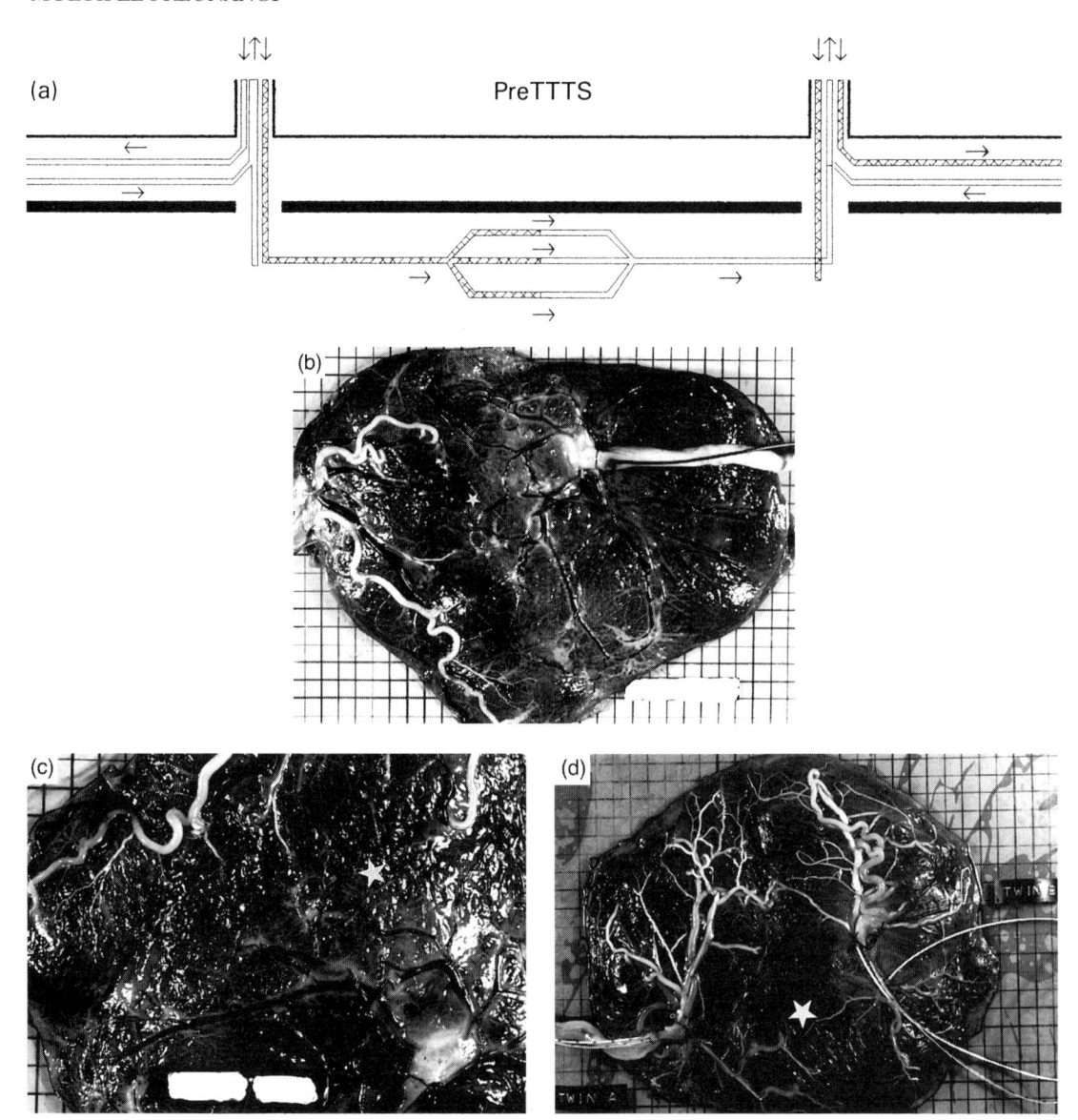

Figure 9 (a) Sketch of lateral view, A–V without superficial anastomoses. *This is the anatomic basis for acute PreTTTS.* (b) Acute PreTTTS, managed conservatively from 20 weeks, with spontaneous regression; both twins survived. Velamentous insertion of cord A. A single, small zone of A–V (asterisk) is present, with B as donor. No superficial anastomoses are present. (c) Close-up view of Figure 9b, showing the area of A–V (asterisk). Gestation was 35 weeks. Diagnosis of acute PreTTTS at 20 weeks, with stuck donor twin, hydramnios, ascites of recipient and growth discordance. One twin subsequently developed cardiomyopathy with tricuspid regurgitation. Twin A female, 2620 g, cardiomyopathy, survived; twin B female, 2540 g, no complications, survived. The postnatal vascular status presumably represented the situation during spontaneous resolution of TTTS. The zone of transfusion involved small vessels. Another zone of transfusion must also have existed; its function may have been modified by onset of hydramnios, but no trace was found postpartum. (d) Acute PreTTTS, successfully treated with indomethacin and therapeutic amniocentesis; both twins survived. Onset of acute PreTTTS at 18 weeks' gestation; stuck twin donor, hydramnios of recipient, growth discordance. Recipient progressed to hydrops, with mitral and tricuspid regurgitation. Two amniocenteses of 500 ml; indomethacin therapy; hydrops resolved. Delivered at 29 weeks. Twin A male, 1075 g; twin B male, 1300 g. The cord of twin B was avulsed. Venous sharing was equal; a zone of A–V (asterisk) was present

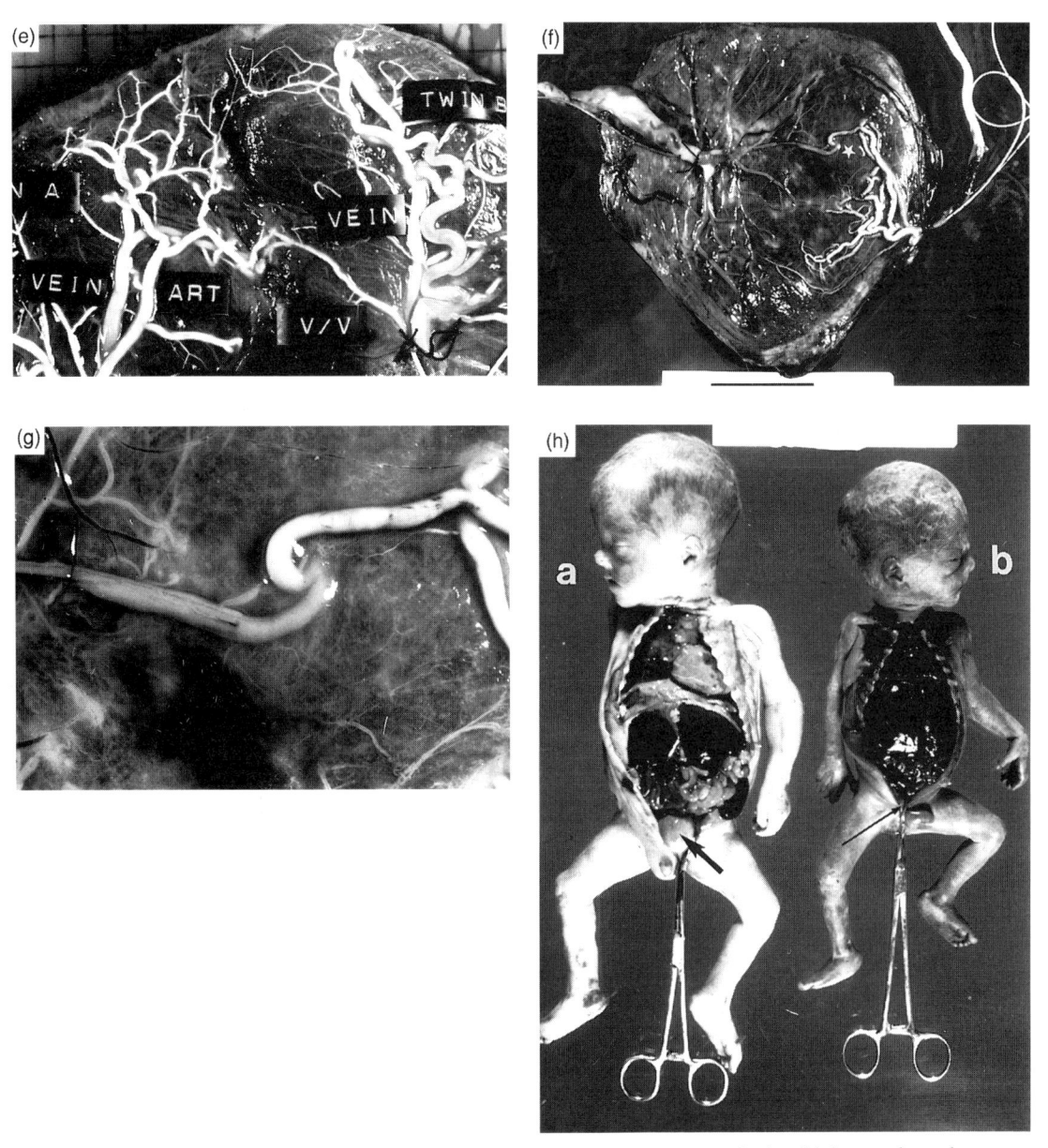

Figure 9 *(continued)* (e) Close-up view of Figure 9d. A small V–V was marked, which may have been occluded by the onset of hydramnios; after amniocentesis, this anastomosis may have functioned again to compensate for the transfusion zone. (f) Acute PreTTTS with death of both twins despite aggressive management. Onset of acute TTTS at 21 weeks of gestation, with stuck donor twin, hydramnios of recipient and growth discordance. Intrauterine fetal death of twin B (donor); twin A (recipient) had multiple complications, including polycythemia and sepsis, dying in the neonatal period. The cord of twin A (recipient) was much thicker than the cord of twin B (donor). Unequal venous sharing was present (A > B). Perfusion of an artery of twin B (donor) and the vein of twin A (recipient) showed a single large A–V (asterisk). No superficial anastomoses were present. (g) Close-up view of Figure 9f, showing zone of A–V. (h) The recipient twin A (left) weighed 1080 g; note large body, heart and urinary bladder (arrow) in comparison with donor twin B (right) which weighed 640 g. Acute reversed PeriTTTS was present. The hydramniotic recipient twin A was born first; after cord clamping, pooled blood in the (single) MC placenta drained into the donor prior to delivery, resulting in paradoxical plethora. *(Continued overleaf)*

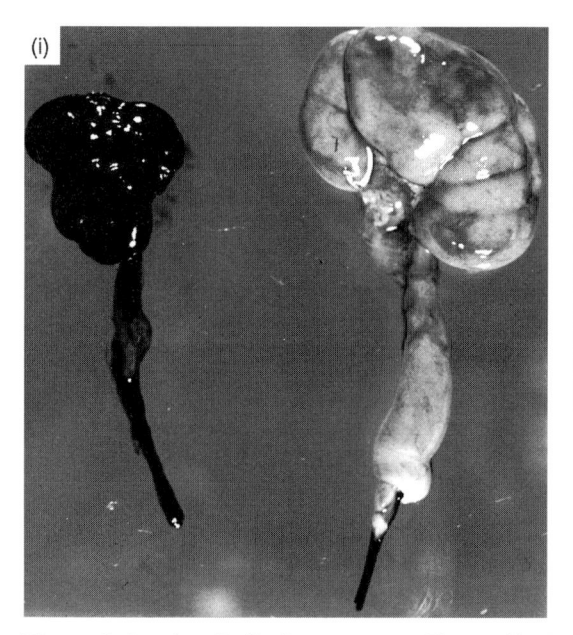

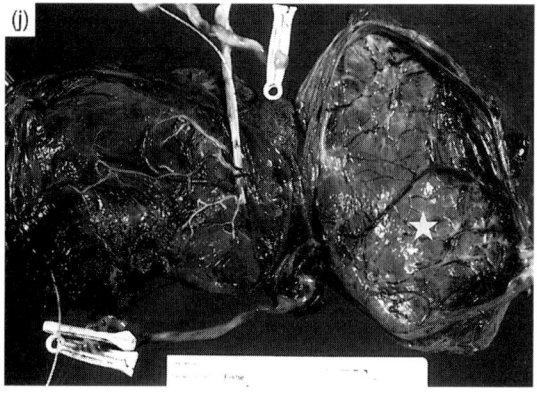

Figure 9 (continued) (i) Same case as Figure 9h. Hydronephrosis and hydroureter of recipient kidney (right), secondary to polyuria, causing hydramnios; the kidney of the oliguric donor (left) was smaller, and was deeply congested because of acute reversed PeriTTTS. (j) Acute PreTTTS in pair of MC twins of a spontaneous MZ triplet pregnancy. Onset was acute, with SPROM at 24 weeks' gestation, affording no opportunity for active management. All three triplets died in the neonatal period. Triplets A and B shared a MC–DA placenta. Triplet C had a separate placenta (asterisk); the triplets were MZ by DNA RFLP testing. Triplet A female, 365 g; triplet B female, 500 g; triplet C female, 735 g. Amnion nodosum was found in the sac of triplet A (donor), indicating chronic oligohydramnios of stuck twin; the cord of triplet B was velamentously inserted and avulsed. This figure demonstrates that the zygosity- and gestation-matched placenta was almost as large as the MCDA twin placenta; likewise, both of the MC twins were growth-retarded in relation to their MZ–DC co-triplet

An approach to monitoring MC twin pregnancies

MC twins are at high risk for any or all of the complications of IFVA listed above. However, diagnosis of PreTTTS is not easy, because of the possible presence of confounding mechanisms that can also give rise to growth discordance, hydramnios, hydrops, anemia and plethora. Therefore, a more general approach to the care of MC twin pregnancies would require early identification and management by intensive prenatal review in order to detect the earliest evidence of complications from IFVA.

MC placentation can be diagnosed reliably by assessing septal membrane thickness using ultrasonography (Table 5)[52–59]. A few cases of DC placentation also have very thin septa, and may be incorrectly diagnosed as MC. Likewise, the septum in MC–DA placentation is very thin and may be difficult to detect; some cases are misdiagnosed as MC–MA. In contrast, MC–DA placentation is seldom misdiagnosed as DC–DA.

The presence of two apparently separate placental disks does not necessarily exclude MC–DA placentation (Figure 4b), but a large succenturiate lobe to an MC placenta can cause difficulty in establishing placental type with accuracy.

No precise figures are available for the prevalence of acute PreTTTS and TRAP among MC twin pregnancies. The frequency of acute PreTTTS may be as much as 10% of MC pregnancies[60] but TRAP is much less common. Acute PeriTTTS can potentially occur in any MC pregnancy.

Without active treatment, the mortality in PreTTTS approaches 100%[22]. Five options for

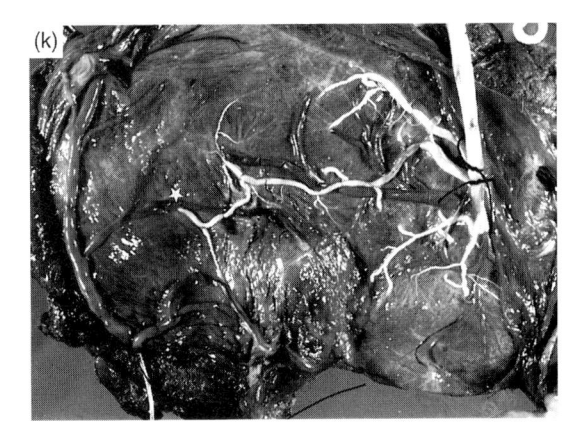

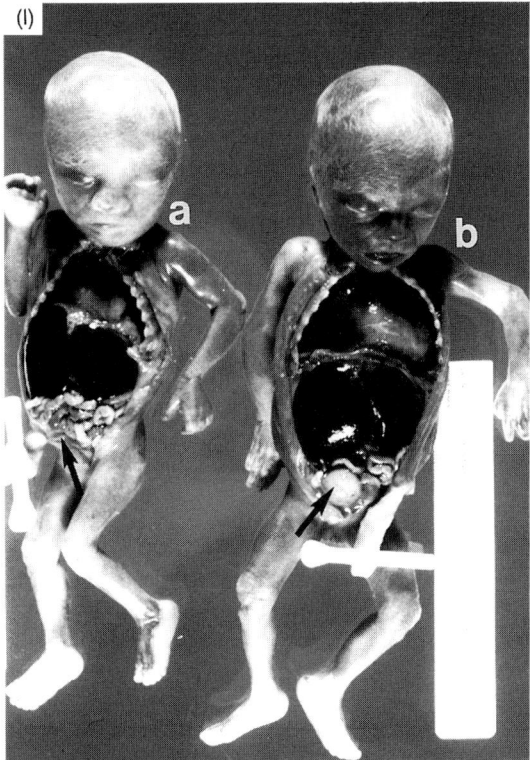

Figure 9 *(continued)* (k) Close-up view of Figure 9j, showing MC–DA placenta; the artery of triplet A (donor) is on the right and the vein of triplet B is on the left. A single A–V zone (asterisk) was present without superficial anastomoses. (l) The MC twins of Figure 9k were discordant for size of bodies, hearts and urinary bladders (arrowed). Twin B (recipient) is on the right. Note the flexed attitude of the stuck donor twin on left. The prognosis for spontaneous higher-order multiple pregnancies is worse than that for products of assisted reproduction, because of a higher frequency of MZ and MC twins. In this case, triplets A and B died of acute PreTTTS, while triplet C, the bystander, died of complications of prematurity

Table 5 Prenatal diagnosis of septal chorionicity: an analysis of 351 reported cases[52–59]

Prenatal diagnosis	DC–DA	MC–DA	MC–MA	Total
Thick septum	233	13	0	246
Thin septum	10	70	0	80
No septum	2	17	6	25
Total	245	100	6	351

In these 351 cases, 'chorionicity' and 'amnionicity' refer to the pathological analysis of the placentas after delivery

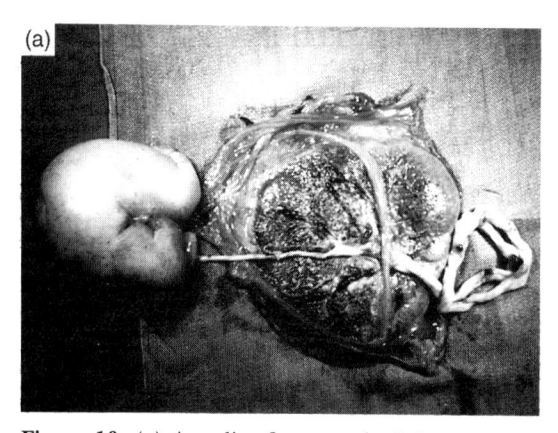

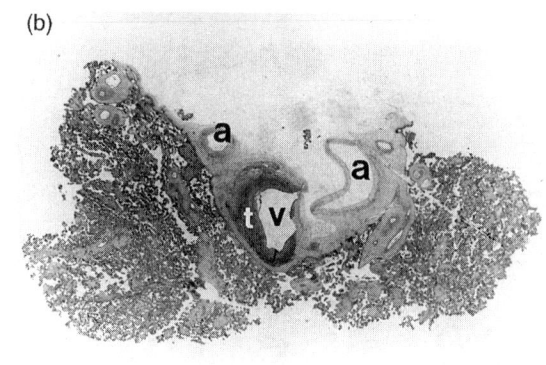

Figure 10 (a) Acardiac fetus on the left was connected to MC–DA placenta by a thin umbilical cord. This was inserted very close to the cord of the pump twin on the right. (b) Histological section of three-vessel cord of pump twin at a point where it inserted into placenta. a, arteries, V, vein; t, thrombosis of the umbilical vein. This was presumably caused by thromboplastic products from the umbilical vein of the acardiac fetus (reversed venous flow from acardiac fetus to placenta) via veno-venous anastomosis to the vein of the pump twin

active management have been reported in recent years:

(1) Maternal digoxin therapy for fetal cardiac failure[61].

(2) Indomethacin therapy. This reduces fetal renal circulation and results in decreased urine formation[62–64]. Such therapy deals with the problem of hydramnios, SPROM and premature labor, but has the side effect of reducing urine production in a donor twin which is already oligohydramniotic.

(3) Selective termination of pregnancy[23,65,66]. The dangers of termination of pregnancy in MC placentation are great in the presence of IFVA, for reasons that have already been discussed with regard to fetal death *in utero* of one twin. Death of the co-twin after selective termination of MC twins has been reported[67,68]. Selective termination of pregnancy has also been used in TRAP[69].

(4) Aggressive therapeutic amniocentesis. Clinical onset of PreTTTS is usually recognized by acute hydramnios in the sac of the recipient. This arises because the recipient is transfused whole blood via an uncompensated A–V anastomosis. Hypervolemia stimulates increased micturition[70–72], probably via atriopeptin production[73]. While the hematocrit of the recipient rises, the amniotic fluid volume increases rapidly. The amniotic fluid pressure also increases in hydramnios regardless of its cause, including PreTTTS[74]. This increased pressure probably modifies flow in various anastomotic vessels. Therapeutic amniocentesis is effective, although the detailed mechanism of its action is not fully understood. Not only does it reduce the risk of SPROM and premature labor, but it also sometimes actually reverses the TTTS. The placenta becomes thicker following therapeutic amniocentesis[75]. From published series and cases of therapeutic amniocentesis[25,26,71,75–85], overall survival following amniocentesis is 48% (96/196).

(5) Selective coagulation of anastomotic vessels. (See Chapter 29.) This method of treatment seems to be the most logical, definitive and specific, although the procedure is associated with risks and complications[86]. The procedure involves the coagulation of all arteries and veins that run near or across the equator, as defined by the point of insertion of the septum onto the fetal surface. Because all of these vessels are likely to be involved in A–V

Table 6 IFVA and clinical outcomes[88]; 164 MC twins (82 pairs) with fully documented IFVA

	Total		Perinatal mortality		Incidence of TTTS	
	No.	%	No.	%	No.	%
Total	164	100	51	31	36	22
A–A only	82	100	8	10	2	2
A–A, A–V	20	100	2	10	8	40
A–A, V–V	38	100	19	50	20	53
V–V only	6	100	5	83	2	33
V–V, A–V	4	100	2	50	0	0
A–V only	14	100	5	36	4	29
All A–A	40	100	29	21	30	21
All V–V	48	100	26	54	22	46
All A–V	38	100	9	24	12	32

Excluded are 28 pairs in which IFVA were recorded as absent or unknown. The prognosis in this group was poor, but there is probably a difference between the undocumented cases and those that lacked IFVA. The definition of TTTS was not given

anastomoses, the procedure is therefore somewhat excessive. It may also ablate some vessels that are important for the nutrition of the twins. Accurate mapping of the sites of A–V anastomoses and acute PreTTTS could allow more selective coagulation. It is not presently clear that results by this method are superior to those from therapeutic amniocentesis. (Editor: This procedure is considered experimental at the time of publication.)

Correlation of vascular anatomy with outcome in twin pregnancy

As mentioned previously, growth discordance, hydramnios and hydrops may occur in MC twins for reasons other than PreTTTS[27]. Cordocentesis samples from twin pairs may give misleadingly similar hemoglobin results in PreTTS[79]; however, others have found that discordant hemoglobin, hematocrit and viscosity values in fetoscopic blood samples are reliable criteria for the diagnosis of PreTTTS[87].

Because the diagnosis of PreTTTS is difficult to make with certainty in the prenatal state, we undertook a study in which the placental vascular anatomy was documented by perfusion studies soon after birth; clinical outcome data were also collected, such as gestational age, mortality, presence of hydramnios and growth discordance. A less detailed study has been reported[88], in which the prevalence

Table 7 University of Alberta series: percentage of DC and MC twins born at various gestational ages

Chorionicity	< 28 weeks	29–36 weeks	> 37 weeks
DC	3	59	37
MC	15	58	27
ALL	8	59	33

Table 8 University of Alberta series: percentage of DC and MC twins having mild, moderate and severe growth discordance

Chorionicity	Mild	Moderate	Severe
DC	53	26	21
MC	52	24	24

Birth weight discordance is expressed as: $\left(\dfrac{L-S}{L}\right) \times 100$

Mild discordance, <10%; moderate discordance, 10–20%; severe discordance, >20%

of TTTS (not otherwise specified) was correlated with placental vascular anatomy (Table 6). In contrast, our clinical data (which did not include hemoglobin measurements) were correlated with the underlying vascular anatomy of the placenta. Our analyses allow us to describe:

(1) The relative frequencies of the vascular anastomotic patterns illustrated in Figures 4–9;

(2) The clinical outcomes with these vascular patterns; and

(3) The most frequent locations of uncompensated A–V anastomoses that could be targeted for specific coagulation in the definitive treatment of acute PreTTTS.

Study material

Our analysis was carried out on a series of 80 consecutive MC twin pregnancies managed at the University of Alberta Hospitals, Edmonton, Canada. Of these 160 twin infants, 26 (16%) died in the perinatal period and hydramnios was present in 19 pairs (24%). The placental vascular anatomy could be analyzed in 69 pairs; in the remaining cases, the placenta was fragmented or had been fixed in formalin, thus precluding perfusion studies. In the group that was studied in detail, perinatal mortality was 16% and hydramnios was present in 20%.

During the same period, the perinatal mortality in DC twins was 4%. Table 7 compares gestational age distribution of the MC and DC twins; Table 8 shows that the frequency and severity of growth discordance is similar in the two types of twins.

Observations

Placental vascularity was classified according to the principles outlined above and illustrated in Figures 3–9. Of the many possible patterns of anastomosis and venous sharing, 15 types were found, and these are illustrated in Figures 11–15. The most common vascular pattern (No.

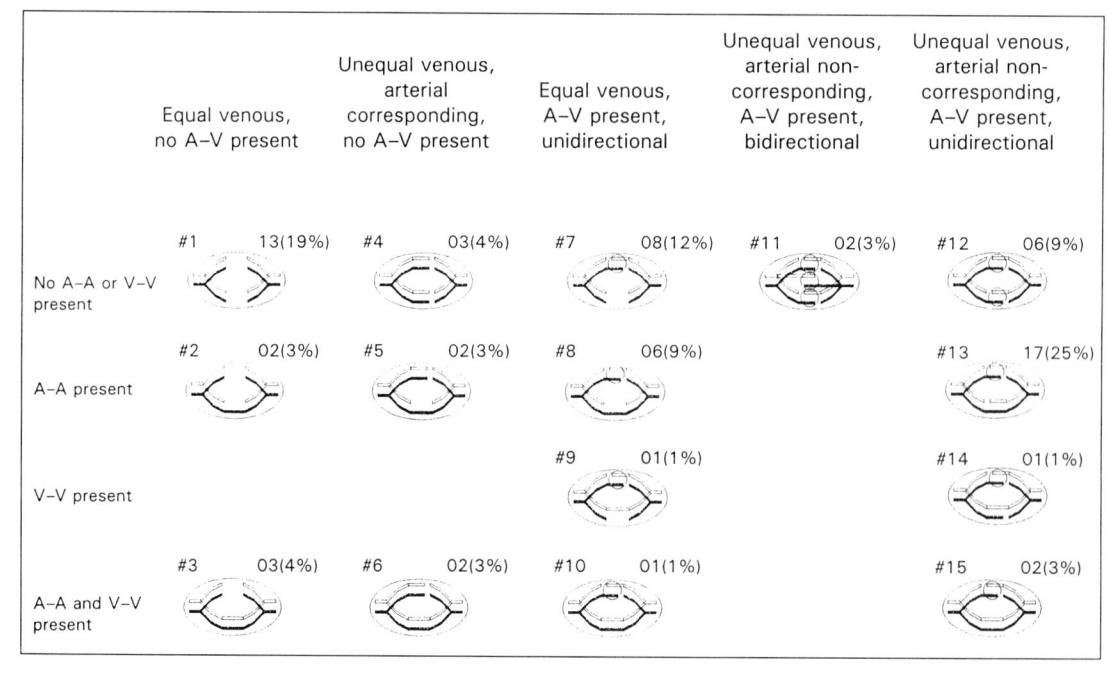

	Equal venous, no A–V present	Unequal venous, arterial corresponding, no A–V present	Equal venous, A–V present, unidirectional	Unequal venous, arterial non-corresponding, A–V present, bidirectional	Unequal venous, arterial non-corresponding, A–V present, unidirectional
No A–A or V–V present	#1 13(19%)	#4 03(4%)	#7 08(12%)	#11 02(3%)	#12 06(9%)
A–A present	#2 02(3%)	#5 02(3%)	#8 06(9%)		#13 17(25%)
V–V present			#9 01(1%)		#14 01(1%)
A–A and V–V present	#3 03(4%)	#6 02(3%)	#10 01(1%)		#15 02(3%)

Figure 11 Clinical outcomes analyzed by placental vascular anatomy. The overall frequency of each type of IFVA pattern is shown on the right side of each pattern form, directly oppisite the number of the anatomic variation

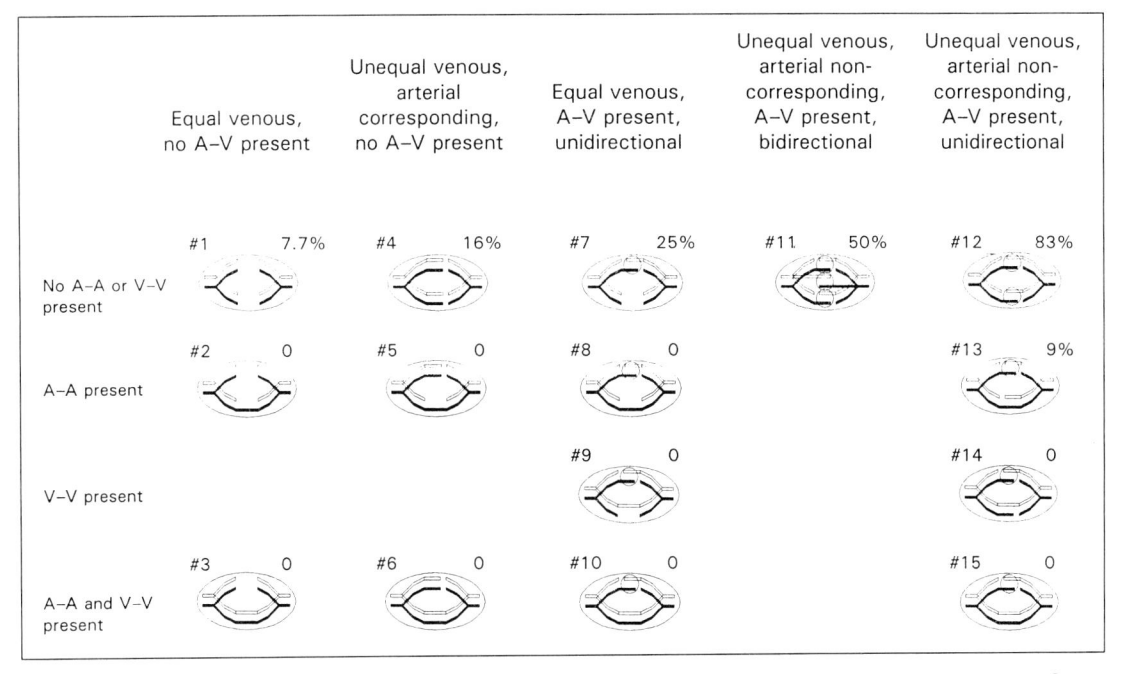

Figure 12 Perinatal mortality (%) in each type of IFVA is shown on the right side of each pattern form, directly opposite the number of the anatomic variation

13) involved A–A and unidirectional A–V anastomoses with unequal venous sharing (Figure 11). Surprisingly, the next most common pattern (No. 1) involved no anastomoses and equal venous sharing; followed by No. 7, in which A–V anastomosis was present with equal venous sharing. The most lethal type (83%) of placenta (No. 12) was seen in 9% of cases, as was No. 8. All other vascular patterns were rare.

Perinatal mortality (Figure 12) Perinatal mortality was highest in the group in which no superficial anastomoses were present (No. 1, 4, 7, 11 and 12). There was 83% mortality in group No. 12, in which the classic pattern for acute PreTTTS was seen, as shown in Figure 9f,g,k. The combination of unequal venous sharing with A–V anastomosis in the absence of superficial anastomoses allows the development of a major transfusion zone supplied by a large artery of the donor and drained by a large vein of the recipient. All the perinatal deaths in group No. 12 were attributable to acute PreTTTS.

Whereas the majority of deaths were caused by TTTS, all of these deaths occurred in groups 4, 11 and 12. Furthermore, all deaths in these groups were caused by TTTS. However, there were other causes of death, as follows:

One pair of twins was born extremely prematurely because of cervical incompetence (Figure 4d), but had no IFVA. These twins accounted for all deaths in group 1. In one monoamniotic pair, one twin was stillborn because of cord knotting and the other twin survived. This stillborn was the one death in group 4. One pair of twins (in group 13) died of acute antepartum hemorrhage with complete placental separation. In another pair in group 13, after a second-trimester fetal death, the co-twin was born with multiple gut atresias. The cause of fetal death could not be determined, but the gut atresias may have presumably resulted from a vascular event that occurred at the time of the fetal death.

Hydramnios (Figure 13) Hydramnios was present in all cases in group 12, and was also seen in groups 9 and 14, in which significant V–V anastomoses were present.

MULTIPLE PREGNANCY

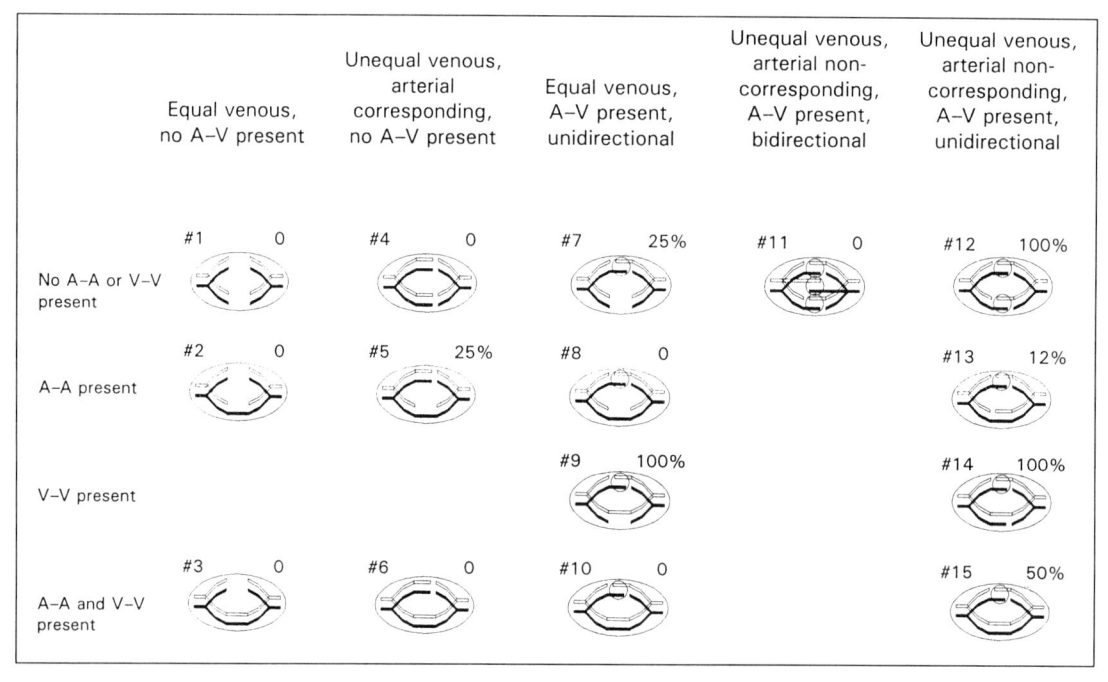

Figure 13 Frequency of hydramnios (%) in each type of IFVA is shown on the right side of each pattern form, directly opposite the number of the anatomic variation

Gestational age at delivery (Figure 14) The acute PreTTTS group (No. 12) had a significantly reduced gestational age, reflecting the onset of hydramnios, SPROM and premature labor. This low gestational age exposed the newborn twins to complications of prematurity, because the majority of newborns were at or below the limit of viability.

Growth discordance (Figure 15) Discordance (%) expressed as

$$\left(\frac{L-S}{L}\right) \times 100$$

i.e. the growth difference as a proportion of the birth weight of the larger twin. Growth discordance was highest in the groups with unequal venous sharing but lacking A–V anastomosis (groups 4 and 5). Even in the presence of A–A anastomosis (group 5), unequal venous sharing caused severe growth discordance but low mortality. Naturally, growth discordance was also high in the acute PreTTTS twins (group 12).

Mapping of A–V anastomoses (Figure 9b, c, d, g, k) The presence of large, significant A–V anastomosis zones is the cause of PreTTTS. This pattern was seen in all cases of untreated or untreatable acute PreTTTS, but was not seen in the one case with spontaneous resolution of acute TTTS. In this case (Figure 9b, c), a small A–V anastomosis was present at the equator. In the remaining ten cases, eight had single, large equatorial A–V anastomoses (Figure 9f, g, j, k). In one instance, an A–V anastomosis arose from a V–V anastomosis (Figure 9b, c). This case was unusual in that spontaneous resolution occurred, and the presence of a V–V anastomosis was significant. The pathophysiology for this disease may have included a change in the function of the V–V anastomosis with time. In one case of acute TTTS, there were multiple small A–V anastomoses scattered across the equator, which, in sum, would have allowed sufficient transfusion to cause TTTS. In one other case, there were two adjacent zones of A–V anastomosis, both of which were smaller than the vessels that are seen when a single major transfusion zone is involved.

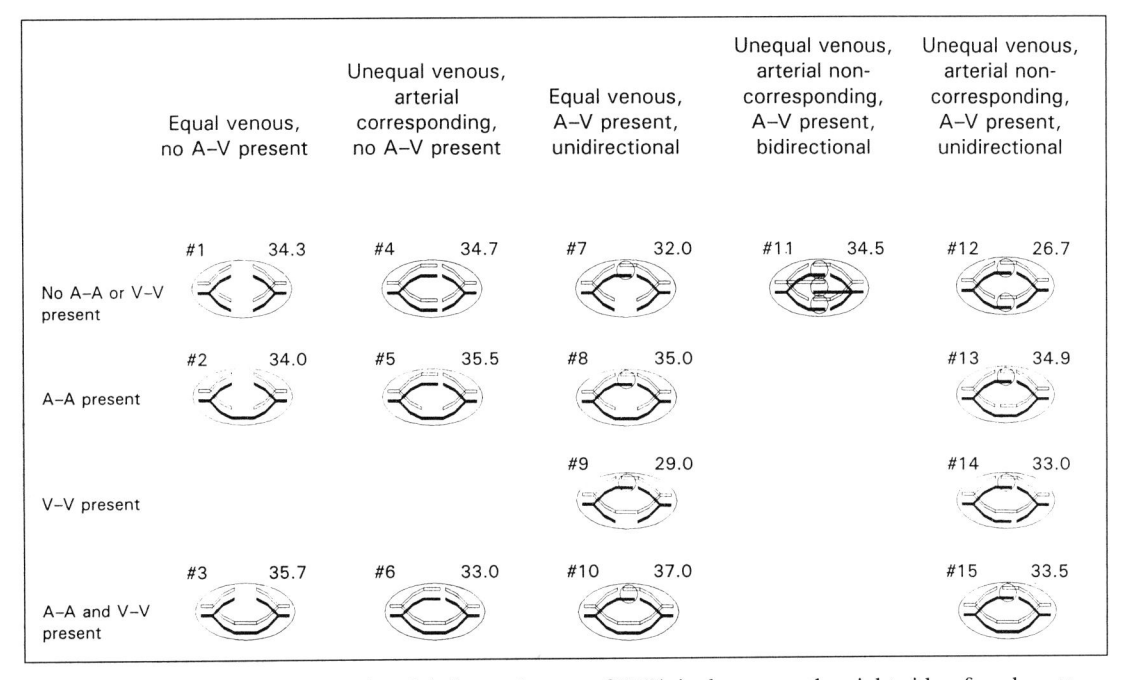

Figure 14 Mean gestational age (weeks) for each type of IFVA is shown on the right side of each pattern form, directly opposite the number of the anatomic variation

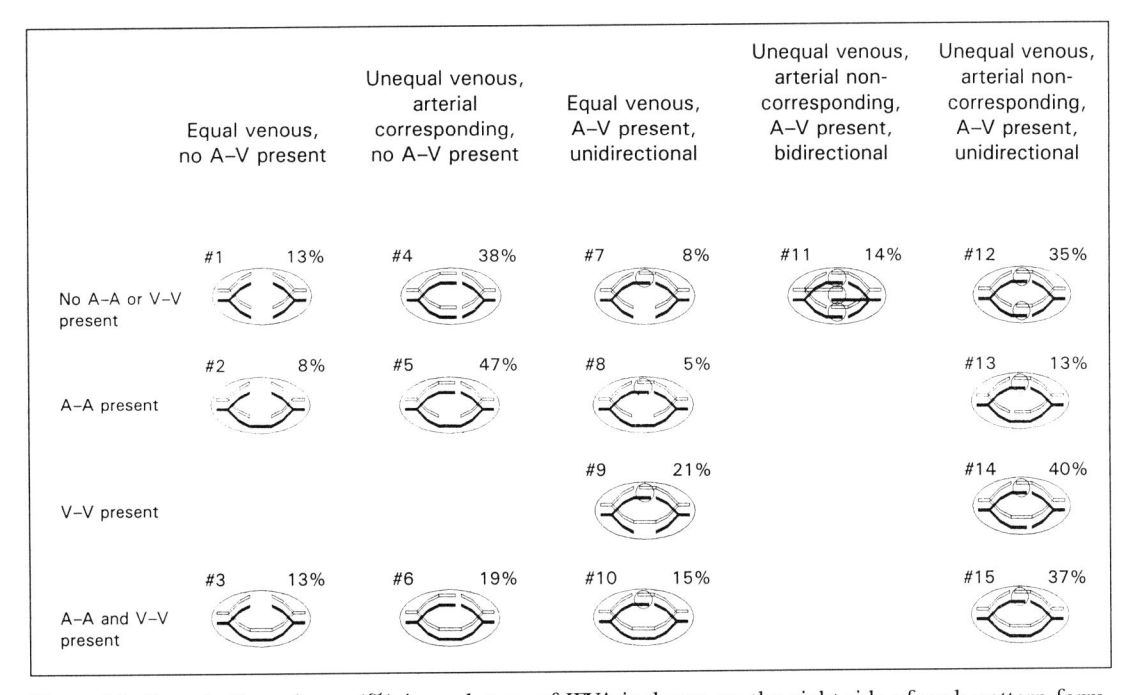

Figure 15 Growth discordance (%) in each type of IFVA is shown on the right side of each pattern form, directly opposite the number of the anatomic variation. Cases with intrauterine fetal death are excluded

Thus, in eight of 11 cases of acute PreTTTS, a single area of A–V anastomosis lay at the edge of the large venous zone of the recipient on the placental equator, not far from a line joining the roots of the two cords.

Comment

This chapter documents the vascular basis for a number of features of MC twin pregnancy which give positive and false-positive indications of the existence of TTTS. In cases of true PreTTTS, the arrangement of vascular anastomoses in the placental parenchyma results in a simple pattern of chorionic vessels in which one large artery of the donor supplies an equatorial zone which is drained by one large vein to the recipient. Although variations on this pattern exist, the most common pattern is simple. *All cases of TTTS occur where there is unequal venous sharing, and the responsible transfusion zone lies at the outer edge of the large venous zone of the recipient, and therefore closer to the donor cord than the recipient cord.* Because most cases of acute PreTTTS involve one transfusion zone only, accurate mapping theoretically would allow specific coagulation in this zone, while other vessels, possibly important in fetal nutrition, could be left undisturbed. The major remaining issue is the position of the septum. This presumably varies in time with the development of hydramnios in the recipient, but it is likely to lie closer to the cord of the donor than of the recipient, making for easier visualization of potential sites of A–V anastomosis. However, if it were possible to perform simultaneous double fetoscopy, with one fetoscope in each sac, this might allow the delineation of the arteriovenous zone from both sides of the septum.

Misleading anatomic features that can lead to a false diagnosis of TTTS include major growth discordance, which is often caused by unequal venous sharing in the absence of TTTS. Such cases probably do not require treatment unless one of the twin fetuses dies.

In order to map the zones of fetal vascularity prenatally, methods are needed to enhance the visibility of these vessels. The presence of transfusion has been confirmed by the use of adult red cells which were injected into the cord of the donor and subsequently appeared in the blood of the recipient[21]. The use of fluorescent dyes, injected into the donor, might identify the particular venous branch which is transfusing blood to the recipient. It is expected that more precise mapping methods will be available in the future, allowing for precise obliteration of the zone or zones of transfusion which are responsible for the development of acute TTTS.

Without doubt, little progress can be made if all cases of TTTS present clinically in the established form of the disease. Progress can only be made if all twin pregnancies are diagnosed early and characterized as MC and DC. The MC pregnancies can then be followed intensively for early evidence of onset of acute TTTS, at which time thorough investigation, including accurate placental vascular mapping, could be carried out in a less urgent clinical setting.

Figure 16 summarizes the events that give rise to acute TTTS, based on placental vascular anatomy. Large volumes of amniotic fluid are usually removed repeatedly in order to control hydramnios and prevent SPROM and/or premature labor. It is clear that the total volume of amniotic fluid removed (which may be several liters) cannot have been transfused to the recipient from the donor. The initial event might be a transfusion of a few milliliters of whole blood sufficient to raise the circulating blood volume and induce polyuria. As the result of polyuria, the blood of the recipient becomes viscous and hyperosmotic[87]; in passage through the placental villi, this fetal blood could absorb water from the maternal space, undergoing hemodilution, and again increasing the circulating blood volume; in turn, polyuria would continue. According to this schema, there is a dynamic equilibrium between the osmolality and volume of the recipient's circulation and available water in the maternal space. This equilibrium is set up at the time of the transfusional event, and would not necessarily require any further transfusion. One of the effects of amniocentesis may simply

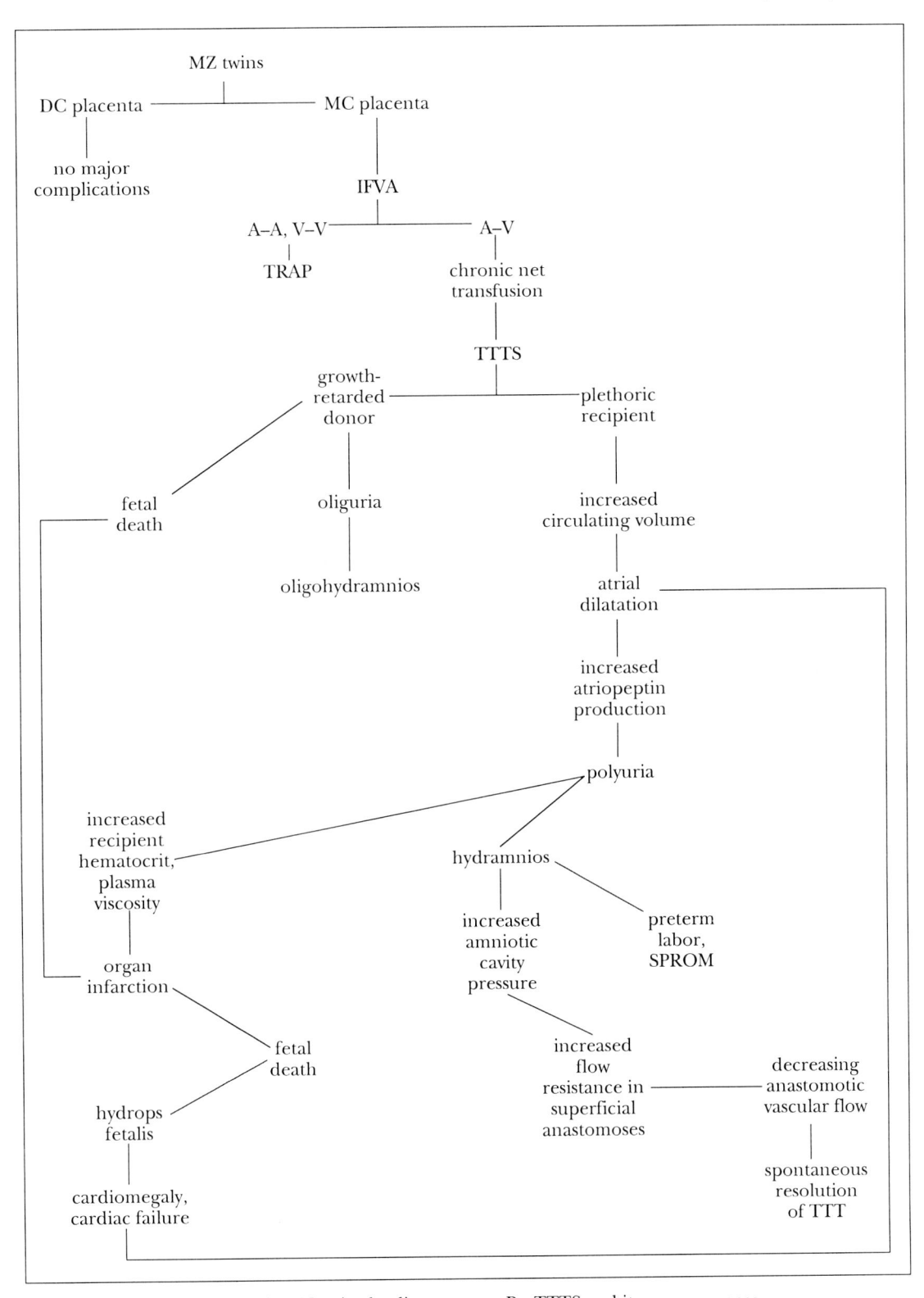

Figure 16 Cascade of events in MC twins leading to acute PreTTTS and its consequences

MULTIPLE PREGNANCY

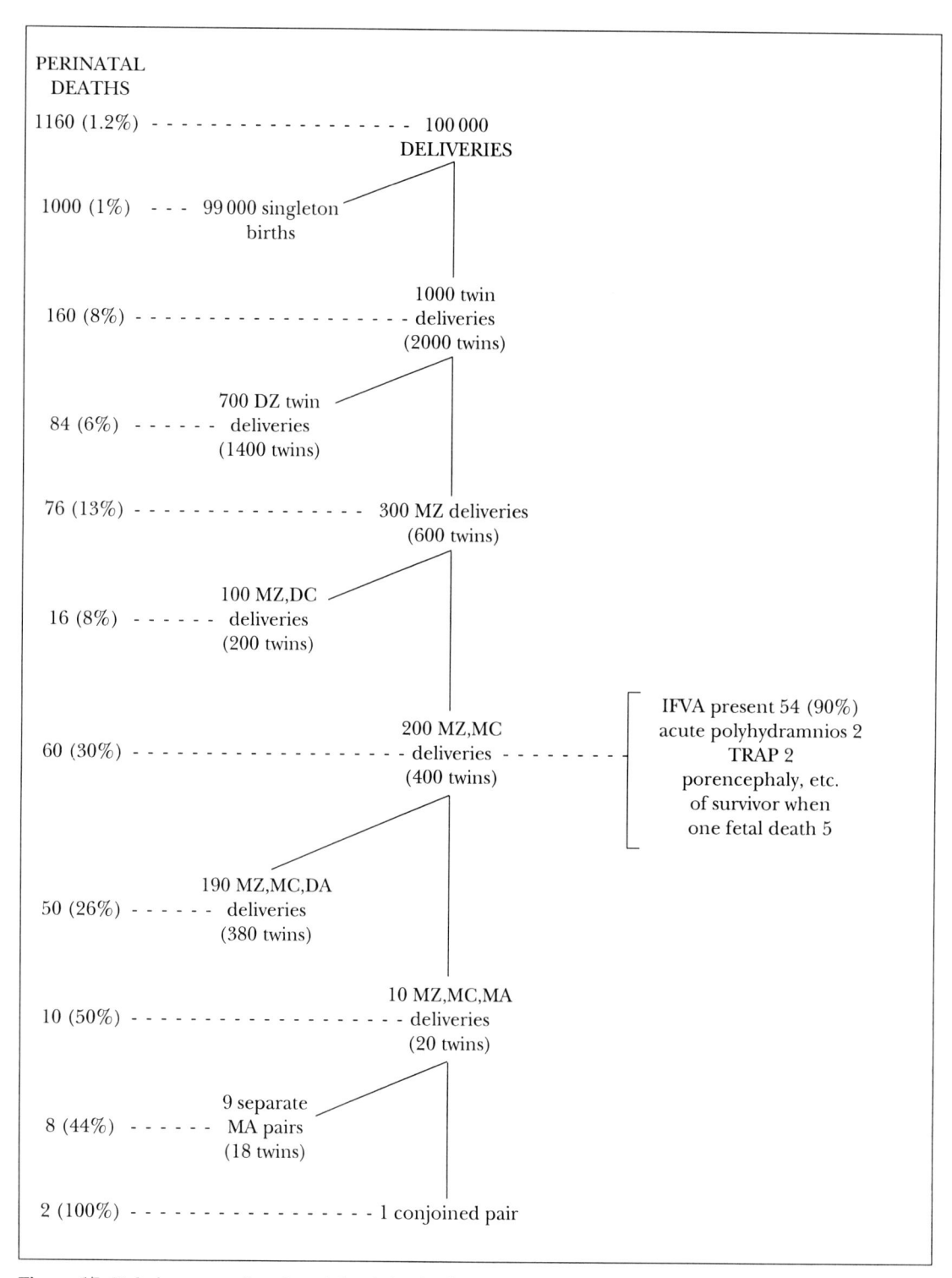

```
PERINATAL
  DEATHS
1160 (1.2%) ----------------- 100 000
                                DELIVERIES

1000 (1%)   --- 99 000 singleton
                      births

                              1000 twin
160 (8%)  ------------------ deliveries
                              (2000 twins)

              700 DZ twin
 84 (6%)  ------ deliveries
                 (1400 twins)

 76 (13%) --------------- 300 MZ deliveries
                              (600 twins)

              100 MZ,DC
 16 (8%)  ------ deliveries
                 (200 twins)

                                                    IFVA present 54 (90%)
                              200 MZ,MC             acute polyhydramnios 2
 60 (30%) ------------------ deliveries  --------   TRAP 2
                              (400 twins)           porencephaly, etc.
                                                    of survivor when
                                                    one fetal death 5

              190 MZ,MC,DA
 50 (26%) ------ deliveries
                 (380 twins)

                              10 MZ,MC,MA
 10 (50%) ------------------ deliveries
                              (20 twins)

              9 separate
  8 (44%) ------ MA pairs
                 (18 twins)

  2 (100%) ---------------- 1 conjoined pair
```

Figure 17 Relative rates of perinatal death in singletons and in twins by chorionicity and zygosity. The frequency of acute PreTTTS, TRAP and vascular disease after fetal death of co-twin are estimated. The perinatal death rate is based on a survey of the literature

be to relieve the hydramnios, and there may also be a slow corrective effect on the osmotic overload of the recipient. Nevertheless, effects of hydramnios on the patency and function of small V–V anastomoses are probably also important.

Figure 17 documents the relative frequencies of birth, perinatal death and other complications in twin pregnancies compared with singletons. The perinatal death rates are much higher in MC twins, and are mostly attributable to TTTS, TRAP and mutual knotting of the umbilical cords.

Acknowledgments

We are grateful to Tasneem Lalani, a student intern, who carried out the statistical analysis that correlated clinical outcomes with placental vascular anatomy. The line drawings in this chapter were made using AutoCAD, a product of Autodesk Inc., Sausalito, California.

References

1. Potter, E.L. (1963). Twin zygosity and placental form in relation to outcome of pregnancy. *Am. J. Obstet. Gynecol.*, **87**, 566–77
2. Benirschke, K. (1961). Twin placenta in perinatal mortality. *NY State Med. J.*, **61**, 1499–508
3. Fujikura, T. and Froehlich, L.A. (1971). Twin placentation and zygosity. *Obstet. Gynecol.*, **37**, 34–43
4. Cameron, A.H., Edwards, J.H., Derom, R. *et al.* (1983). The value of twin surveys in the study of malformations. *Eur. J. Obstet. Gynecol. Reprod. Biol.*, **14**, 347–56
5. Naeye, R.L., Tarafi, N., Judge, D. *et al.* (1978). Twins: causes of perinatal death in 12 United States cities and one African city. *Am. J. Obstet. Gynecol.*, **131**, 267–72
6. Gruenwald, P. (1970). Environmental influences on twins apparent at birth. A preliminary study. *Biol. Neonat.*, **15**, 79–93
7. Myrianthopoulos, N.C. (1970.) An epidemiologic survey of twins in a large prospectively studied population. *Am. J. Hum. Genet.*, **22**, 611–29
8. Benirschke, K. and Driscoll, S.G. (1967). *The Pathology of the Placenta.* (New York: Springer-Verlag)
9. Bleker, O.P., Breur, W. and Huidekoper, B.L. (1979). A study of birth weight, placental weight and mortality of twins as compared to singletons. *Br. J. Obstet. Gynaecol.*, **86**, 111–18
10. Strong, S.J. and Corney, C.T. (1967). *The Placenta in Twin Pregnancy.* (Oxford: Permagon Press)
11. Galea, P., Scott, J.M. and Goel, K.M. (1982). Feto-fetal transfusion syndrome. *Arch. Dis. Child.*, **57**, 781–4
12. Arts, N.F. and Lohman, A.M.M. (1971). The vascular anatomy of monochorionic diamniotic twin placentas and the transfusion syndrome. *Eur. J. Obstet. Gynecol. Reprod. Biol.*, **1**, 85–93
13. Sekiya, S. and Hafez, E.S.E. (1977). Physiomorphology of twin transfusion syndrome. A study of 86 twin gestations. *Obstet. Gynecol.*, **50**, 288–92
14. Bejar, R., Vigliocco, G., Gramajo, H. *et al.* (1990). Antenatal origin of neurologic damage in newborn infants. II. Multiple gestations. *Am. J. Obstet. Gynecol.*, **162**, 1230–6
15. Bendon, R.W. and Siddiqui, T. (1989). Clinical Pathology Conference: acute twin-to-twin transfusion. *Pediatr. Pathol.*, **9**, 591–8
16. Lubinsky, M. and Rappaport, P. (1983). Transient fetal hydrops and 'prune belly' in one identical female twin. *N. Engl. J. Med.*, **308**, 256–7
17. Shaprio, I. and Sharf, M. (1985). Spontaneous intrauterine remission of hydrops fetalis in one identical twin: sonographic diagnosis. *J. Clin. Ultrasound*, **13**, 427–30
18. Tan, K.L., Tan, R., Tan, S.H. *et al.* (1979). The twin transfusion syndrome. Clinical observations on 35 affected pairs. *Clin. Pediatr.*, **18**, 111–14
19. Brant, D.D., Exalto, N., Barnardus, R.E. *et al.* (1985). Twin pregnancy: case reports illustrating variations in twin transfusion syndrome. *Eur. J. Obstet. Gynecol. Reprod. Biol.*, **19**, 383–90
20. Blickstein, I. (1990). The twin–twin transfusion syndrome. *Obstet. Gynecol.*, **76**, 714–22
21. Fisk, N.M., Borrell, A., Hubimont, C. *et al.* (1990). Feto-fetal transfusion syndrome: do

the neonatal criteria apply *in utero?* *Arch. Dis. Child.*, **65**, 657–61
22. Weir, P.E., Pattern, C.T.J. and Beischer, N.A. (1979). Acute polyhydramnios – a complication of monozygous twin pregnancy. *Br. J. Obstet. Gynaecol.*, **86**, 849–53
23. Weiner, C.P. (1987). Diagnosis and treatment of twin to twin transfusion in the mid-second trimester of pregnancy. *Fetal Ther.*, **2**, 71–4
24. Yameda, A., Kasugai. M., Ohno, Y. *et al.* (1991). Antenatal diagnosis of twin–twin transfusion syndrome by Doppler ultrasound. *Obstet. Gynecol.*, **78**, 1058–61
25. Mahony, B.S., Petty, C.N., Nyberg, D.A. *et al.* (1990). The 'stuck twin' phenomenon: ultrasonographic findings, pregnancy outcome, and management with serial amniocenteses. *Am. J. Obstet. Gynecol.*, **163**, 1513–22
26. Bebbington, M.W. and Wittmann, B.K. (1989). Fetal transfusion syndrome: antenatal factors predicting outcome. *Am. J. Obstet. Gynecol.*, **160**, 913–15
27. Danskin, F.H. and Neilson, J.P. (1989). Twin-to-twin transfusion syndrome: what are the appropriate diagnostic criteria? *Am. J. Obstet. Gynecol.*, **161**, 365–9
28. Gibson, J.Y., D'Cruz, C.A., Patel, R.B. *et al.* (1986). Acardiac anomaly: reveiw of the subject with case report and emphasis on practical sonography. *J. Clin. Ultrasound*, **14**, 541–5
29. Van Allen, M.I., Smith, D.W. and Shepard, T.H. (1983). Twin reversed arterial perfusion (TRAP) sequence: a study of 14 twin pregnancies with acardius. *Semin. Perinatol.*, **7**, 285–93
30. Platt, L.D., DeVore, G.R., Bieniarz, A. *et al.* (1983). Antenantal diagnosis of acephalus acardia: a proposed management scheme. *Am. J. Obstet. Gynecol.*, **146**, 857–8
31. Stiller, R.J., Romero, R., Pace, S. *et al.* (1989). Prenatal identification of twin reversed arterial perfusion syndrome in the first trimester. *Am. J. Obstet. Gynecol.*, **160**, 1194–6
32. Simpson, P.C., Trudinger, B.J., Walker, A. and Baird, P.J. (1983). The intrauterine treatment of fetal cardiac failure in a twin pregnancy with an acardiac, acephalic monster. *Am. J. Obstet. Gynecol.*, **147**, 842–4
33. Benson, C.B., Bieber, F.R., Genest, D.R. *et al.* (1989). Doppler demonstration of reversed umbilical blood flow in an arcadiac twin. *J. Clin. Ultrasound*, **17**, 291–5
34. Pretorius, D.H., Leopold, G.R., Moore, T.R. *et al.* (1988). Arcardiac twin: report of Doppler sonography. *J. Ultrasound Med.*, **7**, 413–16
35. Borrell, A., Pecarrodona, A., Puerto, B. *et al.* (1990). Ultrasound diagnostic features of twin reversed arterial perfusion sequence. *Prenat. Diagn.*, **10**, 443–8
36. Donnenfeld, A.E., van de Woestijne, J., Craparo, F. *et al.* (1991). The normal fetus of an acardiac pregnancy: perinatal management based on echocardiographic and sonographic evaluation. *Prenat. Diagn.*, **11**, 235–44
37. Sherer, D.M., Sinkin, R.A., Metlay, L.A. *et al.* (1992). Acute intrapartum twin–twin transfusion. A case report. *J. Reprod. Med.*, **37**, 184–96
38. Fusi, L., McParland, P., Fisk, N. *et al.* (1991). Acute twin–twin transfusion. A possible mechanism for brain-damaged survivors after intrauterine death of a monchorionic twin. *Obstet. Gynecol.*, **77**, 517–20
39. Dimmick, J., Hardwick, D. and Ho-Yueh, B. (1971). A case of renal necrosis and fibrosis in the immediate newborn period. Association with twin-to-twin transfusion syndrome. *Am. J. Dis. Child.*, **122**, 345–7
40. Patten, R.M., Mack, L.A., Nyberg, D.A. *et al.* (1989). Twin embolization syndrome: prenatal sonographic detection and significance. *Radiology*, **173**, 685–9
41. Moore, C.M., McAdams, A.J. and Sutherland, J. (1969). Intrauterine disseminated intravascular coagulation: a syndrome of multiple pregnancy with a dead twin fetus. *J. Pediatr.*, **74**, 523–8
42. Jung, J.H., Graham, J.M., Schultz, N. *et al.* (1984). Congenital hydramencephaly/porencephaly due to vascular disruption in monozygotic twins. *Pediatrics*, **73**, 467–9
43. Mannino, F.L., Jones, K.L. and Benirschke, K. (1977). Congenital skin defects and fetus papyraceus. *J. Pediatr.*, **91**, 559–64
44. Yoshida, K. and Soma, H. (1986). Outcome of the surviving cotwin of a fetus papyraceus or of a dead fetus. *Acta Genet. Med. Gemellol.*, **35**, 91–8
45. Cruikshank, S.H. and Granados, J.L. (1988). Increased amniotic acetylcholinesterase activity with a fetus papyraceus and aplasia cutis congentia. *Obstet. Gynecol.*, **71**, 997–9
46. Markman, L., Sugar, L. and Zuker, R.M. (1982). Association of aplasia cutis congenita and fetus papyraceus in a triplet pregnancy. *Austr. Pediatri. J.*, **18**, 294–6
47. Hoyme, H.E., Higginbottom, M.C. and Jones, K.L. (1981). Vascular etiology of disruptive structural defects in monozygotic twins. *Pediatrics*, **67**, 288–91

48. Fusi, L. and Gordon, H. (1990). Twin pregnancy complicated by single intrauterine death. Problems and outcome with conservative management. *Br. J. Obstet. Gynaecol.*, **97**, 511–16
49. Larroche, J.C., Droulle, P., Delezoide, A.L. *et al.* (1990). Brain damage in monozygous twins. *Biol. Neotnate*, **57**, 261–78
50. Yoshida, K. and Matayoshi, K. (1990). A study on prognosis of surviving cotwin. *Acta Genet. Med. Gemellol.*, **39**, 383–7
51. Enbom, J.A. (1985). Twin preganacy with intrauterine death of one twin. *Am. J. Obstet. Gynecol.*, **152**, 424–9
52. Mahony, B.S., Filly, R.A. and Callen, P.W. (1985). Amnionicity and chorionicity in twin pregnancies: prediction using ultrasound. *Radiology*, **155**, 205–29
53. Barss, V.A., Benacerraf, B.R. and Frigoletto, F.D. (1985). Ultrasonographic determination of chorion type in twin gestation. *Obstet. Gynecol.*, **66**, 779–83
54. D'Alton, M.E. and Dudley, D.K. (1989). The ultrasonographic predicition of chorionicity in twin gestation. *Am. J. Obstet. Gynecol.*, **160**, 557–61
55. Hertzberg, B.S., Murtz, A.B., Choi, H.Y. *et al.* (1987). Significance of membrane thickness in the sonographic evaluation of twin gestations. *Am. J. Radiol.*, **148**, 151–3
56. Winn, H.N., Gabrielli, S., Reese, E.A. *et al.* (1989). Ultrasonographic criteria for prenatal diagnosis of placental chorionicity in twin gestations. *Am. J. Obstet. Gynecol.*, **161**, 1540–2
57. Cheung, A., Wan, M. and Collins, R.J. (1990). Differentiation of monochorionic and dichorionic twin placentas by antenatal ultrasonic evaluation. *Aust. NZ J. Obstet. Gynaecol.*, **30**, 134–6
58. Townsend, R.R., Simpson, G.F. and Filly, R.A. (1988). Membrane thickness in ultrasound prediction of chorionicity of twin gestations. *J. Ultrasound Med.*, **7**, 327–32
59. Watson, W.J., Valea, F.A. and Seeds, J.W. (1991). Sonographic evaluation of growth discordance and chorionicity in twin gestation *Am. J. Perinatol.*, **8**, 342–4
60. Bebbington, M.W. and Wittmann, B.K. (1989). Fetal transfusion syndrome: antenatal factors affecting outcome. *Am. J. Obstet. Gynecol.*, **160**, 913–15
61. DeLia, J.E., Emery, M.G., Sheafor, S.A. *et al.* (1985). Twin transfusion syndrome: successful *in utero* treatment with digoxin. *Int. J. Gynaecol. Obstet.*, **23**, 197–201
62. Lange, I.R., Harman, C.R., Ash, K.M. *et al.* (1989). Twin with hydramnios: treating premature labor at source. *Am. J. Obstet. Gynecol.*, **160**, 552–7
63. Ash, K., Harman, C.R. and Gritter, H. (1990) TRAP sequence – successful outcome with indomethacin treatment. *Obstet. Gynecol.*, **76**, 960–2
64. Demaudt, E., Legins, E., Devlieger, H. *et al.* (1990). Prenatal indomethacin toxicity in one member of monozygous twins; a case report. *Eur. J. Obstet. Gynecol. Reprod. Biol.*, **35**, 267–9
65. Wittmann, B.K., Farquaharson, D.F., Thomas, W.D.S *et al.* (1986). The role of feticide in the management of severe twin transfusion syndrome. *Am. J. Obstet. Gynecol.*, **155**, 1023–6
66. Robie, G.F., Payne, G.G. and Morgan, M.A. (1989). Selective delivery of an acardiac acephalic twin. *N. Engl. J. Med.*, **320**, 512–13
67. Urig, M.A., Simpson, G.F., Elliott, J.P. *et al.* (1988). Twin–twin transfusion syndrome: the surgical removal of one twin as a treatment option. *Fetal Ther.*, **3**, 185–8
68. Golbus, M.S., Cunningham, N., Goldberg, J.D. *et al.* (1988). Selective termination of multiple gestations. *Am. J. Med. Genet.*, **31**, 339–48
69. Donnenfeld, A.E., Glazerman, L.R., Cubillo, D.M. *et al.* (1989). Fetal exsanguination following intrauterine angiographic assessment and selective termination of a hydrocephalic monozygotic co-twin. *Prenat. Diagn.*, **9**, 301–8
70. Achiron, R., Rosen, N. and Zakut, H. (1987). Pathophysiologic mechanism of hydramnios development in twin transfusion syndrome. A case report. *J. Reprod. Med.*, **32**, 305–8
71. Rosen, D.J., Rabinovitz, R., Beyeth, Y. *et al.* (1990). Fetal urine production in normal twins and in twins with acute polyhydramnios. *Fetal Diagn. Ther.*, **5**, 57–60
72. Kirshon, B. (1989). Fetal urine output in hydramnios. *Obstet. Gynecol.*, **73**, 240–2
73. Nageotte, M.P., Hurwitz, S.R., Kaupke, C.J. *et al.* (1989). Atriopeptin in the twin transfusion syndrome. *Obstet. Gynecol.*, **73**, 867–70
74. Nicolini, U., Fisk, N.M., Talbert, G. *et al.* (1989). Intrauterine manometry: technique and applications to fetal pathology. *Prenat. Diagn.*, **9**, 243–54
75. Elliott, J.P., Urig, M.A. and Clewell, W.H. (1991). Aggressive therapeutic amniocentesis for treatment of twin–twin transfusion syndrome. *Obstet. Gynecol.*, **77**, 537–40

76. Brennan, J.N., Diwan, R.V., Rosin, M.G. et al. (1982). Feto-fetal transfusion syndrome: prenatal ultrasonographic diagnosis. *Radiology*, **143**, 535–6
77. Chescheir, N.C. and Seeds, J.W. (1988). Polyhydramnios and olighydramnios in twin gestations. *Obstet. Gynecol.*, **77**, 882–4
78. Montan, S., Jorgensen, C. and Sjoberg, N.O. (1985). Amniocentesis in treatment of acute polyhydramnios in twin preganancies. *Acta Obstet. Gynecol. Scand.*, **64**, 537–9
79. Saunders, N.J., Snijders, R.J. and Nicolaides, K.H. (1992). Therapeutic amniocentesis in twin–twin transfusion syndrome appearing in the second trimester of pregnancy. *Am. J. Obstet. Gynecol.*, **166**, 820–4
80. Wax, J.R., Blakemore, K.J., Blohm, P. et al. (1991). Stuck twin with cotwin nonimmune hydrops: successful treatment by amniocentesis. *Fetal Diagn. Ther.*, **6**, 126–31
81. Feingold, M., Cetrulo, C.L., Newton, E.R. et al. (1986). Serial amniocentesis in the treatment of twin to twin transfusion complicated with acute hydramnios. *Acta Genet. Med. Gemellol.*, **35**, 107–13
82. Urig, M.A., Clewell, W.H. and Elliot, J.P. (1990). Twin–twin transfusion syndrome. *Am. J. Obstet. Gynecol.*, **163**, 1522–6
83. Gonsoulin, W., Moise, K.J., Kirshon, B. et al. (1990). Outcome of twin–twin transfusion diagnosed before 28 weeks of gestation. *Obstet. Gynecol.*, **75**, 214–16
84. Schneider, K.T.M., Vetter, K., Huch, R. et al. (1984). Acute polyhydramnios complicating twin pregnancies. *Acta Genet. Med. Gemellol.*, **34**, 179–84
85. Radestad, A. and Thomassen, P.A. (1990). Acute polyhydramnios twin pregnancy. *Acta Genet. Obstet. Gynecol. Scand.*, **69**, 297–300
86. De Lia, J., Cruikshank, D.P. and Keye, W.R. (1990). Fetoscopic neodymium:YAG laser occlusion of placental vessels in severe twin–twin transfusion syndrome. *Obstet. Gynecol.*, **75**, 1046–53
87. Weiner, C. and Ludomirsky, A. (1992). Diagnosis and treatment of twin to twin transfusion syndrome (TTTS). *Am. J. Obstet. Gynecol.*, **166**, 284 (abstr.)
88. Yoshida, K. and Soma, H. (1984). A study of twin placentation in Tokyo. *Acta Genet. Med. Gemellol.*, **33**, 115–20

The twin–twin transfusion syndrome: three-dimensional modelling of the 'common villous district'

28

A. Schoenfeld, M. Hod, J. Ovadia and R. Amir

Introduction

Twin–twin transfusion syndrome (TTTS) is a severe *in utero* complication of monozygotic twin pregnancies. It occurs as a result of blood transfer through anastomotic vessels in the placenta's 'common villous district'[1]. Schatz was the first to describe the phenomenon of shared circulation between monochorionic twins[2]. Although anastomoses of arteries and veins are present in almost all monochorionic placentas, it is the anastomosis of an artery to a vein that shifts blood from one twin to the other. Schatz demonstrated that this 'third circulation' usually was accompanied by another arteriovenous anastomosis in the opposite direction which tended to balance the flow and minimize hemodynamic shifts. Depending on the net flow between these anastomoses, mild, moderate or severe TTTS may develop[3–7].

Routine examination of placental morphology remains the most important and widely used tool for understanding TTTS. Classical methods of placental examination include histological sections, injection of vessels using colored gelatin with added barium 5%, histomorphology combined with radioangiography and X-ray cinematography. All of these methods, including injection of milk to demonstrate the anastomotic network as described in one recent study[8], are imperfect for one reason or another and may someday be replaced by other types of evaluations which derive from recent technological advances in other branches of science.

This chapter describes preliminary observations based upon three-dimensional imaging of placental vessel architecture in TTTS. These images were created using a computer-assisted three-dimensional interactive application.

Technique of three-dimensional modelling

Placental tissue from the 'villous district' (Figure 1) was examined in histological sections of

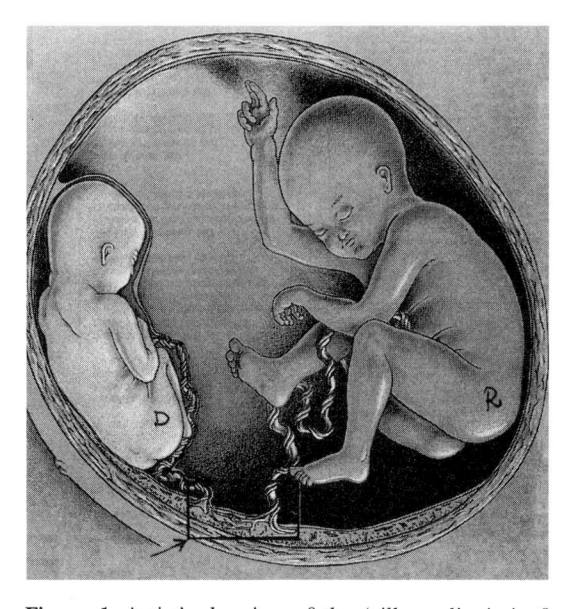

Figure 1 Artist's drawing of the 'villous district' of the TTTS placenta. Histological sections were obtained from this region

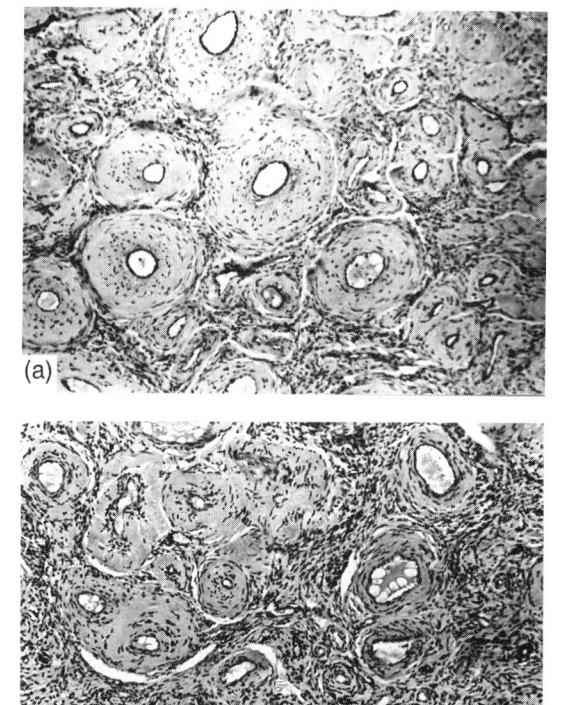

Figure 2 Selected regions of interest of TTTS placenta shows Factor VIII immunohistochemical discrete staining of the donor side (a) and recipient side (b) vessels with various diameters of 30–105 μm. Planar reformatted ultrathin tissue sections (n, 50–75; thickness, 5 μm) were required for the three-dimensional multiplanar reconstruction

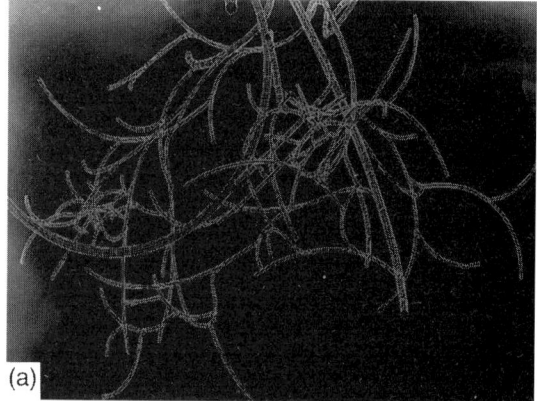

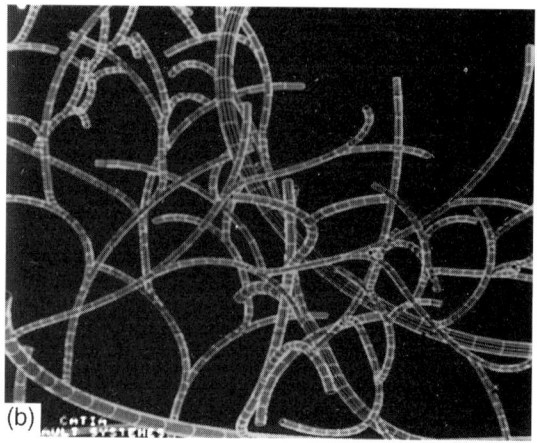

Figure 3 Three-dimensional global displays (a) and (b) of the 'villous district' region of the (TTTS) placenta: chaotic arrangement of the TTTS placental vessels showing shunts, branching, 'flyover' regions of possible turbulence, variability of bifurcation angles and loop formation

5 μm thickness after staining with Factor VIII-related antigen, one of the three functional components of the antihemophiliac factors. This antigen is synthesized in the endothelial cells of blood vessels and is widely used as a nearly specific marker of endothelial cell differentiation. The diameter of the vessels in the tissue sections varies between 30 and 105 μm (mean 70 μm). The dimensions of the selected region of interest were 0.4×0.3 mm (Figure 2a and b).

The global model shown in Figure 3a was reconstructed from 50–75 serial cross-sections using a computer-assisted three-dimensional interactive application on an IBM RISC System/6000 32H platform (CATIA). This design has powerful capabilities in general geometric modelling, rendering it suitable for construction of computer models of any kind of three-dimensional object, be it complex mechanical assemblies, human organs or various mathematically defined geometries. The platform used is a powerful desktop workstation utilizing a reduced instruction set computing architecture. The operating system is AIX, the IBM version of UNIX, which includes numerous extensions beyond the standard UNIX functions.

The three-dimensional architectural patterns of placental vasculature shown in Figure 3b were developed on the basis of the discrete staining with Factor VIII. The vessels are often dilated and tortuous, with arteriovenous shunting, loop formation, variability of bifurcation angles and non-linear branches, all of which indicate the possibility of regular flow patterns combined with chaotic flows.

Comment

As implied by its name, in non-linear dynamic systems, such as those used in human pathophysiology, output is not proportional to input. Two central concepts in non-linear dynamics are fractals and chaos. Of physiological interest is the fractal-like (self-similar) branching architecture of many anatomies, including certain nerve networks, His–Purkinje fibers, gastrointestinal folds and vascular systems[9,10]. The term 'chaos' is used to define the apparently unpredictable behavior that may arise from the internal feedback loops of certain non-linear systems[9,11–13]. This chaotic process generates complex fluctuations that do not have a single or characteristic scale of time. Instead, chaos produces a 'noisy looking' signal that varies in an erratic and unpredictable fashion.

We hypothesized that the bizarre placental vasculature of TTTS, demonstrated by three-dimensional modelling, might be related to the complexity derived from the field of non-linear dynamics (fractals and chaos theory) which may help assess arteriovenous-related flow indices, control of vascular resistance in the human placenta and physiological influence of vascular anastomoses on umbilical artery flow-velocity waveforms. This 'chaotic' vascular architecture may, in part, explain the difficulty of Doppler evaluation to make an antenatal diagnosis of TTTS[14–21].

We plan to evaluate the capabilities of our approach over the next 2–3 years. We hope to determine how accurately the three-dimensional modelling can be used to estimate the spatial distribution of fetal vascular systems, and the three-dimensional anatomy and hemodynamics of complex structures such as the placenta. Once the capabilities have been defined, physiological questions of higher order and more difficult pathophysiological problems can be addressed. We expect some of these studies to indicate that current diagnostic techniques (such as two-dimensional ultrasonography) should be coupled with three-dimensional imaging to obtain more accurate and complete diagnostic information from the patient. The potential advantages of three-dimensional ultrasound will improve visualization of normal and abnormal anatomical structures, evaluation of fetal anomalies, surface structures (e.g. vessels, fetus), volume calculations of the fetus, placenta and ovaries, and standardization of ultrasound examinations.

We also believe that three-dimensional modelling can greatly enhance diagnostic capabilities. However, equipment of considerable complexity and powerful computing and display capabilities will be required. Progress is being made towards attaining these goals, and such technology could well be in clinical use by the end of this decade.

References

1. Benirschke, K. and Kim, C.K. (1973). Multiple pregnancy. *N. Engl. J. Med.*, **288**, 1276
2. Schatz, F. (1875). Zwillinge. *Arch Gynaek.*, **7**, 336
3. Tan, K.L., Tan, R., Tan, S.H. and Tan, A.M. (1979). The twin transfusion syndrome. *J. Pediatr.*, **18**, 111
4. Becker, A.H. and Glass, H. (1963). Twin transfusion syndrome. *Am. J. Dis. Child.*, **106**, 624
5. Corney, G. and Aherne, W. (1965). The placental transfusion syndrome in monozygotic twins. *Arch. Dis. Child.*, **40**, 264
6. Naeye, R.L. (1963). Human intrauterine parabiotic syndrome and its complications. *N. Engl. J. Med.*, **268**, 804
7. Brennan, J.M.N., Diwan, R.V., Mortimer, G.R. and Bellon, E.M. (1982). Fetofetal transfusion

8. Achiron, R., Rabinovitz, R., Aboulafia, Y. et al. (1992). Intrauterine assessment of high-output cardiac failure with spontaneous remission of hydrops fetalis in TTTS. *J. Clin. Ultrasound*, **20**, 271

9. Goldberger, A.L., Rigney, D.R. and West, B.J. (1990). Chaos and fractals in human physiology. *Sci. Am.* **262**, 42

10. West, B.J. and Goldberger, A.L. (1987). Physiology in fractal dimensions. *Am. Sci.*, **75**, 354

11. Mandelbrot, B.B. (1982). *The Fractal Geometry of Nature.* (New York: W.H. Freeman)

12. Goldberger, A.L. and West, B.J. (1987). Applications of nonlinear dynamics to clinical cardiology. *Ann. NY Acad. Sci.*, **504**, 195

13. Goldberger, A.L. (1991). Is the normal heartbeat chaotic or homeostatic? *NIPS*, **6**, 87

14. Giles, W.B., Trudinger, B.J., Cook, C.M. et al. (1990). Doppler umbilical artery studies in the twin–twin transfusion syndrome. *Obstet. Gynecol.*, **76**, 1097

15. Giles, W.B., Trudinger, B.J. and Cook, C.M. (1989). Doppler sonography findings of the umbilical arteries in eight cases of twin transfusion syndrome. *J. Ultrasound Med.*, **8**, 531

16. Formakides, G., Schulman, H., Saldana, L.R. et al. (1985). Surveillance of twin pregnancy with umbilical artery velocimetry. *Am. J. Obstet. Gynecol.*, **153**, 789

17. Erskine, R.L.A., Ritchie, J.W.K. and Murnaghan, G.A. (1986). Antenatal diagnosis of placental anastomoses in a twin pregnancy using Doppler ultrasound. *Br. J. Obstet. Gynaecol.*, **93**, 955

18. Pretorius, D.H., Manchester, D., Barkin, S. et al. (1988). Doppler ultrasound of twin transfusion syndrome. *J.Ultrasound Med.*, **7**, 117

19. Nelson, J.P., Danskin, F. and Hastie, S.J. (1989). Monozygotic twin pregnancy: diagnostic and Doppler ultrasound. *Br. J. Obstet. Gynaecol.*, **96**, 1413

20. Hecher, K., Jauniaux, E., Campbell, S. et al. (1994). Artery-to-artery anastomoses in monochorionic twins. *Am. J. Obstet. Gynecol.*, **171**, 570

21. Kirkinen, P., Kurmanavichius, J., Huch, A. et al. (1993). Blood flow velocities in human intraplacental arteries. *Acta Obstet. Gynecol. Scand.*, **73**, 220

The twin–twin transfusion syndrome: treatment of chorioangiopagus and asymmetry

J.E. De Lia

Introduction

The concept of monozygous (MZ) twins imparts the notion of sameness, both genotypically and phenotypically. Nonetheless, physicians and others with scientific training often demonstrate surprise when informed that a twin pregnancy discordant for an anomalous twin is more apt to be MZ than dizygous (DZ)[1].

Unfortunately, an anomalous twin is but one aspect of the spectrum of developmental and physiological problems that can occur once the MZ twin pregnancy is established. Perhaps the most common is total loss of one twin[2]. Others include the deaths of two normally formed fetuses from prematurity, malformations incompatible with life, or tragically handicapped surviving children. Ironically, despite important research efforts into teratology and significant improvements in prenatal care during the past two decades, many of the risks cited above will persist into the future, because they have no primary prevention. Simply stated, their pathogenesis can be traced to the chance occurrence of the vascular anastomoses in monochorionic placentas that connect twins and arise during the period of placental vasculogenesis (chorioangiopagous vessels).

Placental vascular communications

The nature of the communicating vessels in monochorionic (MC) placentas has been the subject of extensive study during the last century and more recently[3,4]. In the past, this information was used to satisfy clinicians' curiosity or to explain to grieving parents the poor outcome of a twin gestation. In the last several years, I have used the study of these vessels in fresh MC placentas as a groundwork for their early identification and ablation (see below) in an attempt to diminish their potentially lethal impact.

For the most part, the direct surface and indirect deep placental anastomoses vary in size, type and number. According to Bleisch, their diameter is inversely proportional to the distance between the umbilical cords[5]. However, no pattern exists for their frequency or type. Artery-to-artery anastomoses are the most common, followed by artery-to-vein and then vein-to-vein. The number and type of vessels have a profound influence on the outcome of the pregnancy[6]. A single artery-to-vein anastomosis is the most ominous. Although the overwhelming majority of MC placentas have communicating vessels, only a minority of twins suffer significant morbidity as a result of their chorioangiopagus status.

The communicating blood vessels are randomly located along the so-called 'vascular equator' that functionally divides the chorion plate and villous units into two segments, one for each twin. Most often, this equator bears no relationship to the axis of the interfetal bilaminar membranous septum which separates the diamnionic monochorionic (DiMo) twins and is also variably located. Equally variable are the disparate locations of the insertion of each twin's umbilical cord into the discoid MC

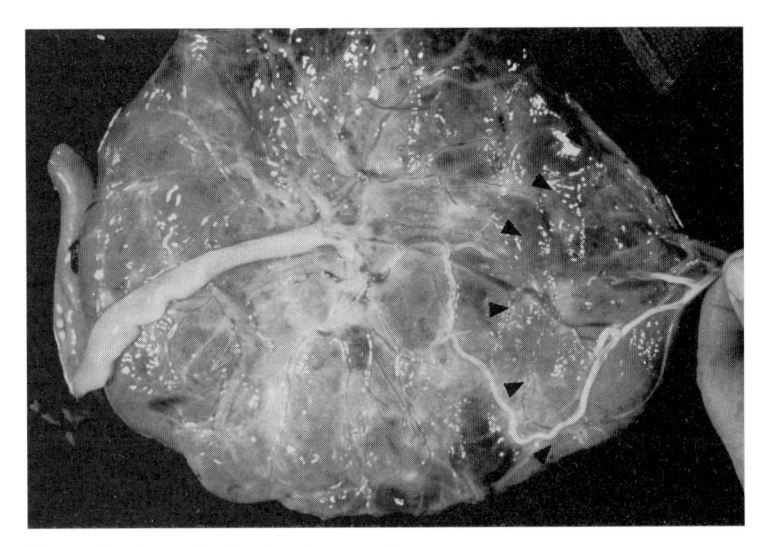

Figure 1 Monochorionic placenta from a 20-week twin loss with A–A and V–V anastomoses. The fetuses had a paradoxical relationship of size to hematocrit. The smaller twin's velamentous cord is being injected. Its small chorionic area is seen outlined with arrows, and may explain the smaller twin's death with subsequent exsanguination of the larger twin via the A–A anastomosis. (From reference 1)

placenta. Various combinations of central and peripheral (velamentous) insertions occur (Figure 1; see Chapter 27).

The presence of either superficial or indirect anastomotic channels between the placental segments potentially allows for the unequal passage of blood between the twins. Depending upon the amount and timing of the passage of blood in the pregnancy, a host of adverse outcomes may result (Table 1)[7].

Table 1 Manifestations of chorioangiopagus pregnancies

Vanishing first-trimester twin

Second-trimester twin loss

Previable/premature twin–twin transfusion with hydrops poly/oligohydramnios

Discordance of weight, hematocrit, organ size in near-term live twins

Concordant term twins with significantly different hematocrits

Acardiac twinning

Structural loss by disruption from DIC or shock after co-twin death

---

The complications of chorioangiopagous vessels listed in Table 1 span the entire duration of pregnancy. Initial studies of early loss of sonographically diagnosed twins did not include placental examination[8]. In 1986, Sulak and Dodson reported pathological confirmation of vanishing sonographic triplets followed by singleton birth after *in vitro* fertilization and transfer of five embryos[9]. This placenta contained four succenturiate/spuriate lobes and a thickening in the membranes which histologically revealed a degenerated pregnancy.

Unlike chromosomal abnormalities, the role of chorioangiopagous vessels in very early fetal loss has yet to be documented. However, since the loss from a transfusion would occur after the 6th week of embryonic life – when fetal–placental circulation becomes established – the use of vaginal ultrasound earlier in the first trimester might some day demonstrate this event as well as provide evidence for the role of 'transfusion' in developmental abnormalities such as acardius. Theoretically, two normal fetuses with cardiac activity are seen at 3–4 weeks; after 6 weeks, one becomes a pump twin and the other an acardius. By this point in pregnancy, ultrasound assignment of chorion type is possible, and these examinations can document further consequences of MC placentation[10].

In the past, the rates of the complications of MC twinnings outlined in the table were unknown. However, it is possible that with the use of early and frequent ultrasound examinations – especially if twins are detected at the initial scan – a more accurate picture will evolve in the future. Regardless, a substantial number of lost twins from pregnancies that reached term without the benefit of early ultrasound examination will go undetected, because most clinicians fail to perform a truly analytic examination of the placenta at the births they attend[11], and because the quality of the placental examinations provided by many anatomic pathologists is less than ideal.

If one accepts the hypothesis that chorioangiopagous vessels can lead to morbidity and malformations, it is easier to understand flaws in the present-day teratology literature (which rarely reports placental findings), and the incongruities that exist in various published series on antenatal management of twin pregnancies as well as behavioral/developmental studies on identical twin children reared apart. These studies can be profoundly biased by the effects of MC placentation *per se*, specifically the chorioangiopagous vessels or extremes of asymmetric sharing of the common placenta[12]. Figure 1 demonstrates an example of profound chorion asymmetry which can lead to growth retardation of the twin with the small chorion. Without placental examination and documentation, this information becomes lost forever.

The acardiac twin

Perhaps the most dramatic example of the effect of vascular communications on the MZ tendency for sameness is the acardiac fetal malformation. This broad class of anomalies is in reality a spectrum of malformations and reduction defects of the entire visceral and somatic structure, although a relative sparing of the lower body is common[13]. Despite their lack of a primary circulation, acardiac twins survive as a consequence of perfusion via an artery-to-artery anastomosis within the chorion which connects to the normal 'pump' twin. In this manner, the acardius receives reversed arterial perfusion and returns blood to the placenta and co-twin via its umbilical vein and a vein-to-vein anastomosis. Since monochorionicity and chorioangiopagous vessels are constant findings in acardiac twins, this type of placentation is believed to be the etiology of the condition. Although some chromosomal aneuploidy has been observed in acardiacs, the majority of their pump twins have normal chromosomes[14]. Regardless of the acardiac's karyotype, the patterns of defects are such that specific chromosomal abnormalities, *per se*, could not explain their appearance.

The risk to the normal pump twin associated with an acardius relates to the vastly expanded cardiac demand, which may lead to cardiac failure (Figure 2). The mortality for the normal twin averages 50–75%. Moore *et al.* reported one of the largest series of such pregnancies, and observed that the relationship of the weight ratio of the acardius to the pump twin was predictive of perinatal complications and outcome[15]. Once hydrops or hydramnios occurs in a previable pregnancy, reducing cardiac load by isolating the acardius may improve the outcome. The precariousness of the pump twin's survival is reflected by recent reports of selective delivery of the acardius by *hysterotomy* in an effort to salvage the normal twin[16,17]. A less invasive approach was suggested by Quintero *et al.*[18] who performed fetoscopic umbilical cord ligation of the acardiac twin. But this technique requires that the acardiac twin has a cord long enough to be identified and tied, and that the diamnionic status of the twins be converted to monoamnionic and risk cord entanglement. Porreco *et al.*[19] successfully placed a thrombogenic metal coil into the umbilical artery of the acardius at 24 weeks and gained 15 additional weeks for the pump twin. This approach – interrupting the communicating vessels – represents less risk to the mother and her future reproductive ability, and simultaneously addresses the pathogenesis of the condition. The section below describes efforts to

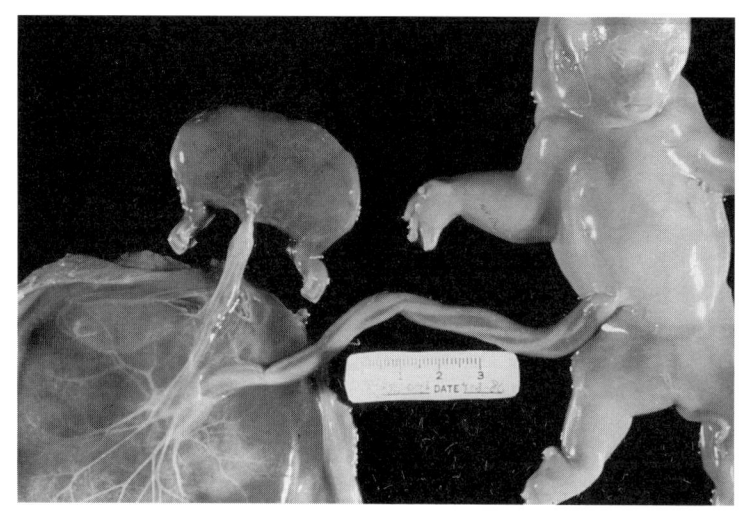

Figure 2 Midpregnancy loss of a normal pump twin and an acardiac twin in a rhesus monkey pregnancy, similar to the experience in humans. The pump twin succumbed from non-immunologic hydrops. The monoamniotic monochorionic placenta, umbilical cords and fetuses were delivered intact. (Courtesy California Regional Primate Center, Davis, CA)

accomplish similar vascular isolation of MC twins utilizing fetoscopy combined with the coagulative properties of laser light.

Sirenomelia

Additional evidence for the vascular etiology of somatic malformations is provided by the equally dramatic sirenomelia. Here a single umbilical artery *of vitelline origin* assumes the function of the umbilical arteries and diverts (steals) blood from the caudal end of the embryo[20]. The fetus's upper body is spared, but the lower extremity remains unipodal from the failure of allantoic structures to cleave the lower limb bud field. The cause of the failure of the allantois to develop normally is unknown. Curiously, sirenomelia is 100 times more common in MZ twins compared to singletons[21].

Comment

Both acardia and sirenomelia are profound examples of abnormalities believed to occur from poor perfusion during development. The etiology of both conditions may lie in the placental vasculature. Additional and significant losses of previously formed structures also occur in normally developing fetuses as a result of decreased vascular flow – from either debris or hypovolemic shock[22,23]. Theoretically, it follows that minor anomalies and malformations of all systems might also occur from such a mechanism and that very subtle clues might be found only by a careful placental examination.

The twin–twin transfusion syndrome

As mentioned elsewhere in this text (Chapter 4), the morbidity and mortality rates associated with identical twinning increase as a function of the time from fertilization to embryo cleavage. The greatest mortality is seen in conjoined twins (split after 14 days), with monoamniotic twins (split during the second week) experiencing a near 50% loss rate, primarily due to umbilical cord entanglement. Diamnionic monochorionic twins (the largest placental group type of MZ twins) experience varying degrees of morbidity and mortality based on the nature of their chorioangiopagus status[24]. Although all DiMo twins have communicating vessels, only approximately 15% develop clinically specific signs and symptoms of a transfusion phenomenon. When this process occurs in anatomically normal previable twins (<26 weeks), an 80–100% mortality rate has been observed[25–27].

Previable twin–twin transfusion syndrome (TTTS) is a presumptive diagnosis made by ultrasound scanning in patients who generally present large for dates[27]. The criteria include like-sex, a single placental disc, a thin (amnions only) interfetal membrane septum, discordant fetal size, discordant amniotic fluid volumes (poly/oligohydramnios, stuck twin), and possible non-immune hydrops from overload or anemia. With the shift of the diagnosis from the pediatric pathologist to the obstetrician, a window of opportunity has now been created to modify the uniformly poor outcome of this subset of MZ twins.

The antepartum diagnosis of TTTS prior to viability presents the clinician with a therapeutic dilemma, because no treatment to date has been associated with a uniformly improved outcome. Expectant management generally results in 100% mortality. Previously reported attempts at therapy have largely been symptomatic or created serious ethical choices for the parents and physician. These included serial reduction amniocenteses for polyhydramnios[28], maternal digitalization for fetal non-immune hydrops[29], feticide by *in utero* ligation of one umbilical cord[1], cardiac injection[30], or surgical removal of one twin[17]. Repeated reduction amniocenteses have produced the best outcomes thus far. Blickstein calculated the overall perinatal mortality rate to be 55% (23 of 42 babies) in a review of reported cases treated by amniocentesis scattered over half a century, but treatment was applied at various gestational ages[6]. Many of these reports, including the publications by Elliott *et al.* and Mahoney *et al.*, do not report placental findings (type or communications)[31,32]; despite this, these authors reported survival rates of 79% and 69%, respectively. Mahoney *et al.* reported a 37% complication rate from amniocenteses, and only three of 12 survivors were intact.

As a 'therapy', selective feticide is indicative of clinicians' general perception of the hopelessness of symptomatic therapy at mid-pregnancy. Hysterotomy *risks the mother's future reproductive capacity*, and cardiac injections place the surviving fetus at risk, because of potential transfer of thromboplastin and blood through the open communications from one twin to the other. The death of one member of an MZ pair with MC placentation, whether spontaneous or induced, has been associated with death or serious neurological and anatomical complications in the survivor[22].

Because TTTS does not exist without chorioangiopagous vessels and passage of blood from one twin to the other, clearly, none of the therapies proposed to date have been directed at the pathogenesis of the condition. Only the interruption of the vascular communication would represent a logical means to (1) halt the one-way transfusion of nutrients between the twins; (2) improve their intrauterine environment; (3) prolong the pregnancy; and (4) prevent the passage of debris or the occurrence of shock and structural loss should one twin die. However, surgical interruption of the communicating vessels must be performed with techniques that, in themselves, do not jeopardize the continuation of the pregnancy or risk the future reproductive capacity of the mother.

The evolution of surgical lasers, especially the neodymium:YAG, has provided a technological capability to photocoagulate placental vessels in a fluid-filled medium. Even when passed through a diminutive fetoscope, sufficient laser energy can be delivered via a fiberoptic cable to destroy the selected parts of the placental vasculature, with minimal risk to the pregnancy and uterus. Preliminary experiments in animals to test this concept were initially performed at the University of Utah and the California Regional Primate Center[33]. These experiments proved that placental vessels could be sealed with minimal placental damage and no ill effects from the laser seen in the fetuses.

Later, a special fetoscope was constructed for use in the overdistended human uterus and to maximize *placental* visualization. The 4 × 2-mm fetoscope sleeve (Bryan Corporation, Woburn, MA) has a 25-cm telescope and a side port to accommodate the 400-μm quartz rod to transmit the laser light. This prototype has performed admirably in the first 25 cases of TTTS in humans treated at the University of Utah and the Medical College of Wisconsin. The details of the first three cases were recently reported[34].

During our ongoing pilot study, we limit treatments of TTTS to patients at 17–24 weeks' gestation, with posteriorly implanted placentas. Not only do these cases have the worst prognosis, but the fetal eyelids are fused at that time, providing the necessary protection from reflected laser light. Upon entering the sac of the polyhydramniotic twin with the fetoscope, it is first necessary to visualize the vascular equator. Here, the twins' arteries and veins, which course on the chorion surface from their respective umbilical cord insertions, terminate, as (a) a normal cotyledon with an artery and a vein diving into the placenta without other vessels nearby; (b) direct communications in which an artery or vein is found to course on the surface from one circulation to the other; or (c) indirect communications. The last appears as an artery from one twin entering a cotyledon without its companion vein, whereas a vein originating from the co-twin's chorion is seen entering this shared cotyledon. Finally, the blood vessels may disappear behind the interfetal membrane septum where their characterization is rendered impossible.

Direct communications, indirect communications, and vessels that disappear behind the interfetal membrane septum are photocoagulated at 60 W over a distance of 1 cm. Questionable vascular relationships can also be coagulated, recognizing the possible risk of rendering a normal cotyledon non-functional. Thus far, our postpartum examination of laser impact sites has verified the long-term occlusion of chorion vasculature and separation of the twins' placental circulations.

Conclusion

Monochorionic placentation has been considered a congenital anomaly *per se*, because of the significant role it plays in the morbidity and mortality of multiple pregnancy. Most of the clinically challenging prenatal risks can be traced to the chorioangiopagus status of the fetuses. Many of the serious developmental abnormalities, such as acardius, may never be treatable and will continue to cause fetal wastage. However, the wastage associated with normal fetuses affected by severe mid-pregnancy TTTS or pump twins in heart failure from supporting an acardius may now benefit from a new therapeutic option[35]. My experience thus far indicates the feasibility of identifying and interrupting the pathological placental vessels with fetoscopic laser surgery. The ethics and superiority of this technique compared to hysterotomy, feticide or symptomatic therapy will be determined by future controlled trials.

References

1. Benirschke, K. and Kaufmann, P. (1990). *The Pathology of the Human Placenta*, 2nd edn., pp. 716–20. (New York: Springer-Verlag)
2. Landy, H.J., Weiner, S., Corson, S.L. *et al.* (1986). The 'vanishing twin': ultrasonographic assessment of fetal disappearance in the first trimester. *Am. J. Obstet. Gynecol.*, **155**, 14
3. Schatz, F. (1882). Eine besondere Art von einseitiger Polyhydramnie mit anderseitiger Olygohydramnie bei eineiigen Zwillingen. *Arch. Gynak.*, **19**, 329
4. Robertson, E.G. and Neer, K.J. (1983). Placental injection studies in twin gestation. *Obstet. Gynecol.*, **147**, 170

5. Bleisch, V.R. (1965). Placental circulation of human twins: constant arterial anastomoses in monochorionic placentas. *Am. J. Obstet. Gynecol.*, **91**, 862
6. Blickstein, I. (1990). The twin–twin transfusion syndrome. *Obstet. Gynecol.*, **76**, 714
7. Naeye, R.L. (1987). Functionally important disorders of the placenta, umbilical cord, and fetal membranes. *Hum. Pathol.*, **18**, 680
8. Landy, H.J., Keith, L. and Keith, D. (1982). The vanishing twin. *Acta Genet. Med. Gemellol.*, **31**, 179
9. Sulak, L.E. and Dodson, M.G. (1986). The vanishing twin: pathologic confirmation of an ultrasonographic phenomenon. *Obstet. Gynecol.*, **68**, 811
10. Barss, V.S., Benacerraf, B.R. and Frigoletto, F.D. (1985). Ultrasonographic determination of chorion type in twin gestation. *Obstet. Gynecol.*, **66**, 779
11. Salafia, C.M. and Vintzileos, A.M. (1990). Why all placentas should be examined by a pathologist in 1990. *Am. J. Obstet. Gynecol.*, **163**, 1282
12. Baldwin, V.J. (1992). Pathology of multiple pregnancy. In Dimmick, J.E. and Kalousek, D.K. (eds.) *Developmental Pathology of the Embryo and Fetus*, pp. 320–40. (Philadelphia: J.B. Lippincott)
13. Van Allen, M.I., Smith, D.W. and Shepard, T.H. (1983). Twin reversed arterial perfusion (TRAP) sequence: a study of 14 twin pregnancies with acardius. *Semin. Perinatol.*, **7**, 285
14. Moore, C.A., Buehler, B.A., McManus, B.M. et al. (1987). Acephalus-acardia in twins with aneuploidy. *Am. J. Med. Genet.* (Suppl.) **3**, 139
15. Moore, T.R., Gale, S. and Benirschke, K. (1990). Perinatal outcome of forty-nine pregnancies complicated by acardiac twinning. *Am. J. Obstet. Gynecol.*, **163**, 907
16. Robie, G.F., Payne, G.G. and Morgan, M.A. (1989). Selective delivery of an acardiac acephalic twin. *N. Engl. J. Med.*, **320**, 512
17. Fries, M.H., Goldberg, J.D. and Golbus, M.S. (1992). Treatment of acardiac-acephalus twin gestations by hysterotomy and selective delivery. *Obstet. Gynecol.*, **79**, 601
18. Quintero, R.A., Reish, M., Puder, K.S. et al. (1994). Umbilical-cord ligation of an acardiac twin by fetoscopy at 19 weeks of gestation. *N. Engl. J. Med.*, **330**, 469
19. Porreco, R.P., Barton, S.M. and Haverkamp, A.D. (1991). Occlusion of umbilical artery in acardiac, acephalus twin. *Lancet*, **1**, 326
20. Stevenson, R.E., Jones, K.L., Phelan, M.C. et al. (1986). Vascular steal: the pathogenetic mechanism producing sirenomelia and associated defects of the viscera and soft tissues. *Pediatrics*, **78**, 451
21. Davies, J., Chazen, E. and Nancy, W.E. (1971). Symmelia in one of monozygotic twins. *Teratology*, **4**, 367
22. Patten, R.M., Mack, L.A., Nyberg, D.A. et al. (1989). Twin embolization syndrome: prenatal sonographic detection and significance. *Radiology*, **173**, 685
23. Okamura, K., Murotsuki, J., Tanigawara, S. et al. (1994). Funipuncture for evaluation of hematologic and coagulation indices in the surviving twin following co-twin's death. *Obstet. Gynecol.*, **83**, 975
24. Benirschke, K. and Kim, C.K. (1973). Multiple pregnancy (first of two parts). *N. Engl. J. Med.*, **288**, 127
25. Moore, T.R., Garret, V. and Benirschke, K. (1991). Prognostic factors for survival in the twin transfusion syndrome. *Am. J. Obstet. Gynecol.*, **164**, 279
26. Gonsoulin, W., Moise, K.J., Kirshon, B. et al. (1990). Outcome of twin–twin transfusion diagnosed before 28 weeks of gestation. *Obstet. Gynecol.*, **75**, 214
27. Brown, D.L., Benson, C.B., Driscoll, S.G. et al. (1989). Twin–twin transfusion syndrome: sonographic findings. *Radiology*, **170**, 61
28. Saunders, N.J., Snijders, R.J. and Nicolaides, K.H. (1992). Therapeutic amniocentesis in twin–twin transfusion syndrome appearing in the second trimester of pregnancy. *Am. J. Obstet. Gynecol.*, **166**, 820
29. De Lia, J.E., Emery, M.G., Sheafor, S.A. et al. (1985). Twin transfusion syndrome: successful *in utero* treatment with digoxin. *Int. J. Gynaecol. Obstet.*, **23**, 197
30. Baldwin, V.J. and Wittman, B.K. (1990). Pathology of intragestational intervention in twin–twin transfusion syndrome. *Pediatr. Pathol.*, **10**, 79
31. Elliott, J.P., Urig, M.A. and Clewell, W.H. (1990). Aggressive therapeutic amniocentesis for treatment of twin–twin transfusion syndrome. *Obstet. Gynecol.*, **77**, 537
32. Mahoney, B.S., Petty, C.N., Nyberg, D.A. et al. (1990). The 'stuck twin' phenomena: ultrasonographic findings, pregnancy outcome, and management with serial amniocenteses. *Am. J. Obstet. Gynecol.*, **163**, 1513

33. De Lia, J.E. (1990). The neodymium:YAG laser in fetal/placental surgery. In Keye, W.R. (ed.) *Laser Surgery in Gynecology and Obstetrics*, 2nd edn., pp. 242–9. (Chicago: Year Book Medical Publishers)
34. De Lia, J.E., Cruikshank, D.P. and Keye, W.R. (1990). Fetoscopic neodymium:YAG laser occlusion of placental vessels in severe twin–twin transfusion syndrome. *Obstet. Gynecol.*, **75**, 1046
35. De Lia, J.E., Kuhlman, R.S., Cruikshank, D.P. *et al.* (1993). Placental surgery: a new frontier. *Placenta*, **14**, 477

The intrauterine demise of one fetus 30

J.A. Lopez-Zeno and J. Navarro-Pando

Introduction

One of the most serious and catastrophic antepartum complications of multiple pregnancy is the intrauterine fetal demise (IUFD) of one or more of the fetuses. This event generates an enormous emotional stress for the patient as well as the obstetric team. Fortunately, this condition is rare, with a reported incidence of 0.5–6.8% of all multiple gestations[1]. Although several case reports and retrospective reviews have been published[2], controversy still exists regarding the ideal management of this complication.

Etiology

The most frequent etiology of IUFD of one fetus is the presence of monochorionic placentation. Indeed, this type of placentation is present in 47–76.5% of all twin gestations complicated by an IUFD, and is also associated with growth discordancy and the twin–twin transfusion syndrome[3]. The risk of IUFD with monochorionic placentation is 3:1 compared with dichorionic placentation[3]. According to Ahn and Phelan, growth discordancy is present in approximately 15% of all twin gestations[4]. If severe, the placental insufficiency of the smaller twin can ultimately result in an IUFD. This process is more frequent with monochorionic placentation and it may be a manifestation of the twin–twin transfusion syndrome[1,5,6]. Some monochorionic placentas are also monoamnionic. The presence of only one gestational sac is associated with the possibility of a catastrophic cord entanglement[7] in as many as 50% of such pregnancies[8].

Although the presence of dichorionic placentation carries a lower probability of an IUFD, this phenomenon may not be construed as protective. In one series of 19 multiple pregnancies complicated by IUFD, Carlson and Towers[1] reported 53% (10 of 19) as having a dichorionic placentation. However, only two of these mothers remained without medical or obstetric complications. Clearly, multiple pregnancies with superimposed medical or obstetric complications should be considered at higher risk and, as such, should be monitored closely for signs of fetal compromise.

Less frequently encountered are problems that may affect only one fetus, including congenital infections[9], chromosomal abnormalities and malformations. One recent large study failed to document a higher incidence of congenital infections or chromosomal abnormalities in twin gestations[10]. The higher incidence of congenital anomalies in twin gestations is documented elsewhere in this book (see Chapter 7).

Management

The management of any IUFD requires close and thorough clinical scrunity, keeping in mind the emotional stress that the IUFD and its resultant scrunity exerts upon both parents. Numerous management decisions are in order when the diagnosis of an IUFD is made in a multiple pregnancy. Different clinical approaches may be considered, depending on chorionicity, gestational age and the condition of the surviving fetus. All are discussed separately in the sections that follow. In the final analysis, the presence of a maternal complication may call for significantly different management.

Table 1 Diagnosis of dichorionic gestation

Separate placentas
Different fetal sexes
Presence of three or more layers in the amniotic membranes
Thickness of the amniotic membranes of ≥ 2 mm

Chorionicity

If a dichorionic placenta is visualized on ultrasound, the possibility of morbidity or mortality in the surviving fetus is lessened (see next paragraph). Chorionicity can be determined by several means (Table 1). All are discussed in detail elsewhere in this book. Once a diagnosis of a dichorionic placentation is made, it is appropriate to consider expectant management with serial antenatal monitoring by ultrasound and non-stress tests (NSTs) (see Chapter 20), along with weekly maternal coagulation profiles to rule out a consumption coagulopathy originating from the placenta of the dead fetus. This complication is often mentioned in texts and articles, but only rarely reported[11]. It is more likely to occur in patients with a dead fetus retained for more than 4 weeks. Using data obtained from the observation of singleton pregnancies, Pritchard[12] estimated the incidence of maternal disseminated intravascular coagulation (DIC) after 4 weeks of retention of a dead fetus to be 25%. In cases in which the death of the twin occurred at a very premature gestational age, delivery may not be an alternative. If during the expectant management the mother develops DIC, heparin has been used successfully, to stop the coagulopathy[13].

Another possible scenario involves a diamniotic monochorionic pregnancy in which a common placenta is identified by ultrasound and none of the findings suggestive of dichorionic placentation are present. In such an instance, it is possible that thrombogenic material from the dead fetus might enter the circulation of the living fetus, causing infarction or coagulopathy through the same placental anastomoses that give rise to the twin–twin transfusion syndrome. This type of embolization is hypothesized as the etiology for what is charcaterized as the fetal coagulopathy syndrome (FCS). A wide range of unusual fetal lesions has been reported as part of this syndrome. Among them are the postpartum cerebellar syndrome[14], multicystic encephalomalacia[15], renal infarcts[16] and neonatal skin slough[17]. The true incidence of these complications is unknown, as is the incidence of maternal DIC, but it is assumed that both complications are rare. Nevertheless, because of their potential severity, an earlier delivery should be considered, because no data exist to suggest how soon after the demise the FCS might develop.

The last (and probably most serious) clinical picture is that of a monoamniotic twin pregnancy. In this situation, it is reasonable to assume that the etiology of the IUFD is cord entanglement. This would place the surviving twin at great risk of undergoing a similar accident. Prevention of these catastrophies is an elusive, if not impossible, task. Usually there are no completely reliable advance indications of complete asphyxiation from entanglement, although recent reports strongly suggest that variable decelerations detected on electronic fetal heart monitoring is suggestive of impending cord occlusion. Should such abnormalities be detected, emergency abdominal delivery may be warranted, depending on the estimated gestational age. The only role for expectant management would be prior to 28 weeks, due to the severe complications attendant on a very preterm delivery. Between 28 and 32 weeks, maternal steroid administration is reasonable to induce lung maturity. After 32 weeks, delivery should be strongly considered, even though complications of prematurity remain a distinct possibility.

A recent article by Liu *et al.*[1] reported a series of 41 sets of multiple gestations (38 twins, three triplets) complicated by fetal demise of one infant. Monochorionic placentation was present in 74% of the cases. To the surprise of the investigators, 49% of the surviving infants had neurological damage. Of these, 21% had a dichorionic placentation. It appears that this damage can also result from mechanisms other than embolization from the dead fetus and/or placenta. Careful attention should be given to any other complications that may be present.

After delivery, a complete postmortem examination of the deceased twin and the placenta is of great importance if any explanation for this complication is to be attempted. Close supervision of the surviving twin is urged, in view of the possibility of the FCS becoming apparent during the neonatal period.

It is important to emphasize that rigid standards of care based on randomized trials do no exist. Rather, this complication requires significant individualization of care, especially if the etiology of the IUFD is one that compromises the possible survival of the remaining live fetus(es). In this circumstance, the clinician may have no other choice but to deliver a premature fetus from its hostile uterine environment.

Gestational age

For all practical purposes, if an IUFD of one twin occurs at term, or if a positive diagnosis of pulmonary maturity has been made for the surviving twin, delivery should be accomplished without hesitation. The route should be indicated by the obstetric circumstances. Automatic Cesarean section is not required. Induction of labor should be considered if the maternal and fetal conditions are appropriate. On the other hand, if the fetal demise is diagnosed far from term or if the surviving fetus(es) has an immature pulmonary profile, the clinical management must be individualized. As a general guideline, the clinician should assume expectant management before 28 weeks, of gestation. Between 28 and 32 weeks, the administration of steroids could accelerate the development of pulmonary maturity in the surviving fetus(es). After 32 weeks, delivery should be accomplished after documentation of pulmonary maturity. At some medical centers, neonatal statistics document ≥95% survival after 32 weeks. Obviously, the clinician will have to judge at which gestational age intensive neonatal care will be better than the intrauterine environment.

Condition of the surviving fetus

Once the diagnosis of IUFD is made in one of the fetuses of a multiple gestation, close surveillance of the surviving fetus(es) is appropriate. The frequency of such surveillance will depend on the resources available to the clinician and to the status of the surviving twin. The non-stress test should be performed a minimum of twice a week. As an alternative, biophysical profiles can be utilized. Frequent sonography is essential. Unfortunately, once sonographic signs of embolization to the surviving fetus are detected, the likelihood of adverse neurological sequelae is high[5,18]. If signs of fetal compromise are evident, immediate delivery should be accomplished even if the gestational age is premature.

Conclusion

The management of multiple gestations complicated with an IUFD remains one of challenging clinical problems in the practice of obstetrics. The possibility of prevention of IUFD by identifying multiple gestations with monochorionic placentation and then increasing the level of antenatal surveillance needs to be explored. Clearly, once the problem is present, close fetal and maternal monitoring are warranted.

References

1. Carlson, N.J. and Towers, C.V. (1989). Multiple gestation complicated by the death of one fetus. *Obstet. Gynecol.*, **73**, 685–9
2. Enbom, J.A. (1985). Intrauterine death of one twin. *Am. J. Obstet. Gynecol.*, **152**, 424–9
3. Benirschke, K. (1961). Twin placenta in perinatal mortality. *NY State J. Med.*, **61**, 1499–508

4. Ahn, M.O. and Phelan, J.P. (1988). Multiple pregnancy: antepartum management. *Clin. Perinatol.*, **15**, 55
5. Liu, S., Benirschke, D., Scioscia, A.L. and Mannino, F.L. (1992). Intrauterine death in multiple gestation. *Acta Genet. Med. Gemellol.*, **41**, 5–26
6. Bebbington, M.W. and Wittmann, B.K. (1989). Fetal transfusion syndrome: antenatal factors predicting outcome. *Am. J. Obstet. Gynecol.*, **160**, 913
7. Lyndrup, J. and Schouenborg, L. (1987). Cord entanglement in monoamniotic twin pregnancies. *Eur. J. Obstet. Gynecol. Reprod. Biol.*, **26**, 275–8
8. Carr, S.R., Aronson, M.P. and Coustan, D.R. (1990). Survival rates of monoamniotic twins do not decrease after 30 weeks' gestation. *Am. J. Obstet. Gynecol.*, **163**, 719–22
9. Vogler, C., Kohl, S. and Rosenberg, H.S. (1986). Cytomegalovirus infection and fetal death in a twin. A case report. *J. Reprod. Med.*, **31**, 207–10
10. Spellacy, W.N., Handler, A. and Ferre, C.D. (1990). A case–control study of 1253 twin pregnancies from a 1982–1987 perinatal data base. *Obstet. Gynecol.*, **75**, 168–71
11. Landy, H.J. and Weingold, A.B. (1989). Management of a multiple gestation complicated by an antepartum fetal demise. *Obstet. Gynecol. Surv.*, **44**, 171–6
12. Pritchard, J.A. (1959). Fetal death *in utero*. *Obstet. Gynecol.*, **14**, 573–80
13. Romero, R., Duffy, T.P., Berkowitz, R.L., Chang, E. and Hobbins, J.C. (1984). Prolongation of a preterm pregnancy complicated by death of a single twin *in utero* and disseminated intravascular coagulation. Effects of treatment with heparin. *N. Engl. J. Med.*, **310**, 772–4
14. Averback, P. and Wiglesworth, F.W. (1977). Monochorionic, monoamniotic, double-battledore placenta with stillborn and postpartum cerebellar syndrome. *Am. J. Obstet. Gynecol.*, **128**, 697–9
15. Yoshioka, H., Kadomoto, Y., Mino, M., Morikawa, Y., Kasubuchi, Y. and Kusunoki, T. (1979). Multicystic encephalomalacia in liveborn twin with a stillborn macerated co-twin. *J. Pediatr.*, **95**, 798–800
16. Moore, C.M., McAdams, A.J. and Sutherland, J. (1969). Intrauterine disseminated intravascular coagulation: a syndrome of multiple pregnancy with a dead twin fetus. *J. Pediatr.*, **74**, 523–8
17. Mannino, F.L., Jones, K.L. and Benirschke, K. (1977). Congenital skin defects and fetus papyraceus. *J. Pediatr.*, **91**, 559–64
18. Patten, R.M., Mack, L.A., Harvey, D., Cyr, D.R. and Pretorius, D.H. (1989). Disparity of amniotic fluid volume and fetal size: problem of the stuck twin – US studies. *Radiology*, **172**, 153–7

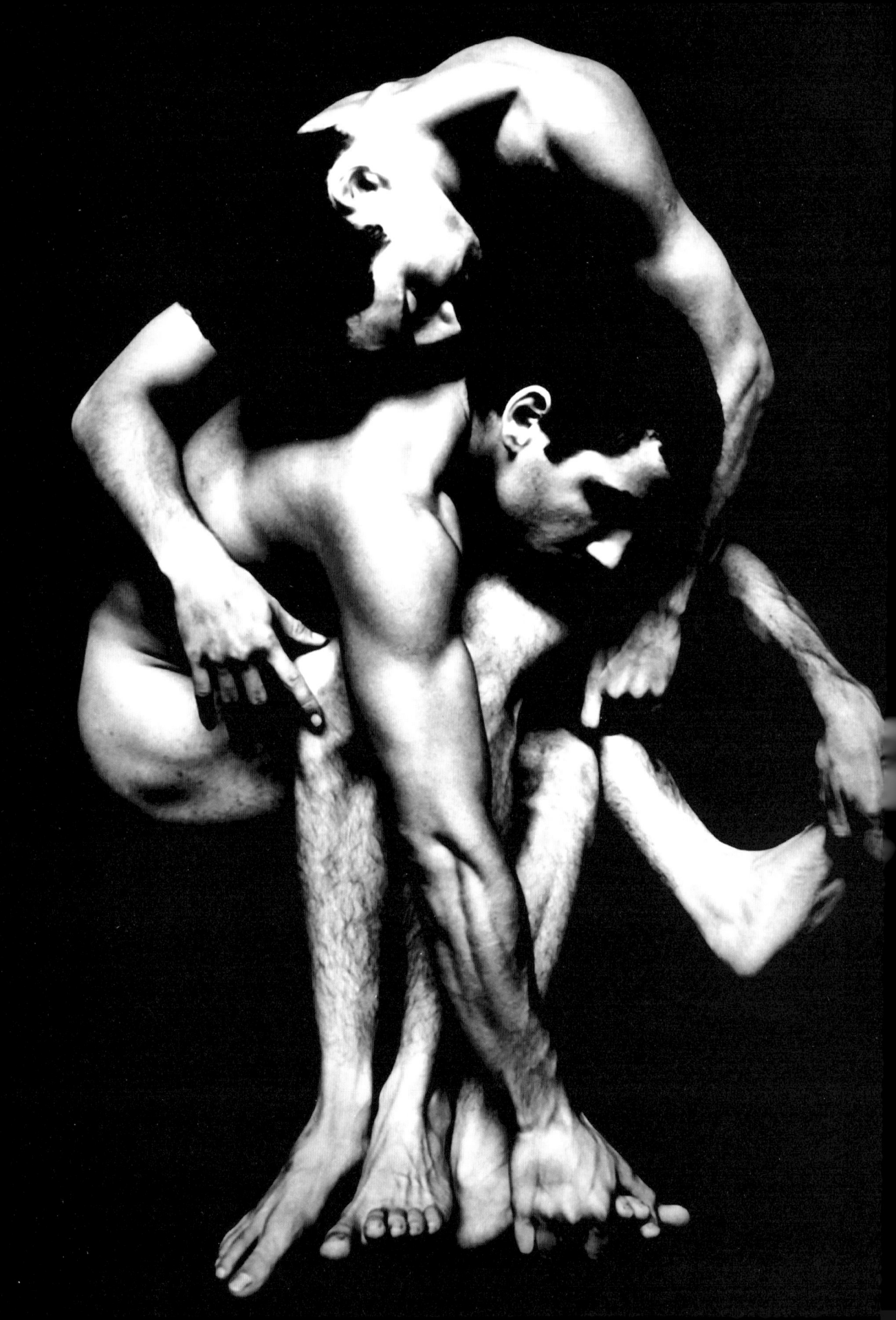

section VI
Antepartum Considerations

Refusion

David Teplica, 1991,
Collection of Harry Drake, Minneapolis, Minnesota

The physiology of preterm labor 31

R.E. Besinger and N.J. Carlson

Introduction

Premature labor contributes substantially to perinatal morbidity and mortality in the multifetal pregnancy. The likelihood of twins being born prior to 37 weeks in the USA during 1985 was 43% compared to 9% for singletons[1]. More importantly, 11.4% of twins are born before the end of 31 weeks' gestation compared to 1.6% of singletons, and 9.1% of twins weighed less than 1500 g at birth compared to 0.9% of singletons in that same year[1]. The incidence of preterm delivery in triplet pregnancies is even more alarming, with over 80% of these pregnancies experiencing premature labor[2].

The causes of the increased rate of preterm labor and delivery in twins (and higher-order multiple gestations) are not entirely clear. (Editor: The term multifetal as used in this chapter refers to twins *and* higher-order gestations.) Not only is the mean weekly frequency of uterine contractions significantly higher in twin compared to singleton pregnancies[3,4], but a gradual increase in the frequency of contractions occurs as twin gestations progress[3]. This increase is accompanied by a gradual increase in low-amplitude high-frequency contractions within the 48 h prior to the onset of overt preterm labor, a phenomenon which is more pronounced in triplet and quadruplet gestations[4,5]. Clinical observations such as these suggest a characteristic pattern of increasing baseline uterine contractility in multifetal pregnancy, followed by a prodromal state of excessive uterine irritability immediately prior to overt preterm labor.

The purpose of this chapter is to characterize a physiological basis for the increased incidence of preterm labor in multifetal gestations and explore potentially associated clinical factors. Whereas scientific investigation into the causes of preterm labor in the singleton pregnancy is progressing, the application of these techniques and findings to multiple gestations has been limited. This circumstance stems at least in part from the preference of investigators to simplify their study designs by excluding multiple gestations. As a result, much of the current understanding of premature labor in singleton gestations necessarily will be extrapolated to the circumstances of multifetal pregnancy. In some situations, hypotheses for future investigation will also be presented.

Physiological factors affecting uterine contractility

A model of myometrial contractility encompassing both term as well as preterm labor has been proposed by Garfield in 1984 (Figure 1)[6]. This model is useful to explore differences in uterine contractility in singleton versus multifetal gestations. Six major factors contribute to uterine contractility in any pregnancy: actin–myosin interactions, intracellular calcium metabolism, local prostaglandin production, oxytocin sensitivity, cellular responses to estrogen/progesterone and the formation of gap junctions. Specific differences in these factors in multifetal compared to singleton pregnancies may explain the increased incidence of preterm labor in multiple gestations.

Actin–myosin interactions

Actin–myosin interactions in uterine smooth muscle form the molecular basis of uterine contractions[7]. The thick filaments containing

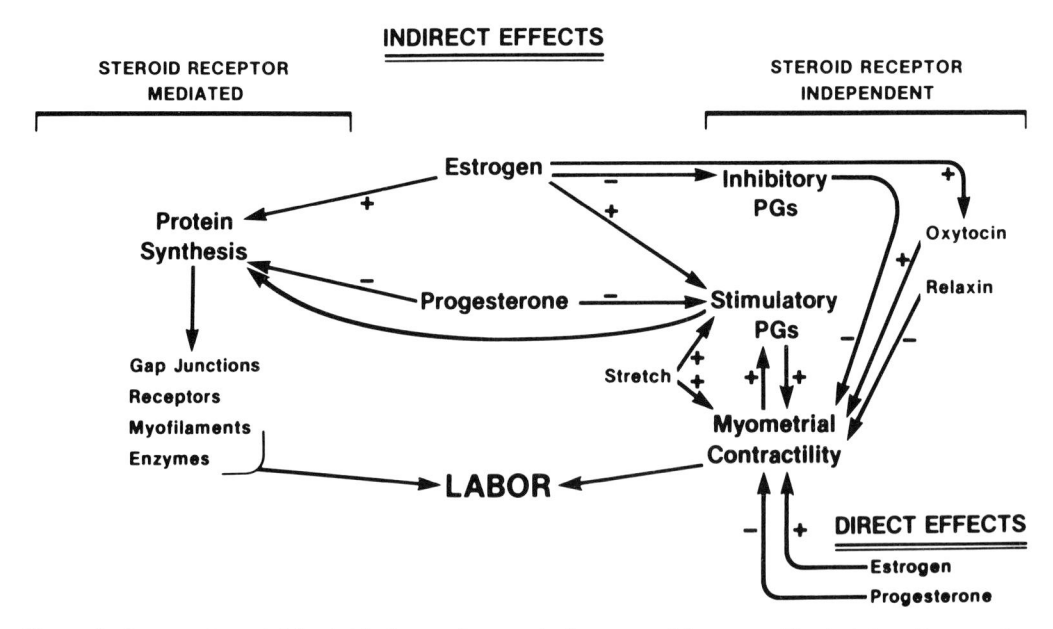

Figure 1 Proposed model for initiation and control of myometrial contractility in labor. From reference 6, with permission

the protein myosin are irregularly aligned and interdigitate with the thin filaments containing actin. The thin filaments are arranged in parallel to the cell axis or in rosettes, and attach to the plasma membranes via dense bodies. This unique arrangement of actin and myosin accounts for the ability of a smooth muscle cell to shorten to less than 50% and lengthen to more than twice its resting length[8]. The contraction–relaxation cycle is initiated by a calcium-dependent phosphorylation of the myosin light chain[9].

The uterine overdistension accompanying multifetal pregnancy places a unique set of physiological demands upon myometrial actin–myosin function. When smooth muscle cells of the uterus are stretched past their resting length, they produce a greater force and lower velocity of contraction[7]. The frequency of spontaneous contractions in these cells also increases as they elongate[10]. *In vitro* observations such as these can be extrapolated to multifetal gestations by which a disproportionate degree of myometrial stretch places these pregnancies at greater risk for spontaneous and forceful contractions prior to term.

Intracellular calcium metabolism

The concentration of intracellular calcium is a major determinant of myometrial contractility[7]. Smooth muscle cellular contractions are initiated either by electrical stimuli or by hormonal binding at the cell membrane. Whereas electromechanical coupling of contractions is characteristic of smooth as well as striated muscle cells, pharmacomechanical coupling is unique to smooth muscle cell function and plays an important role in the initiation of uterine contractions. Myometrial cell membranes possess voltage-operated as well as receptor-operated calcium channels; both allow the influx of calcium into the cell. Intracellular calcium levels are crucial to the regulation of the contraction–relaxation cycle. Receptors in these membrane channels apparently are sensitive to prostaglandins, norepinephrine and calcium channel blocking agents[7]. Calcium channels, along with gap junctions, are vital to the propagation of an action potential among myometrial cells.

Normally, the influx of calcium through membrane channels is insufficient to activate or sustain a cellular contraction. The majority of intracellular calcium for a given contraction are derived from the sarcoplasmic reticulum. Sarcoplasmic reticulum release and the uptake of intracellular calcium is modulated by oxytocin, prostaglandins and magnesium[7]. Thus, the ultimate regulation of intracellular calcium levels occurs in the sarcoplasmic reticulum, whereas the initiation of a contraction sequence in response to a stimulus is attributable to the calcium channels in the myometrial cell membrane.

A wide variety of clinical stimuli have been proposed to explain the onset of preterm uterine contractility. For any of these mechanisms to prove valid, however, they must ultimately alter the intracellular calcium concentration of the myometrial cell. To date, no substantial body of literature investigating the effect of multifetal pregnancy upon the basic intracellular calcium metabolism of myometrial cells has been published.

Local prostaglandin metabolism

Prostaglandins are produced locally in the amnion, chorion and decidua[11] and have profound effects upon uterine contractility. Human fetal membranes store arachidonic acid, the precursor of prostaglandins, which is released by the action of phospholipase A_2. Free arachidonic acid is converted to PGE_2 and $PGF_{2\alpha}$ via the enzyme cyclo-oxygenase[7]. Cyclo-oxygenase activity is stimulated by estradiol[12] and oxytocin stimulates prostaglandin production in the decidua[13]. At the same time, calcium plays a role in mobilization of arachidonic acid in amniotic tissue[14]. *In vitro* studies reveal that human myometrium releases prostaglandins under conditions of progressive stretch[15].

Although certain prostaglandins ultimately regulate intracellular calcium metabolism, and thereby stimulate uterine contractile activity, prostaglandin receptors on the myometrial plasma and sarcoplasmic membranes do not appear to increase in number as gestation progresses[16]. Rather, the onset of labor at term is probably due to an increased local biosynthesis of these agents[7]. The possibility that subclinical infections of the female genital tract stimulate an increased local production of prostaglandins and ultimately are a cause of preterm labor is appealing, but to date has not been adequately substantiated. Some evidence suggests that the fetal fraction of the increasing levels of contractile amniotic prostaglandin production is discordant between the presenting and the second twin as gestation progresses. In one study, higher levels of prostaglandins were present in the amniotic fluid of the presenting twin compared to the aftercoming twin[17].

Increased estrogen production, duplication of amnion/chorion surfaces and the influence of uterine stretch may all be physiological factors that predispose to the increased prostaglandin production associated with preterm labor in the multifetal pregnancy.

Cellular response to estrogen/progesterone

The effects of estrogen and progesterone upon uterine function are derived from the ability of these agents to regulate the myogenic mechanisms of the myometrial cells. Generally, estrogen and progesterone exert opposing effects upon the myogenic properties of the uterus (Table 1)[6]. The effects of both hormones are either acute or delayed. Alterations in plasma membrane excitation and myometrial conduction are acute effects mediated by the influence of estrogen and progesterone on calcium and/or prostaglandin metabolism; the transformation of cellular structures to facilitate contractile activity is a delayed effect, probably mediated through a steroid-receptor system that stimulates (estrogen) or inhibits (progesterone) protein production.

Whereas it is quite possible that the maintenance of pregnancy involves a balance between the levels of progesterone and estrogen, the onset of labor, in contrast, involves an imbalance in which decreasing progesterone levels parallel increasing estrogen and prostaglandin levels[18]. Despite the general unavailability of serial determinations of these hormone levels in multifetal pregnancy prior

Table 1 Effects of estrogen and progesterone on the myogenic properties of the uterus

	Progesterone	Estrogen
Acute effects		
Conduction	increase	decrease
Threshold for stimulation	decrease	increase
Membrane potential	increase	no change
Pacemaker activity	increase	decrease
Spontaneous activity	increase	decrease
Delayed effects		
Adenosine triphosphate	increase	no change
Muscle mass	increase	no change
Sarcoplasmic reticulum	increase	no change
Contractile filaments	increase	no change
Receptors	increase	decrease
Gap junctions	increase	decrease

to the onset of labor, it remains possible that such a regulatory imbalance may play a role in the initiation of preterm contractions in multiple gestations.

Oxytocin sensitivity

It is widely accepted that the myometrium is increasingly sensitive to oxytocin as gestation progresses[7]. The concentration of oxytocin receptors in the myometrium increases toward the end of pregnancy and peaks during labor[19]. This phenomenon appears to be regulated by estrogen and progesterone[20] and mediated by the presence of prostaglandins.

Sensitivity to oxytocin correlates with term as well as preterm delivery. In one investigation, women who delivered preterm had the highest sensitivity to oxytocin[21]. Although the degree of oxytocin sensitivity in multiple gestations has yet to be described in detail, this unknown factor may be central to explaining the increased incidence of preterm labor in multiple gestations. It is quite probable that enhanced oxytocin sensitivity occurs in response to exaggerated local prostaglandin production in multifetal gestations.

Formation of gap junctions

Gap junctions are believed to be the site of electrical coupling between cells and are characterized by regions of approximated plasma membranes with intramembranous proteins forming channels between the cell interiors. The gap junctions between myometrial cells represent a key to the conduction and coordination of myometrial electrophysiological signals[6]. The coordinated propagation of uterine contractions is required to successfully complete the physical work of parturition. Increasing concentrations of gap junctions are observed in humans prior to and during preterm and term labor[7,22]. It appears that the formation of gap junctions is modulated by a variety of hormones, including estrogen, progesterone and prostaglandins[23]. Progesterone inhibits gap junction formation; in contrast, estrogen and prostaglandins promote this process. Fluctuations in the levels of these steroids in late pregnancy probably activates cellular protein synthesis to provide an increased number of gap junctions.

The formation of gap junctions is an early signal that the cellular mechanics of the myometrium are preparing for coordinated uterine contractility and subsequent preterm or term labor. There are no current research data investigating the timing and degree of gap junction formation in multifetal gestations.

Clinical factors associated with preterm labor

Multifetal gestation *per se* is classically described as a cause of preterm delivery. The accompanying explanation generally is as follows: uterine overdistension results in premature activation of the mechanisms responsible for the initiation of labor. Despite the attractiveness of this simplistic explanation, additional etiological factors – infection, premature rupture of membranes, cervical weakness, polyhydramnios, antepartum bleeding, placental hormone production and psychological stress – all must also be considered in any comprehensive approach to understanding preterm labor in multiple gestations (Table 2).

Table 2 Clinical factors associated with preterm labor in multifetal pregnancies

---
Overdistension
Polyhydramnios
Subclinical infections
Antepartum bleeding
Cervical incompetence
Placentation
Psychological stress

Uterine overdistension

A normal characteristic of the human uterus is its ability to distend to hundreds of times its original volumetric capacity. This ability is severely limited, however, when anatomical distortions are present, as is the case with fibromyomata or congenital malformations. In these instances, even singleton pregnancies are at high risk of preterm labor. In other circumstances, the normal uterus can be stretched beyond its usual limits, as is seen with polyhydramnios and/or multiple gestations.

Both *in vitro* and *in vivo* studies have demonstrated that normal myometrial stretch results in the release of prostaglandins which induce cervical softening and initiate labor[15,24]. This increase in prostaglandin production in turn affects calcium metabolism, promotes gap junction formation and increases the sensitivity of the uterus to oxytocin. Excessive stretch may result in an increase of high-frequency, low-amplitude contractions and a higher frequency of stronger uterine contractions. These factors appear to predispose patients with multifetal pregnancy to premature labor. That this is so is suggested by the increasing frequency of preterm labor following the progressive stretching associated with polyhydramnios[25] and an increasing number of fetuses. Despite the reality of these clinical observations, little experimental data specific to multiple gestations are available to confirm this physiological hypothesis.

Acute polyhydramnios is more likely to be associated with preterm labor than a slower accumulation of amniotic fluid[26]. Over time, accommodation to stretch by the uterine musculature may occur, accompanied perhaps by diminished release of prostaglandins and a lessened potential for their subsequent effects. Some authors have shown an increased incidence of preterm labor in primiparous women compared to multigravidas with twin gestations[27]. This suggests that the uterus distended by a previous pregnancy may be able to overdistend for a twin pregnancy with fewer significant contractions.

Polyhydramnios

The increased incidence of polyhydramnios in twin pregnancies is well documented[28]. Polyhydramnios may lead to uterine overdistension and preterm labor. Those pregnancies complicated by twin-to-twin transfusion often are associated with rapid accumulation of amniotic fluid and subsequent preterm labor. It is possible that the rapid distension of the fetal membranes by acute polyhydramnios results in accelerated metabolism of the arachidonic acid stored in the amnion, with subsequent increases in prostaglandin production and stimulation of uterine contractility. A sudden stretch of the fetal membranes may also play a role in weakening the chorion/amnion, hence making them more vulnerable to rupture. Scientific data to support this hypothesis in either singleton or multifetal gestations are not available at this time.

The polyhydramnios associated with monozygotic twinning occurs in the presence of excessive fetal urination in the hyperperfused twin[29]. Fetal urine contains platelet activating factor (PAF) which can stimulate uterine contractions[30]. It is thus possible that the overproduction of fetal urine in multiple gestations with polyhydramnios may predispose to premature contractions, perhaps due to increased amounts of PAF. This hypothesis has yet to be verified.

Subclinical infection

Numerous investigations have focused on the role of micro-organisms ascending from the lower genital tract to cause inflammations and/or infections of the decidua, fetal membranes and amniotic fluid. Colonization of the vagina/cervix with *Gardnerella vaginalis*, *Chlamydia trachomatis*, *Mycoplasma hominis/Ureaplasma urealyticum*, group B streptococcus, *Neisseria gonorrhoea* and other micro-organisms has been implicated as an important factor in preterm delivery[31–34]. Vaginal and endocervical overgrowth of organisms such as those cited above may result in extension into the decidua and fetal membranes, after which subclinical infection traverses the intact membranes and contaminates the amniotic fluid.

A striking association is present between preterm labor and intrauterine, endocervical and urinary tract infections. Many organisms associated with such infections have been shown to have phospholipase A_2 activity[35,36]. In addition, numerous bacteria present in amniotic fluid of women in preterm labor stimulate production of other substances which also initiate myometrial contractions[37,38]. These include:

(1) IgA proteases, neuraminidases and mucinases which facilitate the passage of micro-organisms past the cervical mucus;

(2) Phospholipase A_2 and phospholipase C, which locally augment production of eicosanoids within the uterus; these substances are important in cervical ripening and labor;

(3) Proteases, including collagenase, which weaken the fetal membranes and predispose them to rupture and also ripen the cervix;

(4) Endotoxin, which is capable of stimulating prostaglandin production[39]; and

(5) Platelet activating factor, which causes chemotaxis, increased lysosomal excretion and stimulation of eicosanoid formation and directly stimulates the myometrium to contract[37,38].

Although the factors that initiate these ascending infections are as yet unclear, the presence of these bioactive substances may lead to an increased release of arachidonic acid from the fetal membranes followed by increased prostaglandin biosynthesis and resultant preterm labor. In addition, local inflammatory responses to various micro-organisms may lead to release of similar substances, as well as monokines, which further potentiate the mechanisms involved in preterm contractility.

If the hypothesis that subclinical infection activates the onset of preterm labor is valid, intervention with antibiotic therapy should alter the outcome in these high-risk pregnancies. Indeed, studies using adjunctive antibiotic therapy in preterm labor are provocative and such management schemes need to be evaluated further[40,41]. In particular, a prospective randomized double-blind study in twin gestations would be useful, although it seems reasonable to suppose that the role of infection would be similar to that in singleton gestations.

Several studies support the contention that intra-amniotic infection is an important etiological factor of preterm labor in twin gestations. An ascending route is likely, because no gravida with positive cultures had a second twin with an isolated positive culture[42]. In addition, histological examination of twin placentas has shown that chorioamnionitis is more common in the first than the second twin and isolated chorioamnionitis of the second twin has not been documented[38]. The incidence of twin gestations with positive amniotic fluid cultures was 11%, which is similar to rates observed in singleton gestations with preterm labor and intact membranes[43,44]. As interesting and provocative as these studies are, they do not totally account for the greater incidence of prematurity in multiple pregnancies.

Premature rupture of membranes

Premature rupture of membranes (PROM) occurs in 5–15% of twin pregnancies[28]. The rate of PROM increases progressively with higher-order multiple gestations[45]. Predisposing factors for PROM may include increased vulnerability of the fetal membranes, due to earlier cervical ripening in multiple gestations, exposure to antepartum hemorrhage and overdistension of the fetal membranes by polyhydramnios. Fetal membranes that have ruptured prematurely are thinner in proximity to the rupture site and possess less tensile strength compared to normal specimens. Moreover, the collagen content of the amnion in these membranes is decreased compared to that of gestationally matched controls[46].

Precocious cervical ripening and overt preterm labor have been associated with increased prostaglandin biosynthesis. Stable metabolites of the prostaglandin F series increase concomitantly with cervical ripening in the absence of demonstrable uterine contractions[47]. These metabolites are also significantly increased in pregnancies destined to deliver prematurely after preterm labor[48]. Elevated levels of relaxin are also present in multiple gestations, a phenomenon that may affect the structural integrity of the cervix and predispose it to premature changes[49].

Romero et al.[50] measured concentrations of amniotic fluid prostaglandins in women with preterm PROM without preterm labor or infection and in women with preterm PROM and infection and/or preterm labor. Infection was associated with increased prostaglandin concentrations but PROM alone was not.

Antepartum bleeding

Antepartum bleeding complicates approximately 2–6% of twin gestations[28]. Bleeding results from an increase in the respective incidences of placenta previa and abruption[51]. The higher incidence of placenta previa is related to the greater placental mass in multifetal gestations. The factors leading to an increase in placental abruption are less definite, but probably include uterine overdistension, increased contraction frequency, and increased occurrence of polyhydramnios and premature rupture of membranes. In twins, a maternal serum alpha-fetoprotein (MSAFP) level 4.0 multiples of the median or more is associated with a ten-fold increase in risk of placental abruption and perinatal mortality[52]. It has been postulated that placental abruption may cause an exaggerated release of prostaglandins[53], but this hypothesis has not been evaluated.

Cervical incompetence

It would be logical to presume that, in the absence of contractions, the increased uterine volume and the weight of the uterine contents place a much greater stress on the cervix in a multifetal pregnancy than is the case in a singleton pregnancy. If this were so, these circumstances would theoretically result in a greater incidence of cervical incompetence in women with multifetal pregnancy and placement of a cervical cerclage to provide mechanical support would then improve outcome. The cerclage would also function to isolate the fetal membranes from the vagina and its micro-organisms by keeping the cervix closed. Despite this theoretical advantage, cerclage is not without problems, at least in twin gestations. Placement of a cerclage is associated with a transient increase in prostaglandin levels which then return to normal within 24 h[54,55]. Moreover, cerclage is associated with increased risks of bleeding, chorioamnionitis, premature rupture of membranes and increased contraction frequency[28,56]. In addition, no benefit has been found in twin gestations managed with or without prophylactic cerclage[57,58]. These findings suggest that cervical incompetence probably does not contribute significantly to prematurity in multifetal gestations.

Placental hormone production

Compared to singleton gestations, twin pregnancies produce a proportionately increased amount of estrogen and progesterone by virtue of their increased placental mass[59]. Higher-order multiple pregnancies, particularly quintuplets, apparently produce proportionately more sex steroids following implantation than their singleton counterparts[60]. Whereas estrogen production increases just prior to the onset of term parturition in singletons[61], this process has been poorly studied in multifetal pregnancies; nonetheless, it is reasonable to infer that the phenomenon of increased steroid production may be responsible for the increase in uterine activity observed in multiple gestations via gap junction formation, increases in oxytocin receptors and calcium/prostaglandin metabolism. A relative change in the estrogen/progesterone ratio prior to the onset of preterm contractility in multifetal gestations may be an important etiological factor in the onset of preterm labor, but little data exist to confirm this hypothesis.

Psychological stress

Increased stress has been suggested to be associated with a greater risk of preterm delivery in singletons[62]. The anxiety involved with the anticipation of delivery and care of more than one newborn, let alone more than one preterm newborn, is indeed stressful (see Chapter 20). However, stress is difficult to measure, and further investigation is necessary to determine its significance in multifetal pregnancy.

Conclusions

The higher incidence of preterm labor in the multifetal pregnancy may be attributable to any or all of the hypotheses presented in this chapter. A variety of physiological alterations in myometrial contractility peculiar to the multifetal gestation have been presented. Some of the potential explanations predisposing to preterm labor include maximized myometrial stretch, increased prostaglandin sensitivity, exaggerated cellular response to estrogen/progesterone, increased oxytocin sensitivity and accelerated gap junction formation. Additionally, a variety of clinical circumstances in multifetal gestation also appear to predispose to preterm labor. These include uterine overdistension, polyhydramnios, ascending subclinical infections, antepartum bleeding, cervical weakening and increased psychological stress. The wide-ranging hypotheses underlying the effects of many of these disparate circumstances are preliminary and await further substantiation in the literature. In this light, the use of the multifetal gestation as a research model for investigation of the cause of preterm labor may actually be advantageous to addressing these issues.

References

1. US Department of Health and Human Services (1985). *Vital Statistics for the United States – 1985*, vol. 1. Public Health Services, National Center for Health Statistics
2. Sassoon, D.A., Castro, L.C., Davis, J.L. *et al.* (1990). Perinatal outcome in triplet versus twin gestations. *Obstet. Gynecol.*, **75**, 817
3. Newman, R.B., Gill, P.J. and Katz, M. (1986). Uterine activity during pregnancy in ambulat-

ory patients: comparison of singleton and twin gestations. *Am. J. Obstet. Gynecol.*, **154**, 530
4. Newman, R.B., Gill, P.J., Campion, S. and Katz, M. (1989). The influence of fetal number on antepartum uterine activity. *Obstet. Gynecol.*, **73**, 695
5. Garite, T.J., Bentley, D.L., Hamer, C.A. and Porto, M.L. (1990). Uterine activity characteristics in multiple gestations. *Obstet. Gynecol.*, **76**, 56S
6. Garfield, R.E. (1984). Control of myometrial function in preterm versus term labor. *Clin. Obstet. Gynecol.*, **27**, 572–91
7. Carsten, M.E. and Miller, J.D. (1987). A new look at uterine muscle contraction. *Am. J. Obstet. Gynecol.*, **157**, 1303
8. Marsten, S.B. and Smith, C.W.J. (1985). The thin filaments of smooth muscle. *J. Muscle Res. Cell Motil.*, **6**, 669
9. Janis, R.A., Barany, M., Barany, K. *et al.* (1981). Association between myosin light chain phosphorylation and contractions of rat uterine smooth muscle. *Molec. Physiol.*, **1**, 3
10. Kao, C.Y. (1977). Electrophysiologic properties of uterine smooth muscle. In Wynn, R.M. (ed.) *Biology of the Uterus*, p. 3 (New York: Plenum Press)
11. Okazaki, T., Casey, M.L., Okita, J.R. *et al.* (1981). Initiation of human parturition. XII. Biosynthesis and metabolism of prostaglandins in human fetal membranes and uterine decidua. *Am. J. Obstet. Gynecol.*, **139**, 373
12. Anderson, A.B.M., Webb, R. and Turnbull, A.C. (1981). Oestrogens and parturition. *J. Endocrinol.*, **89**, 103P
13. Fuchs, A.R., Husslein, P. and Fuchs, F. (1981). Oxytocin and the initiation of human parturition. II. Stimulation of prostaglandin production in human decidua by oxytocin. *Am. J. Obstet. Gynecol.*, **141**, 694
14. Bleasdale, J.E. and Johnston, J.M. (1984). Prostaglandins and human parturition: regulation of arachidonic acid mobilization. *Rev. Perinatal. Med.*, **5**, 151
15. Kloeck, F.K. and Jung, H. (1973). *In vitro* release of prostaglandins from the human myometrium under the influence of stretching. *Am. J. Obstet. Gynecol.*, **115**, 1066
16. Giannopoulos, G., Jackson, K., Kredenster, J. *et al.* (1985). Prostaglandin E and $F_{2\alpha}$ receptors in human myometrium during the menstrual cycle and in pregnancy and labor. *Am. J. Obstet. Gynecol.*, **153**, 904
17. Norman, R.J., Bredenkamp, B.L., Joubert, S.M. *et al.* (1981). Fetal prostaglandin levels in twin pregnancies. *Prostaglandins Med.*, **6**, 309
18. Csapo, A.L. (1981). Forces in labor. In Iffy, I. and Kaminetzky, H.A. (eds.) *Principles and Practice of Obstetrics and Perinatology*, p. 761. (New York: John Wiley and Sons)
19. Alexandrova, M. and Soloff, M.S. (1980). Oxytocin receptors and parturition. I. Control of oxytocin receptor concentration in the rat myometrium at term. *Endocrinology*, **106**, 730
20. Fuchs, A.R., Periyasamy, S., Alexandrova, M. *et al.* (1983). Correlation between oxytocin receptor concentration and responsiveness to oxytocin in pregnant rat myometrium: effects of ovarian steroids. *Endocrinology*, **113**, 742
21. Takahashi, K., Diamond, F., Bieniarz, J. *et al.* (1980). Uterine contractility and oxytocin sensitivity in preterm, term and postdates pregnancy. *Am. J. Obstet. Gynecol.*, **136**, 774
22. Garfield, R.E. and Hayashi, R.H. (1981). Appearance of gap junctions in the myometrium of women in labor. *Am. J. Obstet. Gynecol.*, **140**, 254
23. Garfield, R.E., Kannan, M.S. and Daniels, E.E. (1980). Gap junction formation in the myometrium: control by estrogens, progesterone and prostaglandins. *Am. J. Physiol.*, **238**, C81
24. Manabe, Y., Okazaki, A. and Takahasi, A. (1983). Prostaglandins E and F in amniotic fluid during stretch-induced cervical softening and labor at term. *Gynecol. Obstet. Invest.*, **15**, 343
25. Varma, R., Bateman, S., Patel, R. *et al.* (1988). The relationship of increased amniotic fluid volume to perinatal outcome. *Int. J. Gynaecol. Obstet.*, **27**, 327
26. Cardwell, M. (1987). Polyhydramnios: a review. *Obstet. Gynecol. Surv.*, **42**, 612
27. Alexander, S. and Leroy, F. (1978). Gestational length and intrauterine growth in twin pregnancy. In *Twin Research: Clinical Studies*, pp. 129–36. (New York: Alan R. Liss)
28. Newton, E. (1986). Antepartum care in multiple gestation. *Semin. Perinatol.*, **10**, 19
29. Kirshon, B. (1989). Fetal urine output in hydramnios. *Obstet. Gynecol.*, **73**, 240
30. Billah, M.M. and Johnston, J.M. (1983). Identification of phospholipid platelet activating factor in human amniotic fluid and urine. *Biochem. Biophys. Res. Commun.*, **113**, 51
31. Martius, J. and Eschenbach, D. (1990). The role of bacterial vaginosis as a cause of am-

niotic fluid infection, chorioamnionitis and prematurity – a review. *Arch. Gynecol. Obstet.*, **247**, 1
32. Gravett, M., Hummel, D., Eschenbach, D. *et al.* (1986). Preterm labor associated with subclinical amniotic fluid infection and with bacterial vaginosis. *Obstet. Gynecol.*, **67**, 229
33. Romero, R., Mazor, M., Oyarzun, E. *et al.* (1989). Is genital colonization with *Mycoplasma hominis* or *Ureaplasma urealyticum* associated with prematurity/low birth weight? *Obstet. Gynecol.*, **73**, 532
34. Ledger, W. (1989). Infection and premature labor. *Am. J. Perinatol.*, **6**, 234
35. Bejar, R., Curbello, V., Davis, C. *et al.* (1981). Premature labor: II. Bacterial sources of phospholipase. *Obstet. Gynecol.*, **57**, 479
36. Bennett, P., Rose, M., Myatt, L. and Elder, M. (1987). Preterm labor: stimulation of arachidonic acid metabolism in human amnion cells by bacterial products. *Am. J. Obstet. Gynecol.*, **156**, 649
37. MacGregor, J., French, J., Lawellin, D. and Todd, J. (1988). Preterm birth and infection: pathogenic possibilities. *Am. J. Reprod. Immunol. Microbiol.*, **16**, 123
38. Romero, R. and Mazor, M. (1988). Infection and preterm labor. *Clin. Obstet. Gynecol.*, **31**, 553
39. Romero, R., Hobbins, J.C. and Mitchell, M.D. (1988). Endotoxin stimulates prostaglandin E2 production by human amnion. *Obstet. Gynecol.*, **71**, 227
40. McGregor, J., French, J., Reller, L.B. *et al.* (1986). Adjunctive erythromycin treatment for idiopathic preterm labor: results of a randomized, double-blinded, placebo-controlled trial. *Am. J. Obstet. Gynecol.*, **154**, 98
41. Morales, W., Angel, J., O'Brien, W. *et al.* (1988). A randomized study of antibiotic therapy in idiopathic preterm labor. *Obstet. Gynecol.*, **72**, 829
42. Romero, R., Shamma, F., Avila, C. *et al.* (1990). Infection and labor. VI. Prevalence, microbiology, and clinical significance of intraamniotic infection in twin gestations with preterm labor. *Am. J. Obstet. Gynecol.*, **163**, 757
43. Leigh, J. and Garite, T. (1986). Amniocentesis and the management of premature labor. *Obstet. Gynecol.*, **67**, 500
44. Romero, R., Sirtori, M., Oyarzun, E. *et al.* (1989). Infection and labor. V. Prevalence, microbiology and clinical significance of intra-amniotic infection in women with preterm labor and intact membranes. *Am. J. Obstet. Gynecol.*, **161**, 817
45. Knitza, R., Hasbargen, U., Ott, M. *et al.* (1989). Duration of pregnancy in higher degree multiple birth. *Geburtsh. Frauenheilkd.*, **49**, 1070
46. Gazaway, P. and Mullins, L. (1989). Prevention of preterm labor and premature rupture of the membranes. *Clin. Obstet. Gynecol.*, **29**, 835
47. Keirse, M.J.N.C., Thiery, M., Parewijck, W. *et al.* (1983). Chronic stimulation of uterine prostaglandin synthesis during cervical ripening before the onset of labor. *Prostaglandins*, **25**, 671
48. Weitz, C.M., Ghodgaonkar, R.B., Dubin, N.H. *et al.* (1986). Prostaglandin F metabolite concentrations as a prognostic factor in preterm labor. *Obstet. Gynecol.*, **67**, 496
49. Haning, R.V. Jr, Steinetz, B. and Weiss, G. (1985). Elevated serum relaxin levels in multiple pregnancy after metrodin treatment. *Obstet. Gynecol.*, **66**, 42
50. Romero, R., Emamian, M., Wan, M. *et al.* (1987). Prostaglandin concentrations in amniotic fluid of women with intra-amniotic infection and preterm labor. *Am. J. Obstet. Gynecol.*, **157**, 1461
51. Karegard, M. and Gennser, G. (1986). Incidence and recurrence rate of abruptio placentae in Sweden. *Obstet. Gynecol.*, **67**, 523
52. Katz, V., Chescheir, N. and Cefalo, R. (1990). Unexplained elevations of maternal serum alphafetoprotein. *Obstet. Gynecol. Surv.*, **45**, 719
53. Morror, R. and Knox-Ritchie, J. (1988). Uteroplacental and umbilical artery blood velocity waveforms in placental abruption assessed by Doppler ultrasound. *Br. J. Obstet. Gynaecol.*, **95**, 723
54. Toplis, P., Shepherd, J., Youssefmejadian, E. *et al.* (1980). Plasma prostaglandin concentrations after cerclage in early pregnancy. *Br. J. Obstet. Gynaecol.*, **87**, 669
55. Novy, M.J., Ducsay, C.A. and Stanczyk, F.Z. (1987). Plasma concentrations of prostaglandin $F_{2\alpha}$ and prostaglandin E_2 metabolites after transabdominal and transvaginal cervical cerclage. *Am. J. Obstet. Gynecol.*, **156**, 1543
56. Rush, R.W., Isaacs, S., McPherson, K. *et al.* (1984). A randomized controlled trial of cervical cerclage in women at high risk of spontaneous preterm delivery. *Br. J. Obstet. Gynaecol.*, **91**, 724

57. Weekes, A., Menzies, D. and Boer, C. (1977). The relative efficacy of bedrest, cervical suture and no treatment in the management of twin pregnancy. *Br. J. Obstet. Gynaecol.*, **84**, 161
58. Dor, J., Shalev, J., Mashiach, G. *et al.* (1982). Elective cervical suture of twin pregnancies diagnosed ultrasonically in the first trimester following induced ovulation. *Gynecol. Obstet. Invest.*, **13**, 55
59. TambyRaja, R.L. and Ratnam, S.S. (1981). Plasma steroid changes in twin pregnancies. *Prog. Clin. Biol. Res.*, **69A**, 189
60. Muechler, E.K. and Huang, K.E. (1983). Plasma estrogen and progesterone in quintuplet pregnancy induced with menotropins. *Am. J. Obstet. Gynecol.*, **147**, 105
61. Thornburn, G.D. and Challis, J.R.G. (1979). Endocrine control of parturition. *Physiol. Rev.*, **59**, 863
62. Omer, H. (1986). Possible psychophysiologic mechanisms in premature labor. *Psychosomatics*, **27**, 580

Normal and abnormal patterns of labor 32

E.A. Friedman

Introduction

Paradoxical impressions pervade our discipline in regard to the type of labor physicians should anticipate in association with multifetal pregnancies. Conflicting information abounds. Gravidas with twin* pregnancy are expected to have either short labors or unduly long ones, depending on the source of the information. The American College of Obstetricians and Gynecologists, for example, in a publication meant for dissemination to patients, gives the following pessimistic message: 'Because the uterus stretches more in a multiple pregnancy, labor may be slower and may not progress well'[1]. In contrast, the 17th Edition of the renowned textbook, *Williams Obstetrics*, states, '...labor, in general, is shorter with twins...'[2]. These contradictory statements reflect divergent clinical impressions concerning the type of labor obstetricians consider likely to occur in a woman who is carrying more than one fetus in her uterus; some authors expect rapid labors leading to precipitate delivery and others envisage complicated, prolonged and dysfunctional labors. Comparable dicta, reflecting opposing viewpoints, have appeared in the literature from time to time, most often without objective data to support the contention that the labor accompanying multiple pregnancy is unduly short or long.

Resolution of this issue is perhaps of less clinical importance than it may have been in the past, because increasingly greater proportions of women with multifetal pregnancy – 44%[3,4] to 52%[5] – are being delivered by Cesarean section. Nonetheless, it is useful to appreciate the labor patterns commonly encountered with twin pregnancies. Without meaningful information, physicians and other health-care providers will be ill-equipped to quickly recognize when the course of labor is abnormal and deal with it expeditiously and appropriately.

Factors potentially influencing the course of labor

One part of the problem with nearly all prior investigations attempting to characterize labor in multifetal pregnancy was that only the total duration of labor was examined rather than the dynamic progression of labor over time. Another was the fact that simple comparisons with the labors of singleton pregnancies often failed to take into account obvious differences between singleton and multiple gestations. Differences include the propensity for preterm labor and delivery[6,7] and for fetal malpresentation[5,8,9]. Both of these complications are commonly associated with multifetal pregnancy and, at the same time, exert a major impact on the progression of labor[10].

In addition, there are a number of other, perhaps more subtle, factors which may also affect the course of labor in twin and high-order pregnancies and which are less likely to be found in the same frequency among gravidas who carry only a single fetus. These factors are as diverse as differential maternal age, racial and parity characteristics, fetal and uterine malformations, polyhydramnios, intrauterine

---

* Editor: Dr Friedman has used the terms twin and multifetal interchangeably in this chapter. The data presented here are based (almost but not entirely) on the labor patterns of mothers with twins rather than higher-order births.

growth retardation, placenta previa, abruptio placentae, maternal anemia and pregnancy-induced hypertension[11]. Even more esoteric differences have been documented as well, such as fetal sex, which is also said to exert a potential influence on the duration of the labor[7,12]. Further, and of great importance, is the fact that pre-labor cervical dilatation is also common. The factor of initial cervical dilatation has a major bearing on the course of labor in singleton pregnancies[13], but it does not appear to have been taken into account for multifetal pregnancies thus far.

Labor duration studies

When multifetal and singleton cases are matched for factors of this nature, even if only for preterm delivery and fetal malpresentations, the total duration of labor for the two groups is quite comparable on the average[14,15]. This suggests that multifetal pregnancy does not affect the course of labor *per se*, notwithstanding clinical impressions to the contrary, except insofar as it may be affected by the associated factors of prematurity and malpresentation, and perhaps others.

Experiential reports, providing numerical summations of collective data from more or less homogeneous groups of patients with multifetal pregnancy, have not contributed much insight. An example is one that reported the average labor duration of twin pregnancies subgrouped according to parity[16]. This report showed essentially normal lengths of labor as might be expected for nulliparas and multiparas, respectively. However, no data were presented to show that singleton pregnancies with comparable parity distribution fared the same. Recent reviews of this subject merely re-cite pre-existing studies, leaving the issue essentially unresolved[17,18].

These clinical explorations fall short of the mark in three important areas. First, they fail to take into account factors that may confound the analysis, namely those factors which are known to affect the course of labor or may possibly have an impact on labor. Second, they deal only with duration of labor from onset to delivery as the measured end-point. Total duration of labor is a coarse means for assessing the true progress of labor, because it ignores subtle and sometimes not so subtle alterations in the pattern of labor. Such alterations are of importance to the well-being of the mother and her fetus; they are crucial to the obstetric attendants and their ability to gauge whether the labor is normal or not. Merely focusing on total duration without being aware of what may be happening over time is short-sighted at best and hazardous at worst.

Investigation based on graphic analysis of labor

Objective data are required if the question of the effect of multiple pregnancy on labor is to be answered in a manner that will prove satisfactory for direct application to clinical practice. One early attempt used the technique of graphic analysis of cervical dilatation and fetal descent labor patterns of twin and triplet pregnancies[19]. It involved a study of 222 sets of twins and three sets of triplets from among a population of nearly 24 000 gravidas studied over a 5-year period. From this group, 184 multifetal labors could be reconstructed in sufficient detail to provide adequate dilatation and descent patterns. Demographic information from this subset of women showed a normal age distribution. This was unexpected, because natural, as opposed to induced, twinning is an age-related phenomenon[20]. However, the study group presented an excess concentration of multiparas, as anticipated (66 nulliparas and 118 multiparas). Nearly 50% of the infants delivered weighed less than 2500 g. The proportion of small fetuses exceeded by far the prematurity rate for the gravid population at large. Similarly, fetal malpresentations were very common, especially breech presentations, and these were particularly concentrated among those who delivered prematurely.

Of special relevance to the labor pattern in these cases was the distribution of initial cervical dilatation. There were great differences in this regard from what would ordinarily have been expected in women delivering a singleton fetus.

Three-quarters of nulliparas with twins began labor with a cervix already 2 cm dilated, nearly 40% had reached 3 cm or more, and 20% at least 4 cm (as compared with 38%, 7% and 2%, respectively, in nulliparas with singletons). Similar differences were encountered for multiparas as well, with 60% achieving 3 cm or more before labor began (vs. 23% with singletons) (see Chapter 33).

The raw data derived from the graphic analytic technique, previously described in detail[21], are shown in Table 1 for the durations and slopes of the several phases of the labor curves for multifetal and singleton pregnancies, stratified by nulliparas and multiparas. It is clear from these data that the latent phase duration is significantly foreshortened in multifetal gestations in both nulliparas and multiparas. The remainder of the labor course appears to be somewhat slowed, although not significantly so, except for the deceleration phase and second-stage durations among multiparas.

These observations showed a paradoxical dichotomy between the obviously foreshortened latent phase and the apparently prolonged active phase and second stage. Overall, the total duration of labor was a bit shorter in the multifetal pregnancies, because the decrease in latent phase duration overwhelmed the lengthening of the rest of the labor, although the difference in the data for the total duration did not prove to be statistically significant.

Given the fact that so many of the labors began prematurely in this series of cases, it was deemed necessary to make adjustments. On the one hand, it was necessary to account for the factor of prematurity; on the other, it was also necessary to consider that whereas the presenting infant may have had a tendency to be small by virtue of prematurity, uterine overdistension may have been present, because of the presence of two fetuses. Accordingly, the effect on the labor course of the combined fetal weight (the sum of the birth weights in 1000-g increments) was assessed. As seen in Table 2, the combined fetal weight had no relationship to the latent phase duration. However, clearcut trends were encountered, indicating definite prolongation of the active phase duration with slowing of the maximum rate of dilatation (and also to a lesser extent with prolongation of the deceleration phase) in association with increasing combined fetal weight. Overdistension by larger intrauterine fetal (and perhaps amniotic fluid) content thus appears to have a definite adverse impact upon progress in the active phase of labor. A later study of uterine overdistension in singleton pregnancies complicated by polyhydramnios, however, failed to verify any association with prolonged labors[22]. Quite the contrary, nulliparous labor was actually shorter overall on average, although not significantly so. Given this divergence of findings, the apparent impact of the ostensible overdistension caused

Table 1 Comparative labor data for singleton and multifetal pregnancies by parity

	n	Latent phase (h)	Active phase (h)	Maximum slope (cm/h)	Deceleration phase (h)	Second stage (h)
Nulliparas						
Singleton	496	8.6	4.9	3.0	0.90	0.95
Multifetal	66	6.2*	5.4	3.0	1.26	1.05
Multiparas						
Singleton	494	5.3	2.2	5.7	0.23	0.29
Multifetal	118	4.0*	2.6	5.5	0.042*	0.39*

*Statistically significant at $p < 0.05$ level

Table 2 Labor data for multifetal pregnancies by combined fetal weight

Combined infant weight (g)	n	Latent phase (h)	Active phase (h)	Maximum slope (cm/h)	Deceleration phase (h)	Second stage (h)
Nulliparas						
<4000	16	7.1	4.1	3.4	0.54*	0.49*
4000–4999	16	4.5	5.0	3.3	1.71	1.26
5000+	23	7.8	6.7	2.5	1.28	1.14
Multiparas						
<4000	20	5.6	2.2	5.9	0.37	0.53
4000–4999	32	3.8	2.0	6.4	0.24*	0.28*
5000–5999	49	3.3	3.1	5.2	0.48	0.41
6000+	17	4.5	3.0	4.5	0.64	0.11

*Statistically significant at $p < 0.05$ level

Table 3 Labor data for multifetal pregnancies by initial cervical dilatation in multiparas

Initial dilatation (cm)	n	Latent phase (h)	Active phase (h)	Maximum slope (cm/h)	Deceleration phase (h)	Second stage (h)
1.0–1.9						
Singleton	297	5.3	2.2	5.7	0.23	0.29
Multifetal	15	7.1	2.7	7.7	0.36	0.45
2.0–2.9						
Singleton	53	4.0	1.9	6.4	0.18	0.22
Multifetal	30	3.8	2.9	6.0	0.33	0.34*
3.0–3.9						
Singleton	85	4.2	1.9	5.4	0.23	0.24
Multifetal	27	3.9	2.5	6.0	0.36	0.39
4.0+						
Singleton	28	3.4	1.5	5.5	0.19	0.18
Multifetal	44	3.0	1.9	4.3	0.44*	0.39*

*Statistically significant at $p < 0.05$ level

by sizeable combined fetal weights deserves to be re-evaluated by more sensitive means.

With regard to differential pre-labor cervical dilatation, it was necessary to determine if this finding was an adequate explanation for the foreshortened average latent phase observed in this study. Stratifying the data by initial cervical dilatation, as presented in Table 3, effectively obliterated the latent phase distinctions seen earlier. However, it had no effect on the active phase durations. In other words, within each cervical dilatation subgroup, no differences in the latent phase were present between multifetal and singleton labors, but the previously noted differences in the active phase persisted, remaining longer in multifetal gestation than in singleton labor. These observations validate the concept that the multifetal labor is characterized by a short latent phase entirely accountable for by the advanced pre-labor cervical dilatation.

A number of other factors occurred at different rates among multifetal labors than among singletons, such as the administration

Table 4 Labor data for matched pairs of multiparous singletons and twin pregnancies

Group	n	Latent phase (h)	Active phase (h)	Maximum slope (cm/h)	Deceleration phase (h)	Second stage (h)
Singleton	50	5.6	1.8	6.3	0.15	0.16
Twin	50	2.7*	1.8	6.6	0.26*	0.31*

*Statistically significant at $p < 0.05$ level

of oxytocin and sedation. In order to correct for these differences, cases were matched for comparison purposes on the basis of an array of factors, including maternal age, parity, fetal weight (of the presenting fetus), fetal position, analgesic effect, uterotonic stimulation and conduction anesthesia. A total of 50 such matched pairs, all multiparas and all with twins, were available for more intensive comparative study of their labor patterns. The graphic analytic approach was applied to these two parallel series in order to ascertain if the changes seen earlier were indeed due to the multifetal labor and not caused by some hidden influence for which proper analytic safeguards had not been imposed.

The labor data derived from these matched cases (Table 4) showed essentially the same trends as before. Significant foreshortening of the latent phase was very clearly shown among twin pregnancies, as well as prolongation of the average duration of the deceleration phase and second stage. Based on these data, little doubt should remain that these changes were characteristic of labor in gravidas with twin pregnancy.

Further matching of cases to take into account the factor of initial cervical dilatation, the single remaining potentially confounding item for which evidence existed (see above), reduced the number of pairs to a mere 18 in number. As anticipated, this had the effect of completely eliminating the latent phase differences. Correcting for the influence of this factor yielded an average latent phase duration of 2.7 h, which was the same in both singleton and twin labors among this small group of matched multiparas.

The overview conclusion from these data was that the labor associated with twin pregnancy was characterized by a short latent phase resulting from the pre-labor cervical dilatation. The advanced dilatation, in turn, was probably related to or even possibly caused by the associated uterine overdistension of late pregnancy, although often such dilatation appeared to arise before term and thus well before the uterus was truly overdistended. At the same time, the active phase and second stage of twin labor was slower than among singleton pregnancies. Whether this latter slowing was also related to the uterine overdistension was conjectural at best, because comparable overdistension by polyhydramnios did not appear to be associated with the same slowing. Moreover, the relative impact of this slowing was clearly outweighed by the considerably greater latent-phase speeding.

Univariate and multivariate analysis

Despite the insights provided by this type of in-depth analysis, the issue of the labor pattern that one could expect to occur with multifetal pregnancy was not entirely laid to rest. Incompletely resolved was the nagging concern over the pervasive clinical impression of a dysfunctional quality to some of these labors. Supporting this view in the investigation just cited[19], for example, it was determined that there was a significant excess number of dysfunctional labors among the multifetal pregnancies. This was the case despite the fact that this high rate of abnormal labors did not seriously affect the average labor course.

Table 5 Relative frequencies of dysfunctional labor patterns among singleton and multifetal pregnancies

Dysfunction labor pattern	Nulliparas		Multiparas	
	Singleton	Multifetal	Singleton	Multifetal
Prolonged active phase	3.1	7.6*	0.4	5.1*
Protracted active-phase dilatation	4.8	21.2*	0.3	10.2*
Secondary arrest of dilatation	5.2	12.1*	0.4	2.5*
Total	7.1	33.3*	0.8	16.1*

*Statistically significant at $p < 0.01$ level

The relative frequencies of the specific types of disordered patterns are shown in Table 5. All identifiable varieties of abnormal labors occurred in statistically significantly increased frequencies relative to the rates among singleton labors. Thus, there were significantly more prolonged latent phase aberrations (defined by a latent phase duration exceeding 20 h in nulliparas or 14 h in multiparas), more protracted dilatation patterns (defined by a maximum slope of dilatation less than 1.2 cm/h in nulliparas or 1.5 cm/h in multiparas) and more secondary arrest of dilatation abnormalities (defined by arrest in the active phase for at least 2 h). These findings raised scepticism about the real meaning of the data from the graphic analysis data presented earlier.

The hidden implications of the differences shown in Table 5 deserved exploration with more sophisticated tools, which would allow a closer and more penetrating inquiry. One such technique is that of logistic regression analysis. The complexities of using this method for a clinical study such as this are described elsewhere[23]. Suffice it to say that logistic regression has proved especially useful for the purposes of searching for significant risk variables, that is, for quantitating the relative significance of the effects of each of a number of defined factors on a given outcome, while simultaneously taking into account the effects of all other identified factors. The goal of this approach is to determine effect-estimates (measures of the degree of impact of a given factor on the outcome in question) of risk factors, controlling for the effects of all the other possibly relevant risk factors at the same time.

Data from the National Collaborative Perinatal Project (NCPP) pertaining to 1195 twin pregnancies were available for investigation by logistic regression. The epidemiological characteristics of this series of cases have been previously published[24,25]. The clinical observations made during the course of the labors were sufficiently frequent and adequately recorded to permit reconstruction of the labor pattern in regard to cervical dilatation and fetal descent progression in 976 cases. Among them, 62.5% were pregnancies in multiparas, an excessive proportion, as expected. Of the 1952 infants who made up the index population, 87.0% were delivered prematurely and weighed less than 2500 g, an even greater than anticipated excess. Among them, 20.7% had fetal malpresentations, most often breech presentation, consistent with their relatively high rate of prematurity. Major anatomical malformations were detected in 18.3% of cases, and were most common in monozygotic twins, among twins born to black women, and in male offspring. Perinatal mortality was unusually high at 112 per 1000, mostly attributable to the prematurity and the associated congenital malformations. It was clear from examination of these few elemental data that the factors of

Table 6 Logistic regression analysis of factors affecting labor in twin pregnancies

Variable	Regression coefficient	Standard error	Ratio	Relative risk	p-Value
Constant	−2.546	0.090	−28.29		
Birth weight of first twin of 3500 g or more	0.622	0.202	3.08	1.94*	0.0036
Gestational diabetes	0.763	0.240	3.18	2.15*	0.0062
Prematurity	−0.290	0.118	2.46	0.70*	0.018
Polyhydramnios	0.309	0.191	1.61	1.41	0.068
Fetal malpresentation	0.312	0.204	1.53	1.33	0.094

*Statistically significant at $p < 0.05$ level.

maternal race, gestational age, fetal weight, fetal presentation, twin zygosity, fetal malformation and fetal sex all had to be weighed in the balance, at the very least.

Simple univariate screening analysis (non-parametric analytic method using the Freeman–Tukey deviate[26]) was undertaken at the outset to determine which among these and other potentially relevant factors intrinsic to the gravida – in terms of demographics, constitution, past or concurrent illness or pregnancy complication – might have an effect upon the course of labor. Factors examined embraced a wide range of attributes and conditions, such as contributing institution, maternal age, race, parity, gravidity, socioeconomic index, educational background, marital status, hospital payer classification, abnormal labor, previous abortion or premature labor, weight, ponderal index, weight gain, smoking, and so forth. The end point used for analytical purposes was the dichotomy between a normal labor progression pattern and the presence of dysfunctional labor patterns.

The results of this initial analysis indicated that a number of the maternal variables tested might indeed play a role in the development of abnormal labor patterns among twin pregnancies. For example, significant ($p < 0.05$) excesses of abnormal labors were identified in association with factors of race (white over black), age (more than 35 years), parity (high multiparity), socioeconomic index (affluence), weight gain (excessive), pelvic adequacy (cephalopelvic disproportion) and gestational diabetes. Some factors proved 'protective', that is, the frequency of abnormal labor patterns was significantly reduced in their presence; among these were prior premature birth, chronic hypertensive disease, pregnancy-induced hypertension and cigarette smoking.

The impression gained from examining this list was that factors commonly associated with the delivery of large babies appeared to be adverse, whereas those yielding small fetuses were beneficial, insofar as their impact upon the ensuing labor was concerned. This impression was confirmed by the parallel findings of significant association between the occurrence of abnormal labor and certain fetal factors. These factors included first-twin birth weight (over 3500 g), combined birth weight (over 6000 g), fetal malpresentation (breech) and malposition (persistent occiput transverse and posterior) and concurrent polyhydramnios. 'Protective' fetal factors consisted of birth weight (under 2500 g), intrauterine growth retardation, and preterm gestational duration. Thus, not only were large babies associated with abnormal labors in significant numbers, but factors exposing the maternal–fetal unit to the possibility of some form of dystocia had a similar effect. In addition, the question of an influence from uterine overdistension, as reflected in the factors of large combined fetal weight and especially the combination of twin pregnancy and hydramnios, was once again raised.

After these preliminary explorations, it was then possible to proceed with the more sophisticated logistic regression analysis for purposes of determining which of these preselected variables actually had a significant residual relationship with abnormal labor in twin pregnancy if the effects of all the others were considered simultaneously. In other words, the study was conducted to probe for statistically significant relationships while controlling for confounding and interactional effects. All the aforementioned variables were included in the analysis simultaneously. The estimate of relative risk for each variable, controlled for the effect of all others, was derived for each of them from the logistic regression coefficient. The statistical significance was defined by the relationship of the regression coefficient to the standard error.

This analysis yielded the data shown in Table 6, which provides derivative information pertaining to all the variables that yielded documentable associations at or below the 10% level of statistical significance. Two factors were shown to carry the greatest impact in terms of their relationship to the development of abnormal labor in twin pregnancies: the known presence of gestational diabetes mellitus in the mother and a large birth weight of the first twin, specifically 3500 g or greater. When the effect of both of these factors is taken into account, very little else seems to have any discernible adverse influence.

The variables of combined fetal weight and cephalopelvic disproportion showed no significance in this analysis; that is, whatever effect they may have exerted was completely subsumed by some other factor or factors. Polyhydramnios and fetal malpresentation had some degree of residual effect, but only at a marginally significant level of >5%. It is possible that because they were represented in this study by relatively small numbers, their true impact could not be properly documented here, but this is admittedly conjectural.

Of more than passing interest was the significantly 'protective' effect of premature birth, defined for purposes of this study as less than 36 weeks. The logistic regression analysis showed a marked reduction in the relative risk of having an abnormal labor pattern in prematurely delivered twin pregnancy. The factor of prematurity appears to have subsumed the effects of such closely related factors as low first-twin birth weight, intrauterine growth retardation (present in relatively few cases in this series), hypertension and smoking. It appears, therefore, that shortened gestational duration at delivery (that is, premature birth) serves as an adequate proxy for these last factors.

Resolution

It is perhaps now possible to resolve the paradox described earlier concerning the divergence of clinical opinions as to the type of labor one can expect to find in association with twin pregnancy. Both sides of the argument are sometimes correct, although obviously not in regard to the same situations. Those labors occurring at a premature gestational age can be expected to be normal, while those taking place at term, especially if associated with a large-size first twin or some factor which is likely to result in such a large fetus, are much more likely to show an abnormal labor pattern.

This two-tier conclusion is reminiscent of the findings in an investigation of the labor patterns associated with preterm births[10]. Two distinctive groups were found to exist; each represented a separate population of gravidas in premature labor under very different conditions. One group consisted of patients who made rapid progress because there was minimal resistance by maternal soft tissues in the presence of effective, strong contractions. The contrasting group had unfavorable conditions, such as long, closed, resistant cervix and inefficient uterine contractions.

By analogy, multifetal labors appear to be divisible into two comparably distinct categories, namely, those with conditions more or less favoring the development of normal labor (i.e. preterm labor with small fetuses) and those with especially undesirable circumstances (term labor with a large first fetus) likely to lead to disordered labor. Needless to say, those prevailing conditions determine the type of labor that will follow. Favorable factors lead to expeditious labors, while suboptimal factors generate abnormal labor patterns.

References

1. American College of Obstetricians and Gynecologists (1990). *Multiple Pregnancy*, ACOG Patient Education Pamphlet APO92. (Washington, DC: ACOG)
2. Prichard, J.A., MacDonald, P.C. and Gant, N.F. (1985). *Williams Obstetrics*, 17th edn., p. 520. (Norwalk, CT: Appleton-Century-Crofts)
3. Acker, D.B. and Sachs, B.P. (1989). Twin gestation and labor. In Cohen, W.R., Acker, D.B. and Friedman, E.A. (eds.) *Management of Labor*, 2nd edn., p. 435. (Rockville, MD: Aspen Publications)
4. Pritchard, J.A. *et al.* (1985). *Williams Obstetrics*, 17th edn., p. 521. (Norwalk, CT: Appleton-Century-Crofts)
5. Fleming, A.D., Rayburn, W.F., Mandsager, N.T. *et al.* (1990). Perinatal outcomes of twin pregnancies at term. *J. Reprod. Med.*, **35**, 881
6. MacGillivray, I. (1975). Labour in multiple pregnancies. In MacGillivray, I., Nylander, P.P.S. and Corney, G. (eds.) *Multiple Human Reproduction*, p. 147. (Philadelphia: W.B. Saunders)
7. MacGillivray, I., Campbell, D.M., Samphier, M. *et al.* (1982). Preterm deliveries in twin pregnancies in Aberdeen. *Acta Genet. Med. Gemellol.*, **31**, 207
8. Potter, E.L. and Fuller, H. (1949). Multiple pregnancies at the Chicago Lying-in Hospital, 1941–1947. *Am. J. Obstet. Gynecol.*, **58**, 139
9. Zuckerman, H. and Brzezinski, A. (1961). Multiple pregnancies. *Israel Med. J.*, **20**, 251
10. Friedman, E.A. and Sachtleben, M.R. (1969). Preterm labor. *Am. J. Obstet. Gynecol.*, **104**, 1152
11. Burke, L. (1987). Prenatal care in multiple pregnancy. In Friedman, E.A., Acker, D.B. and Sachs, B.P. (eds.) *Obstetrical Decision Making*, 2nd edn., p. 220. (Toronto: B.C. Decker)
12. Newton, W., Keith, L. and Keith, D. (1984). The Northwestern University Multihospital Twin Study: IV. Duration of gestation according to fetal sex. *Am. J. Obstet. Gynecol.*, **149**, 655
13. Friedman, E.A. and Sachtleben, M.R. (1962). The determinant role of initial cervical dilatation on the course of labor. *Am. J. Obstet. Gynecol.*, **84**, 930
14. Bender, S. (1952). Twin pregnancy: a review of 472 cases. *J. Obstet. Gynaecol. Br. Empire*, **59**, 510
15. Garrett, W.J. (1960). Uterine over-distention and the duration of labour. *Med. J. Australia*, **47**, 376
16. Ross, R.C. and Philpott, N.W. (1953). Five-year survey of multiple pregnancies. *Can. Med. Assoc. J.*, **69**, 247
17. Parsons, M. (1988). Effect of twins: maternal, fetal and labor (Symposium on Twin Pregnancy). *Clin. Perinatol.*, **15**, 41
18. Zuidema, L. (1988). The management of labor (Symposium on Twin Pregnancy). *Clin. Perinatol.*, **15**, 87
19. Friedman, E.A. and Sachtleben, M.R. (1964). The effect of uterine overdistention on labor: I. Multiple pregnancy. *Obstet. Gynecol.*, **23**, 164
20. Waterhouse, J.A. (1950). Twinning in twin pedigrees. *Br. J. Soc. Med.*, **4**, 197
21. Friedman, E.A. (1978). *Labor: Clinical Evaluation and Management*, 2nd edn., p 45. (New York: Appleton-Century-Crofts)
22. Friedman, E.A. and Sachtleben, M.R. (1964). The effect of uterine overdistention on labor: II. Hydramnios. *Obstet. Gynecol.*, **23**, 401
23. Friedman, E.A. and Neff, K.R. (1987). *Labor and Delivery: Impact on Offspring*, p 46. (Littleton, MA: PSG Publishing)
24. Myrianthopoulos, N.C. (1970). An epidemiological survey of twins in a large prospectively studied population. *Am. J. Hum. Genet.*, **22**, 611
25. Myrianthopoulos, N.C. (1975). Congenital malformations in twins: epidemiologic survey. *Birth Defects*, **11**, 39
26. Friedman, E.A. and Neff, K.R. (1987). *Labor and Delivery: Impact on Offspring*, p. 40. (Littleton, MA: PSG Publishing)

Reducing the risk of preterm delivery 33

E. Papiernik

Introduction

The major risk of twin pregnancies is the very high rate of preterm delivery. This chapter will discuss four related aspects of this problem: (1) its frequency, compared to singletons; (2) various techniques used to prevent it; (3) their results; and (4) their limitations. This chapter will also describe how and why various preventive programs have been unable to reduce the rate of births prior to 37 weeks, but have been effective in reducing those extremely dangerous births before 28 weeks and from 28 to 31 weeks. Finally, it will be shown how a small change in the distribution of gestational duration, focused on these very early preterm and early preterm births, has been effective in reducing the rates of neonatal deaths related to twin births.

A recent comparison of live births of twins and singletons in the United States illustrates the specific risks of preterm births (Table 1).

Based on the USA vital statistics of live births in the year 1985[1], the risk of being born from 20 to 27 weeks (very early preterm births) is 8.3 times higher for twins than for singletons. The risk of being born from 28 to 31 weeks (early preterm births) is 7.0 times higher for twins than for singletons, and the risk of being born from 32 to 36 weeks (late preterm births) is 5.8 times higher for twins than for singletons. The analogous figures for birth weight are even more striking, as fetal growth retardation is more frequent in twin fetuses than in singletons. Births from 501 to 1000 g are 9.6 times more frequent in twins than in singletons; from 1001 to 1500 g, 11.4 times more frequent; and for 1501 to 2000 g, 14.3 times higher (Table 1).

Data from other countries are in substantial agreement with the American findings. In Germany, for example, the 1989 HEPE report

Table 1 Gestational age and birth weight distribution for 1000 live births of twins vs. singletons – United States, 1985 (from reference 1)

	Singletons	Twins	Odds ratio
Gestational age (weeks)			
20–27 (very early preterm)	6	48	8.3
28–31 (early preterm)	10	66	7.0
32–36 (late preterm)	74	318	5.8
37–41 (term)	611	488	0.6
42+ (post-term)	299	80	0.2
Birth weight (g)			
501–1000	4	37	9.6
1001–1500	5	54	11.4
1501–2000	10	126	14.3
2001–2500	38	278	9.7
2501–3500	528	505	0.95
3501+	415	36	0.05

Table 2 Distributions of twin and singleton births by duration of gestation and birth weight, HEPE 1982–86 (from reference 2)

	Singletons (n = 40 239) (%)	Multiples (n = 2559) (%)
Duration of gestation (weeks)		
≤31	0.8	7.2
32–36	3.3	27.7
37–41	92.5	64.6
42+	3.2	0.3
Unknown	0.2	0.1
Birth weight (g)		
<1000	0.2	2.9
1000–1499	0.6	5.7
1500–1999	0.9	13.5
2000–2499	3.4	31.5
2500–3999	85.3	46.0
4000+	9.7	0.1
Unknown	0.0	0.1

of all births in a geographically defined area showed that, compared to singletons, twins were nine times more likely to deliver prior to 37 weeks and almost ten times more likely to deliver prior to 31 weeks (Table 2)[2]. At the same time, compared to singletons, twins were ten times more likely to have a birth weight of ≤1500 g and almost 15 times more likely to weigh ≤1000 g at birth. This study is of particular interest, because the data were collected during a time (1982–86) when the prevention of preterm birth was proposed for all pregnant women and the effects of this program are demonstrated in the low rate of preterm births in singleton pregnancies.

Other data collected from geographically defined populations show similar results. For example, in a report from the northern region of England describing twin births in 1984[3], a total of 10.5% occurred prior to the 33rd week of gestation, 3.4% before 28 weeks and 7.1% between 29 and 32 weeks (Table 3). Neonatal

Table 3 Perinatal deaths by duration of gestation, twin births, northern region of England, 1984 (from reference 3)

Duration of gestation (weeks)	Births		Stillbirths	Neonatal deaths	Perinatal deaths	Perinatal mortality rate/1000
	n	%				
≤28	24	3.4	2	10	12	500
29–32	50	7.1	2	2	4	80
33–36	234	33.3	5	1	6	25.6
37+	394	56.1	7	6	13	33.1
Total	702	100.0	16	19	35	49.9

Table 4 Stillbirths, neonatal and infant deaths, singletons and multiples, England and Wales, 1982–84 (from reference 4)

	Neonatal death rate	Likelihood ratio
Singletons	7.4	1.0
Twins	43.9	5.9
Triplets	135.0	18.0
Quadruplets	207.5	29.0

deaths were disproportionately high among infants born prior to 28 weeks, in contrast to the stillbirths, which increased steadily with increasing duration of gestation. The lowest perinatal mortality rate was at 33–36 weeks in contrast to 39–40 weeks in singleton gestations.

A comparison of neonatal deaths for singletons, twins, triplets and quadruplets in England and Wales shows that the likelihood of neonatal death is dramatically related to plurality[4] (Table 4). American data from hospital series (Table 5)[5] amplify these findings.

Table 5 Perinatal deaths for twins by different durations of gestation (from reference 5)

	Perinatal deaths/ births	Perinatal mortality rate/1000
Week		
21–24	34/34	
25–28	30/42	
29–32	9/100	
33–36	2/220	
37–42	4/37	
Cumulative from week		
21	79/770	102
25	45/736	61
29	15/694	22

Techniques proposed for prevention of preterm birth

Early diagnosis

The first study to claim success in preventing preterm deliveries in twin pregnancies began in Germany in 1972[6]. The preventive policy was based on several proposals developed from the literature. Although an ultrasound scan was not advocated for every pregnant woman, this policy was effective in recognizing a high percentage of twin pregnancies using the clinical impression of size–date discrepancy to initiate the ultrasound scan in selected women. Commonly unrecognized, however, were the monozygotic twins in which the fundal height may not have been elevated above singleton norms prior to 28 weeks.

Persson et al.[7] first reported a clearcut improvement in the outcomes of twin births in Sweden after routine ultrasound screening was used at the end of the first or the beginning of the second trimester. Subsequently, several other obstetric units developed management policies which used an early ultrasound scan in the first trimester to establish the diagnosis of multiple pregnancies in virtually all instances[8,9].

Since these initial efforts, the rationale for the routine use of ultrasound was confirmed in a controlled trial from Finland[10]. Women who had an early diagnosis of twinning after an ultrasound scan had much better outcomes than women without a scan or for whom the diagnosis of twinning was made at a later date. Outcome was measured in terms of neonatal deaths (27.8 deaths per 1000 twin births in the group with a scan and 65.8 deaths per 1000 twin births for control women without systematic scanning).

Reduction of work load

A major method advocated for the prevention of preterm deliveries in singleton pregnancies has been the modification of life style in an attempt to diminish uterine contractions related to hard work[11]. This proposal was based on a carefully studied relationship between workload and preterm delivery in singleton pregnancies first described by Papiernik in 1969[12], measured by Papiernik and Kaminski in 1974[13,14], and confirmed in a study of 4000 pregnant women in 1984 by Mamelle and coworkers[15]. On this basis, our preventive policy prescribed disability work leave for all pregnant women with twins working outside their homes commencing between 20 and 24 weeks. We first applied this policy at the Clamart Maternity Hospital (outside Paris, France) in the 1970s. Since then, the same preventive policy has become accepted practice in all France. As an example, in a survey conducted in 1990 and 1991 of all twin pregnancies delivered in the Hauts de Seine area west of Paris, the mean week of cessation of work was at 20 weeks, significantly earlier than that of singleton controls (28 weeks). Reduction in workload has also been a major component of the preventive programs proposed in Germany[6] and in Scotland[9].

Bed rest

Bed rest is the oldest proposed method for the prevention of preterm delivery in twin pregnancies, although this has not been properly evaluated[16,17]. An even more recent claim for the effectiveness of this method[18] should also be interpreted with caution. The salutary results and low preterm rates observed in the group of women who accepted bed rest in this latter study are obvious. However, the controls (unrested) were not comparable to the study patients (rested), in that by not accepting the proposal for rest, these women demonstrated a difference in their attitude toward pregnancy. It is therefore not surprising that the rate of preterm deliveries was higher among the controls. Unfortunately, because of the study design, this comparison cannot be accepted as a measure of the effectiveness or lack thereof of bed rest.

Bed rest has been criticized by a group of Swedish investigators who compared historical observations in two Swedish maternity units, the first at Malmö and the second at Lund[19]. In Malmö, bed rest in the hospital was official policy for twin pregnancies from 28 to 32 weeks. In Lund, no systematic hospital bed rest was offered. Because these two communities were located so close to each other, it is unlikely that they differed in important aspects of social class or life style. Given the diametrically opposed treatments, it is remarkable that outcomes were so comparable: 40 perinatal deaths/1000 births in Malmö (18/223) and 35 perinatal deaths/1000 births in Lund (32/409). Moreover, no difference was observed in birth weights or duration of gestation between those two institutions. It was this similarity in outcome that formed the basis of the Swedish authors' criticisms of bed rest beginning at 28 weeks[19]. Other publications have also been critical of bed rest in recent years[20,21].

Controlled trials of this intervention are few indeed. In one, bed rest was prescribed at 28 weeks for half the women randomly chosen; a positive effect was not shown[22]. Furthermore, the women prescribed bed rest at 28 weeks had more preterm deliveries than did the controls.

A key issue in the older studies of bed rest may relate to the time at which bed rest was started. From an epidemiological point of view, it is reasonable to ask why bed rest might be suggested from 28 weeks onward when it is known that all extremely premature births take place before this time? This question has been answered directly by O'Shea[23] in Australia. In this study of 245 pregnancies, 28 of the 42 perinatal deaths occurred in infants delivered before 28 weeks, indicating that bed rest proposed after 28 weeks would have been totally ineffective. This point was also considered by Gilstrap et al.[24], but not in the form of a controlled trial. Of 189 twin gestations delivered at Wilford Hall United States Air Force Medical Center, 57 women had been referred late in gestation and excluded from their analysis. Of the remaining 132 women, 67 (51%) were hospitalized for prophylactic ward rest at or before 28 weeks' gestation. Of these, 55 (42%) were put to rest at 23–26 weeks. The remaining 65 women (49%) were not hospitalized until after 28 weeks' gestation unless a pregnancy complication was detected or labor occurred. Sixty-four of 67 women in the first group were admitted to the hospital for a duration that equalled or exceeded 4 weeks.

The findings in the study by Gilstrap et al.[24] were as follows. No significant difference in gestational age was apparent. Although perinatal mortality was significantly lower in those infants born to mothers admitted for prophylactic rest (three of 134, vs. 11 of 130, $p<0.05$), perinatal morbidity (intracranial hemorrhage, sepsis or respiratory distress syndrome) did not differ significantly between the hospitalized and non-hospitalized group. The eight infants (3%) who weighed less than 1000 g, were all born to women who were not hospitalized for prophylactic ward rest (8/65 vs. zero of 67, $p<0.05$). Although positive results were reported for women with bed rest, a recruitment bias cannot be excluded.

Betamimetics and cerclage

Several authors[25–29] have reported controlled trials to measure the prophylactic effect of betamimetics used during the third trimester. No benefit could be demonstrated. Intravenous administration of betamimetics may be complicated by pulmonary edema, and twin pregnancies can favor its development[30]. In these cases, magnesium sulfate has been suggested as a substitute for betamimetics[31]. The dangers of intravenous administration of betamimetics have been reviewed elsewhere[32]. To date, no published study demonstrates a reduction in the rate of preterm births among twin pregnancies treated with prophylactic betamimetic agents. This statement does not abrogate the need for betamimetic therapy if documented very early preterm labor ensues, but caution is required, as is a reduced-volume perfusion.

Over the years, several authors have proposed cerclage at the end of the first or during the second trimester as a means of preventing premature births in twin gestations[33–36]. Uncontrolled trials report that cerclage has a positive effect in preventing preterm delivery in twin gestations[37]. Goldman et al.[38] investigated triplet and quadruplet births, and compared a group of non-sutured women (referred for complications) with a group of sutured women (with highly different characteristics and followed by their staff for the women's entire pregnancies). Although they claimed a positive effect, the recruitment biases of this study are obvious and conclusions cannot be accepted at face value.

In another study, Sinha et al.[39] concluded that cerclage actually increased the risk of preterm delivery among twin gestations. They compared data from two medical teams in Scotland: a 'cervical suture believer group' and a 'non-believer group'. Patients treated by the latter had fewer premature deliveries.

A randomized survey by Dor et al.[40] on 50 twin pregnancies also failed to show a benefit from cerclage. These authors showed no difference between sutured and non-sutured women with regard to the proportion of late miscarriages in the second trimester (up to 26 weeks), the incidence of severe prematurity, or the number of perinatal deaths (182 perinatal deaths/1000 births for sutured women vs. 152/1000 for non-sutured women).

Progestins and indomethacin

The use of 17α-hydroxyprogesterone for prevention of preterm delivery in twin pregnancies was tested by a controlled trial on 77 patients[41]; no outcome differences were reported. A meta-analysis of 15 published controlled trials on the use of progestational agents for prevention of preterm delivery in singleton and twin pregnancies[42] showed no difference in favor of treated patients in terms of miscarriages, stillbirths and neonatal deaths. Only the preterm delivery vs. the term delivery comparison approached statistical significance. A less pessimistic opinion was expressed by other authors[43] after a similar review of all published controlled trials. Women included in these trials had singleton or twin pregnancies; no specific study was based on twin pregnancies. This analysis suggests that 17α-hydroxyprogesterone caproate reduces the risk of preterm labor (OR 0.43 CI = 0.20–0.89), preterm birth (OR 0.50, CI = 0.30–0.85), and birth weight less than 2500 g (OR 0.46, CI = 0.27–0.80).

Another pharmacological form of progesterone (micronized) available in France was used as an adjunct to betamimetic treatment in preterm labor in one controlled trial. Although the addition of progesterone did not prolong the duration of pregnancy, it significantly reduced the duration of betamimetic treatment, and the mean duration of stay in hospital[44].

The use of indomethacin, first suggested by Zuckerman and co-workers[45] as a treatment for preterm labor, is not without risk, because of premature closure of the ductus arteriosus[33,46]. Despite this, indomethacin is the only effective drug for treatment of acute hydramnios in the second trimester[47]; because of this, it is sometimes used in monochorionic twins with evidence of the twin–twin transfusion syndrome. If used, the shorter the time, the less risk of complications for the newborns.

Home monitoring

Home monitoring of uterine contractions has been advocated as a means of reducing the rate of preterm deliveries in twin pregnancies[48]. Please refer to other sections of this book for full discussions (e.g. Chapter 35).

The twin clinic

Several programs have described special sessions in the outpatient department devoted to twins and other multiples[6–9]. Our twin clinic evolved without the benefit of advanced planning when one of the departmental doctors was placed in charge of all mothers with twin pregnancies and attended them on a special day in conjunction with the ultrasonographer. As the number of patients increased, however, it became apparent that they (the patients) wanted to discuss their problems with other parents as well. Thus, mothers who had delivered were invited to talk with those who were still pregnant about practical items such as returning home with two infants, or long-term issues about growth and development. As time went on, the clinic added a midwife skilled at patient education, and a social worker who helped the women to fully benefit from the French social security network (home help, financial support). Finally, we added a psychologist capable of preparing the parents for the possibility of a preterm delivery and that one or both twins might be admitted to the neonatal intensive-care unit (NICU). This psychologist also studied the postpartum parental adjustments and assessed the need for psychiatric intervention to minimize familial stress.

Results of various prevention efforts

Many authors of twin studies advise that developing a collective interest in twinning is the first and perhaps the most important step in improving the neonatal outcome at a given institution[6,25,49]. The three studies which have compared perinatal death rates between two periods (the first before and the second after developing concerted efforts for twin care) record impressive reductions after institution of specialized care (Table 6). This statement is true even when the various improvements in neonatal care that occurred during these years are fully taken into account.

In addition to comparisons of perinatal death rates, it is equally important to understand whether the program was able to reduce the rate of very early preterm births and, specifically, the number of infants with very low birth weight and extremely low birth weight. The study of Gilstrap et al.[24] described above is relevant to this question. Two groups of women were compared, the first with bed rest (23 to 26 weeks) and the second without (Table 7). Among women who received bed rest, few births occurred before 29 weeks; none of the infants weighed less than 1000 g, and the perinatal death rate was 22/1000. In the group without bed rest from 23 to 26 weeks, however, the outcome measures were not as good. More deliveries occurred before 29 weeks, more infants weighed less than 1000 g and the perinatal death rate was 85/1000.

Another study of interest is a longitudinal observation of all twin births between 1956 and 1983 in the city of Dundee[9] (Table 8). When a new policy of prenatal care was instituted in 1975, three major changes were included: (1) a systematic ultrasound scan was prescribed for all pregnant women in the first trimester; (2) the responsibility for all twin

Table 6 Perinatal death rates (/1000) for twins: comparisons before and after establishing specialized care for twins

	Before	After
Scholtes, 1977[6]	119.5	47
Marivate et al., 1982[25]	70	52
Meehan et al., 1988[49]	98	39

Table 7 Bed rest during the second trimester (23–26 weeks) in twin pregnancies (from reference 24)

	Bed rest	No bed rest	p-value
Birth before 29 weeks	2/67 (3%)	7/65 (11.8%)	0.7
Birth weight of < 1000 g	0/67 (0%)	8/65 (12%)	< 0.05
Perinatal deaths	3/154 (22/1000)	11/130 (85/1000)	< 0.05

Table 8 Historical perspective of duration of gestation, birth weight and neonatal mortality for twins, Dundee, Scotland (from reference 9)

Years	Gestation ≤ 28 weeks (%)	Duration 29/34 weeks (%)	Birth weight (g)		Neonatal deaths (/1000)
			< 1500 (%)	1500–1999 (%)	
1956–60	2.9	16.7	7.7	15.5	51.6
1961–65	2.8	16.6	11.3	15.9	66.7
1966–70	4.9	13.6	10.6	14.7	59.5
1971–75	3.5	18.1	12.1	13.0	64.2
1976–80	0.0	16.4	3.9	15.7	18.4
1981–83	1.6	14.5	4.0	17.7	16.2

pregnancies was given to a single member of the department; and (3) bed rest was advocated, beginning at 28 weeks. Although this new policy failed to produce a reduction in the total preterm birth rate (births before 37 weeks), it was accompanied by two very specific results. The first was a reduction in the rate of births before or at 28 weeks (from 3.5% in the years 1956–75 to 0.8% in 1976–83). The second was a dramatic reduction in the rate of very low birth weight infants from 11% in 1956–75 to 4% in 1976–83. These two changes were sufficient to reduce neonatal death, from 60/1000 in the years 1956–75 to 17/1000 in the years 1976–83 (Table 8).

Experience with the French program at Clamart

Beginning in 1978, we developed a specific program for the prevention of preterm birth in twin pregnancies at the Antoine Béclère Hospital, in Clamart, France. This program included a systematic ultrasound scan for all pregnant women in the first trimester, the provision of specific information on the risks of preterm delivery for all mothers of twins as well as suggestions for prevention of preterm labor and delivery. All mothers of twins were followed in a special twin clinic by the same prenatal care team. All were encouraged to reduce physical efforts associated with paid employment, domestic chores, travel, commuting and professional tasks. A disability work leave was proposed between 20 and 24 weeks for all women with professional jobs. Bed rest was not prescribed except for mothers with documented preterm labor for whom hospital care and perfusion with betamimetic drugs were required.

The results after the first three years showed a small modification in the distribution of gestational duration and, specifically, a reduction in the number of very early preterm births[8]. The proportion of mothers for whom an antenatal hospital stay was required decreased from 88% in 1976–77 to 72% in 1978–80, and the mean lengths of stay (LOS) during pregnancy decreased from 13.6 ± 11 days in 1976–77 to 7.8 ± 9 days in 1978–80. When the results were evaluated in terms of the proportion of newborns who required transfer to an NICU and by LOS in NICU, an important improvement was demonstrated[50], as well as a major reduction in cost related to neonatal intensive care.

The proportion of twin newborns for whom a transfer to the NICU was required decreased from 23.5 to 20.3% (Table 9). However, the reduction in the mean duration of stay of the twin newborns in NICU was far more dramatic. Whereas LOS had been 30.7 ± 25 days in 1976–77, it declined to 11.5 ± 29 days in 1978–80. When costs were calculated in 1980 French Francs[50] in a direct cost analysis from the NICU, the reduction of severity of newborn morbidity translated directly into money saved. Whereas the mean cost of a twin stay in the NICU was 55 700 ± 25 000 FF in 1976–77, it

Table 9 The introduction of a new policy of prevention of preterm delivery at the Teaching Hospital of Clamart-University, Paris-Orsay (from reference 50)

	1976–77	1978–80
Number of twin births	132	226
Transfers to NICU		
n	31	46
%	23.5	20.3
Mean duration of stay (days)	30.7 ± 25	11.5 ± 10
Total cost of NICU (FF)	1 727 400	715 400
Mean cost of stay (FF 1980)	55 700	15 552
Mean cost by transferred newborn (FF)	25 000	14 000
Mean cost by twin birth	13 086	3165

NICU, neonatal intensive care unit; FF, French Francs

declined to 15 552 ± 14 000 FF in 1978–80. If the total cost is divided by the total number of twin births, then it is seen that the mean cost decreased from 13 086 FF in 1976–77 to 3165 FF in 1978, 1979 and 1980 for each twin newborn[50]. The first year of the program produced the best results, when only one physician was in charge of providing prenatal care to all twin mothers[50]. Shortly thereafter, however, other members of the department disagreed with the idea of being excluded from the team. Their admission was followed by reduced programmatic benefits in the second year, and it was only after lengthy discussions with all participants that the program was effectively applied by all members of the department and became a stable force for continuing change.

The department's interest in twin pregnancies had a curious and unexpected effect. The number of twin pregnancies delivered in Clamart increased gradually, either because women chose to come to this clinic as soon as they became aware they were pregnant with twins, or because their doctors referred them with a complication. Regardless, the fact that the maternity unit was associated with a pediatric department and an NICU allowed all women to benefit from delivering in a level III facility. Maternal transfers were explained by medical decisions, but also by direct decisions by the women themselves, acting as well-informed comsumers.

Application of preventive concepts to another locale in France

Gradually, after some years, the program was in place throughout France. We elected to evaluate the effectiveness of the nation's widely applied program on all twin pregnancies in a geographically defined area, the Hauts de Seine district, west of Paris. This district includes the teaching hospital in the city of Clamart, where the initial program was developed. The Hauts de Seine has about 2.5 million inhabitants with about 20 000 births every year. A middle-class population resides mainly in the south, whereas a lower social class predominates in the north. All 27 hospital sites participated in the study. A questionnaire was filled out by a study nurse for every twin birth and for a control singleton birth. Data were collected between October 1, 1990 and September 30, 1991. The aim of the study was to determine if the principles of prevention of preterm births were applied for all women of the Hauts de Seine district.

The study population included 546 twin pregnancies. The results were as follows. The diagnosis of twinning had been established at a mean gestational age of 12 weeks, as the practice of offering an ultrasound scan for all pregnant women in the first trimester has been established since 1985. All women with twins had been informed of the specific risks, especially of the risk of early preterm delivery. These women were also informed of the need for behavior modification to reduce the risk of preterm birth. For women working in paid employment, work leave was prescribed early (20 weeks for twin mothers in contrast to 28 weeks for singleton mothers). All mothers had been advised to reduce their physical activity, running, lifting weights, etc., and were informed of risks related to long automobile

Table 10 Twin Study, Haut de Seine, 1990–91

	Week				
	24–28	29–33	33–36	37+	Total
Live births	16	71	368	547	1088
%	1.4	6.5	33.8	50.2	100.0
Neonatal deaths	4	5	1	1	11
rate/1000	250	70	3	2	10.1

trips and heavy work loads related to moving and household chores.

The application of these measures was not merely provided to women with low incomes or fewer years of schooling; rather, all pregnant women in the district received the same advice. Interestingly, after the diagnosis of twins was established, 20% of the twin mothers changed their mind about the delivery site if the local hospital did not have an NICU.

Table 10 records some of the results. The distribution of gestational age at birth shows no reduction in the total preterm birth rate (49% prior to 37 weeks) even after general application of the prevention proposals to all twin mothers. What is striking, however, is the low rate of extremely preterm births at 24–28 weeks (1.4%). This rate is much lower than all available published series reviewed at the beginning of this chapter. The rate of early preterm births at 29–33 weeks (6.5%) is lower, but not very different in comparison with other published series. There was no reduction in late preterm births at 33–36 weeks. Eleven babies died in the first month of life (10.1/1000 rate of neonatal death); four of these were born between 24 and 28 weeks' gestation.

This study demonstrated that the techniques for prevention of preterm births proposed by us were effectively applied to all women who had a twin pregnancy in this region of France, regardless of their social level, measured either by years of schooling or by income. It also shows that when applied, these techniques resulted in favorable outcome figures with low rates of neonatal deaths, and that a small modification of the distribution of gestation durations can result in a significant decrease in the more dangerous births, i.e. those extreme preterm births at 24–28 weeks, and the early preterm births at 29–32 weeks.

Comment

Our program for women with twin pregnancies was based on the same ideas previously proposed by us and applied in France for the prevention of preterm deliveries in singleton pregnancies[12]. It was based on an early recognition of risk factors[12–14], a consistently applied educational program, and major efforts to reduce the daily work load. The generic prevention program applied progressively throughout France for every pregnant woman from 1971 to 1982, was followed by a significant reduction in preterm births. The effectiveness of this policy was evaluated by means of cross-sectional studies on randomly chosen women. The first was conducted in 1972 at the beginning of the program, and after that in 1976, in 1981 and in 1988[51]. The most important observation was a major reduction in early preterm births, i.e. those before 34 weeks, from 2.4% in 1972 to 1.2% in 1981, and to 0.9% in 1988.

As is discussed in detail in other chapters of this book, the first step in the prevention of preterm birth among twins is to recognize the presence of the twinning phenomenon, at least by the end of the first trimester. If one accepts this concept, all clinical means for the recognition of twin pregnancy are obsolete. Rather, the only effective means to ensure systematic case detection is routine systematic ultrasound screening for every pregnant woman in the first trimester[6–8] (see Chapter 15). These programs, in addition to ours, that have attempted to prevent preterm birth in twin pregnancies have included this strategic point as well[8,9]. Having stated this precept so emphatically, it is reasonable to ask what is so important about early diagnosis and, more pointedly, why or how is it of such great value in preventing early preterm births in twins? In response, the patient who knows she has twins (or higher-order multiples) can be informed of the specific risks for this pregnancy and educated about the modifications of life style that are necessary to minimize these risks. She can also be informed about the warning signs and symptoms of uterine contractions, and about the possible relationships between her work load, travel, domestic activity and signs of significant uterine activity. Prevention can only work if the women are willing to participate and are convinced of the potential benefits. Prevention cannot be prescribed like a drug. The pregnant women's participation is a basic requirement.

The success of any preventive program can be measured by a reduction in the most dangerous births before 28 weeks. This has been the basis of our success and that of others, as measured by a significant reduction in neonatal morbidity and deaths.

The limits of prevention

The fact that the proportion of twin births that take place before 37 weeks cannot be changed (or better said, from 33–36 weeks, as noted above) requires some explanation.

The best hypothesis for explaining this is related to growth retardation among twin fetuses. It is well known that growth retardation is frequent among twins[52] and that the proportion of growth-retarded twins progressively increases after 32 weeks to reach 50% of all twins at 37 weeks. We also know from observations of singletons that the prevention of preterm births only works when the fetus is growing normally. Stated another way, the effective limit of prevention of preterm birth in singletons is the presence of growth retardation[53].

At present we are slowly beginning to understand the physiological relationships between growth retardation and preterm delivery. For example, we now recognize that growth-retarded fetuses mature earlier, as measured by the diminished risk of hyaline membrane disease as a marker of pulmonary maturity, or as measured by neurological signs related to maturity (see Chapter 44). This means that most preterm births in twin pregnancies cannot be prevented, as a major proportion of these twin fetuses are growth retarded. The effectiveness of our preventive program can only be measured very early in twin gestation (at 24–28 weeks), when growth retardation is not yet present. We have to distinguish between 'avoidable preterm births' and 'unavoidable preterm births'. The same distinction was established in France for singleton pregnancies. After 20 years of application of a national program, preterm births are generally babies with lower birth weights, most of them growth retarded. The prevention, as proposed in our program, was only effective in babies with normal growth. These facts have important practical implications for twin pregnancies. Thus, when preterm labor begins between 33 and 36 weeks, the question of whether or not to treat with betamimetics is valid. It could be suggested that a more precise measure of growth is needed at that time. If the fetuses are growth retarded, the treatment will not be effective and may cause iatrogenic complications.

Regardless of one's position on this question, additional epidemiological arguments exist not to treat preterm labor in twin pregnancies if it occurs between 33 and 36 weeks. The first of these relates to the risk of perinatal death by gestational duration, or by birth weight categories; the second to later outcomes of twin infants and the risk of cerebral palsy (CP).

Compared to singletons, the minimum perinatal mortality rates occur earlier in gestation or at lower birth weights for twins. This statement is based on an analysis of 1655 pairs of twins born in the Netherlands between 1952 and 1979. For every twin baby, a paired singleton birth was chosen of the same year of birth, the same gestational duration, the same sex and the same parity of the mother[54]. This Dutch study shows that twins have a lower risk of perinatal deaths between 27 and 37 weeks. A similar observation is available from Belgium[55] and in Britain, where it was shown that the optimum time for births of twins, as measured by the risk of perinatal mortality, is not at term but rather much earlier, because the minimal risk of perinatal death for twins occurs at 33–36 weeks (25.6/1000 births, compared to 31/1000 births at or after 37 weeks[3]. A similar phenomenon appears with the measurement of perinatal deaths when birth weight categories are used instead of gestational duration categories[56]. The comparison of perinatal deaths of twins and singletons shows no difference for birth weights of 500 to 1499 g, or between 1500 and 2400 g. However, twins had a much higher risk of death for birth weights of more than 2500 g (10/1000 for twins compared to 0.5/1000 for singletons). This increase is related to intrauterine growth retardation. A similar finding was noted by Spellacy et al.[57] in the analysis of 1253 twin births compared to 5115 singletons selected at random. The difference between twins and singletons for risk of death is observed in the neonatal period[54–57], but the major difference is in fetal deaths, with a much higher risk for twins than for singletons[58].

Long-term results and the risk for developmental delay

The risk of adverse outcome in twin infants is strongly related not only to preterm birth but also to fetal growth retardation. The earlier it happens, the more severe the outcome observed. The basis of this statement was established on singleton data, and several twin studies have confirmed it[59–67].

Cerebral palsy is more frequently observed in twins compared to singletons[66–71]. The highest risk is for growth-retarded twins born between 34 and 37 weeks[71]. In an Australian study, an attributable risk analysis[71] showed that fetal growth retardation was the major risk factor for CP in 18.5% of CP twin children born at term. In contrast, fetal growth retardation was the major risk factor for 47.7% of CP twin infants born from 34 to 37 weeks.

Induced preterm births in twins

The only available means to prevent the adverse effects of growth retardation is to induce the delivery of the twins, even if this is before 37 weeks.

This decision should be based on a systematic screening of fetal growth by ultrasound at regular intervals. It is also often made on the basis of documented changes in the non-stress tests of one or both fetuses indicating compromise in their condition.

The rationale for induced preterm delivery should be based on the severity of the growth retardation or the fetal compromise. Umbilical artery Doppler flow studies may help in ascertaining the optimal time for delivery[72,73].

Any decision to terminate a twin pregnancy prematurely should also consider their advanced maturity[74,75]. Lung maturity, as measured by lecithin/sphingomyelin ratio, is reached earlier in twins than in singletons[74]. Placental maturity, as assessed by grade, also occurs earlier in twins than in singletons[75].

Neurological performance of newborns related to their gestational age is often accelerated in babies born preterm and growth retarded. This has been documented in singletons and also in twins[76] and confirmed by the physical measurements of auditory evoked responses[77]. Advanced pulmonary maturity is related to advanced neurological maturity[78,79]. The totality of this information is useful in the decision processes required for the care of twin pregnancies.

When only one of the twins is growth retarded and the other is normally growing, the decision to induce preterm delivery will be more difficult, as the reduction of risk for the growth-retarded fetus is accompanied by an increase in the risk for the normally growing fetus. The best time for delivery should be decided based upon the gestation duration and the hospital's experience in caring for preterm infants of various gestational ages.

Conclusion

It is possible to prevent very early preterm births in twin pregnancies, as has been shown by several programs, including measurements of a population study in France. The apparently small reduction in numbers is of major value, as it is addressed to the most endangered babies, those exposed to mortality, severe morbidity and developmental handicap. It is also that small group of very preterm babies that explain the very high cost of the neonatal care of twins. This result is in sharp contrast with the fact that the high proportion of births of twins between 28 and 36 weeks cannot be modified by any of the preventive methods proposed in the published papers.

There is no contradiction between those two statements. It has been shown that prevention is not effective when the fetuses are growth retarded. Those babies develop an earlier maturation process, in which the triggering of labor is related to early maturation of their neurological or pulmonary systems. This is similar to an analagous phenomenon observed in singleton pregnancies, where prevention only works for fetuses not growth retarded.

As a result of this, many practical decisions can be proposed. Prevention of very early preterm deliveries in twins is possible when it is proposed very early. In France, it has been effective in all twin pregnancies recognized at 15 weeks, and also in women pregnant with twins who were included in a preventive program with work leave at 20 weeks of pregnancy.

With decisions similar to these proposed in Sweden, Finland, Germany and the United Kingdom, the same results have been observed: a significant reduction in very early preterm births, and a major decrease in neonatal deaths.

References

1. Luke, B. and Keith, L.G. (1992). The contribution of singletons, twins and triplets to low birth weight, infant mortality and handicap. *J. Reprod. Med.*, **37**, 661
2. Künzel, W. (1989). Problem bei der Uberwachung der Mehrlingsschwangerschaft. *Gynäkologe*, **22**, 190
3. Lowry, M.F. and Stafford, J. (1988). Northern Region Twin Survey, 1984. *J. Obstet. Gynecol*, **8**, 228
4. Botting, B.J., MacDonald Davies, Y. and MacFarlane, A.J. (1987). Recent trends in the incidence of multiple births and associated mortality. *Arch. Dis. Child.*, **62**, 941
5. Chervenak, F.A., Youcha, S., Johnson, R.E. *et al.* (1984). Twin gestation. Antenatal diagnosis and perinatal outcome in 385 consecutive pregnancies. *J. Reprod. Med.*, **29**, 727
6. Scholtès, G. (1977). Uberwachung und Betrevung der Merlingsschwaugerschaften. *Gerburtsh. Frauenheilkd.*, **37**, 747
7. Persson, P.H., Grennert, L., Gennser, G. *et al.* (1979). On improved outcome of twin pregnancies. *Acta Obstet. Gynecol. Scand.*, **58**, 3
8. Heluin, G., Bessis, R. and Papiernik, E. (1979). Clinical management of twin pregnancies. *Acta Genet. Med. Gemellol.*, **28**, 333
9. Osbourne, C.K. and Patel, N.H. (1985). An assessment of perinatal mortality in twin pregnancies, Dundee. *Acta Genet. Med. Gemellol.*, **34**, 193
10. Saari-Kemppainen, A., Karjalainen, O., Ylöstalo, P. *et al.* (1990). Ultrasound screening and perinatal mortality: controlled trial of systemic one-stage screening in pregnancy. *Lancet*, **336**, 387
11. Papiernik, E. (1984). Proposal for a programmed prevention policy of preterm births. *Clin. Obstet. Gynecol.*, **27**, 613
12. Papiernik, E. (1969). Coefficient de risque d'accouchement prématuré. *La Presse Médicale*, **77**, 793
13. Kaminski, M. and Papiernik, E. (1974). Multifactorial study on the risk of prematurity at 32 weeks of gestation. I. A comparison between an empirical prediction and a discriminant analysis. *J. Perinat. Med.*, **2**, 30

14. Papiernik, E. and Kaminski, M. (1974). Multifactorial study on the risk of prematurity at 32 weeks of gestation. II. A comparison between an empirical prediction and a discriminant analysis. *J. Perinat. Med.*, **2**, 37
15. Mamelle, N., Laumon, B. and Lazar, P. (1984). Prematurity and occupational activity during pregnancy. *Am. J. Epidemiol.*, **119**, 309
16. Brown, E.J. and Dixon, H.G. (1963). Twin pregnancy. *J. Obstet. Gynaecol. Br. Emp.*, **70**, 251
17. Barter, R.K., Hsu, I., Erkenbeck, R.V. *et al.* (1965). The prevention of prematurity in multiple pregnancy. *Am. J. Obstet. Gynecol.*, **91**, 787
18. Kappel, B., Hansen, K.B., Moller, J. *et al.* (1985). Bed rest in twin pregnancy. *Acta Genet. Med. Gemellol.*, **34**, 67
19. Rydhström, H., Nordensköld, F., Grennert, L. *et al.* (1987). Routine hospital care does not improve prognosis in twin gestation. *Acta Obstet. Gynecol. Scand.*, **66**, 361
20. Hartikainen-Sorri, A.L. (1985). Is routine hospitalization in twin pregnancy necessary? A follow up study. *Acta Genet. Med. Gemellol.*, **34**, 189
21. Crowther, C.A., Neilson, J.P., Verkuyl, D.A.A. *et al.* (1989). Preterm labour in twin pregnancies: can it be prevented by hospital admission? *Br. J. Obstet. Gynaecol.*, **96**, 850
22. Saunders. M.C., Dick, J.S., Brown, I.M.C.L. *et al.* (1985). The effects of hospital admission for bed rest on the duration of twin pregnancy. Lancet, **2**, 793
23. O'Shea, R.T. (1986). Twin pregnancy: prematurity and perinatal mortality. *Aust. NZ J. Obstet. Gynecol.*, **26**, 165
24. Gilstrap, L.C., Hauth, J.C., Haukins, D.V. *et al.* (1987). Twins: prophylactic hospitalization and ward rest at early gestational age. *Obstet. Gynecol.*, **69**, 578
25. Marivate, M., de Villiers, K.O. and Fairbrother, P. (1977). Effect on prophylactic out patient administration of fenoterol on the time of onset of spontaneous labor and fetal growth rate in twin pregnancy. *Am. J. Obstet. Gynecol.*, **128**, 707
26. O'Connor, M.C., Murphy, H. and Dalrymple, I.J. (1979). Double blind trial of ritodrine and placebo in twin pregnancy. *Br. J. Obstet. Gynaecol.*, **86**, 706
27. Endl, J. and Baumgarten, K. (1982). Uber die Ergagnisse der prophylaktischen oralen Laugzeittokolyse und Cerclage zur Verlangerung der Zwilling. Schwangerschaflen (Eine Multicenterstudie). *Z. Gerburts. Perinat.*, **186**, 319
28. Gummerus, M. and Halonen, O. (1987). Prophylactic tocolysis of twins. *Br. J. Obstet. Gynaecol.*, **94**, 249
29. O'Leary, J.A. (1986). Prophylactic tocolysis of twin. *Am. J. Obstet. Gynecol.*, **154**, 904
30. Elliot, G.R. and Abdulla, U. (1978). Pulmonary oedema associated with ritodrine infusion and betamethasone administration in premature labour. *Br. Med. J.*, **2**, 799
31. Ogburn, P.L., Julian, T.M., Williams, P.P. *et al.* (1986). The use of magnesium sulfate for tocolysis in preterm labor complicated by twin gestation and betamimetic-induced pulmonary edema. *Acta Obstet. Gynaecol. Scand.*, **65**, 793
32. Hadi, H.A. and Albazza, S.J. (1989). Cardiac isoenzymes and electrocardiographic changes during ritodrine tocolysis. *Am. J. Obstet. Gynecol.*, **161**, 318
33. McGowan, G.W. (1970). Cervical incompetence in multiple pregnancy. *Obstet. Gynecol.*, **35**, 589
34. Zakut, H., Insler, V. and Serr, D.M. (1977). Elective cervical suture in preventing premature delivery in multiple pregnancies. *Israel J. Med. Sci.*, **13**, 488
35. Hägele, D., Zahn, B. and Berg, D. (1985). Kann durch die prophylaktische Zervix-cerclage die Frühgebutenvate bei Mehrlingendeseukt werden? Eine retrospektive Statische Analyse über die Effektivität der Cerclage mit Hilfe der BPE von 1978–1980. *Z. Geburtsh. Perinat.*, **189**, 170
36. Kölbl, H. and Gruber, W. (1986). Cerclage bei Mehrlingsgraviditäten. *Wein. Med. Wochenschr.*, **136**, 463
37. Weekes, A.R.L., Menzies, D.N. and West, C.R. (1977). Spontaneous premature birth in twin pregnancy. *Br. Med. J.*, **2**, 16
38. Goldman, C.A., Dicker, D., Peleg, D. *et al.* (1989). Is elective cerclage justified in the management of triplet and quadruplet pregnancy? *Aust. NZ Obstet. Gynaecol.*, **29**, 9
39. Sinha, D.P., Nandakumar, V.C., Brough, A.K. *et al.* (1979). Relative cervical incompetence in twin pregnancy. Assessment and efficacy of cervical suture. *Acta Genet. Med. Gemellol.*, **28**, 327
40. Dor, J., Shalev, J., Mashiach, S. *et al.* (1982). Elective cervical suture of twin pregnancies diagnosed ultrasonically in the first trimester following induced ovulation. *Gynecol. Obstet. Invest.*, **13**, 55
41. Hartikainen Sorri, A.L., Kauppila, A. and Tuimala, R. (1980). Inefficacy of 17α-hydroxypro-

gesterone caproate in the prevention of prematurity in twin pregnancy. *Obstet. Gynecol.*, **56**, 692

42. Goldstein, P., Berrier, J., Rosen, S. *et al.* (1989). A meta-analysis of randomized control trials of progesteronal agents in pregnancy. *Br. J. Obstet. Gynecol.*, **96**, 265

43. Keirse, M.S.N.C. (1991). Progestogen administration in pregnancy may prevent preterm delivery. *Br. J. Obstet. Gynaecol.*, **97**, 149

44. Noblot, G., Andra, P., Dargent, D. *et al.* (1991). The use of micronized progesterone in the treatment of menace of preterm delivery. *Eur. J. Obstet. Gynaecol. Biol. Reprod.*, **40**, 203

45. Zuckerman, H., Reiss, U. and Rubinstein, I. (1974). Inhibition of human premature labor by indomethacin. *Obstet. Gynecol.*, **44**, 787

46. Sharpe, G.L., Thalme, B. and Lorsson, K.S. (1974). Studies on closure of the ductus arteriosus. XI. Ductal closure *in utero* by a prostaglandin synthetase inhibitor. *Prostaglandin*, **8**, 363

47. Lange, I.R., Harman, C.R., Asm, K.M. *et al.* (1989). Twin with hydramnios: treating premature labor at source. *Am. Obstet. Gynecol.*, **160**, 552

48. Morrisson, J.C., Martin, J.N. Jr, Martin, R.W. *et al.* (1987). Prevention of preterm birth by ambulatory assessment of uterine activity. A randomized study. *Am. J. Obstet. Gynecol.*, **156**, 536

49. Meehan, F.P., Magani, I.M. and Mortimer, G. (1988). Perinatal mortality in multiple pregnancy patients. *Acta Genet. Med. Gemellol.*, **37**, 331

50. Tresmontant, R., Heluin, G. and Papiernik, E. (1983). Cost of care and prevention of preterm births in twin pregnancies. *Acta Genet. Med. Gemellol.*, **32**, 99

51. Rumeau Rouquette, C., Du Mazaubran, C. and Rabarizon, V. (1984). Naître en France, 10 ans d'évolution. Doin (ed.). (Paris: Doin-Inserm)

52. McKeown, T. and Record, R.G. (1952). Observations on fetal growth in multiple pregnancy in man. *J. Endocrinol.*, **8**, 386

53. Bouyer, J., Papiernik, E., Gueguen, S. *et al.* (1989). The decline of preterm deliveries in Haguenau. In Papiernik, E., Keith, L., Bouyer, J. *et al.* (eds.) *Effective Prevention of Preterm Birth: The French Experience Measured at Haguenau.* Birth Defects: Original Article Series, vol. 25, number 1, pp. 107–14. (White Plains, NY: March of Dimes Birth Defects Foundation)

54. Bleker, O.P., Breuer, W. and Huidekoper, B.L. (1979). A study of birth weight, placental weight and mortality of twins as compared to singletons. *Br. J. Obstet. Gynaecol.*, **85**, 111

55. Puissant, F. and Leroy, F. (1982). A reappraisal of perinatal mortality factors in twins. *Acta Genet. Med. Gemellol.*, **31**, 213

56. Ghai, V. and Vidyasagar, D. (1988). Morbidity and mortality factors in twins. An epidemiologic approach in pregnancy. *Clin. Perinatol.*, **15**, 123

57. Spellacy, W.N., Handler, A. and Ferre, C.D. (1990). A case–control study of 1253 twin pregnancies from a 1982–1987 perinatal data base. *Obstet. Gynecol.*, **75**, 168

58. Fhegner, J.R.H. (1989). When do perinatal deaths in multiple gestation occur? *Aust. NZ J. Obstet. Gynaecol.*, **29**, 371

59. Bronsteen, R., Goyert, G. and Bottoms, S. (1989). Classification of twins and neonatal morbidity. *Obstet. Gynecol.*, **74**, 201

60. Ruys-Oudot van Heel, I. and de Leeuw, R. (1989). Clinical outcome of small for gestational age preterm infants. *J. Perinat. Med.*, **17**, 77

61. Neligan, G.A., Kalnn, I., Scott, D. *et al.* (1976). *Born Too Soon or Born Too Small, a Follow-up Study to Seven Years of Age.* (London: Spastics International Medical Publications, Heineman)

62. Watt, J. (1989). The consequences of intra-uterine growth retardation: what do we know? *Aust. NZ J. Obstet. Gynaecol.*, **29**, 279

63. McDiarmid, J.M. and Silva, P.A. (1979). Three year old twins and singletons: a comparison of some perinatal, environmental, experimental and development characteristics. *Aust. Paediatr. J.*, **15**, 243

64. Silva, P.A. (1982). Growth and development of twins compared to singletons at ages five and seven: a follow-up on the Dunedin multi-disciplinary child development study. *Aust. Paediatr. J.*, **18**, 35

65. Silva, P.A. (1985). The growth and development of twins compared to singletons at ages nine and eleven. *Aust. Paediatr. J.*, **21**, 265

66. Russel, E.M. (1961). Cerebral palsied twins. *Arch. Dis. Child.*, **36**, 363

67. Illingworth, R.S. and Woods, G.E. (1960). The incidence of twins in cerebral palsy and mental retardation. *Arch. Dis. Child.*, **35**, 333

68. McDonald, A.D. (1963). Cerebral palsy in children of very low birth weight. *Arch. Dis. Child.*, **30**, 579

69. Atkinson, S. and Stanley, F.S. (1983). Spastic dysplasia in children of low and normal birthweight. *Devel. Med. Child. Neurol.*, **25**, 693
70. Stanley, F.S. (1989). Cerebral palsy in multiple births. *Irish Med. J.*, **82**, 97
71. Blair, E. and Stanley, F.S. (1990). Intrauterine growth and spastic cerebral palsy. I. Association with gestational age. *Am. J. Obstet. Gynecol.*, **162**, 219
72. Hastie, S.J., Dauskin, F., Nelson, J.P. *et al.* (1989). Prediction of the small for gestational age twin fetus by Doppler umbilical artery analysis waveforms analysis. *Obstet. Gynecol.*, **74**, 730
73. Giles, V., Trudinger, B.J., Cook, C.M. *et al.* (1988). Umbilical artery flow velocity waveforms and twin pregnancy outcome. *Obstet. Gynecol.*, **71**, 894
74. Leveno, K.J., Quirk, J.G., Whalley, P.J. *et al.* (1984). Fetal lung maturation in twin gestation. *Am. J. Obstet. Gynecol.*, **148**, 405
75. Ohel, G., Grant, N., Zeevi, D. *et al.* (1987). Advanced ultrasonic placental maturation in twin pregnancies. *Am. J. Obstet. Gynecol.*, **156**, 76
76. Amiel-Tison, C. (1980). Possible acceleration of neurological maturity following high risk pregnancies. *Am. J. Obstet. Gynecol.*, **136**, 303
77. Amiel-Tison, C. and Pettigrew, A.G. (1991). Adaptive changes in the developing brain during intrauterine stress. *Brain Dev.*, **13**, 67
78. Pettigrew, A.G., Edwards, D.A. and Henderson-Smart, D.J. (1985). The influence of intrauterine growth retardation on brainstem development of preterm infants. *Dev. Med. Child. Neurol.*, **27**, 467
79. Gould, J.B., Gluck, L. and Koluvich, M.V. (1977). The relationship between accelerated pulmonary maturity and accelerated neurological maturity in certain chronically stressed pregnancies. *Am. J. Obstet. Gynecol.*, **127**, 181

Assessment of cervical change 34

R.B. Newman, R.K. Godsey and J.M. Ellings

Introduction

This chapter discusses the examination of the uterine cervix as part of routine prenatal care provided to women with multifetal pregnancies. An understanding of the evolution of cervical changes in these pregnancies is an issue of particular importance, as this knowledge may help identify women at risk for preterm labor and its subsequent perinatal morbidity and mortality[1-4]. Such knowledge may also identify women at risk for premature rupture of the membranes, assist in the timely diagnosis of cervical incompetence and, finally, enhance the ability to determine the feasibility of labor induction.

The role of antepartum cervical examination as it relates to the processes of preterm and term labor cannot be underestimated. As more information about the relationship between uterine activity and cervical maturation becomes available, information obtained from antepartum cervical examination can only enhance our ability to recognize the onset of preterm labor and to suggest timely and effective interventions.

Anatomy and histology of the cervix

The uterine cervix is divided into vaginal and supravaginal portions. The lowermost boundary of the cervix is the external os, located in the vaginal portion of the cervix, the portio vaginalis. In nulliparous women, the external cervical os is usually small and oval, whereas in multiparous women, it may develop an irregular appearance after scarring of transverse or stellate obstetric lacerations. The upper boundary is the internal os, located in the supravaginal portion of the cervix. The supravaginal portion of the cervix is attached laterally to the transverse cervical ligaments and is separated from the overlying bladder anteriorly by loose connective tissue. The internal cervical os is usually located at the level of the reflection of the uterine serosa onto the bladder. The entire cervix is approximately 4 cm in length and is characterized histologically by the presence of squamous epithelium on the portio vaginalis and proliferative glandular tissue composed of high columnar epithelium located in the endocervix (Figure 1).

The transition zone between the uterine cervix and the muscular fundus occurs over a distance of approximately 1 cm in the lowermost portion of the fundus, an area called the isthmus. Although the isthmus is not considered part of the cervix from a histological point of view, it is considered to be a portion of the anatomical internal cervical os (Figure 2). The uterine isthmus is presumed to have an important role in the retention of the conceptus and is probably involved in the development of the lower uterine segment in late pregnancy[5,6]. *There is no evidence to suggest any differences in the anatomical or histological characteristics of the uterine cervix in either the uncomplicated multifetal gestation or the uncomplicated singleton pregnancy.*

Maturational changes

The uterine cervix contains three principal structural elements: smooth muscle, collagen and connective tissue or 'ground substance'. The smooth muscle component predominates in the muscular fundus but diminishes progressively and dramatically from the isthmus to

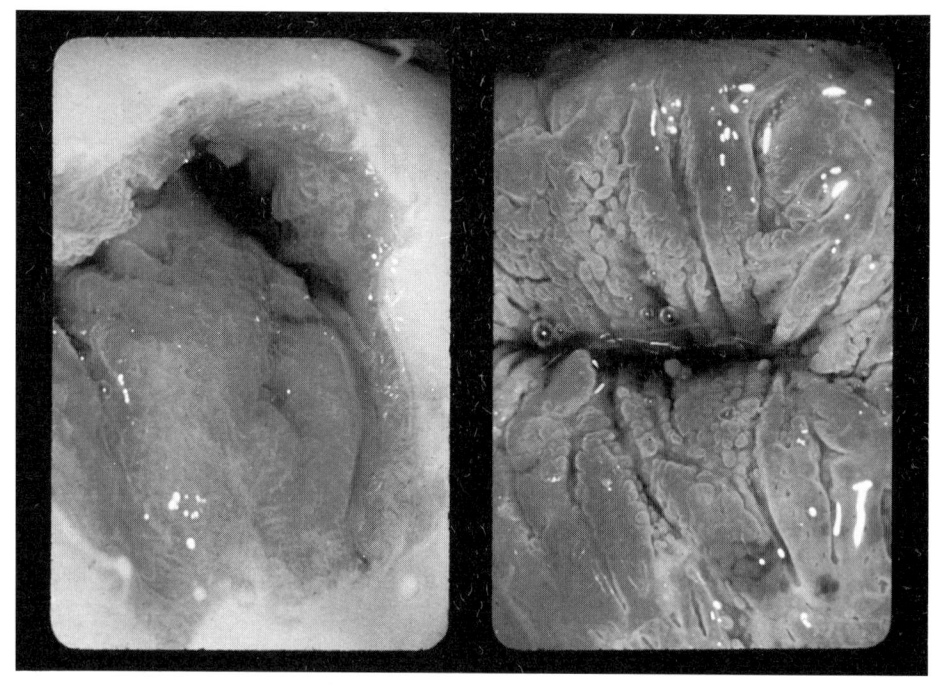

Figure 1 Colposcopic photograph of the portio vaginalis and the normal squamo-columnar junction (left) and proliferative villus-like endocervical glandular tissue (right)

the upper and then to the lower portion of the cervix[7]. Buckingham et al. determined that about 10% of the normal cervix was composed of smooth muscle. Interestingly, however, this percentage was much higher in women diagnosed as having cervical incompetency[8]. However, these investigations did not indicate that the relative proportion of smooth muscle changes appreciably over the course of pregnancy. Therefore, alterations in smooth muscle content are not believed to be major factors in the process of cervical maturation.

Danforth et al. first demonstrated that the major structural changes of cervical maturation primarily involved changes in the collagen and connective tissue components[9]. The triple helix of collagen alpha chains, or tropocollagen, is laid down as ordered fibers embedded in the connective tissue matrix. The ordered arrangement of tropocollagen molecules is the quarter-staggered array stabilized by the formation of both intra-molecular and inter-molecular cross links. The intrinsic stability of the tropocollagen molecule and the binding of the collagen fibrils to the ground substance results in the strength of the non-pregnant cervix. Danforth et al. proposed that the ground substance becomes much more prominent during cervical maturation and that the previously orderly collagen fibrils begin to break apart. The combined changes in the ground substance and the destabilization of the collagen content result in more than a tenfold reduction in mechanical strength of the cervix[10].

The diminution of cervical strength in late pregnancy results from the synthesis of proteolytic and collagenolytic enzymes as well as the activation of preformed zymogens[11,12]. The enzymatic digestion of tropocollagen results in fragmentation, solubilization and elimination of the collagen fragments from the cervical tissue. This process precedes clinical cervical maturation or ripening. Ekman et al. performed cervical biopsies on women in labor at term and identified a close correlation between the clinical course of labor and the biochemical composition of the cervix[13]. Collagen acted as an important regulator of cervical function, and a decline in the collagen content of the cervix was related to a greater

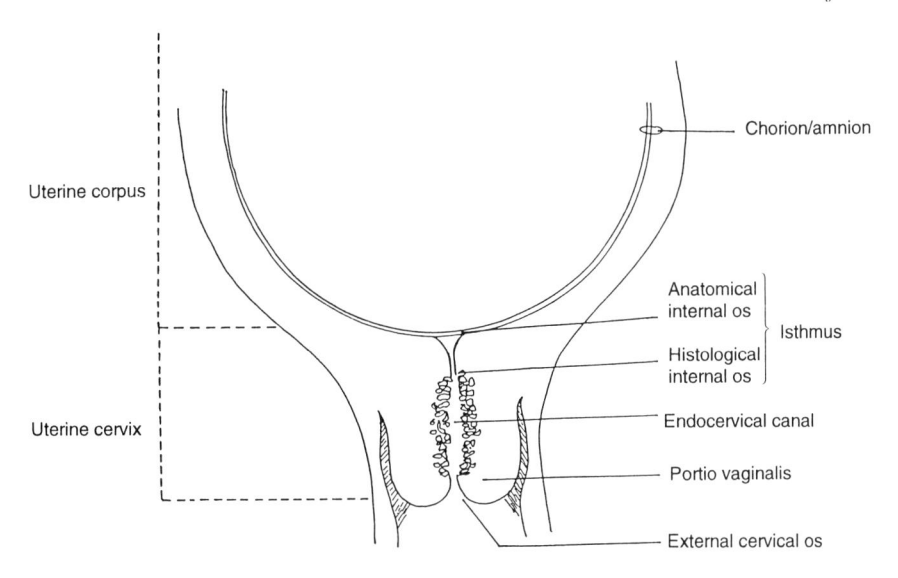

Figure 2 Anatomy and anatomical relationships of the uterine corpus, uterine cervix and isthmus

degree of cervical dilatation and a faster course of labor.

The connective tissue 'ground substance' is composed of cervical glycosaminoglycans, including dermatan sulfate, chondroitin sulfate and hyaluronic acid. As term approaches, alterations in the relative concentrations of these various glycosaminoglycan and glycoprotein complexes influence the arrangement and density of cervical collagen fibers and their water content (Figure 3). Animal investigations indicate that the overall glycosaminoglycan concentrations remains fairly stable during gestation, although the relative proportions of specific glycosaminoglycans varies[13]. Hyaluronic acid concentrations apparently increase significantly near term in conjunction with a simultaneous decline in the concentrations of collagen, dermatan sulfate and chondroitin sulfate in both animal and human cervices[14–18]. A triad of biochemical processes, that is, the degradation of collagen in late pregnancy, the loss of the dermatan and chondroitin sulfates which tend to secure the collagen fibers, and the relative increase in the concentration of hydrophilic hyaluronic acid is primarily responsible for the increased flexibility, distensibility, swelling and softening of the cervix. These changes are considered to represent the process of cervical maturation.

Maturational influences

The mechanism by which the process of cervical maturation is initiated is unknown, as is the case for labor. However, the close temporal relationship between the process of cervical maturation and the initiation of labor suggests that the two processes may be under simultaneous influence. Several possible factors may play important roles.

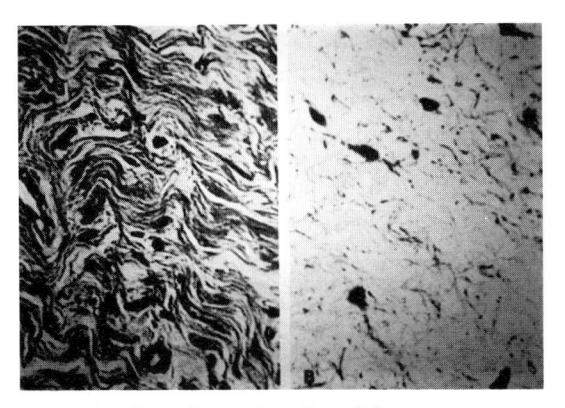

Figure 3 The collagen bundles of the non-pregnant cervix are densely packed and orderly arranged (left). In late pregnancy, these collagen bundles become sparse and more disordered (right). The space between the collagen bundles is filled with ground substance, particularly hydrophilic hyaluronic acid and scattered fibroblasts. (Reproduced with permission from reference 9)

Steroid hormones

An alteration of the steroid hormone environment of the cervix in favor of a rising estrogen/progesterone ratio may initiate collagenolytic activity[19]. Collagenase is synthesized and stored as inactive zymogens which require other proteolytic enzymes for their activation. These enzymes are, for the most part, stored intracellularly in lysosomes whose membranes are stabilized by the high progesterone levels characteristic of pregnancy. A rising estrogen level and a falling progesterone level destabilize these lysosomal membranes and release proteolytic enzymes, such as proteinase, cathepsin-D and peptidase, all of which can then activate tissue collagenases[20]. Progesterone administration prevents collagen breakdown in both animal models and the non-pregnant human cervix[21,22]. Unfortunately, there is no convincing evidence of alterations in the serum concentrations of progesterone in the human pregnancy near term[23]. It remains possible, however, that the actual tissue concentrations of these steroid hormones, their receptor concentrations, or the presence or absence of local inhibitors may play an important role in cervical ripening[24]. Yanaihara *et al.* have identified higher concentrations of free estrone, conjugated estradiol, estriol and dihydroepiendosterone in ripened cervical tissue compared to the unripe cervix[25]. These differences increase as labor progresses. Gordon and Calder demonstrated accelerated cervical ripening with the intra-vaginal application of 150 mg of estradiol valerate gel[26]. The effect of estrogen on cervical maturation is believed to result from its direct action on cervical collagen, rather than being secondary to myometrial contractility[27].

Prostaglandins

The intra-cervical or intra-vaginal application of prostaglandin $F_{2\alpha}$ or prostaglandin E_2 affect cervical maturation in the absence of uterine contractions[28,29]. The action of prostaglandins to induce cervical maturation is likely to be a direct collagenolytic effect[30]. The cervical biopsy studies of Ekman *et al.* demonstrated increased collagenolytic activity and increased collagen extractibility following the local application of prostaglandin E_2 gel in a manner thought to mimic spontaneous cervical ripening[13]. Prostaglandins stimulate uterine contractions with a frequency related to dose and route of administration. However, even when contractions are suppressed by the simultaneous use of betamimetics, prostaglandins still cause significant cervical ripening, thus suggesting a direct effect of prostaglandins on the cervical connective tissue[31].

Relaxin

Several investigators have reported that topical administration of pharmacological doses of porcine relaxin to the human cervix results in cervical softening, effacement and a shortening of the induction–delivery interval[32–34]. In some mammalian species, serum levels of relaxin rise toward the end of pregnancy, and administration of this agent to non-pregnant, estrogen-primed animals results in histological, biochemical and biomechanical changes that mimic spontaneous cervical maturation[35]. Unfortunately, the role of endogenous relaxin in human pregnancy is still unclear, and little evidence exists for a role of this hormone in human pregnancy.

Dilatation and effacement

Whether these or other endocrine factors are solely or only partly responsible for cervical maturation, the end result is a softer, more distensible cervix. Increased cervical compliance does not necessarily result in changes in cervical dilatation or effacement, however. These last two processes result from the contractile activity of the uterine fundus which gradually pulls cervical tissue upward and over the presenting part and incorporates this tissue into the uterine isthmus[36]. The two distinct processes of increasing uterine activity and cervical maturation, which in all likelihood act in concert under endocrine control, are important in the preparation for and the timing of labor in humans.

Although little evidence exists to support the contention that the endocrinological environment is altered in multifetal compared to singleton pregnancies, considerable evidence exists to support the concept that baseline uterine activity is significantly increased in multifetal pregnancies. In what are now considered classic studies of myometrial activity, Caldeyro-Barcia *et al.* introduced intra-myometrial microballoons with pressure catheters, as well as intra-amniotic pressure catheters, and recorded contraction frequency, intensity and uterine tone in the latter half of gestation[37]. These investigators recorded a significant increase in contraction frequency and intensity during the last 2 weeks of pregnancy. These changes were thought to exert an important affect on the cervix in preparation for labor[38]. With regard to twin pregnancies, it was reported that uterine tone and contraction intensity were normal compared to singleton gestations, but no mention was made regarding contraction frequency. It was also shown that uterine over-distension, as is seen with hydramnios, is associated with a rise in uterine tone and a fall in the contraction intensity with an inverse relationship between intensity and frequency. However, Caldeyro-Barcia *et al.* indicated that these findings were not evident with multifetal pregnancies, presumably because the increase in uterine volume was sufficiently gradual to allow time for compensatory hypertrophy and hyperplasia of the myometrial fibers[37,39].

The frequency of antepartum uterine contractions in multifetal gestations has been examined in recent years. Using a lightweight tocodynamometer designed for ambulatory outpatient use, Newman *et al.* monitored uterine activity daily during the latter half of pregnancy in 22 women with one fetus and 18 women with twins. Among these 40 women, all of whom delivered at term, the twins showed a significant increase in contraction frequency before 36 weeks' gestation compared to the singletons[40]. This finding is consistent with the findings of Caldeyro-Barcia *et al.* for the over-distended uterus[37]. For reasons that are not well understood, women with multifetal pregnancies are significantly less likely to perceive their contractions than are the mothers of singletons[41]. This is unfortunate, because uterine activity of this nature and degree may result in early, painless cervical dilatation and effacement. The incorrect diagnosis of this condition (painless cervical dilatation and effacement) as cervical incompetency frequently has led to the unsuccessful use of cervical cerclage for both twin and triplet gestations[3,42,43]. To be effective, the practice of cerclage should be limited to very carefully selected women who have had a classic history of painless, mid-trimester pre-viable loss of a prior singleton gestation.

Preterm labor with documented progressive cervical dilatation and effacement among high-risk singleton and twin pregnancies is often heralded by a sharp increase in the baseline contraction frequency compared to women who labor at term[44,45]. Women with triplet gestations also have an increased baseline contraction frequency similar to twin gestations. Surprisingly, however, no significant increase in the mean contraction frequency occurs immediately prior to pre-term labor. The occurrence of progressive cervical dilatation and effacement in high-risk singleton and twin gestations is, at least in part, contraction-dependent. In contrast, a significant increase in pre-labor uterine contraction frequency may not play as critical a role in affecting cervical change in triplet gestations. Whereas the forces that bring about early cervical change in triplet gestations are not as clear, our own investigations suggest that an increased frequency of low-amplitude, high-frequency contractility may be an important marker for this change[44,46]. Alternatively, a more rapid progression of cervical change in response to an increase in uterine contraction frequency may be obscured by the calculation of a mean weekly contraction frequency, as was the case in our studies. At present, this issue remains unresolved. However, there is no doubt that as the fetal number increases, the duration of gestation decreases. The inverse relationship between fetal number and the duration of pregnancy was reported first in a classic paper by McKowan and Record, confirmed in 1976 by Caspi et al.[47,48], and now is accepted as a clinical reality.

As a result of excessive uterine activity, multifetal gestations experience significant pre-labor cervical dilatation and effacement. In our own review of 166 multifetal gestations presenting in labor between 1977 and 1982, we observed significant pre-labor cervical maturation. Seventy-seven per cent of the women with multiple gestations had cervical dilatation of 3 cm or more at the time of admission in labor, and 82% had cervical effacement of >60%. An additional perspective is provided by graphico-statistical analysis of the effect of multiple pregnancy on the course of labor[49]. Friedman and Sachtleben concluded that 'because of the high incidence of significant pre-labor cervical dilatation, a clearly defined shortening of the latent phase occurs'[49]. These authors also noted that the distribution of the initial cervical dilatation among patients with multifetal gestations was significantly different from that of patients with singleton gestations. Sixty-two per cent of nulliparous singleton pregnancies began labor with less than 2 cm cervical dilatation, and only 7% began labor dilated ≥ 3 cm. A parallel analysis for twin pregnancies revealed that only 26% of nulliparas started labor with < 2 cm cervical dilatation, in contrast to 39% who were dilated ≥ 3 cm. Among multiparous women, 23% of singleton pregnancies began labor with the cervix dilated ≥ 3 cm compared to 60% of the multiparous twin pregnancies[49] (see Chapter 32).

In summary, multiple processes that occur prior to labor in multifetal gestations may result in advanced states of pre-labor cervical maturation. For example, levels of steroid hormones are increased in multifetal compared to singleton gestations. Higher maternal serum levels of various estrogens, progesterone, human placental lactogen, human chorionic gonadotropin, for example, have all been reported in multifetal pregnancies. Whatever role these hormones may have, either to promote or to inhibit the cervical maturation process, certainly they may be magnified in the multifetal pregnancy. In addition, it has been postulated that prostaglandin synthesis may be increased in multifetal pregnancies. It is believed that uterine overdistension may cause a relative decidual ischemia with liberation of lysosomal enzymes. These enzymes include various phospholipases, which initiate the prostaglandin cascade by liberating arachidonic acid from its glycerophospholipid storage forms. Arachidonic acid is the critical substrate for prostaglandin synthesis, particularly of the E_2 and F_2 series. Increased prostaglandin activity may also result from other hormonal or humoral factors. As noted previously, these influences affect collagen integrity and the 'ground substance' content, thereby altering the consistency and distensibility of the cervix. Changes in cervical dilatation and effacement then result in response to the hydrostatic forces generated by the increased pre-labor uterine activity in multifetal pregnancy.

Antepartum examination

A complete and well-documented description of the preterm cervix is essential to determine differences between the normal and abnormal cervical state at any given gestational age. Notable characteristics of the antepartum cervix include the respective amounts and degrees of dilatation and effacement, the station of the presenting part and, finally, the consistency and position of the cervix. Cervical examination was popularized by Bishop, and his scoring system is frequently used by obstetricians to evaluate the inducibility of labor at term[50]. Friedman et al. subsequently evaluated the specific components of the Bishop score and found that cervical dilatation prior to induction exerted the greatest prognostic influence on the course of labor[51]. Other investigators have also critically evaluated the antepartum cervical examination in singleton gestations and concluded that cervical dilatation and effacement are the two most important factors predicting the timing of labor onset or the inducibility of labor at term[52–55].

A particularly interesting aspect of the report by Stubbs et al.[55] was the degree of similarity found between the antepartum evaluation of cervical dilatation and effacement among two blinded examiners. Indeed, intra-examiner differences were minimal, and agreement as to the degree of cervical dilatation was within 1 cm in 98% of the paired examinations. Moreover, intra-examiner differences in the assessment of cervical length were less than 1 cm in over 90% of the examinations. These authors concluded that 'the human hand is a sensitive instrument for investigation'[55]. In contrast to the relatively objective measurement of cervical dilatation and effacement, however, the evaluation of cervical position and consistency is, by its very nature, highly subjective, and provides little prognostic information once cervical dilatation and effacement have been considered[53]. The antepartum evaluation of fetal station in singleton pregnancies is also of limited value, because it is significantly affected by parity, the presenting part frequently being lower in nulliparous patients[54,55]. Houlton et al. reported that in twin pregnancies, station also had limited usefulness, because the presenting part is often high before the onset of labor in parous women and because of the increased incidence of malpresentation[56].

Over and above the process of cervical maturation, the factor that most affects cervical status is maternal parity. Numerous investigations have described the influence of parity on cervical dilatation. These reports have repeatedly identified a greater degree of cervical dilatation at the internal os in multiparous compared to nulliparous singleton pregnancies[54,55,57,58]. However, in the study by Stubbs et al., a significant increase in the amount of cervical dilatation was observed in parous women, but the absolute difference was small (less than 0.5 cm)[55].

In the study by Hendricks et al., nulliparous women with singletons were generally more effaced than parous women during the last 4 weeks prior to delivery[54]. Because parous women have a greater degree of cervical dilatation and nulliparous women have a greater degree of cervical effacement preceding the onset of labor, these authors calculated a cervical coefficient score that represented cervical dilatation in centimeters multiplied by the percentage cervical effacement. Using this system, a progressive increase in the cervical coefficient score preceded labor, and the cervical coefficients were similar for both nulliparous and parous women[51]. Another effort to standardize the differences in cervical status between nulliparous and parous women is the calculated cervical score described by Houlton et al.[56]. The cervical score is derived by subtracting cervical dilatation at the internal os in centimeters from the cervical length in centimeters. For example, a cervix 2 cm long with a closed internal os would give a score of +2. A cervix 1 cm long with a cervix dilated 1 cm at the internal os gives a score of zero. A cervix 1 cm long with an internal os dilated 3 cm would give a score of −2 (Figure 4).

Prediction of preterm delivery

The use of the antepartum cervical examination has been investigated extensively to assess its validity in predicting the onset of preterm labor. The majority of available information derives from studies of high- and low-risk singleton gestations. Many investigators, most notably Papiernik and co-workers, have emphasized the importance of the assessment of cervical status in late pregnancy as a sign of impending preterm labor[59]. In a prospective study of serial changes in cervical status in more than 8000 pregnancies, Papiernik et al. showed that term as well as preterm labor were preceded by cervical changes that were detectable days or weeks before parturition[57]. These authors noted that the early dilatation of the internal cervical os (≥1 cm) predicted the highest relative risk of preterm delivery and that cervical length (≤1 cm) was of secondary importance. The gestational age at which the dilatation of the internal os was identified could be directly related to the gestational age at delivery.

At our institution, Stubbs et al. prospectively evaluated the predictive value of serial antepartum cervical examinations in singletons[55]. Again, the occurrence of abnormal premature cervical change was associated with an increased relative risk of preterm delivery[55]. The

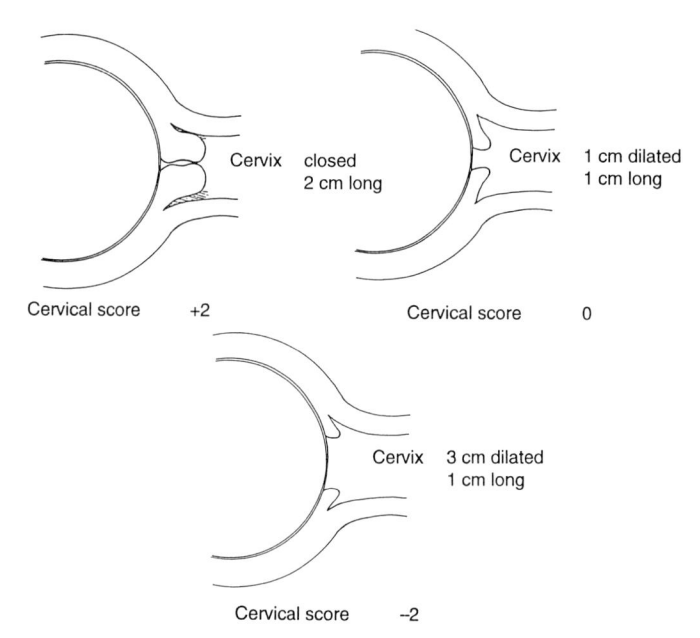

Figure 4 Diagram of various cervical examinations resulting in cervical scores of +2, zero and −2 as described by Houlton et al.[56]. (Cervical score = cervical length (cm) minus cervical dilatation (cm) at the internal os)

positive predictive value for preterm delivery was low, however, but this would be anticipated in a low-prevalence population. In contrast, the negative predictive value of the absence of any preterm cervical change was very high, and this information may be of great value in a higher prevalence population such as that of multiple pregnancy. Leveno et al. performed a single cervical examination between 26 and 30 weeks' gestation in 185 low-risk singletons and found that 15 had cervical dilatation of 2–3 cm. Preterm birth occurred in 27% of these women, in contrast to only 2% of those women with a cervix dilated 1 cm or less[60]. Wood et al. performed cervical examinations every other week from 24 weeks onward in 250 singleton pregnancies. Twelve per cent of the singletons developed cervical dilatation of ≥1 cm or complete effacement prior to 34 weeks' gestation. Premature labor occurred in 28% of these women. Only one of the remaining women without such cervical change went into uncomplicated preterm labor[61].

Despite these observations, the value of the antepartum cervical examination in the prediction of preterm delivery among singleton gestations remains controversial. Anderson and Turnbull evaluated the cervix in the latter half of pregnancy in 90 healthy primigravid women. They found that dilatation of the internal cervical os at 32 weeks' gestation was related to an earlier onset of labor but was not related to the onset of preterm labor[62]. However, this study has limited value in view of the fact that there were only 77 spontaneous deliveries among this very low-risk group. Parikh and Mehta, as well as Schaffner and Schanzer, found that a relatively high percentage of women had an open internal cervical os between 28 and 32 weeks' gestation (38% and 27%, respectively); however, dilatation of the internal cervical os could not be related to an increased risk of preterm delivery[58,63]. These two groups of authors concluded that such changes were anatomical variants related primarily to increased parity.

Most commonly applied risk scoring systems identify multiple gestation as an independent factor classifying a woman as being at risk for preterm labor and delivery. The potential value of the antepartum cervical examination in these pregnancies may lie in developing an ongoing risk assessment tool. Wood et al. first suggested the value of antepartum cervical examination in predicting the risk of preterm delivery among multifetal gestations[61]. Although the authors followed a small number of women (nine), three had dilatation of the internal cervical os of at least one fingerbreadth before the 34th week of gestation and all three delivered preterm. In five of the remaining six women, the cervix was closed until the 36th week of gestation, and labor occurred after the 38th week in all cases. O'Connor et al. instituted routine cervical examination as part of a special antepartum twin clinic and reported their findings in 1981. In their study, a cervical dilatation of 2 cm or more before 30 weeks' gestation predicted preterm delivery with a sensitivity of only 20%[64]. However, such low sensitivity may not be unexpected, given the early gestational age at which these examinations were performed. Of the 28 primigravidas in their study, only two had cervical dilatation before 30 weeks and one delivered preterm. Of the 72 multigravid patients, only 14 had a cervical dilatation of 2 cm on or before 30 weeks' gestation and six delivered prematurely[64].

Since the publication of the study by O'Connor et al., several other investigations have reported the predictive value of the antepartum cervical examination in larger populations of multifetal pregnancies. Houlton, Marivate and Philpott followed 128 twin pregnancies with weekly cervical examinations at the King Edward VIII Hospital in Durban, South Africa. Women were followed in a special clinic with weekly cervical evaluation for the purpose of calculating a cervical score. Examinations continued until the spontaneous onset of labor, without benefit of tocolysis[56]. These authors found that a cervical score of ≤ 0 on any single examination was significantly related to the onset of labor. A cervical score of ≤ 0 or a fall in the cervical score predicted preterm labor within 14 days in 69% of the women with such cervical changes. When only multiparous women were considered, the predictive value rose to 80%, suggesting that the predictive value of the cervical score may be marginally less for nulliparous women. In this study, the false-positive rate for a low cervical score and labor within 2 weeks was only 3% $(1/34)$[56].

In 1988, Neilson et al. followed 223 parous women with twins in a special clinic at the Harare Central Hospital in Zimbabwe and performed frequent cervical examinations to calculate a cervical score. As was the case in the study from Durban, no attempt was made to inhibit preterm labor with tocolytic drugs[65]. The findings of Neilson et al. were similar to those of Houlton et al.. Cervical scores provided valuable predictive information regarding the occurrence of preterm delivery. Neilson et al. focused on the prognostic significance of a cervical score of ≤ 0 on or before 34 weeks' gestation. The positive predictive value of such a score was 66%. As the cervical score became more negative, the predictive value rose. A cervical score of ≤ -2 identified a subgroup of women at a 76% risk for preterm delivery. The occasional patient with a low cervical score who did not develop premature labor was thought to represent a dominance by endocrine factors acting directly on the structure of the cervix rather than contractility which would probably be progressive[65].

In 1988, we established a Twin Clinic at the Medical University of South Carolina and have followed over 100 multifetal pregnancies, including seven triplet gestations[66]. Antepartum visits were conducted at intervals of every one or two weeks. At each clinic visit, a digital examination was performed to calculate a cervical score in the manner described by Houlton et al.[56]. Preterm births occurred following the spontaneous onset of preterm labor or as a consequence of preterm premature rupture of the membranes. Some patients with preterm labor were treated with tocolytic therapy. Those patients successfully tocolyzed were classified as either term or preterm births depending on when spontaneous delivery ultimately occurred. Women who were delivered preterm for maternal or fetal indications were excluded from analysis of results, whereas spontaneous and induced term deliveries are included.

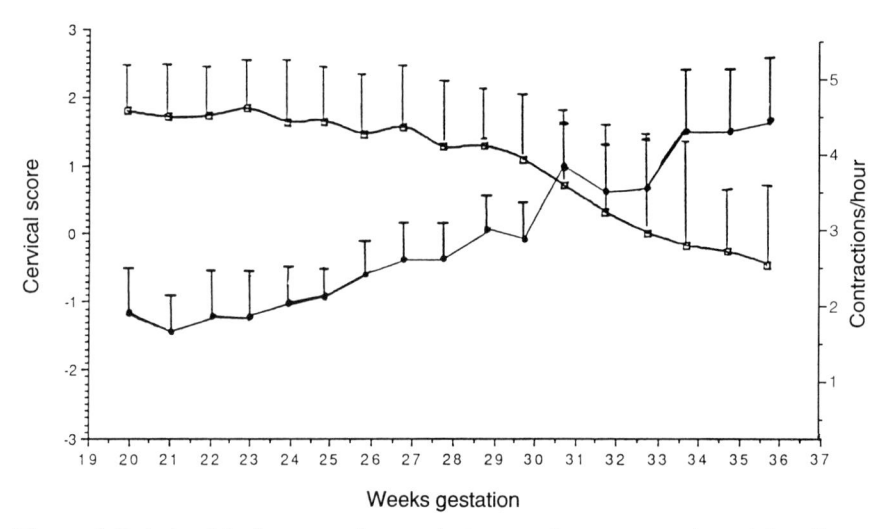

Figure 5 Relationship between the cervical score (open squares) and baseline uterine contraction frequency (filled circles) for multifetal gestations between 20 and 36 weeks' gestation. Bars indicate SD

Weekly cervical assessments of these patients revealed a progressive fall in cervical score throughout the latter half of gestation. This fall in cervical score was most notable after 30 weeks' gestation. The relationship between the decrease in cervical score in multifetal pregnancies and the increase in baseline uterine activity in these gestations is graphically represented in Figure 5. The progressive fall in cervical score with advancing gestation appears to mirror the crescendo of pre-labor uterine activity seen with multifetal gestations. Stated another way, as the cervical score decreases, the mean time until delivery shortens. The time interval until delivery associated with any specific cervical score in our patient population was similar to the findings of Neilson et al. in their study of parous African women with twins (Table 1). The similarities between these two patient populations are clear, despite the use of activity restriction and tocolytic therapy in the racially mixed patient population of South Carolina. Among the women followed in our South Carolina Twin Clinic, there was a very strong correlation ($r^2 = 91\%$) between cervical score and the duration of time until spontaneous delivery. These results suggest a strong relationship between the state of the antepartum cervix and the timing of delivery in the multifetal gestation.

We found that multifetal pregnancies complicated by preterm delivery had lower mean cervical scores compared to the women who delivered at term[66]. These findings are also similar to those of Neilson et al. in that the differences between the groups delivering preterm or at term occurred primarily between 31 and 35 weeks' gestation (Figure 6). In our data, an abnormal cervical score helped define a given patient's risk of preterm labor and delivery. Selecting a cervical score of ≤ 0 on or before 34 weeks' gestation as the definition of an abnormal examination was associated with a positive predictive value of 75% for preterm delivery. Table 2 presents the sensitivity, specificity, predictive values and relative risk of preterm birth associated with a cervical score of ≤ 0 on or before 34 weeks' gestation. In addition, this table also provides the same analysis with respect to gestational age (20–28 weeks and 29–34 weeks) and parity (nulliparous and parous)[66]. The earlier in gestation that a low cervical score is detected, the greater the positive predictive value which can be ascribed to it. In our own patient population, a cervical score of ≤ 0 between 20 and 28 weeks' gestation was associated with a 92% risk of preterm delivery; however, the sensitivity was low, as was the case in the study by O'Connor et al.[64]. Parous women in our population tended to have very similar cervical scores compared to their nulliparous counterparts throughout

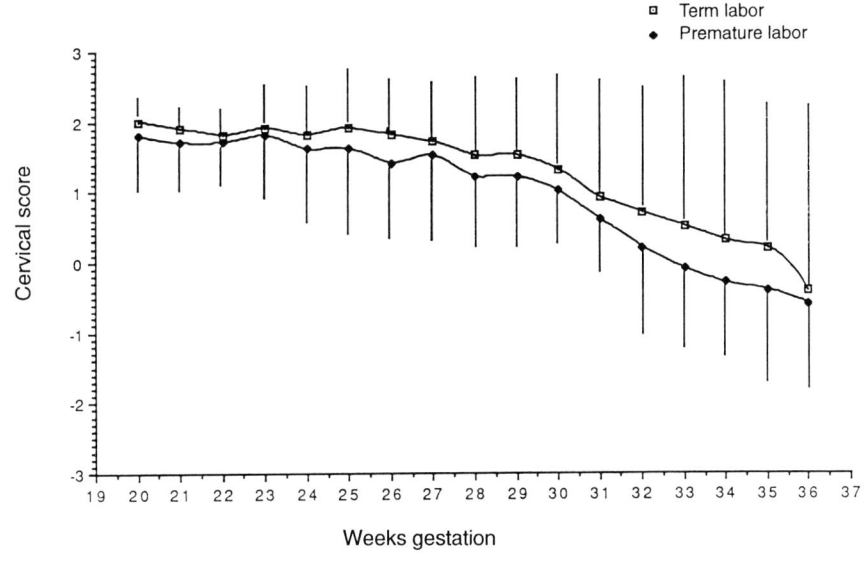

Figure 6 Mean cervical score and the standard deviations from 20 to 36 weeks' gestation for multifetal gestations with term ($n = 34$) and preterm ($n = 44$) delivery

Table 1 Duration (weeks) from the first appearance of a specific cervical score to the spontaneous onset of labor in multifetal gestations

Cervical score	Neilson et al.[65]		Newman et al.[66]	
	n	Duration until labor*	n	Duration until labor*
+2	70	7.9 ± 4.1	66	8.8 ± 4.2
+1	115	4.8 ± 2.5	34	7.0 ± 3.5
0	155	3.6 ± 2.2	25	3.7 ± 1.7
−1	163	2.8 ± 2.1	26	3.2 ± 2.3
−2	159	1.8 ± 1.4	14	2.0 ± 1.3
−3	67	1.3 ± 1.1	12	1.5 ± 0.8

*Mean ± standard deviation

gestation. Slightly lower mean cervical scores were identified after 32 weeks' gestation; however, this did not significantly alter either the positive predictive value (72% vs. 83%) or the relative risk (4.3 vs. 3.3) of preterm delivery[66]. As the cervical score becomes more negative, the positive predictive value for preterm delivery approaches 100%, but the sensitivity is quite low, due to the relative rarity of such abnormal antepartum examinations.

It is reasonable to use a cervical score of ≤0 as a marker of abnormal cervical status and increased preterm delivery risk. A cervical score of ≤0 seems to strike the correct balance between the number of women identified as being at increased risk of preterm delivery and the actual number of jeopardized babies correctly identified. The other important factor to consider is the gestational age at which such an abnormal cervical score is detected. Patients identified as having an abnormal cervical examination at < 30 weeks' gestation are at risk for tragically early preterm delivery associated with a high risk of perinatal morbidity and mortality. The incorporation of serial cervical examinations and the information gained

Table 2 Sensitivity, specificity, predictive values and relative risk of premature delivery (< 37 weeks' gestation) based on a cervical score of ≤ 0 on or before 34 weeks' gestation

Patient groups	Sensitivity (%)	Specificity (%)	Positive predictive value (%)	Negative predictive value (%)	Relative risk*	p-Value
All patients	88	62	75	81	3.9 (1.8 < RR < 8.7)	≤ 0.0001
20–28 weeks	33	96	92	61	2.0 (1.4 < RR < 2.9)	≤ 0.01
29–34 weeks	87	81	73	81	3.8 (1.7 < RR < 8.5)	≤ 0.0001
Nulliparous	83	75	83	75	3.3 (1.0 < RR < 11.4)	≤ 0.02
Parous	91	58	72	83	4.3 (1.5 < RR < 12.4)	≤ 0.001

*Relative risk (RR) with 95% confidence limits

by calculation of the cervical score have helped us to reduce the incidence of very low birth weight deliveries and perinatal mortality among twins followed in a specialized, multidisciplinary clinic[67]. Obstetricians need complete knowledge of the evolution of cervical change in multifetal gestations in order to understand the prognostic significance of any specific cervical score.

Prediction of term delivery

Probably as important as the ability of an abnormal cervical score to predict the premature onset of labor is the reassurance provided by the finding of a normal cervical score. In a series of 223 twin pregnancies reported by Neilson et al.[65], no patient delivered within a week of having a cervical score of > 0. Among our patients, only two of 78 (2.6%) women experienced spontaneous preterm labor or preterm premature rupture of the membranes within one week of being found to have a cervical score of > 0[66]. Women who maintain a cervical score of > 0 appear to be good candidates for continued observation rather than being subjected to controversial obstetric interventions. Better identification of patients at risk for spontaneous preterm labor or preterm premature rupture of the membranes may allow the more specific application of interventions potentially capable of reducing the likelihood of preterm delivery. Unfortunately, the efficacy of interventions such as bed rest, antepartum hospitalization, prophylactic tocolysis, and home uterine activity monitoring have all been questioned. Despite the fact that studies have failed to demonstrate any advantage to routine hospitalized bed rest for twin or triplet gestations, these interventions have been used by practitioners[3,68,69]. Similarly, prophylactic tocolysis has also been extensively applied in multifetal gestations without clear effect[70,71]. Although home uterine activity monitoring has been effective in making the early diagnosis of preterm labor in multifetal gestations, this modality remains an expensive and labor-intensive approach to preterm birth prevention[3,72,73].

Under these circumstances, the ability to differentiate normal from abnormal antepartum cervical examinations may be of enormous value in designing clinical protocols to determine the indications for and effectiveness of a variety of obstetric interventions. The cervical score is recommended as a part of the routine antepartum cervical examination because of its simplicity, quantifiability, reproducibility and focus on cervical dilatation and effacement.

Safety of the antepartum cervical examination

The major impediment to the greater acceptance of antepartum cervical examination is concern over its safety (Table 3). McColgin et al. recently reported that 'membrane stripping' at term results in a lower incidence of post-date pregnancies and an earlier onset of spontaneous labor with no differences in the

Assessment of cervical change

Table 3 Risks (%) associated with antepartum cervical examination in term (>37 weeks' gestation) and preterm singleton gestations

	n	Preterm delivery	PROM	Chorioamnionitis	Endometritis
Term gestations					
McColgin et al.[74]					
examination	286	—	17	3	1
no examination	282	—	17	4	1
Lenihan[75]					
examination	174	—	18	—	—
no examination	175	—	6*	—	—
Preterm gestations					
Holbrook et al.[77]					
examination	133	—	21	3	6
no examination	467	—	30	4	5
Main et al.[78]					
examination	64	25	12	—	—
no examination	68	21	6	—	—

PROM, premature rupture of the membranes
*$p = <0.05$ compared with patients having cervical examinations

rates of premature rupture of the membranes or increase in the infection rate[74]. Lenihan demonstrated an increased risk of premature rupture of the membranes in women undergoing weekly cervical examination after 37 weeks' gestation[75]. More recently, McDuffie et al. were unable to demonstrate any effect of routine cervical examination at term on the rate of premature rupture of the membranes in a controlled randomized trial[76]. Aside from these reports, relatively little information exists regarding the consequences of the preterm cervical examination on the risk of preterm delivery. Investigators in previously cited studies[52,55–58,61,62,65,66] of antepartum cervical examination in singleton and multifetal gestations did not report adverse sequelae. However, none of these studies were specifically designed to assess the risks of antepartum cervical examination.

Holbrook et al. evaluated the role of cervical examination in singleton gestations as a component of the San Francisco Preterm Birth Prevention Program[77]. Compared to a large control group who did not receive antepartum cervical examination, no increase in the rates of premature rupture of the membranes, chorioamnionitis, or endometritis was observed in women who received this examination. Similarly, no relationship was present between the date of the last cervical examination and the ultimate onset of preterm labor[77]. Main et al. reported on an inner city population in which antepartum cervical examination was used as part of an effort to prevent preterm birth[78]. This program was not successful in reducing the rates of preterm delivery, and the rates of premature rupture of the membranes were high in the group of women who had routine cervical asessment. However, the rate of premature rupture of the membranes was similar among the high-risk control group who did not undergo routine cervical examination[78]. Perhaps most importantly, those local and regional programs which have proven to be successful in preventing preterm birth have all emphasized antepartum cervical examination[79–81]. The most notable is the European experience described by Papiernik et al. in Haguenau, France[80]. However, many of the programs which have been successful have been population-based. In other words, cervical

Table 4 Obstetric and neonatal risks potentially associated with routine antepartum cervical examination (Twin Clinic) compared with historical and contemporary controls having cervical examination for indication only

	Twin Clinic		Historical		Contemporary		
	n	%	n	%	n	%	p-Value
Twins	89		237		51		
Delivery < 37 weeks	69	77	155	65	37	73	NS
PROM	11	12	55	23	13	26	$p < 0.05$
Bleeding	2	2	12	5	4	8	NS
IAI	3	3	9	4	3	6	NS
Neonatal sepsis	1	1	14	3	7	7	$p < 0.05$

PROM, premature rupture of the membranes; IAI, intra-amniotic infection

examination was applied to all patients, not only those considered to be at high risk because of historical information or social conditions. The success of these interventions makes it unlikely that routine antepartum cervical examination has a significant adverse effect on the rates of spontaneous preterm labor or preterm premature rupture of the membranes.

Our own experience with the antepartum Twin Clinic has not demonstrated any increased risk of adverse outcome attributable to cervical examination[82]. Obstetric outcome was compared for 89 women attending the Twin Clinic in 1988–90, 237 historical controls delivered in 1981–87, and 51 contemporary controls (1988–90) who did not attend the Twin Clinic. Both the historical and contemporary controls would have undergone cervical examination for indication only. There were no differences between the three groups in terms of preterm delivery, antepartum bleeding, or intra-amniotic infection[82]. The women attending the Twin Clinic actually had a lower risk of premature rupture of membranes (Table 4). Our rate of premature rupture of membranes is consistent with or less than rates reported in other reviews of multifetal gestations not having routine cervical examination[82–85]. These findings suggest that the institution of routine antepartum cervical examination was not associated with any increase in the obstetric or neonatal risks frequently attributed to this procedure.

In conclusion, antepartum cervical examination in multifetal gestations provides valuable information that better defines an individual woman's risk of preterm delivery. *There is no convincing evidence that routine antepartum cervical examination is associated with any adverse obstetric sequelae.* In addition to its clinical value and safety, antepartum cervical examination is generally applicable and inexpensive. An understanding of the prognostic significance of specific quantifiable cervical data will improve the clinical management of multifetal gestations.

References

1. Keith, L., Ellis, R., Berger, G. *et al.* (1980). The Northwestern University multi-hospital twin study. I. A description of 588 twin pregnancies and associated pregnancy loss, 1971 to 1975. *Am. J. Obstet. Gynecol.*, **138**, 781
2. Ho, S.K. and Wu, P.Y.K. (1975). Perinatal factors and neonatal morbidity in twin pregnancy. *Am. J. Obstet. Gynecol.*, **122**, 979
3. Newman, R.B., Hamer, C. and Miller, M.C. (1989). Outpatient triplet management: a

contemporary review. *Am. J. Obstet. Gynecol.*, **161**, 547
4. Hawlaryskin, P.A., Barkin, M., Bernstein, A. *et al.* (1982). Twin pregnancies – a continuing perinatal challenge. *Obstet. Gynecol.*, **59**, 463
5. Aschoff, L. (1906). Das Untere Uterinsegment. *Z. Gebrutschilfe Gyn.*, **58**, 328
6. Danforth, D.N. (1947). The fibrous nature of the human cervix and its relation to the isthmic segment in gravid and non-gravid uteri. *Am. J. Obstet. Gynecol.*, **53**, 541
7. Rorie, D.K. and Newton, M. (1967). Histologic and chemical studies of the smooth muscle in the human cervix and uterus. *Am. J. Obstet. Gynecol.*, **199**, 466
8. Buckingham, J.C., Buethe, R.A. and Danforth, D.N. (1965). Collagen–muscle ratio in clinically normal and clinically incompetent cervices. *Am. J. Obstet. Gynecol.*, **91**, 232
9. Danforth, D.N., Buckingham, J.C. and Roddick, J.W. (1960). Connective tissue changes incident to cervical effacement. *Am. J. Obstet. Gynecol.*, **80**, 939
10. Rechberger, T., Uldbjerg, N. and Oxlund, H. (1988). Connective tissue changes in the cervix during normal pregnancies and pregnancy complicated by cervical incompetence. *Obstet. Gynecol.*, **71**, 563
11. Padykula, H.A. and Tansey, T.R. (1979). The occurrence of uterine stromal and intraepithelial monocytes and heterophils during normal late pregnancy in the rat. *Anat. Rec.*, **193**, 329
12. Woessner, J.F. (1979). Total, latent, and active collagenase during the course of postpartum involution of the rat uterus. *Biochem. J.*, **180**, 95
13. Ekman, G., Malmstrom, A., Uldbjerg, N. and Ulmsten, U. (1986). Cervical collagen: an important regulator of cervical function in term labor. *Obstet. Gynecol.*, **67**, 633
14. Golichowski, A.M., King, S.R. and Mascaro, K. (1980). Pregnancy-related changes in rat cervical glycosaminoglycans. *Biochem. J.*, **192**, 1
15. Kitamura, K., Ito, A., Mori, Y. *et al.* (1980). Glycosaminoglycans of human uterine cervix: heparin sulfate increase with reference to cervical ripening. *Biochem. Med.*, **23**, 159
16. VonMaillot, K., Stuhlsatz, H.W., Mohanaradhakrishnan, V. *et al.* (1979). Changes in the glycosaminoglycans distribution pattern in the human cervix during pregnancy and labor. *J. Obstet. Gynecol.*, **135**, 503
17. Uldbjerg, N., Ekman, G., Malmstrom, A. *et al.* (1983). Ripening of the human uterine cervix related to changes in collagen, glycosaminoglycans, and collagenolytic activity. *Am. J. Obstet. Gynecol.*, **147**, 662
18. Kitamura, K., Ito, A., Mori, Y. *et al.* (1979). Changes in the human uterine cervical collagenase, with special reference to cervical ripening. *Biochem. Med.*, **22**, 332
19. MacDonald, P.C., Porter, J.C., Schwarz, G.E. *et al.* (1978). Initiation of parturition in the human female. *Semin. Perinat.*, **2**, 273
20. Huszar, G. (1981). Biology and biochemistry of myometrial contractility and cervical maturation. *Semin. Perinat.*, **5**, 216
21. Tansey, R.R. and Padykula, H.A. (1978). Cellular responses to experimental inhibition of collagen degradation in the postpartum rat uterus. *Anat. Rec.*, **191**, 287
22. Ward, L.M., Blandau, R.J. and Page, R.C. (1977). Effect of hormones on collagen metabolism and collagenase activity in the pubic symphysis ligament of the guinea pig. *Endocrinology*, **100**, 571
23. Yannone, M.E., Mueller, J.R. and Osborn, R.H. (1969). Protein binding of progesterone in the peripheral 4 plasma during pregnancy and labor. *Steroids*, **13**, 773
24. Schwartz, B.E., Milewich, L., Gant, N.F. *et al.* (1977). Progesterone binding and metabolism in human fetal membranes. *Ann. NY Acad. Sci.*, **286**, 304
25. Nakayama, T., Tahara, K., Yanaihara, T. *et al.* (1982). Ripening human cervix: steroid concentrations and proline hydroxylase activity in cervical tissue. *Program of the 10th World Congress on Obstetric Gynecology, San Francisco, October 17–22*
26. Gordon, A.J. and Calder, A.A. (1981). Estradiol applied locally to ripen unfavorable cervix. *Lancet*, **2**, 1319
27. Tromans, P.M., Beazley, J.M. and Shenouda, P.I. (1981). Comparative study of estradiol and prostaglandin E_2 vaginal gel for ripening the unfavorable cervix before induction of labor. *Br. Med. J.*, **282**, 679
28. Fitzpatrick, R.J. (1977). Changes in cervical function at parturition. *Ann. Rech. Vet.*, **8**, 438
29. Hollingsworth, M. and Isherwood, C.N.M. (1977). Changes in the extensibility of the cervix of the rat in late pregnancy produced by prostaglandin F_2 alpha, ovariectomy and steroid replacement. *Br. J. Pharmacol.*, **61**, 501
30. Uldbjerg, N., Ekman, G., Malmstrom, A. *et al.* (1981). Biochemical and morphological changes

in the human cervix after local application of prostaglandin E$_2$ in pregnancy. *Lancet*, **1**, 267

31. Goeschen, U., Fuchs, A.-R., Fuch, F. *et al.* (1985). Effect of betamimetic tocolysis on cervical ripening and plasma prostaglandin F$_2$ alpha metabolite after endocervical application of prostaglandin E$_2$. *Obstet. Gynecol.*, **65**, 166
32. MacLennan, A.H., Green, R.C., Bryant-Greenwood, G.D. *et al.* (1980). Ripening of the human cervix and induction of labor with purified porcine relaxin. *Lancet*, **1**, 220
33. Evans, M.I., Dougan, M.B., Moawad, A.H. *et al.* (1983). Ripening of the human cervix with porcine ovarian relaxin. *Am. J. Obstet. Gynecol.*, **147**, 410
34. Porter, D.G. (1980). Relaxin and cervical ripening. In Anderson, A.M. and Ellwood, D.A. (eds.) *The Cervix in Pregnancy and Labour*. (Edinburgh: Churchill Livingston)
35. Steinetz, B.G., O'Byrne, E.M. and Kroc, R.L. (1980). The role of relaxin in cervical softening during pregnancy in mammals. In Naflolin, F. and Stubblefield, P.G. (eds.) *Dilation of the Uterine Cervix. Connective Tissue Biology and Clinical Management*, pp. 157–77. (New York: Raven Press)
36. Liggins, G.C. (1978). Ripening of the cervix. *Sem. Perinat.*, **2**, 261
37. Caldeyro-Barcia, R., Alvarez, H. and Poseiro, J.J. (1954). Normal and abnormal uterine contractility in labour. *Triangle*, **2**, 41
38. Alvarez, H. and Caldeyro, R. (1950). Contractility of the human uterus recorded by new methods. *Surg. Gynecol. Obstet.*, **91**, 1
39. Caldeyro-Barcia, R. and Poseiro, J.J. (1960). Physiology of uterine contraction. *Clin. Obstet. Gynecol.*, **June**, 386
40. Newman, R.B., Gill, P.J. and Katz, M. (1986). Uterine activity during pregnancy in ambulatory patients: comparison of singleton and twin gestations. *Am. J. Obstet. Gynecol.*, **154**, 530
41. Newman, R.B., Gill, P.J., Wittreich, W. *et al.* (1986). Maternal perception of prelabor uterine activity. *Obstet. Gynecol.*, **68**, 765
42. Weekes, A.R.L., Menzies, D.N. and DeBoer, C.H. (1986). The relative efficacy of bed rest, cervix suture and no treatment in the management of twin pregnancy. *Br. J. Obstet. Gynaecol.*, **154**, 530
43. Marivate, M. and Norman, R.J. (1982). Twins. *Clin. Obstet. Gynaecol.*, **9**, 723
44. Newman, R.B., Gill, P.J., Campion, S. *et al.* (1989). The influence of fetal number on antepartum uterine activity. *Obstet. Gynecol.*, **73**, 695
45. Garite, T.J., Bentley, D.L., Hamer, C.A. *et al.* (1990). Uterine activity characteristics in multiple gestations. *Obstet. Gynecol.*, **76**, 56S
46. Newman, R.B., Gill, P.J., Campion, S. *et al.* (1987). Antepartum ambulatory tocodynamometry: the significance of low amplitude, high frequency contractions. *Obstet. Gynecol.*, **70**, 701
47. McKowan, T. and Record, R.G. (1952). Observations on foetal growth in multiple pregnancy in man. *Endocrinology*, **8**, 386
48. Caspi, E., Ronen, J., Schreyer, P. *et al.* (1976). The outcome of pregnancy after gonadotropin therapy. *Br. J. Obstet. Gynaecol.*, **83**, 967
49. Friedman, E.A. and Sachtleben, M.R. (1964). The effect of uterine overdistention on labor: I. Multiple pregnancy. *Obstet. Gynecol.*, **23**, 164
50. Bishop, E.H. (1964). Pelvic scoring for elective induction. *Obstet. Gynecol.*, **24**, 266
51. Friedman, E.A., Niswander, K.R., Bayonet-Rivera, N.P. *et al.* (1966). Relation of prelabor evaluation to inducibility and the course of labor. *Obstet. Gynecol.*, **28**, 495
52. Bouyer, J., Papiernik, E., Dreyfuss, J. *et al.* (1986). Maturation signs of the cervix and the prediction of preterm birth. *Obstet. Gynecol.*, **68**, 209
53. Lange, J.P., Secher, N.J., Westergaard, J.G. *et al.* (1982). Prelabor evaluation of inducibility. *Obstet. Gynecol.*, **60**, 137
54. Hendricks, C.H., Brenner, W.E. and Kraus, G. (1970). Normal cervical dilation pattern in late pregnancy and labor. *Am. J. Obstet. Gynecol.*, **106**, 1065
55. Stubbs, T.M., Van Dorsten, J.P. and Miller, M.C. (1986). The preterm cervix and preterm labor: relative risks, predictive values, and change over time. *Am. J. Obstet. Gynecol.*, **155**, 829
56. Houlton, M.C.C., Marivate, M. and Philpott, R.H. (1982). Factors associated with preterm labor and changes in the cervix before labor in twin pregnancy. *Br. J. Obstet. Gynaecol.*, **89**, 190
57. Papiernik, E., Bouyer, J., Collin, D. *et al.* (1986). Precocious cervical ripening and preterm labor. *Obstet. Gynecol.*, **67**, 238
58. Schaffner, F. and Schanzer, S.N. (1966). Cervical dilation in the early third trimester. *Obstet. Gynecol.*, **27**, 130
59. Papiernik, E. and Kaminski, M. (1974). Multifactorial study of the risk of prematurity at 32 weeks' gestation. *J. Perinat. Med.*, **2**, 30

60. Leveno, K.J., Cox, K. and Roark, M.L. (1986). Cervical dilatation and prematurity revisited. *Obstet. Gynecol.*, **68**, 434
61. Wood, C., Bannerman, R.H.O., Booth, R.T. *et al.* (1965). The prediction of premature labor by observation of the cervix and external tocography. *Am. J. Obstet. Gynecol.*, **91**, 396
62. Anderson, A.B.M. and Turnbull, A.C. (1969). Relationship between length of gestation and cervical dilatation, uterine contractility and other factors during pregnancy. *Am. J. Obstet. Gynecol.*, **105**, 1207
63. Parikh, M.N. and Mehta, A.C. (1961). Internal cervical os during the second half of pregnancy. *J. Obstet. Gynaecol. Br. Commonw.*, **86**, 818
64. O'Connor, M.C., Arias, E., Royston, J.P. *et al.* (1981). The merits of special antenatal care for twin pregnancies. *Br. J. Obstet. Gynaecol.*, **88**, 222
65. Neilson, J.P., Verkuyl, D.A.A., Crowther, C.A. *et al.* (1988). Preterm labor in twin pregnancies: prediction by cervical assessment. *Obstet. Gynecol.*, **72**, 719
66. Newman, R.B., Godsey, R.K., Ellings, J.M. *et al.* (1991). Quantification of cervical change: relationship to preterm delivery in the multifetal gestation. *Am. J. Obstet. Gynecol.*, **165**, 264
67. Ellings, J.M., Newman, R.B., Hulsey, T.C. *et al.* (1993). Reduction in very low birth weight deliveries and perinatal mortality in a specialized multidisciplinary twin clinic. *Obstet. Gynecol.*, **81**, 387
68. Saunders, M.C., Dick, J.S., Brown, I.M.V. *et al.* (1985). The effects of hospitalized admission for bedrest on the duration of twin pregnancy: a randomized trial. *Lancet*, **2**, 793
69. Hartikainen, A.L. and Jouppila, P. (1984). Is routine hospitalization needed in antenatal care of twin pregnancy. *J. Perinat. Med.*, **12**, 31
70. Marivate, M.M., deVilliers, K.Q. and Fairbrother, P. (1977). Effect of prophylactic outpatient administration of fenoteral on the time of onset of spontaneous labor and fetal growth rate in twin pregnancy. *Am. J. Obstet. Gynecol.*, **128**, 707
71. O'Connor, M.C., Murphy, H. and Dalrymple, I.J. (1979). Double blind trial of ritodrine and placebo in twin pregnancy. *Br. J. Obstet. Gynaecol.*, **86**, 706
72. Knupple, R.A., Lake, M.F., Watson, D.L. *et al.* (1990). Preventing preterm birth in twin gestation: home uterine activity monitoring and perinatal nursing support. *Obstet. Gynecol.*, **76**, 24S
73. Katz, M., Gill, P.J. and Newman, R.B. (1986). Detection of preterm labor by ambulatory monitoring of uterine activity: a preliminary report. *Obstet. Gynecol.*, **68**, 773
74. McColgin, S.W., Hampton, H.L., McCaul, J.F. *et al.* (1990). Stripping membranes at term: can it safely reduce the incidence of post-term pregnancies? *Obstet. Gynecol.*, **76**, 678
75. Lenihan, J.P. (1984). Relationship of antepartum pelvic examinations to premature rupture of the membranes. *Obstet. Gynecol.*, **63**, 33
76. McDuffie, R.S., Nelson, G.E., Osbourn, C.L. *et al.* (1992). Effect of routine weekly cervical examinations at term on premature rupture of the membranes: a randomized controlled trial. *Obstet. Gynecol.*, **79**, 219
77. Holbrook, R.H., Falcon, J., Herron, M. *et al.* (1987). Evaluation of the weekly cervical examination in a preterm birth prevention program. *Am. J. Perinat.*, **4**, 240
78. Main, D.M., Gabbe, S.G., Richardson, D. *et al.* (1985). Can preterm deliveries by prevented? *Am. J. Obstet. Gynecol.*, **151**, 892
79. Herron, M.A., Katz, M. and Creasy, R.K. (1982). Evaluation of a preterm birth prevention program: preliminary report. *Obstet. Gynecol.*, **59**, 452
80. Papiernik, E., Bouyer, J., Dreyfuss, J. *et al.* (1985). Prevention of preterm births: a perinatal study in Haguenau, France. *Pediatrics*, **76**, 154
81. Meis, P.J., Ernest, J.M., Moore, M.L. *et al.* (1987). Regional progam for prevention of premature birth in northwestern North Carolina. *Am. J. Obstet. Gynecol.*, **157**, 550
82. Bivins, H.A., Newman, R.B., Ellings, J.M. *et al.* (1993). Risks of antepartum cervical examination in multifetal gestations. *Am. J. Obstet. Gynecol.*, **169**, 22
83. O'Grady, J.P. (1987). Clinical management of twins. *Cont. Obstet. Gynecol.*, **29**, 126
84. Pussant, F. and Leroy, F. (1982). A reappraisal of perinatal mortality factors in twins. *Acta Genet. Med. Gemellol.*, **31**, 213
85. Tucker, J.M., Goldenberg, R.L., Winkler, C.L. *et al.* (1991). Etiologies of preterm birth in twin gestation. *Am. J. Obstet. Gynecol.*, **164**, 426

Ambulatory tocolysis

F. Lam and P.J. Gill

Introduction

Since the early 1980s, many clinicians have appreciated the need to distinguish between the traditional but imprecise term 'prematurity' and two additional terms: 'preterm labor' and 'low birth weight' (<2500 g). The former terminology had been used loosely for decades to describe without distinction preterm births and infants whose birth weights were less than 2500 g. As a result of this imprecision, present day readings of the older literature and major textbooks is often limited by an inability to distinguish between these entities and retrospective comparisons are often difficult, if not impossible.

In the 1990s, it is widely accepted that the term 'preterm labor' in a pregnancy between 20 and 36 weeks' gestation should be based upon the presence of regular uterine contractions (4/20 min, 8/60 min) that result in cervical change. In addition, to strengthen the precision of this diagnosis, it is deemed appropriate that cervical change be documented by the same examiner who evaluates cervical dilatation, effacement, consistency, position and station of the presenting part at two different examinations[1]. Thus, a reliable diagnosis of preterm labor can be established if progressive cervical change occurs in the presence of regular uterine activity. Further, the diagnosis of advanced preterm labor can be established in the presence of cervical dilatation of ≥2 cm *or* effacement of ≥80%, although the likelihood of successful tocolysis is decreased in this latter circumstance[2].

For the past 20 years, a variety of drugs (tocolytic agents) have been used to treat preterm labor. To date, no large prospective study of the use of systemic tocolytics for the management of preterm labor in multiple gestations has been published, and the use of prophylactic oral tocolytic therapy in these circumstances is of no proven benefit[3]. Most of the investigations of therapy for preterm labor have been conducted on singletons and/or mixed (singleton and twins) populations, and the results often must be extrapolated to multiple gestations. It is clear, however, that tocolytics alone are by no means a panacea for preventing preterm birth[4].

Individualization of tocolytic therapy is critical for success and for preventing complications. The management of preterm labor in multiple gestation poses several challenges. First, among multiples, there is an increased frequency of premature labor, with a marked tendency for onset at earlier gestational ages. Second, the latency period before which tocolysis becomes effective is greater than for singletons. Third, patients with multiple pregnancies are less likely to perceive uterine contractions and often present with advanced cervical dilatation or preterm, premature rupture of the amniotic membranes. Fourth, the risk of complications from tocolytic treatment is greater[3]. For example, because of the increased workload on the heart that results from increased blood volume and anemia, patients are more susceptible to fluid overload and pulmonary edema. In addition, increased plasma volume and increased renal clearance may make tocolytic dosing and titration erratic. Fifth, and finally, any therapeutic failure results in more than one infant being exposed to the potential morbidity and mortality of preterm birth.

Two decades ago, only a small percentage of cases were considered suitable candidates for inhibition of preterm labor[5]. More recently, however, increasing numbers of patients are deemed suitable candidates for long-term inhibition of preterm labor. This chapter discusses ambulatory tocolysis as it has been used for multiple gestations since 1976. Because bed rest is an integral part of most therapeutic regimens that attempt to treat preterm labor, a brief discussion of bed rest in patients with multiple gestations is also provided.

Prophylactic bed rest

The concept of providing bed rest prophylactically is controversial, although few authorities question the wisdom of limiting physical activity after the 20th week of gestation, especially if the patient is gainfully employed outside the home. Theoretically, bed rest offers the unique advantage of improving uterine blood flow and relieving mechanical pressure on the cervix, two features not provided by activity reduction alone. Unfortunately, the specific effects of increased uterine perfusion (from bed rest) or the diminished tendency for contractions (from reduced activity) on the incidence of preterm labor is difficult to quantitate in humans.

The concept of hospitalizing women with multiple pregnancy near term was proposed as early as 1952, when Russell[6] noted that middle-class women in the United Kingdom generally delivered heavier and more mature twins compared to working class mothers. Russell postulated that privileged patients had 'more leisure and consequently more rest during their pregnancies'[6]. His ideas in this regard clearly followed those articulated by Adolphe Pinard in France in 1895. Pinard had advocated termination of hard physical work. Russell extended this concept and proposed that patients with twins be hospitalized at the 30th week in order to ensure the health of their infants at a time when delivery might have disastrous consequences. As a result of Russell's recommendation, women with multiple pregnancies were provided hospital bed rest in the third trimester. The economics of this practice were not at issue, as the government of the United Kingdom had previously nationalized its health service. Economics were also not at issue in similar decisions taken in the late 1950s and 1960s in Sweden and some Eastern European nations (Poland and Hungary). Data from early studies of rested mothers in these nations confirmed that their infants weighed, on the average, 400–500 g more than the infants of unrested mothers with multiple gestations. Comparisons were not made on the basis of randomization, however, in these initial investigations, but rather were made with the help of historically constituted control groups.

Numerous research workers have subsequently either supported or refuted the value of prophylactic bed rest for patients with multiple pregnancy. Controversial issues surrounding its application include when it should begin, where it should take place, how long it should continue and whether it is cost effective[3]. The prophylactic hospitalization of all patients with multiple gestation is presently considered prohibitively expensive in most well-developed countries, regardless of the nature and type of the existing health care system. Elsewhere in the world, it is logistically impossible.

In general, the cost effectiveness of bed rest in twin gestation has received only modest attention. In 1979, Powers and Miller concluded that the cost of prophylactic bed rest for all twin gestations between 27 and 34 weeks' gestation would be two to four times the costs for neonatal intensive-care units (NICU) provided for the infants delivered early because of non-intervention[7]. This study may not be relevant today, however, because NICU costs have escalated enormously since 1979, and the total number of infants with low birth weights has increased as a result of the 'epidemic' of higher-order multiples. In the mid-1980s, Newton observed that the type of cost analysis performed by Powers and Miller could only evaluate short-term costs, i.e. hospital costs[8]. Newton further cautioned that the long-term cost of handicap would profoundly affect any analysis of cost effectiveness[8]. A 1992 analysis by Luke et al. cites a lifetime cost of $106 000 per child with moderate handicap and $413 000 per child with severe handicap. These calculations were based on data published by the Office of Technological Assessment[9].

In theory, prophylactic hospitalization has the following theoretical benefits: (1) enforced bed rest; (2) improved nutrition; (3) access to maternal–fetal surveillance modalities and access to other therapeutic modalities; (4) exposure to patient education programs; and (5) sequestration from a potentially hostile home environment. The disadvantages of routine prophylactic rest in the hospital include: (1) considerable financial costs; (2) major life disruption for the patient and her family; and (3) increased risk of thromboembolism. Other authors have discussed prophylactic bed rest in their respective chapters (see Chapter 33). Later in this chapter, we will discuss therapeutic bed rest as it is used in programs to prevent recurrent preterm labor.

Ambulatory tocolysis

Early diagnosis and immediate intervention are *the essential prerequisites* for halting preterm labor. The initial hospital process for the observation of a patient with preterm labor should include the following components: (1) bed rest in left lateral position; (2) assessment of uterine activity by electronic monitoring; (3) elimination of the possibility of infection as an inciting cause of contractions by obtaining cultures and diagnostic tests from the urine and the cervix; (4) hydration; and (5) performance of a cervical examination, if not otherwise contraindicated.

After admission to labor and delivery, several circumstances may ensue. First, the patient may present with complaints of uterine contractions or other symptoms, without evidence of regular uterine activity documented by electronic monitoring. If serial examinations of the cervix by the same individual indicate no change after 2–4 h, these patients may return home. However, they should be encouraged to watch for further symptoms and to notify the health care provider should they reappear. Second, regular uterine contractions may be present, in the absence of cervical change after a 2–4 h period of monitoring. Sedation and hydration may be prescribed to these patients to decrease uterine activity, and monitoring should continue over the next 24 h. These patients may be discharged if uterine activity either diminishes or is determined to be within normal limits (fewer than six contractions per hour). Finally, if regular uterine activity and progressive cervical change are both documented and the former cannot be controlled with bed rest and hydration alone, then tocolytic therapy should be initiated.

As currently practiced, established preterm labor (using the criteria described above) should be promptly treated with intravenous tocolytics. When uterine activity is stabilized, the patient can be gradually weaned to an oral tocolytic agent for maintenance on an ambulatory basis. Therapy is continued either until term or recurrent preterm labor ensues. The goal of ambulatory tocolysis is the prevention of recurrent preterm labor and its early detection should it occur.

Over the years, tocolysis has been advocated for three principal indications in the treatment of preterm labor in multiple pregnancies: (1) prophylaxis – that is, therapy based on the presence of a risk factor or uterine activity alone (in the absence of documented cervical change) – in an effort to prevent preterm labor; (2) therapy – that is, administration of parenteral agents for prompt control of the acute episode of preterm labor for varying durations of 24–72 h; and (3) maintenance – that is, the use of oral or subcutaneous medications for long-term tocolysis after cessation of preterm labor to prevent the recurrence of uterine activity.

Of the three principal indications cited above, the use of beta-sympathomimetic drugs for prophylaxis in twin gestations has received the most rigorous scientific evaluation[8]. Double-blinded randomized studies using placebo control have evaluated oral fenoterol[10], terbutaline[11] and ritodrine[12,13]. All trials failed to demonstrate a significant increase in the length of gestation or increased birth weight in the treated patients[8].

In contrast, the initiation of tocolytic therapy has been predicated upon the assessment

Table 1 Indications and contraindications of tocolysis

Indications
Gestational age between 20 and 36 weeks
Fetal weight less than 2500 g
Documented fetal lung immaturity
Regular uterine contractions
Labor progressing with documented cervical change

Contraindications
Active vaginal bleeding
Eclampsia or severe pre-eclampsia
Fetal demise or any condition incompatible with life
Intrauterine infection
Any obstetric or medical condition that is a contraindication to the prolongation of pregnancy
Conditions limiting the chance of success, e.g. cervical dilatation greater than 4 cm, rupture of membranes

Table 2 Receptor stimulation by betamimetic agents

Beta-1
Heart rate increased
Heart force increased
Lipolysis increased
Intestinal motility decreased

Beta-2
Uterine relaxation
Arteriolar relaxation
Bronchiolar relaxation
Muscle and liver stimulation – glycogenolysis
Pancreatic stimulation – hyperinsulinism
Cell stimulation – hypokalemia

Table 3 Side-effects of betamimetic agents

Maternal
Minor
  nausea and vomiting
  tremors
  anxiety
  flushing
  headache
  palpitations
  heartburn
  constipation

Major
  angina
  dyspnea
  pulmonary edema
  myocardial ischemia
  cardiac arrythmias
  myocardial infarction
  ileus
  hyperglycemia
  hyperinsulinism
  ketosis
  hypokalemia

Fetal
  tachycardia, 5–10 beats above baseline

Neonatal
  hypoglycemia
  hyperinsulinism
  hypocalcemia
  ketoacidosis
  ileus

of its potential benefits vs. the possibility of adverse maternal or fetal complications. The general criteria which support or refute this basic decision are listed in Table 1. The subsections that follow discuss specific therapeutic modalities.

Beta-adrenergic receptor stimulators (betamimetics)

Physiology Betamimetic agents stimulate the beta receptors of the sympathetic nervous system. Interactions with the receptor sites cause an increase in intracellular production of cyclic adenosine monophosphate (cAMP). This phenomenon results in the reduction of intracellular calcium concentrations in the smooth muscle. The lower level of calcium inhibits activation of the contractile proteins actin and myosin which in turn results in relaxation of the myometrium. There are two types of beta receptors: beta-1 and beta-2. Each type is associated with a different set of physiological responses (see Table 2). Because ritodrine and terbutaline individually possess beta-2 specific properties, they are the drugs of choice when uterine relaxation is desired. Table 3 lists the major adverse effects from betamimetic stimulation.

Precautions Prior to initiation of betamimetic therapy for acute-onset preterm labor, baseline evaluations should include vital signs, electronic monitoring of the fetal heart rate and uterine activity pattern, laboratory assessment (complete blood count (CBC), blood glucose, electrolytes, urinalysis with culture and sensitivity, and cervical culture), EKG to identify any previously unrecognized cardiac irregularity and, finally, a thorough pulmonary auscultation.

Therapeutic plan Initiation of therapy may consist of only a fluid bolus (500 ml of isotonic crystalloid over 30 min) administered via an indwelling catheter (18-gauge). If hydration is unsuccessful, therapy with intravenous ritodrine or terbutaline can be started. If ritodrine is selected, it should be prepared according to approved protocol (see package insert) and the infusion begun using a controlled infusion pump at 100 μg/min. The dose should be increased by 50 μg/min every 10 min until regular contractions cease or the apical pulse rate is greater than 130 beats per minute. The maximum dose should not exceed 350 μg/min. Once an effective dose has been established, this rate can be maintained for 12–24 h. Oral ritodrine maintenance therapy may begin 30 min prior to discontinuing the intravenous infusion using a dose of 10–20 mg every 2–4 h. If terbutaline is selected, administration can begin at 10 μg/min intravenous and be increased by 10 μg every 20–30 min to a maximum dose of 80 μg/min. After stabilization (less than six contractions per hour with no further cervical change) for 4–6 h, terbutaline 0.25 mg may be given subcutaneously every 2–4 h. The oral maintenance dose is 2.5–5 mg every 2–4 h. Oral therapy is generally initiated after 6–12 h of subcutaneous therapy.

Nursing intervention Nursing care should aim toward achieving the desired effect and preventing or avoiding serious side-effects.

(1) Reinforce the physician's prior discussion about potential adverse reactions;

(2) Monitor vital signs every 15 min during initial intravenous titration and for 1 h after the effective dose is reached; this activity may be reduced to every hour after stabilization;

(3) Use a cardiac monitor during the initial period of treatment. The maternal heart rate should not exceed 130 beats per minute and any irregularities should be noted;

(4) Maintain the systolic blood pressure above 90 mmHg;

(5) Repeat the EKG 24 h after initiation of therapy;

(6) Monitor the fetal heart rate and uterine activity closely. The fetal heart rate should not exceed 180 beats per minute; and

(7) Repeat pulmonary auscultation frequently. Pulmonary edema is a serious side-effect.

Comment Patients at highest risk for pulmonary edema include women with multiple gestations, those with fluid overload or those with underlying infection. Initial symptoms may include shortness of breath, coughing or wheezing. Maximum fluid administration should not exceed 3000 ml per 24 h. Monitoring of intake and output must be strictly maintained. Oral fluid intake should also be monitored, and a positive fluid balance should be avoided. Patients should be weighed each day. The monitoring of metabolic status during therapy includes repeated evaluations of glucose levels, CBC and electrolyte status.

After successful treatment, patients with preterm labor can be discharged home on oral beta-sympathomimetic therapy[3]. The potential advantages of oral therapy at home include reduced risks, reduced costs, decreased stress and ease of administration.

Prevention of recurrent preterm labor is the goal of long-term tocolysis. During episodes of recurrent preterm labor, patients are at risk for premature rupture of membranes (PROM), further cervical change and preterm delivery. Among the many potential causes of tocolytic failure are patient non-compliance, drug side-effects, PROM and the emergence of drug tolerance. In addition, oral medications are poorly absorbed during pregnancy.

Perhaps the major cause of recurrent preterm labor is the desensitization of myometrial β2-adrenergic receptor sites by prolonged and continuous exposure to high-dose betamimetic agents such as terbutaline and ritodrine. This down-regulation phenomenon may also explain the failure of betamimetic tocolytics when used for the prophylactic treatment of preterm labor[10,13–18].

If the diagnosis of recurrent preterm labor is made prior to advanced cervical dilatation (> 2 cm), tocolysis will be successful in 90% of cases if a sequential approach is taken[19]. Patients in preterm labor with tocolytic breakthrough from terbutaline or ritodrine should be treated with magnesium sulfate ($MgSO_4$). Because $MgSO_4$ acts differently from the betamimetic agents, a betamimetic-free period allows the myometrial receptor sites to recover their sensitivity[20]. Patients who are treated with a betamimetic agent after a betamimetic failure have less than a 25% chance of success[19]. The minimum period for this 'drug holiday' should be 24–48 h; once stable, the patient can be considered a candidate for ambulatory tocolysis again[21].

Magnesium sulfate

Alternative tocolytic agents such as $MgSO_4$ have been proposed because of the high frequency of maternal side-effects and tachyphylaxis associated with betamimetic agents.

Physiology Magnesium sulfate is a major cation in the intracellular fluid. Elevated levels diminish the release of acetylcholine, thereby decreasing sensitivity at the motor end plates. At the cellular level, magnesium competes with calcium, leading to impairment of light-chain phosphorylation of myosin and decreased contractility of uterine smooth muscle. The inhibitory effect on skeletal muscle results in hyporeflexia and hypotonia, chiefly due to the inhibition of acetylcholine release at the neuromuscular junction. Magnesium acts directly on the central nervous system, resulting in depressant effects.

Precautions The normal plasma concentration of magnesium is 1.5–2.25 mg/dl. Therapeutic levels effecting uterine relaxation are 4–8 mg/dl. However, the patient may experience flushing, feelings of warmth, headaches, lethargy, drowsiness, blurred vision, decreased reflexes, decreased gastrointestinal motility, nausea and vomiting after therapeutic levels have been established and before toxicity is reached. Toxicity results in loss of patellar reflexes at concentrations of 10 mg/dl, loss of respiration at 12–15 mg/dl, and cardiac arrest at 15 mg/dl. Clinical studies have demonstrated that $MgSO_4$ is equally efficacious as is intravenous terbutaline and intravenous ritodrine, albeit with fewer side-effects[22–24].

Magnesium sulfate passes the placental barrier and causes central nervous system depression in the fetus, frequently manifest as changes in beat-to-beat variability. Neonatal depression is reflected by a lower Apgar score of 1–2 points due to loss of tone, decreased respirations and decreased reflex irritability. High magnesium levels and low calcium levels may be observed. Gastrointestinal motility may be decreased. Supportive care for the neonate may include intubation, intravenous fluids, intravenous calcium and exchange transfusion. These effects are transient and usually resolve within 3–4 days.

Therapeutic plans Baseline physical parameters should be assessed prior to the initiation of $MgSO_4$ treatment, as is the case with betamimetic therapy. Magnesium is delivered intravenously and is mixed according to hospital protocol. An initial bolus of 4–6 g is given slowly over 20 min via additive set, and then followed by a maintenance dose of 1–3 g/h via infusion pump. Oral maintenance on a betamimetic agent can be initiated after stabilization on intravenous $MgSO_4$. Patients who were previously unable to tolerate intravenous betamimetic therapy (e.g. diabetics, or those with multiple gestations) and received $MgSO_4$ instead, should be monitored carefully during the transition to an oral agent. In a diabetic pregnancy, oral ritodrine may be better tolerated, due to terbutaline's greater hyperglycemic effects.

Nursing interventions The nursing implications are similar to those of betamimetic therapy with additional attention placed on neurological assessment.

(1) Inform the patient of the expected side-effects, prior to the initiation of therapy;

(2) Monitor vital signs every 5 min during the loading dose and every 15–30 min during the maintenance dose until stable, then hourly. Observe respiratory rate and notify physician if respirations are depressed or below 15/min;

(3) Evaluate the fetal heart rate. $MgSO_4$ can decrease the beat-to-beat variability;

(4) Evaluate deep tendon reflexes hourly;

(5) Check the intravenous injection site frequently. Magnesium is extremely irritating to the vein. If infiltration occurs, the needle site should be changed immediately. The preferred site is a large vein in the forearm, rather than the hand;

(6) Monitor intake and output. Magnesium is cleared almost entirely via the kidney. Fluid retention may result in magnesium toxicity, and pulmonary edema may occur. Notify the physician if the urine output is less than 30 ml/h. Daily weights will aid in evaluating fluid retention;

(7) Monitor bowel sounds and function. Gastrointestinal relaxation may develop into an ileus;

(8) Laboratory assessment should include frequent magnesium levels, CBC with differential, and electrolytes;

(9) Prepare emergency equipment and maintain a 10 ml syringe of calcium gluconate (10 ml of 10% solution) at the bedside to reverse magnesium toxicity; and

(10) Provide additional emotional support, due to depressive effects of magnesium.

Comment Oral magnesium preparations can be used for long-term tocolysis. Magnesium gluconate can be administered 1 g every 2–4 h or magnesium oxide 250–450 mg every 3 h. Some have suggested that oral magnesium preparations may be as effective as oral terbutaline or ritodrine for the maintenance of tocolysis, with fewer side-effects and at lower cost[25,26]. Therapeutic serum levels of magnesium have not been achieved, however, via oral administration[27].

Prostaglandin synthetase inhibitors (indomethacin)

Physiology In pregnancy, PGE_2 and $PGF_{2\alpha}$ stimulate uterine contractility by increasing free intracellular calcium levels in the myometrium. Prostaglandins stimulate the formation of gap junctions between myometrial cells facilitating the synchronization of uterine contractions. They may also play a role in cervical maturation before the onset of labor. Prostaglandins are produced by the synthesis and metabolism of the compounds of the arachidonic cascade. Prostaglandin synthetase inhibitors (non-steroidal anti-inflammatory compounds) act by inhibiting the enzyme cyclo-oxygenase from converting arachidonic acid into PGG_2 and PGH_2, and then ultimately to PGE_2 and $PGF_{2\alpha}$. Prostaglandin synthetase inhibitors also directly inhibit calcium influx into the cells and the storage of calcium within the sarcoplasmic reticulum. The decrease in free intracellular calcium inhibits myosin light-chain kinase, thereby causing uterine relaxation[28].

Precautions Side-effects of prostaglandin synthetase inhibitors include gastric irritation resulting in nausea, vomiting, epigastric pain, rectal irritation and peptic ulceration. Inhibition of platelet aggregation may result in maternal bleeding. Water and sodium retention may occur. An increased pressor response to angiotension II may affect maternal blood pressure and cause headaches and dizziness. Transient elevations in the liver enzymes SGOT, SGPT, bilirubin and alkaline phosphatase may occur during treatment.

Fetal effects are of primary significance with possible increased pulmonary vasculature, ductal constriction and case reports of premature closure of the ductus arteriosis *in utero*. Water excretion from the fetal kidney may be inhibited and result in oligohydramnios. Neonatal pulmonary hypertension may result from therapy and is usually associated with other causes, such as hypoxia, acidosis and hypovolemia. The adverse effects of indomethacin seem to be related to dose, length of therapy and gestational age of administration.

No significant difference in the incidence of neonatal complications is found when indomethacin has been administered for tocolysis over a short term (1–2 days) and to infants less than 34 weeks' gestational age[29–31]. However, a relationship exists between total daily maternal indomethacin intake and fetal renal inhibition[32]. Oligohydramnios, transient neonatal anuria and renal insufficiency have been reported after maternal indomethacin administration in doses of 150–300 mg/day[33]. No significant adverse fetal or neonatal effects of maternal indomethacin exposure were observed, however, when the daily maternal dosage was 125 mg or less per day[32]. Contraindications to therapy include hypertensive disease, renal disease, oligohydramnios, bleeding disorders and liver disease.

Therapeutic plan Indomethacin may be administered as rectal suppositories or in oral tablets. An initial dose of 50–100 mg is recommended, followed by 25 mg every 4–6 h for a maximum of 48 h. The medication should be titrated until uterine activity is reduced. The lowest effective dose (not greater than 125 mg/day) should be used for no longer than 48 h. The drug should not be administered at a gestational age of more than 32 weeks. Serial ultrasonographic evaluations of amniotic fluid volume are recommended. Indomethacin is of limited value for outpatient tocolytic treatment, because of these restrictions.

Indomethacin may be administered in conjunction with betamimetic therapy. Alternating these drugs may aid in decreasing the risk of betamimetic desensitization and the risk of fetal vascular effects during betamimetic stimulation.

Nursing interventions The nursing activities specific to indomethacin therapy include:

(1) Continuous monitoring of the fetal heart rate for signs of compromise. Observation for cardiac irregularities. Variable decelerations may be an indication of oligohydramnios;

(2) Assessment for maternal side-effects, e.g. headaches, dizziness, intestinal disorders, bleeding. Inform the patient of these potential effects prior to the onset of treatment;

(3) Monitoring of intake and output. Evaluate fundal height measurement and observe for signs of decreasing amniotic fluid. Evaluate lung sounds and observe for signs of pulmonary edema;

(4) Monitoring of maternal blood pressure; and

(5) Betamimetic therapy, possibly received by patients receiving indomethacin.

Calcium channel blockers (nifedipine)

Physiology Calcium blockers inhibit the influx of extracellular calcium across the cell membrane. As a result, calcium is not available as a component with myosin light-chain kinase. Nifedipine selectively inhibits uterine tension, making it the drug of choice among the calcium channel blockers. Nifedipine may also interact with calcium binding proteins, thereby inhibiting uterine contractions[34].

Precautions Side-effects of calcium channel blockers include vasodilatation and direct cardiovascular effects – specifically, slowed atrioventricular node conduction. Nifedipine has little direct cardiac effect compared to other similar agents (e.g. verapamil). Its major side-effects are reflex tachycardia and hypotension secondary to the vasodilatory effect.

Therapeutic plan The recommended dose is nifedipine 30 mg orally, followed by 20 mg

Table 4 Discharge teaching plan for patients with preterm labor in whom home care is anticipated

---

On-going patient teaching
Signs and symptoms of preterm labor
Self monitoring of preterm labor
Tocolytic therapy
   dose schedule
   potential side-effects
   adjustment of therapy within specific guidelines,
     according to uterine activity and vital signs
Activity restrictions
   definition of bed rest
   activities to pass the time while on bed rest
   physical discomforts associated with bed rest
   plan for finding help with childcare,
     housekeeping, meal preparation, etc.

Points for emphasis prior to discharge
When to call the physician regarding problems
How to take tocolytic agents at home
Importance of maintaining bed rest
How to contact members of the interdisciplinary
   team, e.g. social worker, nutritionist, nurse and
   physician

---

three times daily for three days, then twice a day during the remainder of treatment. An effect is noted 20 min after ingestion of the drug, with facial flushing, an increase in maternal heart rate of 10–25 beats per min and a decrease in uterine activity. The plasma half-life is 2–3 h, with a duration of 6 h. As is the case with $MgSO_4$ and indomethacin, the mode of action of nifedipine is independent of interaction with the beta-receptor, allowing for its use in sequential tocolysis.

Nursing interventions Nursing considerations specific to calcium channel blockers include:

(1) Inform patients of potential side effects prior to the onset of treatment;

(2) Nifedipine may be contraindicated in patients with a history of migraine headaches;

(3) Monitor maternal vital signs, specifically pulse rate and blood pressure;

(4) Observe maternal side effects, including headaches and flushing;

(5) Monitor fetal heart rate to assess fetal well-being; and

(6) Position the patient in the lateral recumbent position to enhance uterine blood flow.

Management of preterm labor in the home

The success of hospital therapy for preterm labor provides a subset of patients who require long-term maintenance therapy. The need for home care is supported by the high cost of hospitalization and the emotional stress of being away from home and family[35]. Patients who achieve the most benefit from home care include those whose uterine contraction pattern is greatly affected by increased activity and in whom cervical change occurs with a minimal number of uterine contractions or increased pressure.

Preparation for discharge and continued home therapy should begin at the time of admission for the treatment of preterm labor. It is important to remember that home therapy may not be feasible if the patient is in advanced preterm labor with a high degree of cervical dilatation and/or spontaneous rupture of membranes and delivery is deemed inevitable. For home care to be successful, the patient must have a clear understanding of the potential adverse consequences of preterm labor, the nature of the management plan, including the proposed tocolytic therapy, and the degree of activity restrictions that she will be expected to maintain. A teaching plan must be developed and followed (Table 4 is an example of such a plan).

Prior to discharge, the home care nurse should obtain a thorough medical and obstetric history and be knowledgeable of the treatment plan to be initially followed in the home. In addition, the home environment should be evaluated to determine if adequate resources are available to make bed rest or activity restriction feasible. *The entire family should be included in the plan of care. Without their cooperation and support, chances of success are diminished.*

MULTIPLE PREGNANCY

Home visits should take place on a weekly or more frequent basis as dictated by the patient's status. The initial visit should be planned within 2 days after discharge, to aid in the transition from hospital to home care. All nursing care provided during the home visit should be based upon specific protocols and physician orders.

Vital signs Notify the physician if the pulse is consistently over 120 beats per minute, the diastolic blood pressure is greater than 15 mmHg above baseline or systolic pressure is 30 mmHg above baseline.

Lung assessment Notify physician at the slightest sign of congestion, regardless of whether it is in association with dyspnea or chest pain.

Weight Refer for nutrition counselling if weight gain is inadequate. If weight gain is rapid, assess lung sounds and palpate for the presence of edema.

Fetal heart tones/fetal movement Notify physician if fetal heart rate is less than 120 beats per min or greater than 160 beats per min and/or if decreased fetal movement is discerned.

Fundal height Notify physician if fundal growth exceeds or falls behind expected growth.

Urine dipstick for sugar, acetone or protein If glucose is present, check serum glucose levels. A glucose loading test should be obtained in all patients at 28 weeks' gestation. Patients on oral betamimetic therapy have a higher incidence of glucose intolerance and should have another glucose testing after tocolytic therapy has been initiated. If acetone is present, the patient's nutritional status should be evaluated as well. If protein is present, the blood pressure should be evaluated.

Deep tendon reflexes If reflexes are greater than 2+, the patient should be examined for the presence of clonus, edema and elevated blood pressure.

Uterine activity pattern When the patient is resting in bed, the cervical status should be evaluated if more than four contractions per hour are present. The physician should be notified if contraction pattern persists.

Cervical status The physician should be notified of any change in cervical status: dilatation, effacement, consistency, position or station of the presenting part.

Gastrointestinal/nutrition The patient should be offered a bowel program consisting of stool softeners and a diet high in fiber and protein. Consultation with a trained dietician is beneficial.

Bed rest Activity reduction and therapeutic bed rest are major components of the home management of preterm labor. The nurse must reinforce the importance of bed rest, lying in a lateral position and possible elevation of the foot of the bed or the use of pillows under the hip to reduce pressure on the cervix. The guidelines regarding time allowed for activities such as showers and sitting up for meals should be clear and depend on patient status and physician orders. The home environment should be comprehensively evaluated to determine if the patient is receiving adequate help with child care, meal preparations and housekeeping. If home help is required, the patient should be assisted in her search for adequate service. If necessary, the patient should be referred to a hospital-based or independent social service program. Rehospitalization may be required if the patient is not able to maintain adequate activity reduction and bed rest at home.

Oral tocolysis The dosage of oral tocolytic agents and the uterine activity pattern should be assessed concomitantly to ascertain effectiveness of the maintenance dose. Adjustments should be made accordingly.

Psychosocial Community services and parent support groups are often available to aid women on bed rest and should be contacted. Insurance companies often cover costs for help in the home (see Appendix).

Properly planned and initiated, the home environment can provide an atmosphere conducive to meeting the specific needs of each patient. A major focus in home care is educating the patient and allowing her to participate in her care.

Uterine activity monitoring

All patients should be instructed in self-monitoring of uterine activity and observation of signs and symptoms of preterm labor as a part of their initial prenatal teaching. In addition, objective monitoring of uterine activity can provide two types of particularly useful information in assessing patient status at home: (1) the identification of regular uterine contractions as soon as possible in order to make a prompt diagnosis of preterm labor and initiate effective tocolytic therapy[36], and (2) the identification of recurrent preterm labor and the prompt adjustment of tocolytic treatment regimens[37]. Use of a home uterine activity monitor has also been shown to be useful in titrating tocolysis at home and reducing unnecessary hospital admissions, unless they are required to institute or re-institute intravenous tocolysis[37,38].

In general, a home monitor is worn by the patient during two 1-h sessions per day and during periods of perceived increases in uterine activity. The monitor tracing is then transmitted via the telephone to a nursing service where the data are evaluated. Regardless of the level of uterine activity, the patient has daily contact with the nurse to discuss any of the other possible signs or symptoms of preterm labor or any problems or concerns. At present, it is not clear if the device is more effective in the identification of preterm labor than the nursing contact, and this question is under intense investigation.

Low-amplitude high-frequency uterine activity and the onset of preterm labor

The guard-ring tocodynamometer introduced by Smyth[39] in 1957 was the basis for the identification of a specific pattern of uterine activity in which contractions occur frequently, with low amplitude (Figure 1). Previously, these low-amplitude high-frequency (LAHF) contractions had been characterized either as 'uterine irritability' or as 'Braxton–Hicks contractions' and their importance had been minimized, because they were regarded as physiological. However, more recent reports suggest that the LAHF contractility pattern may have a causative role in the occurrence of preterm labor[40–43].

LAHF contractions were originally described by Alvarez and Caldeyro. Often characterized as 'Alvarez waves' in the past, they are defined as uterine contractions with intensity of <5 mmHg and a frequency of $1-2/\text{min}^{40}$. Alvarez and Caldeyro ascribed LAHF uterine activity to asynchronic local contractions occurring randomly in different parts of the uterus and characterized this activity as 'uterine fibrillation'. These contractions are generally not perceived by the woman, but can be detected by internal tocodynamometers[43] or external guard-ring tocodynamometers[39,42,43]. Many years later, Nakae classified each waveform of the external tocograph and observed that 'small waves' were increased in women with preterm labor and who were receiving tocolytic treatment[44].

The significance of the LAHF contraction has not always been appreciated. According to Warkentin, LAHF contractions account for 70–80% of the total contractions recorded in normal pregnancies. On this basis, he concluded that they were not associated with preterm labor or poor outcome[45]. However, after these contraction patterns were subject to intense clinical scrutiny, Creasy and more recent observers all concluded that they served as the prodromal events that lead to the development of more synchronous contractions of greater intensity and subsequently to preterm labor[41,46].

Newman et al. concluded that parity and gestational age had no effect on the occurrence of LAHF contractions, based on a study of 50 women at low risk and 92 women at high risk of preterm labor, including 20 twin pregnancies. Patients destined to develop preterm labor exhibited an LAHF contractility pattern significantly more frequently than their counterparts who delivered at term (13.5 vs. 9.2%, respectively). Newman and co-workers subsequently studied the influence of fetal number on uterine

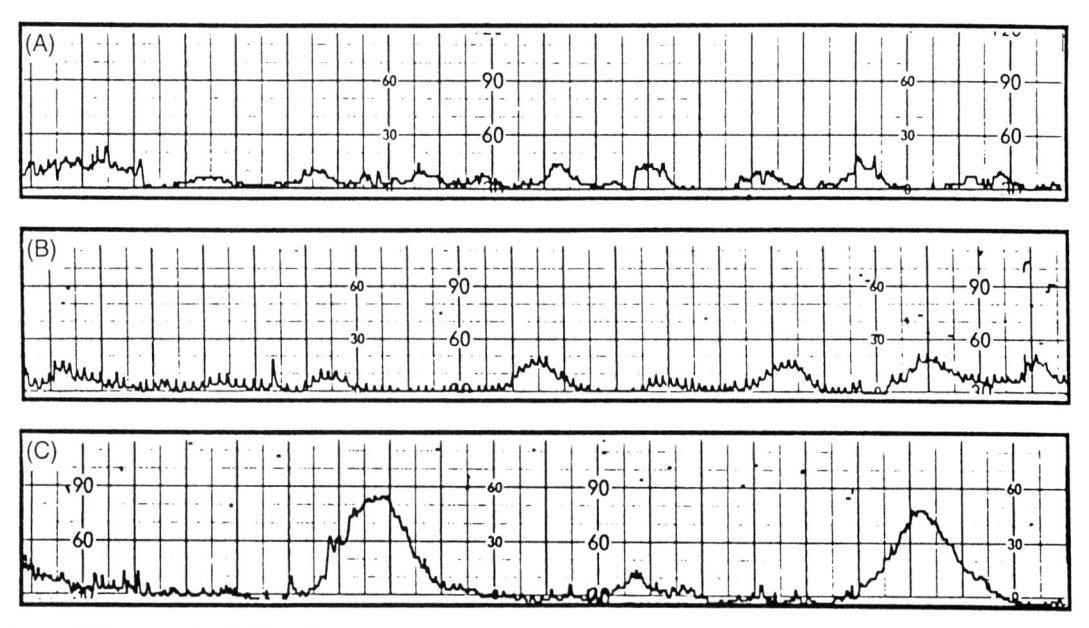

Figure 1 Low-amplitude high-frequency (LAHF) contractions (A and B) may be the precursors to the organized uterine contractions (C) that can cause preterm birth

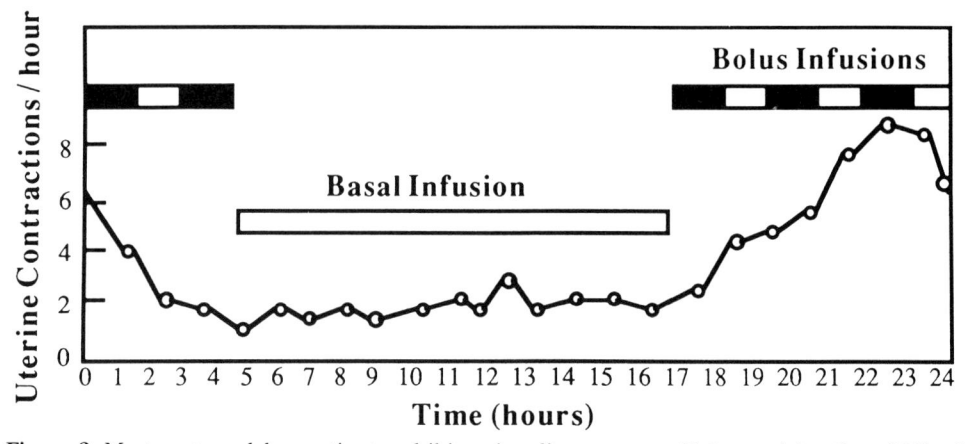

Figure 2 Most preterm labor patients exhibit a circadian pattern of labor activity. Over 80% of all contractions occur during a 6-h nocturnal period in the late evening. Subcutaneous terbutaline pumps are programmed to infuse a low dose (0.05–0.09 mg/h) basal rate during periods of low-amplitude high-frequency uterine activity. During the nocturnal period of organized contractions, intermittent boluses of 0.25 mg of terbutaline are infused. The overall result is a low total daily dosage (3–4 mg/day) of terbutaline, reducing the chance of side effects and tachyphylaxis

activity. They concluded that although fetal number had no impact on the intensity of pre-labor contractions, triplet gestations had a significantly higher incidence of increased LAHF uterine activity[42]. These authors additionally suggested that LAHF contractions played a role in bringing about the 'silent' cervical changes so often seen in triplet gestation[47].

Kawarabayashi et al.[43] studied 6363 cardiotocographs obtained from 578 patients and observed: (1) the presence of small wave (LAHF) activity in 7.5% of the patients; (2) a decrease in the rate of LAHF activity as the pregnancy progressed; (3) an increase in small wave (LAHF) activity in 42.3% of patients in preterm labor; and (4) patients with increased LAHF activity had relatively poor obstetric parameters and fetal outcomes. Their observations suggest that small wave LAHF activity is a real manifestation of a specific type of uterine contractility, and its presence is ominous for the outcome of the pregnancy in general. Stated another way, LAHF activity may indicate the presence of a state of high excitability and poor coordination of the uterine muscle before the onset of large phasic contractions.

If LAHF contractions indeed are precursors to more organized, phasic contractions that precede cervical change and preterm delivery, three important clinical questions immediately arise: (1) can the detection of increased LAHF wave activity be used as a screening tool to diagnose preterm labor at an earlier stage? (2) can LAHF contractions be suppressed with tocolytic agents? and (3) can suppression of this activity be achieved with smaller doses of tocolytic agents? With regard to the first question, the diagnostic role of LAHF activity has not been substantiated. In the Newman study[42], an analysis of the last 7 days before the onset of labor in the group of patients who developed preterm labor failed to show an increasing frequency of LAHF activity. The response to the second question is much more promising. Newman et al. observed a 50% decrease of LAHF contractions during tocolysis[42]. Moreover, Kawarabayashi et al. suggested that the appearance of LAHF activity does not lead to a poor prognosis in preterm labor if large phasic contractions could be abolished by beta-2-stimulant treatment[43]. Finally, in response to the third question, preliminary studies suggest that LAHF contractions can be suppressed by low-dose subcutaneous infusions of terbutaline[21].

Circadian patterns of uterine activity

In 1982, Schwenzer and co-workers described a circadian pattern of uterine contractions in resting pregnant women who were monitored with a stationary tocodynamometer[48]. A nocturnal increase in uterine activity was noted between 2300 and 0300 h and a diurnal increase between 1100 and 1300 h. The period of least uterine activity was between 1300 and 0900 h. Zahn subsequently evaluated 57 women with normal pregnancies by continuous 24-h tocodynamometry[49]. He observed a circadian pattern of contraction frequency with peaks between 2200 and 0200 h, followed by a decrease in uterine activity. A similar pattern was also noted in normal women by Arakai[50], with a frequency of distribution similar to that of Zahn's. In patients with recurrent preterm labor, we observed a nocturnal frequency distribution pattern of organized contractions, with 80% of all uterine activity occurring during a 6-h peak period in the late evening[21,46,51]. This nocturnal pattern of increased uterine activity was observed in singleton and multiple gestations. Although individuals exhibited different patterns, any given patient's pattern of uterine activity was usually consistent over time and repetitive. The appearance of LAHF contractions generally preceded the onset of organized uterine contractions.

The existence of a circadian pattern of uterine activity suggests that treatment of preterm labor can be planned on an individual basis (Figure 2). The tocolytic dose can be increased during the nocturnal peak of uterine activity and decreased during periods of uterine quiescence. Such patient-specific regimens not only reduce overall medication requirements but also minimize the risk of tachyphylaxsis and toxicity.

Prior to initiation of this variable dose therapy, individual patterns of uterine activity should be determined by 24-hour continuous in-hospital tocodynamometry. In addition, any perceived uterine activity detected by self papation should be recorded on a preterm labor log (Figure 3). Medication dosage or frequency can be adjusted accordingly, based on changes of uterine activity.

Subcutaneous pump therapy

Subcutaneous (SQ) pump therapy was developed as an alternative to intravenous tocolysis

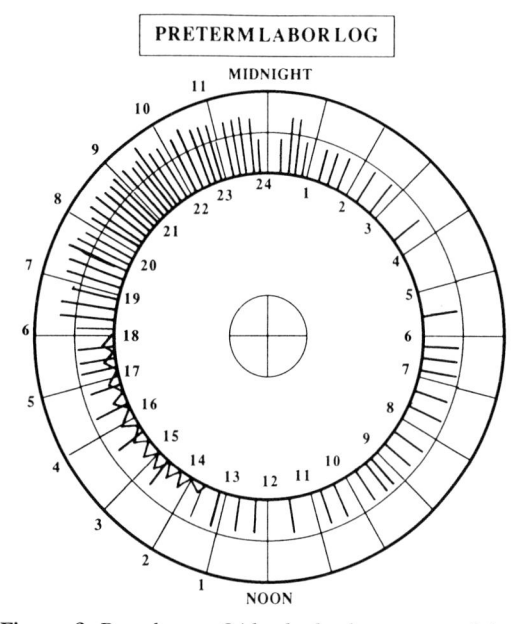

Figure 3 Based on a 24-h clock, the preterm labor log provides a graphic record of uterine activity. Records are made daily based on tocodynamometry, palpation and self-perception of uterine contractions. The solid lines represent uterine contractions and the serrated line represents periods of uterine irritability (low-amplitude high-frequency uterine contractions)

in patients who failed oral treatment due to recurrent preterm labor[21]. Subcutaneous pump therapy delivers a continuous low basal rate of terbutaline and scheduled boluses of 0.25 mg of this agent during identified periods of increased uterine activity. The total average daily dose (including basal and bolus infusions) is 3–4 mg/day and this dose is titrated according to changes in uterine activity. Essential to the success of this therapy is the re-sensitization of the beta-receptors. Patients are first maintained on intravenous $MgSO_4$ for 24–48 h as a 'drug holiday' to allow the beta-receptors to regain their sensitivity.

Patients who could not otherwise be discharged to home care because of inadequate response to oral therapy may be successfully maintained on pump therapy. Not unexpectedly, nursing care plays a significant role in patient education prior to discharge and the subsequent management of pump therapy in the home[52–54]. Nursing actions include those listed above for betamimetic therapy at home, plus several interventions specific to subcutaneous terbutaline pump therapy:

(1) Elucidate the patient regarding the use and mechanics of the pump;

(2) Teach the care and changing of the infusion site;

(3) Monitor the titration of the dose according to uterine activity as ordered by the physician. Deliver basal and bolus doses according to specific protocol. Set criteria for notifying the physician of changes in contraction patterns; and

(4) Instruct patient to monitor her radial pulse rate prior to emergency bolus doses.

Basal infusion rates should be adjusted to minimize periods of low-amplitude high-frequency uterine activity. Our dose–response studies demonstrated that continuous basal terbutaline infusion rates of 0.05–0.08 mg/h were most effective in suppressing LAHF waves and subsequent uterine contractions. In multiple gestations, basal infusion rates of 0.06–0.09 mg/h may be required. Higher basal infusion rates should be avoided, because they not only result in more medication than is necessary to control LAHF waves, but also fail to provide significant additional suppression of organized uterine contractions. Our experience has shown that tocolytic breakthrough occurs much more rapidly at basal infusion rates above 0.09 mg/h often within 3 weeks. With multiple gestataions, however, basal rates near the 0.09 mg/h maximum may be needed, because of the higher maternal blood volume.

Bolus schedules are determined according to the patient's individual contraction pattern. Bolus doses of 0.25–0.30 mg are given to suppress organized uterine contractions. These are scheduled every 2 h during the established peak period of uterine activity and less frequently during the periods of minimal uterine activity. The typical patient requires 6–8 bolus doses distributed over a 24-h period, for a total infusion of less than 4 mg/day[24,51]. This dose level compares very favorably with the typical oral dosages of 40–60 mg/day and typical intravenous dosages of 60–80 mg/day.

We start the majority of our patients with multiple pregnancy who are in preterm labor on a standard dosage schedule: a basal infusion of 0.06 mg/h and boluses of 0.25 mg at 09.00, 12 noon, 15.00, 18.00, 20.00 and 22.00 h[51]. Patients are instructed to use supplemental demand boluses if they experience more than 4–6 contractions per hour and to record these on their preterm labor log. Demand bolus histories are of particular value in making adjustments to the patient's routine bolus schedule. Boluses should not be given if the maternal pulse rate is greater than 110 beats per min and, in any case, no more frequently than every hour. Whereas the currently accepted practice for titrating dosage levels of oral betamimetic agents relies on measuring maternal tachycardia (a secondary beta-1 cardiac effect), patient-specific dosing with the terbutaline pump is directed toward a reduction of uterine activity (a direct beta-2 end organ effect)[51]. Current investigations involving pharmacokinetic dosing will further enhance the ability to effectively titrate tocolytic administration.

The schedule of intermittent boluses can be adjusted if the patient's pattern of uterine activity changes either during the hospital stay or after discharge home. Adjustments may include increasing the frequency of boluses, adding additional boluses, increasing the individual bolus doses up to a maximum of 0.3 mg or shifting the cluster of boluses to coincide with a shift in the period of peak uterine activity.

The basal rate may be increased if there is an increase in uterine LAHF waves or a persistent increase in uterine contractions of greater than 4–6/h despite repeated boluses. It is best to maintain the basal infusion at the lowest rate possible, however, to prevent beta-2 receptor site desensitization. After the patient has been stabilized on terbutaline pump therapy, she can be discharged home on bed rest and monitored intermittently with a portable tocodynamometer.

Monitoring is scheduled for one hour during the peak period of contractions and one hour during the 'quiet' period to determine LAHF wave activity. Additional monitoring may be needed if periods of increased uterine activity occur. A home care perinatal nurse should visit the patient on a weekly basis to check blood pressure, pulse rate, fundal height and fetal heart rate, and perform a urinalysis and perform cervical exams, as indicated.

Our prior studies of recurrent preterm labor in patients with singleton or multiple pregnancies who were receiving betamimetic therapy demonstrated the following patterns (Figure 4): (1) a return of excessive levels of low-amplitude high-frequency (LAHF) contractions; (2) a return of a circadian, generally nocturnal pattern of organized high-amplitude uterine contractions; (3) a rapidly increasing need for increased frequency and dosing of terbutaline or ritodrine[51]; and (4) a 'crescendo' effect or acceleration of the frequency of uterine contractions 48–72 h prior to the episode of active recurrent preterm labor[55].

Although infrequent, breakthrough does occur in patients receiving terbutaline pump therapy. Should this take place, the patient should be readmitted to the hospital and stabilized on intravenous $MgSO_4$ for 24–48 h after discontinuation of terbutaline pump therapy (both basal and bolus infusions). This 'drug holiday' allows the myometrial receptors to regain their sensitivity to terbutaline (Figure 5). When stable, the patient can be restarted on terbutaline pump therapy and discharged home. Tocolytic therapy is generally discontinued at 36–37 weeks and at this point, patients may resume normal activity until delivery.

The combined use of home uterine activity monitoring and the subcutaneous terbutaline pumps to prevent the recurrence of preterm labor has been evaluated in a large number of patients at very high risk of preterm labor. Allbert and associates retrospectively reviewed 992 patients (including 206 patients with twins) who were prescribed home uterine activity monitoring as well as terbutaline pump therapy[56]. Therapy extended the duration of gestation a mean of 38 ± 23 days; and the average gestational age at delivery was 36.3 ± 2.6 weeks with a mean birth weight of 2759 ± 681 g.

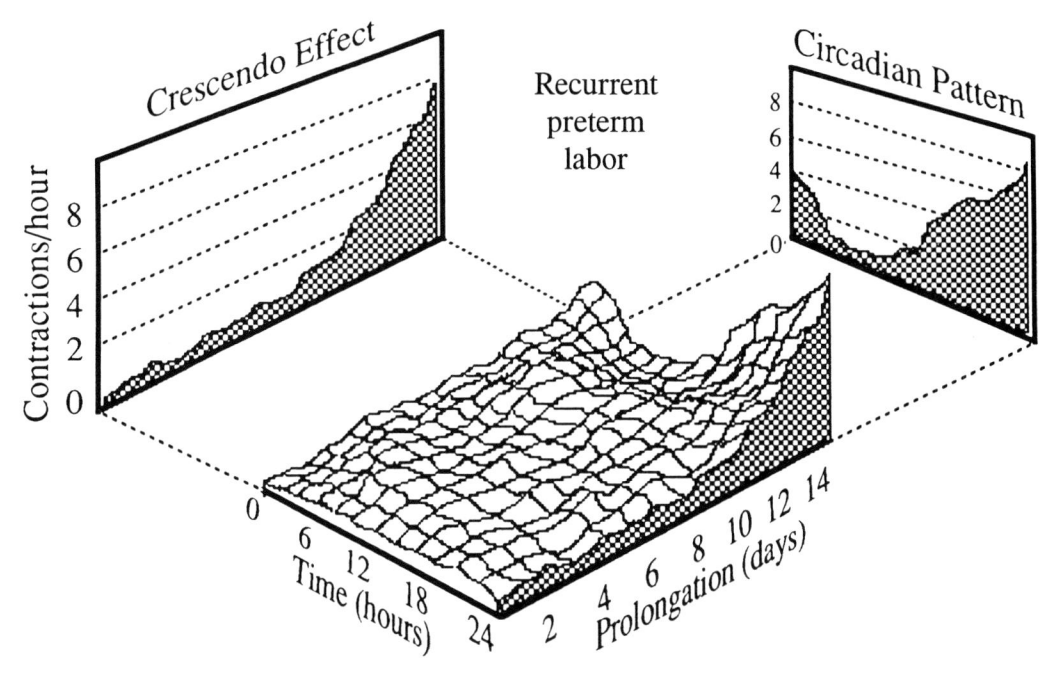

Figure 4 Three-dimensional plot of uterine activity in a twin gestation leading to recurrent preterm labor. Continuous monitoring of patient on oral terbutaline therapy: x-axis, time of day; y-axis, number of contractions per hour; z-axis, number of days of tocolytic treatment. Recurrent preterm labor is characterized by (1) a return of excessive levels of low-amplitude high-frequency (LAHF) precursor uterine contractions; (2) a return of a circadian, generally nocturnal pattern of organized high-amplitude uterine contractions; (3) a rapidly increasing need for increased frequency and dosage of terbutaline or ritodrine; and (4) a 'crescendo' effect of acceleration of frequency of uterine contractions 48–72 h prior to the episode of active recurrent preterm labor

Elliott and Radin[57] combined home monitoring and infusion pumps in their management protocol for ten quadruplet pregnancies. These authors achieved a mean gestational age at delivery of 32.5 weeks compared to 30.2 weeks in a control group.

The preliminary clinical experience at our hospital with the combined use of home monitoring and infusion pumps has been equally favorable. Nineteen twin pregnancies in the monitor/pump treatment group were compared to 54 twin pregnancies in the control group. Figure 6 shows that the treatment group achieved a significantly greater mean gestational age of delivery than the control group (36.7 weeks vs. 34.9 weeks). Notably, the treatment group also had significantly less recurrent preterm labor resulting in a tighter clustering of deliveries at a gestational age when fetal lung maturity can be achieved, and adverse neonatal outcomes potentially avoided. Despite these salutary results, the number of patients studied have been small. Additional prospective randomized trials are warranted.

Recommendations

The early diagnosis of preterm labor and immediate intervention may be essential components in halting the process of preterm labor in multiple pregnancy. However, the early recognition of preterm labor only results in successful inhibition of the labor process if patients at risk are identified and comprehensive antepartum management is applied. In this regard, practitioners should be prepared to:

(1) Regard all multifetal gestations as at high-risk for preterm labor and delivery;

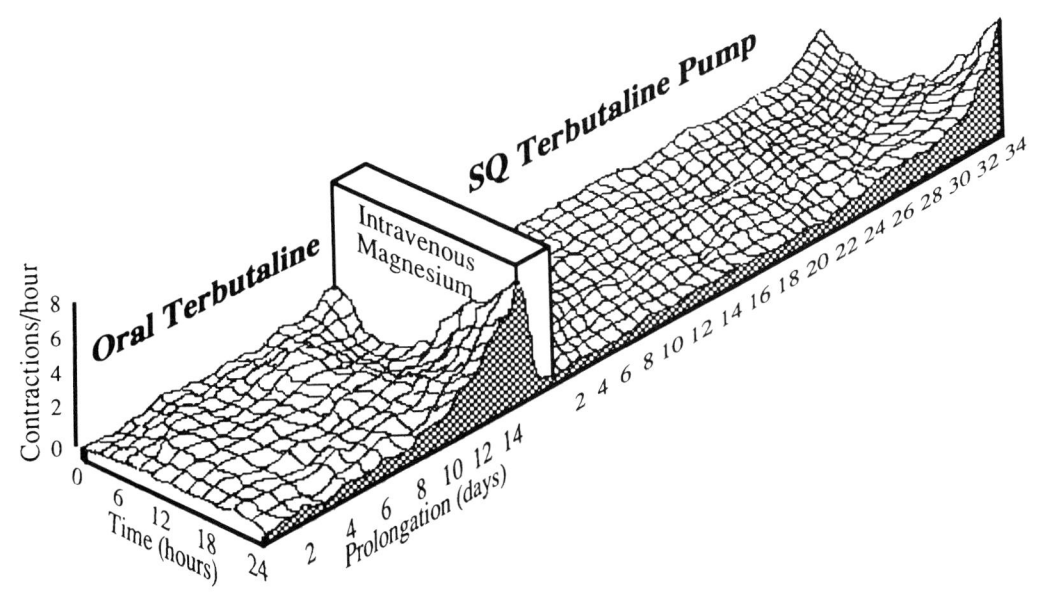

Figure 5 Recurrent preterm labor may be secondary to down-regulation of the uterine beta-receptors. Intravenous magnesium sulfate is initiated in a sequential fashion to provide a 'drug holiday'. It requires at least 24–48 h for the uterine beta-receptors to up-regulate and regain their sensitivity to terbutaline or ritodrine. At this point, subcutaneous (SQ) terbutaline pump therapy can be started to prevent the recurrence of preterm labor

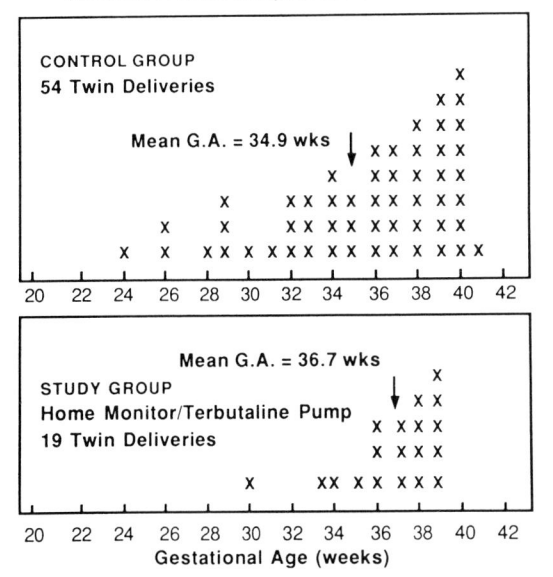

Figure 6 Preliminary clinical trials at California–Pacific Hospital (San Francisco, California) suggest that the use of home uterine activity monitoring and terbutaline pump tocolytic therapy in twin pregnancies can significantly reduce preterm births that result from recurrent preterm labor

(2) Enrol all patients with multifetal gestation in preterm labor/education programs by 20 weeks' gestation;

(3) Evaluate cervical status on a weekly basis after 22–24 weeks;

(4) Consider ambulatory tocodynamometry;

(5) Avoid prophylactic tocolysis with oral beta-mimetic agents because this leads to down-regulation of the beta-receptors;

(6) Advise bed rest and hydrate moderately if increased uterine activity becomes evident;

(7) When cervical change is documented, hospitalize and treat aggressively with parenteral tocolytic agents before advanced cervical dilatation (≥ 2 cm);

(8) Rule out pathological causes of preterm labor: infection, abruption, polyhydramnios and congenital anomalies;

(9) Consider using intravenous $MgSO_4$ as a primary tocolytic agent, because it is associated with fewer maternal side effects and does not down-regulate the

beta-receptors which may later be needed for long-term tocolysis;

(10) Consider ambulatory tocolysis only after the patient has been stabilized on parenteral tocolytic agents;

(11) Fully respect the contraindications to tocolytic use;

(12) Select a tocolytic agent to maximize efficacy and minimize toxicity on an individualized patient-specific basis;

(13) Titrate tocolytic dosage to end-organ effect (decrease of uterine activity) not to toxicity (tachycardia or other side effects);

(14) Monitor for signs of recurrent preterm labor;

(15) Provide close nursing support;

(16) Re-admit patients with recurrent preterm labor for re-infusion with parenteral tocolysis;

(17) Use a sequential approach for tocolysis in recurrent preterm labor. Alternate beta-adrenergic agents (ritodrine or terbutaline) with tocolytic agents that do not bind to the beta-2 receptor ($MgSO_4$) to allow the beta-receptors to regain their sensitivity;

(18) Provide a 24–48 h intravenous $MgSO_4$ 'drug holiday' in patients who experience a betamimetic tocolytic breakthrough;

(19) Consider terbutaline pump therapy for patients with recurrent preterm labor or for those who cannot tolerate oral therapy;

(20) Continue all required prenatal testing on an ambulatory basis; and

(21) Intensify maternal and fetal surveillance at 34 weeks to determine the best time for delivery.

The ultimate goal of achieving a term delivery with reduction in the incidence of low birth weight infants will provide the greatest contribution to improving perinatal outcome in the future.

References

1. Creasy, R.K. and Katz, M. (1984). Basic research and clinical experience with β-adrenergic tocolytics in the United States. In Fuchs, F. and Stubblefield, P.G. (eds.) *Preterm Birth: Causes, Prevention and Management*, pp. 150–70. (Toronto: MacMillan)
2. Downey, L.J. and Martin, A.J. (1983). Ritodrine in the treatment of preterm labour: a study of 213 patients. *Br. J. Obstet. Gynaecol.*, **90**, 1046–53
3. Nageotte, M.P. (1990). Prevention and treatment of preterm labor in twin gestation. *Clin. Obstet. Gynecol.*, **33**, 61–8
4. Hollander, D. and Stefanelli, J. (1989). Prematurity and preterm labor: a review. *Clin. Consult. Obstet. Gynecol.*, **1**, 77–88
5. Zlatnick, F.J. (1972). The applicability of labor inhibition to the problem of prematurity. *Am. J. Obstet. Gynecol.*, **113**, 704–6
6. Russell, J.K. (1952). Maternal and fetal hazards associated with twin pregnancies. *J. Obstet. Gynaecol. Br. Emp.*, **59**, 208
7. Powers, W.F. and Miller, T.C. (1979). Bedrest in twin pregnancy: identification of a critical period and its cost implications. *Am. J. Obstet. Gynecol.*, **134**, 23
8. Newton, E.R. (1986). Antepartum care in multiple gestation. *Semin. Perinatol.*, **10**, 19–29
9. Luke, B., Keith, L. and Witter, F. (1992). Theoretical model for reducing neonatal morbidity and mortality and associated cost among twins. *J. Matern. Fet. Med.*, **1**, 14–19
10. Marivate, M., De Villiers, K.Q. and Fairbrother, P. (1977). Effect of prophylactic outpatient administration of fenoterol on the time of onset of spontaneous labor and fetal growth rate in twin pregnancy. *Am. J. Obstet. Gynecol.*, **128**, 707

11. Skjaerris, J. and Aberg, A. (1982). Prevention of prematurity in twin pregnancy by orally administered terbutaline. *Acta Obstet. Gynecol. Scand.* (Suppl.), **108**, 39
12. Cetrulo, C.L. and Freeman, R.K. (1976). Ritodrine HCL for the prevention of premature labor in twin pregnancies. *Acta Genet. Med. Gemollol.*, **25**, 321
13. O'Connor, M.C., Murphy, H. and Dalymple, I.J. (1979). Double blind trial of ritodrine and placebo in twin pregnancy. *Br. J. Obstet. Gynaecol.*, **86**, 706
14. Berg, G., Andersson, R.G.G. and Rygen, G. (1985). β-Adrenergic receptors in human myometrium during pregnancy: changes in the number of receptors after β-mimetic treatment. *Am. J. Obstet. Gynecol.*, **151**, 392
15. Fredholm, B.B., Lunell, N., Persson, B. *et al.* (1982). Development of tolerance to the metabolic actions of β$_2$-adrenoceptor stimulating drugs. *Acta Obstet. Gynecol. Scand.* (Suppl.), **18**, 53–9
16. Mickey, J., Tate, R. and Lefkowitz, R.J. (1975). Subsensitivity of adenylate cyclase and decreased β-adrenergic receptor binding after chronic exposure to (−) isoproterenol *in vitro*. *J. Biol. Chem.*, **250**, 5727
17. Ryden, G., Rolf, G., Andersson, G. *et al.* (1982). Is the relaxing effect of β-adrenergic agonists on the human myometrium only transitory? *Acta Obstet. Gynecol. Scand.* (Suppl.), **108**, 47
18. Swillens, S., Lefort, E., Barber, R. *et al.* (1980). Consequences of hormone-induced desensitization of adenylate cyclase in intact cells. *Biochem. J.*, **188**, 169
19. Beall, M., Edgar, B., Paul, R. *et al.* (1985). A comparison of ritodrine, terbutaline, and magnesium sulfate for the suppression of preterm labor. *Am. J. Obstet. Gynecol.*, **153**, 857–9
20. Valenzuela, G. and Cline, S. (1982). Use of magnesium sulphate in premature labor that fails to respond to β-mimetic drugs. *Am. J. Obstet. Gynecol.*, **143**, 718
21. Lam, F., Gill, P., Smith, M. *et al.* (1988). Use of the subcutaneous terbutaline pump for long-term tocolysis. *Obstet. Gynecol.*, **72**, 810–13
22. Miller, J.M., Keane, M. and Horger, E.O. (1982). A comparison of magnesium sulphate and terbutaline for the arrest of premature labor: a preliminary report. *J. Reprod. Med.*, **27**, 348–51
23. Hollander, D., Nagey, D. and Pupkin, M. (1987). Magnesium sulphate and ritodrine hydrochloride: a randomized comparison. *Am. J. Obstet. Gynecol.*, **156**, 631
24. Elliot, J.P. (1983). Magnesium sulfate as a tocolytic agent. *Am. J. Obstet. Gynecol.*, **147**, 277
25. Ridgway, L.E., Muise, K., Wright, J.W. *et al.* (1990). A prospective randomized comparison of oral terbutaline and magnesium oxide for the maintenance of tocolysis. *Am. J. Obstet. Gynecol.*, **163**, 879–82
26. Martin, R.W., Martin, J.N., Morrison, J.C. *et al.* (1988). Comparison of oral ritodrine and magnesium gluconate for ambulatory tocolysis. *Am. J. Obstet. Gynecol.*, **158**, 1440–5
27. Martin, R.W., Gaddy, D.K., Morrison, J.C. *et al.* (1987). Tocolysis with oral magnesium. *Am. J. Obstet. Gynecol.*, **156**, 433–4
28. Repke, J. and Niebyl, J. (1985). The role of prostaglandin synthetase inhibitors in the treatment of preterm labor. *Semin. Reprod. Endocrinol.*, **3**, 259
29. Niebyl, J.R. and Witter, F.R. (1986). Neonatal outcome after indomethacin treatment for preterm labor. *Am. J. Obstet. Gynecol.*, **155**, 747–9
30. Dudley, D. and Hardie, M. (1985). Fetal and neonatal effects of indomethacin used as a tocolytic agent. *Am. J. Obstet. Gynecol.*, **151**, 181–4
31. Zuckerman, H., Reiss, U. and Rubinstein, I. (1974). Inhibition of human premature labor by indomethacin. *Obstet. Gynecol.*, **44**, 787–92
32. Wurtzel, D. (1990). Prenatal administration of indomethacin as a tocolytic agent: effect on neonatal renal function. *Obstet. Gynecol.*, **76**, 689–92
33. Kirshon, B., Moise, K.J., Wasserstrum, N. *et al.* (1988). Influence of short-term indomethacin therapy on fetal urine output. *Obstet. Gynecol.*, **72**, 51–3
34. Read, M.D. and Wellby, D.E. (1986). The use of calcium antagonists (nifedipine) to suppress preterm labour. *Br. J. Obstet. Gynaecol.*, **93**, 933
35. Dahlberg, N.L. (1988). A perinatal center based antepartum homecare program. *J. Obstet. Gynecol. Neonatal Nurs.*, **17**, 30–4
36. Katz, M., Gill, P.J. and Newman, R.B. (1986). Detection of preterm labor by ambulatory monitoring of uterine activity: a preliminary report. *Obstet. Gynecol.*, **68**, 773–8
37. Katz, M., Gill, P.J. and Newman, R.B. (1986). Detection of preterm labor by ambulatory monitoring of uterine activity for the management of oral tocolysis. *Am. J. Obstet. Gynecol.*, **154**, 1253–6

38. Knuppel, R.A., Lake, M.F., Watson, D.L. *et al.* (1990). Preventing preterm birth in twin gestation: home uterine activity monitoring and perinatal nursing support. *Obstet. Gynecol.*, **76**, 24S–27S
39. Smyth, C.N. (1957). The guard-ring tocodynamometer: absolute assessment of intra-amniotic pressure by a new instrument. *J. Obstet. Gynaecol. Br. Commonw.*, **64**, 59
40. Alvarez, H. and Caldeyro, R. (1950). Contractility of the human uterus recorded by new methods. *Surg. Gynecol. Obstet.*, **91**, 1
41. Creasy, R.K. (1984). Preterm labor and delivery. In Creasy, R.K. and Resnick, R. (eds.) *Maternal–Fetal Medicine, Principles and Practice*, pp. 415–43. (Philadelphia: W.B. Saunders)
42. Newman, R.B., Gill, P.G. and Campion, S. (1987). Antepartum ambulatory tocodynamometry: the significance of low-amplitude, high-frequency contractions. *Obstet. Gynecol.*, **70**, 701
43. Kawarabayashi, T., Kuriyama, K. and Kishikawa, T. (1988). Clinical features of small contraction wave recorded by an external tocodynamometer. *Am. J. Obstet. Gynecol.*, **158**, 474–8
44. Nakae, S. (1978). Analysis of uterine contraction in late pregnancy and premature labor. *Acta Obstet. Gynaecol. Jpn*, **30**, 1637
45. Warkentin, B. (1976). Die uterine aktivitat in der spatschwangerschaft. *Z. Geburtsh. Perinat.*, **180**, 225
46. Scheerer, L. and Katz, M.M. (1989). Home monitoring for preterm labor. In Parer, J.T. (ed.) *Antepartum and Intrapartum Management*, pp. 32–52. (Philadelphia: Lea and Febiger)
47. Newman, R.B., Gill, P.J., Campion, S. *et al.* (1989). The influence of fetal number on antepartum uterine activity. *Obstet. Gynecol.*, **73**, 695
48. Schwenzer, T.H., Schumann, R. and Halberstadt, E. (1982). The importance of 24 hour cardiotocographic monitoring during tocolytic therapy. In Jung, H. and Lamberti, G. (eds.), *Beta-mimetic Drugs in Obstetrics and Perinatology*, p. 60. (New York: Thieme-Stratton)
49. Zahn, V. (1984). Uterine contractions during pregnancy. *J. Perinat. Med.*, **12**, 107
50. Arakai, R. (1984). The investigations of the effect of daily activity on the uterine contractions during pregnancy. *Acta Obstet. Gynecol. Jpn.*, **36**, 589
51. Lam, F. (1989). Miniature pump infusion of terbutaline – an option in preterm labor. *Contemp. Obstet. Gynecol.*, **33**, 53
52. Gill, P., Smith, M. and McGregor, C. (1989). Terbutaline by pump to prevent recurrent preterm labor. *Matern. Child. Nurs*, **14**, 163–7
53. Sala, D.J. and Moise, K.J. (1989). The treatment of preterm labor using a portable subcutaneous terbutaline pump. *J. Obstet. Gynecol. Neonat. Nursing*, **19**, 108–15
54. Stanton, R.J. (1991). Comanagement of the patient on subcutaneous terbutaline pump therapy. *J. Nurse-Midwifery*, **36**, 204–8
55. Garite, T.J., Bentley, D.L., Hamer, C.A. *et al.* (1990). Uterine activity characteristics in multiple gestations. *Obstet. Gynecol.*, **76**, 56S–59S
56. Allbert, J.R., Wise, C.A., Lou, C.H. *et. al.* (1992). Subcutaneous tocolytic infusion therapy for patients at very high risk for preterm birth. *J. Perinatol.*, **12**, 28–31
57. Elliott, J.P. and Radin, T.G. (1992). Quadruplet pregnancy: contemporary management and outcome. *Obstet. Gynecol.*, **80**, 421–4

The optimum route of delivery 36

F.A. Chervenak

Introduction

The optimum route of delivery of multiple gestations remains a matter of controversy. Currently, the role of elective Cesarean delivery for certain subsets of twin gestation is a matter of debate. Any delivery plan for twins requires consideration of the varied possible presentations for twin A and twin B.

Figure 1 illustrates these varied combinations for a population of twins, but Figure 2 illustrates a clinically more useful classification of twin presentations, with all combinations of twin presentations classified into three groups: (1) twin A, vertex with twin B, vertex (42.5% of the total twin population); (2) twin A, vertex with twin B, non-vertex (38.4% of the total twin population); and (3) twin A, non-vertex (19.1% of the total twin population)[1]. This chapter presents an intrapartum management plan for each of these groups, based upon analysis of outcome, and discusses controversial issues associated with the choice of the route of delivery.

Twin A, vertex with twin B, vertex

Vaginal delivery (or, at least an attempt at vaginal delivery) is appropriate for vertex–vertex twins[1-9]. Although Cesarean delivery has been proposed for vertex–vertex twins of $<1500\,\text{g}$[10], few data support this proposition. Indeed, some series[2,3] show that 70–80% of vertex–vertex twins can safely deliver vaginally.

Previously, it was accepted clinical practice that the time interval between twin deliveries

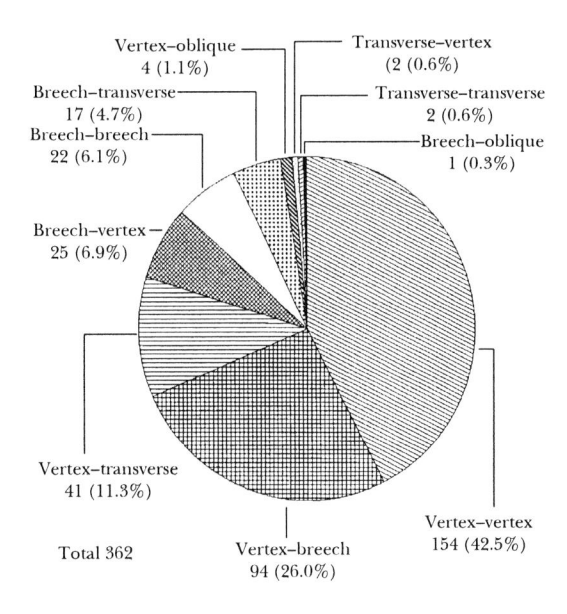

Figure 1 Diagram showing occurrence of intrapartum presentations for 362 consecutive twin gestations. (Reprinted with permission from reference 2)

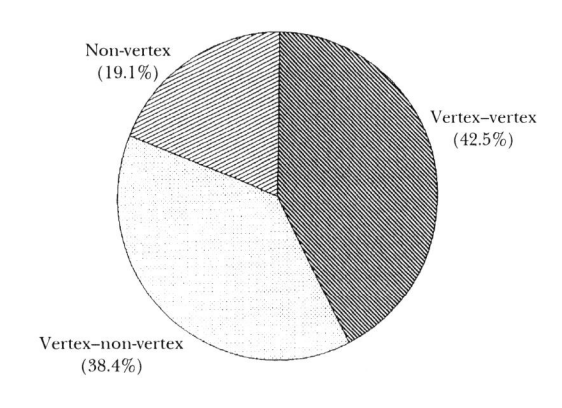

Figure 2 Diagram showing occurrence of twin A, vertex with twin B, vertex; twin A, vertex with twin B, non-vertex; and twin A, non-vertex for 362 consecutive twin gestations. (Reprinted with permission from reference 51)

should be no more than 30 min to avoid asphyxia to the second twin, cord prolapse, uterine inertia, placental abruption and retraction of the cervix[1-13]. More recently, however, 5-min Apgar scores have been shown not to correlate with the time interval between twin deliveries in several studies[2,3,9]. Indeed there is no urgency to deliver twin B after delivery of twin A if electronic fetal heart rate monitoring or sonographic visualization of the fetal heart if reassuring.

Although uncommon, intervals between deliveries of multiples of up to 131 days have been reported in patients with normal or bicornuate uteri[13-16]. For this to be contemplated, however, especially after delivery of a very premature twin, the membranes of the second twin must be intact, and if the placenta is retained, the umbilical cord of the first twin should be tied and cut close to the cervix. Cervical suture and tocolysis may not be indicated in this setting[15]. The risks and benefits of this form of management will probably be more clearly defined in the future as more cases are reported in detail.

With vertex–vertex presentations, oxytocin augmentation with careful surveillance of fetal heart function may be useful if labor has not resumed within 10 min of delivery of the first twin[8]. Once the vertex of the second twin is in the pelvic inlet, amniotomy is recommended. No modern series exists demonstrating the safety of internal podalic version in cases of fetal distress. If the fetal heart rate tracing of twin B deteriorates before atraumatic vaginal delivery is possible, Cesarean delivery is the management of choice. Because of this possibility, delivery of twins should always take place in clinical settings where it is possible to perform immediate Cesarean delivery. Indeed, such a setting should be considered the standard of care for all twins (see Chapter 37). The very rare possibility of spontaneous conversion of a vertex second twin to a non-vertex presentation does not, in my opinion, warrant the routine use of pelvimetry for all cases. If this rare situation occurs, the intrapartum management of the second twin can proceed as described in the sections that follow.

For both twins and singletons, a growing body of literature supports vaginal delivery of even the very low birth weight fetus (VLBW) in the vertex presentation[17-19]. In the past, it was commonly believed that labor and subsequent vaginal delivery led to head compression and intraventricular hemorrhage (IVH) with its attendant complications. However, the incidence and severity of IVH are no longer thought to be affected by mode of delivery[17,18]. Although I agree with other authors that vaginal delivery is appropriate for the vertex–vertex twin gestation, even in the VLBW group[1-3], this recommendation is not universally accepted[10].

Twin A, vertex with twin B, non-vertex

The management of twin gestations in vertex–breech (Figure 3) or vertex–transverse presentation is particularly controversial. Several

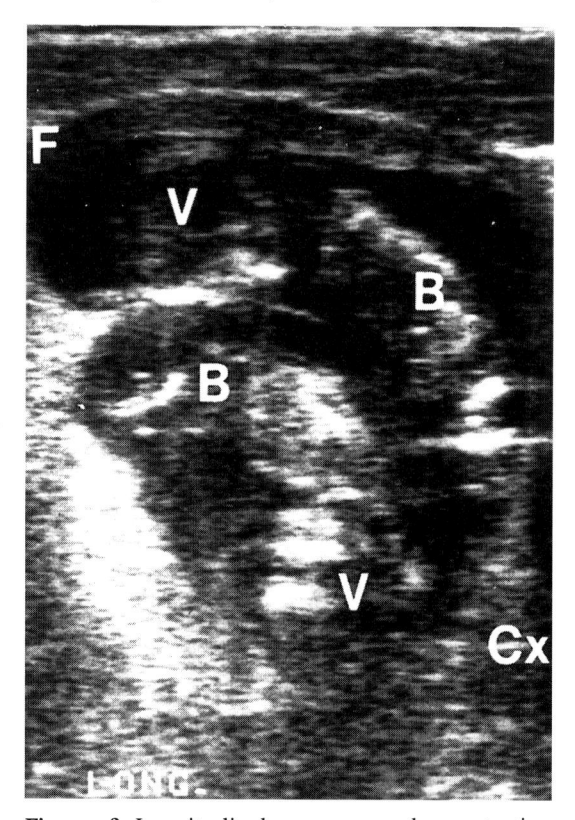

Figure 3 Longitudinal sonogram demonstrating twin gestation in vertex–breech presentation. F, uterine fundus; Cx, cervix; V, vertex; B, breech. (Reprinted with permission from reference 51)

investigators have advocated Cesarean delivery as the management of choice when the second twin is in a breech presentation or transverse lie[3–8]. This approach originally was justified by reports of increased perinatal mortality[20–22] and depressed Apgar scores[22,23] with breech delivery of the second twin. Cetrulo has reviewed experience at St Margaret's Hospital in Boston, where almost all vertex–non-vertex twins are delivered by Cesarean section. He found that the usual differential mortality and morbidity for twin B vs. twin A was virtually eliminated[3]. Regardless, I do not believe that route Cesarean delivery is always necessary in order to achieve an atraumatic birth.

The options of intrapartum external version and breech delivery of the second twin will now be discussed, and the effects of using these options on the neonatal morbidity and mortality of the vaginally delivered second twin in malpresentation will be analyzed.

Intrapartum external version

Several investigators have proposed external cephalic version for delivery of the singleton breech[24–27]. This position is not universally accepted, however, as others note[28,29] that the risk of cord accident or placental abruption is substantial. This question was addressed in one prospective randomized study, in which external cephalic version was found to be a safe and effective manner to manage breech presentation late in singleton pregnancy[30].

Over the years, several reports have advocated external cephalic version of the second twin[31–34]. Ranney reported successful version with subsequent vaginal delivery in nine transverse and two breech second twins[31]. In our series, in ten of 14 (71%) transverse presentations, and eight of 11 (73%) breech presentations, version was successful and resulted in vertex vaginal delivery (Figure 4). The success of version was not related to gestational age or birth weight, or parity. All eight versions attempted under peridural anesthesia were successful, thus suggesting that relaxation of the abdominal wall musculature may be helpful for the successful performance of version. In this series the 5-min Apgar score was depressed in only two cases (Apgar = 6 in each case). Because the time interval between delivery of

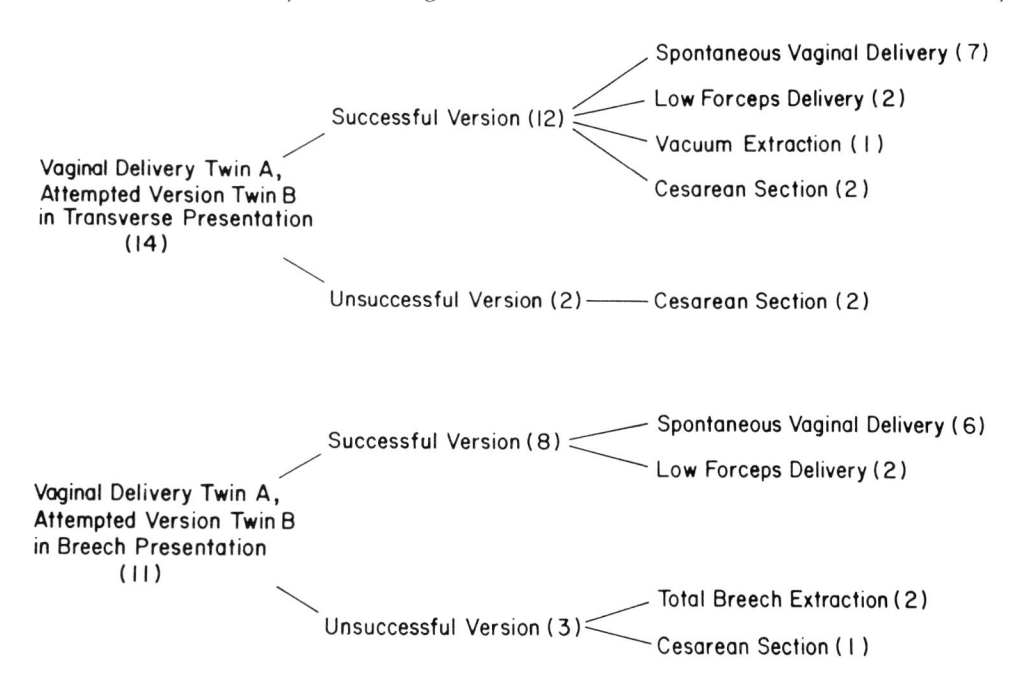

Figure 4 Mode of delivery after attempted external version of second twins in transverse or breech presentation. (Reprinted with permission from reference 34)

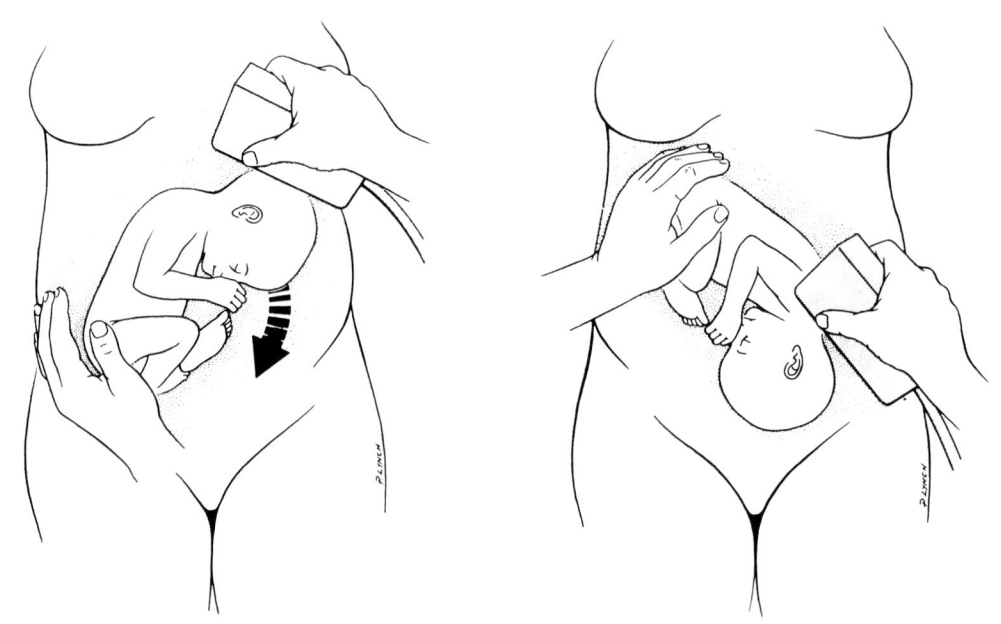

Figure 5 Method of using ultrasound transducer to guide vertex into pelvis. (Reprinted with permission from reference 34)

twin A and twin B was not related to either 1- or 5-min Apgar scores, the time spent in version apparently did not exert a detrimental effect. The maternal morbidity in this small series was not excessive. There were two cases of endometritis requiring antibiotics and one case of uterine atony managed by uterine massage and oxytocin administration[34].

The following guidelines are recommended for performance of intrapartum external version of the second twin: An initial sonographic assessment of the size of each fetus should be made. If twin B is larger than twin A and a great disparity exists, version with attempts at vaginal delivery is best avoided. Epidural anesthesia is advisable before delivery, to provide abdominal wall relaxation. Intact membranes are required for consideration of a version. Version should be performed only if immediate Cesarean section is possible. The version should be attempted immediately after, or even during, delivery of the first twin while the uterus is most relaxed. A real-time ultrasound machine should be present in the delivery room to accurately determine fetal presentation after delivery of the first twin. The fetal heart rate should be monitored continuously thereafter. Gentle pressure with the transducer may be used to guide the infant's head into vertex presentation above the birth canal (Figure 5). If this is not successful, external version can be attempted either as a forward or as a backward roll. The shortest arc between the vertex and the pelvic inlet should be attempted first. Undue force should always be avoided. If version to vertex presentation is successful, membranes then should be ruptured and oxytocin augmentation may be used. If version is unsuccessful, if the fetal heart tones of twin B show evidence of fetal distress, or if twin B fails to descend after successful version, Cesarean delivery or breech extraction would be necessary[34].

Breech delivery

Acker et al.[35] found no increase in perinatal mortality or depressed 5-min Apgar scores when the second twin was delivered vaginally as a breech. Our experience is in agreement with this. In a series of 60 breech-delivered second twins with a birth weight of 1500 g or greater, no 5-min Apgar scores were recorded in the low range: three infants (5%) had scores

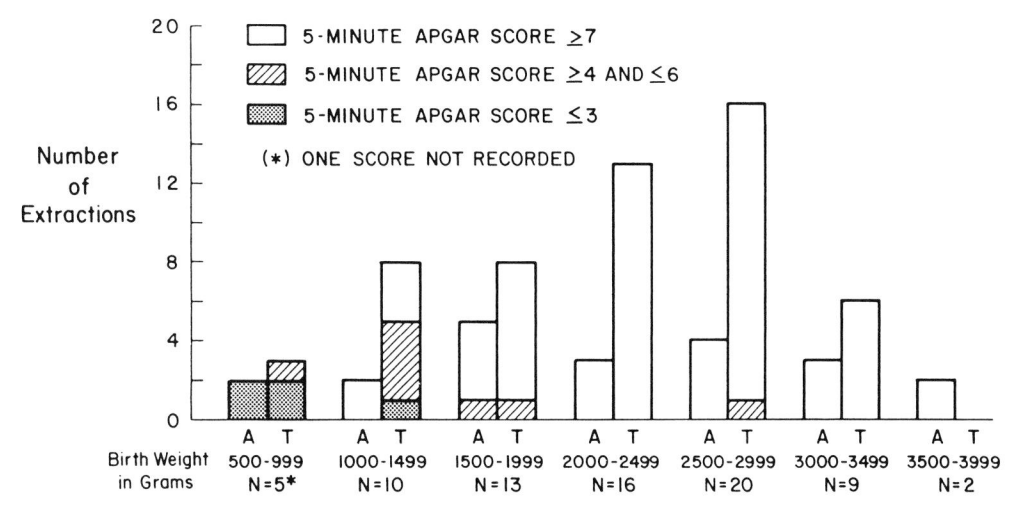

Figure 6 Five-minute Apgar scores of extracted second twins by birth weight. (Reprinted with permission from reference 36)

Table 1 Significant birth trauma for 362 consecutive twin gestations

Birth trauma	Presentation	Birth weight (g)	Mode of delivery
Neonatal death, 12 h, perinatal asphyxia	breech–breech; twin B	1000	Cesarean section with low vertical uterine incision
Erb's paralysis, paralysis left hemi-diaphragm	vertex–vertex; twin A	2100	vertex vaginal delivery (mid-forceps, prolonged second stage of labor)
Greenstick fracture right clavicle; non-displaced fracture, right humerus	vertex–breech; twin B	3420	vaginal delivery; total breech extraction
Large cephalohematoma, resultant anemia and hyperbilirubinemia	vertex–breech; twin A	2640	vertex vaginal delivery (vacuum extraction, prolonged second stage of labor)

Reprinted with permission from reference 2

in the midrange, and 55 infants (95%) had scores in the high range. One of the three twins with 5-min Apgar scores in the midrange was not diagnosed until after delivery of the first twin. The second infant had a monoamniotic placenta and its cord was intertwined with that of twin A. The third midrange score occurred in a 32-week gestation in which the first twin also had a depressed Apgar score[36]. Our data suggest that there is no excessive risk of asphyxia for the vaginally delivered breech second twin above 1500 g (Figure 6).

Examination of a large twin population in which 71% of 139 twins in vertex–non-vertex presentation delivered vaginally fails to document a high rate of birth trauma due to

Table 2 Neonatal mortality and morbidity of twin B in vertex–vertex* and vertex–non-vertex vaginal deliveries according to birth weight

Birth weight (g)	Neonatal death		RDS		IVH		5-min Apgar score < 6		Total	
	Vertex–vertex	Vertex–non-vertex	Vertex–vertex	Vertex–non-vertex	Vertex–vertex	Vertex–non-vertex	Vertex–vertex	Vertex–non-vertex	Vertex–vertex	Vertex–non-vertex
500–999		5/7 (71.4%)		2/7 (28.6%)		1/7 (14.3%)		6/6† (100%)	0	7
1000–1499	1/7 (14.3%)	2/12 (16.7%)	5/7 (71.4%)	8/12 (75%)	2/7 (28.6%)	4/12 (33.3%)	1/7 (14.3%)	4/12 (33.3%)	7	12
1500–1999			6/32 (18.8%)	5/18 (27.8%)	1/32 (3.1%)		3/32 (9.4%)	3/18 (16.7%)	32	18
2000–2499			1/31 (3.2%)						31	17
>2500								1/45 (2.2%)	49	45
Summary										
500–1499	1/7 (14.3%)	7/19 (36.8%)	5/7 (71.4%)	10/19 (52.6%)	2/7 (28.6%)	5/19 (26.3%)	1/7 (14.3%)	10/18 (55.6%)	7	19
	($p > 0.1$)		($p > 0.1$)		($p > 0.1$)		($p > 0.1$)			
			7/112 (6.3%)	5/80 (6.3%)	1/112 (0.9%)		3/112 (2.7%)	4/80 (5%)	112	80
			($p > 0.1$)				($p > 0.1$)			

RDS, respiratory distress syndrome; IVH, intraventricular hemorrhage; *Six cases not included, in which the second twin of vertex–vertex pairings was delivered by internal podalic version; †One 5-min Apgar score not recorded. Reprinted with permission from reference 2

vaginal breech delivery. The four cases of significant birth trauma for the entire twin population are summarized in Table 1[2].

The one instance of neonatal death clearly related to birth trauma occurred in a 1000-g second twin of a breech–breech pair. Both were delivered by Cesarean delivery through a low vertical uterine incision. The uterus clamped down around the head of the second twin during breech extraction, and extension of the uterine incision was necessary for delivery. Neonatal death occurred at 12 h. The three remaining cases of significant birth trauma occurred during vaginal delivery. One was related to a difficult total breech extraction of a second twin, and the other two were associated with operative vertex deliveries. In all three cases, follow-up examinations revealed no residual deficits in the infants. In addition to the four cases of significant birth trauma, there were two infants with transient facial nerve palsies and ten infants with small uncomplicated cephalohematomas. Of these, eight occurred in first twins, and four occurred in second twins. In this series, there were seven additional cases of neonatal death in which birth weight was > 1000 g. Six of these (two, twin A; four, twin B) were due to complications of prematurity, and one was due to complications resulting from a severe fetomaternal transfusion. The last occurred in association with bradycardia and placental abruption in the first twin of a vertex–transverse pair delivered by Cesarean delivery. Finally, there were 20 deaths among neonates with birth weights between 500 and 1000 g (12, twin A; 8, twin B). All of these deaths were due to complications of prematurity[2].

Comparison of the outcome of vaginally delivered second twins in the vertex and non-vertex presentations in this series is enlightening[2]. Table 2 shows neonatal morbidity and mortality for Twin B of vertex–vertex and vertex–non-vertex vaginal deliveries. Seven non-vertex vaginal deliveries were in the 500–999-g range; there were no vertex vaginal deliveries in this group. For infants below 1500 g, the occurrence of 5-min Apgar score <7 in twin B was 14.3% for vertex–vertex presentations vs. 55.6% for vertex–non-vertex presentations, and the rate of neonatal death was 14.3% and 36.8%, respectively, for these two combinations. However, neither difference was statistically significant ($p>0.1$). For infants above 1500 g, there were no neonatal deaths and no significant differences ($p>0.1$) between twin B of vertex–vertex and vertex–non-vertex presentations in any of the measures of outcome[2]. Due to rarity of adverse outcomes, the statistical power of this lack of meaningful difference is weak. Thus, it is quite possible that a type-2 statistical error is present, especially in the subgroup of twins of <1500 g. For non-vertex second twins with a birth weight of >1500 g, however, the rarity of adverse outcomes, both in absolute terms and relative to the vertex second twin, is reassuring. It should be emphasized once again that only one of the four cases of significant birth trauma in this series occurred in the second twin of a vaginally delivered vertex–non-vertex pair[2].

In this same series, only 4.7% of these twin gestations were undiagnosed before the delivery of twin B[2]. The low incidence of neonatal morbidity and mortality series is probably related to the high rate of antepartum and intrapartum diagnosis of twin gestation[2]. Antenatal diagnosis is essential to prepare for proper intrapartum monitoring (see Chapter 37) and to avoid a difficult operative vaginal delivery when twin B is distressed. The lack of intrapartum monitoring for twin B and breech delivery in the presence of undetected fetal distress may explain the poorer outcome of vaginally delivered non-vertex twins reported in some other series[21–23].

Recently, Blickstein et al. reported on their experience with 39 vertex–breech twin pairs delivered vaginally. These authors found no difference in outcome between the breech second twin delivered vaginally and a control group of vertex second twins delivered by the same route[37]. In addition, Rabinovici et al. reported no differences in outcome in a randomized trial of breech delivery vs. elective Cesarean delivery for the second non-vertex twin[38].

Goecke et al. prospectively studied modes of delivery for the non-vertex second twin weighing >1500 g[39]. They compared three approaches: Cesarean delivery, external version and breech extraction. Breech delivery had the best results, with no increase in maternal or neonatal morbidity, and was associated with the shortest postpartum stay. External version was successful in 46% of cases, but this procedure necessitated an emergency Cesarean delivery in six of 41 cases. The authors concluded that breech extraction of the second twin is both safe and efficient. They also suggested that breech delivery is, at least, a reasonable secondary approach to vaginal delivery for the non-vertex second twin if version is unsuccessful.

The documented ill effects of vaginal delivery for low birth weight (<1500 g) singleton breech presentation[17,18], although controversial, should be considered in any plan of intrapartum management for vertex–non-vertex twin gestations. Neither our series, nor those of others, demonstrated any protection against the hazards of breech delivery for the low birth weight non-vertex second twin. Because of the lack of data demonstrating its safety, I believe that vaginal breech delivery currently is not warranted when birth weight is <1500 g. Fortunately, the fetal weight can be estimated with fair reliability using antenatal sonography[40–42]. With current methods, sonographic estimations of fetal weight are very accurate within ±20% of actual weight. Under this circumstance, the use of a cutoff of 2000 g for estimated fetal weight would be highly unlikely to result in an infant with a birth weight of <1500 g.

A schematic plan for the intrapartum management of vertex–non-vertex twins is presented in Figure 7. Nevertheless, in view of the divergent opinions expressed in the currently available data, a more liberal Cesarean delivery

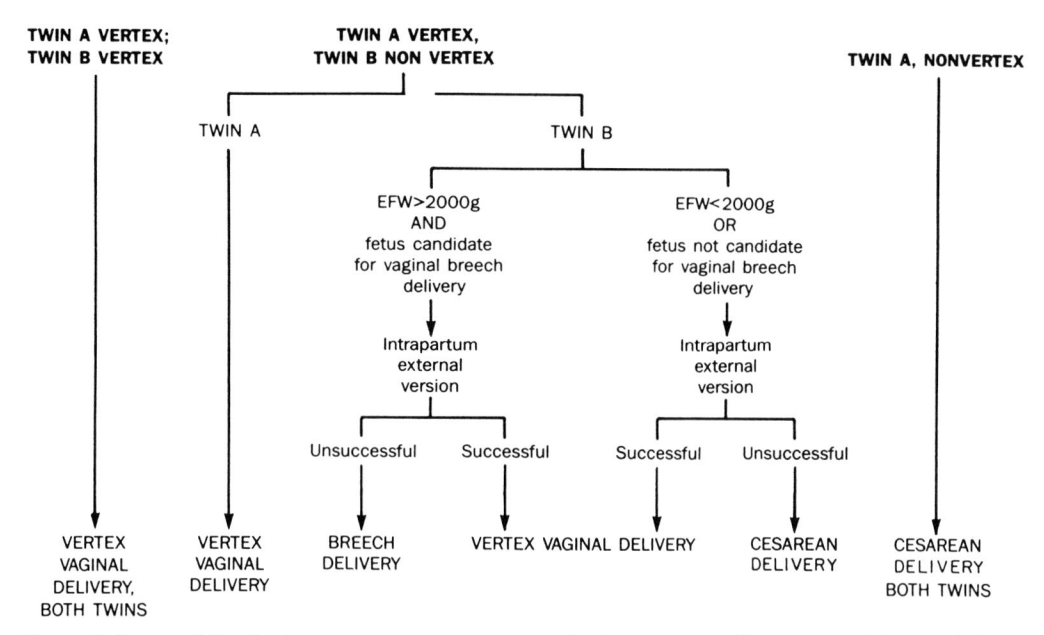

Figure 7 Protocol for the intrapartum management of twin gestation. (Reprinted with permission from reference 2)

policy as described by Cetrulo[4] or the avoidance of external version in favor of breech delivery as described by Goecke et al.[39] are also acceptable. During the intrapartum period, it is possible and advisable to obtain sonographic estimation of fetal weight and to use this in the context of the standard criteria for vaginal breech delivery (i.e. an adequate pelvis[43], flexed fetal head and estimated fetal weight of < 3500 g). If the sonographic estimation of fetal weight is > 2000 g and the criteria for vaginal breech delivery are satisfied, external cephalic version can be attempted; if unsuccessful, a breech delivery is performed.

If the sonographic estimation of fetal weight is < 2000 g or the criteria for vaginal breech delivery are not satisfied, external cephalic version is attempted. If this is unsuccessful, a Cesarean section should be performed. Even in those hospitals where breech delivery is not acceptable under any circumstance, routine Cesarean delivery may not be necessary for vertex–non-vertex twin gestations, if intrapartum external cephalic version of the second twin is successful[34,44].

It must be emphasized that Cesarean section is not a panacea[45] and does not preclude the possibility of birth injury. The only neonatal death clearly related to intrapartum asphyxia from birth trauma in our series occurred in a second twin of 1000 g delivered by breech extraction at the time of a low vertical Cesarean section[2]. Note: when Cesarean delivery is performed, an adequate uterine incision is mandatory if birth injury is to be avoided.

Twin A, non-vertex

Currently, Cesarean section seems to be the delivery method of choice when the first twin is non-vertex, because there are no studies to document the safety of vaginal delivery for this group of infants. External cephalic version of a non-vertex first twin would be difficult, if not impossible. Interlocking of fetal heads is a potentially disastrous complication of vaginal breech delivery of the first twin[46]. It is not inconceivable that the second twin might also interfere with breech vaginal delivery of the first twin in more subtle ways, such as deflexion of the descending vertex. Having said this, however, I also recognize that my concern about non-vertex vaginal delivery of the first twin may not be shared by others[1], and that vaginal delivery may be safe in specific cases.

Final considerations

There are special circumstances for which the plan of management cited above are not appropriate. For example, monoamniotic twin pregnancies have such a high risk for cord entanglement and subsequent intrauterine death[47] that elective Cesarean section should be performed after documentation of lung maturity (see Chapter 39). Likewise, conjoined twins for whom there is some hope of survival or for whom dystocia is likely should be delivered by elective Cesarean section[48] (see Chapter 8).

Growth retardation frequently occurs in a twin pregnancy. Some fetus(es) are unable to withstand the stress of labor. Cesarean delivery is then necessary. Rarely, the position of a dead twin or of an acardiac fetus may affect the mode of delivery. Some indications for Cesarean delivery, such as placenta previa, prolapsed cord, and dysfunctional labor of cephalopelvic disproportion occur with increased frequency in twins.

Lastly, in the rare instance when three or more fetuses are present, Cesarean delivery is judicious. Although Loucopolos and Jewelewicz[49] suggest that Cesarean delivery does not improve outcome in multifetal pregnancies, the difficulties associated with intrapartum surveillance and atraumatic vaginal delivery demand that only the most experienced operator[49,50] attempt vaginal delivery for higher-order multiples (see Chapters 37 and 40).

References

1. Hays, P.M. and Smeltzer, J.S. (1986). Multiple gestation. *Clin. Obstet. Gynecol.*, **29**, 264–85
2. Chervenak, F.A., Johnson, R.E., Youcha, S. *et al.* (1985). Intrapartum management of twin gestation. *Obstet. Gynecol.*, **65**, 119–24
3. Cetrulo, C. (1986). The controversy of mode of delivery in twins: the intrapartum management of twin gestation. *Semin. Perinatol.*, **23**, 533–48
4. Cetrulo, C.L., Ingradia, C.J. and Sbarra, A.J. (1980). Management of multiple gestation. *Clin. Obstet. Gynecol.*, **23**, 533–48
5. Taylor, E.S. (1976). Editorial. *Obstet. Gynecol. Surv.*, **31**, 535–6
6. Taylor, E.S. (1983). Editorial. *Obstet. Gynecol. Surv.*, **38**, 272
7. Keith, L. and Hughey, M.J. (1981). Twin gestation. In Gerbie, A.B. and Sciarra, J.J. (eds). *Gynecology and Obstetrics*, 2nd edn., pp. 1–10. (New York: Harper & Row)
8. Pritchard, J.A. and MacDonald, P.C. (1980). *Williams Obstetrics*, 16th edn., pp. 660–1. (New York: Appleton-Century-Crofts)
9. Rayburn, W.F., Lavin, J.P., Miodovnik, M. *et al.* (1984). Multiple gestation: time interval between delivery of the first and second twin. *Obstet. Gynecol.*, **63**, 502–6
10. Barrett, J.M., Staggs, S.M., Van Mooydonk, J.E. *et al.* (1982). The effect of type of delivery upon neonatal outcome in premature twins. *Am. J. Obstet. Gynecol.*, **143**, 360–7
11. Faroqui, M.O., Grossman, J.H. and Shannon, R.S. (1973). A review of twin pregnancy and perinatal mortality. *Obstet. Gynecol. Surv.*, **28**, 144
12. Ferguson, W.F. (1964). Perinatal mortality in multiple gestations. A review of perinatal deaths from 1609 multiple gestations. *Obstet. Gynecol.*, **23**, 861–70
13. Simpson, C.W., Olatunbosun, O.A. and Baldwin, V.J. (1984). Delayed interval delivery in triplet pregnancy: report of a single case and review of the literature. *Obstet. Gynecol.*, **64**, 8–11S
14. Banchi, M.T. (1984). Triplet pregnancy with second trimester abortion and delivery of twins at 35 weeks gestation. *Obstet. Gynecol.*, **64**, 728–30
15. Woolfson, J., Fay, T. and Bates, A. (1983). Twins with 54 days between deliveries. Case Report. *Br. J. Obstet. Gynaecol.*, **90**, 685–6
16. Mikkelsen, A.L. and Hansen, P.K. (1986). Survival of second twin 37 days after abortion of the first. *Acta Gynecol. Scand.*, **65**, 795–6

17. Kauppila, O., Groncoos, M., Aro, P. *et al.* (1981). Management of low birth weight breech delivery: should cesarean section be routine? *Obstet. Gynecol.*, **57**, 289–94
18. Duenmoelter, J.H., Wells, C.E. and Reisch, J.S. (1979). A paired controlled study of vaginal and abdominal delivery of the low birth weight breech fetus. *Obstet. Gynecol.*, **54**, 310–13
19. Pritchard, J.A. (1985). Cesarean section and cesarean hysterectomy. In Pritchard, J.S., MacDonald, O.C. and Gant, N.F. (eds.) *Williams Obstetrics*, 17th edn., pp. 867–86. (Norwalk: Appleton-Century-Crofts)
20. Kauppila, A., Jouppila, P., Koivisto, M. *et al.* (1975). Twin pregnancy: a clinical study of 335 cases. *Acta Obstet. Gynecol. Scand.*, **54** (Suppl.), 5–11
21. Brown, E.J. and Dixon, H.G. (1963). Twin pregnancy. *Br. J. Obstet. Gynaecol.*, **70**, 251–7
22. Kelsick, F. and Minkoff, H. (1982). Management of the breech second twin. *Am. J. Obstet. Gynecol.*, **144**, 783–6
23. Ho, S.K. and Wu, P.Y.K. (1975). Perinatal factors and neonatal morbidity in twin pregnancy. *Am. J. Obstet. Gynecol.*, **122**, 979–87
24. Stine, L.E., Phelan, J.P., Wallace, R. *et al.* (1985). Update on external cephalic version performed at term. *Obstet. Gynecol.*, **65**, 642–6
25. Fall, O. and Nilsson, B.A. (1979). External cephalic version in breech presentation under tocolysis. *Obstet. Gynecol.*, **53**, 712–15
26. Ylikorkala, A. and Hartikainen-Sorri, A. (1977). Value of external version in fetal malpresentation in combination with use of ultrasound. *Acta Obstet. Gynecol. Scand.*, **56**, 63–7
27. Saling, E. and Mueller-Holve, W. (1975). External cephalic version under tocolysis. *J. Perinatol. Med.*, **3**, 115–22
28. Bradley-Wason, P.J. (1975). The decreasing value of external version in modern obstetric practice. *Am. J. Obstet. Gynecol.*, **123**, 237–40
29. Berg, D. and Kunze, U. (1977). Critical remarks on external cephalic version under tocolysis: report of a case of antepartum fetal death. *J. Perinatol. Med.*, **5**, 32–8
30. Van Dorsten, J.P., Schifrin, B.S. and Wallace, R.L. (1981). Randomized control trial of external cephalic version with tocolysis in late pregnancy. *Am. J. Obstet. Gynecol.*, **141**, 417–24
31. Ranney, B. (1973). The gentle art of external cephalic version. *Am. J. Obstet. Gynecol.*, **116**, 239–51
32. Ganesh, V., Apuzzio, J. and Iffy, L. (1981). Clinical aspects of multiple gestation. In Iffy, L. and Kaminetsky, H.S. (eds.) *Principles and Practice of Obstetrics and Perinatology*, pp. 1183–92. (New York: Wiley)
33. Camilleri, A.P. (1963). In defense of the second twin. *Br. J. Obstet. Gynaecol.*, **70**, 258–62
34. Chervenak, F.A., Johnson, R.E., Berkowitz, R.L. *et al.* (1983). Intrapartum external version of the second twin. *Obstet. Gynecol.*, **62**, 160–5
35. Acker, D., Leiberman, M., Holbrook, H. *et al.* (1982). Delivery of the second twin. *Obstet. Gynecol.*, **59**, 710–11
36. Chervenak, F.A., Johnson, R.E., Berkowitz, R.L. *et al.* (1984). Is routine cesarean section necessary for vertex–breech vertex–transverse twin gestation? *Am. J. Obstet. Gynecol.*, **148**, 1–5
37. Blickstein, I., Schwartz-Shoham, Z., Lancet, M.D. and Borenstein, R. (1987). Vaginal delivery of the second twin in breech presentation. *Obstet. Gynecol.*, **69**, 774–6
38. Rabinovici, J., Barkai, G., Reichman, B. *et al.* (1987). Randomized management of the second nonvertex twin: vaginal delivery or cesarean section. *Am. J. Obstet. Gynecol.*, **156**, 52–6
39. Goecke, S.E., Nageotte, M.P., Garite, T., Towers, C.V. and Dorcester, W. (1989). Management of the nonvertex second twin: primary cesarean section, external version, or primary breech extraction. *Am. J. Obstet. Gynecol.*, **162**, 111–14
40. Shepard, M.J., Richards, V.A., Berkowitz, R.L. *et al.* (1982). An evaluation of the two equations for predicting fetal weight by ultrasound. *Am. J. Obstet. Gynecol.*, **142**, 47–54
41. Deter, R.L., Hadlock, F.P., Harrist, R.B. *et al.* (1981). Evaluation of three methods for obtaining fetal weight estimates using dynamic image ultrasound. *J. Clin. Ultrasound*, **9**, 421–5
42. Hadlock, F.P., Harrist, R.B., Carpenter, R.J. *et al.* (1984). Sonographic estimation of fetal weight. The value of femur length to head and abdomen measurements. *Radiology*, **150**, 535–54
43. Collea, J.V., Rabin, S.C., Weghorst, G.R. *et al.* (1978). The randomized management of term frank breech presentation: vaginal delivery vs cesarean section. *Am. J. Obstet. Gynecol.*, **131**, 186–95
44. Tchabo, J. and Tomain, T. (1992). Selected intrapartum external cephalic version of the second twin. *Obstet. Gynecol.*, **79**, 421

45. Olofsson, P. and Rydhstrom, H. (1985). Twin delivery. How should the second twin be delivered? *Am. J. Obstet. Gynecol.*, **153**, 479–81
46. Nissen, E.D. (1958). Twins: collision, impaction, compaction, and interlocking. *Obstet. Gynecol.*, **11**, 514–26
47. Sutter, J., Arab, H. and Manning, F.A. (1986). Monoamniotic twins: antenatal diagnosis and management. *Am. J. Obstet. Gynecol.*, **155**, 836–7
48. Filler, R.M. (1986). Conjoined twins and their separation. *Semin. Perinatol.*, **10**, 82–9
49. Loucopoulos, A. and Jewelewicz, R. (1982). Management of multifetal pregnancies: sixteen years experience at the Sloane Hospital for Women. *Am. J. Obstet. Gynecol.*, **143**, 902–5
50. Ron-El, R., Caspi, E., Schreyer, P. *et al.* (1981). Triplet and quadruplet pregnancies and management. *Obstet. Gynecol.*, **57**, 458–63
51. Chervenak, F.A. (1986). The controversy of mode of delivery in twins: the intrapartum management of twin gestation (Part II). *Semin. Perinatol.*, **10**, 44–9

Labor and delivery

L.G. Keith, T.R.B. Johnson, J.A. Lopez-Zeno and M. Creinin

Introduction

The high-risk nature of twin pregnancy has been documented in several preceding chapters. These chapters have also described various methods of reducing risk in the antepartum period, starting with early diagnosis, continuing with careful assessment of fetal well-being, and progressing to specific therapies designed to minimize the potential for preterm delivery. The delivery itself, though, still poses great challenges to the skill of the obstetrician, as well as to the team of assistants he or she should assemble to assist at the moment of birth. The delivery of twins is a high-risk event, regardless of whether it occurs at term or preterm[1]. Planning for delivery should begin during pregnancy, and these plans should reflect various changes in patient or fetal status that might occur as the pregnancy progresses.

Prerequisites for delivery of multiples

Hospital and obstetric units providing maternity service to mothers of twins should have a full range of personnel and equipment to reduce the potential sequelae of preterm delivery, minimize the risk of birth trauma and optimize the quality of resuscitation provided to the newborn infants. At the minimum, the requisite personnel for the delivery of twins should include the following: two qualified physicians, an anesthesiologist (and assistant), two neonatal resuscitation teams, and a qualified sonographic assistant. Equipment should include sufficient clamps for two umbilical cords, ultrasound, monitoring equipment, oxytocic agents, methergine and prostaglandin and, finally, a complete set-up for emergency Cesarean section in the delivery room.

At times, patients and their healthcare providers are faced with the difficult decision of whether it is better to arrange an antenatal transfer and delivery miles away from family and support systems or to risk complications that may occur in a hospital setting inadequately prepared to effect delivery of a high-risk pregnancy. The capacity to transfer newborns to a neonatal intensive care unit (NICU) is not a substitute for timely antepartum transfer of the mother and her fetus(es) to an optimal facility prior to delivery. Not only is the immediate prognosis for transferred newborns less salutary, but the maternal–infant bonding process may be abruptly shortened or never take place.

Five areas of obstetric practice (fetal monitoring, fetal imaging, anesthesia, Cesarean section and immediate neonatal care) impact on the management of labor and delivery in twin pregnancies. They are mentioned briefly in the next paragraphs. Detailed discussions of each follow later, or are found in other chapters of this book.

Fetal monitoring

Monitoring the fetal heart rate is essential throughout labor and delivery. Continuous electronic external and internal fetal monitoring systems with the capacity to monitor both fetuses simultaneously are commercially available and is the preferable monitoring system. Auscultation of the fetal heart rate with a stethoscope or a hand-held Doppler can be used in the absence of monitoring technology, but this system is not sufficiently precise to detect subtle changes in heart rate of both fetuses at the same time even when two examiners are present simultaneously.

Fetal imaging

Facilities and technical capability for diagnostic real-time ultrasound should be available at all times. A great measure of the success of the skilful intrapartum management of twin gestations is related to an accurate assessment of gestational age and fetal presentation.

Anesthesia

A skilled anesthesiologist should be available throughout labor in the event that circumstances require immediate operative intervention. Adequate anesthetic is mandatory should the delivery of the second twin require intrauterine manipulation or Cesarean section.

Cesarean section

Patients with twin gestation should be cared for in an institution capable of providing an emergency Cesarean section should circumstances warrant. Institutions that cannot provide the means and personnel to deliver an infant of a high-risk mother by Cesarean section in 30 min or less should not attempt to provide care for these patients.

Immediate neonatal care

The first few minutes of extrauterine existence are of paramount importance to perinatal morbidity and mortality. Ideally, an experienced pediatrician or neonatologist should be present at the delivery. Whereas it may be acceptable for the obstetrician, anesthesiologist or delivery room nurse to provide emergency pediatric stabilization with low-risk patients, this is less than ideal for deliveries of twins.

The conduct of labor

Initial concerns

Several precautions should be observed when the patient is admitted to the labor and delivery unit. Blood should be drawn and sent for type and screen to ensure rapid availability of blood in the event of life-threatening hemorrhage. Isotonic crystalloid solution should be infused intravenously, to prevent dehydration that would otherwise decrease uterine perfusion. The intravenous line should be of sufficient diameter to allow therapy with blood or blood products. The patient should be maintained nil per os throughout her labor and the delivery to decrease the likelihood of aspiration of stomach contents. She should also be given medication to reduce the level of gastric acidity and reduce the risk of aspiration of gastric contents (see below and Chapter 38).

Vaginal delivery after previous Cesarean section

Vaginal delivery of twins after Cesarean section was reported in the 1960s[2,3], well before the trend to permit vaginal delivery of singletons after Cesarean section. Indeed, some of the early cohorts that examined the safety of this concept specifically excluded twins[4,5]. In 1988, the American College of Obstetricians and Gynecologists (ACOG) released a committee opinion stating that data were insufficient to assess the safety or dangers associated with this type of delivery in twins[6]. In the same year, however, Derom *et al.* reported successful vaginal delivery in patients with twins after previous Cesarean section[7]. Since then, other authors have followed suit[8,9].

Depending on the circumstances of the case, the risk for maternal trauma in association with vaginal delivery is always present, especially if an intrauterine manipulation is required to affect an emergency delivery with internal podalic version and total breech extraction. In one reported case, the uterus ruptured[3], but this patient was delivered before ultrasound became available and might have had a different outcome if it had been present and appropriately utilized. In the absence of data from comparative randomized trials, any assessment of the safety of vaginal delivery of twins after previous Cesarean section must be evaluated on an individual case basis. Diverse elements that merit consideration include the patient's desires (and potential fears), the obstetrician's experience and, finally, the ability of the hospital to provide for a safe vaginal or abdominal delivery on a 24-h basis, 365 days of the year. Informed consent should be obtained whatever the plan for delivery.

Dual-channel monitoring

As noted above, continuous monitoring of both fetal heart rates is essential. Newer monitors are capable of monitoring both twins externally. Two caveats are associated with dual channel recording, however. First, it is possible to monitor one twin twice; and second, it is possible to confuse the maternal heart rate with bradycardia in one of the twins[10].

Some monitors (Corometrics, Wallingford, CT and Hewlett-Packard, Toitu) use a single longitudinal scale for monitoring both twins. The presence of a solitary fetal heart rate (FHR), however, may be an indication that one twin is being recorded by both transducers. In contrast, other monitors (Litton and PPG, Lenexa, KS) use paper with separate fetal heart scales for each fetus[10]. If the tracings are absolutely identical, the transducer requires adjustment until two distinct tracings appear[10]. It is important to remember that synchronous tracings are possible, but the presence of absolute identicality is not, and should alert the examiner to the possibility of system malfunction or simultaneous monitoring of one twin by two transducers (Figure 1) (see Chapter 24).

The acute onset of bradycardia in one twin should alert the care-giver to immediately check the maternal pulse. If this is identical to the rate of bradycardia, the transducers can then be adjusted until the two FHRs reappear. If not, immediate steps must be undertaken to ascertain the reason for the change in FHR in one twin. In either circumstance, all assessments and evaluations should be documented on the monitor strip and in the concurrent description of labor located in either the nurse's or doctor's notes. If appropriate, the mother and her support person should be reassured that technical problems are not indicative of fetal compromise. On the other hand, it is inappropriate to ascribe FHR changes to technical difficulties unless the care-giver is absolutely certain that this is the fact.

After the birth of the first twin, monitoring should continue. The position of the second twin and its umbilical cord can quickly be assessed using real-time ultrasound. When the second twin enters the pelvis and it is deemed safe to perform amniotomy without undue risk of cord prolapse, a spiral electrode can be applied to the second twin's scalp. Prior to that, the FHR can be assessed by a cardiotransducer and/or a hand-held Doppler. Regardless of whether labor is then augmented or allowed to progress spontaneously, the use of a tocotransducer permits assessment of the strength and frequency of contractions.

A comprehensive protocol for monitoring twins in labor has recently been described by Eganhause, and is shown in Figure 2. Rather than the dual channel monitoring described above, this protocol advocates two monitors from different manufacruers to improve signal quality.

The intrapartum use of ultrasonography

The presence of ultrasonography in the labor–delivery suite allows: (1) documentation of the positions of both twins at the onset of labor; (2) early detection of locked twins; (3) reassurance that the cord is not in front of the presenting head (this is especially useful in cases of hydramnios); (4) immediate detection of any change in the second twin's position during and after delivery of the first twin; (5) visual guidance in the event that an internal podalic version and/or breech extraction is deemed appropriate; and (6) visual assurance of the position of the cord of the second twin during the inter-twin delivery interval. For all these reasons, ultrasonography is presently considered an indispensable requisite to the safe delivery of twins.

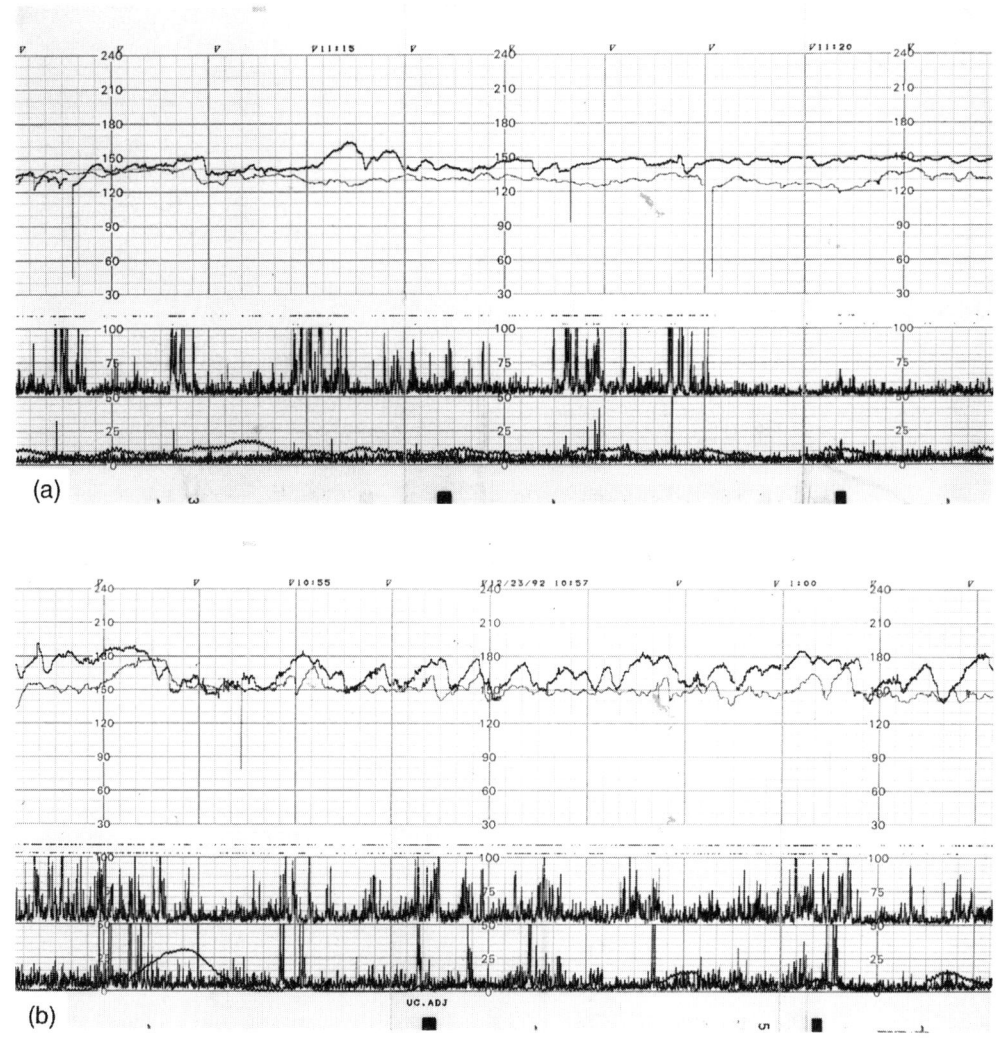

Figure 1 Simultaneous but non-synchronous dual-channel monitoring in two patients (a and b). Courtesy Dr Timothy R.B. Johnson

Additionally, according to Chervenak et al.[11,12] ultrasonography is indispensable for the external version of a second twin after delivery of the first twin. These authors reported success in ten of 14 transverse lies and eight of 11 breech presentations, respectively. Epidural anesthesia appeared to enhance the likelihood of success in these two small series. In two of the failures, however, the weight of twin B exceeded that of twin A by 500 g or more. Without ultrasound, such procedures would be deemed potentially unsafe by many.

Deciding on a delivery route

Controversy exists about the preferable mode of delivery in twins. In the past, the decision to practice abdominal or vaginal delivery was often dogmatic and based on the personal preference of the physician or the clinic director in charge[13]. More recently, this decision has been made based upon an analysis of case outcomes (see Chapter 36). In addition to the pioneer work by Chervenak[14], others have also addressed this issue[15,16]. Figure 3, taken from

Protocol for the use of monitors with twins

(1) Apply EFM externally with mother in the lateral position or semi-Fowler's.
   (a) Use two different brands of monitors to improve signal quality.
   (b) Synchronize internal clocks of both monitors.
   (c) Auscultate twin A and apply the cardiotransducer.
   (d) Apply the tocotransducer.
   (e) Auscultate twin B and discriminate from A's tracing. Apply cardiotransducer for twin B.
   (f) Adjust belts to hold transducers in place. Try to accomplish monitoring with two or three belts rather than four.
   (g) Observe FHR tracings carefully to ascertain that both fetuses are being monitored.
   (h) Document location of FHR's.

(2) Apply a spiral electrode to twin A as soon as possible.
   (a) Ascertain that U/S and spiral electrode produce different tracings. (It is possible to monitor the twin A using two modes.)
   (b) If only one tracing appears, reauscultate and readjust the cardiotransducer for twin B.

(3) Observe for non-reassuring FHR patterns, including decreased variability, late, severe variable, or prolonged decelerations.
   (a) Watch for non-reassuring patterns.
   (b) Institute appropriate interventions for non-reassuring FHR patterns as needed.

Figure 2 A protocol for the use of monitors with twins, from reference 10

Protocol for route of delivery

Vertex A/vertex B → vaginal delivery

Vertex A/non-vertex >1800 g → vaginal delivery of A with management of B as follows:

Twin B
- Breech (or) transverse with feet dependent → vaginal delivery
- Transverse with back dependent → external version to vertex (Cesarean if failed)

Vertex A/non-vertex B >1800 g → Cesarean section

Breech A → Cesarean section

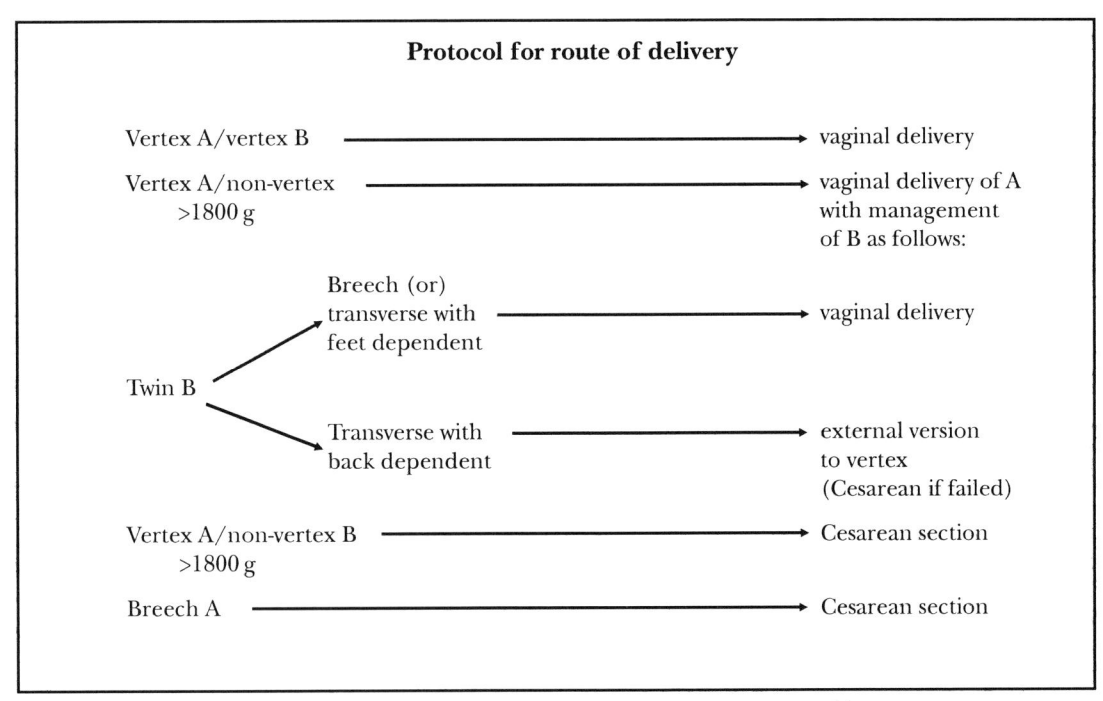

Figure 3 A protocol for route of delivery proposed by Warenski and Kochenauer[16]

VV	BB	TT
VB	BV	TV
VT	BT	TB

Figure 4 The nine possible combinations for twins. V, vertex; B, breech; T, transverse

Warenski and Kochenaur[16], is presented for comparison with that of Chervenak in Chapter 36. This schema, and others like it, are of particular use of the vertex–non-vertex presentation or when the first twin is breech. It is important to remember, however, that nine combinations of positions are possible for twins (Figure 4). Unless specific obstetric conditions mitigate against vaginal delivery, it is appropriate for the VV combinations. Many experienced clinicians are also comfortable with the vaginal delivery route for the combinations of VB, BV, BB or vaginal traverse (VT); others are not. As noted above, delivery route may depend on institutional policy, practice and experience.

Regardless of the data in the case series cited above[14–16], the delivery mode for the remaining five combinations of fetal positions in Figure 4 depends greatly on the circumstances of the individual case (e.g. gestational age, estimated fetal weight, etc.), the skill and experience of the operator, and the skill of the team of assistants available to help with the delivery and resuscitation, both under the best of circumstances, and at other times, such as nights, holidays and weekends. A safe and atraumatic delivery is of paramount importance.

Those clinicians contemplating vaginal delivery of malpositioned twins should carefully consider that much of the morbidity and mortality associated with breech delivery is a function of physician intervention, particularly in the premature breech birth. Regardless of method of delivery, the premature fetus in breech or vertex presentation may have less respiratory reserve and less mature cardiovascular reflexes. Such fetuses are more likely to suffer long-lasting effects if subjected to the stress of asphyxia.

If a decision is made to proceed with a Cesarean section, either a low vertical or a low transverse cervical incision may be appropriate. The larger intrauterine bulk of a twin gestation usually leads to development of the lower uterine segment earlier in the pregnancy. Generally, little difficulty attends the extraction of smaller fetuses one at a time through a low transverse incision. An exception may occur if the second fetus is transverse, however. In this instance, a vertical incision may be preferred because it can be extended superiorly if circumstances warrant.

A full discussion of anesthetic considerations for delivery is presented in Chapter 38 by Cohen and Brunner. These authors note that a successful delivery is dependent on a number of factors, not the least of which is an early consultation between the anesthesiologist, the patient and her doctor. Although Cohen and Brunner acknowledge that both general and regional anesthetics can be given with safety (provided the anesthesiologist is familiar with the risks of both as they relate to twins), other authors[17,18] prefer epidural anesthesia for the following reasons:

(1) It eliminates the need for maternal narcotics and sedatives, thus avoiding the fetal respiratory and depressant effects of such drugs;

(2) Perineal anesthesia prevents reflex bearing down by the mother and permits a more controlled delivery of the infant over a relaxed perineum;

(3) Operative delivery, more common with twins, is easier to accomplish in the presence of epidural anesthesia; and

(4) Epidural anesthesia facilitates uterine examination postpartum, by providing good pain relief without compromising uterine contractility.

If primary Cesarean section becomes necessary, the block is merely extended to provide abdominal anesthesia. Similarly, if Cesarean section is performed for the second twin, an additional dose may be all that is required to provide sufficient pain relief for surgery. Opponents of continuous lumbar epidural anesthesia consider the loss of the bearing-down sensation a detrimental factor that leads to a higher incidence of operative intervention in the form of forceps deliveries (owing to malposition of the head in a persistent transverse position) and breech extractions. The use of continuous lumbar epidural anesthesia in the management of twin gestation is enhanced when anesthesiologists are skilled in its use, when appropriate safeguards are followed, and when anesthesiologists are immediately available to manage complications.

Two factors are of over-riding importance with any anesthesia: the fetuses must be monitored throughout delivery, and the anesthesiologist must be present and prepared to give general endotracheal anesthesia at a moment's notice should circumstances require this. The course of labor should progress smoothly in patients selected for vaginal delivery. Careful attention to information obtained from the fetal monitor is important, because it may provide the first indication of an unexpected intrapartum complication, such as cord prolapse or fetal distress. Finally, the anesthesia plan for delivery must be flexible. Continuous lumbar epidural anesthesia, if used successfully for first-stage pain relief, may be renewed to provide good anesthesia for delivery. Pudendal block or local infiltration may also be used.

Whatever anesthetic modality is chosen, and even when none is contemplated, it is necessary to provide prophylaxis against aspiration of gastric acid. The most popular combination of medications used for reducing the risk of aspiration of gastric acid is 30 ml of an oral non-particulate antacid such as sodium bicitrate. This can be administered with 10 mg of intravenous metoclopramide to enhance stomach emptying and increase the tone of the gastroesophageal sphincter. The administration of an H_2 blocker, such as ranitidine, 50 mg intravenously, decreases the acidity of subsequent gastric secretions. No adverse maternal or neonatal side effects have been described following the use of these agents. Metoclopramide and ranitidine (repeated every 6 h) may be administered as soon as the patient is in active labor.

In recent years, psychoprophylactic methods of pain relief have become popular in North America. They not only are harmless, as far as obstetric outcome is concerned, but also appear to be of benefit to many patients. In patients with twin gestation, in whom premature labor is common (and thus the provision of analgesia represents a significant therapeutic concern), psychoprophylaxis should be encouraged in order to minimize analgesic needs (see Chapter 20).

Systemically administered narcotics may be given safely early in labor if due regard is given to their potential respiratory depressant effect on the fetuses. Should delivery occur unexpectedly or at any time when drug activity may still be present, naloxone (Narcan®) should be administered to the mother to reverse these narcotic effects prior to delivery. The use of paracervical block has fallen into disfavor, because of its association with fetal bradycardia.

Delivery of the second twin

After delivery of the first twin, monitoring of the second twin continues. One obstetrician should attend to the second infant, while the other assumes primary responsibility for the mother and the neonatologist cares for the first twin. Continuous fetal monitoring, regardless of the elapsed time since the delivery of the first twin, provides reassurance about the continued intrauterine health of the second twin. If the fetal heart rate pattern is normal, there should be no reason to intervene prematurely. Indeed, dilute oxytocin may be given with safety to effect delivery. Operative intervention is not necessary in the presence of a normal FHT tracing and the obstetrician should await the natural processes of labor. If, on the other hand, the fetal monitor tracing indicates a sudden, serious abnormality, a fetal scalp pH determination should be made if the clinician is of the opinion that the time required for this would not place the fetus in jeopardy. If sufficient time is present and if the result shows fetal acidosis, a decision must be made to undertake immediate vaginal or abdominal delivery. In other instances, this decision will be made on other grounds, such as the type of tracing and a clinical assessment of the fetal condition. If the decision is to proceed with a vaginal delivery, in order for this to be advantageous over a Cesarean section it should be accomplished within a reasonable amount of time and at no added risk of maternal or fetal trauma. Adequate expertise and supervision are required for the safe performance of an operative vaginal delivery. If Cesarean section is to be performed, haste is required to achieve the maximum fetal benefit. Significant delay may neutralize or obviate these efforts.

There is no agreement as to when membranes should be ruptured for the second twin. Some physicians advocate leaving membranes unruptured as long as possible to maintain a dilating wedge against the cervix; others favor administration of oxytocin by infusion pump to stimulate contractions and accelerate labor; still others favor artificial rupture of membranes after a specific arbitrary time (e.g. 5 or 10 min) has elapsed. Adequate prospective studies have yet to demonstrate conclusively the value of any of these maneuvers.

Similarly, it is not clear which method of delivery of the second twin is safest, especially if the second twin is non-vertex. There are three options: primary Cesarean section, external version or primary breech extraction. Reports in the early 1980s by Chervenak et al. noted an 80% success rate after version in 25 cases[11,12]. A later report by Gocke and Nageotte was able to document only a 66% success rate and a total section rate of 40% in those patients in whom version was attempted[19]. It is important to remember that if the version attempt fails, breech extraction may be more difficult[16].

The combined method of vaginal delivery followed by a Cesarean section no longer raises eyebrows. Despite this, the decision to conduct an abdominal delivery of the second twin should be based on documented indications that are clearly recorded in the progress notes. Most such operations are based on objective evidence of a decline in the status of the second twin. The potential benefit to the fetus should always be considered in light of the risks of Cesarean delivery in terms of maternal morbidity and/or mortality.

The inter-twin delivery interval

Older texts and clinical aphorisms suggested a need to deliver the second twin within a relatively short interval (i.e. 20 min or less). Undoubtedly, these dicta contributed in some part to the use of interventions that were unnecessary. The basis of the obstetrician's concern no doubt relates to the risk of hypoperfusion of the placenta or abruption, when the uterine size is rapidly reduced after the delivery of the first twin. Other concerns include the possibility of uterine inertia, cord prolapse and constriction of the cervical os, thus making rapid delivery of the second twin difficult if not near impossible without undue trauma in the event that fetal distress occurs.

The length of time for delivery of the second twin was reviewed at Prentice Women's Hospital. Intervals varied from 30 to 300 min without adverse fetal consequences[20]. It should be clearly understood, however, that in all instances the second twin was carefully monitored by internal or external tocodynamometry during this interval. Moreover, ultrasound was available to make an initial assessment of the second twin's position after the first twin had delivered and to document the fact that this position did not change. Furthermore, anesthesia personnel were present to assist in supporting the mother, and an operating room was ready in the event circumstances changed and required an immediate delivery by Cesarean section.

Other authors also suggest that time alone is not the major consideration in effecting a rapid delivery of the second twin[21,22].

Developing protocol for delivery management

Preparing for the delivery of twins should not be left to chance. Prior sections of this chapter cite specific areas of care that must be planned and provided for. Specific attention should go into the selection of the delivery team and the set-up of the room. The patient should be amply forewarned of the following four points. First, she and her support person will be surrounded by a multitude of hospital personnel in the moments preceding, during and immediately after the delivery. Second, once it is determined that she and her babies are in stable postpartum condition, most of these individuals will disappear, leaving the mother, her support person and her babies time to become acquainted in private. Third, even if all goes well, low infant birth weight or any number of unforeseen possibilities may necessitate a 24-h stay for one or both infants in the NICU. Finally, should this last eventuality take place, the bonding process will not be irrevocably disrupted.

Higher-order multiples

The care and delivery of higher-order gestations presents great challenges to obstetricians. The majority of these pregnancies are complicated by malpresentation, the need for either abdominal or vaginal operative delivery and the likelihood that one or more newborns will require immediate specialized care. The recent published American literature[23,24] clearly states a preference for abdominal delivery. In contrast, European clinics[25,26] tend to prefer vaginal delivery, at least for triplets. In one recent review of triplet series, the cited rate of Cesarean delivery ranged from a low of 14% to a high of 94%[23].

The low rate of 14% was recorded in South Africa between 1967 and 1987[27]. The majority of cases were diagnosed during labor. The two patients scheduled for elective Cesarean delivery (due to prior Cesarean delivery) both presented in active labor and delivered vaginally. The indication for the solitary Cesarean delivery was obstructed labor. However, vaginal manipulation was required in the great majority (67.6%) of cases, and data in the report were insufficient to calculate morbidity or mortality secondary to these procedures[27]. Despite this, the authors recommended elective Cesarean section on all triplets if the leading twin is not vertex.

A later series of 78 triplets, reported in 1989, described deliveries occurring between 1975 and 1988, and reported a 78% Cesarean rate[28]. Whereas these authors were of the opinion that after 26 weeks of gestation no difference was discernible in the perinatal mortality associated with either vaginal or abdominal delivery, the vaginally born third triplets had a higher incidence of low Apgar scores and respiratory disorders. Because of this, these authors concluded, 'we find little justification to attempt vaginal delivery in these high-risk patients'[28].

Olofsson[26] reported a series of 14 triplet and quadruplet pregnancies. He recommended vaginal delivery for triplets from 34 weeks onward, even if the leading infant was in the breech position. Not all attempts at vaginal delivery were successful, however, in Olofsson's hands. Three pregnancies underwent emergency Cesarean section for fetal distress while attempting a vaginal delivery.

The Cesarean section rate was 42% in another series involving 27 sets of triplets, seven quadruplets and one set of quintuplets[29]. For triplets, the only improvement provided by Cesarean section over vaginal delivery was improvement of the 1-min Apgar score for the third-born triplet (6.8 vs. 5.0). The relevance of these findings are questionable, however, in view of the enormous changes that occurred during the 16-year period in which the cases were collected prior to publication in 1982. Other, albeit much older, reports suggest a higher mortality for breech triplets delivered vaginally[30].

The largest and most recent triplet review encompassed 198 sets delivered in 24 regional centers[23]. Almost all (94%) of the 186 patients were delivered abdominally. Of the 12 attempts at vaginal delivery, three patients required emergency Cesarean section after the vaginal delivery of the first triplet, due to an intrapartum complication.

Because of the controversy surrounding the ideal method for the delivery of triplets, one group of investigators designed a historical cohort study to evaluate the merits of both

Table 1 Possible triplet presentation

Combinations of triplets			Keith[35]		Michlewitz[36]		Syrop[37]		Holcberg[38]		Total	
A	B	C	n	%	n	%	n	%	n	%	n	%
VTX	BR	BR	3	23.08	1	6.67	7	35	4	13	15	18.1
VTX	VTX	BR	2	15.38	2	13.3	4	20	5	16	13	16.4
VTX	VTX	VTX	2	15.38	3	20	2	10	5	16	12	15.2
BR	BR	BR	1	7.69	2	13.3	2	10	5	16	10	12.7
VTX	BR	VTX	0		0		0		6	20	6	7.6
BR	VTX	BR	1	7.69	1	6.67	1	5	1	3	4	5.1
VTX	VTX	Trans	2	15.38	1	6.67	0		1	3	4	5.1
BR	BR	Trans	0		0		2	10	0		2	2.5
VTX	Trans	Trans	0		2	13.3	0		0		2	2.5
BR	VTX	VTX	0		1	6.67	0		1	3	2	2.5
BR	VTX	Trans	0		0		0		2	7	2	2.5
BR	Face	VTX	0		0		1	5	0		1	1.3
VTX	Trans	BR	0		0		1	5	0		1	1.3
—	Unknown	—	1	7.69	0		0		0		1	1.3
VTX	Brow	Trans	1	7.69	0		0		0		1	1.3
CMP	BR	VTX	0		1	6.67	0		0		1	1.3
VTX	VTX	N/A	0		1	6.67	0		0		1	1.3
BR	BR	VTX	0		0		0		1	3	1	1.3
Total			13		15		20		31		79	

From Lopez-Zeno, J.A. and Keith, L. (1993). Higher order multiple gestations. In Sciarra, J.J. (ed.) *Gynecology and Obstetrics*, Chapter 74. (Harper and Row)

possibilities[31]. The study group (delivered abdominally) had significantly higher Apgar scores at 1- and 5-min, respectively. In addition, no differences were present within the study group, when combined mortality and morbidity were compared between first-, second- and third-born triplets. In contrast, among the vaginally born control, this figure increased from 21% in the first-born triplet to 31% in the second to 43% in the third. Based on these findings, a more liberal approach toward Cesarean section was advocated. Unfortunately, this study was confounded by selection bias and the possibility that different levels of medical care had been afforded the two groups, because the controls delivered during an earlier period than the study group (1954–76 vs. 1977–86, respectively), and the concepts of prenatal and intrapartum care had changed vastly in this 20-year interval.

More recently, the biochemical parameters of triplets born at term were evaluated. The first study from New York University reported on six sets of triplets delivered by Cesarean section[32]. Apgar scores, umbilical artery and venous pH, pO_2, pCO_2, lactate and base deficit were compared in the third-born triplet with the first two neonates, respectively. No differences were found. A similar analysis was performed at Northwestern University on 11 sets of triplets, only one of which was delivered vaginally[33]. Even though the 1-min Apgar score was lower in the group of third-born triplets, no difference was seen in the 5-min Apgar score or in any of the umbilical arterial and venous cord gas analyses. Nevertheless, the only acidotic pH (7.08) occurred in the third-born triplet of the only set born vaginally.

The problems associated with deliveries in quadruplets and higher-order pregnancies indicate the value of elective Cesarean section as the ideal route of delivery[34]. The possible presentations for triplets from four of ten quoted studies are listed in Table 1. The VTX–BR–BR combination was most common (18.1%), followed by VTX–VTX–BR (16.4%). After these, wide variations are apparent.

Aside from malpresentation, a broad spectrum of obstetric complications face the obstetrician attempting vaginal delivery of a higher order gestation. Cord prolapse, fetal heart rate deceleration and placental abruption with hemorrhage are all possible. An additional but absolutely crucial factor in favor of delivering all higher-order gestations by elective Cesarean section is the nature of the neonatal team that must be assembled. Usually, teams are staffed by one pediatrician/neonatologist, two nurses and one respiratory technician for each infant. Additional support staff may be required, especially if the delivery is preterm. An elective scheduled operation permits sufficient time to assemble such a team and arrange other optimal conditions at the moment of delivery, including the provision of three beds (or more) in the neonatal intensive care unit or nursery.

If it is decided to perform Cesarean delivery, the operation should be executed by a team of experienced obstetricians capable of performing a hysterectomy in the event of an intractable postpartum hemorrhage. Moreover, an experienced anesthesiologist with sufficient support staff should be available. Epidural or general anesthesia are appropriate. Blood products should be readily available in case of severe hemorrhage. Uterotonics, such as ergonovine derivatives or injectable prostaglandins, should also be available and used without hesitation.

If, after considering all factors, a decision is made to attempt vaginal delivery, an equally prepared neonatal team must be assembled for each infant. The delivery should not be conducted by a single obstetrician. At least two scrubbed obstetricians should be present, and both should be highly proficient in performing intrauterine manipulations on a malpresenting fetus. A third obstetrician or similarly skilled technician should be present to perform real-time sonography during the second stage of labor to plan the delivery and assist with manipulation if required.

Delivery complications in multiple pregnancy

The most serious complication is not knowing that the pregnancy is multiple. At one time, delivery room diagnoses were common (25% or more)[39]. Since the advent of ultrasonography, however, this phenomenon is not as frequent. Indeed, in many American hospitals, delivery room diagnosis is a rare circumstance, especially among patients who have received prenatal care. Regardless, it is disquieting not to know how often the diagnosis occurs only at the moment of delivery or how often the patient is erroneously told she is having a singleton, when in fact she is carrying twins. In this regard, it is particularly unfortunate that no reliable data exist to document the rate of undiagnosed twins among the large number of poor and under-served minority women who come to the hospital in labor without ever having one prenatal visit. It is equally unfortunate that no reliable measures exist to quantitate the contribution that indigent women who have received no prenatal care and their newborns make to the overall neonatal morbidity and mortality of twins compared to singletons.

Locking

Fetal locking is a rare condition. Bryan suggests its occurrence is only one in 1000 twin deliveries[40]. A review of the literature prior to the use of ultrasonography divided cases into four groups according to the type of locking[41]. The first is *collision* (Figure 5), which describes the fact that the contact of the fetal parts (generally the heads) prevents engagement of either. The second is *impaction*. In this case, both twins partially engage, because the fetal parts of one impact into the body of the other. The third is *compaction*, in which the presenting parts of both fetuses become fully engaged in the pelvis and prevent further descent. Finally, in *interlocking* (Figure 6), the chins of

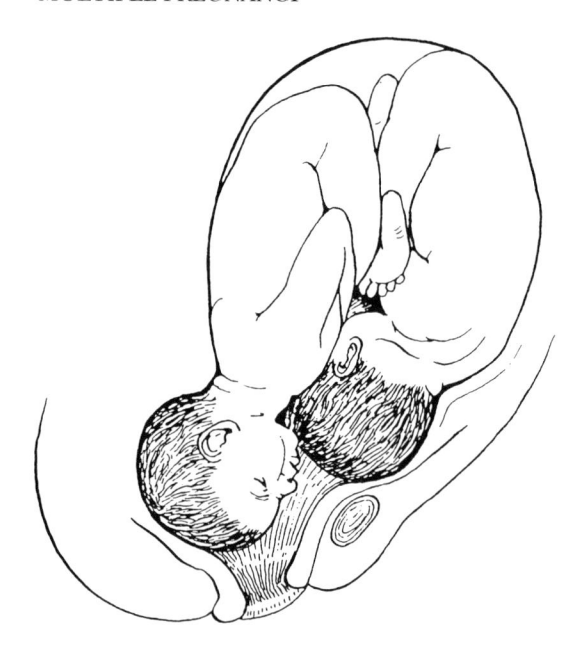

Figure 5 Collision of two heads causing a form of locked twins. (Reproduced with permission from MacGillivray, I., Nylander, P.P.S. and Carney, G. (eds.) (1975). *Human Multiple Reproduction*, p. 162. (London, Philadelphia, Toronto: W.B. Saunders Company Ltd.)

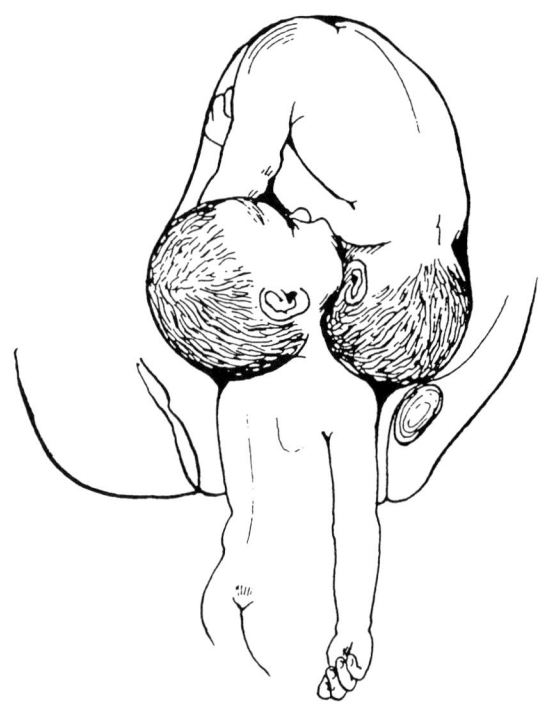

Figure 6 Chin-to-chin locking in twins. (Reproduced with permission from MacGillivray, I., Nylander, P.P.S. and Carney, G. (eds.) (1975). *Human Multiple Reproduction*, p. 161. (London, Philadelphia, Toronto: W.B. Saunders Company Ltd.)

both fetuses are in such close proximity that the delivery of the first breech is prevented. This condition is probably more common in monochorionic, monoamniotic pairs[41], but also probably relates to small fetal size, oligohydramnios and uterine hypertonicity[40].

Acute twin–twin transfusion syndrome and exsanguination of the second twin

Two other chapters of this book (Chapters 27 and 29) discuss the chronic variety of twin–twin transfusion syndrome (TTS), and Lopez-Zeno (Chapter 23) also notes the possibility of acute TTS at the time of delivery. When this occurs, blood is transferred from the donor twin to the recipient twin as a result of a hemodynamic imbalance in the fetoplacental unit. Presumably this is due to changes in intravascular pressures across large-vessel anastomoses secondary to the changing uterine pressures of labor. Both fetuses may die, one of exsanguination and the other of cardiac failure.

Vasa previa and velamentous insertion

Both vasa previa and velamentous insertion have been described in twin pregnancy. Whereas vasa previa insertion may be associated with disastrous consequences (fetal exsanguination), velamentous insertion is not (see Chapter 9).

Reducing parental anxiety

Several chapters throughout this book discuss parental anxiety as it relates to twin pregnancy and advise various means to diminish it. The very act of going into labor may precipitate another set of concerns that ideally should be addressed at the onset of labor or in the discussions held in the months before delivery. The first is the concern that the labor will be doubly painful (it is not). The second is the concern that labor will last twice as long (it does not; see Chapter 32). The third is that there will not be sufficient personnel to care for the mother and her infants (this should not be the case if the pregnancy has been diagnosed beforehand and the appropriate delivery site is selected). Other concerns relate to abdominal distension, difficulty in achieving a comfortable position while recumbent and the potential effect of vena caval compression if the patient rolls over onto her back. Even if the patient has been advised that her delivery will be something special in terms of equipment and personnel, the medical staff are well advised not to accentuate the potential for anxiety by conducting prolonged discussions at the bedside. A bedside lecture of great anatomic detail replete with quotations from the literature may only inspire a feeling of increasing dread among couples who had, until that moment, been quite comfortable. Care should be taken to emphasize to the family what is to be the joy of childbirth and parenting (see Chapters 20, 48, 50 and 51).

References

1. Keith, L. and Luke, B. (1993). Multiple gestation. In *Textbook of Prematurity: Antecedents, Treatment and Outcome*, pp. 115–20. (Boston: Little, Brown)
2. Allanbadia, N. (1963). Vaginal delivery following Cesarean section. *Am. J. Obstet. Gynecol.*, **85**, 241
3. Browne, A. and McGrath, J. (1965). Vaginal delivery after previous Cesarean section: a survey of 800 cases at the Rotunda Hospital, Dublin. *J. Obstet. Gynaecol. Br. Emp.*, **72**, 557
4. O'Connel, W. (1982). Vaginal delivery following Cesarean section: a two-year experience. *Am. J. Obstet. Gynecol.*, **144**, 671
5. Lavin, J.P., Stephens, R.J., Miodovnik, M. *et al.* (1982). Vaginal delivery in patients with a prior Cesarean section. *Obstet. Gynecol.*, **59**, 135
6. American College of Obstetricians and Gynecologists (1988). *Committee Opinion*, No. 64, October
7. Derom, C., Vlietinck, R., Derom, R. *et al.* (1988). Vaginal delivery of twins after previous Cesarean section. *N. Engl. J. Med.*, **319**, 117
8. Strong, T.H., Phelan, J.P., Ahn, M.D. *et al.* (1989). Vaginal birth after Cesarean delivery in twin gestation. *Am. J. Obstet. Gynecol.*, **161**, 29
9. Brady, K. and Read, J.A. (1988). Vaginal delivery of twins after previous Cesarean section. (Letter) *N. Engl. J. Med.*, **319**, 118
10. Eganhouse, D. (1992). Fetal monitoring of twin. *J. Obstet. Gynecol. Nursing*, **21**, 17
11. Chervenak, F.A., Johnson, R.E., Berkowitz, R.L. *et al.* (1983). Intrapartum external version of the second twin. *Obstet. Gynecol.*, **62**, 160
12. Chervenak, F.A., Johnson, R.E., Youcha, S. *et al.* (1985). Intrapartum management of twin gestation. *Obstet. Gynecol.*, **65**, 119
13. Depp, R., Keith, L.G. and Sciarra, J.J. (1988). The Northwestern University twin study VII: the mode of delivery in twin pregnancy, North American considerations. *Acta Genet. Med. Gemellol.*, **37**, 111
14. Chervenak, F.A., Johnson, R.E., Berkowitz, R.L. *et al.* (1984). Is routine Cesarean section necessary for vertex-breech and vertex-transverse twin gestations? *Am. J. Obstet. Gynecol.*, **148**, 1
15. Rabinovich, J., Barkai, G., Reichman, B. *et al.* (1987). Randomized management of the second nonvertex twin: vaginal delivery or Cesarean section. *Am. J. Obstet. Gynecol.*, **156**, 52
16. Warenski, J.C. and Kochenour, N.K. (1989). Intrapartum management of twin gestation. *Clin. Perinat.*, **16**, 4
17. James, F.M., Crawford, J.S., Davies, P. *et al.* (1977). Lumbar epidural analgesia for labor and delivery of twins. *Am. J. Obstet. Gynecol.*, **127**, 176
18. Crawford, J.S. (1987). A prospective study of 200 consecutive twin deliveries. *Anesthesia*, **42**, 33
19. Gocke, S. and Nageotte, M.P. (1988). Management of the nonvertex second twin: primary Cesarean section, external version or primary breech extraction. *Eighth Annual Meeting of the Society of Perinatal Obstetricians*, Las Vegas

20. Depp, R. and Keith, L.G. (1984) Unpublished data
21. Chitkara, U. and Berkowitz, R.L. (1992). Multiple gestations. In *Multiple Gestation in Obstetrics: Normal and Problem Pregnancy*, pp. 881–920. (New York: Churchill Livingstone)
22. Rayburn, W.F., Lavin, J.P. Jr, Miodovnik, M. *et al.* (1984). Multiple gestation: time interval between the delivery of the first and second twins. *Obstet. Gynecol.*, **63**, 502
23. Newman, R.B., Hamer, C. and Miller, M.C. (1989). Outpatient triplet management: a contemporary review. *Am. J. Obstet. Gynecol.*, **161**, 547
24. Collins, M.S. and Blyel, J.A. (1990). Seventy-one quadruplet pregnancies: management and outcome. *Am. J. Obstet. Gynecol.*, **162**, 1384
25. Vervliet, J., DeCleyn, K., Reiner, M. *et al.* (1989). Management and outcome of 21 triplet and quadruplet pregnancies. *Eur. J. Obstet. Gynecol. Reprod. Biol.*, **33**, 61
26. Olofsson, P. (1990). Triplet and quadruplet pregnancies – a forthcoming challenge also for the 'general' obstetrician. *Eur. J. Obstet. Gynecol. Reprod. Biol.*, **35**, 159
27. Pheiffer, E.L. and Golan, A. (1979). Triplet pregnancy: a 10-year review of cases at Baragwanath Hospital. *S. Afr. Med. J.*, **55**, 843
28. Lipitz, S., Rechman, B., Paret, G. *et al.* (1989). The improving outcome of triplet pregnancies. *Am. J. Obstet. Gynecol.*, **161**, 1279
29. Loucopoulos, A. and Jewelewicz, R. (1982). Management of multifetal pregnancies: sixteen years' experience at the Sloane Hospital for Women. *Am. J. Obstet. Gynecol.*, **143**, 902
30. Daw, E. (1978). Triplet pregnancy. *Br. J. Obstet. Gynaecol.*, **85**, 505
31. Feingold, M., Cetrulo, C., Peters, M. *et al.* (1988). Mode of delivery in multiple birth of higher order. *Acta Genet. Med. Gemellol.*, **37**, 105
32. Antoine, C., Kirshenbaum, N.W. and Young, B.K. (1986). Biochemical differences related to birth order in triplets. *J. Reprod. Med.*, **31**, 330
33. Creinin, M., MacGregor, S., Socol, M. *et al.* (1988). The Northwestern University triplet study IV. Biochemical parameters. *Am. J. Obstet. Gynecol.*, **159**, 1140
34. Petrikovsky, B.M. and Vintzileos, A.M. (1989). Management and outcome of multiple pregnancy of high fetal order: literature review. *Obstet. Gynecol. Surv.*, **44**, 578
35. Keith, L.G., Ameli, S., Depp, O.R. *et al.* (1988). The Northwestern University triplet study II. Fourteen triplet pregnancies delivered between 1981 and 1986. *Acta Genet. Med. Gemellol. (Roma)*, **37**, 65
36. Michlewitz, H., Kennedy, J., Kawada, C. *et al.* (1981). Triplet pregnancies. *J. Reprod. Med.*, **26**, 243
37. Syrop, C.H. and Varner, M.W. (1985). Triplet gestation: maternal and neonatal implications. *Acta Genet. Med. Gemellol. (Roma)*, **34**, 81
38. Holcberg, G., Biale, Y., Lewenthal, H. *et al.* (1989). Outcome of pregnancy in 31 triplet pregnancies. *Am. J. Obstet. Gynecol.*, **161**, 1279
39. Keith, L., Ellis, R., Berger, G. and Depp, R. (1980). The Northwestern University multi-hospital twin study I. Description of 588 twin pregnancies and associated pregnancy loss, 1970 to 1975. *Am. J. Obstet. Gynecol.*, **138**, 781
40. Bryan, E. (1992). *Twins and Higher Multiple Births: a Guide to their Nature and Nurture.* (London: Edward Arnold)
41. Nissen, E.D. (1958). Twins: collision, impaction, compaction and interlocking. *Obstet. Gynecol.*, **11**, 514

Analgesic and anesthetic considerations 38

H. Cohen and E.A. Brunner

Introduction

Women with multiple pregnancies present unique challenges to all the members of the perinatal team. These challenges relate to potential complications in the mother and/or her infants. Many potential problems impact on anesthetic management and may be crucial to determining maternal and/or fetal outcome.

Without doubt, expertly administered analgesia and anesthesia facilitate any delivery, thus benefiting the mother and her infants. On the other hand, improperly administered analgesia and anesthesia may contribute to maternal and perinatal morbidity and/or mortality. To provide optimal care, the anesthesiologist must understand the pathophysiology of multiple gestations, the potential complications that may occur during pregnancy, the processes of labor and delivery, and the various modalities by which the obstetrician commonly manages these problems and complications. Many of the concepts presented below have been discussed in detail elsewhere in this volume; it is useful, however, to summarize them as they relate to analgesia and anesthesia.

Non-anesthetic problems that may affect anesthesia and analgesia

Maternal

The more common maternal complications include pregnancy-induced hypertension (eclampsia, pre-eclampsia), anemia, preterm labor, prolonged labor, hemorrhage (antepartum, intrapartum, postpartum) and premature separation of the placenta.

Cardiovascular changes of pregnancy, as shown in Table 1, are enhanced in multiple pregnancy. These changes also tend to occur earlier. The maternal blood volume reaches levels approximately 40% greater than in singleton gestation; hence, relative anemia occurs more frequently and is more severe. The considerably larger uterus predisposes the parturient to more severe hypotension, with increased aortocaval compression, and additionally, leads to more frequent nausea and vomiting, edema of lower extremities and varicosities. Blood loss at delivery is twice that of a singleton gestation and manual extraction of the placenta is required twice as often. The risk of pulmonary aspiration of acidic gastric contents, normally present in all parturients, is exacerbated because of the presence of the greatly enlarged uterus.

The respiratory physiological changes with multiple pregnancy are summarized in Table 2. Total lung capacity is minimally reduced as patients approach near-term. However, functional residual capacity, expiratory reserve volume and residual volume decrease more than

Table 1 Cardiovascular changes (%)

Variable	Increase	Decrease
Total blood volume	40	—
Plasma volume	50	—
Red cell volume	30	—
Cardiac output	40	—
Renal blood flow	15	—
Hepatic blood flow	5	—
Hematocrit	—	6
Total proteins	—	10
Albumin concentration	—	20

Changes with multiple gestation tend to be increased and occur earlier in pregnancy than in singleton pregnancy

Table 2 Respiratory changes

Variable	Average change	
	Singleton	Twins
Total lung capacity (%)	0–5	–5
Functional residual capacity (%)	–20	–25
Expiratory reserve volume (%)	–20	–25
Residual volume (%)	–20	–25
Minute ventilation (%)	+50	+55
Alveolar ventilation (%)	+70	+75
Tidal volume (%)	+40	+40
Respiratory rate (%)	+15	+15
Oxygen consumption (%)	+20	+25
Blood gases		
arterial pO_2	+10 mmHg	same
arterial pCO_2	–8 mmHg	same
arterial pH	no change	same
serum bicarbonate	–3 mEq/l	same
MAC, inhalation agents (%)	–10	same

MAC, minimal alveolar concentration

in singleton pregnancies, because of the increased size of the uterus and its contents. Minute ventilation may increase moderately. Patients often complain of increased shortness of breath and difficult breathing, especially in the supine position. Respiratory distress requires adjustment in maternal position during labor, and particularly during induction of anesthesia for Cesarean section.

The neonate

Preterm delivery occurs 6–10 times more frequently in multiple gestations. The etiology is unknown; however, it has been attributed to over-distension of the uterus plus an increased incidence of maternal complications – such as pregnancy-induced hypertension. Fetal growth is independent of the number of fetuses until the 30th week of gestation, at which point, progressive lag develops compared to singleton gestation. Neonatal death rates rise progressively as birth weight decreases. The impact of prematurity on outcome can be assessed not only by mortality rates, but also by morbidity measurements.

During vaginal delivery, the second and/or additional fetuses are likely to be more depressed and asphyxiated, and require resuscitation more frequently than the first. The most significant risk factor for the second twin is the period of hypoxemia caused by decreased volume and capacity of the uterine cavity, effecting the surface area of uteroplacental exchange and/or by premature separation of the placenta after delivery of the first fetus.

The increased morbidity and mortality for the second twin may also be partly explained by the more frequent occurrence of malpresentations and, hence, the more frequent occurrence of operative deliveries[1]. Graves et al. reported that operative intervention was required in 16% of first twin deliveries as compared to 24% for the second twin. Of all operative obstetric procedures, version, version and extraction, and breech extraction commanded the most attention, because of their association with fetal morbidity and mortality[2].

Obstetric considerations that affect analgesia and anesthesia

Twins present in one of nine possible combinations: vertex–vertex; vertex–breech; vertex–transverse; breech–vertex; breech–breech; breech–transverse; transverse–transverse; transverse–vertex; transverse–breech. At any period of gestation, vaginal delivery offers a poorer outcome for the second twin than for the first. The first twin usually delivers without incident, while uterine atony, malpresentation and operative–manipulative maneuvers often complicate the second twin's birth. In the past, it was believed and taught that optimal results occurred when the second twin delivered within 15 min of the first. We now know that this dictum is not valid if the second twin is continuously monitored and ultrasound equipment is present to assess the fetal lie and, at the same time, to seek evidence of placental detachment. Unmonitored prolonged delivery intervals may result in poor outcome due to obstetric complications (placental separation, hemorrhage, prolapsed cord), adverse maternal effects (prolonged aortocaval compression, supine lithotomy position and lengthy exposure to general anesthesia). Most obstetricians administer intravenous oxytocin to shorten delivery intervals by promoting uterine contractility. The mothers should be positioned in left lateral tilt to prevent aortocaval compression until after delivery. A wedge placed under the right hip before institution of lithotomy position will tilt the mother's pelvis to the left. In all instances, the heart rate of the undelivered fetuses should be continuously monitored on the delivery table for early detection of fetal distress.

Management for parturition

There should be enough personnel in the delivery room to care for the mother as well as all infants. Specifically, an experienced neonatal team should be present to provide resuscitation for each infant. Also, extra resuscitation equipment should be available. The more recently conceived 'labor/delivery room' is not an ideal site for delivery of multiples. Rather, a high-risk delivery room with operating room anesthesia equipment and/or a Cesarean section operating room is needed. A minimum of two units of packed red blood cells or whole blood should be available in advance of delivery, and stored in the vicinity of the labor/delivery suite. For specific recommendations on obstetric management, the reader should refer to the appropriate chapters within this text.

In about half of all mothers with twins, delivery is preterm; this figure is much higher for triplets and quadruplets. In any case, if a vaginal delivery is anticipated, it can be conducted in a manner similar to that for a single premature infant. If the first infant presents in the cephalic position, vaginal delivery will, for the most part, be uncomplicated. Specific recommendations for the delivery of the second, third, and perhaps fourth fetus will vary, and will be largely dictated by specific circumstances: presentation, status of membranes, cord factors, placental bleeding and fetal heart rates. The management of labor and choice of delivery will often dictate the choice of anesthesia.

Anesthetic considerations for vaginal delivery

The anesthetic management of multiple births is similar in many respects to that of breech delivery. The successful culmination of a multiple pregnancy requires expert anesthetic care. Ideally, the patient with multiple pregnancy should be scheduled for an initial evaluation by a member of the anesthesia team early in the third trimester, keeping in mind the risk of preterm labor. The anesthesia team should evaluate the physical status of the mother again prior to or early during labor, have equipment prepared, and remain in proximity to the labor/delivery suite.

Due to the high incidence of maternal complications in multiple pregnancies, anesthesia care must be individualized for each case. Even in uncomplicated twin pregnancies, the cardiovascular response to anesthesia may be exaggerated, due to the greater increases in blood volume, cardiac index and total peripheral resistance, greater combined fetal weights and hydramnios, all of which increase the severity of aortocaval compression. This phenomenon fosters development of severe hypotension in supine gravidas when they are administered lumbar epidural or spinal (intrathecal) blocks.

The presence of multiple pregnancy can produce marked lordosis and increased abdominal girth, and may complicate the initiation of spinal blocks. Lumbosacral edema, which frequently results from prolonged bed rest, further adds to the problem. Before deciding upon an anesthetic technique, the mother's dorsal spine must be examined to identify potential problems such as scoliosis or extreme lordosis, and to determine the mother's ability to flex her lumbodorsal spine.

The anesthesiologist must remain constantly aware of the depressant effects of narcotics and sedatives of the infants, especially if labor is premature. The superimposition of depressant drugs in neonates that have been

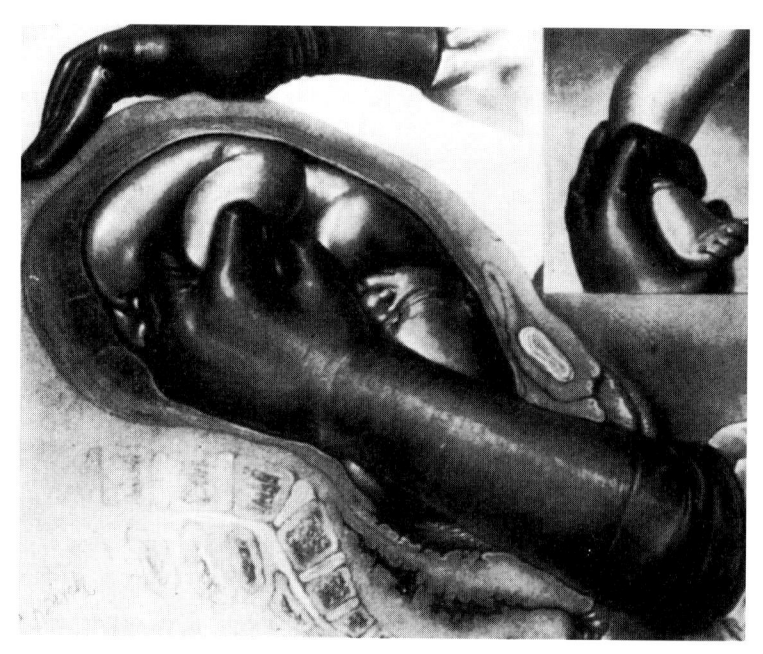

Figure 1 Internal podalic version. Both feet are grasped, thus facilitating turning of the infant. Reprinted with permission from reference 5

subjected to asphyxia may decrease their chance for survival.

No single analgesic or anesthetic technique is ideal for delivery of all multiple pregnancies. After the spontaneous delivery of a first twin in cephalic presentation with local infiltration or pudendal block, the obstetrician not infrequently requests the anesthesiologist to administer a general anesthetic for completion of delivery of one or more additional fetuses. It is reasonable to assume that some risk occurs when providing general anesthesia to any mother who presents with a second fetus in breech or shoulder presentation or where a cord prolapse occurs (Figures 1 and 2). Occasionally, internal podalic version and extraction are performed with the second twin delivered vaginally in the breech position. This procedure is best performed under general endotracheal anesthesia. The risk of postpartum hemorrhage from uterine atony complicated by the depressant effect of general anesthetics on uterine contractility must be anticipated. There should be no hesitation in providing deep general anesthesia in this situation, provided the anesthesiologist is qualified and aware of the risks involved. Following completion of delivery of the fetuses and prior to extraction of the placenta, a skilled anesthesiologist can retrieve a potent inhalational anesthetic agent rapidly from the mother by hyperventilation – and administer an accepted dose of oxytocic drug to promote effective uterine contractility. With evidence of contractility, the obstetrician may then elect to manually extract the placentae followed by active uterine massage to effect complete hemostasis. In most circumstances, a continued infusion of oxytocin is indicated. It is important that the mother be closely monitored in the immediate postpartum period to observe for any evidence of uterine relaxation and active hemorrhage. The mother should not be transferred to the recovery area after a major anesthetic until assurance is reached of stability of all vital signs.

General principles of anesthesia management

The preferred anesthetic techniques for the first fetus may be totally inappropriate for the

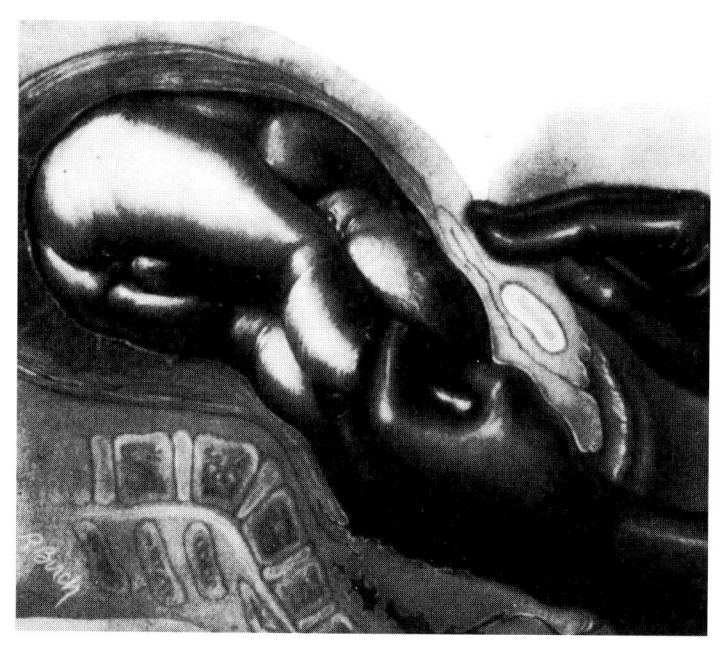

Figure 2 Internal podalic version. Upward pressure on the head is exerted as downward traction is exerted on the feet. Reprinted with permission from reference 5

other(s). Moreover, what is preferable for the mother may not be the safest for either or all of the infants. Finally, the maximum benefits from analgesia and anesthesia for infants and mother can be achieved only if the method of pain relief is applied specifically for each circumstance.

In selecting the initial technique for analgesia and anesthesia, consideration must be given to the possibility that the obstetrician may need to change obstetric management unexpectedly, because of a need for prompt anesthesia and/or uterine relaxation for version and extraction, breech delivery, mid-forceps delivery, or for Cesarean section. Regardless of the initial techniques used, the mother is exposed to the increased risk of aspiration of gastric contents associated with general anesthesia if she has eaten within the preceding 6–8 h.

The anesthesiologist ought to be consulted as soon as the patient enters the hospital, in order to develop clinical rapport, to assess the patient's physical and emotional status, to discuss alternative anesthetic and analgesic techniques and their attendant risks and benefits, and finally to make specific preparations for the initial analgesia and anesthetic management plan. This consultation should be requested even if the patient has had an earlier evaluation by the anesthesia team, because changes in the patient's condition, the fetal assessment, or the duration of pregnancy may necessitate a change from the original care plan.

The anesthesiologists, obstetrician and neonatologist should concur on the proposed care plan for the early stages of labor, recognizing that abrupt changes may be necessary based on changes in the clinical picture. Any existing problems should be discussed, and a well-coordinated plan of overall care should be developed. It should be emphasized that all current analgesia and anesthesia techniques can be used for multiple delivery with good results, provided they are skilfully administered and properly applied. Each agent and technique has its own advantages, limitations and disadvantages, and may produce certain complications. A skilled anesthesiologist can manipulate a combination of various techniques to the maximum advantage of mother and infants. One cannot dogmatically indicate what should be the given anesthetic management for multiple pregnancy. When making management decisions, one of the most important considerations is to recognize the level of skill and expertise of the obstetrician, the pediatrician and the anesthesiologist, as well as their awareness of outcomes within their own medical center, as compared to currently published standards.

Management for labor and vaginal delivery

The pre-anesthetic preparations for vaginal delivery of multiple gestations include:

(1) Administer intravenous fluids through a large bore cannula (either 16- or 14-gauge);

(2) For pre-load or volume expansion, use glucose-free fluids to prevent prolonged neonatal hypoglycemia;

(3) Type, screen and crossmatch a minimum of two units of packed red blood cells;

(4) Withhold liquids and solid food if the mother is in prodromal or active labor;

(5) Monitor both fetal heart rates and uterine activity continuously;

(6) Evaluate the mother's lumbothoracic spine in the sitting position to facilitate insertion of the epidural needle;

(7) Evaluate the patient's airway in the event that a rapid induction of general anesthesia is necessary;

(8) Determine the use of all current medication (magnesium sulfate, ritodrine, hydralazine) that may impact on the anesthetic;

(9) Prepare to resuscitate the newborn; and

(10) Prevent acid gastric aspiration syndrome by using H-2 blocking drugs, e.g. ranitidine (Zantac®) or cimetidine (Tagament®), metaclopromide (Reglan®), sodium citrate, (Bicitra®).

Analgesic techniques during active-phase labor

Many obstetricians are reluctant to use major regional blocks (e.g. continuous lumbar epidural analgesia) for patients with multiple gestations and prefer systemic analgesics (e.g. low-dose narcotics and sedatives) in combination with local anesthetic infiltration of the perineum or pudendal block for vaginal delivery. These latter techniques can provide adequate analgesia for vaginal delivery with minimal depression of the neonates. Unfortunately, however, they provide inadequate analgesia for the first and second stages of labor. They also provide no degree of uterine relaxation, should it prove necessary.

Prior to 1975, regional analgesia and anesthesia were thought to be contraindicated for multiple gestation. It was thought that regional blocks prolonged the duration of labor as well as increased the risk of aortocaval compression with resulting maternal hypotension and reduced placental perfusion. In addition, because of the increased need for forceps extraction, regional analgesia was often avoided. Crawford noted that labor was not significantly prolonged by the use of lumbar epidural analgesia, and that the interval between the birth of the first and second twin could be shortened[3]. The safety of this technique in multiple gestation was later confirmed by others. Crawford and Weaver later reported that in vaginal delivery with epidural analgesia, the acid–base status of the second twin was as good as or better than that of its sibling[4]. This was not the case in the deliveries conducted without epidural analgesia. Crawford also reported an apparent benefit to both twins when the bearing down reflex was abolished during terminal labor[4].

When properly administered, regional anesthesia is an excellent method for pain relief during labor and delivery of multiple gestations. It provides continuous and near-complete pain relief for the mother without direct depression of the fetus – provided that the complications of regional analgesia are avoided. It should be emphasized that regional blocks should not be administered by the 'occasional' anesthetist or any other physician unless he/she has had extensive experience in the administration of epidural analgesia for normal deliveries. For multiple pregnancy, proper application requires that analgesic blocks not be started until obstetric conditions are 'right'; that is, frequent, strong, uterine contractions which produce an adequate rate of cervical dilatation.

Analgesia can be provided by the careful titration of 0.125–0.25% bupivacaine with epinephrine added in a concentration of 1:300 000 to 1:400 000. Note that epinephrine is best avoided in patients who have recently received betamimetic therapy (ritodrine or terbutaline). Improved analgesia may be achieved by the addition of the narcotic Sublimaze® (fentanyl) in a concentration of 5 µg/ml to the infusate. Optimally, an infusion rate of local anesthesia–narcotic solution 7–10 ml/h through the epidural catheter will maintain excellent, continuous analgesia for the first and second stages of labor. To prevent premature 'bearing down' through an incompletely dilated cervix, the block may be extended to the sacral segments by the use of an increased rate of infusion and by the use of a slight head-up position.

Anesthesia either for a forceps delivery or for intrauterine manipulation may be achieved rapidly by infusing either 2% lidocaine, 3% chloroprocaine, or 0.5% bupivacaine with or without the use of epinephrine into the epidural catheter with the patient in a semi-Fowlers position. The resulting level of sensory block should be closely monitored and titrated to the desired effect.

After birth of the first infant, the overdistended uterus is usually sufficiently relaxed to permit intrauterine manipulation between contractions. If further relaxation is required, a small intravenous bolus of nitroglycerine (50–100 µg) often is sufficient. This appropriate dose can be rapidly achieved by the double dilution technique utilizing a 10-ml syringe – injecting 1.0 ml of the final solution (equivalent to 50 µg)[6–8]. An emergency rapid induction of general anesthesia to achieve uterine relaxation should be an exception rather than the rule at this time, but the managing anesthesiologist must be prepared to administer it should this need arise.

Anesthetic technique for Cesarean section

To date, no studies compare general vs. regional anesthesia for Cesarean section in multiple pregnancy, with regard to either maternal safety or neonatal outcome. The choice of technique depends entirely upon the experience and expertise of the anesthesiologist and the wishes of the obstetrician and the patient. At our institution, epidural anesthesia is the preferred technique.

Before induction of either regional or general anesthesia for Cesarean delivery, one or two large-bore intravenous cannulae must be inserted and the mother carefully rehydrated with at least 1500 ml of a dextrose-free solution. Maternal protection from acid gastric aspiration syndrome *must* be provided, regardless of whether regional or general anesthesia is selected. Depending upon circumstances (twins, triplets, quadruplets), 2–4 units of blood must be cross-matched in advance – and should be immediately available in the vicinity of the labor/delivery suite. One must anticipate significantly greater blood loss during Cesarean delivery with multiples than with a single fetus, due to marked uterine overdistension and postpartum uterine atony.

During the operation, one should consider administering an oxytocin infusion as soon as the fetuses have been delivered and prior to manual extraction of the placentae. Massage of the uterus at this time induces initial contractility and helps to reduce uterine size prior to delivery of the placenta or its manual extraction. If the oxytocin infusion fails to promote sufficient uterine contractility and hemorrhage is profuse, prostaglandin $F_{2\alpha}$ can be injected directly into the uterine muscle as well as intravenously[9]. The contents of the vial should be diluted to a concentration of 0.2 mg/ml. This is then injected slowly in 1–3 ml increments to a total dose not exceeding 25 ml (equivalent to 5 mg).

In some patients, the excessive enlargement of the uterus requires early delivery before term. For indicated scheduled Cesarean sections, regional anesthesia is considered safer than general anesthesia for the following reasons: (1) premature infants are more sensitive to the depressant effects of narcotics and other general anesthetic agents; (2) maternal gastric emptying may be significantly delayed; (3) gastric activity is likely to be increased, because of the extremely large uterine mass; (4) although pulmonary aspiration is generally not a problem following regional blockade, protection must, nevertheless, be provided, because occasionally general anesthetic supplementation may be required; (5) post-operative pain can be more easily managed after epidural block; and (6) mothers are far more alert during the recovery period than after general anesthesia.

Epidural anesthesia

Although epidural anesthesia is considered safe, one cannot ignore the risk of hypotension consequent to aortocaval compression produced by the massively enlarged uterus and further compounded by sympathetic blockade. However, epidural anesthesia allows for careful titration of the local anesthetic solution in small incremental doses and permits a more gradual onset of the block, with better control of the mother's blood pressure. In contrast, spinal anesthesia (intrathecal block) has a much more rapid onset of action with less control of level of blockade, and profound hypotension is more likely to occur; this anesthetic method should, therefore, be avoided.

General anesthesia

General anesthesia is occasionally required for emergency Cesarean section as well as in the occasional patient for whom regional anesthesia is contraindicated. General anesthesia should be induced with the uterine mass carefully displaced laterally and to the left. Pre-oxygenation and nitrogen wash-out are essential, because of the rapid maternal oxygen desaturation expected to occur after induction and prior to endotracheal intubation and controlled ventilation. It is important to recognize that, because the intravenous anesthetic agent redistributes so rapidly within the maternal venous pool, only a minimal amount of drug is transported across the uteroplacental barrier and into the fetal circulation. In contrast, the amount of potent inhalational agent transported into the fetal compartment is time- and dose-related, and these agents must be administered to the mother with caution. High concentrations are administered only to achieve uterine relaxation and are rarely necessary during the operation itself.

Summary

Parturients with multiple gestation challenge all members of the perinatal team. Satisfactory maternal and fetal outcome require the experience and expertise of the obstetrician, anesthesiologist and neonatologist, all of whom must be well informed in terms of the total care and management plan. No single anesthetic approach can be expected to produce perfect results in all cases. The obstetrician and the anesthesiologist must work together to plan for optimal results.

Acknowledgements

We wish to gratefully acknowledge the assistance of Dr Louis G. Keith and Ms Toni Sallis for the editing and preparation of this manuscript.

References

1. Ware, H.H. (1971). The second twin. *Am. J. Obstet. Gynecol.*, **110**, 865
2. Graves, L.R., Adams, J. *et al.* (1962). The fate of the second twin. *Obstet. Gynecol.*, **19**, 246
3. Crawford, J.S. (1974). An appraisal of lumbar epidural blockade in patients with a singleton fetus presenting by the breech. *J. Obstet. Gynaecol. Br. Commonw.*, **81**, 867
4. Crawford, J.S. and Weaver, J.B. (1982). Anesthetic management of twin and breech deliveries. *Clin. Obstet. Gynecol.*, **9**, 291
5. Pritchard, J.A., MacDonald, P.C. and Gant, N.F. (1985). *Williams Obstetrics*, 17th edn, p. 865. (New York: Appleton-Century-Crofts)
6. Peng, A.T.C., Gorman, R.S. *et al.* (1989). Intravenous nitroglycerin for uterine relaxation in the post-partum patient with retained placenta. *Anesthesiology*, **71**, 172
7. DiSimone, C.A., Norris, M.C. and Leighton, B.L. (1990). Intravenous nitroglycerin for manual extraction of retained placenta. *Anesthesiology*, **73**, 787
8. Rolbin, S.H., Hew, E.M. *et al.* (1991). Uterine relaxation can be life saving. *Can. J. Anesth.*, **38**, 939
9. Jacobs, M.M., Arias, F. (1989). Intramyometrial prostaglandin F_2 alpha in treatment of severe postpartum hemorrhage. *Obstet. Gynecol.*, **55**, 665

Clinical management of monoamniotic twins

M. Motew and N.A. Ginsberg

Introduction

Monoamniotic (MA) twins are generally reported to occur in about 2% of twin pregnancies, although their relative proportion among all types of twins differs from country to country. Compared to diamniotic (DA) twins, MA twins are associated with significantly higher morbidity and mortality. The first review to emphasize this point appeared in 1935[1]. Since that time, until 1986, reported mortality rates have ranged from 40 to 70%[2-4]. A clear understanding of the reasons for this high fetal wastage is critical to developing a rational plan of management for these pregnancies.

Simply stated, the high mortality of MA twins is related to a combination of factors: congenital anomalies, cord entanglement, prematurity, twin–twin transfusion syndrome (TTTS) and adverse outcome of term delivery[4]. Most often, fetal death of one or more of the fetuses occurs before the last trimester, and two recent reports suggest that after 30–32 weeks' gestation the fetal loss rate is comparable to that of DA twins[4,5].

Given these circumstances, the early diagnosis of the MA condition and the appropriate monitoring of these pregnancies during the first and second trimesters may help to reduce early fetal loss. Although no prospective studies have been reported on the management of MA twins using modern technology, such as high resolution ultrasound[6], home monitoring[7] and non-stress testing (NST), the use of these technological innovations has the potential to lower fetal wastage[5,8].

Antepartum diagnosis and care

First trimester

As noted in other chapters in this volume, the diagnosis of multiple gestation may be inferred on clinical grounds by a discrepancy between the gestational age and the size of the uterus or by auscultating two distinct fetal heart rates. This latter method, however, cannot be implemented until the clinician at least considers the possibility of multiple gestation. Nevertheless, no type of clinical examination can be used to discern zygosity. Moreover, and of far greater importance, no type of clinical examination can distinguish between MA and DA twins. The most commonly used means to make this distinction antenatally is real-time ultrasound. Zygosity is best evaluated by ultrasound during the first trimester, because the pregnancy does not fill the entire uterine cavity before the 10th week of gestation and the separation between dizygotic sacs is more readily visualized (see Chapters 14 and 16).

Ideally, first-trimester ultrasound assessment should include transabdominal as well as transvaginal scans. The transabdominal scan provides a far better panoramic picture than the transvaginal scan, and is therefore more useful for orientation. For example, the fundus of the uterus is more easily visualized using this approach. In contrast, with the transvaginal scan, the fundus becomes the far field and may be difficult to visualize in proper focus. Very occasionally, the presence of a dividing amniotic or chorionic membrane may be more readily visible using a transabdominal scan. Because of

apparent with a transvaginal approach, even if it is not visualized with the abdominal scan.

Finally, the different acoustic properties of the amniotic and chorioamniotic spaces are best appreciated if a transvaginal scan is used. This difference can be accentuated by increasing the gain. Even though a dividing membrane may still be difficult to visualize, the contrast between the fluids in the different spaces will highlight the separate nature of the amniotic sacs.

The yolk sac is located in the chorioamniotic space and is best visualized during the first trimester, before the chorioamniotic space becomes obliterated (Figure 1). The allantoic vessels are most easily visualized during the 7th and 8th weeks of gestation, when fluid can be seen rushing through them. One can trace the allantoic vessel from the fetus to the yolk sac. *When both allantoic vessels insert into a single yolk sac, this finding provides conclusive evidence of the presence of MA twins.* MA twins can have two separate yolk sacs or a single fused yolk sac, depending upon the time when the germinal disc split (see Figure 1, Chapter 9).

It is always important to rule out conjoined twins in the presence of presumed MA twins. This distinction can generally be accomplished with ease, because both fetuses normally are clearly seen to move separately and as two distinct entities by the 9th week of gestation. Before this time, however, their activity level is not as great and the conjoined state may be more difficult to classify (see Chapter 8).

After the 9th week, the relative ratio of amniotic fluid to the fetus is greater than later in gestation, and at this time it is not uncommon to witness the two umbilical cords intertwine within a single MA sac. Color flow Doppler may assist in demonstrating this phenomenon. Color flow Doppler is also worthwhile if conjoined twins are suspected, especially if they are joined at the chest and share a common circulation.

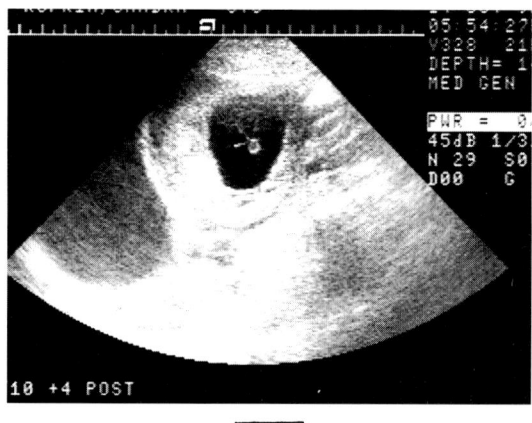

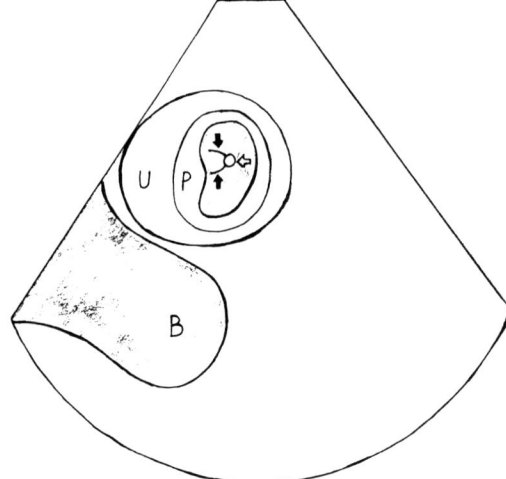

Figure 1 Ultrasound image (a) and diagram (b) in a 10-week monochorionic monoamniotic twin pregnancy, showing two allantoic vessels (dark arrows) inserting into a single yolk sac. The open arrow points to the yolk sac. P, placenta; U, uterus; B, bladder. Artistic rendition of the ultrasound image provided by Melinda Ginsberg

considerations such as these, the path of the dividing membrane should ideally be the determining factor for selection of a scanning method that allows for better resolution.

A particular advantage of transvaginal scanning is its ability to accommodate higher-frequency transducers, which provide excellent resolution. Indeed, crown–rump lengths of smaller magnitude can be visualized more readily and fetal cardiac activity can be seen at an earlier gestational age, if the vaginal transducer is used[9,10]. Often a dividing membrane becomes

Second trimester

For a number of reasons, once the second trimester has begun, it is more difficult to make the diagnosis of MA twins. Most importantly, abdominal scans used for the detection of a dividing membrane may be limited by non-correctible factors, such as obesity or prior abdominal surgery. At the same time, vaginal scans often are limited by the depth of field of the higher-frequency transducers.

Fortunately, abdominal scans can be enhanced by using non-standard examination positions. These include having the woman sit up or scanning a spectrum of lateral angles. Increasing the number of angles through which the scanning is performed increases the probability that the sound beam will become perpendicular to a membrane. These maneuvers are also useful to take advantage of the fact that the axial resolution of the ultrasound is greater than lateral resolution.

Second-trimester ultrasound examinations of known twin pairs also should include evaluation for umbilical cord entanglement, TTTS, growth discrepancy, placental implantation abnormalities, fetal anomalies and, when indicated, guidance for amniocentesis. In particular, following the umbilical cords back to their insertion into the placenta may demonstrate entanglement, a finding confirmatory of MA twins. The umbilical cords can be more easily followed at this stage, especially when color Doppler is not available.

In contrast to the potential difficulty in establishing the diagnosis of MA twins, genetic amniocentesis is much easier once this diagnosis has been made, because only one tap is required and genetic information from both twins can be pooled within that single sample. After removing a satisfactory amount of fluid, it is useful to inject indigo carmine dye into the gestational sac. Before injecting this dye, however, the syringe should be vigorously agitated to create microbubbles, which then diffuse throughout the entire gestational sac. The presence of the microbubbles throughout the sac thus provides confirmation of the presence of MA twins. If, on the other hand, the diagnosis of MA twins has been in error, a marker is present to assist in sampling the sac of the other twin.

Having stated that genetic sampling from MA twins may be technically more simple on some occasions, this determination may also be more challenging on others, because, for example, amniotic fluid from MA twins represents the sum of the secretions of both fetuses. Thus, a high alpha-fetoprotein secretion from one twin might be obscured by a low level from its co-twin and thereby fail to suggest the presence of an open neural tube defect in the rare occurrence of discordance for this anomaly. Just as challenging is the fact that difficulty may arise if the chromosomal analysis is mosaic (see Chapter 7). In this circumstance, one is uncertain if true mosaicism exists or if one of the twins is genetically discordant. If genetic discordance exists, then it must be determined in which fetus the abnormality lies.

It is important to remember that when TTTS occurs in DA twins, the dividing membrane may be obscured and a false-positive diagnosis of MA twinning may be made. Commonly, one twin has oligohydramnios and the other polyhydramnios[11]. In the presence of the full-blown manifestations of these disparate findings, it is often difficult to visualize the amniotic membrane surrounding the fetus with the oligohydramnios. The first indication that this syndrome may be present may be derived from the observation that one of the twins maintains itself in a constant location within its sac (sometimes called the 'cocoon effect') despite the fact that there appears to be sufficient amniotic fluid for free movement. Marked discordance in size at this time may also be suggestive of TTTS. Amniocentesis may help clarify this situation[12] by mechanically bringing the membrane into a better focal plane or by differentiating it from the limb–body wall complex.

Third trimester

The third trimester is probably the most difficult time to establish the diagnosis of MA twins by ultrasound, because the relative ratio of fetus to amniotic fluid is at its greatest. In addition, the two fetuses create a greater amount of shadowing, making it more difficult to find a dividing membrane if it is present. Increased shadowing also may interfere with any attempted evaluation for fetal anomalies.

It is particularly important to evaluate placental position at this late stage of pregnancy. Placenta previa is more likely with twins, because the two placentas possess a greater surface area[13]. When this condition is suspected, it should be confirmed by transvaginal or transperineal ultrasound examination. MA twins are no exception to this rule. True placenta previa should be relatively easy to diagnose, because the lower segment is usually well developed in multiple pregnancies by the third trimester. Attention should also be paid at this time to the site of cord insertion, in order to discern a velamentous insertion.

The slope of twin growth is increased during the last trimester, but at a lesser rate than in singleton pregnancies[14]. Discordant growth may become more pronounced as the pregnancy progresses. If serious discordance develops, it may become necessary to effect a delivery (albeit iatrogenically preterm) for the sake of the well-being of the more growth-retarded fetus. When early delivery is contemplated, one generally should determine the state of lung maturity of both twins. In the case of MA twins, this is a problem, because the amniotic fluid reflects the sum of the pulmonary secretions of both twins and is not particularly reliable to reflect either twins' state of lung maturity.

As term approaches, the fetal position becomes a crucial consideration relating to the advisability of vaginal delivery. If the fetuses are in the breech/vertex position, a greater potential exists for locking (see Chapter 36) of the fetal heads at the level of the bony pelvis while the first fetus is being delivered, because no dividing membrane separates the MA twins[15]. Ultrasound examination of the internal cervical os for premature dilatation or membrane protrusion can alter management of either imminent preterm labor or premature rupture of the membranes.

Patient preparation

Once the diagnosis of MA twinning has been made, it is essential to explain all potential risks to the patient so that she will be prepared for the care she will receive. The potential for fetal loss, fetal anomalies, prematurity, preeclampsia, and the requirements for limited activity, bed rest and frequent antenatal visits and testing all should be explained to the patient and her partner. The possibility of Cesarean section, transfusion and prolonged hospitalization should also be extensively discussed. At the same time, commentary on the joys of raising twins and watching their growth should be offered, along with mention of the improvements and progress in reducing complications. Finally, the patient needs to be reminded of the encouragement that she can receive from other mothers of twins. Prenatal education classes should always be encouraged, even if they must be at home (see Appendix).

Specific treatment

In addition to the usual prenatal evaluation, additional blood work could include a SMA-20 baseline and close serial monitoring of the patient's hemoglobin. Cervical cultures should be obtained for group B beta-hemolytic streptococci and mycoplasma, because of the higher incidence of premature rupture of the membranes. At 18 weeks, a Smith–Hodge pessary could be inserted into the vagina to provide mechanical support of the cervix[16]. Visits should be scheduled every 2 weeks and serial ultrasound evaluations should be performed at each visit. Bed rest starting at 20–22 weeks should be suggested and home tocodynomometry can be initiated with any cervical change or symptomatology which does not require hospitalization. Once viability has been established, serial NSTs should be performed to assess the presence of variable deceleration patterns. Autologous blood donation is recommended, even if the patient's complete blood count is normal. Initially, extra iron supplementation should be advised.

Intrapartum management

Preparing the team
Consultative discussions with additional obstetricians, pediatricians, anesthesiologists and nursing staff should occur well in advance of anticipated delivery. Each member of the team should be familiar with his/her planned role in the management of labor and delivery.

Management of labor
If vaginal delivery is deemed appropriate, the management of labor is no different than with DA twins. Constant fetal monitoring of both fetuses, tocodynomometry and evaluation of vital signs should begin at the onset of labor just as if the patient was in the active phase of labor.

Upon admission, an ultrasound examination should determine fetal positions, estimated fetal weights and placental site. If technically possible, detailed assessment of the umbilical cord status should look for knotting or entwinement, proximity to each fetus and position with regard to the presenting part. Labor curves common to twin pregnancy are described by Friedman in Chapter 32 of this book. Early amniotomy is not advisable because of the higher likelihood of cord entanglement and/or compression or prolapse. Blood should be drawn for type and screen, and the patient should be kept nil per os. The choice of anesthetic during labor should depend on a joint decision of the patient, her obstetrician and the anesthesiologist (see Chapter 38). During the second stage, however, local blocks are preferable, so that the patient is awake and alert and can use all possible expulsive efforts to assist in a vaginal delivery.

A vaginal trial of labor may be attempted at term, or if the fetuses weigh more than 1500 g, if the following criteria are met:

(1) A reassuring heart rate pattern with no significant variable decelerations;

(2) Little chance of locked twins (i.e. vertex first);

(3) The patient is cooperative and capable of assisting in the delivery;

(4) Ultrasound is available in the delivery room; and

(5) Sufficient ancillary staff are present.

If any of the above conditions cannot be met, a Cesarean section should be performed.

Techniques of delivery

The dictum of De Lee '*primum non nocere*' applies to twins as well. In the case of MA twins, however, this dictum can be split into a series of precautionary maxims:

(1) Be patient with the first twin;

(2) Monitor the second twin constantly after delivery of the first;

(3) Determine with ultrasound and manual examination the position of the second twin and, if possible, the cord;

(4) Do not cut the nuchal cord of the first twin until it is identified as the cord of that twin;

(5) Be prepared for emergency delivery of the second twin by breech extraction or Cesarean section; and

(6) Support and inform the patient and the father during the delivery.

Examples of clinical management
Two illustrated cases of MA twins with vaginal delivery are presented.

Patient R.K.

The patient was a 30-year-old white female, gravida 4 para 1021. The patient's first two pregnancies had resulted in spontaneous abortions, but her last pregnancy was uneventful. Ultrasound examination at gestational age of

12 weeks and 4 days (by dates) documented two fetuses with no apparent dividing membrane; however, the gestational ages of twins A and B were assessed as 1.5 and 2 weeks less, respectively, than the age by dates. At gestational age of 14 weeks and 3 days, a second ultrasound examination was performed, because of a small amount of vaginal bleeding, and a small clot was noted in the lower uterine segment. At this time, a single sac was observed, and the umbilical cords were noted to have separate insertions. A Smith–Hodge pessary was prophylactically placed in the vagina at 22 weeks to provide mechanical support of the cervix, and was subsequently removed at 37 weeks' gestation. Serial ultrasound examinations were performed. Ultrasonically assigned gestational age was consistently 1–2 weeks less than the age by dates; each of the later ultrasound examinations confirmed the absence of a dividing membrane. Weekly NSTs were performed at 36–39 weeks' gestation and were reactive.

At 39 weeks' gestation, the patient was admitted in labor. Ultrasound examination for presentation showed twin A to be vertex and twin B to be breech. The membranes ruptured approximately 50 min prior to delivery and the fluid was clear. Both infants were delivered vaginally over a midline episiotomy with pudendal and local anesthesia. Fetal heart tracings on both twins at the time of the first delivery were normal and reactive. Twin A was a 2510-g female with Apgar scores of 9 and 9, an umbilical arterial blood gas of 7.25/49/−5, and required no resuscitative efforts by the neonatologists who were present in the delivery room. Twin B was delivered approximately 3 min after twin A as an incomplete breech by assisted breech extraction. Time of delivery from the umbilicus to the head was approximately 1 min, and delivery proceeded without difficulty. A nuchal cord with one revolution was untwisted at delivery. Twin B was a 2960-g female with 1- and 5-min Apgar scores of 4 and 9, respectively, and an umbilical arterial blood gas of 7.28/49/−3. She required resuscitation with mask O_2 and stimulation. When the umbilical cord of twin B was clamped and cut, a true knot was noted where the two cords were intertwined (Figure 2).

The placenta was manually removed 23 min after delivery of twin B and the uterus was explored. Pathological examination confirmed intact monochorionic, monoamniotic placentation. Each umbilical cord was inserted eccentrically, 2.5 cm apart. The length of each umbilical cord was not noted. The placenta weighed 771 g.

The postpartum course was uncomplicated and both infants were discharged with their mother at 3 days of age.

Patient M.K.

The patient was a 24-year-old white female, gravida 2 para 0010. An initial ultrasound examination at 8 weeks' gestation showed a single fetus with size equivalent to dates. Because the patient's mother was born with spina bifida, an ultrasound-guided amniocentesis was performed at 17 weeks' gestation, at which time twins were noted with no apparent dividing membrane. Fetal size was equivalent to dates, no congenital abnormalities were noted and the amniocentesis was unremarkable. The remainder of the antepartum course was complicated by premature cervical effacement at 18 weeks, for which the patient was hospitalized for cerclage. The cervix reformed after admission and the patient was discharged after 3 hospital days, to be managed on bed rest. A Smith–Hodge pessary was prophylactically placed in the vagina 2 weeks later and removed at approximately 37 weeks' gestation. Serial ultrasound examinations performed every 2–4 weeks for the duration of the pregnancy were unremarkable, except for increased amniotic fluid volume noted at 32 weeks and 4 days, for which strict bed rest was initiated. All ultrasound examinations documented appropriate fetal growth and confirmed the absence of a dividing membrane. The three NSTs performed in the last trimester were all reactive.

At 38 weeks' gestation, the patient was admitted in the latent phase of labor. Ultrasound

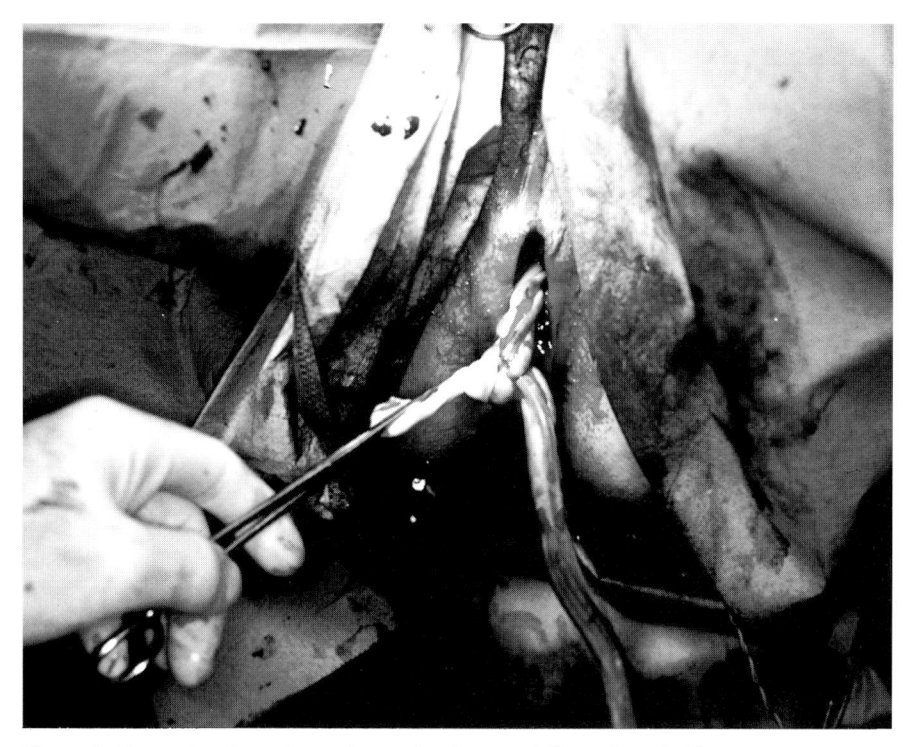

Figure 2 Example of true knots in cords of a case delivered vaginally

examination showed both infants in the vertex position. Labor progressed smoothly and artificial rupture of membranes was undertaken 3.5 h before delivery. The fluid had light meconium staining. Both infants were spontaneously delivered over a midline episiotomy with pudendal and local anesthesia. Twin A was a 2825-g female with 1- and 5-min Apgar scores of 9 and 9, respectively, and an umbilical arterial blood gas of 7.32/43/−3. No resuscitative efforts were required by the neonatologists who were present in the delivery room. Twin B, delivered approximately 3 min after twin A, was a 3375-g female with 1-, 5- and 10-min Apgar scores of 3, 8 and 9, respectively, and an umbilical arterial blood gas of 7.26/58/−2. This infant required supplemental oxygen by mask. No intertwining of the umbilical cords or true knots were observed.

The placenta delivered spontaneously, measured 21 cm in diameter, and weighed 1100 g. Pathological examination confirmed monochorionic, monoamniotic placentation. Each umbilical cord contained three vessels and they measured 21 and 25 cm in length.

The postpartum course was uncomplicated and both infants were discharged with their mother at 2 days of age.

Epilogue

We are aware that many practitioners prefer to avoid vaginal deliveries in these cases. At the same time, we believe it is important to provide another point of view, as well as to describe the optimal outcome in such instances.

References

1. Quigley, J.K. (1935). Monoamniotic twin pregnancy – a case record with review of the world literature. *Am. J. Obstet. Gynecol.*, **29**, 354
2. Paul, F. (1969). Monoamniotic twin pregnancy – review of the world literature and a report of two new cases. *Can. Med. Assoc. J.*, **100**, 254
3. Raphael, S.L. (1961). Monoamniotic twin pregnancy: review of the literature and a report of five new cases. *Am. J. Obstet. Gynecol.*, **81**, 323
4. Carr, S.R., Aronson, M.P. and Coustan, D.R. (1990). Survival rates of monoamniotic twins do not decrease after 30 weeks' gestation. *Am. J. Obstet. Gynecol.*, **163**, 719
5. Tessen, J.A. and Zietnik, F.J. (1991). Monoamniotic twins – a retrospective controlled study. *Obstet. Gynecol.*, **77**, 832
6. Townsend, R.R. and Filly, R.A. (1988). Sonography of non-conjoined monoamniotic pregnancies. *J. Ultrasound Med.*, **7**, 665
7. Knuppel, R.R., Lake, M.F., Watson, D.L. *et al.* (1990). Preventing preterm birth in twin gestation: home uterine activity monitoring and prenatal nursing support. *Obstet. Gynecol.*, **76**, 245
8. Chang, L. (1992). Management of monoamniotic twins diagnosed by ultrasound. *Am. J. Gynecol. Health*, **6**, 17
9. Cadkin, A.V. and McAlpin, J. (1984). Detection of fetal cardiac activity between 41 and 43 day of gestation. *J. Ultrasound Med.*, **3**, 499
10. Cadkin, A. (1992). Crown–rump length dating of pregnancy at less than nine weeks' gestation. *Am. J. Obstet. Gynecol.*, **166**, 269
11. Mahony, B., Filly, R. and Callen, P. (1985). Amnionicity and chorionicity in twin pregnancies: prediction using ultrasound. *Radiology*, **155**, 205
12. Brennan, J., Diwan, R., Rosen, M. *et al.* (1982). Fetofetal transfusion syndrome: prenatal ultrasonographic diagnosis. *Radiology*, **143**, 535
13. Laing, F.C. (1985). Ultrasound evaluation of obstetric problems relating to the lower uterine segment and cervix. In Sanders, R.C. and Jame, A.E. Jr (eds.) *The Principles and Practice of Ultrasonography in Obstetrics and Gynecology*, 3rd edn., pp. 355–67. (Norwalk, CT: Apple-Century-Crofts)
14. Socol, M.L., Tamura, R.K., Sabbagha, R.E. *et al.* (1984). Diminished biparietal diameter and abdominal circumference growth in twins. *Obstet. Gynecol.*, **64**, 235
15. Cohen, M., Kohl, S.G. and Rosenthal, A.H. (1965). Fetal interlocking complicating twin gestation. *Am. J. Obstet. Gynecol.*, **91**, 407
16. Oster, S. and Javert, C.T. (1966). Treatment of the incompetent cervix with the Hodge pessary. *Obstet. Gynecol.*, **28**, 206

Management of triplet and higher-order pregnancies

J.-C. Pons, Y. Laurent, D. Selim and E. Papiernik

Introduction

In 1960, Lacomme[1] commented on triplet, quadruplet and higher-order pregnancies in the following terms: 'These rarities don't present extraordinary problems; their delivery presents the same difficulties as twin pregnancies'. Today, this statement is no longer valid, because most obstetricians recognize that higher-order pregnancies do present extraordinary problems, not the least of which results from their increasing frequency.

As a result of recent improvements in infertility treatment, conceptions of this type have taken on 'epidemic' proportions in many countries (e.g. USA, UK, France, Belgium, Canada and Japan). More importantly, the remarkable advances in neonatal care in the past 20 years have ensured that a significant number of the newborns survive, albeit with some degree of handicap. Unfortunately, the degree of handicap is substantial for many[2].

This chapter presents an overview of the literature on the epidemiology and management of higher-order (more than two) multifetal pregnancies.

Epidemiology

Frequency

The frequency of multiple pregnancies has been investigated since the end of the 19th century. According to Hellin's law, the rate of twin deliveries is $1/80$, $1/80^2$ for triplets, $1/80^3$ for quadruplets, etc. In 1921, Zeleny[3] suggested the following derivative equation: if the rate for twins is $1/n$, the rate for triplets is $1/n^2$, and the rate for quadruplets is $1/n^3$. Perhaps neither equation describes the clinical reality, because Miettinen[4] in 1954 reported a vast range of published reported rates of higher-order multiple births: twins: between 1/83 and 1/89 births; triplets: 1/6400 to 1/7910 births; and quadruplets: 1/371 124 to 1/778 690 births.

As shown in Table 1, both twin and triplet births vary considerably from country to country and by year of report. In general, studies have reported low rates of higher-order multiples among Asiatic populations[4–6], and high rates among black populations[7–13]. Notwithstanding the fact that the general rate for triplets is three times lower in Japan than in the UK, the rate for monozygotic triplets is three times higher[5,12].

Using the Hellin hypothesis for quintuplets yields a frequency of 1/41 million births. This figure unfortunately does not correspond to clinical reality, because investigators report ranges between 1/20 million and 1/57 million births[4]. Nichols[11] reported two quintuplet births out of 72 000 births in the USA. Miettinen[4], in a 1954 study, found only 72 reported cases, in the literature, 56 of which seemed reliable. Prior to 1974, there were only two reported instances in which all five infants survived[14], one being the Dionne monozygotic quintuplets in Canada. A later case was reported by Berbos *et al.* in 1984[15]. (Editor: In 1990, one of the Editors (LK) attended a private reunion of more than a dozen surviving sets of quintuplets. All had resulted from ovulation induction or assisted reproductive technologies. The incidence of higher-order births

MULTIPLE PREGNANCY

Table 1 Frequency of multiple pregnancies (per 1000 deliveries)

Country	Years	Twin	Triplet	Quadruplet	Authors
Switzerland		12.3	0.116	0.0018	Miettinen[4]
Chile		21.3	0.070		Miettinen[4]
Japan		3.3	0.024		Komai and Fukuoka[143]
	1955–67	6.4	0.056	0.0014	Imaizumi and Inouye[5]
	1974	5.8	0.058	0.0039	
Osaka		6.7	0.029		Miettinen[4]
USA	1915–48				
	total	11.11	0.109	0.0015	
	white	10.41			Nichols[11]
	black	12.61			
	1922–36				
	total	11.61	0.1189	0.00203	
	white	11.29	0.1089	0.00175	Guttmacher[10]
	black	14.15	0.1970	0.00420	
	1928–49				
	total	11.2	0.1095		
	white	10.8	0.101		Guttmacher[10]
	black	13.5	0.177		
Scotland		9.70	0.112		Daw[82]
England	1938–62		0.109		Bulmer[144]
	1971–75	10.4	0.101		Brown and Daw[96]
	1982–85	10.1	0.14		Botting et al.[22]
Poland	1950	12.0	0.12		Rola-Janichi[25]
South Africa	1967–76		0.42		
	white		0.12		Deale and Cronje[8]
	black		0.44		
	colored		0.13		
Nigeria	1963–69	45.0	1.62		Nylander[12]
Finland	1881–63	14.53	0.17	0.0037	Miettinen[4]
Sweden	1881–40	14.37	0.16	0.0020	Miettinen[4]
	1921–50	13.6	0.13	0.0016	Nylander[12]
Hungary	1960–70		0.29		Czeizel[23]
Australia	1920–60		0.100		Brackenbridge[145]
Italy	1933–54		0.48		Bulmer[144]

has been skewed by these developments, and the vital records of many nations fail to reflect this by listing all multiples as a general category without reference to specific types. Furthermore, the Editors are unaware of any vital records (USA included) which differentiate natural from induced multiple gestations.) (Additional discussion on quintuplet and higher-order births is found later in the chapter.)

Natural multiple pregnancies with five or more fetuses doubtless exist[4,14,16–21], but it is difficult to separate real from apocryphal cases. Miettinen[4] and Nichols[11] each reported two cases of what appeared to be sextuplets. Mayer[17,18] provided a review of the literature which cited data from the Middle Ages and antiquity; this review described a large number of cases of sextuplets (22), septuplets (14), octuplets (23), nonuplets (15), and more; most must be assumed to be folklore.

Predisposing factors

Aside from ethnicity, several other factors also predispose to higher-order multiple pregnancies. These include: (1) high age of the mother[4,5,10,22–25] (the rate is 4 and 10 times higher at 15–20 and 35–40 years of age, respectively); (2) multiparity (a 1909 study reported that most (264/429) mothers of triplets already had six children or more (Editor: Obviously these mothers also aged in the years they had their children.); and (3) hereditary factors. According to Miettinen[4], the rate of multiple pregnancies is ten times higher in families with triplets. The hereditary maternal contribution to this phenomenon apparently is much stronger than the paternal[4,12,26–29], although some recent evidence suggests that the paternal contribution may be higher than previously believed (see Chapter 2).

Exceptional families of multiples have been described[4,30]. A classic case cited in Russian folklore is that of Vassilief, who had 84 children with his two successive wives (four cases of quadruplets and seven cases of triplets)[26]. In this instance the circumstances were reported to Czarina Ekaterina Maximova, the Empress Catherine by the Abbott of a remote monastery and the patient and Vassilief's children were examined by competent physicians attached to the Imperial Court. More recently, Nichols[11] and Waksman et al.[20] have cited similar cases.

Other factors that reputedly predispose to multifetal pregnancies include the following: maternal marital status (pregnancies in or out of wedlock)[4,29]; rural vs. city residency[4,25,29]; prior high fertility of the couple[29,31–33]; maternal anthropometric factors (tall, heavy, high level of gonadotropin)[29]; discontinuation of oral contraception[34–36]; and finally, seasonal and climatic variations (more pronounced for triplets than for twins)[13,23,31,37].

Current trends in rates

After a decline in the rate of multiple pregnancies between 1940 and 1970, most probably due to a general decrease in parity and maternal age[5,22–25,38–40], the impact of ovulation stimulants in France, Great Britain and Japan resulted in a 2- to 3-fold increase in the number of triplet pregnancies and a 10- to 20-fold increase in quadruplet pregnancies[24,38,41,42]. In the United States between 1978 and 1988, the number of twin pregnancies increased by 33% and triplets by 101%. This increase was attributed to the large numbers of women over age 35 who were having children and the fact that many of them also used ovulation-enhancing agents (B. Luke, personal communication, 1993).

A survey conducted in France between 1985 and 1989 reported 298 cases of triplet pregnancies after medically assisted reproduction (as compared to roughly 80 natural triplet pregnancies per year in France). These figures do not take into account the effect of embryo reduction, which has been estimated to occur in one case out of three of higher-order multiples[43].

A review of published data provides the following rates of higher-order multiple pregnancies after various treatments to induce ovulation[44–50]: clomiphene: 0.5% triplet pregnancies and 0.5% higher-order pregnancies; hMG–hCG: 5–10% of pregnancies equal to or higher than three; *in vitro* fertilization (IVF): roughly 6% triplet pregnancies after replacing three embryos[43,51-55]; gamete intra-fallopian transfer (GIFT): roughly 8.5% pregnancies with three or more embryos[27,56-59]. In France the rate of triplet or higher-order pregnancies obtained by medically assisted procreation (MAP) (Editor: This term is assisted reproductive technology (ART) in US literature) is 6% before reduction[43].

Management of triplet and quadruplet pregnancies

No consensus exists regarding management of triplet or quadruplet gestations. Indeed, the literature is relatively scant, especially considering the increased numbers of these pregnancies in recent years (see above), and their important contribution to perinatal morbidity and mortality (see Chapters 10 and 12). The published literature comprises only 22 small studies, which vary in size from 8 to 61 cases, and four multicentric studies with 65 to 454 cases. Most were conducted over a 15–20-year period, during which time numerous important changes occurred in medical practice, thus making their interpretation difficult by present-day standards.

Diagnosis

The major advantage provided by the early diagnosis of multifetal gestation is the ability to instigate preventive measures to reduce the likelihood of preterm delivery as soon as possible. In older studies, the diagnosis of multiple pregnancy was either made at delivery or by taking X-rays of the uterus[49,60-62]. More recently, the use of ultrasound has made early diagnosis possible in virtually 100% of cases. In one report, for example, the mean gestational age for ultrasound diagnosis was around 9 weeks for 29 triplet pregnancies[49].

Botting et al.[63] reported that when an ultrasound scan is performed before 12 weeks of amenorrhea, multiple pregnancies can be diagnosed in 96% of the cases, and the precise number of embryos can be determined in 64% of the cases. In this study, however, only 26% of the triplet pregnancies and 38% of the quadruplet pregnancies, respectively, were recognized as multiple pregnancies before 12 weeks of amenorrhea. Correct diagnosis was made before delivery by ultrasound in 87% of the triplet pregnancies and 64% of the quadruplet pregnancies, and by X-ray in 6.6% and 20% of the cases, respectively. Even when ultrasound is used to establish the diagnosis, a repeat examination is advised prior to the 20th week, to ensure that the original number was not underestimated or that one or more embryos of a triplet or higher-order gestation was not spontaneously resorbed (see Chapters 5, 6 and 14 for further discussion).

Fetal complications

The over-riding problem of triplet and higher-order multiple gestations is preterm delivery. In the case of triplet gestations, the rate of preterm delivery varies between 75 and 100%. The average length of gestation is 34 weeks. In two recent multicentric studies[63,64], 20% and 37% of the triplet pregnancies ended before 32 weeks, respectively. Three studies report a lower mean length of gestation for primiparae[65-67].

As early as 1982, Holcberg et al.[60] suggested that women who received ovulation induction treatment delivered significantly later than women who conceived spontaneously. A similar observation was made by Luke et al.[68] in a 10-year review of twin births at The Johns Hopkins Medical Institutions in the USA. In both reports, however, patients who underwent ovulation induction had earlier diagnosis, more intensive antenatal care and more frequent hospitalization. In contrast, Syrop and Varner[62] as well as Ron-el et al.[67] reported that birth was significantly later in cases of natural multiple pregnancies. These latter authors also indicated that the mortality rate was lower for spontaneous cases compared to induced triplets[67].

In the study of triplets reported from Clamart, France[69], induced pregnancies were found to have significantly longer gestation lengths than spontaneous pregnancies. In a study by Blanc et al.[70] this difference did not appear to be significant. For quadruplet pregnancies, the rate of prematurity is 100% and the mean length of gestation is 31 weeks[32].

Mortality In a study conducted between 1975 and 1983, Botting et al.[22] reported a 5% stillbirth and a 15% neonatal mortality rate, among triplets. This represents a neonatal risk 19 times higher than that of singletons. In this study, 76% of the triplets born in 1983 in England survived, compared to 69% in 1975. An unpublished compilation of the literature indicates that overall mortality is 17%. This figure includes 8.5% miscarriages before 28 weeks and 3.5% deaths *in utero*[71].

Prolonged pregnancies may be associated with fetal demise, presumably due to placental incompetence. This problem was first pointed out by Berg et al.[72] and confirmed by Botting et al.[22]. Newman et al.[64] and Blanc et al.[70] reported low mortality rates. In the study by Blanc et al., 2/61 000 deaths were due to loss *in utero*, and neonatal mortality was 80.3% for 1000 births. These authors reported an overall mortality of 67/1000, including miscarriages before 24 weeks. After 24 weeks, the rate of stillbirths was 22/1000 and neonatal mortality 28/1000[70]. These findings were obtained despite a mean length of gestation and a mean birth weight which did not differ from other cohorts. These results probably reflect the best outcomes reported by 1991. The study by Newman et al.[64] differs from the study by Blanc et al.[70] with fewer births before 28 weeks (6.6% vs. 11.1%) and a length of gestation ranging from 28 to 32 weeks (12.6% vs. 24.7%).

Botting et al.[22] reported that mortality in terms of birth weight was much lower for triplet pregnancies than for singletons: 48 per 1000 vs. 117 per 1000 between 1500 and 2500 g and 13.5 per 1000 vs. 32 per 1000 between 1000 and 1500 g.

Growth retardation Average triplet birth weight varies between 1474 and 2011 g; this range is primarily dependent on whether calculation includes late miscarriages or not. A global estimate of the frequency of growth retardation can be obtained by comparing the birth weight for triplet pregnancies with birth weights for singletons. Growth retardation (below the 10th percentile) occurs in 50% of all triplet-birth infants, and 25% exhibit severe growth retardation (below the 3rd percentile).

Blanc et al.[70] proposed some causes for the severe (25% <3rd percentile) growth retardation in triplets, namely maternal high blood pressure and malformations. However, the vast majority of their cases of growth retardation were not related to these problems. In the study by Blanc et al.[70] the percentage of growth-retarded infants was lower for natural pregnancies (21%) than for induced pregnancies (31.7%) or MAP pregnancies (47.3%). Growth retardation increases with gestational age and diminishes with parity.

Respiratory complications Hyaline membrane disease (HMD) is the main cause of mortality and morbidity in preterm infants[49,60,67,72]. Corticoids have generally been suggested as a treatment to reduce the morbidity and mortality from HMD[22,73]. A number of investigators have also used corticoids to prevent HMD in multiples[6,49,60,67,72,74–76]. In one published study, Pons et al.[69] compared 12 patients treated by corticoids and 12 untreated patients. Length of gestation was identical, and no hyaline membrane disease was observed in the group receiving treatment. Although the groups were not randomized, respiratory distress was significantly higher among the untreated patients.

Malformations Of 19 published studies, only seven reported severe lethal malformations. The overall rate of congenital malformations reported in these studies was 2.5%. These include: two pairs of conjoined twins[62,77], four hydrocephalic infants[71,78,79], three anencephalic infants[71,77,78], one spina bifida[77], one multiple hemangioma[77] and two unspecified lethal malformations[60,65].

Waksman et al.[20] and Onyskowova et al.[80] reported higher rates of overall malformations (6.8% and 5.75%, respectively), but Blanc et al.[70] presented a rate of 1.92% for major malformations in a triplet series. In the study reported by Botting et al.[63], the malformation rate for triplets was the same as that of the twin reference group, i.e. 4.47%.

Maternal complications

Toxemia Toxemia is described in 10–45% of cases in reported cohorts. In a recent multicenter study by Newman et al.[64], 28 (14%) of 198 women had Cesarean sections because of high blood pressure. Blanc et al.[70] reported a 16.6% rate of toxemia and a single case of eclampsia. Botting et al.[63] reported more cases of severe toxemia in quadruplet compared to triplet pregnancies.

Iron deficiency anemia Available data vary considerably. Kurtz et al.[81] reported anemia in 100% of the cases. Egwuatu[9] indicated 75%; other recruitments reported less than 50%[60,62,66,67,77,78,82].

Complications related to betamimetics Publications dealing with multifetal pregnancies have reported four cases of acute pulmonary edema[64,70,76] and one case of heart failure[70] after prolonged treatment with betamimetics. In these series, only five maternal complications were reported, despite the frequent use of betamimetics[20,60,61,64,66,67,70,74,76,83–85]. Of interest, articles describing problems related to betamimetics also reported other cardiovascular complications in women with multifetal pregnancies[83,85–93]. Indeed, according to some authors, the risk of cardiovascular complications is higher in cases of multiple pregnancies[94,95].

Other complications Several other complications have been reported. Some are secondary to ovulation induction; others are the problems of pregnancy in general. Reported complications include: ectopic pregnancies, hyperstimulation[59], cholestasis[70,96], urinary infections[20,30], renal insufficiency[81], bowel obstruction[70,97], thrombocytopenia[70] and respiratory distress[9,82]. Although severe maternal complications are fairly infrequent, many patients exhibit a variety of somatic complaints toward the end of pregnancy, including shortness of breath, weight gain, varices, stretch marks, pain in fingers and joints, hemorrhoids, etc.

Obstetric complications

Hydramnios is commonly cited as an obstetric complication, although percentages differ widely, from 6% for Blanc et al.[70] to 60% in the report by Daw[82]. Only a few studies reported problems of coagulation, placenta previa, or abruptio placenta[77,78,81]. In contrast, the frequency of postpartum hemorrhages ranged from lows of 5–10%[60,74], to highs of 25–30%[9,49,63]; three hysterectomies have been reported for uncontrollable bleeding[25,60,63]. In the postpartum period, Botting et al.[63] reported two hysterectomies out of 149 cases, postpartum complication rates of 8% for anemia, and 5% and 25% transfusions, respectively, in triplet and quadruplet pregnancies. These authors also reported 7% and 17% postpartum infection rates, in triplet and quadruplet pregnancies, respectively.

Prevention of prematurity

In the UK, vaginal examinations are not always routine. This situation also exists in other countries, including the USA. Despite this, Keith et al.[98] and other American authors[64] recommend routine vaginal examinations after 22 weeks in order to detect premature or 'precocious' dilatation and effacement of the cervix that may precede the onset of overt preterm labor. They also recommend external monitoring of 'silent' contractions, which also often increase in intensity and frequency prior to the onset of overt preterm labor (see Chapters 34 and 35).

Rest and hospitalization Studies on prophylactic bed rest show that this intervention does not appear to reduce the incidence of preterm labor in twin pregnancies[23,99,100]; neither does routine hospitalization[8,101,102]. However, a drop in rate of prematurity in infants born with birth weights of < 2500 g and a concomitant decline in perinatal morbidity have both been reported for women on regimens of strict bed rest[62,78], and these changes have been viewed as being valuable by themselves. The literature on the management of higher-order pregnancies (>2) provides no consensus on bed rest. A number of writers advise bed rest[20,62,67,78,81] or routine hospitalization[49,61,67,72,74,85]. Others propose that these methods should be replaced by close surveillance at home[20,64]. For example, in the report by Newman et al.[64] on home monitoring, hospitalization was not prescribed systematically and was only used in cases of complication or threatened preterm delivery. In this report, the use of home monitoring reduced hospital admissions in the third trimester by 83%. This dramatic change was accompanied by equally dramatic reductions in antenatal costs. Whereas the mean length of gestation and mean birth weight remained comparable to other cohorts, fetal prognosis was improved[64].

Cervical suture Opinions differ as to the usefulness of cerclage in the case of higher-order multiple pregnancies. Some authors argue for its use[20,61]; others report no improvement in length of gestation and believe this operation to be useless or even harmful, except in cases in which true cervical incompetence is present[49,67,77].

Two controlled trials show no advantage of cerclage in singleton pregnancies[103,104], and neither contained multiple pregnancies beyond twins. Controlled trials of cerclage in twin pregnancies are not in agreement. Weekes et al.[102] and Dor[105] reported that cerclage was not beneficial, whereas Zakut et al.[106] advise it.

Goldman et al.[74] compared 12 triplet pregnancies with cerclage against ten without it. These authors reported a significant difference in length of gestation (35 vs. 30.7 weeks), birth weight (2022 g vs. 1416 g), mortality and Apgar scores. Better results were obtained in the sutured group despite the fact that the non-sutured group had higher mean hospital stays than the sutured group. The study, however, was not a controlled trial.

Lipitz et al.[30] and Newman et al.[64] independently reported that the use of suture in the second trimester in cases of cervical alteration helped prolong pregnancy several weeks to reach a mean length of gestation between 29 and 30 weeks.

Tocolytic treatments with betamimetics Several authors advise betamimetics to prolong pregnancy in cases of threatened preterm delivery[60,98]. In Clamart[66], betamimetics are used in high-risk patients, but are monitored carefully with special precautions, such as restriction of intravenous fluid load and the use of flow regulators. No complications have been observed to date. Several other writers also use betamimetics in cases of true threatened preterm delivery[6,20,49,60,61,64,67,74,76,78,85], but rarely are these agents advised for prophylactic reasons[64,74].

Aside from the use of betamimetics in threatened preterm delivery, they are not recommended and have been shown to be inefficient for prophylaxis against preterm labor in twin pregnancies[100,107–111]. Newman et al.[64] reported no advantage in using prophylactic tocopherol treatment in multiple pregnancies.

A few publications mention the use of progestins[20,67,74], Indomethacin[76,112] or magnesium sulfate[64,112] as tocolytics for higher-order multifetal pregnancy.

Additional concerns

Supplements Systematic prescription of iron supplements, folic acids[25,66,74,76,112–114] as well as vitamins B and C[67,74,114] and high-calorie, high-protein diets[6,66,67,106] are often recommended, although none of these has been tested in controlled trials.

Ultrasound scans All recent publications recognize the diagnostic value of early ultrasound examinations. Surprisingly, little attention has been given to the major role of ultrasound scans in repetitive analyses of fetal biometry[115–117], morphological examinations for malformations, assessment of fetal well-being, and Doppler effect in higher-order multiples (see Chapters 14, 16 and 17).

Delivery

Vaginal delivery is characterized by a high number of operative maneuvers for abnormal fetal presentation. Review of the literature shows that a quarter of first triplets, as well as two out of five of second and third triplets, respectively, are in the breech presentation. Moreover, one out of ten of second triplets and one out of seven of third triplets are in irregular or transverse presentations.

Commonly used operative maneuvers include the following: forceps 30%, breech extractions 50% and internal podalic version 20%. One out of five of second or third triplets, respectively, is subject to breech extraction and one out of seven third triplets receives internal podalic version.

Several writers stress the sharp increase in mortality between the second and third triplets and the even sharper rise between the first and the third triplet in instances of vaginal delivery[9,60,62,77,81,82]. The nature of these differences was shown by Deale and Cronje[8] in a study of 367 triplet pregnancies: first triplet mortality 13%, second triplet mortality 15.4%, third triplet mortality 26.2%. These authors also report a significant difference in Apgar score as a function of birth rank. In contrast, this difference in mortality as a function of birth rank is not observed in the cases of Cesarean deliveries[20,64,66,78,118]. Similarly, Apgar scores and blood gas determinations do not differ as a function of birth rank[8,49,63,119,120].

Interestingly, the rate of Cesarean sections varies between 1.6%[61] and 94%[64] as a function of date of publication. The increase in Cesarean delivery has reduced morbidity and neonatal mortality[21,22,60,64,72,85,98]. Neonatal mortality ranges from 15 to 20% in older publications in which vaginal delivery was the general rule[49,60,62,67,77,82] to 3–10% for Cesarean deliveries.

In more recent reports on vaginal delivery, several authors stress the importance of reducing the interval between the births[49,61,65,81], because of the potential for decreased placental blood flow as a result of the progressive reduction in uterine size following the delivery of the first and second infant, respectively. The value of general anesthesia has been stressed to facilitate operative maneuvers[49,61,65,81], but some authors[20,61,65] prefer spinal over general anesthesia (see Chapters 37 and 38).

In practice, our group tries to schedule Cesarean sections as much as possible at 37 weeks using epidural analgesia. This is also the policy at the Pitié hospital[71] and in the patient population described by Keith *et al.*[78]. As in many institutions, we utilize newborn management systems formed by three teams of neonatologists. Neonatal prognosis is almost uniformly linked to complications from prematurity or to growth retardation. This is true at other institutions around the world as well as ours.

Quintuplet and higher-order pregnancies

Although the increased rate of these pregnancies has also been spectacular since the introduction of ovulation induction treatments, they are, nevertheless, rare. Whereas quintuplet pregnancies were practically unknown in France prior to 1971, 32 were recorded in the following 15 years (a rate of 1/4 000 000), as was one sextuplet pregnancy. In France, the exact number of pregnancies higher than four is not known, because the numbers of embryo reductions and miscarriages are not linked to the number of higher-order conceptions. This situation also exists in other industrialized nations such as the UK, USA, Belgium and Japan.

In 1966, Turksoy *et al.*[121] reported a septuplet pregnancy after hMG–hCG treatment for a woman with the Budd–Chiarri–Fromel syndrome; this pregnancy ended by miscarriage at 23 weeks. In the same year, Liggins and Ibbertson[122] reported an induced pregnancy with the same treatment in another woman with this condition. In this case, however, pregnancy was terminated at 34 weeks by vaginal delivery of five infants who survived.

Between 1966 and 1989, a total of 19 quintuplet pregnancies[19,49,71,84,87,90,122–126], five sextuplet[71,127–129], two septuplet[121,130], one octuplet[131] and one nonuplet[132] were reported. Of these, only one quintuplet pregnancy ensued after treatment by clomiphene alone; all the others occurred after ovulation induction with gonadotropins. Under-reporting of higher-order multiple pregnancies is common, although the successful conduct of such high-risk gestations at tertiary medical centers increases the likelihood that they are recorded in the literature. Whether the number of grand multiple pregnancies that deliver remains static or declines in the future is an open question, since the introduction of techniques for selective fetal reduction (see Chapters 25 and 26).

Diagnosis

The diagnosis of multifetal pregnancy is generally established by clinical or ultrasound examination at the end of the first trimester or the start of the second trimester. The diagnosis of the exact number of fetuses is often difficult and requires repeated examinations. Prior to 1980, diagnosis was generally performed by radiography, but doubt often existed as to the exact number of fetuses[125,127,129]. More recently, several ultrasound observations have occasionally been required to determine the precise number of fetuses[124,128,133]. Currently, early ultrasound scans most easily indicate the correct number of embryos[42,134-138] and these are almost invariably obtained after ovulation induction treatments (see Chapter 14 for further comments).

Whereas systematic ultrasound examination has long been advocated in Sweden to detect spontaneously occurring twin gestations (see Chapter 15), no such policies have been advocated for the detection of spontaneous triplet or higher–order gestations, as they could not be justified as being cost-effective. On the other hand, close attention to discrepancy between uterine size and the date of the last menstrual period is highly effective in suggesting which patients should have ultrasound examination, if such examinations are not routinely obtained.

Obstetric management

In all articles which provide detail, authors recommend bed rest and reduction of physical activity almost as soon as the diagnosis is made. Those who advise hospitalization do so between the 17th and the 25th week. The only exception is Tran-Ngoc et al.[133] who hospitalized a woman for a quintuplet pregnancy at 30 weeks for a delivery at 31 weeks. It is a matter of speculation whether gestation length could have been prolonged had bed rest been instituted earlier. Although the patients in the report by Newman et al.[64] were only hospitalized for obstetric indications, they were put to bed rest at home and a program of home uterine activity monitoring started. Many of those patients also had regular examinations of cervical status.

Routine treatment includes vitamin supplements[127,139], iron[15,49,90,119,123,127,129], sedatives[124,128,129,139], and a high-calorie, high-protein diet[124,139]. Early and adequate weight gain is important, because the majority of these pregnancies deliver preterm. Monnier et al.[124] describe the unusual case of a sextuplet pregnancy which had to be terminated at 22 weeks, because of maternal loss of weight. Cerclage is uncommonly reported[124,125], but many authors recommend tocolysis by betamimetics[125,126,128,129,133,139] and corticoids to prevent hyaline membrane disease[124-126,128,138,139].

Complications of quintuplet and sextuplet pregnancies

No published data exist on the number of early miscarriages in these pregnancies, although Shenker et al.[125] reported two late miscarriages out of five quintuplet pregnancies (see Chapter 25).

Out of 16 detailed reports in the literature[84,90,122-129,133,139], only seven instances of hyperstimulations are described. Much more commonly, these pregnancies are characterized by high rates of maternal anemia and minor discomforts of pregnancy, including insomnia, abdominal and back pains, dependent edema not related to toxemia, difficulty in breathing[90,122,126,128] and maternal toxemia[90,123,125,127].

Delivery

Vaginal delivery has occasionally been reported[84,90,122], albeit accompanied by various operative maneuvers. Most authors advocate planned Cesarean delivery to lessen fetal risk due to potential trauma of obstetric maneuvers, hypoxia, hemorrhage due to placental detachment during delivery, and to decrease maternal risks of hemorrhage due to atony and postpartum infection. Cesarean sections are, however, not entirely risk-free[127], as postpartum atony may be so severe as to require multiple transfusion and/or hysterectomy. Several authors describe the need to provide for a pediatric team consisting of a minimum of two persons per newborn. Teams such as these must develop elaborate plans for notification of all personnel in the event of an unplanned preterm birth. During operations, the mother of a grand multiple pregnancy may find herself surrounded by as many as 20 or more physicians, ten or more nurses, three or four anesthesiologists and numerous technicians. It is little wonder that many women are exhausted and depressed when the delivery is over and they are left to recover.

Gestation, birth weight and mortality

The mean length of gestation for quintuplet and sextuplet pregnancies as reported in the literature is 32.8 weeks and ranges between 31 and 35 weeks. Of seven women who received betamimetic tocolysis, the mean length of gestation was 33.2 weeks compared to five others not administered drugs, who had a mean gestation length of 32 weeks. Three women who had cerclage had gestation lengths of 32, 33 and 34 weeks. The mean birth weights for the 12 quintuplet and sextuplet pregnancies (63 infants) was 1370 g and ranged from 1050 to 1800 g for live infants.

Botting *et al.*[22] evaluated the mortality rates for higher-order pregnancies lasting beyond 28 weeks. There were 16 survivors out of 20 quintuplet infants. One septuplet pregnancy had six surviving infants, and in another similar case, no infant survived. This last pregnancy ended at 23 weeks by a miscarriage. The one reported octuplet pregnancy[131] was treated by bed rest, hospitalization at 28 weeks, repeated transfusions and corticoid treatments, and terminated by Cesarean section at 33 weeks. Five infants survived, and three were stillborn. At the age of 2, the five survivors were developing normally. The one reported nonuplet pregnancy[132] was complicated by severe anemia and pre-eclampsia and terminated by a miscarriage at 25 weeks.

Numerous authors call attention to the difficult management of these pregnancies, of the high degree of parental anxiety, long hospital stays, and invasion of privacy by the media if the pregnancy is not kept secret.

Prevention of higher-order gestations

Currently most higher-order multiple pregnancies are iatrogenic and their frequency can be reduced. Several groups[45,71,140,141] advocate that close monitoring of ovulation by ultrasound and hormone assays could successfully avoid the majority of these pregnancies.

With regard to MAP (ART), the dilemma lies between the risk of a multiple pregnancy and the increase in success rate as a function of the number of embryos transferred. The 1989 French statistics document that one embryo transfer results in 9% pregnancies, whereas with five or more embryos transferred, the rate of pregnancies is 33%[43]. Factors favorable to multiple pregnancies include maternal age under 35, rate of fecundation higher than 75% and IVF with donor[142]. By considering these data, along with the possibility of embryo freezing, a transfer strategy can be developed that should make it possible to restrict or eliminate the risk of triplet or higher-order pregnancies[142]. In any case, it is crucial to inform couples who request these technologies of the risks related to higher-order pregnancies. Couples should also be informed of the possibility of embryo reduction (see Chapters 25, 26 and 49).

References

1. Lacomme, M. (1960). *Pratique Obstétricale.* (Paris: Masson)
2. Luke, B. and Keith, L. (1992). The contribution of singletons, twins and triplets to low birthweight, infant mortality and handicap in the United States. *Int. J. Obstet. Gynaecol.*, **37**, 661
3. Zeleny, C. (1921). The relative number of twins and triplets. *Science*, **53**, 262
4. Miettinen, M. (1954). On triplet and quadruplet pregnancies in Finland. *Acta Paediatr. (Suppl.)*, **99**, 23
5. Imaizumi, Y. and Inouye, E. (1984). Multiple birth rates in Japan. Further analysis. *Acta Genet. Med. Gemellol.*, **33**, 107
6. Shennan, A.T., Milligan, J.E. and Yeung, P.K. (1979). Successful management of a quadruplet pregnancy in a perinatal unit. *Can. Med. Assoc. J.*, **22**, 741
7. Cox, M.L. (1963). Incidence and aetiology of multiple births in Nigeria. *J. Obstet. Gynaecol. Br. Commonwlth.*, **70**, 878
8. Deale, C.J.C. and Cronje, H.S. (1984). A review of 367 triplet pregnancies. *S. Afr. Med. J.*, **66**, 92
9. Egwuatu, V.E. (1980). Triplet pregnancy: a review of 27 cases. *Int. J. Gynaecol. Obstet.*, **18**, 460
10. Guttmacher, A.F. (1953). The incidence of multiple births in man and some of other unipara. *Obstet. Gynecol.*, **2**, 22
11. Nichols, J.B. (1953). Plural births in the United States. *West J. Surg.*, **61**, 229
12. Nylander, P.S. (1971). The incidence of triplets and higher multiple births in some rural and urban populations in Western Nigeria. *Ann. Hum. Genet.*, **34**, 409
13. Rehan, N. and Tafida, D.S. (1980). Multiple births in Hausa women. *Br. J. Obstet. Gynaecol.*, **87**, 997
14. Davies, P.A. and Davis, J.P. (1970). Very low birth-weight and subsequent head growth. *Lancet*, **2**, 1216
15. Berbos, J.N., King, B.F., Janusz, A. *et al.* (1984). Quintuplet pregnancy. *J. Am. Med. Assoc.*, **188**, 813
16. Ahlgren, M., Kallen, B. and Rannevik, G. (1976). Outcome of pregnancy after clomiphene therapy. *Acta Obstet. Gynecol. Scand.*, **55**, 371
17. Mayer, C.F. (1952). Sextuplet and higher multiparous birth, a critical review of history and legend from Aristotle to the 20th century, Part 1. *Acta Genet. Med. Gemellol.*, **1**, 118
18. Mayer, C.F. (1952). Sextuplet and higher multiparous birth, a critical review of history and legend from Aristotle to the 20th century, Part 2. *Acta Genet. Med. Gemellol.*, **1**, 242
19. Waksman, S., Bouchard, P. and Monnier, J.C. (1990). Les grossesses multifoetales. 1. Mythes et réalités. *J. Gynecol. Obstet. Biol. Reprod.*, **19**, 261
20. Waksman, S., Bouchard, P., Patey-Savatier, P. *et al.* (1990). Les grossesses multifoetales. II. Epidémiologie, aspects cliniques. *J. Gynecol. Obstet. Biol. Reprod.*, **19**, 383
21. Waksman, S., Bouchard, P., Fonteyne, G. *et al.* (1990). Les grossesses multifoetales. III. Aspects thérapeutiques, psychologiques et sociaux. *J. Gynecol. Obstet. Biol. Reprod.*, **19**, 667
22. Botting, B.J., MacDonald Davies, I. and MacFarlane, A.J. (1987). Recent trends in the incidence of multiple births and associated mortality. *Arch. Dis. Child.*, **62**, 941
23. Czeizel, A. (1973). Unexplainable demographic phenomena of multiple births in Hungary. *Acta Genet. Med. Gemellol. (Suppl.)*, **22**, 214
24. Elwood, J.M. (1985). Maternal and environmental factors affecting twin birth in Canadian cities. *Br. J. Obstet. Gynaecol.*, **26**, 351
25. Rola-Janichi, A. (1973). Multiple births in Poland in 1949–1971. *Acta Genet. Med. Gemellol. (Suppl.)*, **22**, 202
26. *Le Livre des Records Guinness 1990* (1989). Edition numéro 1. (Paris)
27. Craft, I., Al-Shawaf, T., Lewis, P. *et al.* (1988). Analysis of 1071 gift procedures – the case for a flexible approach to treatment. *Lancet*, **1**, 1094
28. Derom, R., Cameron, A.H., Edwards, J.H. *et al.* (1983). Zygosity and genetic anomalies in twins. *Eur. J. Obstet. Gynaecol. Reprod. Biol.*, **15**, 261
29. MacGillivray, I. (1986). Epidemiology of twin pregnancy. *Semin. Perinat.*, **10**, 4
30. Lipitz, S., Reichman, B., Paret, G. *et al.* (1989). The improving outcome of triplet pregnancy. *Am. J. Obstet. Gynecol.*, **162**, 1279

31. Kamimura, K. (1976). Epidemiology of twin births from a climatic point of view. *Br. J. Prev. Soc. Med.*, **30**, 175, .
32. Petrikovski, B.M. and Vintzileos, A.M. (1989). Management of multiple pregnancy of high foetal order: literature review. *Obstet. Gynecol. Surv.*, **44**, 578
33. Shelden, R., Kemman, E., Boherer, M. *et al.* (1988). Multiple gestation is associated with the use of high sperm numbers in the intrauterine insemination specimen in women undergoing gonadotropin stimulation. *Fertil. Steril.*, **49**, 607
34. Bracken, B.M. (1979). Oral contraception and twinning: an epidemiologic study. *Am. J. Obstet. Gynecol.*, **133**, 432
35. Hemon, D., Berger, C. and Lazar, P. (1981). Twinning following oral contraceptive discontinuation. *Int. J. Epidemiol.*, **10**, 319
36. Rothman, K.J. (1977). Fetal loss, twinning and birth weight after oral-contraceptive use. *N. Engl. J. Med.*, **297**, 468
37. Selvin, S. and Janerich, D.T. (1972). Seasonal variations in twin births. *Nature (London)*, **237**, 289
38. Blondel, B. and Kaminski, M. (1988). Les accouchements multiples en France. *J. Gynecol. Obstet. Biol. Reprod.*, **17**, 1106
39. Elwood, J.M. (1983). The end of the drop in twinning rates. *Lancet*, **1**, 470
40. James, W. (1982). Second survey of secular trends in twinning rates. *J. Biosoc. Sci.*, **14**, 481
41. Imaizumi, Y. (1987). Recent trends in multiple births and stillbirth rates in Japan. *Acta Genet. Med. Gemellol.*, **36**, 325
42. Martenne-Duplan, J., Aknin, A.J. and Alamowitch, R. (1983). Aspiration embryonnaire partielle au cours de grossesses multiples. *Contr. Fert. Sex.*, **11**, 745
43. Buvat, J., Buvat-Herbaut, M. and Dancoine, F. (1990). Bilan des PMA en France en 1989 (enquête GEFF). *Contr. Fert. Sex.*, **18**, 583
44. Andrews, M.C., Muasher, S.J., Levy, D.L. *et al.* (1986). An analysis of the obstetric outcome of 125 consecutive pregnancies conceived *in vitro* and resulting in 100 deliveries. *Am. J. Obstet. Gynecol.*, **154**, 848
45. Cabau, A. and Bessis, R. (1982). Surveillance échographique de l'induction de l'ovulation par HMG–HCG. *Contr. Fert. Sex.*, **10**, 859
46. Caspi, E., Ronen, J., Schreyer, P. *et al.* (1976). The outcome of pregnancy after gonadotrophin therapy. *Br. J. Obstet. Gynaecol.*, **83**, 967
47. Hack, M., Brish, M., Serr, M. *et al.* (1970). Outcome of pregnancy after induced ovulation. *J. Am. Med. Assoc.*, **211**, 791
48. Konefa, H. (1973). Multiple pregnancy induced by ovary hyper-stimulation. *Acta Genet. Med. Gemellol.* (Suppl.), **22**, 193
49. Loucopoulos, A. and Jewelewicz, R. (1982). Management of multifetal pregnancies: sixteen years' experience at the Sloane Hospital for Women. *Am. J. Obstet. Gynecol.*, **143**, 902
50. Schenker, J.G., Kaern, J. and Hansen, P.K. (1985). Intrauterine growth in twin pregnancies: prediction of fetal growth retardation. *Obstet. Gynecol.*, **66**, 63
51. Australian *In Vitro* Fertilisation Collaborative Group. (1988). *In-vitro* fertilisation pregnancies in Australia and New Zealand, 1979–1985. *Med. J. Austr.*, **148**, 429
52. Australian *In Vitro* Fertilisation Collaborative Group. (1985). High incidence of preterm births and early losses in pregnancy after *in vitro* fertilisation. *Br. Med. J.*, **291**, 1160
53. F.I.V.N.A.T. (1990). Bilan 1989 et bilan général 1986–89. *Contr. Fert. Sex.*, **18**, 558
54. Speirs, A.L., Lopata, A., Gronow, M.J. *et al.* (1983). Analysis of the benefits and risks of multiple embryo transfer. *Fertil. Steril.*, **39**, 468
55. Walters, D.E., Edwards, R.G. and Meistrich, M.L. (1985). A statistical evaluation of implantation after replacing one or more human embryos. *J. Reprod. Fertil.*, **74**, 557
56. Craft, I., Brindsen, P., Lewis, P. *et al.* (1988). Multiple pregnancy, selective reduction, flexible treatment. *Lancet*, **2**, 1087
57. Craft I., Brindsen, P., Simons, E.G. *et al.* (1988). Limitations of GIFT. *Lancet*, **1**, 183
58. Craft, I., Brindsen, P., Simons, E.G. *et al.* (1987). How many oocytes/embryos should be transferred? *Lancet*, **2**, 109
59. Zorn, J.R., Barata, M., Brami, C. *et al.* (1988). Transfert intratubaire de gamètes (GIFT). Résultats d'une série continue de 105 cycles avec stimulation programmée associant D-Trp-6-LH-RH et gonadotrophines. *Contr. Fert. Sex.*, **16**, 367
60. Holcberg, G., Biale, Y., Lewenthal, H. *et al.* (1982). Outcome of pregnancy in 31 triplet gestations. *Obstet. Gynecol.*, **59**, 472
61. Pheiffer, E.L. and Golan, A. (1979). Triplet pregnancy. A 10 year review of cases at Baragwanath hospital. *S. Afr. Med. J.*, **55**, 843
62. Syrop, C.H. and Varner, M.W. (1985). Triplet gestation: maternal and neonatal implications. *Acta Genet. Med. Gemellol.*, **34**, 81

63. Botting, B.J., MacFarlane, A.J. and Price, F. (1991). *Three, Four and More; A Study of Triplet and High-order Birth*. (London: Her Majesty's Stationery Office)
64. Newman, R.B., Hamer, C. and Miller, C. (1989). Outpatient triplet management: a contemporary review. *Am. J. Obstet. Gynecol.*, **161**, 547
65. Michlewitz, H., Kennedy, J., Kawada, C. *et al.* (1981). Triplet pregnancies. *J. Reprod. Med.*, **26**, 243
66. Pons, J.C., Fernandez, H., Diochin, P. *et al.* (1989). Prise en charge des grossesses triples. *J. Gynecol. Obstet. Biol. Reprod.*, **18**, 72
67. Ron-el, R., Caspi, E., Schreyer, P. *et al.* (1981). Triplet and quadruplet pregnancies and management. *Obstet. Gynecol.*, **57**, 458
68. Luke, B., Damewood, M. and Keith, L.G. (1995). Maternal characteristics in women delivered of twins, natural vs induced. *Int. J. Fertil.*, in press
69. Pons, J.C., Mayenga, J.M., Plu G. *et al.* (1988). Management of triplet pregnancy. *Acta Genet. Med. Gemellol.*, **37**, 99
70. Blanc, B., Boubli, L. and Nadal, F. (1991). Grossesses triples en France. In Papiernik, E. and Pons, J.C. (eds.) *Les Grossesses Multiples*, pp. 283–99. (Paris: Doin)
71. Laurent, Y. (1989). Etude d'une série de 17 grossesses triples et 2 quadruples. Revue de la littérature. Unpublished data
72. Berg, G., Finnstrom, O. and Selbing, A. (1983). Triplet pregnancies in Linköping, Sweden, 1973–1981. *Acta Genet. Med. Gemellol.*, **32**, 251
73. Liggins, C.G. and Howie, R.N. (1972). A controlled trial of antepartum glycocorticoid treatment for prevention of the respiratory distress syndrome in premature infants. *Pediatrics*, **50**, 515
74. Goldman, G., Dicker, D., Peleg, D. *et al.* (1989). Is elective cerclage justified in the management of triplet and quadruplet pregnancy? *Austr. NZ J. Obstet. Gynecol.*, **29**, 9
75. Goldman, J.A., Felberg, D., Ashkenasi, J. *et al.* (1987). Multiple pregnancy after *in-vitro* fertilisation and embryo transfer: report of a quadruplet pregnancy and delivery. *Hum. Reprod.*, **2**, 511
76. Vervliet, J., De Cleyn, K., Renier, M. *et al.* (1989). Management and outcome of 21 triplet and quadruplet pregnancies. *Eur. J. Obstet. Gynecol. Reprod. Biol.*, **33**, 61
77. Itzkowic, D. (1979). A survey of 59 triplet pregnancies. *Br. J. Obstet. Gynaecol.*, **86**, 23
78. Keith, L.G., Ameli, S., Depp, O.R. *et al.* (1988). The Northwestern University Triplet Study II: fourteen triplet pregnancies delivered between 1981 and 1986. *Acta Genet. Med. Gemellol.*, **37**, 65
79. Ogburn, P.L., Julian, T.M., Williams, P.P. *et al.* (1986). The use of magnesium sulfate for tocolysis in preterm labor complicated by twin gestation and betamimetic induced pulmonary edema. *Acta Obstet. Gynecol. Scand.*, **65**, 793
80. Onyskowova, Z., Dolezal, A. and Jedlicka, V. (1971). The frequency and the character of malformations in the multiple birth (a preliminary report). *Teratology*, **4**, 496
81. Kurtz, G.R., Davis, L.L. and Loftus, J.B. (1958). Factors influencing the survival of triplets. *Obstet. Gynecol.*, **12**, 5
82. Daw, E. (1978). Triplet pregnancy. *Br. J. Obstet. Gynaecol.*, **85**, 505
83. Berland, M., Rudigoz, R.C., Partensky, E. *et al.* (1980). Ischémie myocardique après ingestion de salbutamol au cours du troisième trimestre de la grossesse. *J. Gynecol. Obstet. Biol. Reprod.*, **9**, 397
84. Bienarz, J., Shah, N., Dmowski, P. *et al.* (1978). Premature labor treatment with ritodrine in multiple pregnancy with three or more fetuses. *Acta Obstet. Gynecol. Scand.*, **57**, 25
85. Boulot, P., Hedon, B., Pelicia, G. *et al.* (1990). Comparaison des données obstétricales de 33 grossesses triples non réduites à 28 grossesses triples réduites. *Contr. Fert. Sex.*, **18**, 668
86. Blum, M. and Belhassen, R. (1981). Un cas de complication du traitement par Ritodrine chez une cardiaque non diagnostiquée hospitalisée pour contractions prématurées. *Rev. Fr. Gynecol. Obstet.*, **75**, 251
87. Crosby, E.T. and Elliot, R.D. (1988). Anaesthesia for Caesarean section in a parturient with quintuplet gestation, pulmonary oedema and thrombocytopenia. *Can. J. Anaesth.*, **35**, 417
88. Edouté, Y., Blumenfeld, Z., Bronstein, M. *et al.* (1987). Peripartum congestive cardiomyopathy and endocardial fibroelastosis associated with Ritodrine treatment. *J. Reprod. Med.*, **32**, 793
89. Elliot, H.R. and Abdulla, U. (1978). Pulmonary oedema associated with ritodrine infusion and betamethasone administration in premature labour. *Br. Med. J.*, **2**, 799
90. Jewelewicz, R., James, S.L., Finster, M. *et al.* (1972). Quintuplet gestation after ovulation induction with menopausal gonadotropins and pituitary luteinizing hormone. *J. Obstet. Gynecol.*, **40**, 1

91. Katz, M., Robertson, P.A. and Creasy, R. (1981). Cardiovascular complications associated with terbutaline treatment for preterm labor. *Am. J. Obstet. Gynecol.*, **139**, 605
92. Parer, S., Jullien, Y., Rochette, A. *et al.* (1983). Cardiomyopathie du post partum attribuée à l'usage des betamimetiques. *Ann. Fr. Anesth. Réanim.*, **2**, 86
93. Stubblefield, P.G. (1978). Pulmonary edema occurring after therapy with dexamethasone and terbutaline for premature labor: a case report. *Am. J. Obstet. Gynecol.*, **132**, 341
94. Benedetti, T.J. (1983). Maternal complications of parenteral β-sympathomimetic therapy for premature labor. *Am. J. Obstet. Gynecol.*, **145**, 1
95. Monod, J.F. and De Grandi, P. (1981). Tocoluse par les betamimetiques et cardiopathies. *J. Gynecol. Obstet. Biol. Reprod.*, **10**, 493, .
96. Brown, G. and Daw, E. (1990). Some aspects of triplet pregnancies in England and Wales, 1971–1975. *Br. J. Clin. Pract.*, **34**, 134
97. Dan, U., Rabinovici, J., Koller, M. *et al.* (1988). Iatrogenic mechanical ileus due to over-distended uterus. *Gynecol. Obstet. Invest.*, **25**, 143
98. Keith, L.G., Ameli S. and Keith, D.M. (1988). The Northwestern University Triplet Study I: overview of the international literature. *Acta Genet. Med. Gemellol.*, **37**, 55
99. Fitzhardinge, P. and Senterre, J. (1983). The very-low-birthweight infants: challenges and dilemmas. *Eur. J. Obstet. Gynecol. Reprod. Biol.*, **15**, 281
100. Newton, E.R. (1986). Anterpartum care in multiple gestation. *Semin. Perinat.*, **10**, 19
101. Saunders, M.C., Dick, J.S., McLBrown, I. *et al.* (1985). The effects of hospital admission for bed rest on the duration of twin pregnancy: a randomised trial. *Lancet*, **2**, 793
102. Weekes, A.R.L., Menzies, D.N. and De Boer, C.H. (1977). The relative efficacy of bed rest, cervical suture, and no treatment in the management of twin pregnancy. *Br. J. Obstet. Gynaecol.*, **84**, 161
103. Lazar, P., Gueguen, S., Dreyfus, J. *et al.* (1984). Multicentred controlled trial of cervical cerclage in women at moderate risk of preterm delivery. *Br. J. Obstet. Gynaecol.*, **91**, 731
104. Rush, R.W., Isaacs, S., McTerhon, K. *et al.* (1984). Randomised controlled trial of cervical cerclage in women at high risk of spontaneous preterm delivery. *Br. J. Obstet. Gynaecol.*, **91**, 724
105. Dor, J. (1982). Elective cervical suture of twin pregnancies diagnosed ultrasonically in the first trimester following induced ovulation. *Gynecol. Obstet. Invest.*, **13**, 55
106. Zakut, H., Insler, V. and Seer, D.M. (1977). Elective cervical suture in preventing premature delivery in multiple pregnancies. *Isr. J. Med. Sci.*, **13**, 488
107. Gummerus, M. and Halonnen, O. (1987). Prophylactic long term oral tocolysis of multiple pregnancies. *Br. J. Obstet. Gynaecol.*, **984**, 249
108. Marivate, M., De Villiers, K.Q. and Fairbrother, P. (1977). Effects of prophylactic outpatient administration of fenoterol on the time of spontaneous labor and fetal growth rate in twin pregnancy. *Am. J. Obstet. Gynecol.*, **128**, 707
109. O'Connor, M.C., Murphy H. and Dalrymple, I.J. (1979). Double blind trial of ritodrine and placebo in twin pregnancy. *Br. J. Obstet. Gynaecol.*, **86**, 706
110. Prescott, P. (1980). Sensitivity of a double-blind trial of ritodrine and placebo in twin pregnancy. *Br. J. Obstet. Gynaecol.*, **87**, 393
111. Skjaerris, J. and Aberg, A. (1982). Prevention of prematurity in twins by orally administered Terbutaline. *Acta Obstet. Gynecol. Scand.*, **108**, 39
112. Thiery, M., Kermans, G. and Derom, R. (1988). Triplet and higher order birth: what is the optimal delivery route? *Acta Genet. Med. Gemellol.*, **37**, 89
113. MacFee, J.G., Lord, E.L., Jeffrey, R.L. *et al.* (1974). Multiple gestations of high fetal number. *Obstet. Gynecol.*, **44**, 99
114. Wu, I.H., Kenneweg, W. and Langer, A. (1983). Successful management of a quadruplet pregnancy, a case report. *J. Reprod. Med.*, **28**, 163
115. Nylander, P.T.S. (1983). *The Phenomenon of Twinning.* (London: Academic Press)
116. Secher, N.J., Kaern, J. and Hansen, P.K. (1985). Intrauterine growth in twin pregnancies: prediction of fetal growth retardation. *Obstet. Gynecol.*, **66**, 63
117. Tournaire, M., Breart, G., Papiernik, E. *et al.* (1980). Apport de l'échographie en obstétrique. *Med. Hyg.*, **38**, 1717
118. Feingold, R. (1986). Mode of delivery in multiple birth of high order. Presented at *5th International Congress of the International Society for Twins and Twin Studies*, Amsterdam, The Netherlands, September
119. Antoine, C., Kirshenbaum, N.W. and Young, B.K. (1986). Biochemical differences related

to birth order in triplets. *J. Reprod. Med.*, **31**, 330

120. Collins, J.W., Merrick, D., David, R.J. et al. (1988). The Northwestern University Triplet Study III: neonatal outcome. *Acta Genet. Med, Gemellol.*, **37**, 77
121. Turksoy, R.N., Toy, B.L., Rogers, J. et al. (1967). Birth of septuplets following human gonadotropin administration in Chiari–Frommel Syndrome. *Obstet. Gynecol.*, **30**, 692
122. Liggins, G.C. and Ibbertson, H.K. (1966). A successful quintuplet pregnancy following treatment with human pituitary gonadotrophin. *Lancet*, **1**, 114
123. Campbell, S. and Dewhurst, C.J. (1970). Quintuplet pregnancy diagnosed and assessed by ultrasonic compound scanning. *Lancet*, **1**, 101
124. Monnier, J.C., Lanciaux, B., Boulogne, M. et al. (1980). Problèmes posés par la surveillance d'une grossesse quintuple. *Rev. Fr. Gynecol.*, **75**, 4
125. Schenker, J.G., Laufer, N., Weinstein, D. et al. (1980). Quintuplet pregnancy. *Eur. J. Obstet. Gynecol. Reprod. Biol.*, **10**, 257
126. Vafai, J. and Shapiro, D.L. (1985). Perinatal aspects of high multiple gestation. *NY State J. Med.*, **85**, 560
127. Aiken, R.A. (1969). An account of the Birmingham sextuplet. *J. Obstet. Gynaecol. Br. Commonwlth.*, **76**, 684
128. Gutowitz, H.E., Ballie, P., Harrison, V. et al. (1974). Sextuplet gestation, a case report. *S. Afr. Med. J.*, **48**, 1449
129. Lachelin, G.C.L., Brandt, H.A., Swier, G.I.M. et al. (1972). Sextuplet pregnancy. *Br. Med. J.*, **1**, 787
130. Fedorkow, D.M., Corenblum, B., Pattinson, H.A. et al. (1988). Septuplet gestation following the use of human menopausal gonadotropin despite intensive monitoring. *Fertil. Steril.*, **49**, 364
131. Serreyn, R., Thiery, M. and Vandekerckove, D. (1984). Outcome of an octuplet pregnancy. *Arch. Gynecol.*, **234**, 283
132. Garrett, W.J., Carey, H.M., Stevans, L.H. et al. (1988). A case of nonuplet pregnancy. *Aust. NZ J. Obstet Gynecol.*, **71**, 289
133. Tran-Ngoc, T., De Watteville, H., Beguin, F. et al. (1980). Grossesse quintuple. *Méd. Hyg.*, **38**, 1717
134. Berkowitz, R.L., Lynch, L., Chitkara, U. et al. (1988). Selective reduction of multifetal pregnancies in the first trimester. *N. Eng. J. Med.*, **318**, 1043
135. Evans, M.I., Fletcher, J.C., Zador, I.E. et al. (1988). Selective first-trimester termination in octuplet and quadruplet pregnancies: clinical and ethical issues. *Obstet. Gynecol.*, **71**, 289
136. Itzkovitz, J., Boldes, R., Thaler, I. et al. (1989). Transvaginal ultrasonography guided aspiration of gestational sacs for selective abortion in multiple pregnancy. *Am. J. Obstet. Gynecol.*, **160**, 215
137. Jeny, R. and Leroy, B. (1983). Réduction sélective en cas de grossesse multiple. *Ann. Radiol.*, **25**, 446
138. Salat-Baroux, J., Aknin, J., Antoine, J.M. et al. (1988). The management of multiple pregnancies after induction for superovulation. *Hum. Reprod.*, **3**, 399
139. Nerl, A., Ovadia, Y., Friedman, S. et al. (1981). Medical, social and psychological aspects of quintuplet pregnancy and delivery. *Isr. J. Med. Sci.*, **17**, 5
140. Ritchie, W.G.M. (1985). Ultrasound in the evaluation of normal and induced ovulation. *Fertil. Steril.*, **43**, 167
141. Stone, S.C., Schimberni, M. and Schuster, P.A. (1987). Incidence of multiple gestations in the presence of two or more mature follicles in the conception cycle. *Fertil. Steril.*, **48**, 503
142. Arnal, F. and Cohen, J. (1990). Stratégie de transfert des embryons en FIV. *Contr. Fert. Sex.*, **18**, 598
143. Komai, T. and Fukuoka, G. (1936). Frequency of multiple births among the Japanese and related peoples. *Am. J. Phys. Anthropol.*, **21**, 433
144. Bulmer, M.G. (1970). *The Biology of Twinning in Man.* (Oxford: Clarendon Press)
145. Brackenbridge, C.J. (1978). Aspects of the increasing triplet rate in Australia. *J. Biosoc. Sci.*, **10**, 183

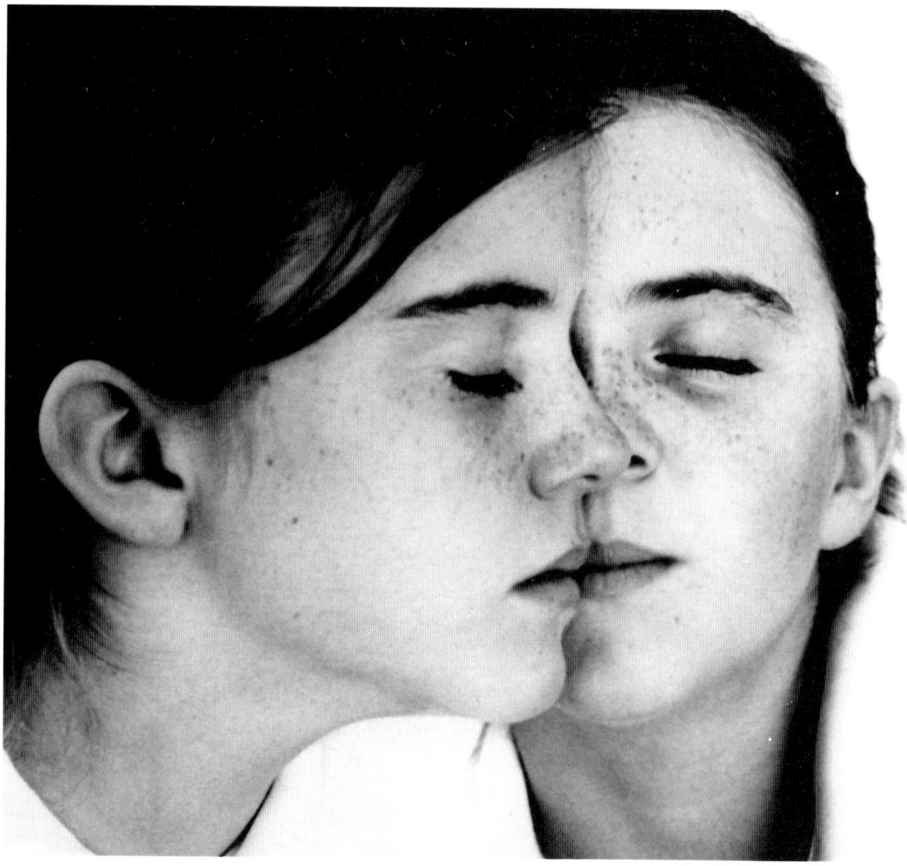

section VII
Postpartum Considerations

Monozygotic Fusion

David Teplica, 1989,
Collection of Lisa Jackley Dayton, Minneapolis, Minnesota

Breast feeding multiples

41

J.M. Wilton

Introduction

The benefits of breast feeding are well known. Despite this, current national data indicate that of the 54% of singleton mothers who initiate breast feeding in the United States, only 20% continue through 5–6 months[1]. Similarly, data indicate that, whereas 48% of mothers of twins initiated breast feeding in the hospital, only 13% continued through 6 months[1]. A recent published report observed that mothers of multiples generally breast fed at a lower rate and supplemented sooner than mothers of singletons[2]. Another report describing 28 mothers who gave birth to twins or triplets found that 42% began breast feeding, but that more than half stopped after the first few days and only 20% still breast fed their infants at 5 weeks of age[3].

Unfortunately, many mothers of multiples choose not to breast feed, because they incorrectly believe that it will take too much time or because they have been inadequately or inappropriately informed about proper breast feeding techniques and the comparable time required for feeding two infants with bottles. Indeed, many women who initially considered breast feeding change their minds after the diagnosis of twins is made, solely as a result of concerns about time. Although the actual time involved in breast feeding twins has been calculated as 5–7 h a day, a mother needs the same time to feed if she uses bottles and also needs another hour for warming bottles as well as two more for washing and sterilizing the bottles and preparing formula[4]. Moreover, whereas nursing support is generally available immediately after delivery for help with bottle feeding, once the mother leaves the hospital, she (and those at home with her) will need to feed the two infants at once. Understandably, any decision to breast or bottle feed should be based upon facts and well-founded information. Happily, mothers can breast feed both twins at the same time with safety. In contrast, she can only bottle feed them at the same time if their bottles are propped, and this technique is not considered safe. This chapter describes various issues surrounding the breast feeding of multiples and the best techniques to accomplish it.

Prenatal preparation

The advantages of breast feeding multiples are exactly the same as they are for singletons. These benefits should repeatedly be addressed in the antenatal period by every obstetrician or nurse-midwife. Repetition of this information, along with instruction, encouragement and support, not only helps the mother with breast feeding, but also goes a long way toward allaying her anxiety and that of her significant other[5,6].

In virtually all instances, the primary health care providers' instructions on breast feeding should be augmented by lay literature. Examples of recommended patient handouts and books are given in the Appendix.

A referral to Mothers or Parents of Twins Clubs (see Appendix) allows parents to obtain additional information on the process of breast feeding[7]. The La Lèche League can provide contact with other mothers of multiples who have breast fed successfully. Such contacts not only help simplify the decision-making process but also provide the expectant mother with realistic expectations of what can take place after delivery. Often a home visit can be arranged for firsthand observation of a mother breast feeding her multiples.

Many hospitals provide patients prenatal breast feeding classes and contact with a lactation consultant. A lactation consultant is a health care professional (usually a nurse) with advanced certification in the field of lactation. These individuals assist mothers, both in the hospital and at home, to initiate and maintain breast feeding. These experiences positively affect the duration of breast feeding[5,6].

If the mother is hospitalized or on bed rest at home and is unable to attend classes, it is especially important to ensure that she has access to proper information. Many excellent videotapes on breast feeding are available (see Appendix). In addition, it is possible to arrange a home or hospital visit by a lactation consultant for specific and personalized instruction. Regardless of whether the patient is ambulatory or hospitalized, fathers and other family members should be involved with the educational process, because they will become the primary source of breast feeding support for the mother. It is also useful to encourage parents to select a pediatrician or neonatologist who is supportive of breast feeding.

The initial prenatal physical examination should always include a thorough assessment of the mother's nipples. It is important to remember that sore nipples may occur, even with careful attention to nipple preparation[8–10]. Women who have flat or inverted nipples (about 10–15% of the population) may have difficulty breast feeding. A simple procedure of pinching the tissue on the edges of the areola will positively identify a nipple that is truly flat or inverted. If the nipple is not truly flat or inverted, it will become erect when pinched.

The mother who has flat/inverted nipples should be counselled to wear breast shells or milk cups (see Figure 1) regularly for increasing lengths of time. These provide negative pressure that helps evert the nipple. Referral to a lactation consultant may also help these women anticipate problems that might arise after delivery.

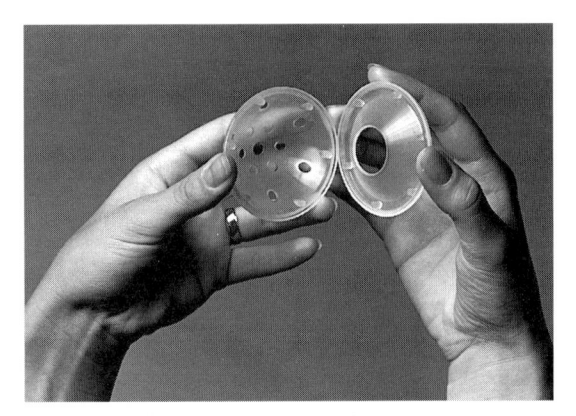

Figure 1 Breast milk cups or shells. Courtesy of Medela, Inc.

Immediate postpartum concerns

Supply/timing

The most common reason women discontinue breast feeding is a perception that their milk supply is inadequate[11]. With appropriate education and support, the majority of women can produce sufficient milk even for multiples. Indeed, mothers who breast feed their twins have been shown to produce twice as much milk as mothers of singletons[12].

The key to establishing a good milk supply is early and frequent breast feeding. If the babies are full-term and/or stable, they should be put to breast in the delivery or recovery room within the first hour of life. Infants who are put to breast early exhibit better weight gains and continue to breast feed longer[13,14].

A full-term singleton generally feeds every 2–3 h for 8–12 feedings in 24 h. The duration of feedings ranges from 5–30 min per breast. Because the milk changes during each feeding from a watery foremilk to hindmilk with a higher fat content, limited feeding times can decrease weight gain and cause colic[15].

If a mother of twins were to nurse one infant at a time, she could spend almost all of her waking hours breast feeding. Accordingly, simultaneous feedings are recommended. They not only save time, but also increase the milk supply[16]. Often one baby suckles more strongly than the other, and stimulates the milk let-down for both breasts. With simultaneous nursing, the baby that awakens first is put to breast and sets the feeding pace; then the second baby is awakened and positioned.

Unfortunately, simultaneous feeding may not allow individual attention to each child. Many mothers choose one or two feedings each day when they nurse each baby individually in an attempt to avoid this situation. Other mothers assign each baby to a breast. However, it may be advantageous to alternate breasts. If one baby is not a good nurser, he or she may decrease the supply on one side, whereas an adequate milk supply will be ensured if the more vigorous infant regularly stimulates both breasts[17]. Older twins often choose a favorite side. If weight gain is appropriate, this does not pose a problem, because regular breast feeding and adequate draining of both breasts is crucial to establishment of an adequate milk supply. On the other hand, if engorgement persists and the breast remains full, involution can rapidly follow[16].

Positioning

Proper positioning of both babies on the breast not only is important for the mother's comfort, but also promotes an adequate milk flow[10]. The mother should be provided with ample opportunity to practice both single and simultaneous feeding in the hospital before discharge. Some mothers find it difficult at first to position both infants without assistance, and the breast(s) may require support through the entire feeding, particularly if a baby is small and/or the breasts are large. Rolling a washcloth or towel under the breast can provide sufficient support. Most staff nurses are capable of assisting the mother to position her infants. If a lactation consultant is available, the extra attention provided by this individual often helps the mother feel more confident. In the author's experience, premature infants are more difficult to position, and their mothers can rarely breast feed simultaneously until each infant reaches what would have been full-term size by dates.

Nursing can begin soon after delivery, even if the mother has had a Cesarean birth. Most pain medications are safe for the mother to take while breast feeding. If taken 20–30 min before a nursing session, they help the mother deal with uterine contractions without permitting an undue amount of drug to be transferred to the babies[18].

The mother's back should be supported by the head of the bed, a chair back or pillows during nursing. Support should also be provided for her knees, elbows, shoulders and neck. A 'twin pillow' is helpful to many mothers for simultaneous feedings (Figure 2 and Appendix). Both infants should be brought to the mother so she can comfort one while the other is nursing if she does not plan to nurse both infants simultaneously during a specific feeding.

Five general positions are useful for simultaneous feedings – football hold, cradle/football hold, crisscross, 'V' and parallel hold. The most common is the football hold (Figure 3). In this position, the head and neck of each infant are supported by the mother's hands while the infants' bodies are tucked under each of the mother's arms. If pillows are properly placed or a twin pillow is used, it is possible for the mother to free her hands in this position once the babies learn how to suckle well. Then she will be able to control their heads, and both infants will be in a flexed position that is optimal for suckling.

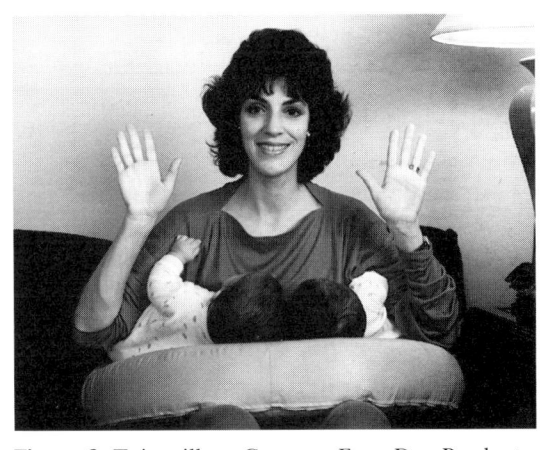

Figure 2 Twin pillow. Courtesy Four Dee Products, Inc.

MULTIPLE PREGNANCY

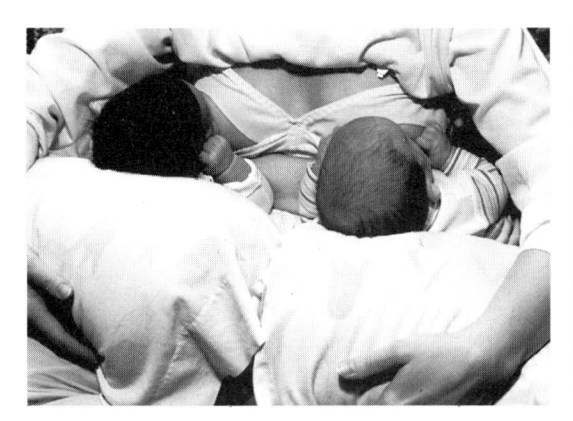

Figure 3 Football hold. Courtesy Virginia Brackett, RN, PNP, IBCLC

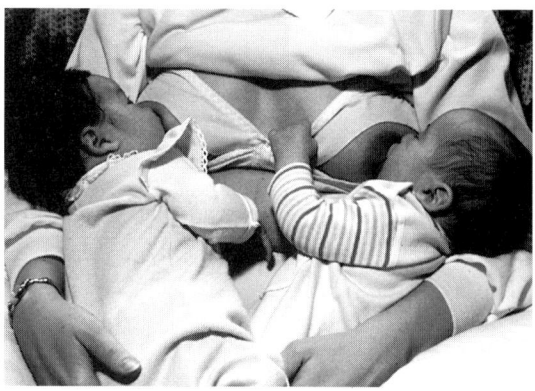

Figure 5 Crisscross hold. Courtesy Virginia Brackett, RN, PNP, IBCLC

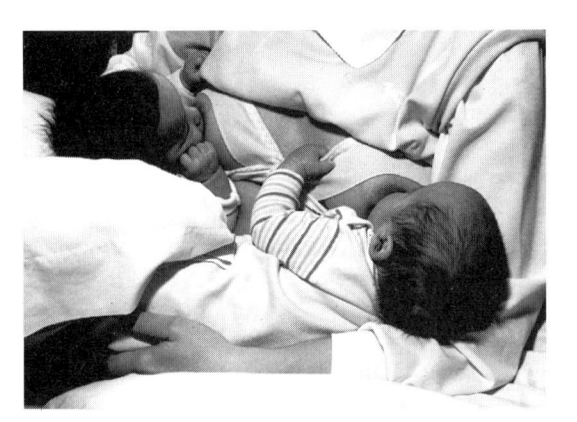

Figure 4 Cradle/football hold. Courtesy of Virginia Brackett, RN, PNP, IBCLC

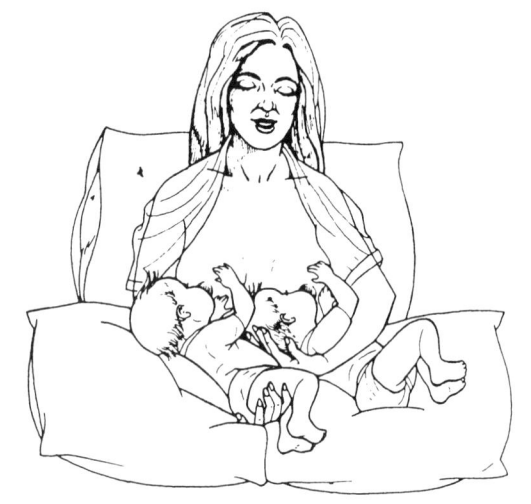

Figure 6 Parallel hold. Courtesy Keith, D.M., McInnes, S. and Keith, L.G., reference 4, p. 35

In the cradle/football position (Figure 4), one infant is held in the football hold and the other is on its side across the mother's abdomen in the cradle hold. A pillow underneath the cradled infant helps bring it to the mother's breast.

The third position is the crisscross hold (Figure 5). In this position, both infants are cradled with their legs crossing. A modification of this hold is the V-position, in which the infants' legs do not cross but their bodies are parallel. Both positions require an infant to have more head control, and the positions become more difficult as the infants attain higher weights.

The fifth and final position is the parallel hold (Figure 6). Both infants are angled in the same direction, but one infant's legs actually help support the other's head. By alternating positions from feeding to feeding, the pressure of the baby's jaws is directed to different points on the breast. This helps decrease the potential for nipple soreness and the incidence of clogged milk ducts. Most mothers settle into one comfortable position after a period of experimentation.

Nutrition

Malnourished women initially supply nutritionally adequate milk for their infants, but eventually milk quantity diminishes[19]. In adequately nourished women, on the other hand, the fat stores that have accumulated during pregnancy supply the increased caloric need for the first 3 months of lactation[19]. Although specific caloric needs are not as high as once thought, dieting is not recommended and it is crucial for the mother to drink when thirsty and eat whenever she is hungry[19]. Most women are surprised how hungry they are during nursing and can eat to abandon without gaining weight.

Prematurity and breast pumping

Twins are 4–5 times more likely to be born preterm than singletons. If born before 36 weeks, one or both infants is likely to require hospitalization in a neonatal intensive care unit (NICU). Because the ingestion of human milk decreases the incidence of neonatal sepsis and necrotizing enterocolitis, it is important to encourage mothers of twins to provide milk for their twins, even when the infants are in the NICU[20]. Many neonatal intensive care units request that mothers pump their breasts to provide breast milk for their hospitalized babies, even if it is anticipated that breast feeding will be discontinued at a later date.

The most efficient pumps are the piston-powered electric variety (Figure 7). The pumping action of these machines simulates the infant's suck. Double-pumping systems are available, and their use increases serum prolactin levels[16]. They also save the mother time; she needs only to pump for 10–15 min in total rather than 10–15 min per side[21]. Such pumps can be rented for use at home (see Appendix), and insurance companies may reimburse the mother for this expense if a prescription or letter is provided by the attending obstetrician or neonatologist. Some hospitals have loaner programs for low-income mothers. To maintain an adequate milk supply, the mother should pump a minimum of 8–10 times every 24 h, until one or both of the preterm infants are ready to suckle[16]. Babies should be put to breast for a short 'acquaintance time' once they are stable and able to come out of the isolette. Feeding times of preterm twins (while in the NICU) should not be scheduled at the same time in order to provide the mother sufficient opportunity to be with each baby individually and establish a bond with each child[3].

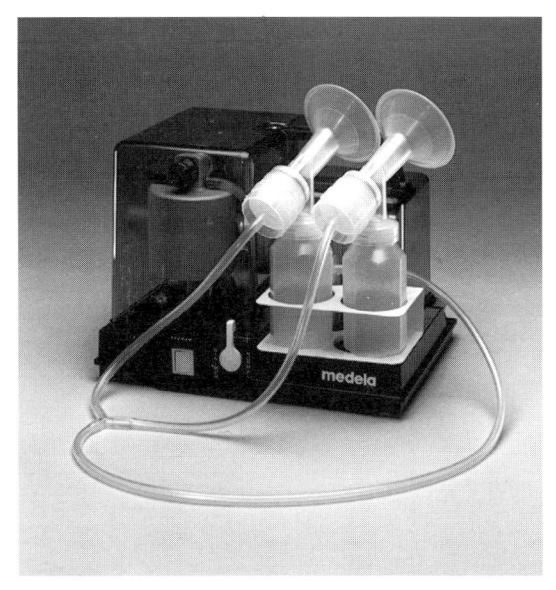

Figure 7 Piston-powered electric breast pump

The criteria for initiating breast feeding no longer rely merely on an absolute weight (i.e. 1800 g) or the ability to bottle feed[22,23]. Rather, studies utilizing 'kangaroo care' show that infants so treated gain better and breast feed sooner if put chest-to-chest at an earlier gestational age[24].

If one infant is discharged before the other, an individual care plan for breast feeding should be developed collaboratively with the mother. If possible, she should breast feed the infant at home regularly and pump in between feedings or simultaneously for the infant who has remained in the hospital. One to two breast feedings per day thus may be maintained with the infant that is still hospitalized. Other alternatives include increasing pumping frequency the week before the hospitalized infant goes home or increasing the frequency of feedings for the infant at home prior to discharge of the hospitalized infant.

The health care team taking care of a mother with separated infants should never underestimate the enormous stresses these families experience[25]. The delivery of multiples may precipitate a family crisis under the best of circumstances. If one or both infants are sick, the financial burden, and possibly the responsibility for more children at home, increases dramatically. Realistically, many mothers do not breast feed exclusively. Whereas they can rely on other family members to help bottle feed the babies, the efforts behind breast feeding rely on the mother alone.

Home support

The mothers who are most successful at breast feeding multiples have adequate home support. Some state 'a body for every baby' is a necessity. Efforts should be made before delivery to help the mother find home help either through relatives, home health aides or volunteer groups[26]. Fatigue is the most common complaint of mothers of multiples and adequate home support can diminish this concern[2,3]. If friends offer to help, doing a load of laundry or preparing a meal that can be put in the freezer for later use can be the best gift parents can receive.

Common concerns and their resolution

Most women are concerned with adequate milk supply, and it is necessary to re-emphasize that in the vast majority of cases the milk supply is simply related to frequency of feeding. The addition of supplemental bottles contributes to decreased milk supply[27]. The health care team should assist the mother to formulate goals regarding breast feeding if the issue of early supplementation arises. Anticipatory guidance regarding growth spurts also helps. Typically, growth spurts occur around 5 days, 10–14 days, 6 weeks, 12 weeks, 6 months and 9 months. At these times, the babies want to nurse more frequently for a few days. This can be especially difficult for mothers with twins, because the growth spurts may be longer and more demanding. Many women commonly stop breast feeding during growth spurts, because they misinterpret the increased demand and begin to supplement.

Maternal fatigue decreases the milk supply. New mothers need to sleep when their babies sleep or keep them in bassinets during rest breaks. Many parents prefer that the father give one or two bottle feedings per day so that the mother can obtain more rest. If the mother prefers to use breast milk for this feeding, she can pump in between her normal feedings.

Parents should be encouraged to keep a simple record of feedings, wet diapers and stools for each baby. The babies are getting enough milk if they have at least 6–8 wet diapers and at least two stools each 24 h during the first month of life. This use of an objective record also provides objective data regarding individualized care and eases parental anxiety. Such records are also helpful during discussions with the pediatrician.

Almost half of all mothers who breast feed complain of sore nipples[9]. Proper positioning can prevent or minimize this problem. A baby should have at least one inch (in diameter) of the areola in its mouth and be positioned with its body facing the mother's and its head at breast level. If breast feeding hurts or there are signs of trauma or overt nipple damage, the mother should try repositioning. Other causes of sore nipples include improper use of a breast pump, wearing breast pads with plastic liners, or a baby who has thrush. Expressing some breast milk by hand and letting it dry on the nipples promotes healing. If sore nipples persist, advice should be obtained from the physician, a lactation consultant or through the La Leche League.

Engorgement is another common postpartum concern. One recent study noted that longer durations of feedings in the first few days decreased the incidence of engorgement on the 3rd to 5th day postpartum[28]. Engorgement is more likely if feeding frequency decreases or feedings are skipped. Unresolved engorgement may lead to clogged ducts, mastitis and decreased milk supply[29]. If engorgement occurs, counsel the mother to use warm compresses or a hot shower, gentle massage to promote let-down and, most importantly, to nurse frequently and long. If the mother develops flu-like symptoms, red streaking or patches on the breast and fever (usually greater than

101°F), mastitis is likely. Frequent and long feedings on the affected breast accompanied by rest, increased fluids, antipyretics, heat and gentle massage may resolve the infection in 24 h. If not, consultation with the obstetrician and antibiotic therapy may be necessary. A penicillin derivative effective against staphylococcus is preferable and should be prescribed for 7–10 days[17]. Sudden weaning or simply pumping the affected side is not recommended, because both may increase the incidence of abscess[30].

Triplets/quadruplets

All the techniques and concerns mentioned above apply to mothers who breast feed triplets or quadruplets. In these instances, however, feedings require more time, because the mother can only nurse two of her infants at once. Obviously, home help and support are even more important.

Because higher-order multiple gestations are very likely to deliver preterm, it is virtually certain that the infants will be admitted to the NICU, at least initially. It is therefore essential that frequent pumping be initiated and maintained so that the milk flow will not be inhibited and the supply will not diminish. Feeding schedules may require frequent readjustment once the infants are put to breast. The mother can pick one to two feeding times for each infant and pump after feedings when time allows.

About half of the mothers of triplets and quadruplets who responded to a survey in England attempted to breast feed their infants[31]. However, many of these women stated that they had been discouraged from breast feeding by health care providers, who believed it would be too tiring. This concern is probably unwarranted, however. In the study reported by Saint, et al., one mother of triplets produced nutritionally adequate milk (3.08 kg milk per 24 h), and was able to breast feed each infant nine times in 24 h[12].

A case study of a mother who breast fed quadruplets has also been reported[32]. This mother successfully breast fed her children by combining direct breast feeding with expressed breast milk in a bottle. The babies were born at 34 weeks and ranged in weight from 1820 to 2240 g. Two were able to breast feed and gavage feed initially, whereas the other two required ventilatory assistance for 7 days. Two babies were discharged at 14 days of age and weighed 2140 and 2120 g, respectively. The remaining two were discharged at 18 days of age and weighed 2000 and 2010 g, respectively. In the first 28 days at home, the infants were breast fed 12–34 times per day and bottles ranged from a total of 4–28 per day. This mother did not often feed two infants simultaneously, because she observed that the infants distracted each other. If she was nursing one and another awakened, it would be given a bottle if it became fussy. All infants gained well. The husband and a homemaker were present for 8 h daily for the first 8 weeks postpartum. The mother also received intensive, individualized support from the authors of the case study and successfully breast fed these infants until 12 months, 15 months (two infants) and 18 months of age, respectively.

One mother of triplets who breast fed successfully offered the following comments: '(1) teach each baby (one at a time) to nurse; (2) when you have established a good milk supply and your babies are nursing effectively, begin to conserve time and energy... (she suggested feeding two simultaneously); (3) when the two babies finish nursing, burp them and pick up the remaining baby(ies) and repeat the process'[33]. Mothers have also recommended: (1) rotating the babies, so each one has one breast and the third is bottle fed; in this manner, a different baby is bottle fed each time; (2) allowing the home help to do the work so the mother can rest; (3) increasing food and fluid consumption; and (4) using a care chart as mentioned previously[4].

One final point should not be overlooked, and that is the extreme marital and financial stress that these parents endure. In one report, 42% of mothers of multiples complained of depression, compared to 7% of mothers of singletons[3]. In another, half the parents (mother or father) required psychiatric help by the childrens' first birthday[34]. Support groups are extremely useful. The Parents of Multiple Birth Association (POMBA) of Canada has a Parents of Triplets and Quadruplets Council. In the USA, the Triplet Connection and the National Organization of Mothers of Twins Clubs, Inc. both have a 'supertwin' referral system. These organizations provide valuable information and support for parents (see Appendix).

Weaning

Women who breast feed multiples wean at nearly the same rate as the general population. According to a survey of 1000 breast feeding mothers of multiples, 25% wean at less than 6 months, 26% at 6 months to less than a year, 26% at a year or more and 25% were still nursing at the time of the survey[25]. Mothers who breast fed longer than 6 months had more support from both a husband and homemaker, worked less and initiated solid feedings at a later stage of development[25]. Thirty-seven per cent of mothers let their babies lead the weaning process.

Whenever the mother of multiples decides to wean, she should be supported in that decision by her family and the health care team. Regardless of duration, breast feeding benefited her infants. Gradual weaning is recommended to avoid engorgement, clogged ducts and mastitis. The mother can either reduce the length of feedings or drop one feeding every three to seven days for each infant. No hard and fast rule applies. Weaning should be directed by maternal comfort levels. Many mothers feel sad, because a special time is ending. To facilitate the process of weaning, the American Academy of Pediatrics recommends using infant formula until the infants are 1 year old, because cow's milk is not adequately digested. Solid foods are not usually offered until 4–6 months of age.

Summary

Breast milk is the ideal food for all babies in the first year of life. Breast feeding multiples is a rewarding experience for mothers, despite its challenges. The health care team can provide support, anticipatory guidance and education to families, to assist them become successful with breast feeding.

References

1. Martinez, G.A. (1990). Ross Laboratories National Mothers Surveys. Columbus, OH: Ross Laboratories, unpublished data
2. Sollid, D.T., Evans, B.T., McClowry, S.G. *et al.* (1989). Breastfeeding multiples. *J. Perinat. Neonat. Nurs.*, **3**, 46
3. Broadbent, B. (1985). Twin trauma. *Nurs. Times.*, **81**, 28
4. Keith, D.M., McInnes, S. and Keith, L.G. (eds) (1982). *Breastfeeding Twins, Triplets, and Quadruplets: 195 Practical Hints for Success.* (Chicago: The Center for Study of Multiple Birth)
5. Jones, D.A. and West, R.R. (1986). Effect of a lactation nurse on the success of breastfeeding: a randomized controlled trial. *J. Epid. Comm. Health.*, **40**, 45
6. Wiles, L.S. (1984). The effect of prenatal breastfeeding education on breastfeeding success and maternal perception of the infant. *J. Obstet. Gynecol. Neonatal Nurs.*, **13**, 253
7. Spiro, A. (1992). Supporting parents who wish to breastfeed twins. *Health Visitor*, **65**, 197–8
8. Hewat, R. and Ellis, D. (1987). A comparison of the effectiveness of two methods of nipple care. *Birth*, **14**, 41
9. Walker, M. and Driscoll, J.W. (1989). Sore nipples: the new mother's nemesis. *Am. J. Matern. Child Nurs.*, **14**, 260
10. Woolridge, M.W. (1986). Aetiology of sore nipples. *Midwifery*, **2**, 172
11. Hill, P. (1991). The enigma of insufficient milk supply. *Am. J. Matern. Child Nurs.*, **16**, 312
12. Saint, L., Maggiore, P. and Hartman, P.E. (1986). Yield and nutrient content of milk in eight women breastfeeding twins and one

woman breastfeeding triplets. *Br. J. Nutrit.*, **56**, 49
13. Thompson, M.E., Hartsock, T.G. and Larson, C. (1979). The importance of immediate postnatal contact. Its effect on breastfeeding. *Can. Fam. Physician*, **25**, 1374
14. Taylor, P.M., Maloni, J.A. and Brown, D.R. (1986). Early suckling and prolonged breastfeeding. *Am. J. Dis. Child.*, **140**, 151
15. Woolridge, M.W. and Fisher, C. (1988). Colic, 'overfeeding', and symptoms of lactose malabsorption in the breastfed baby: a possible artifact of feed management? *Lancet*, **2**, 382
16. Neifert, M. and Seacat, J. (1985). Milk yield and prolactin rise with simultaneous breast pumping. Presented at *the Annual Meeting of the Ambulatory Pediatric Association*, Washington, DC, May 9
17. Neifert, M. and Thorpe, J. (1990). Twins: family adjustment, parenting, and infant feeding in the fourth trimester. *Clin. Obstet. Gynecol.*, **33**, 102
18. AAP Committee on Drugs. (1989). Transfer of drugs and other chemicals into human milk. *Pediatrics*, **84**, 924
19. Worthington-Roberts, B. and Williams, S.R. (eds.) (1989). *Nutrition in Pregnancy and Lactation*. (St Louis: Times Mirror/Mosby)
20. Barlow, B., Santulli, T.V. and Heird, W.C. (1974). Experimental necrotizing enterocolitis. The importance of breast milk. *J. Pediatr. Surg.*, **9**, 587
21. Auerbach, K.G. (1990). Single or double pumping: which method works best? *Rental Roundup*, **7**, 1
22. Meier, P. and Pugh, E. (1985). Breastfeeding behavior of small pre-term infants. *Am. J. Matern. Child Nurs.*, **10**, 396
23. Meier, P. (1988). Bottle and breast-feeding. Effects on transcutaneous oxygen pressure and temperature in preterm infants. *Nurs. Res.*, **37**, 36
24. Anderson, G.C. (1989). Skin to skin: kangaroo care in western Europe. *Am. J. Nurs.*, **89**, 662
25. Brewster, D. (1989). Breastfeeding twins. Part 1. *Twins*, **5**, 18
26. Gromada, K.K. (1992). Breastfeeding more than one: multiples and tandem breastfeeding. *NAACOG's Clinical Issues in Perinatal and Women's Health Nursing*, **3**, 656–66
27. Beske, E.J. and Garvis, M.S. (1982). Important factors in breastfeeding success. *Am. J. Matern. Child Nurs.*, **7**, 174
28. Moon, J.L. and Humenick, S.S. (1989). Breast engorgement: contributing variables and variables amenable to nursing intervention. *J. Obstet. Gynecol. Neonatal Nurs.*, **18**, 309
29. Applebaum, R.M. (1970). The modern management of successful breastfeeding. *Pediatr. Clin. N. Am.*, **17**, 202
30. Marshall, B.R., Hepper, J.K. and Zirbel, C.C. (1975). Sporadic puerperal mastitis. An infection that need not interrupt lactation. *J. Am. Med. Assoc.*, **233**, 1377
31. Botting, B.J., Macfarlane, A.J. and Price, F.V. (eds.) (1990). *Three, Four and More. A Study of Triplet and Higher Order Births*. (London: HMSO)
32. Mead, L.G., Chuffo, R., Lawlor-Klean, P. *et al.* (1992). Breastfeeding success with preterm quadruplets. *J. Obstet. Gynecol. Neonatal Nurs.*, **21**, 221
33. Bleyl, J.L. (1988). Breastfeeding supertwins: can I do it? *Twins*, **4**, 49
34. Robin, M. (1989). Personal communication to L. Keith, Paris

Bonding and attachment

R. Theroux and J.F. Tingley

Introduction

A bond is a unique relationship between two people that is specific and endures through time. Parent–infant bonding is the phenomenon in which adults become committed by a one-way flow of concern and affection toward children whom they have cared for during the first months or weeks of life[1].

Attachment differs from bonding in that the activity is reciprocal. This interactive behavior is a prerequisite for infant survival. According to Bowlby, human infants are born with a predisposition to seek close contact with adults through attachment behaviors such as crying, smiling and clinging[2]. The goal of these behaviors is to initiate or maintain proximity between the infant and its mother or primary care giver. Not only does the infant derive comfort from this contact, but the mother or father and the infant become active partners in a reciprocal relationship which develops during the first year of life and is influenced by the quality and timing of parent–infant encounters. The power of this attachment is so great that it enables parents to make sacrifices necessary for the care of their infant. Moreover, the strength of this attachment influences all future ties to other individuals, regardless of gender[2].

Bonding and attachment

Although it has been recognized since Biblical times that maternal–infant attachment is of an exceptional nature (e.g. King Solomon's decision about disputed parenthood), the descriptive literature available to health professionals is relatively new. The first experimental study of maternal–infant contact appeared in the *New England Journal of Medicine* in 1972[3]. Diverse nursing, pediatric or psychiatric journals reported subsequent studies. With a few notable exceptions, this subject has failed to capture interest, despite the fact that obstetricians are present during many of the initial bonding encounters.

The initial study of bonding by Klaus *et al.*[3] contrasted parent–infant separation with parent–infant contact. These authors postulated that a variety of parenting disorders were due to parent–infant separation after birth. Because mothers who experienced extra contact with their infants at the time of delivery and during the early postpartum period displayed more attachment behaviors, Klaus *et al.*[3] suggested that early and extended mother–infant contact facilitated maternal–infant bonding.

The initial presentation of the theory of parent–infant bonding postulated that a brief 'maternal sensitive' period exists within the first minutes and hours after birth and that this time is optimal for parent–infant bonding[4]. Bonding is facilitated by the physical contact between the mother and her newborn through skin-to-skin contact, suckling, mutual visual regard and fondling. These interactions help bind mother and infant together. The infant is in a quiet alert state during the first hour after delivery, and is able to respond to his/her environment. Parenting behaviors, such as fondling, fingertip touching, massage and stroking, kissing, cuddling, prolonged gazing and 'en face' contact are indicators of attachment and reflect the parent–infant bond. The traditional hospital practice of separation of mothers and infants at birth fails to recognize this period, and impairs the establishment of an effective parent–infant bond.

According to Rubin[5], the phenomenon of 'binding in' follows delivery. This process has three mutually dependent phases. During 'identification', the mother has a need to know her child through tactile and visual methods. Following this, she 'claims' her child, and includes it in her sphere. It is at this time that a mother may remark that the child looks like herself or its father. During 'polarization', the third and final phase, the mother begins to see her infant as a separate person, someone whom she views affectionately.

Some writers suggest that an emotional attachment to the fetus starts shortly after conception and deepens as the pregnancy progresses[6–8]. Prenatal attachment behaviors include talking to the fetus, naming it and mentally visualizing what it looks like. Even women with high-risk pregnancies develop these feelings of attachment[9]. This observation is important, because multifetal pregnancies are classified as high-risk, despite what may be a benign prenatal course, and it might be anticipated that mothers of multiples would possibly avoid becoming deeply attached to their infants because of anxiety about the high-risk condition.

Since its publication, questions have arisen regarding specific aspects of the study by Klaus et al.[3]. These include concerns about research design, sampling procedures, long-term follow up and variables such as social support, intervention in labor, and maternal education and age. Some investigators[10] support the early work, whereas others believe that early contact has no enduring effect on maternal attachment[11,12]. Regardless of one's personal position, additional research is needed to define appropriate medical or nursing interventions that support and facilitate the vital processes of parent–infant bonding and attachment during the prenatal through postpartum phases.

Changes in hospital practices that have facilitated bonding and attachment

Hospitals began to modify their practices following the publication of the initial bonding research and the papers that followed. Changes included allowing support persons to be present during labor, giving parents more time with their infants after delivery and in the hospital, and altering what had previously been absolutely rigid feeding schedules. What had been considered avant-garde, i.e. birthing rooms and family-centered care, soon became standard hospital practice. These efforts were generally positive, in that they created more humane and family-oriented care, but in the process the theory of bonding became distorted by the mass media. This misinterpretation resulted from the characterization of bonding as a 'rapid glue' process that, if missed, would be followed by permanent detrimental effects to the infant's psychological development. Parents of sick or premature infants who had little early contact often felt guilty or worried about their lack of bonding time. A backlash soon developed against hospital practices in which professionals pressured parents to instantly relate to their infants in a specific manner which was described as if it were unique and all-encompassing. It soon became apparent, however, that not all mothers had the desire or the capacity to have their infants at the bedside and assume all caretaking duties immediately after birth[13].

The early contact theory was tempered in a subsequent work by Klaus and Kennell[14]. This study recognized that: (1) parents who had little or no early mother–infant contact were still able to form a bond with their infants; and (2) not every parent was able to develop a close tie to the infant at birth. This later paper proposed that early and extended contact should still be provided if a mother wished it, but if the health of the mother or infant made it impossible, reassurance should be given to the parents that they could attach to their infant at a later time[14]. Because this middle-of-the-road policy was reassuring to parents as well as professionals, it soon became widely accepted.

Many maternity services gradually evolved to provide different models of care. One provided parents and families who requested or were able to accept unlimited contact with their newborn an opportunity to do so, along with appropriate support and preparation for parenthood. Alternative models were available when circumstances dictated their use. As an example, the labor/delivery/recovery/postpartum (LDRP) concept provides clients with home-like birth settings, full participation of support-people during the birth and hospital stay, facilities for infants and fathers to 'room in', and flexibility with infant care and contact. In this setting, the same nurse provides care for the woman and her family from the initial phase of labor through the postpartum period. All care, from admission through discharge, is provided in one room. The single-room concept of care facilitates privacy for parents and infants as they become acquainted. This care model recognizes bonding and attachment as a complex reciprocal process that gradually evolves over time rather than a single event that occurs with the first contact between mother and infant. Bonding and attachment depends on many variables, only one of which is a supportive hospital environment[15,16].

Bonding and attachment with multiples

The bonding and attachment literature contains scant information relevant to multiples. Many of the available studies report observations on small numbers of patients. Others provide twin data in the absence of control singleton data. Nonetheless, we will attempt to summarize these studies in the paragraphs that follow. In addition, we will present our opinions, which have developed as mothers (of twins and singletons), as authors of the first and most widely read book on the care of twin children[17], and as health-care providers to parents and their multiples.

Klaus and Kennell's[4] observation in 1976 that a higher incidence of child abuse occurred to the smaller twin when it was discharged from the hospital later than its larger co-twin led them to suggest that a close attachment could optimally be formed to only one person at a time. In reality, monotrophy, or optimal one-on-one mother–child attachment is the norm in humans. When more than one infant is involved, attachment theoretically becomes more difficult and the process requires a longer duration[18]. To date, the theory of monotrophy is neither supported nor refuted by the twin literature.

When the behavior of mothers of twins, triplets and quadruplets was studied through a series of home observations, Goshen-Gottstein[19] found that none of the infants exhibited signs of an insecure attachment at one year of age, regardless of their number. Despite this, the mothers of twins expressed having had negative feelings and fears prenatally which may have positively influenced their ability to form a warm relationship with their children in a short time. In contrast, the mothers of 'supertwins' (triplets, quadruplets or higher-order births) noted that their negative emotions continued after the birth. Moreover, many of these latter mothers felt that they were pressed into treating their children as a unit in an effort to diminish stress and increase efficiency. Because getting used to more than one infant requires a long period of acclimatization, some mothers had difficulty in becoming fully invested in all their infants at the same time, especially in the case of triplets and quadruplets. These mothers tended to relate to their infants by degrees.

A retrospective survey of 18 mothers of twins investigated how proximity and timing influenced the bonding process. Abbink *et al.*[20] found that early affectional relationships developed with both twins, although many mothers did not have equal opportunity to hold both infants at birth. Despite this, mothers did not perceive that the early separation from one or both twins was detrimental to the long-term relationship.

Twenty-eight mothers of twins were queried in another retrospective study to determine the effect of multiple birth on the family and how this effect differed from that of a singleton birth[21]. Compared to mothers of singletons, fewer of the mothers of twins (71% vs. 50%) felt 'immediate love' for their infants, and over 25% of mothers of twins encountered some obstacles in establishing bonds with their babies. Initial bonding difficulty was associated with a variety of factors, including: (1) a difficult delivery followed by maternal exhaustion;

(2) delay in establishing physical contact with the babies (only 50% of the mothers held their twins after delivery); (3) prematurity (37% of the twin infants were admitted to special-care nursery); (4) unequal contact with each twin; (5) lack of assistance with feeding and infant care by hospital staff; and (6) maternal feelings of inadequacy in infant care.

Anderson and Anderson studied ten mothers of twins to determine how mothers developed a relationship with their twins during their first year of life[22,23]. Individuation or recognition that each twin was an individual was influenced by considerations of polarization, differentiation, maternal justice and support. These authors concluded that a mother must first compare the differences in the babies' appearance and behavior in order to relate to them as distinct individuals. Stated another way, at times twins need to be treated as a team and at others as individuals.

In our opinion, the early diagnosis of a multiple pregnancy is an extremely important part of the attachment process[24]. Early use of ultrasound allows parents the opportunity to view their babies several times before delivery and sufficient time to discuss birthing plans and prepare for infant care. In contrast, mothers who first discover they are carrying twins in the delivery room are more likely to undergo great emotional stress. Many experience ambivalent emotions and/or are completely overwhelmed. Subsequently such feelings may be followed by guilt. These mothers require time alone to resolve these feelings and may also need to express them to a supportive, non-judgmental person who can understand their point of view. All too often, mothers are congratulated for having a 'bonus baby', and told that they should be thrilled. In reality, these women may feel frightened, angry, scared, depressed, or just numb. Indeed, they may regard their second baby as a 'tagalong', whereas the firstborn is considered the baby they had attached to prenatally[25].

The presence of the father or a requested support-person during labor and delivery provides the mother with more tolerance for the increased numbers of personnel who may be present at the birth of twins or higher-order multiples. After the delivery and viewing of baby A, the mother can then shift her attention to the delivery of baby B, while the father or supporter can interact with baby A. In the absence of the father or supporter, the mother may remain so attentive to baby A as to fail to recall the birth of baby B[18].

Gromada[25] suggests that mothers should first bond with the twins as 'a unit', then later with each child as an individual. Maternal–child attachment is the focal point in promoting the individuality of each child. With ideal conditions prevailing (vaginal delivery of two full-term infants), bonding with twins may take longer than with a single infant. Initial contact should be with both babies together to achieve and reinforce the reality of twins.

Difficulties with bonding can arise when complications occur during or after delivery. Long periods of separation in special-care nurseries or different medical facilities may then ensue. Mothers of premature twins are often depressed and experience a sense of failure when the need for special-care nursery arises[26]. Sick infants who are attached to medical equipment may frighten parents and deter them from holding, touching, or nursing. Some parents may distance themselves from their newborns because of fear of death, and these individuals need active encouragement by health-care providers to hold or touch their twins. In this regard, placing the isolettes side by side reinforces the reality of having twins.

Comparisons of the two infants are necessary at first, in order to learn and recognize each baby's differences. Even identical children have distinguishing features and behavioral characteristics that mothers can discern from the first day of life[19]. The more physically alike the babies appear, however, the longer will be the process of individuation. This is particularly true for identical twins if the mother has trouble distinguishing each baby initially. Indeed, mothers who treat their children as a unit while meeting their physical needs have more difficulty in becoming acquainted with each child as a distinct individual. The process of differentiation is facilitated by dressing the babies differently so that their differences are accentuated.

Twins often exhibit 'role switching', or personality changes during the first year of life and occasionally later as well, and mothers need time to adjust to this phenomenon[17]. The recognition of the uniqueness of each child aids in the development of a distinctive mother–child relationship. It is necessary to spend time alone with each infant to identify its personal characteristics so that the mother can establish two intimate and separate mother–infant relationships[27,28]. Such a process assists mothers to consider each baby as an individual apart from his/her co-twin.

Death of one or both members of a twin pair is a serious impediment to bonding. Klaus and Kennell[4] correctly observe that the process of attachment and detachment cannot occur simultaneously. In such a circumstance, parents who have lost one of a twin pair experience difficulty in attaching to the other baby. They are faced with simultaneous and conflicting emotions of grief and happiness. Because the death of an infant is difficult to accept, focus is turned to the living baby, without fully acknowledging the loss of its sibling. Friends and family may erroneously believe that the living child somehow lessens the grief of the parents. This is wrong, however, and parental attempts to deal simultaneously with these two divergent emotions are often met by a silent conspiracy of non-support. It is imperative that these conflicting emotions be addressed, to prevent parents from feeling guilty and having low self-esteem if they experience difficulty attaching to the surviving baby(ies)[29,30]. The inability of the health-care team members to react in an appropriate and caring way at this extraordinary moment should never be an additional burden to the parents[31]. (Editor: This feeling of ambivalence will continue for years and may be particularly evident on the birthday of the survivor. The parents never forget their loss although the pain diminishes with time.)

The time immediately after hospital discharge is crucial to the process of bonding and attachment. A major consideration is adequate help during the first weeks at home. The mother's need for rest is often overlooked. A mother who is sick, depressed, fatigued, or lacks social contacts cannot give her babies or other family members proper care. Although the father can be an important source of help and support, many families need additional help from outside sources, such as a visiting nurse association[21].

Sleep deprivation, stress and chaotic home conditions limit the attachment process and greatly increase the likelihood of child abuse and neglect. One study which compared mothers of singletons and twins from the same backgrounds, ages and socioeconomic standings found that child abuse was nine times more prevalent in twin households[32].

Some mothers admit to feeling closer to one infant than the other and develop guilt about this. To compensate, they often give extra attention to the one perceived as the non-favorite. If mothers tend to favor one twin over the other, the favorite tends to shift. According to Brazelton, it is unlikely that a parent will attach to one twin to the total exclusion of the other. Rather, they may attach differently to each twin and this difference may wax and wane over time[33].

Often the smaller, less healthy baby who was admitted to the special-care nursery is the sole object of negative feelings, at least initially, when this infant is perceived as being more vulnerable. Because mothers tend to attach to the baby who came home first, this circumstance can be devastating to the child who remains behind. Fortunately, if mothers come to realize that these feelings are natural, they can make an extra effort to spend time with the other twin[25,34].

Neifert and Thorpe[35] have characterized the time spent adjusting and assimilating multiples into the family structure as the 'fourth trimester'. Because this can be a time of intense stress and crisis, health-care providers must help families cope by providing realistic suggestions on the care of twin children. Referral to a parent-support group is an absolute necessity.

Brazelton[32] has aptly noted that 'bonding' is sometimes looked upon as 'magical' or instantaneous, instead of as an ongoing and natural process, with few guidelines to follow. Most mothers eventually attach to their children, if a nurturing environment is maintained. Parents of twins need to enjoy their children, since a great deal of extra work is involved in rearing them. Davis[35] sums it up by stating that it may take many months, even years, for parents of twins to finally realize that 'we're all in love with each other the way we should be'.

Practical experience with bonding and attachment

We conducted a survey with the Massachusetts Mothers of Twins Clubs in 1990 in an effort to obtain additional insights about the process of twin bonding and attachment[36]. A total of 137 respondents (100% of those surveyed) who had singleton and twin children returned the questionnaires. The twin pairs were distributed as follows: identical males 23%, identical females 20%, fraternal females 20%, fraternal males 11%, and boy/girl fraternals 27%. The average age of the twins was 4 years (ranging from 3 months to 28 years) and of singleton siblings, 8 years (ranging from 5 months to 40 years).

Prenatal considerations

The diagnosis of twins was accomplished in the 3rd month of pregnancy, on the average, by ultrasound in the majority (84%) of instances. Later ultrasound examinations determined the sex of one or both twins in 41% of cases. Individual movement patterns of each twin were identified by 66% of the mothers. The immediate feelings after learning that the forthcoming delivery would be twins ranged from happiness and elation to shock, a sensation of feeling overwhelmed and emotionally numb. The majority of mothers remembered a combination of ambivalent feelings, such as being excited and worried, happy and nervous, or elated and frightened, all at the same time.

Postpartum considerations

Two-thirds of mothers thought they had bonded/attached to each twin in the hospital; slightly more than half breast fed their twins; of these latter mothers, 83% believed that breast feeding aided in the attachment process. Nonetheless, only 40% of mothers felt the hospital staff were sufficiently sensitive to their needs for bonding. Of those who felt that the staff were *not* responsive to their needs, the reasons cited were:

(1) The staff did not provide enough assistance in handling both infants after delivery. Some babies were taken away with no explanation.

(2) There was not enough consistent help with breast feeding of twins.

(3) There was insufficient specific information given about postpartum care of twins and/or the condition of the babies from the special-care nursery staff.

(4) There was lack of privacy during the delivery.

(5) The infants were always brought to the mother together, with no time with each baby to learn the individuality of each one.

Over half of the babies (61%) were brought to their mothers together for feeding. This caused anxiety in some mothers who wanted to give special attention to each child. Sixty-nine per cent of the twins went home with the mother. Thirty per cent of mothers reported feeling closer to one twin in the hospital, and 80% experienced guilt about this. Half of the mothers of identicals reported difficulty in distinguishing each baby.

The following characteristics distinguished mothers who reported that they did not bond to either both or one twin in the hospital (25% of all respondents): 70% had Cesarean section; 30% of the children were premature; 71% did not hold or touch their twins after delivery; and 68% of the twins were diagnosed as being in fair or critical condition immediately after birth.

Sixty-five per cent of the respondents reported that it was easier to attach to their singletons than their twins, and 63% thought that having twins adversely affected the bonding process. Twin attachment time ranged from 2 weeks to 12 months, with an average of 7 weeks. Attachment times were longer for those twins who remained in special-care nursery. In these cases, the attachment process usually began when the twins came home. At the time of the survey, only 17% of the mothers felt closer to one twin than the other, but 40% remembered the bonding process as more difficult than with their singleton children. Thirty-five per cent were closer to their singleton children than their twins. Despite this, within the first year of life, all of the mothers reported attachment.

Although any interpretation of these findings is hampered by the retrospective nature of the survey, its limited numbers and the absence of a singleton-only comparison group, the fact that all mothers bonded and attached to their twins as well as to their singletons makes these findings of interest, because they have implications for health-care providers.

Implications for health-care providers

Health-care providers should not regard the processes of bonding and attachment with multiples as a one-time event, but rather as an evolving process. The process of parental attachment is more complex with multiples and may take longer to achieve than with singletons. Attachment involves both maternal and infant variables, and depends on a supportive environment in both the hospital and at home. Health-care providers should assist parents at all stages of the pregnancy to achieve and strengthen parent–twin bonds.

To do this, parents of multiples should be prepared for the possibility of prematurity and complications at delivery, prenatal hospitalization, infant resuscitation at delivery, admission of one or both infants to special-care nurseries, operative delivery, and maternal–infant separation, by assuring them that a satisfactory relationship can develop even in the absence of early prolonged contact.

Suggestions to enhance bonding and attachment

Prenatal

(1) Perform an ultrasound examination whenever multiple gestation is suspected, to assist in prenatal attachment.

(2) Refer parents to a counsellor if they express negative feelings when informed about having twins, so that they can verbalize their fears and concerns.

(3) Request a perinatal clinical nurse specialist to provide additional education and support, if antenatal hospitalization is required.

(4) Refer parents of multiples to nurse practitioners, nurse midwives and childbirth educators who are knowledgeable about multiple births, for a discussion of their emotional concerns and assistance in planning for the arrival of twins.

(5) *Refer all parents to local Mothers of Twins Clubs for practical information, advice and long-term support, concerning upcoming adjustments in the family.*

(6) Suggest that parents try to set up some type of plan for additional household help after delivery by the seventh month of pregnancy, in the event of preterm delivery.

(7) Refer families with few resources or those under stress to hospital social-service departments or local visiting-nurse associations for provision of resources and follow-up home visits.

Intrapartum

(1) Inform the parents immediately if twins are discovered during labor. Even a few minutes helps to prepare mothers to accept and attach to the second baby.

(2) Allow parents to see both babies together, as soon as possible. If one baby is transported to another facility for special care, provide a picture to the parents.

(3) Limit the numbers of personnel at the delivery, and allow parents a quiet private time to hold the twins after delivery.

Postpartum

(1) Provide a picture of both twins if babies are admitted to special-care nursery. This is vital for the parents until they can visit the babies. Provide reassurance that bonding and attachment will still take place.

(2) Provide constant information to parents about the condition of each baby when twins are in special-care nursery. They need to visit and touch both babies as soon as is feasible. Isolettes should be placed next to each other.

(3) Provide information to the mother about that baby, if one twin is in special care, and allow her adequate time with both babies.

(4) Assess how much contact the mother desires with her babies, and plan individualized care based on this. Mothers need time with both babies at feedings, but also need time with each baby individually.

(5) Assess the mother's ability to recognize each twin if the babies are identical, and assist the mother in identifying individual characteristics of each baby. Comparisons of the physical and behavioral differences are natural during this process.

(6) Provide more assistance, education and support to mothers who have had Cesarean birth or who are breast feeding. Mothers who are exhausted or overwhelmed by twin care are less likely to develop early bonding and attachment.

(7) Assess maternal–infant attachment during feedings, and make an assessment of the mother's behavior with each twin, especially if the mother attends more to one than to the other, or directs negative comments to one twin. Mothers may normally favor one twin, with the favorite changing almost daily. In situations where one baby remains in special-care nursery, the mother may preferentially attach to the other baby. If mothers are aware of this, they can make efforts to interact with the less-favored twin.

(8) Discharge both babies at the same time if possible. If this is not possible, encourage parents to make regular visits to the remaining baby. If parents cannot visit, provide phone contact or letters from their baby through the staff.

(9) Allow parents to start the grieving process when one twin dies at birth or soon after. They need to work through their loss and make it real, by naming the dead child, holding a memorial service and openly expressing their grief. It is important to realize that they will always think of themselves as parents of twins. In these cases, attachment to the living baby may take longer and referral to a support group may be needed.

References

1. Klaus, M. and Kennell, J. (1982). *Parent–Infant Bonding*, 2nd edn., pp. 85–7. (St Louis: C.V. Mosby)

2. Bowlby, J. (1969). *Attachment & Loss*, Vol. 1. – Attachment, pp. 350–3. (New York: Basic Books)

3. Klaus, M., Jerauld, R., Kreger, N. *et al.* (1972). Maternal attachment: importance of the first postpartum days. *N. Engl. J. Med.*, **286**, 460
4. Klaus, M. and Kennell, J. (1976). *Maternal–Infant Bonding*, pp. 8–12. (St Louis: C.V. Mosby)
5. Rubin, R. (1977). Binding-in in the postpartum period. *Matern. Child Nurs. J.*, **6**, 67
6. Cranley, M. (1981). Development of a tool for the measurement of maternal attachment during pregnancy. *Nurs. Res.*, **30**, 281
7. Leifer, M. (1977). Psychological changes accompanying pregnancy and motherhood. *Genet. Psychol. Monogr.*, **95**, 55
8. Rubin, R. (1970). Cognitive style in pregnancy. *Am. J. Nurs.*, **70**, 502
9. Kemp, V. and Page, C. (1987). Maternal prenatal attachment in normal and high-risk pregnancies. *J. Obstet. Gynecol. Neonat. Nurs.*, **16**, 179
10. Ainsfield, E. and Lipper, E. (1983). Early contact, social support, and mother–infant bonding. *Pediatrics*, **72**, 79
11. Lamb, M. (1982). Early contact and maternal–infant bonding: one decade later. *Pediatrics.*, **70**, 763
12. Mitchell, K. and Mills, N. (1983). Is the sensitive period in parent–infant bonding overrated? *Pediatr. Nurs.*, **9**, 91
13. Nelson, S. (1985). Attachment theory. *Nurse Pract.*, **10**, 34
14. Klaus, M. and Kennell, J. (1984). Bonding – another view. *Perinatol–Neonatol.*, **8**, 72
15. Stainton, C. (1986). Parent–infant bonding: a process, not an event. *Dimensions Health Serv.*, **63**, 19
16. Campbell, S. and Taylor, S. (1980). *Bonding and Attachment: Theoretical Issues in Parent–Infant Relationships*, pp. 365–8. (New York: Grune and Stratton)
17. Theroux, R. and Tingley, J. (1984). *The Care of Twin Children: A Commonsense Guide For Parents*, 2nd edn., p. 59. (Chicago: Center For Study of Multiple Birth)
18. Spillman, J. (1987). Emotional impact of multiple pregnancy. *Midwife Health Visitor and Community Nurse*, **23**, 58
19. Goshen-Gottstein, E. (1980). The mothering of twins, triplets, & quadruplets. *Psychiatry*, **43**, 189
20. Abbink, C., Dorsel, S., Flores, J. *et al.* (1982). Bonding as perceived by mothers of twins. *Pediatr. Nurs.*, **8**, 411
21. Broadbent, B. (1985). Postnatal care: twin trauma. Part 3. *Nurs. Times*, **81**, 28
22. Anderson, A. and Anderson, B. (1987). Mothers' beginning relationship with twins. *Birth*, **14**, 94
23. Anderson, A. and Anderson, B. (1990). Toward a substantive theory of mother–twin attachment. *Am. J. Matern. Child Nurs.* **15**, 373
24. Theroux, R. (1989). Multiple birth: a unique parenting experience. *J. Perinat. Neonat. Nurs.*, **3**, 35
25. Gromada, K. (1981). Maternal–infant attachment: the first step in individualizing twins. *Am. J. Matern. Child Nurs.*, **6**, 129
26. Tingley, J. (1983). Premature twins. In Keith, D. and Keith, L. (eds.) *Research Reports.* pp. 1–4. (Chicago: Center for Study of Multiple Birth)
27. Frazer, E. (1977). The work of a multigravida in becoming the mother of twins. *Matern. Child Nurs. J.*, **6**, 87
28. Dickerson, P. (1981). Early postpartum separation and maternal attachment to twins. *J. Obstet. Gynecol. Neonat. Nurs.*, **10**, 120
29. Johannsen, L. (1989). As birth and death coincide. *Am. J. Matern. Child Nurs.*, **14**, 89
30. Swanson-Kaufman, K. (1988). There should have been two: nursing care of parents experiencing the perinatal death of a twin. *J. Perinat. Neonat. Nurs.*, **2**, 78
31. Hradek, C. (1993). *Managing Multiple Birth Families – Prenatal – Postpartum*, p. 12. (Albuquerque: The National Organization of Mothers of Twins Clubs, Inc.)
32. Groothuis, J., Altemeir, W., Robarge, J. *et al.* (1982). Increased child abuse in families with twins. *Pediatrics*, **70**, 769
33. Simons, H. (1987). Infant–parent bonding: an interview with T. Berry Brazelton, MD. *Twins Magazine*, **4**, 36
34. Bryan, E. (1983). Twins in the family. *Nurs. Times*, **79**, 50
35. Neifert, M. and Thorpe, J. (1990). Twins: family adjustment, parenting and feeding in the fourth trimester. *Clin. Obstet. Gynecol.*, **33**, 102
36. Davis, E. (1988). Bonding with multiples: a process, not an event. *Twinline Reporter*, **5**, 1
37. Theroux, R. and Tingley, J. (1990). Maternal perceptions of twin and singleton attachment. (Unpublished research)

Psychiatric considerations after the birth of multiples

K.E. Merenkov

Introduction

> I cannot bear a mother's tears
> Virgil[1]

Humans frequently seek continuity between the past and the future in an attempt to give meaning to their lives. Procreation is a universal means to contribute to the interwoven fabric of generations by producing one's own thread. Thus, fertility has a special, albeit variable, place in almost all cultures[2]. The knowledge that a woman is able to bear children is 'critical in the development of [a] sense of femininity, gender identity, and self-esteem...'[2]. Comparable concerns probably also exist for men, although men generally have other culturally sanctioned opportunities for enhancing self-esteem, such as career development (Editor – or waging war). Until recently, these alternatives almost universally have not been open to women, no matter what their social status. An exception to this statement is the entrance of increasing numbers of women into the work force of modern industrialized nations.

Just as infertility may be a threat to a woman's self-esteem and identity, 'excess evidence of fertility, as occurs in multifetal pregnancies, may be just as threatening. The extent of this threat often is influenced by the value that society, as well as individuals, place on multiples. Clearly, reactions to multiple births throughout the ages and in various cultures have varied from ecstatic enthusiasm to ritualistic abandonment (or death) of the mother and children[3]. Negative reactions to plural birth in past centuries centered around their resemblance to other animal species (in which litters are the norm) or the suspicion that the mother had been unfaithful either with another man or with an evil spirit[3].

In more recent times, multiples and their mothers have been viewed somewhat more positively. Thus, twins on occasion have been associated with good luck and fertile influences. To heighten prospects of a fertile union, for example, their presence was in demand at Welsh weddings in the early part of this century[3]. Even more recently, multiples have become media events and at times have been exploited to promote consumerism[4]. Banishment was replaced by the uncomfortable intrusiveness of the media which quickly turned to forgetfulness as the novelty wore off. More importantly, perhaps, multiples were no longer regarded merely as an unpredictable act of nature, but could now be produced by direct medical intervention for infertility problems.

Overall, what had previously been emphasized in either positive or negative ways is now perceived as 'differentness'. To be different can be a positive factor in an individual's search for uniqueness, but this quality must often be balanced against simultaneous longing to belong. Unfortunately, the constantly changing perspective of multiples probably continues to exert an influence in even subtler manners than I have suggested and makes maintaining a balance difficult, both for parents and for their children.

The reality of conflicting individual and societal perceptions, coupled with the very real stressful nature of child care, may provide an additional negative influence on a woman's vulnerability to certain psychiatric disorders, such as depression. Whether multiples truly increase the risk for postpartum psychiatric disorders compared to singleton births is not clear from a scholarly review of the literature. Comparisons may be biased by the relatively rare occurrences of multiples. However, in light of the often very serious stresses associated with multiple pregnancy and later parenting (especially parenting of iatrogenic higher-order multiples by previously infertile couples), it is imperative to clarify the biopsychosocial risks to the mother's well being in the postpartum period in order to initiate timely and effective psychiatric interventions if required.

The purpose of this chapter is to review postpartum psychiatric concerns and to show that these may apply to mothers with multiple births. An integrated biopsychosocial understanding of the impact of a multiple on the woman's psyche and its aftermath is necessary to promote quality care.

Implications of high risk pregnancy

The postpartum period is a discrete time after birth. Nonetheless, it is influenced by a variety of factors that arise during the pregnancy itself. Opinions are varied about the extent to which pregnancy should be viewed as a combination of physiological, psychological and social phenomena[5], although recent comments in the literature provide greater emphasis on psychosocial perspectives (see also Chapter 20). As Cox has aptly observed[6],

> [the] present increased interest [in postnatal depression] is a consequence of the greater awareness in Western society that childbirth is a social process involving a major change of role and so cannot be construed solely as a biological event.

In contrast to the postpartum period, pregnancy 'may even offer protection against major mental illness'[5]. This vast difference may in reality only reflect the multitude of distracting factors occurring during pregnancy that partially or totally obscure any focus on psychiatric concerns. Such factors include Western society's implicit belief in the 'joys of motherhood'[7] – a belief that often appears more valid during the period of anticipation of the birth and only later is modulated when the woman is faced with the realities of mothering. Another important consideration is that pregnant women with psychiatric disorders may not present as often for prenatal care and therefore may not come to medical (or psychiatric) attention until near or after childbirth. The high-risk nature of a multiple pregnancy may serve to heighten maternal awareness of physical stressors during pregnancy which affect psychological adjustment then, as well as later, in the postpartum period. Unfortunately, these stressors at times may detract from the formal identification of psychiatric disorders.

As Wohlreich has observed[8]:

> Sociocultural and economic pressures have created a trend toward 'natural' deliveries, shorter hospitalizations, at home and birthing center deliveries, midwife assisted birth, and increased involvement by fathers.

Sadly, many of these expectations are unrealized in multiple pregnancies with their prolonged hospitalizations, technologically assisted deliveries (and often conception), increased medical risks, and the accompanying toll on marital and family structures.

The particular stresses[9,10] associated with multiple pregnancy (preterm delivery, low birth weight, likelihood of an operative delivery and potential for birth defects) often impede the pregnant mother of multiples from successfully completing the developmental tasks of pregnancy. These include: '...the acceptance of the reality of the pregnancy, development of an emotional attachment to the fetus, acceptance and resolution of the relationship with her own mother, and separation of the fetus as a person with his own identity'[11]. On an individual level, the implied 'abnormality' of a multifetal pregnancy (derived from its 'high-risk' nature), especially when it involves higher numbers, may interfere with acceptance of the pregnancy and bonding to the fetuses. Often, the expectation of a single birth and the fantasies for this single child come to an abrupt end and must be mourned, so to speak. However, this process often is not discussed openly with patients, because health care providers assume that they (the patients) readily accept the reality of a multiple birth and can immediately focus on that prospect.

On the contrary, this abrupt transition may engender anger towards the fetuses and/or the health professionals, especially if medical technology has assisted in their creation. The mother may feel isolated and may perceive that the real patients are the 'jeopardized fetus(es)'[8], whereas she is but a 'living intensive care incubator required to endure emotionally and physically taxing medical routines...'[8]. Even if the outcome is excellent, the fetuses may have been associated with real or perceived suffering and fear of loss. Should this be the case, these feelings may have long term implications for the new mother's relationship with her children[12]. Advanced maternal age and previous obstetric losses also may affect the current pregnancy and make it even more likely to be 'overvalued and anxiety laden', secondary to an increased risk for medical complications or poor outcome[8]. The hospital environment, with its depersonalized setting and White, middle class values, now must attempt to support many individuals with a variety of psychological and medical vulnerabilities who come from different cultural backgrounds.

Any differences from what is perceived as a 'normal pregnancy' can act as an enormous threat to a patient's self-esteem. Often, pregnancy serves as a catalyst to rework relationships with past parental figures, especially with one's mother[8]. Any comparisons to mother, especially if the relationship was a troubled one, may stir up feelings of inadequacy. Such feelings may be heightened by the increased need to depend on others for help during the pregnancy and the implied loss of control that accompanies such a need. 'False alarms' resulting in admission to labor and delivery may stir up feelings of 'demotion [and] banishment' and guilt about competency to carry the pregnancy[8]. Special population groups, such as single mothers or adolescents, may be particularly vulnerable to threats to self-esteem. A prior history of a difficult or persistent need for assisted reproductive technology procedures with its confrontation of the issues of loss or 'failure' (since that even repetitive procedures are not a guarantee of success) may stir up old issues of 'unresolved grief, guilt, or uncertainties about...[the] ability to become a mother...'[8]. This is especially true because of the 'medicalization of what is usually the most intimate aspect of a couple's relationship'[13]. This circumstance may further erode the mastering of a 'more natural' role so intimately connected with the concept of motherhood.

The susceptibility to anxiety and depression may be increased because of personal and external stressors[14]. Psychoactive side-effects of medications such as ritodrine that are occasionally used in high-risk pregnancies also may increase anxiety and depression, especially in women with a history of infertility or obstetric losses[8]. It is also possible that the high-risk pregnancy *per se* does not allow for adequate emotional and physical preparation for the care of multiples in the postpartum period[8]. This is especially true if prolonged hospitalization has been necessary, along with its imposed separation from the usual sources of physical and psychological support. Individual coping styles may vary from distancing and fear of attachment to being overly optimistic. Either behavior may make adjustment in the postpartum period more difficult. 'Self-esteem, health status, and social support were predicted to have direct positive effects on sense of mastery...'[14] and may serve a protective function against poor postpartum adjustments. The roles of the spouse, other family members, and friends may decrease or increase stress to the new mother, and are colored by these individuals' own expectations and difficulties adjusting to such a pregnancy and postpartum realities.

Postpartum psychiatric disorders

General considerations

Little doubt exists that the postpartum period is 'the time of highest risk of serious emotional disorder'[15]. Rates of mental illness in the first 6 months postpartum average 3–4 times higher than the rates during pregnancy (although the latter may be underestimated)[15]. Even the ancients were conversant with this problem. Hippocrates attempted to distinguish psychological disturbances after pregnancy by linking them to problems with lactation. (We now know[15] his hypothesis that milk was being diverted to the brain is incorrect.) More recently, in the mid-nineteenth century, a French physician by the name of Marce also focused on psychological disturbances after pregnancy, and his term 'morbid sympathy' became a precursor for postpartum disorders[16]. In the early part of the twentieth century, nosologists claimed that 'any psychiatric disorder can be precipitated by childbirth'[7,16] and therefore asserted that nothing was specific to postpartum disorders. As a result of these nihilistic points of view, even today postpartum psychiatric disorders are not recognized as unique categories in the *Diagnostic and Statistical Manual of Mental Disorders* (DSM III-R)[17] or by the International Code of Diseases as devised by the World Health Organization. Regardless, the idea that postpartum psychiatric disorders are unique has gained increasing recognition since the early 1980s[16].

To date, study designs that investigate postpartum psychiatric disorders are often wanting in comparisons to controls, controlling for variables, and adequate sample sizes (although more recent studies are larger). They also suffer from the limited validity of depression screening scales for pregnant and postpartum groups of women[18]. The infrequent occurrence of multiple births and the resulting lower numbers of potential candidates for inclusion into published studies further compound the difficulties in focusing on the risk of postpartum psychiatric disorders in mothers of multiples. Finally, the number of actual fetuses may, in itself, change the experience and risks to psychological well-being and make generalizations among types of multiples rather limited.

Postpartum blues

Postpartum blues is often a mild and transitory syndrome with an estimated prevalence that varies from 40 to 85%[7]. Symptoms seldom occur before the 3rd and usually peak by the 5th day[7,16]. Common complaints include dysphoria, mood lability, crying, anxiety, insomnia, poor appetite and irritability. The major predictors for the blues include a history of depressive symptoms during pregnancy, at least one previous episode of depression or premenstrual depression, or a history of a depressed, first-degree relative[19]. Obstetric stresses apparently have no association with postpartum blues[19]. Stresses associated with child care apparently increase risk[19]. Symptoms may overlap with early signs of a developing depression or psychosis[16]. The unique implications for multiples is unclear, except that, as is the case for singletons, recognizing the symptoms and acknowledging them as common, may help to reassure an already maximally stressed mother.

Severe postpartum syndromes

The more severe postpartum disorders include postpartum psychosis, depression and depression with psychotic features. All are characterized as 'severe', because they imply a significant disruption in functioning with a higher risk of suicide, infanticide and child abuse[15,16]. The etiology of severe postpartum disorders is multifactorial, although those forms involving psychosis tend to be viewed as organically based. It is estimated that 2–8% of female psychiatric admissions are for postpartum illnesses[20]. The overall incidence for these syndromes has been reported to be 1 per 1000 births[16]. Interestingly, this estimated rate of morbidity has been fairly consistent in a variety of studies from the 18th century to current times and in a variety of countries, including Japan and those in Europe, North America and Africa[16]. According to Hamilton, 'improvement or changes in obstetric care have had no apparent effect on morbidity'[16,21,22].

The incidence of postpartum psychosis ranges from 1.1 to 4 per 1000 deliveries[7]. Symptoms center around extreme difficulty with reality testing including the emergence of auditory ('hearing voices') and/or visual hallucinations, delusions and bizarre acts. Symptoms tend to occur earlier than with postpartum depression (often within 2–3 weeks after childbirth) and can last for months, and sometimes become chronic[7,16]. The literature describes a characteristic fluctuation in mental status that mimics an organic brain syndrome[7,16]. These fluctuating symptoms can include: '...inability to sustain attention, distractibility, poor recent memory, labile mood, confusion, bewilderment and transient delirious states'[7]. Risk factors include a personal or family history of an affective disorder, first baby, being single, Cesarean section and perinatal death[22]. Of course, a subgroup of mothers is at particular risk by nature of having had a history of schizophrenic or bipolar (manic-depressive) illness. Social class, other obstetric factors and situational stresses do not appear to be important[22]. There is 'no evidence to support that stillbirths or twin births are associated with an increased risk of psychosis'[21]. Although no substantial direct comparisons of risk for mothers of higher order births are available, reported studies support a major role for 'constitutional predisposition'[21], which can cut across all groups, regardless of whether the birth had been single or multiple. Treatment often includes hospitalization in a psychiatric facility and use of medications, such as antipsychotics, sedative–hypnotics and/or lithium, or electroconvulsive treatment (ECT). With the appropriate treatment, complications such as suicide, infanticide and child abuse have been significantly reduced[7].

A substantial risk of depression is present for women in the general population, increasing with age until the fifth decade[23]. Postpartum depression tends to occur in approximately 10% of new mothers[15]. Symptoms can occur at different times – either early (within a few months) or up to one year after delivery[15]. Symptoms are similar to those for major depression as outlined by DSM III-R[17]. These include crying spells, depressed, irritable or labile mood, fatigue, feelings of hopelessness and helplessness, significantly decreased functioning (which can impair child care), significantly decreased enjoyment of usual interests and guilt centered around the forthcoming role as a mother. Additional symptoms are ambivalent feelings towards the newborn, anxiety, medically unfounded somatic complaints, sleep and appetite disturbances, suicidal ideation and, less commonly, psychotic features. The extreme variety of these presentations has led several authors to distinguish subgroups of patients with milder symptoms (postnatal depression) from those with the most severe symptoms (postpartum psychotic depression)[16]. Whether such distinctions are truly part of a broad spectrum of a single syndrome or deserve to be separate entities is controversial. Such distinctions partially support legal purposes in cases of infanticide. Postpartum psychotic depression may mimic organic brain syndrome with fluctuating symptoms, particularly an increased risk of unpredictable recurrence of psychotic elements. An increased risk for suicide, infanticide and child abuse is present along with the more severe presentations[16].

Symptoms may last a few weeks to a few months, or have a more chronic course. There may be an increased risk for depression after subsequent deliveries[15]. As part of a broader definition of moderate to severe psychiatric illness after childbearing, the recurrence risk may be as high as 1 to 3 or 1 to 4[16]. A variety of treatments for severe depression are used, including antidepressant medications, possibly in combination with antipsychotics for psychotic features, psychiatric hospitalization, ECT and psychotherapy.

The varied time of the first presentation and the multitude of symptomatic possibilities suggest a rather complex etiology that goes beyond mere constitutional factors. Suggested biological considerations have included the changing levels of diverse hormones, such as estrogen, progesterone, prolactin and cortisol in the postpartum period. However, results of hormonal investigations have been inconclusive[7,24]. Anecdotal reports of alleviation of symptoms with progesterone and pyridoxine have appeared, once again suggesting a biological etiology[16]. The confusing results from hormonal studies may reflect laboratory limitations in measuring the active form of these hormones, however.

Speculation on etiology has also included thyroid or pituitary dysfunction, with the latter being associated with adrenal insufficiency – reminiscent of concerns about Sheehan's syndrome in the postpartum period[16].

The dissatisfaction with a strictly biological explanation of postpartum depression has led to further elaboration of potential psychosocial factors. In general, the postpartum period has been described as 'comparable to, but greater than, the psychobiological stress of puberty and menopause...'[20]. Issues that threaten self-esteem, such as pregnancy, produce variable responses depending on the level of individual vulnerability. The combined reworking of personal identity, relationships with past authoritarian figures such as the woman's mother, and dependency issues all are aggravated by the demands of the newborn. On a social level, major adjustments must be made in marital and sibling relationships as well. Postpartum depression has been associated with 'a lack of support of friends, parents, and spouse...' which may also be 'a powerful predictor of parenting difficulties'[20]. The contribution of 'support' may be more complex than previously estimated, because such support has been 'strongly linked in an inverse manner to depressive mood in homemakers but not in employed women or those on maternity leave'[25]. The particular overt and hidden meanings of childbearing and expectations of child care – an irritable infant, poverty and adolescence – may also predispose to depression[20,26]. In this manner, postpartum depression may reflect a 'synergism' among basic but, as yet, unspecified organic factors, adverse psychologically and socially derived meanings centered around motherhood and childcare, and a uniquely 'psychologically or biologically vulnerable individual'[15].

The implications for mothers of multiples suggests a possible increased risk for postpartum disorders. The Australian LaTrobe Twin study conducted over a 12-year period has suggested that mothers of twins are 'more anxious [and] depressed' in the initial postpartum period than mothers of singletons[27]. Hay et al. also reported high rates of anxiety and depression as related by mothers of multiples, suggesting a rate of anxiety at three times the rate for singleton mothers and a rate of 'extreme depression' at five times the rate for singleton mothers[28].

Higher-order multiples may bring even greater risk to new mothers for depression. According to Robin et al., mothers of triplets and quadruplets differed from those of twins by being 'particularly ambivalent and depressed'[29]. Whether such reports of 'depression' equate with the seriousness of symptoms formally attributed to postpartum depression is unclear. Nonetheless, the literature supports the concept that adverse psychosocial factors associated with higher-order births are similar to those associated with postpartum depression. In fact, the demands of an often even higher risk pregnancy (i.e. triplets or quadruplets), coupled with problems associated with parenting of multiples, places the new mothers and their families at a higher risk for infant mortality, child abuse, alcohol and/or drug abuse, financial problems and marital problems including divorce[10]. The child abuse rate has been reported to be 2.5 times higher than the general population[10] and more likely to be associated with older siblings[28].

Families of multiples may underestimate the actual work load involved and its psychological toll. They are often overwhelmed by the sheer amount of investment in time and money, the lack of sleep, extreme fatigue, and disruption in marital bonds, their relationships with other children, and their employment. Individual reactions of shock may occur at the degree of compromise regarding ideals of child care and the myth of being a 'perfect mother'. This is poignantly seen in the adjustment in bonding to multiples (see Chapter 42). Our ideals of bonding are based on a 'dyadic exchange'[30]. Mothers of multiples tend to oscillate between viewing their infants as a unit (which may facilitate organization and a reduction of stress) and emphasizing behavioral differences, which may impose early 'personality labels'[30]. Either tendency may impede a more 'natural' exchange that allows for individualized development. Bonding may be further impaired by medical complications. Mothers of preterm twins often prefer the less ill child[31]. This preference may reflect on the sick infant's level of responsiveness to the mother that is impaired in a neonatal intensive care setting[12]. Such difficulties may further threaten maternal self-esteem. The all-too-demanding infants may now be perceived as reminders of the mother's inadequacy. The expectation of motherhood as being a 'joyous' time is culturally sanctioned, but it may lead to guilt over ambivalent feelings and can predispose the patient to depression.

The important preventive measure against depression – social support – may be less available for mothers of multiples and their families in the USA[10]. American society generally emphasizes self-sufficiency. Nuclear and fragmented families do not provide the extended social network that is so important in coping with multiples. The growing movement of Parents of Twins Clubs may partially address the special educational and psychosocial support needs of this group[10]. However, this support cannot be total and problems may exist at the individual family level.

Family support for the mother may be difficult, because the other members are also adjusting to the realities of taking care of multiples. Fathers of multiples tend to help out more and may even become the 'second mother'[27]. This activity often is greater in the initial postpartum period and diminishes significantly by the end of the second month[27]. Perhaps one reason for declining paternal support may be increasing financial pressures that demand a focus on career development. Some fathers may withdraw as a reaction to feeling excluded from the spouse's attention. Still others may withdraw as a buffer against overwhelming stress. Gender role stereotypes further influence these outcomes. Older children, like their fathers, often feel excluded, especially when their parents', relatives' and friends' attention is focused solely on the newborns. In less traditional family settings, such as those involving single mothers, reliance on extended family members is even greater. The single mother may need to rely on her own parent or other relative to help with child care, but these associations may be difficult to maintain at times, because the new mother's relatives often have personal obligations or are limited by age. No matter whether in a traditional setting or not, mothers of multiples may eventually feel isolated within their own families.

Of extreme importance to the emergence of depression is the tendency of American society to deny death[32]. This may greatly interfere with the grieving process for losses that commonly occur among multiples. The more immediate demands of the 'survivor' infant or infants may not allow adequate time to mourn those lost[33]. Because bonding begins during pregnancy, a definite sense of missing the forever lost possibilities can develop and ultimately threaten the woman's self-esteem, especially if she has already suffered previous losses or experienced difficulty in conceiving[33]. Any such feelings make it difficult to enjoy surviving children, because they also serve as reminders of their lost siblings. The tendency for medical staff and others to encourage focusing on the survivors without acknowledging the unique meaning of those lost may unintentionally imply that multiples are seen more as abstract numbers rather than potential individuals. (See Chapters 20 and 50.)

Guidelines

The following suggestions may be helpful to health care providers in assisting mothers of multiples and decreasing their risk for depression or its more serious sequelae:

(1) History taking should include a careful assessment of risk factors for postpartum psychiatric disorders and a current mental status examination.

(2) If depressive or anxious symptoms are present, an assessment of suicide risk and/or other forms of aggression towards others should be made with appropriate action taken, if necessary, to prevent harm.

(3) If more severe symptoms of depression or psychosis are present, possible organic etiologies such as infections or other post-surgical complications, thyroid dysfunction, drug side-effects, etc., should be assessed.

(4) Patient education should include psychological adjustment to high-risk pregnancy and realities of postpartum life. Although optimism is important, it must be tempered with acknowledgement of anticipated difficulties.

(5) Patients find it reassuring to talk about negative or ambivalent feelings. These feelings should be validated as part of a 'normal reaction' to a difficult situation. Such discussions help maintain self-esteem and facilitate an accurate assessment of potential postpartum psychological difficulties.

(6) The mother-to-be should be prepared for 'not being prepared' and this experience should be normalized. The impact of caring for multiples cannot be fully appreciated ahead of time.

(7) Availability should be maintained in the postpartum period, because most postpartum psychiatric disorders manifest themselves after the hospital stay.

(8) Consultation with a psychiatrist may be beneficial early in a high-risk pregnancy for monitoring the interplay of psychological adjustment, medical concerns and risk factors for postpartum psychiatric disorders and for facilitating appropriate follow-up in the postpartum period. Consultation is imperative if manifestations of psychosis or more serious depressive symptoms are present.

(9) The mother of multiples should be encouraged to seek extended support and maintain social contacts. The mother should be given 'permission' to take time alone and time with her spouse as an important requisite for her mental well-being. Individual time with other children, as well as shared time as a family, should be encouraged.

Conclusion

Delayed motherhood, technology-assisted conception, fertility drugs, obstetric care and neonatology advances have all contributed to an increase in the numbers of multiple-birth babies who are born and survive[10]. Yet, the understanding of the implications for the individual mother and her society may lag behind our eagerness to thwart nature's limitations. Despite this apparent confusion, there is much to be celebrated in the resiliency of many mothers of multiples faced with incredible physical, psychological and social adjustments. Although there may be an increased risk for psychological maladjustment, this is not meant to detract from the positive outcomes that do occur. Yet, to ignore the difficulties can have grave consequences for both the mother and future generations. Society needs to assist these mothers by expanding its norms to include more respect for differences. After all, despite our focus on technology, our humaneness rests on psychological understanding.

References

1. Virgil, Aeneid, bk IX. In Bartlett, J. (ed.) (1968). *Bartlett's Familiar Quotations*, 14th edn, p. 119. (Boston: Little, Brown)
2. Notman, M.T. (1990). Reproduction and pregnancy: a psychodynamic development perspective. In Stotland, N.L. (ed.) *Psychiatric Aspects of Reproductive Technology*. pp. 13–24. (Washington, DC: American Psychiatric Press)
3. Corney, G. (1975). Mythology and customs associated with twins. In MacGillivray, I., Nylander, P.P.S. and Corney, G. (eds.) *Human Multiple Reproduction*, pp. 1–15. (London: W.B. Saunders)

4. Clay, M.M. (1989). *Quadruplets and Higher Multiple Births*, pp. 1–29. (London: MacKeith Press)
5. Kramer, P.D., Coustan, D. and Krzeminski, J. et al. (1986). Hospitalization on the high-risk maternity unit: a pilot study. *Gen. Hosp. Psychiatr.*, **8**, 33–9
6. Cox, J.L. (1988). Childbirth as a life event: sociocultural aspects of postnatal depression. *Acta Psychiatr. Scand.*, **78**, (Suppl.), 75–83
7. Steiner, M. (1990). Postpartum psychiatric disorders. *Can. J. Psychiatr.*, **35**, 89–95
8. Wohlreich, M.M. (1986). Psychiatric aspects of high-risk pregnancy. *Psychiatr. Clin. N. Am.*, **10**, 53–68
9. Malmstrom, P.E., Flaherty, T. and Wagner, P. (1988). Essential nonmedical prenatal services for multiple birth families. *Acta Genet. Med. Gemellol.*, **37**, 193–8
10. Malmstrom, P.M. and Biale, R. (1990). An agenda for meeting the special needs of multiple birth families. *Acta Genet. Med. Gemellol.*, **39**, 507–14
11. Kemp, V.H. and Page, C. (1987). Maternal self-esteem and prenatal attachment in high-risk pregnancy. *Matern. Child Nurs. J.*, **16**, 195–206
12. Davidson, C.S., Barglow, P. and Sripada, B. (1991). Psychological intervention in high-risk pregnancy. In Sciarra, J.J. (ed.) *Gynecology and Obstetrics. Maternal and Fetal Medicine.*, vol. 3, pp. 1–12. (New York: J.B. Lippincott)
13. Dennerstein, L. and Morse, C. (1985). Psychological issues in IVF. *Clin. Obstet. Gynecol.*, **12**, 835–46
14. Mercer, R.T., Ferketich, S.L., DeJoseph, J. et al. (1988). Effect of stress on family functioning during pregnancy. *Nurs. Res.*, **37**, 268–75
15. Casiano, M.E. and Hawkins, D.R. (1987). Major mental illness and childbearing. *Psychiatr. Clin. N. Am.*, **10**, 35–51
16. Hamilton, J.A. (1989). Postpartum psychiatric syndromes. *Psychiatr. Clin. N. Am.*, **12**, 89–103
17. *Diagnostic and Statistical Manual of Mental Disorders.* (1987). 3rd edn, revised. (Washington, DC: American Psychiatric Association)
18. Cox, J.L., Holden, J.M. and Sagovsky, R. (1987). Detection of postnatal depression. *Br. J. Psychiatr.*, **150**, 782–6
19. O'Hara, M.W., Schlechte, J.A., Lewis, D.A. et al. (1991). Prospective study of postpartum blues. *Arch. Gen. Psychiatr.*, **48**, 801–6
20. Landy, S., Montgomery, J. and Walsh, S. (1989). Postpartum depression: a clinical view. *Matern. Child Nurs. J.*, **18**, 1–29
21. Kendall, R.E. (1985). Emotional and physical factors in the genesis of puerperal mental disorders. *J. Psychosom. Res.*, **29**, 3–11
22. Gitlen, M.J. and Pasnau, R.O. (1989). Psychiatric syndromes linked to reproductive function in women: a review of current knowledge. *Am. J. Psychiatr.*, **146**, 1413–22
23. Frank, E., Kupfer, D.J., Jacob, M. et al. (1987). Pregnancy related affective episodes among women with recurrent depression. *Am. J. Psychiatr.*, **144**, 288–93
24. O'Hara, M.W., Lewis, D.A., Schlechte, J.A. et al. (1991). Controlled prospective study of postpartum mood disorders: psychological, environmental, and hormonal variables. *J. Abn. Psychol.*, **100**, 63—73
25. Richman, J.A., Raskin, V.D. and Gaines, C. (1991). Gender roles, social support, and postpartum depressive symptomatology: the benefits of caring. *J. Nerv. Ment. Dis.*, **179**, 139–47
26. McKenry, P.C., Browne, D.H., Kotch, J.B. et al. (1990). Mediators of depression among low-income, adolescent mothers of infants: a longitudinal perspective. *J. Youth Adolesc.*, **19**, 327–47
27. Robin, M., Josse, D. and Tourrette, C. (1991). Forms of family reorganization following the birth of twins. *Acta Genet. Med. Gemellol.*, **40**, 53–61
28. Hay, D.A., Gleeson, C., Davies, C. et al. (1990). What information should the multiple birth family receive before, during and after the birth? *Acta Genet. Med. Gemellol.*, **39**, 259–69
29. Robin, M., Bydlowski, M., Cahen, F. et al. (1991). Maternal reactions to the birth of triplets. *Acta Genet. Med. Gemellol.*, **40**, 41–51
30. Robin, M., Josse, D. and Tourrette, C. (1988). Mother–twin interaction during early childhood. *Acta Genet. Med. Gemellol.*, **37**, 151–9
31. Bennett, D.E. and Slade, P. (1991). Infants born at risk: consequences for maternal postpartum adjustment. *Br. J. Med. Psychol.*, **64**, 159–72
32. Kubler-Ross, E., Wessler, S. and Avioli, L.V. (1972). On death and dying. *J. Am. Med. Assoc.*, **221**, 174–9
33. Sainsbury, M.K. (1988). Grief in multifetal death. *Acta Genet. Med. Gemellol.*, **37**, 181–5

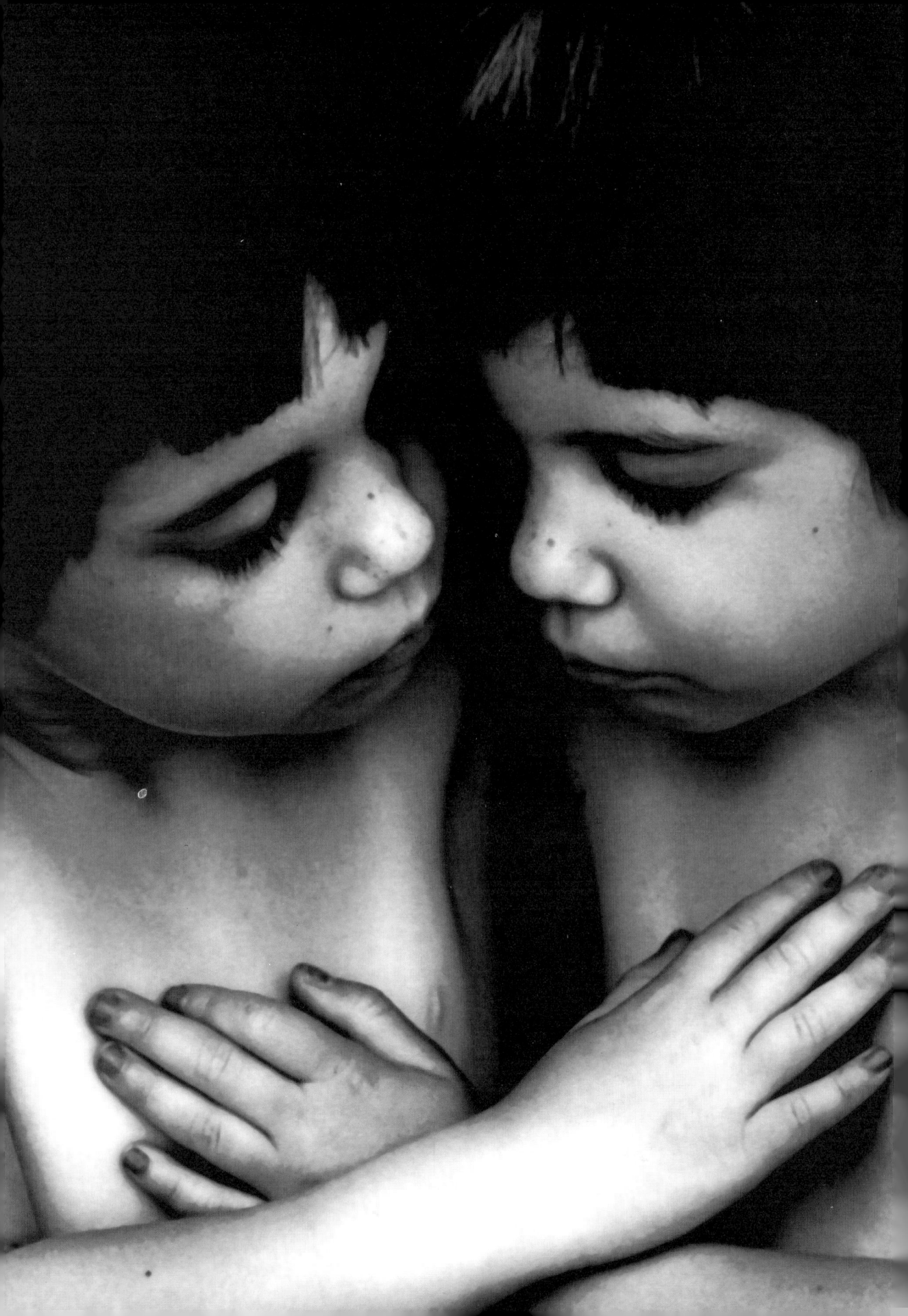

section VIII
Childhood Growth and Development

Difference

David Teplica, 1990,
Collection of Jane and Stephen Lorch, Boston, Massachusetts

Fetal brain and pulmonary adaptation in multiple pregnancy

C. Amiel-Tison and L. Gluck

Introduction

Despite recent advances in care provided to women with multiple pregnancies, the following statements are valid: (1) if twin *birth weights* are compared to singleton standards, a high percentage of twins are identified as small for gestational age (SGA); (2) the *perinatal death rate* is much higher in twins than in singletons; and (3) complications of prematurity represent the most important cause of death in twins. These observations are even more valid for higher-order multiple pregnancies. This situation does not seem surprising, however, in view of the increased incidence of pregnancy complications, early delivery and relatively low birth weight in these gravida.

If one closely examines the maturational processes of multiples, it becomes clear that these fetuses exhibit two major types of adaptive changes that are favorable for survival. The first, an acceleration of the maturation of the developing brain, is of great potential value for multiples destined to be born preterm. The second, an acceleration of the maturation of the developing lung, allows these fetuses to prepare for premature birth and extrauterine life.

In this chapter we examine the maturation of dizygotic (DZ) twins as a model to illustrate the propositions set forth above. We chose this model because it is the most common deviation of fetal number in humans. Of course, the same changes can also be observed in monozygotic (MZ) twins and in higher-order multiple pregnancies. However, the associated complications of very low birth weight (VLBW) often mask the favorable influence of these adaptive changes.

Moderate intrauterine nutritional deprivation appears to be the stimulus for the adaptive changes noted above[1]. In contrast, severe intrauterine starvation may overwhelm these adaptive changes and allow secondary deterioration to set in. Modern obstetric practice tends to take advantage of these adaptive changes and to intervene only at the very end of this favorable period. Thus, any investigation which helps to clarify the exact point in time at which the fetal situation begins to deteriorate has a favorable effect on the outcome, i.e. survival with an intact brain.

The brain

Historical background

After describing a method to test lung maturity by measuring lecithin/sphingomyelin (L/S) ratios in the amniotic fluid[2], Gluck and Kulovich[3] studied patterns of lung maturation according to gestational age (GA) in normal and abnormal pregnancies. Later, new data were reported by the same group[4]: The first of two studies was designed to screen a variety of unselected high-risk pregnancies in order to determine those conditions with intrauterine stress in which an accelerated clinical neurological maturation was present. The authors found eight infants in a cohort of 51 from high-risk pregnancies with neurological maturation that was 3 or more weeks in advance of that predicted from the GA assignment. In their second study, 25 infants with documented early pulmonary surfactant development (L/S ratio of 2 or more at GA 32 weeks or less) were evaluated. All these infants also exhibited an accelerated neurological maturation ranging from 3 to 8 weeks. Of interest, the infants with advanced neurological maturation were from pregnancies complicated by premature rupture of membranes (PROM), placental infarction, toxemia and amnionitis.

In a subsequent study conducted at the Port-Royal Maternity Hospital in Paris[5], Amiel-Tison described 16 infants who exhibited neurological development more than 4 weeks ahead of their GA (which was known with precision). Unfortunately, the L/S ratio was not routinely obtained in these cases). Among these 16 infants, seven came from uterine malformation and/or multiple pregnancies.

The concept that advanced neurological maturation was present in infants from multiple pregnancies was not well accepted until electrophysiological data[6] were presented to support these clinical observations. These very important findings renewed clinical interest in this adaptive phenomenon.

Fetal adaptation in dizygotic twins

DZ twins represent a homogenous group in which intrauterine growth retardation (IUGR), when present, usually begins around 28 weeks, and only rarely earlier. The nutritional support of DZ twins is often unequal, and one twin has an advantage over the other. In fact, the average birthweight difference between twins is statistically greater for DZ pairs than for MZ pairs[7]. As the pregnancy proceeds, both twins may become growth retarded compared to singleton standards, but often one twin exhibits this earlier and is more severely affected than the other. Because of this, DZ twins represent a unique model to study adaptive changes that result from inadequate placental nourishment during the last trimester of pregnancy. Hereditary difference in growth potential for each infant could be proposed as an alternative mechanism; however, asymmetrical growth retardation suggests a nutritional explanation in most of the cases.

Clinical data based on neurological criteria

Identification of maturational stages The process of neurological assessment of maturation in preterm infants is based upon the very rapid changes in motor activity that are manifest during the last trimester. Neurological maturational stages (from 28 to 40 weeks' gestation) were first described by Saint-Anne Dargassies in 1955[8]. From her clinical observations, it became clear that increases in passive as well as active tone proceed in a caudocephalic direction. At the same time, the primary reflexes, present from very early in life, are reinforced according to the progress of tone. The determination of these stages is based upon two distinct physiological processes. The first is the caudocephalic progression of postural tone in the axis and of flexor tone in the limbs. The second is the delay observed between active flexion in the axis (cortical function) compared with extension (sub-cortical function). Consequently, the ascending wave of reinforcement of tone does not affect the whole body at the same time and, therefore, precise markers of neurological maturation exist during the third trimester of fetal life.

Because this process proceeds very rapidly, with few individual variations, it has been possible to separate development in the preterm period into successive intervals of 2 weeks each[9–11]. However, this separation implies that most of the responses are clustered around one of the successive stages. Figure 1 helps the observer in his/her visualization of each stage. In using this form, one or three responses deviating from a line are acceptable. If, on the other hand, more than three responses deviate from a vertical line, then no conclusion can be obtained, as the assessment is invalid. The development of the preterm fetus is quite uniform in that the neurological abilities progress in all categories simultaneously. Correlations exist between this ascending pattern of motor activity and the ascending myelination of the subcorticospinal tracts, as recently reviewed[11,12].

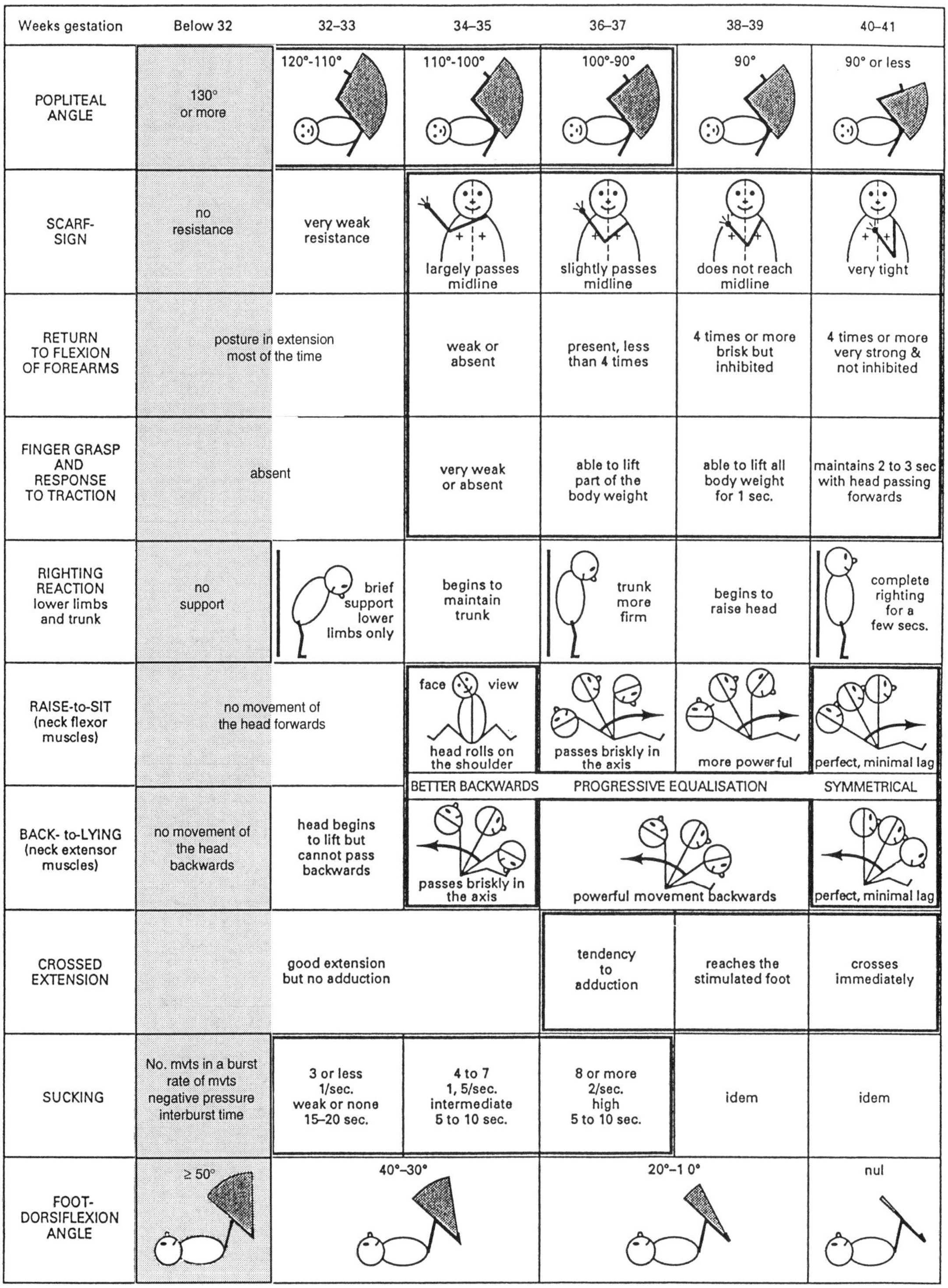

Weeks gestation	Below 32	32–33	34–35	36–37	38–39	40–41
POPLITEAL ANGLE	130° or more	120°–110°	110°–100°	100°–90°	90°	90° or less
SCARF-SIGN	no resistance	very weak resistance	largely passes midline	slightly passes midline	does not reach midline	very tight
RETURN TO FLEXION OF FOREARMS	posture in extension most of the time		weak or absent	present, less than 4 times	4 times or more brisk but inhibited	4 times or more very strong & not inhibited
FINGER GRASP AND RESPONSE TO TRACTION	absent		very weak or absent	able to lift part of the body weight	able to lift all body weight for 1 sec.	maintains 2 to 3 sec with head passing forwards
RIGHTING REACTION lower limbs and trunk	no support		brief support lower limbs only	begins to maintain trunk	trunk more firm	begins to raise head	complete righting for a few secs.
RAISE-to-SIT (neck flexor muscles)	no movement of the head forwards			head rolls on the shoulder	passes briskly in the axis	more powerful	perfect, minimal lag
				BETTER BACKWARDS	PROGRESSIVE EQUALISATION		SYMMETRICAL
BACK-to-LYING (neck extensor muscles)	no movement of the head backwards	head begins to lift but cannot pass backwards		passes briskly in the axis	powerful movement backwards		perfect, minimal lag
CROSSED EXTENSION		good extension but no adduction			tendency to adduction	reaches the stimulated foot	crosses immediately
SUCKING	No. mvts in a burst rate of mvts negative pressure interburst time	3 or less 1/sec. weak or none 15–20 sec.	4 to 7 1, 5/sec. intermediate 5 to 10 sec.	8 or more 2/sec. high 5 to 10 sec.	idem	idem
FOOT-DORSIFLEXION ANGLE	≥ 50°	40°–30°		20°–10°		nul

Figure 1 Neurological criteria described at 2-week intervals. Taken from reference 11 with permission

Limitations of neurological assessment The use of neurological data has some limitations, most commonly due to the clinical instability of VLBW infants. Thus, *prior to 32 weeks* it often is deemed inadvisable to perform a full evaluation of active tone. In addition, when an infant is on assisted ventilation, most of the maneuvers are impossible to assess, and even if respiration is spontaneous, the number of manipulations that one can perform is not always unlimited. Other limitations arise from the inherent nature of the maturation process. By this we mean the rate of neurological maturation slows down by 37 weeks' gestation. Thus, *between 38 and 42 weeks*, only minimal change can be recorded in neurological tone. At this GA, the evaluation process becomes less precise.

Given these circumstances, our clinical abilities to determine the level of neurological maturation are at their best between 32 and 37 weeks. This period correlates very well with anatomical data related to the process of rapid myelination in subcorticospinal pathways. As will be seen below, this period also correlates well with the timing of the maturation of brain auditory evoked responses (BAERs) which become fairly stable by 37 weeks.

Additional limitations of the neurological assessment relate to the lack of space *in utero* in the weeks or months preceding birth. In case of PROM, oligohydramnios, uterine malformation, or the 'crowding' common to multiple pregnancies, the 'communicated tone'[13] that derives from these constraints must not be interpreted as a higher level of maturation. For this reason, it is advisable to perform the maturative assessment 2 or 3 days after birth. If assessed earlier, the infant will appear older than he or she actually is.

Interferences as a result of neurological abnormalities must also be considered. When signs of cerebral dysfunction are present at the time of birth, one cannot be confident in the validity of the maturational assessment[10]. The most common example is mild asphyxia in a term newborn infant in which a transient hypotonia is present, but restricted to upper limbs and neck flexors. In such instances the infant will appear younger than it really is. Eliminating cases with neurological abnormalities creates some bias, however, when a series of multiple births is studied.

Interobserver variability and interval of confidence Interobserver variability is considered the main cause of poor reproducibility in neonatal assessment[14]. Another problem relates to the natural variability of maturation. Because an advance of 4 weeks is probably outside the 95% confidence limits of an estimate based on a neurological examination[14], the diagnosis of accelerated maturation in the Port-Royal study[5] was established only when the neurological development was found to be 4 weeks or more ahead of the GA. Ethnic variations in neurological maturation may also occur. A few studies[15–20] reported accelerated maturation in African populations, but the data are still fragmentary. Moreover, the mechanism of any possible ethnic advance is still debated. In addition to genetic influence, many environmental factors may also play an important role[20].

Deleterious effects of the use of neurological scores Among the numerous pediatric assessments of maturation the Dubowitz score is widely used[16,21]. The external criteria derive from Farr and co-workers[22,23] and the neurological criteria from Saint-Anne Dargassies[8] and Amiel-Tison[9]. The neurological part of the score relies mainly on an estimation of passive tone (eight out of ten criteria are passive). Passive tone is easier to quantify with apparent precision, but is often contaminated by the residual effects of posture *in utero* if the examination is performed in the delivery room or in the first 3 days of life. Moreover, the two criteria selected to define active tone (raise-to-sit and ventral suspension) do not allow comparison of the respective strength of neck flexor and extensor muscles. It was therefore predictable that the neurological criteria selected for the Dubowitz score would overestimate the pediatric age of the premature newborn infant by at least 2 weeks. This lack of reliability is even more marked with the Ballard score[24,25], in which the neurological criteria are reduced to six passive tone responses and ignore all aspects of active tone. Maturational overestimation due to the use of these scoring systems was first demonstrated by Spinnato et al.[26]; subsequently, other studies have confirmed these findings[27–29]. Overestimation in the very preterm group and underestimation in late pregnancy has been recently documented when the Ballard score was used[30].

Electrophysiological data based on BAERs

Brain auditory evoked responses (BAERs), as investigated by Pettigrew et al.[6], confirm the clinical observations of advanced neurological maturation in some preterm SGA infants. In their study of appropriate-for-GA (AGA) and SGA preterm infants, these authors have recorded BAERs believed to be associated with activity at different levels of the brainstem auditory pathways. The interval between waves I and V provides a convenient, objective measure of neural performance in the auditory pathways of the brainstem. The decrease of the I–V interval is particularly sharp between the 30th and 36th week gestation. The I–V interval was significantly shorter in many SGA infants, including multiples, compared to in AGA infants up to term.

Recognition of adaptive acceleration incidence and short-term outcome

Despite the confirmation by BAERs and diverse clinical data, the concept of adaptive acceleration of brain maturation is still not widely accepted, especially by those who favor a more rigid, independent pattern of neurological maturation in the fetus. Apart from methodological difficulties that arise on clinical grounds, two main sources of confusion influence this state of affairs. The first is the lack of clinical recognition of two separate periods when DZ twins face nutritional deprivation in the third trimester. When the initial adaptive mechanisms are overwhelmed, then deterioration occurs. Within a few days, the fetus may show a dramatic reduction in tone and spontaneous movements. At this time, adaptive phenomena may be masked by sufficient fetal distress that an emergency Cesarean section (CS) may be indicated.

The second source of confusion arises from the absence of certainty about GA in a high percentage of cases. This was the case all over the world in the 1970s when our data were gathered[4,5]. It is still the case in many countries where prenatal care is unevenly distributed or registration for care occurs too late. In a large measure resistance toward accepting these adaptive phenomena as real derives from this uncertainty. Although it is acknowledged that neurological scoring is unreliable, the perpetuation of the pediatric custom of 'dating' newborns will probably last until more accurate gestational dating is available and used on a widespread basis.

New studies should be performed in maternity wards in which both accuracy of last menstrual period (LMP) and early confirmation of the dates by ultrasound measurements are routinely available. Until we have sufficient epidemiological data to resolve these issues, a few relevant comments emerge from the continuing study of newborn infants at the Baudelocque Maternity Hospital in Paris.

First, advanced maturation of neurologic performances is not an all or none phenomenon. Rather it is a progressive response of variable degree. Second, it is common that the smallest infant in sets of twins or triplets is more advanced than its sibling(s); however, the siblings may also be advanced with respect to most normally grown infants. In other words, the occurrence of advanced maturation is not restricted to those fetuses labelled as SGA, but may be demonstrated in AGA fetuses as well. In these cases, acceleration of maturation comes first, followed by definite growth retardation. A very elegant demonstration of this possibility is found in the study by Henderson-Smart et al.[31] concerning pregnancies with hypertension. The mean I–V interval in AGA infants of hypertensive mothers lay between the values of AGA controls (infants of non-hypertensive mothers) and SGA infants from hypertensive mothers. Both clinical observation in multiples and electrophysiological observation in hypertensive disorders of pregnancy appear to ascertain a continuum of effects on maturation of the nervous system associated with placental insufficiency.

Third, in our recent data[32], 75% of all twins demonstrate advanced neurological maturation.

Unfortunately, we remain far too ignorant of the mechanisms which induce these adaptive changes to be able to predict them with accuracy, and the data on short term outcome are insufficient to demonstrate the favorable effects of these adaptive changes. Once again, this is due to the fact that infants born during the initial phase of adaptation and those born during the secondary phase of deterioration are pooled together in follow-up studies. In our experience, when either spontaneous or induced birth occurs during the adaptive phase, both immediate and late outcomes are excellent.

Experimental data and possible mechanisms

Using various animal models, numerous investigators have demonstrated the advanced maturation of BAERs[33-37]. In a series of experiments, Chanez et al.[38] examined the structural and biochemical development of various regions of the brain in rats whose growth was restricted after the 16th day of fetal life by ligation of uterine blood vessels. Na/K–ATPase activity that occurs during postnatal development was examined in different regions of the brain. The Na/K–ATPase activity was found to be significantly higher in the brainstem of growth-retarded rats compared to controls at postnatal days 15 and 21. However the development of enzyme activity in the forebrain, cerebellum and hippocampus of growth-retarded animals was delayed compared to that of normal animals. These observations highlight the differential sensitivity of different parts of the brain to adverse conditions which occur at particular stages of development.

The possible mechanisms of advanced brain maturation have been described[39]. Many recent investigations have studied placental function based on umbilical artery velocimetry[40,41]. Investigations on pregnant sheep in which placental vascular resistance was decreased by umbilical placental embolization serves as a model for study of placental insufficiency[42,43]. These studies suggest that fetuses have a considerable capacity to adapt to chronic oxygen deficiency secondary to decreased placental blood flow. This fetal adaptation is characterized at first by a decreased rate of growth and, therefore, reduced oxygen requirement. At later stages of placental insufficiency, however, when the decrease in total placental blood flow exceeded 50%, both the placental circulatory reserve capacity and the capacity of the fetus to produce an adequate circulatory response to hypoxic stress was exceeded. These new data are consistent with the opinion expressed in 1985 by Warshaw[44] that IUGR, secondary to placental insufficiency, can be viewed as an adaptive response of the fetus rather than pathology. Of interest, all these data are applicable to the physiopathology of growth retardation in DZ twins.

At this point, it is reasonable to inquire what are the mechanisms involved in the early fetal adaptation to inadequate nutrition and, more specifically, what are the mechanisms involved in the acceleration of brainstem maturation? The answers to these questions exceed the scope of our chapter and have been detailed elsewhere[39]. To summarize, however, various avenues of research show the following:

(1) The levels of corticosteroids and other steroid hormones can be elevated in 'stressed pregnancies'; the influence of steroids on brain development and function is exerted in many ways and has been reviewed recently[45].

(2) Recent reports have established that the levels of fetal catecholamines can be elevated in 'stressed pregnancies. The influence of catecholamines on the level of synaptic and neuronal activity is reviewed elsewhere[39].

(3) Synaptic maturation seems dependent on the levels of activity in neurons[39]. As a result, enhanced neuronal activity could itself exert a powerful indirect effect on

the maturation of nerve pathways in different regions of the developing brain.

Limits of fetal adaptation in DZ twin pregnancy and consequences on obstetric management

Three different clinical situations may be characterized among DZ twin pregnancies according to the gestational age at which some degree of placental insufficiency begins and according to the division of placental blood flow to each of the twins.

Late growth retardation in both twins The course of the third trimester when nutritional inadequacy affects both fetuses can be described as follows: by 28 to 30 weeks' gestation, growth begins to fall off from the singleton standards as the nutritional demands exceed supply. This undernutrition usually does not reach a significant level before 34–35 weeks, however. Ultrasound measurements of weight, femoral length and head circumference should be performed at about 2-weekly intervals; these may show asymmetric growth retardation in which head circumference is spared. Fetal well-being can be assessed by evaluating tone, spontaneous movements and habituation to sound (the biophysical assessment). It is relatively rare that undernutrition becomes threatening, and birth any time after 36 weeks should be optimal. Not uncommonly, a spontaneous delivery occurs around 37 weeks, with both twins behaving as fullterm newborn infants. In most cases, the two twins do fine with an easy adaptation to extrauterine life and a short stay in the intermediate care nursery.

Severe growth retardation in one twin In some DZ twin pregnancies, nutritional inadequacy affects one of the fetuses sooner and more severely than the other. The use of Doppler velocimetry permits evaluation of decreased or even absent diastolic umbilical blood flow. Modifications of fetal heart rate (FHR) variability, measured by repeated non-stress tests (NST) (30 min, 2–3 times a day) can indicate when fetal deterioration begins. Because fetal acidosis and hypoxemia may develop subsequently, cerebral blood flow may dangerously alter and the risk for cerebral damage is more threatening each day; fetal death may occur any time under these circumstances. At the present time, no better marker exists than the loss of variability of FHR to indicate the end of the adaptive phase and the beginning of the deterioration phase. When this takes place, Cesarean section is indicated in order to save the smallest of the twins. This decision, however, is at the same time, somewhat unfair for the heavier of the twins, as it places it at high risk for respiratory distress syndrome (RDS) and intraventricular hemorrhage (IVH). The truth of the matter is that timing of delivery in these circumstances, in order to obtain the best possible adaptation to extrauterine life, is very different for each of the co-twins, and the situation has to be handled to the best of our ability on a case-to-case basis in light of our knowledge.

Early growth retardation When growth retardation begins within the second trimester, the deterioration phase for one or both fetuses begins sooner in the gestation, i.e. by 30 weeks or earlier. In this situation, the physician has no choice but to accept a very premature birth with its high risk of RDS, IVH and necrotizing enterocolitis. In such infants, the prognosis is dominated by immaturity, and the chance to observe adaptive changes, if any, is small. It is important to remember to check for chromosomal abnormalities in both amniotic sacs; when first or second trimester growth retardation is present trisomy 18 should be sought[46].

Fetal adaptation in MZ twins and higher multiples

The gestation of twins and higher multiples is complicated by many risk factors which limit the favorable effects of adaptive changes. Despite this, these changes take place frequently and must be considered in obstetric decisions.

Monozygotic twins In MZ twins, the situation for both fetuses is often complicated by vascular anastomosis in the placenta. As described elsewhere in this book, both twins are at risk, the small one being growth retarded and anemic and the larger one being plethoric.

The prognosis is usually described as more favorable in the small twin in which adaptive changes may have had time to take place, as these hemodynamic changes are generally not acute but chronic. Moreover, because the risk of malformations is higher in discordant MZ twins, chromosomal abnormalities and multiple malformations should be considered in any case in which the twins differ markedly.

Higher multiples In higher-order multiples, the mean duration of pregnancy decreases sharply with increasing fetal number, and preterm birth (spontaneous or induced) dominates the outcome. An elegant study on quadruplets[47] has shown that the outcome is more favorable in the smallest of the set compared with the 'other' siblings. This series of 47 quadruplets demonstrated that more adaptive changes took place in the most SGA infant. Both survival and short-term outcome were improved. This does not mean that the 'other' fetuses were not adapted at all, but clearly at a somewhat lesser level. The mother should be aware of this circumstance so as not to be surprised to see that her biggest triplet or quadruplet remains longer in the NICU. One mother expressed her understanding and her admiration for her tiniest daughter who was doing so well by saying 'she had to fight'.

In conclusion, more studies are needed to explore adaptive changes. Prospective studies should include the evaluation of placental function, biochemical markers present at birth, the assessment of brain maturity, and evaluation of long-term outcome. Even lacking such data, we already know enough at this time to take adaptive changes into account during obstetric management[48].

The lung

For generations, developmental biologists have taught that embryonic and fetal development proceeded along fixed timelines. They described a natural developmental sequence that did not vary. In their opinions, aberrations of growth and development were considered as outlying phenomena. That these concepts are not totally true should have been realized following the demonstration by Moog in 1953 that enzymes can be induced either early or out of sequence with normal development[49]. From this observation, it additionally should have been realized that enzymatic inductions outside the normal timed cycle of development might cause major changes in structure, function, size, development and maturation of the fetus.

Early in the course of our studies on fetal lung maturation, it became clear that a sizeable percentage of fetuses violated the concept of the immutability of developmental processes. Most of these fetuses had significant *acceleration* of maturation of their lungs, although a smaller proportion exhibited delayed pulmonary maturation[2,3,50–51]. Many of these fetuses from whom this initial information was obtained were identical twins. Indeed, the best natural laboratory for understanding those factors that most influence fetal maturation is the identical twin pair in which one co-twin has had a significant difference in the degree of pulmonary maturation compared with the other[3,50–56].

Of the several clinical situations associated with differences in fetal lung development between twins, the extremes noted in disparate sized twins are particularly startling. In such circumstances, one twin might weigh 1700 or 1800 g or less, whereas the other might weigh 3000 g or more. Usually, this disparity results from a twin-to-twin transfusion in which the smaller of the pair is the donor who is bleeding chronically into its larger co-twin. Such pairs appear significantly different, the smaller donor baby being pale compared to the plethoric, but larger recipient baby. Of the two infants, the smaller always is the more developed physically and shows increased pulmonary maturation compared to the larger. Sometimes the plethoric infant actually has a delay in lung development.

Careful evaluation of infants born after accelerated fetal lung maturation has shown that almost every organ and function of their bodies commonly were accelerated in development, although the degree of this accelerated development varied according to the stress to which the fetus was subjected. The brain often demonstrated the greatest functional acceleration[4,5,57].

It is important to remember that the chronic stresses associated with accelerated pulmonary maturation usually also cause growth problems in fetuses. This is particularly evident with regard to various degrees of placental infarction. When placental compromise is sufficient to limit the flow of oxygen and nutrients to the fetus, some degree of growth failure may be manifest as inappropriately small growth for the length of gestation. In these fetuses, maturation is related in direct proportion to the chronicity and severity of the stress[58,59]. For example, chronic retroplacental bleeding with low-grade progressive placental infarction appears to be the most profound stimulus to overall fetal maturation. Maturations of brain and other functions have been seen in excess of 10 weeks of development[4,57].

Another major stimulus is infection, either chronic or acute. An example of a chronic infection would be villitis of the placenta, which decreases the functional capacity of the placental unit with resultant undergrowth of the fetus. An example of an acute stress is an often surprisingly low-grade chorioamnionitis. This condition can be associated with a dramatic increase in fetal pulmonary maturation. Chronic and acute infections exert significantly different clinical effects on maturation. The greatest acceleration in maturation occurs with those stimuli producing compromise of the uteroplacental unit and growth delay; here general body and organ maturation takes place alongside special acceleration of maturation of the brain. Acute infections, however, particularly chorioamnionitis, are frequently associated with dramatically rapid acceleration of maturation of the lung in the absence of any appreciable effect on other organs or on growth[58,59].

Other causes of accelerated fetal lung maturation include chronic maternal degenerative disease such as advanced diabetes mellitus with renal and other vascular problems, some long standing hypertensive/cardiac/renal disorders, although toxemia of pregnancy and pre-eclampsia, appear to have little or no effect on maturation, and, finally, prolonged (48–72 h or longer) rupture of the membranes.

The biochemical steps that might be associated with accelerated maturation of the brain are presently unknown. We can only offer with certainty a descriptive summary of the clinical effects. On the other hand, the biochemical sequences in the acceleration of pulmonary maturation are relatively straightforward, and much is known and explainable. To understand this process, however, requires a brief review of the anatomical, physiological and biochemical development of the fetal lung.

The lung is a derivative of the primitive gut. It appears at about 24 days of gestation as an outpouching that first bifurcates, then elongates, and finally begins a series of subdivisions to form the tubular airways to the level of the respiratory bronchioles. These are the last part of the respiratory tract that still has cartilage. To this point, the lung basically is an endodermal derivative. It grows into mesodermal buds that form into alveoli and their adjoining blood vessels and begins this differentiation from about 26 weeks' gestation onward.

Alveoli are lined by two kinds of cells. One is an elongated, flat, sheet-like epithelial cell known as a type I cells. These cells function as instruments of diffusion of gases into and out of the blood. The second major cell type is a large cuboidal epithelial cell, which differentiates into highly glandular type II cells, which manufacture, store, and then secrete surfactant.

In the weeks following the 24–26th week of gestation, when functional alveoli first form, the progressive development of surfactant, both qualitatively and quantitatively, is the determinant of pulmonary maturity. Surfactant is a complex material that lines the alveoli, stabilizing them by preventing their collapse on breathing out. Collapse on expiration occurs in lungs that have immature formation of surfactant, as is the case in the very prematurely born infant. In the absence of adequate surfactant, either in amount or in composition, the fluid lining the lung develops a surface tension so high that it collapses the alveoli at low lung volumes, on expiration. Mature surfactant, on the other hand, acts as a detergent and lowers this surface tension, thus stabilizing the lung.

Surfactant consists of about 90% lipids (primarily phospholipids), about 10% protein, and almost no carbohydrate. Although surfactant contains a large number of phospholipids, only four have a significant ability to lower surface tension and are therefore considered 'active' phospholipids. These include a small percentage of sphingomyelin, the major component, lecithin or phosphatidylcholine (PC), and the acidic phospholipids, phosphatidylglycerol (PG) and phosphatidylinositol (PI). Although lecithin comprises as much as 70% of the phospholipids, it is by itself not a sufficiently competent surfactant and depends upon being stabilized by the acidic phospholipids. Prior to about 36–37 weeks, PI is the stabilizer of lecithin. From about 36 weeks on, PG appears and becomes the major phospholipid that stabilizes lecithin in the alveoli[58,59]. The appearance of PG marks the actual biochemical maturation of the lung. In some conditions, such as diabetes mellitus, the baby is not considered ready for delivery without significant risk of RDS until PG appears in the surfactant mixture. Since the use of PG as the signal for infants of diabetic mothers to be able to be delivered safely, RDS in diabetes, once a serious problem, has all but disappeared.

Lecithin is synthesized primarily by a pathway that combines CDP-choline + diglyceride, whereas PG is synthesized from the competitive relationship between glycerol and myoinositol (INO) for CDP-diglyceride. Early, fetal tissues are saturated with INO[60], so that PI is formed by competitive inhibition of glycerol. When INO levels fall normally at about 36 weeks, PG synthesis increases. The competitive relationship of INO and glycerol is the key not only to the normal maturation of the lung but also to the accelerated maturation of the lung[58,59].

Although the CDP-choline + diglyceride pathway to form lecithin is fairly conservative, there is some ability for an early increase in lecithin synthesis, but only by a few weeks at most. The accelerated increase in lecithin synthesis is not nearly as dramatic as the ability to induce the formation of PG extremely early and thereby effect the very early maturation of the fetal lung.

The biochemical processes determining both normal and accelerated fetal lung maturation appear to be closely related, if not identical, to those that regulate the growth of the fetus. Fetal blood and tissue levels of INO are extremely high. Whether the INO functions as a growth substance or reflects increased concentrations of glucose is not entirely clear. The fetal tissue and blood levels of INO remain very high during the normal, natural growth spurt of the fetus between 32 and 36 weeks. At 35–36 weeks, INO is metabolized by formation by the kidney of cyclo-oxygenase, an enzyme converting INO to glucuronide. As the blood and tissue levels of INO fall, the glycerol combines with CDP-diglyceride to form PG[62–64].

When fetal stress is sufficient to accelerate maturation, the mechanism appears to be the induction of cyclo-oxygenase enzyme in the kidney metabolizing INO to glucuronide; the INO levels drop with increasing proportionate PG synthesis. PG synthesis can occur extremely early. In our own studies, PG has been detected in amniotic fluid and in lung aspirates as early as 25–26 weeks, with a resultant competent, mature lung. Significantly, maturation occurring this early with formation of PG is accompanied by significantly slowed fetal growth. The functional (metabolic) maturation of the fetus, however, is accelerated by many weeks, including recorded accelerated maturation of the brain by as much as 10 weeks. The earlier the fetal stress, the earlier and more dramatic the acceleration[58,59].

In summary, a variety of fetal stresses are known to affect the acceleration of the maturational process of the lung and other organs, notably the brain. How early lung maturation occurs and whether the maturation of other organs is affected depends upon the particular stress and when in the course of gestation the stress takes place. In general, chronic stresses, such as chronic retroplacental infarctions that create impairments in transfer of nutrients across the placenta, appear to have the most profound effects on fetal growth and maturation.

Whereas chorioamnionitis appears to have the most acute and rapid effects on pulmonary maturation, it has little or no detectable maturational effects on other organs.

The identification of fetal stresses and their effects are understood best from studies of identical twins. These investigations have been particularly helpful where only one twin has undergone a stress and shows changes in accelerated maturation consistent with those seen in singletons subjected to the same stresses. This phenomenon has helped verify the effects of chorioamnionitis, other infections, prolonged rupture of membranes, and placental infarctions. The problem of twin-to-twin transfusion also is seen uniquely with identical twins.

References

1. Economides, D.L. and Nicolaides, K.H. (1989). Blood glucose and oxygen tension levels in small-for-gestational-age fetuses. *Am. J. Obstet. Gynecol.*, **160**, 385
2. Gluck, L., Kulovich, M.V., Borer, R.C. *et al.* (1971). Diagnosis of the respiratory distress syndrome by amniocentesis. *Am. J. Obstet. Gynecol.*, **109**, 440
3. Gluck, L. and Kulovich, M.V. (1973). Lecithin/sphingomyelin ratios in amniotic fluid in normal and abnormal pregnancy. *Am. J. Obstet. Gynecol.*, **115**, 539
4. Gould, J.B., Gluck, L. and Kulovich, M.V. (1977). The relationship between accelerated pulmonary maturity and accelerated neurological maturity in certain chronically stressed pregnancies. *Am. J. Obstet. Gynecol.*, **127**, 181
5. Amiel-Tison, C. (1980). Possible acceleration of neurological maturity following high risk pregnancy. *Am. J. Obstet. Gynecol.*, **138**, 303
6. Pettigrew, A.G., Edwards, D.A. and Henderson-Smart, D.J. (1985). The influence of intrauterine growth retardation on brainstem development of preterm infants. *Dev. Med. Child. Neurol.*, **27**, 467
7. MacGillivray, I., Campbell, D.M. and Thompson, B. (1988). *Twinning and Twins*, p. 321. (New York: John Wiley)
8. Saint-Anne Dargassies, S. (1955). La maturation neurologique des prématurés. *Etudes Néonatales*, **4**, 71
9. Amiel-Tison, C. (1968). Neurological evaluation of the maturity of newborn infants. *Arch. Dis. Child.*, **43**, 89
10. Amiel-Tison, C. (1974). Neurological evaluation of the small neonate: the importance of head straightening reactions. In Gluck, L. (ed.) *Modern Perinatal Medicine*, pp. 347–57. (Chicago: Year Book Medical Publishers)
11. Amiel-Tison, C. (1995). Clinical assessment of the infant nervous system. In Levene, M.I., Lilford, R.J., Bennett, M.J. and Punt, J. (eds.) *Fetal and Neonatal Neurology and Neurosurgery*, 2nd edn., pp 83–104. (London: Churchill Livingstone)
12. Amiel-Tison, C. and Stewart, A. (1994). *The Newborn Infant: One Brain for Life*. (Paris: Inserm)
13. Saint-Anne Dargassies, S. (1974). Le développement neurologique du nouveau-né à terme et prématuré, p. 350. (Paris: Masson)
14. Finnström, O. (1972). Studies on maturity in newborn infants. IV. Comparison between different methods for maturity estimation. *Acta Paediatr. Scand.*, **61**, 33
15. Parkin, J.M. (1971). The assessment of gestational age in Ugandan and British newborn babies. *Dev. Med. Child. Neurol.*, **13**, 784
16. Dubowitz, L.M. and Dubowitz, V. (1977). *Gestational Age of the Newborn*, p. 139. (London: Addison-Wesley)
17. Agbo, Y.H., Diekonalio, K., Konan, A.M.T. *et al.* (1981). Corrélation entre âge gestationnel et maturation neurologique du prématuré africain. *Med. Afr. Noire*, **28**, 573
18. Marpeau, L., Gauchet, F., Bouillé, J. *et al.* (1988). Variations ethniques de la durée de la gestation. *J. Gynecol. Obstet. Biol. Reprod.*, **17** (Suppl.), 51
19. Stevens-Simon, C., Cullinan, J., Stinson, S. *et al.* (1989). Effects of race on the validity of estimates of gestational age. *J. Pediatr.*, **115**, 1000
20. Papiernik, E., Alexander, G.R. and Paneth, N. (1990). Racial differences in pregnancy dura-

tion and its implications for perinatal care. *Med. Hypotheses*, **33**, 181
21. Dubowitz, L.M., Dubowitz, V. and Goldberg, C. (1970). Clinical assessment of gestational age in the newborn infant. *J. Pediatr.*, **77**, 1
22. Farr, V., Mitchell, R.G., Neligan, G.A. et al. (1966). The definition of some external characteristics used in the assessment of gestational age in the newborn infant. *Dev. Med. Child. Neurol.*, **8**, 507
23. Farr, V., Kerridge, D.F. and Mitchell, R.G. (1966). The value of some external characteristics in the assessment of gestational age at birth. *Dev. Med. Child. Neurol.*, **8**, 657
24. Ballard, J.L., Novak, K.K. and Driver, M. (1979). A simplified score for assessment of fetal maturation of newly born infants. *J. Pediatr.*, **95**, 769
25. Ballard, J.L., Khoury, J.C., Wedig, K. et al. (1991). New Ballard score expanded to include extremely premature infants. *J. Pediatr.*, **119**, 417
26. Spinnato, J.A., Sibac, B.M., Shaver, D.C. et al. (1984). Inaccuracy of Dubowitz gestational age in low birth weight infants. *Obstet. Gynecol.*, **63**, 491
27. Constantine, N.A., Kraemer, H.C., Kendall-Tackett, K.A. et al. (1987). Use of physical and neurologic observations in assessment of gestational age in low birth weight infants. *J. Pediatr.*, **110**, 921
28. Shukla, H., Atakent, Y.S. and Ferrara, A. (1987). Postnatal overestimation of gestational age in preterm infants. *Am. J. Dis. Child.*, **141**, 1106
29. Sanders, M., Allen, M., Alexander, G.R. et al. (1991). Gestational assessment in preterm neonates weighing less than 1500 grams. *Pediatrics*, **88**, 542
30. Alexander, G.R., de Caunes, F., Hulsey, T.C. et al. (1992). Validity of postnatal assessments of gestational age: a comparison of the method of Ballard et al. and early ultrasonography. *Am. J. Obstet. Gynecol.*, **166**, 891
31. Henderson-Smart, D.J., Pettigrew, A.G. and Edwards, D.A. (1985). Prenatal influences on the brainstem development of preterm infants. In Jones, C.T., Mott, J.C. and Nathanielsz, P.W. (eds.) *Physiological Development of the Fetus and Newborn*, p. 627. (Oxford: Academic Press)
32. Amiel-Tison, C., Maillard, F., Lebrun, F. et al. (1994). Acceleration of neurologic and physical maturity in multiple pregnancies. Presented at 14th European Congress of Perinatal Medicine, Helsinki, Finland, 5–8 June 1994, C 36
33. Plantz, R.G., Williston, J.S. and Jewett, D.L. (1981). Effects of undernutrition on development of far-field auditory brainstem responses in rat pups. *Brain Res.*, **213**, 319
34. Nakamura, H., Kawai, S., Nakazawa, S. et al. (1987). Evolution of auditory brainstem responses (AER) in undernourished newborn rats. *Pediatr. Res.*, **21**, 371
35. Kawai, S., Nakamura, H. and Matsuo, T. (1989). Effects of postnatal undernutrition on brainstem auditory evoked potentials in weanling rats. *Biol. Neonate*, **55**, 268
36. Pettigrew, A.G. and Morey, A.L. (1987). Changes in the brainstem auditory evoked response of the rabbit during the first postnatal month. *Dev. Brain Res.*, **33**, 267
37. Cook, C.J., Gluckman, P.D., Williams, C. et al. (1988). Precocious neural function in the growth-retarded fetal lamb. *Pediatr. Res.*, **24**, 600
38. Chanez, C., Flexor, M.A. and Hamon, M. (1985). Long lasting effects on intrauterine growth retardation on basal and 5-HT stimulated Na^+K^+ ATPase in the brain of developing rats. *Neurochem. Int.*, **2**, 319
39. Amiel-Tison, C. and Pettigrew, A.G. (1991). Adaptive changes in the developing brain during intrauterine stress. *Brain. Dev.*, **13**, 67
40. Trudinger, B.J., Giles, W.B. and Cook, L.M. (1985). Flow velocity wave-forms in the maternal uteroplacental and fetal umbilical placental circulations. *Am. J. Obstet. Gynecol.*, **152**, 155
41. Fleischer, A., Schulman, H., Farmakides, G. et al. (1986). Uterine artery Doppler velocimetry in pregnant women with hypertension. *Am. J. Obstet. Gynecol.*, **154**, 806
42. Trudinger, B.J., Stevens, D., Connelly, A. et al. (1987). Umbilical artery flow velocity waveforms and placental resistance: the effects of embolization of the umbilical circulation. *Am. J. Obstet. Gynecol.*, **157**, 144
43. Block, B.S., Schlafer, D.H., Wentworth, R.A. et al. (1989). Intrauterine growth retardation and the circulatory responses to acute hypoxemia in fetal sheep. *Am. J. Obstet. Gynecol.*, **161**, 1576
44. Warshaw, J.B. (1985). Intrauterine growth retardation: adaptation or pathology. *Pediatrics*, **76**, 998
45. Baethmann, A. (1985). Steroids and brain function. In James, H.E., Anas, N.G. and Perkins, R.M. (eds.) *Brain Insults in Infants and*

46. Lynch, L. and Berkowitz, R.L. (1989). First trimester growth delay in trisomy 18. *Am. J. Perinatol.*, **6**, 237
47. Rhein, R., Knitza, R., Fendel, T. *et al.* (1990). Outcome of 47 quadruplets and quintuplets. In Duc, G., Huch, A., and Huch, R. (eds.) *The Very Low Birthweight Infant.* pp. 242–5. (Stuttgart: Thieme Verlag)
48. Amiel-Tison, C. (1994). When is it best to be born? A pediatric perspective on behalf of the fetus. In Amiel-Tison, C. and Stewart, A. (eds.) *The Newborn Infant: One Brain for Life*, pp. 11–22. (Paris: Inserm)
49. Moog, F. (1953). The influence of the pituitary–adrenal system in the differentiation of phosphatase in the duodenum of the suckling mouse. *J. Exp. Zool.*, **124**, 329
50. Gluck, L., Kulovich, M.V., Borer, R.C. *et al.* (1974). The interpretation and significance of the lecithin/sphingomyelin ratio in amniotic fluid. *Am. J. Obstet. Gynecol.*, **120**, 1
51. Obladen, M. and Gluck, L. (1977). RDS and tracheal phospholipid composition in twins: independent of gestational age. *J. Pediatr.*, **90**, 5
52. Leveno, K.J., Quirk, J.G., Whalley, P.J. *et al.* (1984). Fetal lung maturation in twin gestation. *Am. J. Obstet. Gynecol.*, **148**, 405
53. Dyson, D., Blake, M. and Cassady, G. (1975). Amniotic fluid lecithin/sphingomyelin ratio in complicated pregnancies. *Am. J. Obstet. Gynecol.*, **122**, 6
54. Parkinson, C.E. (1976). The lecithin/sphingomyelin (L/S) ratio in twin pregnancies. *Br. J. Obstet. Gynaecol.*, **83**, 447
55. Sims, C.D., Cowan, D.B. and Parkinson, C.E. (1976). The lecithin/sphingomyelin (L/S) ratio in twin pregnancies. *Br. J. Obstet. Gynaecol.*, **83**, 451
56. Spellacy, W.N., Cruz, A.C., Buhl, W.C. *et al.* (1977). Amniotic fluid L/S ratio in twin gestation. *Obstet. Gynecol.*, **50**, 68
57. Gould, J.B., Gluck, L. and Kulovich, M.V. (1972). The acceleration of neurological maturation in high stress pregnancy and its relation to fetal lung maturity. *Pediatr. Res.*, **6**, 408
58. Kulovich, M.V., Hallman, M.B. and Gluck, L. (1979). The lung profile I – normal pregnancy. *Am. J. Obstet. Gynecol.*, **135**, 64
59. Kulovich, M.V. and Gluck, L. (1979). The lung profile II – complicated pregnancy. *Am. J. Obstet. Gynecol.*, **135**, 71
60. Campling, J.D. and Nixon, D.A. (1954). The inositol content of foetal fluids. *J. Physiol.*, **126**, 71
61. Hallman, M. and Epstein, B.L. (1980). Role of myoinositol in the synthesis of phosphatidylinositol and phosphoglycerol in the lung. *Biochem. Biophys. Res. Commun.*, **92**, 1151
62. Hallman, M., Kulovich, M.V., Kirkpatrick, E., Sugarman, R.G. and Gluck, L. (1975). Phosphatidylinositol (PI) and phosphatidylglycerol (PG) in amniotic fluid: indices of lung maturity. *Am. J. Obstet. Gynecol.*, **125**, 613
63. Quirk, J. and Bleasdale, J. (1983). Myo-inositol homeostasis in the human fetus. *Obstet. Gynecol.*, **62**, 41
64. Lewin, L., Melmed, S., Passwell, J.H. *et al.* (1978). Myo-inositol in human neonates: serum concentrations and renal handling. *Pediatr. Res.*, **12**, 3

Factors affecting developmental outcome

45

M.C. Allen

Introduction

Multiple gestations are associated with increased infant mortality and morbidity. As a result, considerable concern has been expressed about the developmental outcomes of the infants of these high risk pregnancies[1-11]. Unfortunately, any evaluation of the effect of multiple gestation on developmental outcome is complicated by numerous confounding factors, including, but not limited to, their higher rates of prematurity, intrauterine growth retardation, and complications of pregnancy, labor and delivery, as well as the increased rate of congenital anomalies.

A number of outcome studies have capitalized on the unique opportunity that twins present for comparing the relative effects of genetics and environment on the processes of development. Twins have been compared to singletons; monozygotic twins have been compared to dizygotic twins; and within twin-set comparisons of twins reared together or apart have been made with respect to differences in birth weight, perinatal complications and, in some cases, postnatal environment. The range and breadth of these comparisons have contributed to an understanding of the effects of zygosity, birth weight, length of gestation, prenatal and perinatal complications, and socioeconomic status and environmental factors on final outcome. Because of this, studying the development of twins not only helps to answer specific questions for parents and clinicians, but also helps to advance our understanding of the complexities of human development.

This chapter discusses the cognitive and neurological outcome of multiple births, the many biological and environmental factors that affect these processes, and some of the issues that these data raise. Most outcome studies have focused on twins, whereas only a few have reported the outcome of higher-order multiples.

Developmental outcome: twins vs. singletons

The vast majority of twins develop normally[12-23]. A number of studies have raised the question, however, whether the incidence of neurological and cognitive abnormalities is higher in twins than in singletons[3,9,10,13,14,18,19,24-37]. In general, the differences noted between twins and singletons are relatively small, and are not always statistically significant.

Neurological outcome

The majority of twins have no neurological problems, and most prospective cohort studies have not found an increased incidence of cerebral palsy or seizure disorder in twins. However, many retrospective studies of children with cerebral palsy demonstrate an excess of twins: approximately 5–10% of children with cerebral palsy are twins, whereas only 1% (range 0.7–5%) of children in the general population are twins[3,10,24-26,28,30,32,36,37] (Table 1). A population-based study in northern California of children with moderate to severe cerebral palsy found that twins had a 6.7 per 1000 chance of developing cerebral palsy, compared to a 1.1 per 1000 chance for singletons[29].

Table 1 Twins as a percentage of total cases of cerebral palsy

Source	Total cases	Twins (% of all cases)	% of twins with co-twin fetal death
Asher and Schonell (1950)[26]	349	5.4	53
Illingworth and Woods (1960)[32]	651	8.4	NA
Russell (1961)[37]	488	9	18
Eastman et al. (1962)[28]	686	7.4	14
Alberman (1964)[24]	436	10.4	20
Griffiths (1967)[30]	400	9	9
Petterson et al. (1990)[36]	932	6.4	24
Grether et al. (1992)[29]	192	10.4	NA
Al-Rajeh et al. (1991)[25]	100	5	NA

NA, not available

Another population-based study of cerebral palsy in Australia found a prevalence rate for cerebral palsy of 2.4 per 1000 for singletons, 6.3 per 1000 for twins and 32 per 1000 for triplets[36].

One study of 78 multiple pregnancies in which at least one child had cerebral palsy found that 73% of the twins with cerebral palsy had spasticity (13% hemiplegia, 32% diplegia, 27% quadriplegia) and 27% had athetoid cerebral palsy[30]. Of four sets of triplets, seven had spastic cerebral palsy, two were stillborn and three did not develop cerebral palsy.

The incidence of seizure disorders in twins is approximately 1–4%, similar to the incidence in singletons[38,39]. Ghai and Vidyasagar found an increased incidence ($p<0.001$) of neonatal seizures in fullterm twins compared to singletons[3]. Although most studies of children and/or adults with seizure disorders have not found an excess of twins, Ottman found that twins had an odds ratio for seizures of 1.4 vs. singletons (the odds ratio was 2.5 for monozygotic twins vs. singletons)[35,40–42]. Among twins, monozygotic twins are more likely to be concordant for seizure disorder than dizygotic twins[39].

Cognition

More twins than expected are found among children with mental retardation (both with and without cerebral palsy)[27,32]. Nevertheless, the majority of twins have normal intelligence[12–23]. In one longitudinal study, twins demonstrated a mean intelligence quotient/developmental quotient (IQ/DQ) during infancy that was depressed by about 10 points, but this normalized by 4–7 years[23].

Studies published between 1970 and 1992 comparing mean IQ/DQs of twins to singletons are listed in Table 2[13,14,16,18,19]. An early study that evaluated verbal reasoning in a large number of children born in 1950–54 in Birmingham, England found a difference in the means among singletons, twins (4.4 points lower) and triplets (8.5 points lower than singletons)[16]. However, statistical calculations were not used to evaluate these differences.

Another early study found that 39 4-year-old twins had a lower mean IQ on the Stanford–Binet test and were more dependent on their mothers than singletons matched for race, sex, birth date, birth weight, maternal age and socioeconomic status[14]. The most recent is a study of children from *in vitro* fertilization (IVF) pregnancies, in which Brandes *et al.* found that twins and triplets had significantly lower mean mental developmental indices on the Bayley scale of infant intelligence at 12–30 months[13]. However, no differences were present between multiples and singletons (or between products of IVF and controls) on the Stanford–Binet at 30–45 months.

Table 2 Intelligence of twins vs. singletons

Study	Years of birth	Age when tested	Test	Twins n	Twins IQ	Singletons n	Singletons IQ
Record et al. (1970)[16]	1950–54	11 y	Verbal reasoning	2164	100.1	48,913	95.7
Kranitz and Welcher (1970)[14]	1958–64	4 y	Stanford–Binet	39	79.8*	39	89.3
Silva et al. (1982)[18]	1972–73	5 y	Stanford–Binet	24	98.3*	960	106.1
		7 y	WISC-R	24	100.0†	924	107.1
Silva and Crosado (1985)[19]	1972–73	9 y	WISC-R	24	97.4*	929	104.6
		11 y	WISC-R	24	101.8*	893	108.4
Brandes et al. (1992)[13]	1985–89	12–30 m	Bayley	51	113.4†	34	106.6
IVF	1985–89	12–30 m	Bayley	51	110.9†	34	98.6
	1985–89	30–45 m	Stanford–Binet	15	104.8	16	104.2
IVF	1985–89	30–45 m	Stanford–Binet	15	106.3	16	106.3

IVF, in vitro fertilization; * $p < 0.05$; † $p < 0.01$

A longitudinal study of a population of 24 twins and 900 singletons published in the mid-1980s noted persistent, statistically significant ($p < 0.05$) differences in IQ on two different tests (Stanford–Binet and Weschler intelligence scale for children – revised; WISC-R) and at a variety of ages (5, 7, 9 and 11 years)[18,19]. At age 3, these twins had been found to be smaller and they demonstrated slower language development[9]. Differences between twins and singletons with respect to WISC-R full scale and verbal IQ persisted at ages 7, 9 and 11 years. Although twins had significantly lower performance IQs (101.4 vs. 107.0, $p < 0.05$) at age 7, this difference in performance IQs was no longer present at ages 9 or 11. Despite an early language delay and lower verbal and full scale IQs, twins performed the same as singletons with respect to language comprehension, reading and spelling at ages 7, 9 and 11, respectively.

On 8 of 9 subtests of the Illinois Test of Psycholinguistic Abilities (a comprehensive test of language skills), 200 4-year-old twins had lower scores than 100 singleton controls[34]. Twins were generally 6 months behind their singleton peers, but they failed to demonstrate any specific pattern of language disorder. Language delay occurred with dizygotic as well as monozygotic twins, and was related more to social class and family size than to biological variables.

Hay et al. found language delay primarily in twin boys[31]. At 30 months, twin boys were 8 months behind singletons and twin girls in expressive language, and 6 months behind in verbal comprehension and 5 months behind on a test of symbolic play, respectively. In addition, twin boys had more articulation problems on entry into preschool at 38–53 months.

Factors that influence developmental outcome

It is reasonable to question why twins and higher-order multiples appear to have a higher incidence of neurological and cognitive problems than singletons. As noted throughout this book, multiples are vulnerable to a wide range of complications and problems during prenatal, perinatal, neonatal and even postnatal life[1–11]. In addition, because twinning is an aberrant event for humans, this process carries with it an increased chance of malformation or pregnancy loss (see Chapter 7).

Although multiples are more likely to face adverse intrauterine and extrauterine conditions than singletons[3,5–7,11,43], it is not clear if they also are more vulnerable, and therefore more likely to sustain damage, when faced with such circumstances. At least some authors suggest that twins have a higher risk than singletons for death[7,8]. Most outcome studies, however, propose that it is the higher complication rate (e.g. prematurity, intrauterine growth retardation, difficulties related to pregnancy and/or delivery) that accounts for the differences seen between multiples and singletons. Indeed, many studies that have controlled for differences in birth weight, gestational age, perinatal complications and/or socioeconomic status between twins and singletons (either by appropriate selection of controls or during data analysis), found no (or much less) difference between twins and singletons with respect to developmental outcome[14,15,22,23,28,30,33,37,44].

As detailed in other chapters, twins and other multiples have higher rates of congenital anomalies than singletons[45–51]. Some monozygotic twins demonstrate brain abnormalities that may well be the result of placental vascular communications and vascular disruption, especially when their co-twin dies *in utero*[4,10,27,47,51,52–64].

Some investigators have compared the developmental outcome of monozygotic to dizygotic twins, and a few have studied twins who have been reared apart[12,20–23]. These studies have attempted to understand the complex interplay between genetics and environment. However, some degree of caution must be used in interpreting specific findings. Even monozygotic twins of similar birth weights reared in the same home may have had different intrauterine and extrauterine experiences. Nevertheless, the striking similarities between monozygotic twins, whether reared together or apart, suggests a very strong role for genetics, not only in neurological development but also in the development of cognition and behavior.

The following section will explore the relationship of a variety of genetic, prenatal, perinatal, neonatal and postnatal variables that impact on development (Table 3). This discussion will include comparisons of monozygotic to dizygotic twins and of twins to each other, reports of twins whose co-twin died *in utero* and a review of studies that evaluate the many factors that influence the development of children (twins, higher multiples and/or singletons).

Genetic factors

Genetic factors include those traits that are inherited as well as chromosomal disorders and dysmorphic syndromes.

Inherited contribution to cognition and behavior
Longitudinal studies of monozygotic and dizygotic twins reared together or apart provide evidence of a strong role for genetics in the development of intelligence[12,20–23,65–67]. The Louisville Twin Study followed nearly 500 pairs of twins and their siblings with serial cognitive assessments throughout childhood[20–23]. Individual differences in mental development during infancy and early childhood were prominent, with each child demonstrating a distinctive pattern of spurts and lags[21–23]. Whereas the intercorrelations of IQ/DQs from age to age were modest in infancy, they progressively improved and subsequently stabilized by school age.

Within twin pairs, twins demonstrate a high degree of concordance in IQ/DQ (initially 0.66–0.67)[21]. Whereas concordance in IQ among monozygotic twin pairs increases over time (to 0.80–0.87), in contrast concordance in IQ among dizygotic twin pairs decreases over time to an intermediate level (0.05) characteristic of sibling–twin and twin–parent pairs. A higher concordance in IQ in monozygotic twins (0.84–0.88) than in dizygotic twins (0.54) was also present in another study, and this finding was true whether twin sets were tested by the same or different examiners[65]. Wilson

Table 3 Factors implicated in the development of twins

Genetic
Inherited contribution to intelligence – monozygotic vs. dizygotic twins; twins reared apart
Chromosomal disorders

Prenatal
Congenital anomalies and vascular disruptions
Maternal factors – maternal illness and drug use
Obstetric factors – polyhydramnios, oligohydramnios, pre-eclampsia, abruption
Intrauterine growth retardation – from intrauterine crowding and limited nutrient supply, discordant twins, subsequent complications
Placenta and cord problems – discordant growth, vascular communications, twin–twin transfusion, fetal demise of co-twin, vascular disruption, 'stuck twin' phenomenon, cord entanglement, velamentous insertion of cord, cord prolapse

Perinatal/neonatal
Factors related to delivery – abruptio placenta, dystocia, mode of delivery, birth sequence
Hypoxia/asphyxia – low Apgar scores, hypoxic–ischemic encephalopathy, neonatal seizures
Prematurity and complications related to prematurity – respiratory distress syndrome, chronic lung disease, metabolic complications, intraventricular hemorrhage, periventricular leukomalacia

Postnatal
Environment
Postnatal insults – meningitis, head trauma, hypoxia, apparent life-threatening events

---

concluded, 'The overall results pointed to a strong developmental thrust in the growth of intelligence, which was principally guided by an intrinsic genetic ground plan' (reference 21, p. 298).

Monozygotic twins demonstrate a high degree of concordance (0.69–0.78) in IQ even when reared apart and tested as adults[12,66]. The Minnesota Study of Twins Reared Apart intensively studied over 100 sets of adult twins or triplets reared apart[12]. Monozygotic twins reared apart and reared together demonstrated not only a similar degree of concordance in IQ, but also in a variety of measurements of aptitude, personality, temperament, leisure time and vocational interests and social skills[12,67].

Although these observations suggest a strong role for genetics, with respect to intelligence and even behavior, the interplay between genetics and environment remains extremely complex. For example, monozygotic twins are more alike than dizygotic twins with respect to infant motor activity level and some aspects of infant and toddler temperament[68,69]. It is possible that similar genotypes may prompt monozygotic twins to elicit similar responses from their environment (e.g. parenting responses) and to seek out comfortable environments that subsequently help elicit similar interests and performance, despite having been reared apart[12]. However, the higher concordance for seizures and cerebral palsy in monozygotic vs. dizygotic twins is attributed more to adverse intrauterine circumstances and/or increased incidence of congenital anomalies than it is to genetics[38,39].

Chromosomal disorders Although twins and other multiple births do not have a higher risk of syndromes of chromosomal abnormalities than singletons, the chance of one fetus being affected is greater than for singletons[70]. For the most part, infants with major chromosomal disorders demonstrate abnormalities of development[71]. Dysmorphic syndromes are characterized by specific physical characteristics as well as known patterns of inheritance and outcome[71].

Prenatal factors

A variety of prenatal characteristics contribute to the developmental outcome of twins, either by directly affecting their central nervous system, or by predisposing them to other adverse perinatal and/or neonatal factors.

Congenital anomalies and vascular disruptions (See also Chapters 7 and 26). Twins and other products of multiple gestation commonly are described as having a higher incidence of congenital anomalies than singletons[11,45-51]. Although some studies have failed to find a higher incidence of malformations in twins compared to singletons, higher incidences of specific types of malformations were present in twins[72,73], including malformations of the central nervous system, and cardiovascular and gastrointestinal systems[45,47,48,50,72,73]. A few abnormalities, such as indeterminate sex, positional foot deformities and kidney malformations are inconsistently reported to occur more frequently in twins[45,48,72], and lower incidences of some anomalies in twins (e.g. polydactyly, syndactyly, congenital dislocation of the hip, Down's syndrome) are also reported[45,72,73]. Even in the absence of a diagnosed syndrome, chromosomal disorder or known central nervous system anomaly, the presence of congenital anomalies carries a higher risk of abnormal neurological and/or cognitive development[74].

Monozygotic twins have a higher incidence of congenital anomalies than dizygotic twins, and this alone may account entirely for the increased incidence of congenital anomalies found in twins[45,47,49,50,51,73,75]. Because concordance rates for monozygotic twins are not high (0-30%), the higher rate of malformations is probably not genetic[73,75]. Some malformations result from the twinning process itself (e.g. conjoined twins, acardiac twins, amorphous twins)[51] (see Chapter 7). Other early malformations in monozygotic twins may also result from aberrant morphogenesis related to the twinning process[51]. Such malformations include sacrococcygeal teratoma, sirenomelia, exstrophy of the cloaca, anencephaly, holoprosencephaly, renal agenesis, anal atresia and tracheoesophageal atresia[47,51].

Monozygotic twins may also demonstrate an increased incidence of disruptive structural defects[1,47,51]. The majority of monochorionic placentas have vascular anastomoses, which may result in twin-twin transfusion syndrome, with hypovolemia and shock in the donor twin, polycythemia and vascular sludging in the recipient twin[1,4,47,51,52,54,55,76]. This circumstance can lead to central nervous system damage or death of either or both twins. If one twin dies, the surviving twin may be damaged by disseminated intravascular coagulation or transfer of thromboemboli from the dead twin into the circulation of the surviving twin, or as a result of acute hemodynamic and ischemic changes at the time of the intrauterine death[1,2,4,47,51,52,54,57,59,62,77]. Antenatal necrosis of white matter is more common in monochorionic than in dichorionic twins (30% vs. 3%; $p<0.01$) whose co-twin died *in utero* and when there are multiple placental vascular connections[52]. Other major central nervous system defects in survivors of a monozygotic pair whose co-twin has died include cerebellar necrosis, cortical infarcts, hydranencephaly, porencephaly, multicystic encephalomalacia, hydrocephalus, microcephaly and spinal cord transection[47,51,54,57-59,62-64]. Disruptive structural defects of other organs include renal cortical necrosis, horseshoe kidney, small bowel or colonic atresia, terminal limb defects, pulmonary infarcts and aplasia cutis[47,51,57,58,63].

Many infants with these abnormalities die or demonstrate severe multiple handicaps[51,52,54,57–59,62–64]. In children with cerebral palsy, not only is there an excess of twins, but also an excess of twins whose co-twins have died *in utero* (Table 1) [10,24,26,28,30,36,37]. Nevertheless, many surviving twins do not manifest these complications, and develop normally[54,59,62,77]. These vascular disruptions appear to be a rare phenomenon, but may account for a fair number of twins who develop cerebral palsy. Recent ultrasound evidence has suggested that more twins are conceived than deliver (the 'vanishing twin')[78,79]. One report has raised the question whether twinning, fetal demise (and subsequent resorption) of one twin and subsequent brain damage to the surviving twin may account for some of the unexplained cases of cerebral palsy seen in (presumed) singletons[10].

Maternal factors Maternal illness and drug use can result in intrauterine growth retardation, congenital anomalies, preterm birth and abnormal developmental outcome in singletons, twins or higher-order multiples[80]. Multiple pregnancy may be more common in mothers addicted to narcotics[81]. Recent studies suggest that cocaine use during pregnancy may lead to fetal vascular disruption with central nervous system lesions (as well as to increased incidence of intrauterine growth retardation, prematurity and abruptio placenta)[82,83].

Obstetric factors Polyhydramnios and oligohydramnios occur more frequently in twins and may signal the presence of congenital malformations (e.g. positional deformities, Potter's syndrome), preterm labor or death of a fetus[6,84]. Twin pregnancies are more likely to be complicated by hypertension, pre-eclampsia, abruption, hyperemesis, urinary tract infection and anemia[6,9,11]. In addition, pre-eclampsia, disseminated intravascular coagulation, fetal distress, abnormal presentation and dystocia are more likely to occur during pregnancies when one twin dies[56,78].

Maternal and obstetric factors affect twin developmental outcome only if they affect the fetus. The majority of infants born to mothers with these problems (e.g. pre-eclampsia, abruption, polyhydramnios, anemia) do well, but some fetuses tolerate the adverse intrauterine environment poorly and develop longterm sequelae.

Intrauterine growth retardation Twins tend to have lower birth weights than singletons, and monochorionic twins have lower birth weights than dichorionic twins[5,8,9,43,85]. This phenomenon is presumably an adaptive response to intrauterine crowding and limited nutrient supply, and the effect of lower birth weight (adjusted for gestational age) on developmental outcome is controversial. A number of studies have found that birth weight influences newborn neurological status, cerebral palsy and behavioral abnormalities in twins[14,33,37,86]. In the Louisville Twin Study, Wilson found that two subgroups of twins, small-for-gestational-age twins and twins with birth weights below 1750 g (regardless of gestational age), had significant but very small deficits in mental development at age 6[22].

The vast majority of full-term infants with intrauterine growth retardation have normal intelligence and do not develop cerebral palsy[81,87–89]. However, they do have a high incidence of minimal cerebral dysfunction, including speech and language problems, minor neuromotor dysfunction, learning disabilities, and attention and behavior problems. Major handicap (cerebral palsy and/or mental retardation) occurs in as many as 10–30% of premature infants with intrauterine growth retardation[80,87,90,91]. The risk of developmental disability appears to be additive for intrauterine growth retardation and prematurity[87,90].

Growth retarded fetuses and neonates are more vulnerable to a number of complications, including fetal distress during labor, perinatal asphyxia, meconium aspiration, persistent pulmonary hypertension, hypothermia, hypoglycemia, polycythemia, hypocalcemia and pulmonary hemorrhage[80,87]. A spectrum of abnormalities is thus seen in children with intrauterine growth retardation, and subsequent developmental outcome appears to be related to etiology, timing of the growth retardation and the presence or absence of perinatal complications.

A number of studies have evaluated the developmental outcome of twins discordant for birth weight by comparing the heavier to the lighter twin[22,44,92–98]. In the National Collaborative Perinatal Project, no differences were found between the heavier and lighter twin on the 8-month Bayley scale of infant intelligence or on the 4-year Stanford–Binet, either in children with ≥15% discordance in birth weight or in children with <15% discordance[94]. Wilson also found no difference in IQs at age 6 in 12 pairs of discordant twins[22].

Nevertheless, seven other studies of discordant twins found that the heavier twin had a higher IQ than the lighter twin[22,44,92–97]. One study found no significant differences when all twins were studied, but found that among 27 pairs of monozygotic twins with large birth weight differences, the heavier twin had a higher IQ ($p<0.05$)[96].

Placenta and cord problems Twins manifest unique or more frequent placental problems, including discordant growth, vascular communications, twin–twin transfusion, 'stuck' twins, vascular disruption anomalies, cord entanglement, velamentous insertion of the cord, cord prolapse and abruption[11,45–51,54,55,60]. These adverse conditions may have catastrophic consequences leading to fetal death or serious insult to the fetal central nervous system.

Perinatal/neonatal factors

The combination of intrauterine growth retardation, prematurity and perinatal complications appears to account for much of the difference in developmental outcome between twins and singletons[14,15,22,23,28,30,33,37,44].

Factors related to delivery Abruption may occur more frequently in twin pregnancies, and fetal distress, abnormal presentation and dystocia are more likely to occur when one twin dies[11,56]. Some controversy exists as to the optimal mode of delivery of twins, especially with respect to abnormal presentations and preterm twins[5,15,17,99] (see Chapter 36). Although birth sequence has been implicated as a factor in mortality and morbidity in twins, its effect on developmental outcome has not been established[3,5,6,17,30,37,44,87,100].

Hypoxia/asphyxia Twins, and perhaps especially the second-born twin, tend to have lower Apgar scores and a lower umbilical cord pH than singletons[3,5,11]. Grothe and Ruttgers found that Apgar score and umbilical cord pH reflected the birth weight (maturity) of twins more than did the intrapartum management[5]. In a longitudinal study of twins, more twins experienced hypoxia at birth than did singletons (8% vs. 1%; $p<0.019$).

Two retrospective studies of twins with cerebral palsy found that they demonstrated neonatal symptoms of asphyxia more than twins who did not develop cerebral palsy[30,37]. Although Apgar scores are not very predictive of outcome in infants (unless they are very low for a long time), symptoms of severe hypoxic–ischemic encephalopathy (including neonatal seizures) are highly associated with severe multiple developmental disability[101,102].

Prematurity Griffiths found that 85% of twins with cerebral palsy were born prematurely[30]. Infants born prematurely are vulnerable to a wide range of perinatal and neonatal complications that can affect their development[7,8,15,103–105]. These complications include respiratory distress syndrome, bronchopulmonary dysplasia, retinopathy of prematurity, infection, hypoxia/asphyxia, apnea of prematurity, metabolic problems (e.g. hypoglycemia, hyponatremia), intraventricular hemorrhage and intraparenchymal hemorrhage and/or cysts. Severe intraventricular and/or intraparenchymal hemorrhage carries a high (40–90%) risk of major handicap in preterm survivors[106,107]. Intraparenchymal cysts, or periventricular leukomalacia, carry a very high risk of major handicap (50–100%), especially if the cysts are large and/or bilateral[108,109].

As a group, preterm infants have a higher incidence of developmental disabilities than the general population[7,103–105,110–114]. Major handicaps (cerebral palsy and/or mental retardation) occur in 5–20% of infants with birth weight <1500 g and in 10–40% of infants with birth weight <800 g[7,104–106,110,111–115]. Sensory impairments, including blindness from retinopathy of prematurity, myopia, strabismus and hearing loss, continue to be a problem for preterm infants, especially the most immature infants.

Two meta-analyses of the developmental outcome of preterm infants have been published recently[114,116]. Aylward *et al.* analyzed results regarding the intelligence (intelligence or developmental quotient) of low birth weight infants from studies published in the last decade[116]. He found that infants with low birth weight (<2500 g) had a lower mean IQ/DQ than full-term controls (97.8 vs. 103.8). This difference was statistically significant, but is clinically significant only in that it reflects more children with mental retardation and borderline intelligence. Escobar *et al.* found that the mean incidence of cerebral palsy in preterm infants with birth weight <1500 g was 7.7% and the mean incidence of disability was 25.0%[114].

In addition to an increased incidence of major handicaps and sensory impairments, preterm infants have an increased incidence of subtle central nervous system dysfunction[103–105,112,113]. Even preterm infants with no major handicap, no sensory impairment and normal intelligence demonstrate more speech and language delay, visual perceptual problems, minor neuromotor dysfunction, learning disabilities and behavior problems, and require more special education. Up to 50% of preterm infants with birth weight <1000 g require special education[105,113].

Given that more twins deliver prematurely and that preterm infants have an increased incidence of complications and developmental disability, it is reasonable to ask if twins and other multiples are more vulnerable to these adverse circumstances than singletons. In a population of preterm infants (gestational age <32 weeks), no differences were present between twins and singletons with respect to neurodevelopmental outcome at 18 months from due date, after adjusting for confounding social, obstetric and neonatal factors[15]. Hoffman and Bennett evaluated the outcome over time (1977–85) of preterm infants with birth weights <800 g[7]. Twins, especially males, were more likely to die: only 7% (1 of 15) of male twins survived, in contrast to 56% of female singletons. Of the survivors, two thirds of twins developed major handicaps vs. 13% of singletons ($p=0.003$). This suggests greater vulnerability of twins born at the limit of viability.

Postnatal factors

Twin studies have generated a great deal of interest regarding the relative effects of genetics vs. environment on cognitive development and behavior. Because the human central nervous system continues to develop postnatally, the infant remains vulnerable to environmental, nutritional and biological influences.

Environment In the Louisville Twin Study, Wilson found that parental education and socioeconomic status had increasing influence on cognition as the child matured[21]. Whereas the relationship was weak at 6 months, it became stronger by 24 months and highly significant from 3 years on. In addition, socioeconomic status and biological risk factors seemed to interact[22]. In infants with birth weight <1750 g, gestational age correlated highly with cognition initially, but the correlation was much weaker by 18 months. Not only did socioeconomic status demonstrate a stronger effect over time, but it also affected the degree of recovery over time. Twins with high socioeconomic status and low birth weight fully recovered by 6 years (their IQs were the same as those of the full twin sample), whereas twins with low socioeconomic status improved between 3 and 6 years, but their IQs remained lower than those of the full twin sample. Studies of language abilities in twins also have suggested that environmental factors play a role in their language development[31,34].

In an intriguing study, Minde *et al.* studied maternal preference for preterm twins[117]. These authors found that not only did mothers demonstrate a preference within 2 weeks, but the preferred twin had a higher IQ and fewer behavior problems at age 4.

Studies of monozygotic vs. dizygotic twins suggest that, although environment greatly influences neonatal temperament, genetics appears to play a stronger role than environment in many aspects of infant and toddler temperament[68,118]. In a study of hyperactivity in 13-year-old twins, adverse family factors demonstrated only a weak relationship with hyperactivity, whereas genetic effects accounted for about half the variance[119]. After controlling for the effects of IQ on reading ability, family size and some aspects of the parent–child relationships predicted their reading ability[120].

Postnatal insults Since the infant and child's central nervous system continues to mature, nutritional and health status remain important contributors to the child's development. Postnatal insults, such as meningitis, head trauma and/or hypoxia can cause or contribute to developmental disability. Twins and other multiples have a higher incidence of apparent life threatening events (sudden infant death syndrome)[121].

Conclusions

Intrauterine growth retardation and preterm delivery, with their subsequent perinatal and neonatal complications, exert a profound affect on development in twins and other multiples. Twins may be especially vulnerable to death and central nervous system injury when born at the limit of viability.

The majority of twins who survive do well. The mean IQ for a given population of twins and triplets is in the normal range, and the majority are free of major handicap, despite having increased incidence of developmental disability, cerebral palsy, mental retardation, sensory impairments, language delays, learning disability, and attention and behavior problems.

Twins have taught us a great deal about the complex interactions between genetics and environment. Rather than framing it solely in terms of the genetics vs. environment controversy, we have been helped by twins to appreciate the continuous interactions between the genome, the developing organism, the intrauterine and the extrauterine environment and the forces that drive development and shape both the organism and the environment.

References

1. Benirschke, K. and Kim, C.K. (1973). Multiple pregnancy (first of two parts). *N. Engl. J. Med.*, **288**, 1276
2. Benirschke, K. and Kim, C.K. (1973). Multiple pregnancy (second of two parts). *N. Engl. J. Med.*, **288**, 1329
3. Ghai, V. and Vidyasagar, D. (1988). Morbidity and mortality factors in twins: an epidemiologic approach. *Clin. Perinatol.*, **15**, 123
4. Bryan, E.M. (1986). The intrauterine hazards of twins. *Arch. Dis. Child.*, **61**, 1044
5. Grothe, W. and Ruttgers, H. (1985). Twin pregnancies: an 11-year review. *Acta Genet. Med. Gemellol.*, **34**, 49
6. Herruzo, A.J., Martinez, L., Biel, E. *et al.* (1991). Perinatal morbidity and mortality in twin pregnancies. *Int. J. Gynecol. Obstet.*, **36**, 17
7. Hoffman, E.L. and Bennett, F.C. (1990). Birth weight less than 800 grams: changing outcomes and influences of gender and gestation number. *Pediatrics*, **86**, 27
8. Kleinman, J.C., Fowler, M.G. and Kessel, S.S. (1991). Comparison of infant mortality among twins and singletons: United States 1960 and 1983. *Am. J. Epidemiol.*, **133**, 133
9. McDiarmid, J.M. and Silva, P.A. (1979). Three-year-old twins and singletons: a comparison of some perinatal, environmental, experiential, and developmental characteristics. *Aust. Paediatr. J.*, **15**, 243

10. Scheller, J.M. and Nelson, K.B. (1992). Twinning and neurologic morbidity. *Am. J. Dis. Child.*, **146**, 1110
11. Spellacy, W.N., Handler, A. and Ferre, C.D. (1990). A case–control study of 1253 twin pregnancies from a 1982–1987 perinatal data base. *Obstet. Gynecol.*, **75**, 168
12. Bouchard, T.J., Lykken, D.T., McGue, M. *et al.* (1990). Sources of human psychological differences: the Minnesota study of twins reared apart. *Science*, **250**, 223
13. Brandes, J.M., Scher, A., Itzkovits, J. *et al.* (1992). Growth and development of children conceived by *in vitro* fertilization. *Pediatrics*, **90**, 424
14. Kranitz, M.A. and Welcher, D.W. (1971). The Johns Hopkins Collaborative Perinatal Project – Part III. Bevahioral characteristics of options. *Johns Hopkins Med. J.*, **129**, 1
15. Morley, R., Cole, T.J., Powell, R. *et al.* (1989). Growth and development in premature twins. *Arch. Dis. Child.*, **64**, 1042
16. Record, R.G., McKeown, T. and Edwards, J.H. (1970). An investigation of the difference in measured intelligence between twins and single births. *Ann. Hum. Genet. Lond.*, **34**, 11
17. Rydhstrom, H. (1990). Prognosis for twins with birth weight <1500 gm: the impact of Cesarean section in relation to fetal presentation. *Am. J. Obstet. Gynecol.*, **163**, 528
18. Silva, P.A., McGee, R.O. and Powell, J. (1982). Growth and development of twins compared with singletons at ages five and seven: a follow-up report from the Dunedin Multidisciplinary Child Development Study. *Aust. Paediatr. J.*, **18**, 35
19. Silva, P.A. and Crosado, B. (1985). The growth and development of twins compared with singletons at ages 9 and 11. *Aust. Paediatr. J.*, **21**, 265
20. Wilson, R.S. (1978). Synchronies in mental development: an epigenetic perspective. *Science*, **202**, 939
21. Wilson, R.S. (1983). The Louisville twin study: developmental synchronies in behavior. *Child Dev.*, **54**, 298
22. Wilson, R.S. (1985). Risk and resilience in early mental development. *Dev. Psychol.*, **21**, 795
23. Wilson, R.S. (1986). Growth and development of human twins. In Falkner, F. and Tanner, J.M. (eds.) *Human Growth: a Comprehensive Treatise*, 2nd edn., pp. 197–211. (New York: Plenum Press)
24. Alberman, E. (1964). Cerebral palsy in twins. *Guy's Hosp. Rep.*, **113**, 285
25. Al-Rajeh, S., Bademosi, O., Awada, A. *et al.* (1991). Cerebral palsy in Saudi Arabia: a case–control study of risk factors. *Dev. Med. Child. Neurol.*, **33**, 1048
26. Asher, P. and Schonell, F.E. (1950). A survey of 400 cases of cerebral palsy in childhood. *Arch. Dis. Child.*, **25**, 360
27. Durkin, M.V., Kaveggia, E.G., Pendleton, E. *et al.* (1976). Analysis of etiologic factors in cerebral palsy with severe mental retardation. I. Analysis of gestational, parturitional and neonatal data. *Eur. J. Pediatr.*, **123**, 67
28. Eastman, N.J., Kohl, S.G., Maisel, J.E. *et al.* (1962). The obstetrical background of 753 cases of cerebral palsy. *Obstet. Gynecol. Surv.*, **17**, 459
29. Grether, J.K., Cummins, S.K. and Nelson, K.B. (1992). The California Cerebral Palsy Project. *Paediatr. Perinat. Epidemiol.*, **6**, 339
30. Griffiths, M. (1967). Cerebral palsy in multiple pregnancy. *Dev. Med. Child Neurol.*, **9**, 713
31. Hay, D.A., Prior, M., Collett, S. *et al.* (1987). Speech and language development in preschool twins. *Acta Genet. Med. Gemellol.*, **36**, 213
32. Illingworth, R.S. and Woods, G.E. (1960). The incidence of twins in cerebral palsy and mental retardation. *Arch. Dis. Child.*, **35**, 333
33. Kragt, H., Huisjes, H.J. and Touwen, B.C.L. (1985). Neurological morbidity in newborn twins. *Eur. J. Obstet. Gynecol. Reprod. Biol.*, **19**, 75
34. Mittler, P. (1970). Biological and social aspects of language development in twins. *Dev. Med. Child Neurol.*, **12**, 741
35. Ottman, R. (1992). Genetic and developmental influences on susceptibility to epilepsy: evidence from twins. *Paediatr. Perinat. Epidemiol.*, **6**, 265
36. Petterson, B., Stanley, F. and Henderson, D. (1990). Cerebral palsy in multiple births in western Australia: genetic aspects. *Am. J. Med. Genet.*, **37**, 346
37. Russell, E.M. (1961). Cerebral palsied twins. *Arch. Dis. Child.*, **36**, 328
38. Berkovic, S.F., Howell, R.A. and Hay, D.A. (1991). Twin birth is not a significant risk factor for epilepsy. *Epilepsia*, **32**, 70
39. Corey, L.A., Berg, K., Pellock, J.M. *et al.* (1991). The occurrence of epilepsy and febrile seizures in Virginian and Norwegian twins. *Neurology*, **41**, 1433
40. Rocca, W.A., Sharbrough, F.W., Hauser, W.A. *et al.* (1987). Risk factors for complex partial

seizures: a population-based case–control study. *Ann. Neurol.*, **21**, 22

41. Rocca, W.A., Sharbrough, F.W., Hauser, W.A. *et al.* (1987). Risk factors for generalized tonic–clonic seizures: a population-based case–control study in Rochester, Minnesota. *Neurology*, **37**, 1315

42. Rocca, W.A., Sharbrough, F.W., Hauser, W.A. *et al.* (1987). Risk factors for absence seizures: a population-based case–control study in Rochester, Minnesota. *Neurology*, **37**, 1309

43. Tessen, J.A. and Zlatnik, F.J. (1991). Monoamniotic twins: a retrospective controlled study. *Obstet. Gynecol.*, **77**, 832

44. Stauffer, A., Burns, W.J., Burns, K.A. *et al.* (1988). Early developmental progress of preterm twins discordant for birthweight and risk. *Acta Genet. Med. Gemellol.*, **37**, 81

45. Hay, S. and Wehrung, D.A. (1970). Congenital malformations in twins. *Am. J. Hum. Genet.*, **22**, 662

46. Hendricks, C.H. (1966). Twinning in relation to birth weight, mortality, and congenital anomalies. *Obstet. Gynecol.*, **27**, 47

47. Jones, K.L. and Benirschke, K. (1983). The developmental pathogenesis of structural defects: the contribution of monozygotic twins. *Semin. Perinatol.*, **7**, 239

48. Kallen, B. (1986). Congenital malformations in twins: a population study. *Acta Genet. Med. Gemellol.*, **35**, 167

49. Layde, P.M., Erickson, J.D., Falek, A. and McCarthy, B.J. (1980). Congenital malformation in twins. *Am. J. Hum. Genet.*, **32**, 69

50. Myrianthopoulos, N.C. (1976). Congenital malformation in twins. *Acta Genet. Med. Gemellol.*, **25**, 331

51. Schinzel, A.A.G.L., Smith, D.W. and Miller, J.R. (1979). Monozygotic twinning and structural defects. **95**, 921

52. Bejar, R., Vigliocco, G., Gramajo, H. *et al.* (1990). Antenatal origin of neurologic damage in newborn infants. II. Multiple gestations. *Am. J. Obstet. Gynecol.*, **162**, 1230

53. Burke, M.S. (1990). Single fetal demise in twin gestation. *Clin. Obstet. Gynaecol.*, **33**, 69

54. D'Alton, M.E., Newton, E.R. and Cetrulo, C.L. (1984). Intrauterine fetal demise in multiple gestation. *Acta Genet. Med. Gemellol.*, **33**, 43

55. Dudley, D.K.L. and D'Alton, M.E. (1986). Single fetal death in twin gestation. *Semin. Perinatol.*, **10**, 65

56. Enbom, J.A. (1985). Twin pregnancy with intrauterine death of one twin. *Am. J. Obstet. Gynecol.*, **152**, 424

57. Fusi, L., McParland, P., Fisk, N. *et al.* (1991). Acute twin–twin transfusion: a possible mechanism for brain-damaged survivors after intrauterine death of a monochorionic twin. *Obstet. Gynecol.*, **78**, 517

58. Hoyme, H.E., Higginbottom, M.C. and Jones, K.L. (1981). Vascular etiology of disruptive structural defects in monozygotic twins. *Pediatrics*, **67**, 288

59. Larroche, J.C.L., Droulle, P., Delezoide, A.L. *et al.* (1990). Brain damage in monozygous twins. *Biol. Neonate*, **57**, 261

60. Mahony, B.S., Petty, C.N., Nyberg, D.A. *et al.* (1990). The 'stuck twin' phenomenon: ultrasonographic findings, pregnancy outcome, and management with serial amniocenteses. *Am. J. Obstet. Gynecol.*, **163**, 1513

61. Moore, C.M., McAdams, A.J. and Sutherland, J. (1969). Intrauterine disseminated intravascular coagulation: a syndrome of multiple pregnancy with a dead twin fetus. *J. Pediatr.*, **74**, 523

62. Melnick, M. (1977). Brain damage in survivor after *in-utero* death of monozygous co-twin. *Lancet*, **2**, 1287

63. Szymonowicz, W., Preston, H. and Yu, V.Y.H. (1986). The surviving monozygotic twin. *Arch. Dis. Child.*, **61**, 454

64. Yoshioka, H., Kadomoto, Y., Mino, M. *et al.* (1979). Multicystic encephalomalacia in liveborn twin with a stillborn macerated co-twin. *J. Pediatr.*, **95**, 798

65. Segal, N.L. and Russell, J. (1991). IQ similarity in monozygotic and dizygotic twin children: effects of the same versus different examiners: a research note. *J. Child Psychol. Psychiatry*, **32**, 703

66. Shields, J. (1962). *Monozygotic Twins: Brought Up Apart and Brought Up Together.* (New York: Oxford University Press)

67. Lykken, D.J., Bouchard, T.J. Jr, McGue, M. *et al.* (1990). *Acta Genet. Med. Gemellol.*, **39**, 35

68. Cyphers, L.H., Phillips, K., Fulker, D.W. *et al.* (1990). Twin temperament during the transition from infancy to early childhood. *J. Am. Acad. Child Adolesc. Psychiatry*, **29**, 392

69. Saudino, K.J. and Eaton, W.O. (1991). Infant temperament and genetics: an objective twin study of motor activity level. *Child Dev.*, **62**, 1167

70. Rodis, J.F., Egan J.F.X., Craffey, A. *et al.* (1990). Calculated risk of chromosomal abnormalities in twin gestations. *Obstet. Gynecol.*, **76**, 1037
71. Jones, K.L. (1988). *Smith's Recognizable Patterns of Human Malformation*, 4th edn. (Philadelphia: W.B. Saunders)
72. Doyle, P.E., Beral, V., Botting, B. *et al.* (1990). Congenital malformations in twins in England and Wales. *J. Epidemiol. Commun. Health*, **45**, 43
73. Windham, G.C. and Bjerkedal, T. (1984). Malformations in twins and their siblings, Norway, 1967–79. *Acta Genet. Med. Gemellol.*, **33**, 87
74. Drillien, C.M. (1970). The small-for-date infant: etiology and prognosis. *Pediatr. Clin. N. Am.*, **17**, 9
75. Fogel, B.J., Nitowsky, H.M. and Gruenwald, P. (1965). Discordant abnormalities in monozygotic twins. *J. Pediatr.*, **66**, 64
76. Urig, M.A., Clewell, W.H. and Elliott, J.P. (1990). Twin–twin transfusion syndrome. *Am. J. Obstet. Gynecol.*, **163**, 1522
77. Hanna, J.H. and Hill, J.M. (1984). Single intrauterine fetal demise in multiple gestation. *Obstet. Gynecol.*, **63**, 126
78. Gindoff, P.R., Yeh, M.N. and Jewelewicz, R. (1986). The vanishing sac syndrome. Ultrasound evidence of pregnancy failure in multiple gestations, induced and spontaneous. *J. Reprod. Med.*, **31**, 322
79. Landy, H.J., Weiner, S., Corson, S.L. *et al.* (1986). The 'vanishing twin': ultrasonographic assessment of fetal disappearance in the first trimester. *Am. J. Obstet. Gynecol.*, **155**, 14
80. Allen, M.C. (1984). Developmental outcome and followup of the small for gestational age infant. *Semin. Perinatol.*, **8**, 123
81. Rementeria, J.L., Janakammal, S. and Hollander, M. (1975). Multiple births in drug-addicted women. *Am. J. Obstet. Gynecol.*, **122**, 958
82. Bandstra, E.S. and Burkett, G. (1991). Maternal–fetal and neonatal effects of *in utero* cocaine exposure. *Semin. Perinatol.*, **15**, 288
83. Hoyme, H.E., Lyons, K.L., Dixon, S.D. *et al.* (1990). Prenatal cocaine exposure and fetal vascular disruption. *Pediatrics*, **85**, 743
84. Chescheir N.C. and Seeds, J.W. (1988). Polyhydramnios and oligohydramnios in twin gestations. *Obstet. Gynecol.*, **71**, 882
85. Naeye, R.L., Benirschke, K., Hagstrom, J.W.C. *et al.* (1966). Intrauterine growth of twins as estimated from liveborn birth-weight data. *Pediatrics*, **37**, 409
86. Matheny A.P. and Brown, A.M. (1971). The behavior of twins: effects of birth weight and birth sequence. *Child Dev.*, **42**, 251
87. Allen, M.C. (1992). Developmental implications of intrauterine growth retardation. *Infants Young Child.*, **5**, 13
88. Fitzhardinge, P.M. and Steven, E.M. (1972). The small-for-date infant. II. Neurological and intellectual sequelae. *Pediatrics*, **49**, 50
89. Westwood, M., Kramer, M.S., Munz, D. *et al.* (1983). Growth and development of full-term nonasphyxiated small-for-gestational-age newborns: follow-up through adolescence. *Pediatrics*, **71**, 376
90. Pena, I.C., Teberg, A.J. and Finello, K.M. (1988). The premature small-for-gestational-age infant during the first year of life: comparison by birth weight and gestational age. *J. Pediatr.*, **113**, 1066
91. Vohr, B.R. and Oh, W. (1983). Growth and development in preterm infants small for gestational age. *J. Pediatr.*, **103**, 941
92. Babson, S.G., Kangas, J., Young, N. *et al.* (1964). Growth and development of twins of dissimilar size at birth. *Pediatrics*, **33**, 327
93. Churchill, J.A. (1965). The relationship between intelligence and birth weight in twins. *Neurology*, **15**, 341
94. Fujikura, T. and Froehlich, L.A. (1974). Mental and motor development in monozygotic co-twins with dissimilar birth weights. *Pediatrics*, **53**, 884
95. Henrichsen, L., Skinhoj, K. and Andersen, G.E. (1986). Delayed growth and reduced intelligence in 9–17 year old intrauterine growth retarded children compared with their monozygous co-twins. *Acta Paediatr. Scand.*, **75**, 31
96. Kaelber, C.T. and Pugh, T.F. (1969). Influence of intrauterine relations on the intelligence of twins. *N. Engl. J. Med.*, **19**, 1030
97. O'Brien, P.J. and Hay, D.A. (1987). Birthweight differences, the transfusion syndrome and the cognitive development of monozygotic twins. *Acta Genet. Med. Gemellol.*, **36**, 181
98. Willerman, L. and Churchill, J.A. (1976). Intelligence and birth weight in identical twins. *Child Dev.*, **38**, 623
99. Trofatter, K.F. Jr (1988). Management of delivery. *Clin. Perinatol.*, **15**, 93
100. Young, B.K., Suidan, J., Antoine, C.L. *et al.* (1985). Differences in twins: the importance of birth order. *Am. J. Obstet. Gynecol.*, **151**, 915

101. Nelson, K.B. and Ellenberg, J.H. (1981). Apgar scores as predictors of chronic neurologic disability. *Pediatrics*, **68**, 36
102. Robertson, C. and Finer, N. (1985). Term infants with hypoxic–ischemic encephalopathy: outcome at 3–5 years. *Dev. Med. Child Neurol.*, **27**, 473
103. Allen, M.C. and Jones, M.D. Jr (1986). Medical complications of prematurity. *Obstet. Gynecol.*, **67**, 427
104. Allen, M.C. (1991). Prematurity. In Capute, A.J. and Accardo, P.J. (eds.) *Developmental Disabilities in Infancy and Childhood*, pp. 87–99. (Baltimore: Paul H. Brookes)
105. Allen, M.C. (1993). An overview of longterm outcome. In Witter, F. and Keith, L. (eds.) *Prematurity: Antecedents, Treatment and Outcome.* (Boston: Little, Brown)
106. Williamson, W.D., Desmond, M.M., Wilson, G.S. *et al.* (1983). Survival of low-birth-weight infants with neonatal intraventricular hemorrhage. *Am. J. Dis. Child.*, **137**, 1181
107. Papile, L.-A., Munsick-Bruno, G. and Schaefer, A. (1983). Relationship of cerebral intraventricular hemorrhage and early childhood neurologic handicaps. *J. Pediatr.*, **103**, 273
108. Guzzetta, F., Shackelford, G.D., Volpe, S. *et al.* (1986). Periventricular intraparenchymal echodensities in the premature newborn: critical determinant of neurologic outcome. *Pediatrics*, **78**, 995
109. Hansen, N.B., Kopechek, J., Miller, R.R. *et al.* (1989). Prognostic significance of cystic intracranial lesions in neonates. *Dev. Behav. Pediatr.*, **10**, 129
110. Saigal, S., Rosenbaum, P., Stoskopf, B. *et al.* (1982). Follow-up of infants 501 to 1,500 gm birth weight delivered to residents of a geographically defined region with perinatal intensive care facilities. *J. Pediatr.*, **100**, 606
111. Saigal, S., Rosenbaum, P., Stoskopf, B. *et al.* (1984). Outcome in infants 501 to 1000 gm birth weight delivered to residents of the McMaster Health Region. *J. Pediatr.*, **105**, 969
112. Saigal, S., Szatmari, P., Rosenbaum, P. *et al.* (1990). Intellectual and functional status at school entry of children who weighed 1000 grams or less at birth: a regional perspective of births in the 1980's. *J. Pediatr.*, **116**, 409
113. Saigal, S., Szatmari, P., Rosenbaum, P. *et al.* (1991). Cognitive abilities and school performance of extremely low birth weight children and matched term control children at age 8 years: a regional study. *J. Pediatr.*, **118**, 751
114. Escobar, G.J., Littenberg, B. and Petitti, D.B. (1991). Outcome among surviving very low birthweight infants: a meta-analysis. *Arch. Dis. Child.*, **66**, 204
115. Hack, M. and Fanaroff, A.V. (1989). Outcomes of extremely-low-birth-weight infants between 1982 and 1988. *N. Engl. J. Med.*, **321**, 1642
116. Aylward, G.P., Pfeiffer, S.I., Wright, A. *et al.* (1989). Outcome studies of low birth weight infants published in the last decade: a metaanalysis. *J. Pediatr.*, **115**, 515
117. Minde, K., Corter, C., Goldberg, S. *et al.* (1990). Maternal preference between premature twins up to age four. *J. Am. Acad. Child Adolesc. Psychiatry*, **29**, 367
118. Riese, M.L. (1990). Neonatal temperament in monozygotic and dizygotic twin pairs. *Child Dev.*, **61**, 1230
119. Goodman, R. and Stevenson, J. (1989). A twin study of hyperactivity-II. The aetiological role of genes, family relationships and perinatal adversity. *J. Child Psychol. Psychiatr.*, **30**, 691
120. Stevenson, J. and Fredman, G. (1990). The social environmental correlates of reading ability. *J. Child Psychol. Psychiatr.*, **31**, 681
121. Beal, S. (1989). Sudden infant death syndrome in twins. *Pediatrics*, **84**, 1038

The long-term development of twins: anthropometric factors and cognition

46

F. Falkner and A.P. Matheny, Jr

Introduction

A key question in any discussion of the long-term outcome of twins is what effect does the twin pregnancy have on infant size at birth and on the subsequent growth and development of each twin? Simply put, fetal growth in singletons begins to slow at 34–36 weeks of gestation because the uterine space becomes restricted. In contrast, twin growth slows earlier – when their combined weight approaches that of a 36-week singleton fetus. What is not clear, however, is exactly when twin growth rate deviates from the singleton growth rate, because various studies (using different methodological approaches) have reported these changes differently.

In contrast, it is absolutely clear that low birth weight (LBW) is as common among twins as is preterm delivery. Given these circumstances, it might be expected that any prenatal restrictions in growth would result in twins being permanently smaller in size compared to singletons. Fortunately, this is not the case and, as Tanner[1] has postulated, an individual's growth is under a self-regulating control mechanism. Thus, any temporary insult or deficit can be overcome by aiming or restoring the child back onto his or her genetic curve of growth. This concept holds true for twins, as it does for singletons.

Clearly, self-regulating control of growth must be considered for each member of a monozygous (MZ) pair, both of whom carry the same genetic material, as well as for members of dizygous (DZ) pairs, in which this is obviously not the case. In this regard, twins are particularly important sources for research on human growth patterns. The role of several antenatal factors that impact on long-term growth is discussed in the sections that follow.

Antenatal factors

Birth size

Surprisingly, DZ twins are more concordant at birth than are MZ twins. As shown by Wilson[2], the within-pair correlation at birth for size in DZ pairs exceeds that of MZ pairs: $r=0.77$, vs. $r=0.66$, respectively. However, the genetically similar MZ pairs quite rapidly become increasingly concordant, so that at 4 years, $r=0.94$. In contrast, DZ pairs move further apart, so that by 9 years, $r=0.49$.

Placental influences

Without dwelling upon the placental factor as an important influence on birth size and early postnatal growth, it is necessary to reiterate certain points as they relate to later growth.

In monochorionic (MC) placentas of MZ twins (various estimates show a minority of MZ twins have dichorionic (DC) placentas), vascular anastomoses occur between the placental segments supplying each twin. Benirschke and Driscoll[3] maintain that: (1) if carefully sought, vascular shunts of some kind can be found in virtually all MC placentas; and (2) the twin–twin transfusion syndrome may be present, to some degree, in one-third of all MC placentas. In contrast, vascular anastomoses are not found between DC placentas, even when these are fused. The implication of this essential difference is that the growth of MZ twins with MC placentas should be viewed differently from MZ twins with DC placentas and also from like-sexed DZ twins, who always have DC placentas.

Maternal–fetal nutrition influences

With regard to MZ twins with MC placentation, anastomoses most often occur in a central plane, known as the vascular equator. Functionally, placental segments are joined at this equator; each is considered as having 'supplied' one of the twins. It could be hypothesized that placental tissue mass and its nutritive content might be thought of as a type of marker for postnatal growth; in other words, one twin's placenta or placental segment is related to its subsequent growth. In MZ twins with a MC placentation, nutritive substances might be transferred from one twin's segment to the other and subsequently affect growth.

The wet and dry weights of the placentas or the respective placental segments are significantly correlated with each corresponding twin's birth weight; this is true for MZ and DZ twins, whether they have MC or DC placentas[4]. For example, in a series of 92 twin pairs, the within-pair birth weight differences had a mean of about 326 g for MZ–MC twins, and a mean of 228 g for MZ–DC twins. This finding demonstrates that separated placental segments among MZ twins are related to a greater tendency among MZ twins for the infants to be more similar in birth weight[5].

A strong positive relationship between birth weight and placental weight is clear, as is the relationship between placental function and placental mass. Differing long-term outcome for MZ twins may well be related to these interrelations. In one study[5] that examined such differences, the percentage components of several biochemical and nutritional substances were the same in both placentas or placental segments, and the subsequent postnatal growth of each twin could not be related to any postulated differences. When one placenta or placental segment is small, albeit possessing the same levels of nutritional substances found in a larger placenta or segment, it is conceivable that a 'critical level' of placental mass exists, below which postnatal growth deficit occurs. The deficit may be reversible or irreversible.

Babson and Phillips[6] and Falkner[5] examined MZ twins with grossly different birth weights. These investigators found that, although the smaller twin (in birth weight) exhibited early good postnatal 'catch-up' growth, this growth was not sufficient to achieve the later size of the larger co-twin. In contrast, Buckler and Robinson[7] followed the postnatal growth of a group of smaller twins (MZ–MC) and found that rapid catch-up growth occurred, so much so that both twins were of similar size and mental ability by age 10 years.

A pair of male infant twins (MZ–MC) from the Louisville Twin Study are illustrative of many features relevant to this discussion. Their birth weight difference was such that the smaller twin (twin A) was 52% of the birth weight of his larger co-twin (twin B). Their subsequent growth followed the pattern described above by Babson and Phillips[6] rather than that of Buckler and Robinson[7]. Nevertheless, the following points are of interest: the smaller twin described by Buckler and Robinson was 45% of the birth weight of the larger twin, whereas the Louisville twin A (just described) was 52% of twin B's birth weight. In sharp contrast, however, is the fact that Buckler and Robinson's smaller twin was supplied by a placental segment that was 87% of the weight of the segment supplying his larger co-twin, whereas our twin A's placental segment only represented 46% of that of his larger co-twin. This observation reinforces our recommendation to strongly consider the specific aspects of placentation as an important factor in the long-term outcome for twins.

Returning to the twins from the Louisville study, twin A exhibited marked catch-up growth in length during the first 9 months to 1 year as he attempted, hypothetically, to eliminate his birth length difference-deficit of 7.0 cm. Thereafter, both twins grew at approximately the same rate even to the timing of their adolescent growth spurt, which they reached at the expected point for MZ pairs at

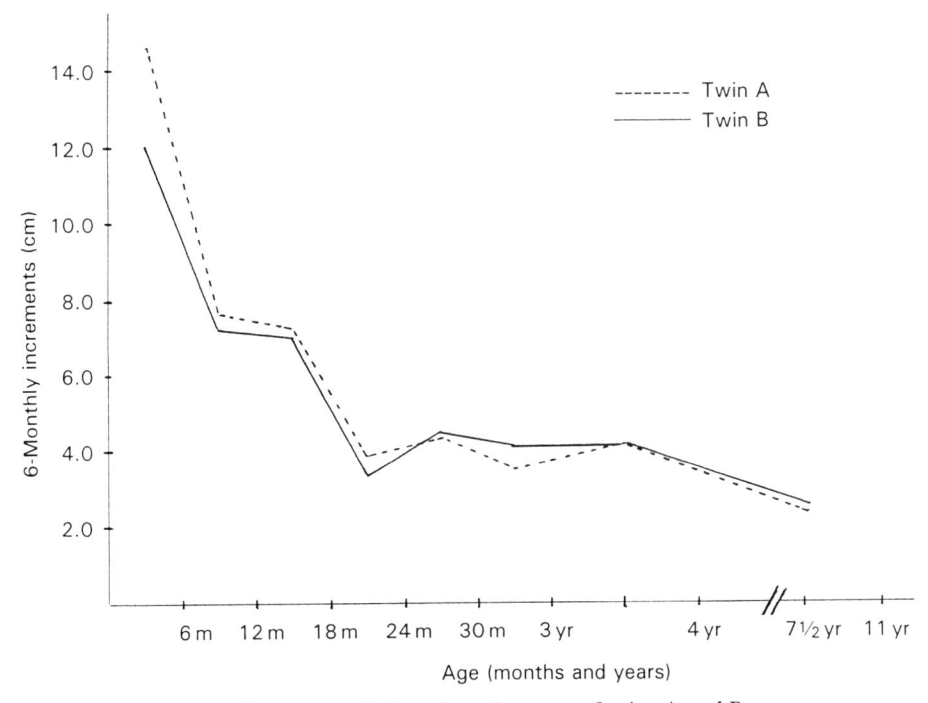

Figure 1 Six-monthly increments in length and stature of twins A and B

the same age. Figure 1 shows this in a velocity growth curve of length and stature. Despite this, twin A never exhibited sufficient catch-up growth to reach his co-twin. At 16 years of age, the within-pair difference was 8.0 kg in weight and 5.4 cm in stature. Although both boys enjoyed good health, markedly different environmental considerations started to 'overwhelm' their genetic target size. After 25 years, a summary was obtained of their growth (Table 1).

The weight difference is of particular interest, and suggested a 'lean and mean' habitus for twin A (the former Marine) that was not adopted by his brother.

Table 1 Summary of growth after 25 years of a twin pair in the Louisville study. Twin A had served in the Marines, and twin B was serving in the US postal service

	Twin A	Twin B
Stature (cm)	165.9	172.3
Weight (kg)	66.02	77.84
Head circumference (cm)	56.0	56.3

Brain size

In the case discussed in the preceding section, head circumference measurements were similar and remained so from about 1 year onwards. As the twins were born at 39 weeks, twin A was characterized as a small-for-gestational-age (SGA) infant. Recently, it was shown[8] that SGA infants are not homogeneous as a group, and that fetuses born SGA with 'normal' head sizes (so-called disproportional or asymmetric intrauterine growth retardation (IUGR)) exhibit better growth postnatally than proportional or symmetrically grown newborns with IUGR. In this latter instance, head size is comparably small with the rest of the small fetal body. Because head circumference is a good indicator of brain mass[9,10], it is important to note this factor in any discussion of twins and, in particular, when one of the pair is SGA.

Postnatal growth

In 1979, Wilson used a large sample of twins to construct distribution curves of length–height and weight as reference values from birth to 9 years. A gender difference in growth was apparent. Whereas male twins were not significantly heavier than their female counterparts at birth, they exhibited notably faster rates of gain until 18 months–2 years and were significantly heavier at those ages. After this point, however, female twins exhibited greater weight gains, so that parity for both genders occurred by 6 years. A similar pattern was apparent for length. Gender differences in birth length were insignificant; later, males had a much faster rate of growth until 18 months. Thereafter, females grew faster, so that by 5 years, parity of height was achieved between the two genders.

The twin reference value curves show that, for weight, up until 3 years of age, the distribution is more or less Gaussian; after that, a skew occurs leading to progressively greater spread or heavier weight distribution among the upper centiles. This is not seen in the lower centiles, however, as is the case with singleton children[11]. The above findings may reflect differences in dietary habits or in patterns of feeding between genders, but admittedly this explanation is speculative.

The length–height curves for male and female twins are much more Gaussian (again, as in singletons[11]). This fact no doubt reflects the basic genotypes for height in the population. The upper centile skew does not occur in height as it does in weight.

Comparing the total twin sample with singleton reference values, Wilson[12] demonstrated that twins had notable deficits in both weight and length at birth. A dramatic reduction in the weight deficit then occurred, particularly in the first 3 months. After this, the reductions became progressively smaller and disappeared by 8 years. Although the birth–length deficit was nowhere near as severe, it paralleled the progressive diminution in weight deficit until it, too, disappeared at later ages.

Weight was by far the more sensitive indicator of intrauterine growth failure and responded well to early postnatal catch up. After the first year of life, the various dimensions of growth moved together toward later and full recovery from deficit.

To summarize, the retardation of growth in twins which was present at birth was notably offset by accelerated growth in the early years, followed by a lowering of rate of gain, but eventually, by 8 years, reached parity with singletons of that age.

Growth and zygosity

As might be expected, the strong genetic role in growth is reflected by the convergence of the growth curves of each dissimilar MZ twin over time. Compared to DZ twins, MZ twins clearly demonstrate the effects of zygosity on twin growth.

In the twin sample investigated by Wilson[12], MZ twins became increasingly concordant throughout childhood. For example, within-pair length correlations were $r=0.66$ at birth. By 4 years, the correlation for height was $r=0.94$. These correlations remained almost constant thereafter. For weight, the corresponding correlations were $r=0.64$ at birth, and from 3 years onward they became essentially constant at $r=0.86$ to 0.89.

Of interest, like-sexed DZ twins grew in a totally opposite pattern. For birth length, $r=0.77$ (more concordant than MZ twins); at 2 years, height $r=0.59$, and at 9 years, $r=0.49$. Weight followed the pattern for length–height. In view of these observations, it is clear that, although DZ twins are more concordant than MZ twins at birth, they rapidly move in divergent directions until they attain an intermediate concordance level in later childhood. The greater concordance at birth of DZ twins (over and above any of the factors previously discussed that explain MZ discordance at birth) was inflated somewhat by linkage with gestational age and a common prenatal environment. Once these effects were taken into account, however, correlations appeared to stabilize at approximately the $r=0.50$ level. The later MZ correlations of $r=0.90$ clearly demonstrate the very strong genetic influence on growth exemplified by analysis of length–height–weight data.

The findings described above from the Louisville Twin Study are similar to those found by Fishbein[13] among adolescent twins in a longitudinal study in Sweden. This investigation suggests the effects of zygosity continue over the whole growth period. Importantly, too, the Swedish study showed a much higher concordance in MZ twins with regard to the timing of the adolescent growth spurt. This finding confirms prior opinions that the appearance of this growth phase was strongly influenced by genetic factors.

Obstetric factors

The paradoxical finding that the survival rate is better among low birth weight twins than among low birth weight singletons has attracted considerable interest of late[14]. Buekens and Wilcox[15] were challenged by this paradox and analyzed data from vital statistics in very large samples of low birth weight singletons and firstborn and secondborn twins. When birth weight distributions were adjusted to a single/mean (and standard deviation) and weight-specific perinatal mortality rates of twins and singletons were compared, mortality rates at every weight were higher for twins than singletons. The paradoxical finding of better survival of small twins over small singletons disappears if the variable of birth weight is brought into the analysis. In the final analysis, a large outcome risk due to twinning falls on all twins, regardless of their weight.

Mental development

The developmental risks of twins generally are attributed to intrauterine growth retardation secondary to crowding and inadequate intrauterine nutrition and to shorter gestations and lower birth weight[16,17]. These factors have been examined in numerous studies of twins to determine: (1) if mental developmental delays are typical for twins; (2) if these delays remain chronic or are offset during childhood; and (3) if the medical and social factors are associated with either chronic lag or eventual recovery?

Although the general trend in the literature suggests that infant twins, relative to singletons, are at increased risk for a lag in the development of cognitive functioning, it is difficult to pinpoint the magnitude of this risk for several reasons. First, the twin samples studied to date are quite small and do not represent a wide range of socioeconomic status (SES) or parental education; second, the twins were not followed systematically for long periods of time; and finally, the studies overly sampled twins with acute or chronic illnesses[18–20].

Despite evidence that twins continue to lag beyond infancy[19,21], data from the Louisville Twin Study suggest that there is a gradual increase in cognitive skills so that twins essentially reach parity with singletons by school age[22]. Wilson examined the mental test scores obtained for approximately 900 twins followed from 6 months to 6 years of age[23]. The twins' mental test scores remained in the range from 85 to 95 throughout infancy. The scores then gradually increased so that by 6 years they reached the level expected for the general population, i.e. an IQ score of 100. Moreover, during this 6-year interval, the mental test scores stabilized, so that the relative ranking of individual differences among all twins for 1-year test–retest correlations increased from $r = 0.48$ at age 1 year to $r = 0.86$ by 6 years. In effect, this series of assessments documented a gain in mental achievement and a stabilization of the individual differences for that gain.

Wilson[23] also examined various neonatal and family characteristics that might be associated with twins' initially suppressed mental test scores and their later recovery. He was able to show that the twins' birth weight and gestational age were modestly correlated with mental test scores (r between 0.35 and 0.55) during the first year, but that these correlations declined to less than $r = 0.20$ by 6 years. In contrast, parental SES and parental education progressed from no association with infant mental test scores to a moderate level of association (r between 0.40 and 0.50) by 6 years. Clearly, the twins' advance over the preschool years was predicted more by family characteristics than by neonatal characteristics.

Wilson[22] further documented the relative effect of SES by examining the 6-year recovery of twins with birth weights ≤ 1750 g who respectively belonged to the highest and lowest of levels of family SES. Among the twins from the lowest SES, mental test scores increased from 73 to 86.5 from 6 months to 6 years. In contrast, the scores of the twins from the highest SES increased from 76.8 to 101.1. These findings documented two trends: (1) the tendency for twins' mental test scores to increase from infancy to school age; and (2) the differential increase associated with impartial demographic characteristics of the twins' families.

Subsequent to Wilson's initial report[22], the number of participants in the Louisville Twin Study has increased, particularly for ages past 6 years. As a result, the long-range outcome of twins' cognitive development can be examined more fully beyond the preschool years. Although the twin sample and research program of the Louisville Twin Study have been described elsewhere[23,24], a brief description is necessary at this point to provide background for these more recent analyses.

Louisville Twin Study

The Louisville Twin Study is an ongoing longitudinal study of twins initiated more than 30 years ago[25]. From the onset, twins were recruited from families of all social levels in the metropolitan area of Louisville, Kentucky. Special efforts were made to recruit and retain families from lower SES and with a lower level of parental education. The distribution of twin families by SES (indexed by Duncan's scale[26] and its later revision[27]) places approximately 30% of families in the first two deciles of the 100-point rating scale. The remaining families are distributed somewhat equally among the other deciles (8–11% each), except for the highest two deciles (about 11%). Maternal and paternal education levels range from 8th grade to completion of a professional degree (e.g. M.D.); approximately 65% of mothers have high school diplomas or a lower level of educational attainment. The mean educational levels for mothers and fathers are approximately 12 and 13 years, respectively. A high degree of assortative mating exists ($r = 0.68$).

The twins are recruited as newborns and their respective birth sizes and gestational age are obtained from medical records. The total sample now includes approximately 700 pairs of twins, whose ages range from infancy to 15 years. Sample sizes vary by specific ages for three reasons: (1) recruitment is ongoing; (2) some families miss visits; and (3) some visits have been altered to comply with changes in research objectives. Nevertheless, sample sizes for annual assessments consist of at least 500 twins at each year of age from 1 to 9 years, and approximately 400 twins at 15 years of age.

At birth, the twins' mean birth weight was 2.6 kg (range: 1.0–4.1 kg), and the mean gestational age was 37.9 weeks (range: 29.3–43.3 weeks). By the singleton standards of Battaglia and Lubchenco[28], 23% of the twins were classified as SGA, with mean birth weight of 2.2 kg and a mean gestational age of 38.6 weeks.

After recruitment, the annual assessments of mental development were based upon the most thoroughly constructed tests or their subsequent revisions as they became available. These tests included the Bayley Scales of Infant Development[29] for infants, the Stanford–Binet[30] for 3-year-olds, the Wechsler Preschool and Primary Scale of Intelligence (WPPSI)[31] for ages 4, 5 and 6 years (until the McCarthy Scales of Children's Abilities[32] was introduced for 4-year-olds), and finally the Wechsler Intelligence Scale for Children (WISC)[33] for ages 7–15 years.

The full-scale mental test scores – either the Mental Development Index (MDI) for the Bayley Scales of Infant Development or the Intelligence Quotient (IQ) for tests thereafter – are shown by age in Table 2. The progressive increase in mental test scores documented by Wilson[23] is evident in this expanded sample. By 6 years of age, the twins essentially reach the level of IQ scores obtained by singletons. With the exception of a slight downturn at 7 years, perhaps because of the introduction of the novel and more difficult WISC, the twins' level of mental test scores remains close to 100 from 6–15 years.

Table 2 Mental test scores for twins tested yearly at ages 1–9 and retested at age 15 years

Age (years)	Test: Full Scale Score	MDI/IG (mean)	Correlation with age 15 years
1	Bayley: MDI	88.2	0.28
2	Bayley: MDI	93.1	0.42
3	Stanford–Binet: IQ	91.0	0.58
4	WPPSI/McCarthy: IQ/GCI	90.7	0.62
5	WPPSI: IQ	96.5	0.71
6	WPPSI: IQ	100.6	0.78
7	WISC: IQ	97.9	0.81
8	WISC: IQ	101.7	0.84
9	WISC: IQ	101.4	0.86
15	WISC: IQ	99.6	—

Description of tests provided in text. Sample at each age between 500 and 800 twins. Range of standard deviations for mental tests: Bayley, Stanford–Binet and McCarthy, 14.9–17.0; WPPSI and WISC, 13.6–14.7

Table 2 also shows the correlation between the mental test scores obtained for each of the 9 ages prior to 15 years and the mental test scores obtained at the criterion age of 15 years. At age 1 year, mental test scores correlate 0.28 with 15-year mental test scores. After 1 year, there is a progressive increase in the magnitude of the correlations. By school age, the predictive correlations become stable. Thus, the initially large reordering of individual differences in infant twins' mental test scores slackens during the preschool years, the same period when the twins made up the deficit in mental test scores shown during infancy.

Newborn characteristics

Many studies assert that a strong association exists between newborn characteristics and later deficits in cognitive development. For example, the incidence of mental retardation and CNS deficits are higher among samples of infants classified by weight or gestation[34]. In this regard, twins constitute a special risk group, because the percentage of twins with lower birth weights and shorter gestations is higher than those for singletons[35] (see Section III, Epidemiology).

Table 3 shows correlations between gestational age and birth weight and the mental test scores obtained at each age are shown in Table 2. The correlates for both of these characteristics indicate that the smaller or earlier born infant is likely to score lower at the first year, but the correlations for both characteristics decline progressively in their importance thereafter. By 15 years, measures of newborn characteristics are essentially uninformative for the twin sample as a whole. For most twins, it is evident that being small at birth or being born after a shorter pregnancy is not sufficient in itself to account for individual differences in mental test scores at 15 years.

Family characteristics

If newborn characteristics do not rank order twins for their developmental progress to adolescence, it is reasonable to ask what might? Maternal education and the SES of the family, also shown in Table 3, represent moderately strong candidates for the ordering of twins' mental test scores. By 2 years, for example, the education of the mother becomes a significant predictor of mental development, whereas it had provided no prediction during the first year. As previously noted by Wilson[2], the latent effect of family attributes, indirectly assessed by maternal education and SES, becomes manifest from age

Table 3 Correlations between twins' mental development scores and characteristics of newborn family

Twin test age (years)	Gestational age	Birth weight	Mother's education	SES
1	0.32	0.33	0.02	0.05
2	0.19	0.21	0.35	0.33
3	0.14	0.16	0.39	0.43
4	0.07	0.18	0.39	0.39
5	0.12	0.19	0.43	0.43
6	0.08	0.21	0.42	0.45
7	0.11	0.23	0.41	0.43
8	0.08	0.20	0.38	0.41
9	0.09	0.22	0.39	0.42
15	−0.11	0.07	0.39	0.41

SES, socioeconomic status

2 years and remains markedly persistent thereafter.

Infant risk and family characteristics

The data presented in Table 3 indicate that family characteristics, globally represented by education and SES, are more informative than newborn characteristics for predicting long-term cognitive developmental outcome. When these characteristics are considered one by one, however, they do not explain the outcome of twins who are defined by multiple risks; that is, twins who differ both by birth characteristics and by family characteristics. For example, does an SGA twin born to a less-educated set of parents display developmental gains for mental test scores that are different from an SGA twin born to a more highly educated set of parents? To assess these potential interactions, if present, the twins in the Louisville study were classified into two groups: SGA and average-for-gestational age (AGA). They were further classified by maternal education, represented by less than high school (< 12 years), college higher education (> 16 years), and more than high school but less than college (12–15 years). Maternal education was used in this classification, because it correlates highly with both paternal education and family SES[36].

The mental test scores in Table 4, and Bonferroni Test of Significance (Table 5), show several interesting trends. Mental test scores systematically increase according to a combination of SGA and maternal education, the latter characteristic providing a larger effect. Twins who are most disadvantaged (SGA and delivered to mothers with less education) obtained no gain over the 15-year period and had only minimal gains of 5 points or less from 1 to 9 years. In contrast, SGA twins of more highly educated mothers gained 11 points and 17 points, when the mothers' education was at least high school and college level, respectively. Mental test scores from the AGA twins show the same general pattern. AGA twins whose mothers had less than a high school diploma gained 8 points from infancy to 15 years. When mothers of AGA twins had at least a high school diploma, the twins gained 12 points; finally, when mothers had at least a college degree, the AGA twins gained 27 points. Over the course of 15 years, mental test scores are apparently conditioned by a combination of the initial deflections marked by size for gestation and recoveries marked by mothers' educational attainments.

To exemplify the general trends provided by these longitudinal data, we can compare two pairs of identical twin girls followed from infancy to 9 years. One pair was born to a

Table 4 Mental test scores for twins to 15 years according to mother's education and size for gestational age

Mother's education	Size for gestational age (%)		MDI/IQ scores for age									
			1 y	2 y	3 y	4 y	5 y	6 y	7 y	8 y	9 y	15 y
< 12 y	SGA	(4.6)	82	84	80	77	83	86	83	85	87	81
	AGA	(12.8)	83	84	82	84	87	91	87	90	92	91
12–15 y	SGA	(13.7)	87	89	90	87	95	98	93	97	98	98
	AGA	(44.9)	87	93	92	91	97	101	97	101	102	99
≥ 16 y	SGA	(4.6)	91	101	99	97	106	107	104	107	111	108
	AGA	(19.4)	87	98	102	101	108	113	108	113	115	114

See Table 5 for significance
Mother's education: < 12 y, less than high school diploma; 12–15 y, from high school diploma to 3 years past high school; ≥ 16 y, college degree or higher education; SGA, small for gestational age; AGA, average for gestational age

Table 5 Bonferroni Test for Significance ($p < 0.05$) between groups for each age

Group	Group		Significant at
< 12 y, SGA	< 12 y	AGA	no ages
	12–15 y	SGA	4, 5, 6, 7, 9, 15 y
	12–15 y	AGA	2, 3, 4, 5, 6, 7, 8, 9, 15 y
	≥ 16 y	SGA	2, 3, 4, 5, 6, 7, 8, 9, 15 y
	≥ 16 y	AGA	2, 3, 4, 5, 6, 7, 8, 9, 15 y
< 12 y, AGA	12–15 y	SGA	5, 8 y
	12–15 y	AGA	2, 3, 4, 5, 6, 7, 8, 9, 15 y
	≥ 16 y	SGA	2, 3, 4, 5, 6, 7, 8, 9, 15 y
	≥ 16 y	AGA	2, 3, 4, 5, 6, 7, 8, 9, 15y
12–15 y, SGA	12–15 y	AGA	no ages
	≥ 16 y	SGA	2, 5, 6, 7, 9 y
	≥ 16 y	AGA	2, 3, 4, 5, 6, 7, 9, 15 y
12–15 y, AGA	≥ 16	SGA	9 y
	≥ 16 y	AGA	3, 4, 5, 6, 7, 8, 9, 15 y
≥ 16 y, SGA	≥ 16 y	AGA	no ages

mother with 10 years of schooling and a father with 11 years of schooling. These twin girls had birth weights of 1.5 kg and 1.2 kg, respectively, after a pregnancy of 37 weeks. A second pair of twins, born about four years later, had parents with college degrees. These girls weighed 1.3 kg and 1.2 kg, respectively, after a pregnancy of 37 weeks. Neither mother smoked during pregnancy; after delivery, both pairs of twins were released from the hospital nursery at about two months of age. Gains in stature were more rapid for the twins born to the less-educated parents; by 9 years, they were above the 60th percentile for weight and above the 75th percentile for height. In contrast, the twins born to the better-educated parents only reached the 50th percentile for weight and height by 9 years. At 1 year, the pair whose parents were less educated had a pair-mean mental score of 68; the pair-mean score for the twins of better-educated parents was 55. At 3 years, however, this situation reversed itself, in that the mental test scores were 66 and 81 for the 'low education' and 'high education' pairs, respectively. Finally, at 6 and 9 years the 'low education' pair-mean scores were 81 and 87, respectively, compared with pair-mean scores of 100 and 103 for the 'high education' pair at the same ages. This example indicates that, although at early ages both twin pairs would have been classified as at risk for mental retardation (i.e. initial scores ≤70), both pairs recovered over time and the recovery was more pronounced for the pair with more highly educated parents.

Mental retardation

If it is possible for twin infants to recover from the effects of prenatal growth suppression, it is reasonable to ask how many twins classified as significantly delayed or retarded in development at one age would retain the same classification at a later age. The literature on infant and toddler twins implies that the higher rates of delay or retardation are likely to be preserved well past infancy and on through the school years. However, our longitudinal data indicate that these deficits are offset to some degree over time. Therefore, it is possible to state that some twins classified as significantly delayed or retarded during their infancy will not be similarly characterized when tested at later ages.

A complete longitudinal panel of mental test scores from infancy to 6 years was examined for 367 twins, representing 184 pairs of twins selected from the total twin sample of identical pairs, same-sex fraternal pairs and opposite-sex pairs, regardless of birth weight, gestational age, or parental education and SES. (One twin was deleted from the sample, because a test was not obtained at one age.) The target age of 6 years was selected, because at this age the gain in scores for twins had reached the full recovery level. At 1 year, 12.8% of the twin sample obtained mental scores equal to or less than 70 with the Bayley test. This percentage is about five times greater than that expected in the general population of infants assessed with the same test. From 1 to 3 years, the percentage of delayed/retarded twins decreased to 5.4, and from 3 to 6 years, it continued to decline to 1.4%. Translated into actual numbers of delayed/retarded twins, the frequency of 47 delayed/retarded twins at 1 year declined to a frequency of 5 delayed/retarded twins by 6 years.

Among the twins initially classified as delayed/retarded, more twins were boys, MZ and SGA, and had mothers with lower levels of education. It was not unexpected that monozygosity would characterize some of the delayed/retarded twins, because a higher developmental risk has been noted for monozygotics[37]. Except for this feature, however, the relative developmental risks associated with gender, SGA and parental education are not unique to multiple births.

These results, which extend previous reports on the physical and mental development of twins[2,38], indicate that the apparent developmental risks to twins are tempered by important parental and family characteristics. As a group, twins certainly seem to be at much higher risk than singletons during the infant and toddler periods. Nevertheless, the regulatory processes that program growth and development appear to provide a remarkable recovery for twins who seemingly are seriously compromised during their infancy. From a clinical perspective, the prediction of developmental handicaps in individual sets of young twins who are born too small and/or too soon may be difficult, in view of the mediating effects of the twins' postnatal life, as broadly gauged by parental attainments in education and SES.

Acknowledgements

We would like to dedicate this chapter to the late Ronald S. Wilson, admired good friend and colleague, who was Director of Louisville Twin Study between our tenureships. We have drawn heavily on his important contributions.

The research for this chapter was supported, in part, by the National Institute of Child Health and Human Development (HD22637).

References

1. Tanner, J.M. (1990). *Fetus into Man*. (Cambridge, MA: Harvard University Press)
2. Wilson, R.S. (1986). Growth and development of human twins. In Falkner, F. and Tanner, J.M. (eds.) *Human Growth*, 2nd edn., Vol. 3, pp. 197–211. (New York, London: Plenum Press)
3. Benirschke, K. and Driscoll, S.G. (1967). *The Pathology of the Human Placenta*. (Berlin: Springer-Verlag)
4. Falkner, F. (1966). General considerations in human development. In Falkner, F. (ed.) *Human Development*, pp. 197–211. (Philadelphia: W.B. Saunders)
5. Falkner, F. (1986). Twin growth and placentation. In Falkner, F. and Tanner, J.M. (eds.) *Human Growth*, 2nd edn., Vol. 3. (New York: Plenum Press)
6. Babson, S.G. and Phillips, D.S. (1973). Growth and development of twins dissimilar in size at birth. *N. Engl. J. Med.*, **289**, 937
7. Buckler, J.M.H. and Robinson, A. (1974). Matched development of a pair of monozygous twins of grossly different size at birth. *Arch. Dis. Child.*, **49**, 472
8. Villar, J., Smeriglio, V., Martivell, R. *et al.* (1985). Heterogeneous growth and mental development of intrauterine growth-retarded infants during the first three years of life. *Pediatrics*, **74**, 783
9. Brandt, I. (1986). Growth dynamics of low birth weight infants with emphasis on the perinatal period. In Falkner, F. and Tanner, J.M. (eds.) *Human Growth*, 2nd edn., Vol. 1, pp. 415–68. (New York: Plenum Press)
10. Dobbing, J. and Sands, J. (1978). Head circumference, biparietal diameter, and brain growth in fetal and postnatal life. *Early Hum. Dev.*, **2**, 81
11. Hamil, P.V.V., Drizd, T.A., Johnson, C.L. *et al.* (1972). *NCHS Growth Curves for Children. Vital and Health Statistics*, series 11, no. 165. DHEW Pub. No. (PHS) 78–1650. (Washington, DC: US Government Printing Office)
12. Wilson, R.S. (1979). Twin growth: initial deficit, recovery and trends in concordance from birth to nine years. *Ann. Hum. Biol.*, **6**, 205
13. Fishbein, S. (1977). Intra-pair similarity in physical growth of monozygotic and dizygotic twins during puberty. *Ann. Hum. Biol.*, **4**, 417
14. Kiely, J. (1990). The epidemiology of perinatal mortality in multiple births. *Bull. NY Acad. Med.*, **66**, 618
15. Buekens, P. and Wilcox, A. (1992). Why do small twins have a lower mortality rate than small singletons? Paper, Nat. Inst. Environ. Hlth. Sci. Research Triangle Park, N.C., 1992. *Am. J. Obstet. Gynecol.*, in press
16. Fujikara, T. and Froelich, L.A. (1974). Mental and motor development in monozygotic co-twins with dissimilar birth weights. *Pediatrics*, **53**, 884
17. Naeye, R.L., Benirschke, K., Hagstrom, L. *et al.* (1966). Intrauterine growth of twins as estimated from live born birth-weight data. *Pediatrics*, **37**, 409
18. Field, T., Walden, T., Widmeyer, S. *et al.* (1982). The early development of preterm, discordant twin pairs: bigger is not always better. In Lipsett, L.P. and Fields, T. (eds.) *Infant Behavior and Development: Perinatal Risk and Newborn Behavior*, pp. 153–63 (Norwood, NJ: Ablex)
19. Hay, D.A. and O'Brien, P. (1982). The La Trobe Twin Study: a genetic approach to the structure and development of cognition in twin children. *Child Develop.*, **54**, 317
20. Myrianthopoulus, N.C., Nichols, P.L., Broman, S.H. *et al.* (1972). Intellectual development of a prospectively studied population of twins and comparison with singleton. In de Grouchy, J., Ebling, F.G. and Henderson, I.W. (eds.) *Human Genetics*. (Amsterdam: Excerpta Medica)
21. Mittler, P. (1971). *The Study of Twins*. (Harmondsworth, England: Penguin)
22. Wilson, R.S. (1985). Risk and resilience in early mental development. *Dev. Psych.*, **21**, 795
23. Wilson, R.S. (1983). The Louisville Twin Study: Developmental synchronies in behavior. *Child Develop.*, **54**, 298
24. Matheny, A.P. (1990). Developmental behavior genetics: contributions from the Louisville Twin Study. In Hahn, M.E., Hewitt, J.K., Henderson, N.D. and Benno, R. (eds.) *Developmental Behavior Genetics: Neural, Biometrical, and Evolutionary Approaches*. (New York: Oxford University Press)
25. Falkner, F. (1957). An appraisal of the potential contribution of longitudinal twin studies.

In *The Nature and Transmission of the Genetic and Cultural Characteristics of Human Populations*, Proc. 1956 Annual Conference, 1956, pp. 122–41. (Philadelphia: Milbank Memorial Fund)

26. Reiss, A.J. Jr (1961). *Occupations and Social Status*. (New York: Free Press of Glencoe)
27. Stevens, G. and Featherman, D.L. (1981). A revised socioeconomic index of occupational status. *Soc. Sci. Res.*, **10**, 364
28. Battaglia, F.C. and Lubchenco, L. (1967). A practical classification of newborn infants by weight and gestational age. *J. Pediatr.*, **71**, 159
29. Bayley, N. (1969). *Bayley Scales of Infant Development*. (New York: Psychological Corporation)
30. Thorndike, R.L. (1973). *Stanford–Binet Intelligence Scale*, 3rd rev. *Norms Tables*. (Boston: Houghton-Mifflin)
31. Wechsler, D. (1967). *Wechsler Preschool and Primary Scale of Intelligence*. (New York: Psychological Corporation)
32. McCarthy, D. (1972). *McCarthy Scales of Children's Abilities*. (New York: Psychological Corporation)
33. Wechsler, D. (1974). *Wechsler Intelligence Scale for Children – Revised.* (New York: Psychological Corporation)
34. Broman, S.H., Nichols, P.L. and Kennedy, W.A. (1975). *Preschool IQ: Prenatal and Early Developent Correlates.* (Hillsdale, NJ: Lawrence Erlbaum)
35. MacGillivray, I (ed). (1979). *Proceedings of workshop of International Society of Twin Studies on twin pregnancy. Acta Genet. Med. Gemellol.*, **4**, 249
36. Wilson, R.S. and Matheny, A.P. Jr (1983). Mental development: family environment and genetic influences. *Intelligence*, **7**, 195
37. Ackerman, B.A. and Fischbein, S. (1991). Twins: are they at risk? A longitudinal study of twins and nontwins from birth to 18 years of age. *Acta Genet. Med. Gemellol.*, **40**, 29
38. Wilson, R.S. (1977). Mental development in twins. In Oliverio, A. (ed.) *Genetics, Environment, and Intelligence*, pp. 305–27 (Amsterdam: Elsevier)

Postnatal zygosity determination

E. Pergament

Introduction

A long-standing challenge of those interested in multiple births has been the need to develop a flawless method to distinguish between monozygotic and dizygotic twins. Not only physicians but parents and the twins themselves frequently wish to know zygosity for a variety of reasons, including the need to establish 'identity'. In addition, important social as well as medical reasons for determining zygosity without equivocation often exist.

Practical and informative methods of zygosity diagnosis can be applied prenatally if there is a need for intervention in the twin-to-twin transfusion syndrome, for example, or postnatally for investigating the etiology of major malformations in discordant twins or obtaining a better understanding of the pathogenesis of genetic diseases. Despite these possibilities, critical review of numerous twin studies clearly shows that their conclusions are weakened because zygosity was never determined definitively or was merely assumed on the basis of inadequate criteria and analysis. This chapter describes several statistical and laboratory methods for assessing zygosity after birth.

Zygosity of twins in populations

A simple method is often used to calculate how many twins in a given population are monozygotic and how many are dizygotic. Originally developed by Bertillon and later improved by Weinberg, this method is based on the fact that sex is genetically determined. Since unlike-sexed twins undoubtedly originate from two separate zygotes, the number of like-sexed dizygotic twins should bear a simple relationship to that of the unlike-sexed ones; that is, the combined number of like-sexed dizygotic male and female twin pairs should be the same as the number of the unlike-sexed twins. In other words, the total number of dizygotic twins (males and females) should be two times that of the observed number of unlike-sexed twins. The number of monozygotic twins can then be calculated by subtracting the number of dizygotic twins from the total number of all twins. This approach is commonly referred to as the Weinberg 'differential method', because the number of monozygotic twins is derived from the difference between all twins and the number of dizygotic pairs. Because the sex ratio in most populations deviates from equality, a more accurate formulation of the differential method has been proposed using the specific values of female and male births[1]. This formula is not without criticism, however, because some investigators are of the opinion that it relies on invalid assumptions (see Chapters 2 and 4).

Regardless of these criticisms, these formulations can be applied to total populations. Thus, in the United States, approximately one out of three sets of twins born are monozygotic, whereas in Japan, with its low frequency (0.7%) of twin births, the differential method indicates that a much larger fraction (60%) of the twins are monozygotic. The main difference between the overall frequencies of twin births among Japanese, Americans and Africans, for that matter, is primarily due to differences in the frequency of dizygotic twins. Unfortunately, the Weinberg method and its later refinements accounting for differences in the sex ratio cannot be applied to differentiate zygosity of a specific set of twins.

The zygosity of twin pairs based on embryology

As late as the 1950s, the attribution of mono- or dizygotic origin in a given pair of twins was generally made by means of the 'similarity diagnosis', i.e. a detailed study of the twins' phenotypes. Indeed, one of the most eminent human geneticists of that era described this approach as 'nothing more than a refinement of the inspection method often used by the layman to conclude that a specific pair is so similar as to be called identical, or another one sufficiently dissimilar as to be nonidentical'[1].

Some years later, however, the method of similarity diagnosis was applied to one of the most successful methods of assessing zygosity. The accurate examination of placental form and structure by the obstetrician at the moment of birth was advocated as the method of choice for the determination of zygosity, most probably as a result of the seminal work of the renowned perinatal pathologist, Kurt Benirschke. Accordingly, the placentas of twin pregnancies can be classified by the number of chorions and amnions. Two classes of placentas are recognized: dichorionic and monochorionic. In the former, the dividing membrane consists of two chorions and two amnions. Two subclasses of dichorionic–diamniotic placentas are found: (1) separate dichorionic–diamniotic placentas, including completely separate placentas as well as partially fused placentas, in which the placental tissues are separated on the marginal surface and the membranes are loosely adherent; and (2) completely fused dichorionic–diamniotic placentas, making it impossible to separate the two placentas.

In the latter type of placenta (monochorionic), there are also two subclasses: (1) monochorionic–diamniotic placentas, in which the dividing membranes consist of two amnions; and (2) monochorionic–monoamniotic placentas, in which the twin gestations are contained within a single amniotic cavity. Based on these observations, certain categorizations of twin pregnancies are possible.

Twins with a single amnion, chorion and placenta are unequivocally monozygotic. This placentation, however, characterizes a small minority of twins, so that the number of amnions usually is of little help in diagnosis. However, twins with separate amnions and single chorion and placenta are also unequivocally monozygotic. However, twins with separate amnions and chorions and fused placentas may be either monozygotic or dizygotic, as well as those with separate placentas. *Obstetricians attempting to determine zygosity by means of single or double placenta should remember that the presence of a single placenta does not invariably mean monozygosity; it may simply represent the fusion of two placentas. Alternatively, the presence of two placentas is not diagnostic of dizygosity; it may represent separate implantations of two blastocysts derived from the cleavages of a single zygote.* (Editor: Italics added.) A concise review of examining and evaluating the placenta and chorion is presented in Chapter 9.

Diagnosis of twin zygosity by the similarity method

During the past half-century, a number of approaches for determination of zygosity based on similarity or dissimilarity have been proposed, but found to be of limited value: fingerprint analysis of ridge counts and palmar angles[1], morphological similarity with regard to hair, eye and skin color and shape of nose, lips and eyes[2] and tissue grafts between twins[3]. The similarity method of diagnosis, as elaborated by Siemens[4] and von Verschuer[2], has also been applied to blood group and histocompatibility antigens, serum proteins and enzyme polymorphisms, in order to classify a particular twin pair as mono- or dizygotic. Using these systems, any twin pair discordant for one or more blood groups is dizygotic. To determine the probability of a set of twins being monozygotic, on the other hand, the possibility of dizygotic twins being alike for a series of blood groups must be calculated. To accomplish this, the probabilities for each blood group being similar is determined separately; this is based on their frequency in the population, which, in turn, varies with ethnicity. It is possible to construct probability tables with respect to different blood-group systems for any one of the three possible genotypic combinations of two siblings, i.e. AA, Aa, aa. These probabilities are then combined with the initial probability of a twin pair being dizygotic and that of a dizygotic pair being like-sexed. Using eight different blood-groups, ABO, MNSS, Rh, P, Kell, Kidde, Duffy, and Lewis A and B antigens, there is a 97% probability that the assignment of the twins to the monozygotic class is correct if all eight blood groups are alike in both twins; on the other hand, the probability of the two twins being dizygotic remains as high as 3%[5]. If other blood group systems and serum proteins, e.g. haptoglobins, are added to the calculations, the probability of being monozygotic can be increased to 99.3%[6]. Nevertheless, these probabilities, while highly suggestive, are not sufficient to unequivocally establish the zygosity of individual twin sets. To reach this goal required the introduction of the newer technologies involving the analysis of DNA.

The nature of DNA

DNA, or deoxyribonucleic acid, is the chemical substance that comprises genes. DNA is composed of a chain (sequence) of basic units called nucleotides, each of which contains a sugar (deoxyribose), phosphate, and one of four nitrogenous bases, adenine, guanine, cytosine and thymine. In nature, DNA usually consists of two tightly coiled helical chains of nucleotide bases, the backbone of each chain being formed by deoxyribose and phosphate. The two chains of DNA are complementary and held together by hydrogen bonding between the four bases, with adenine in one chain always being bonded to thymine in the other and guanine always bonded to cytosine. During replication, the two DNA chains come apart and each chain acts as a template for the synthesis of a complementary strand. This can be easily and reproducibly performed in the laboratory. By simply heating DNA sufficiently, the two strands separate, exposing the four nitrogenous bases. Each strand of DNA can act as a template, a critical element in the technique to identify and compare the nucleotide sequences of different individuals. It is thus possible to synthesize short segments of DNA ('probes') which can hybridize with complementary sequences only if present in the DNA sample undergoing analysis. Labelling the DNA probes with radioactive phosphorus or fluorescent moieties provides reliable and easily verifiable documentation that a specific sequence complementary to the DNA probe is present. Failure of the probe to hybridize documents an absence of the complementary sequence.

Genes have several fundamental functions in living systems: first, they are units of inheritance, physically passed from parent to offspring via oocyte and spermatozoa; second, genes are units of function, responsible for directing the synthesis of enzymes and other proteins based on the sequence of nucleotides comprising the DNA of each gene; and, third, genes are also units of mutation, which represent changes in the structure of DNA that lead to phenotypic differences between individuals.

It is estimated that there are between 50 000 and 100 000 genes in each of the 14 billion cells directing the development and functioning of a human being. About one-third of these genes differ from individual to individual, so that the number of possible gene combinations is inestimable! This means that each human is a genetically distinct individual and, therefore, based solely on DNA gene content, each individual is distinguishable from all the other 5 billion individuals comprising the total world population. Because the variation within certain gene sequences is so great, the chance of two individuals simultaneously possessing the same sequence may be in the order of less than 10^{-10}, two to twenty times greater than the number of people presently inhabiting the earth[7]. Monozygotic twins then represent a singular exception to the genetic uniqueness of each individual.

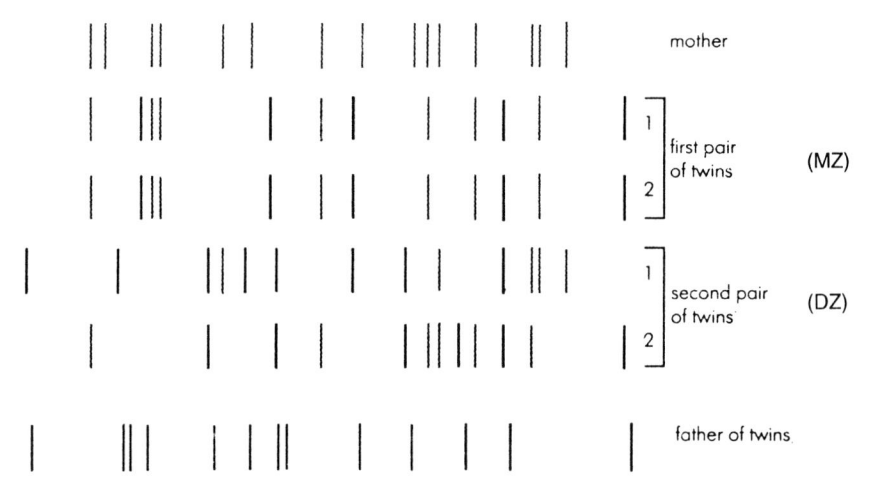

Figure 1 DNA fingerprinting using a minisatellite probe. A hypothetical example of two sets of twins, one monozygotic and the other dizygotic

In addition to determining differences between individuals in the nucleotide sequences of their functioning genes, another approach analyzes DNA copy number. No more than 3–5% of the DNA in the human genome has a known function of coding for protein. Present evidence suggests that mammalian genomes have evolved rather untidily with little pressure for economy or neat organization. Most of the DNA appears to have no function. Nevertheless, molecular techniques used to identify and characterize DNA are completely independent of whether or not the DNA has any function. The human genome contains both unique and repetitive sequences. Unique sequences occur once, or only a few times, in the genome. They include most genes. Repetitive sequences are present in many copies per genome and consist of two families, satellite DNA and minisatellites. Satellite DNA is the most highly repetitive class; it consists of short sequences repeated in tandem hundreds of thousands of times and is mostly located at centromeres of chromosomes. Minisatellites are tandem repeats of, perhaps, 100 copies of some short sequence, each comprising one to a few dozen clusters randomly spread in the human genome. Minisatellites have become extremely valuable tools for genetic analysis, especially for establishing biological relationships, e.g. paternity, zygosity, source of DNA. An alternative name for minisatellites is 'VNTR sequences' (variable number of tandem repeats).

VNTR sequences are very informative genetic markers, because, as their name suggests, they show a high degree of polymorphism in the general population, are very useful in unequivocally distinguishing the DNA of different individuals, and, therefore, are directly applicable to assess the origin of twin zygosity (Figure 1). The application of VNTR analysis to determine personal identity is so precise that the term 'DNA fingerprinting' was coined[8].

DNA fingerprinting

It is reasonable for clinicians to ask molecular geneticists just how accurate is the technique of 'DNA fingerprinting' and how does it work? The ability to correctly identify dizygotic twins is directly related to the number and type of DNA probes applied to the DNA samples. For example, a single probe representing one set of VNTR sequences may produce a pattern that is unique to one person in one hundred (1:100). A second probe with the same discriminatory power would produce a combined pattern that is unique to one person in ten thousand, i.e. the product of their separate probabilities ($1/100 \times 1/100 = 1/10\,000$).

The application of just two independent DNA probes could result in a DNA pattern in which the probability of complete DNA fingerprinting concordance between two siblings is $0.5^{60} = 9 \times 10^{-19}$ [7,9–11]. Even when two multi-allelic probes with the lowest number of discriminating bands are used[7], a false positive rate of less than 1 in 50 billion (5×10^{-10}) can be achieved for siblings (who have half of their genomes in common). This number indicates that zygosity can be determined with near certainty.

Several reports concerning the determination of twin zygosity have used Jeffrey's minisatellite probes[8]. Hill and Jeffreys[12] correctly analyzed DNA from 12 sets of twins in which zygosity was known in seven instances by sex or placental arrangement. Azuma et al.[13], analyzing DNA from two sets of triplets, identified different DNA profiles in all three males of one set and monozygotic male twins in the second set coupled with a female sibling. Finally, Jones et al.[14] used DNA testing to confirm monozygosity for the purpose of syngeneic bone marrow transplants in three patients with chronic myelogenous leukemia. In two of the three cases, previously administered blood transfusions precluded zygosity identification by conventional serology analysis. Numerous other applications of a similar nature undoubtedly exist.

New developments in DNA fingerprinting

A new form of hypervariable VNTR markers has been described in the human genome: short repeat units composed of a small number of DNA nucleotides[15]. These short tandem repeats, termed 'STR', are dimeric, trimeric, or tetrameric and it will soon become possible to run a single reaction for zygosity testing which will make possible the simultaneous identification of STRs differing only in one or two bases in length[16]. This form of DNA fingerprinting will be accomplished through a high-resolution, fluorescence-based, semi-automated method of DNA analysis. DNA profiles produced with these extraordinary variable sequences will make the analysis of zygosity almost infallible.

Another novel approach to individual identification is based not on copy number but on the internal sequence variation within minisatellites[17]. This additional level of polymorphism can be used to discriminate minisatellites of indistinguishable copy number but with diverged internal sequences. It will be of great interest to investigate apparent homozygotes, especially monozygotic twins, at well-characterized minisatellites to determine how labile is DNA and what the DNA spontaneous mutation rate may be at the single nucleotide base level.

Summary

The use of DNA methods to analyze variable numbers of tandem repeat (VNTR) sequences dispersed in the human genome has become a powerful tool for the postnatal determination of twin zygosity. DNA techniques have proven to be reliable, reproducible and relatively simple to perform. Moreover, they provide an unprecedented degree of accuracy in determining monozygosity. The probability that two individuals will share, by chance, all DNA sequences detected by a single probe is related to the mean population frequency of alleles detected by the probe. Using hypervariable markers at a single gene locus, it is now possible to demonstrate statistically that the

---

Editor: The phenotypic similarity of identical twins is shown in the photographs of Steven and Joel Dworkin. Figure 2 is Steven. Figure 3 is Joel. Figure 4 represents the composite figure of both young men made by superimposing the negatives. Aside from difference in arm position, pectoral hair pattern and facial expression, the overlay is nearly exact. By using a magnifying glass, examination of Figure 4 will demonstrate minor differences in postnatal umbilical scarring. Figure 5 shows their hair whorls and Figure 6 illustrates their respective index fingers. Figure 7 is the DNA fingerprints of Steven and Joel Dworkin. All photographs provided courtesy of David Teplica, MD, MFA

MULTIPLE PREGNANCY

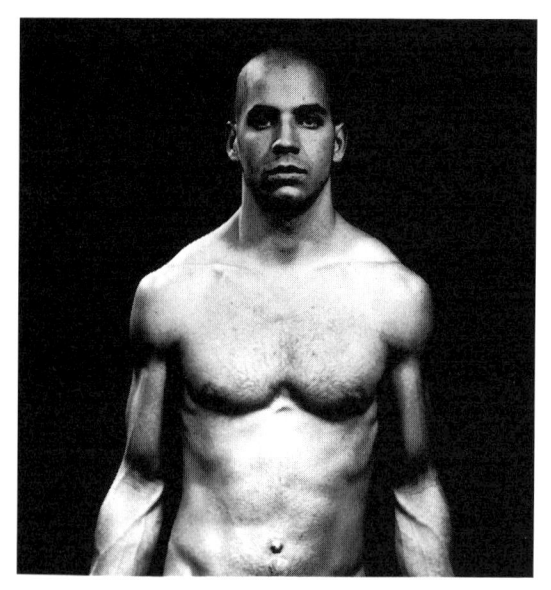

Figure 2 Steven Dworkin. Original in color (36 × 44 in Cibachrome)

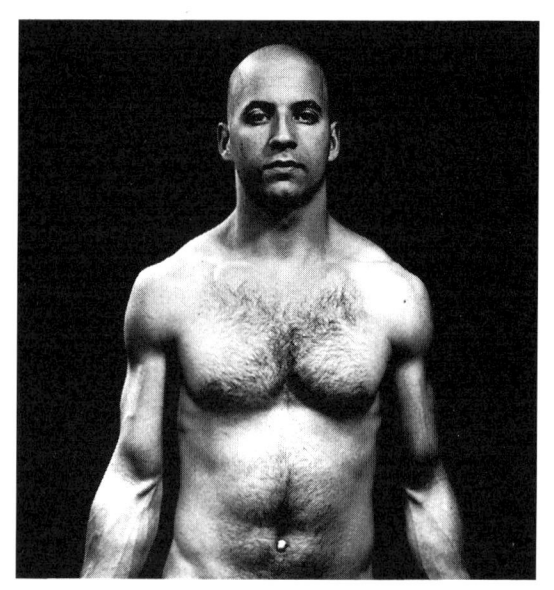

Figure 3 Joel Dworkin. Original in color (36 × 44 in Cibachrome)

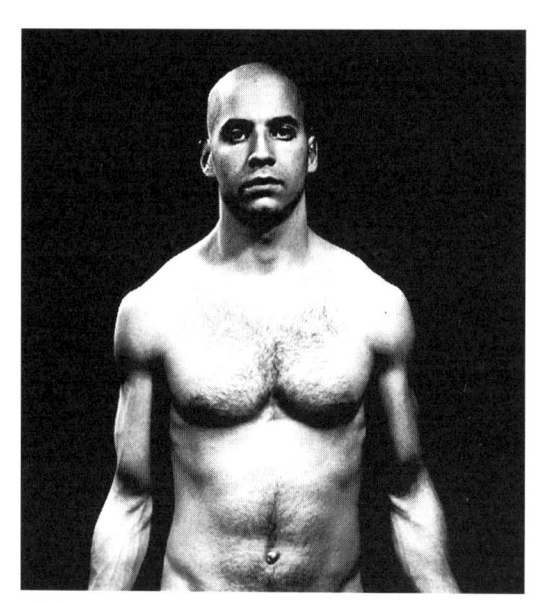

Figure 4 Composite picture of Steven and Joel Dworkin. Original in color (36 × 44 in Cibachrome)

Postnatal zygosity determination

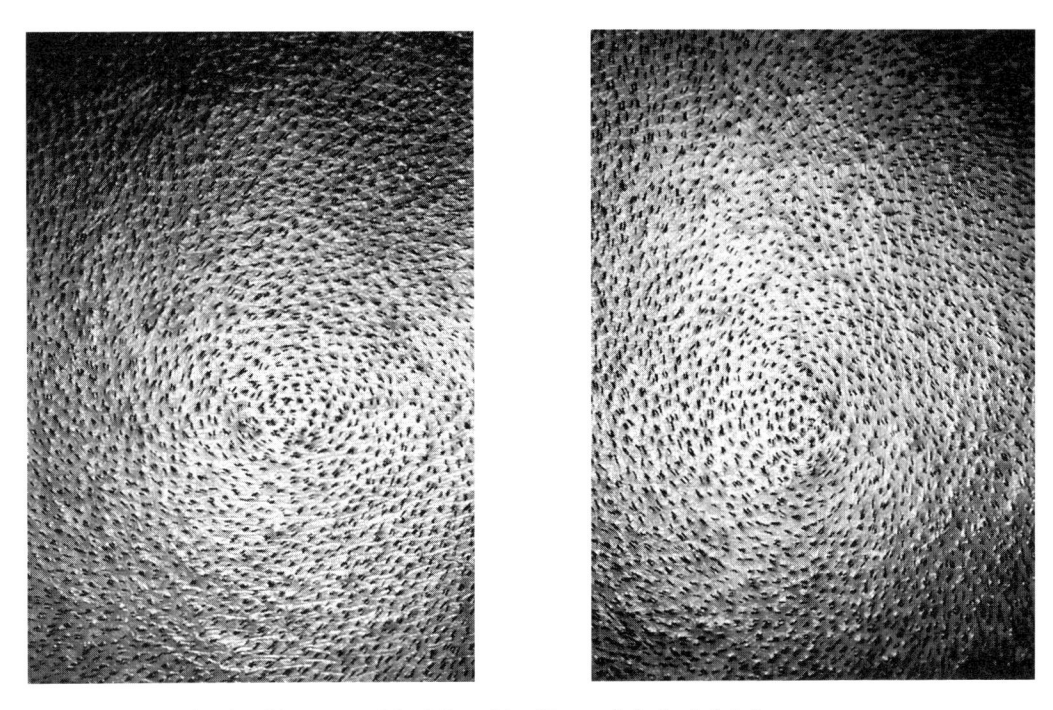

Figure 5 Hair whorls of Steven and Joel Dworkin (Steven left; Joel right)

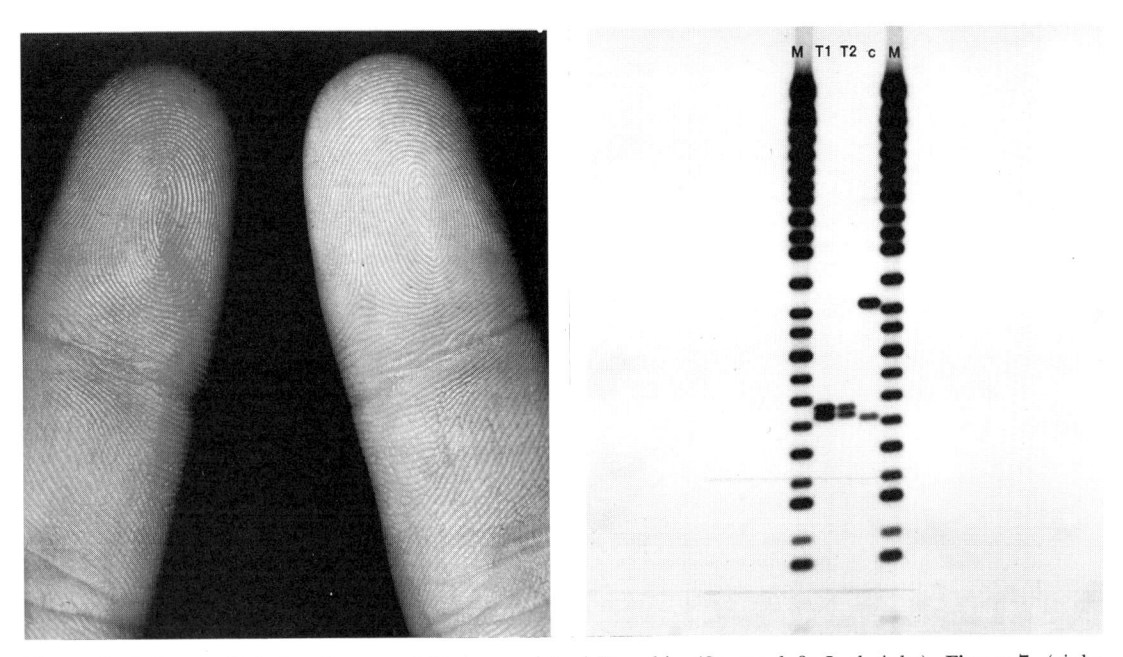

Figure 6 (left panel) Index fingers of Steven and Joel Dworkin (Steven left; Joel right). **Figure 7** (right panel) Zygosity determination of twins Steven and Joel Dworkin by DNA testing. Four independent VNTR loci (probes) were used: D2S44 (YNH24) (shown above); D10S28 (TBQ7); D17S26 (EFD52); and D6S132 (PAC424). Probabability of monozygosity = 99.3%. M, molecular weight marker; T1 and T2, Steven and Joel Dworkin; c, control DNA. Studies conducted by Fairfax Identity Laboratories, A Division of Genetics and IVF Institute, Fairfax, VA, Joel Schulman, MD, Medical Director. Probability determinations made by D. Lemers, PhD, Laboratory Director

probability of any two unrelated persons having identical patterns is about one in 300 billion; for siblings this number is reduced to one in 300 000, as a result of sharing DNA sequences[18]. Using probes from two independent multiallelic loci, the probability that two first-degree relatives (parents and offspring) will have identical DNA fingerprints is estimated to be one in 300 trillion[19]. The use of hypervariable gene loci virtually eliminates the possibility of incorrectly distinguishing between monozygotic and dizygotic twins.

Finally, it should be noted that other markers employed for twin zygosity determination, such as placentation, HLA typing, and blood group antigens, should not be so easily discarded, despite the analytical powers of DNA technology. Although these markers may not be uniformly informative, their potential contribution to the rapid and relatively inexpensive delineation of dizygosity from monozygosity should not be minimized.

References

1. Stern, C. (1960). *Principles of Human Genetics*, 2nd edn., p. 535. (San Francisco: W.H. Freeman)
2. v. Verschuer, O. (1939). Twin research from the time of Francis Galton to the present day. *Proc. R. Soc. B.*, **128**, 62
3. Franceschetii, Baxmatter, Klein (1948). *Bull. Acad. Suisse Sc. Med.*, **4**,
4. Siemens, H.W. (1924). *Die Zwillingspathologie*, p. 103. (Berlin: Springer)
5. Wilson, R.S. (1970). Blood typing and twin zygosity. *Hum. Hered.*, **20**, 30
6. Juel-Nielsen, N. and Hauge, M. (1958). On the diagnosis of zygosity in twins and the value of blood groups. *Acta Genet.*, **8**, 256
7. Jeffreys, A.J., Turner, M. and Debenham, P. (1991). The efficacy of multilocus DNA fingerprint probes for individualization and establishment of family relationships, determined by extensive casework. *Am. J. Hum. Genet.*, **48**, 824
8. Jeffreys, A.J., Wilson, V. and Thein, S.L. (1985). Hypervariable 'minisatellite' regions in human DNA. *Nature (London)*, **314**, 67
9. Jeffreys, A.J., Wilson, V., Thein, S.L. *et al.* (1986). DNA 'fingerprints' and segregation analysis of multiple markers in human pedigrees. *Am. J. Hum. Genet.*, **39**, 11
10. Lynch, M. (1988). Estimation of relatedness by DNA fingerprinting. *Mol. Biol. Evol.*, **5**, 584
11. Orrego, C. and King, M.-C. (1990). Determination of familial relationships. In Ennis, M., Gelfand, D., Sninksy, J. and White, T. (eds.) *PCR Protocols: A Guide to Methods and Applications*, pp. 416–26. (New York: Academic Press)
12. Hill, A.V.S. and Jeffreys, A.J. (1985). Use of minisatellite DNA probes for determination of twin zygosity at birth. *Lancet*, **2**, 1394
13. Azuma, C., Kamiura, S., Nobunaga, T. *et al.* (1989). Zygosity determination of multiple pregnancy by deoxyribonucleic acid fingerprints. *Am. J. Obstet. Gynecol.*, **160**, 734
14. Jones, L., Thein, S.L., Jeffreys, A.J. *et al.* (1987). Identical twin marrow transplatation for 5 patients with chronic myeloid leukemia: role of DNA fingerprints to confirm monozygosity in 3 cases. *Eur. J. Haematol.*, **37**, 144
15. Edwards, A., Civitello, A., Hammond, H.A. *et al.* (1991). DNA typing and genetic mapping with trimeric and tetrameric tandem repeats. *Am. J. Hum. Genet.*, **49**, 746
16. Carrano, A.V., Lamerdin, J., Ashworth, L.K. *et al.* (1989). A high-resolution, fluorescence-based, semi-automated method for DNA fingerprinting. *Genomics*, **4**, 129
17. Monckton, D. and Jeffreys, A.J. (1991). Minisatellite allele discrimination using internal mapping of variant repeat units and single strand mobility polymorphisms (SSMP) on agarose gels. *Proc. 8th Int. Congr. Hum. Genet. Am. J. Hum. Genet.*, **49**, A2789
18. Kovacs, B., Shahbahrami, B., Platt, L.D. and Comings, D.E. (1988). Molecular genetic prenatal determination of twin zygosity. *Obstet. Gynecol.*, **72**, 954
19. Jeffreys, A.J. (1987). Highly variable minisatellites and DNA fingerprints. *Biochem. Soc. Trans.*, **15**, 309

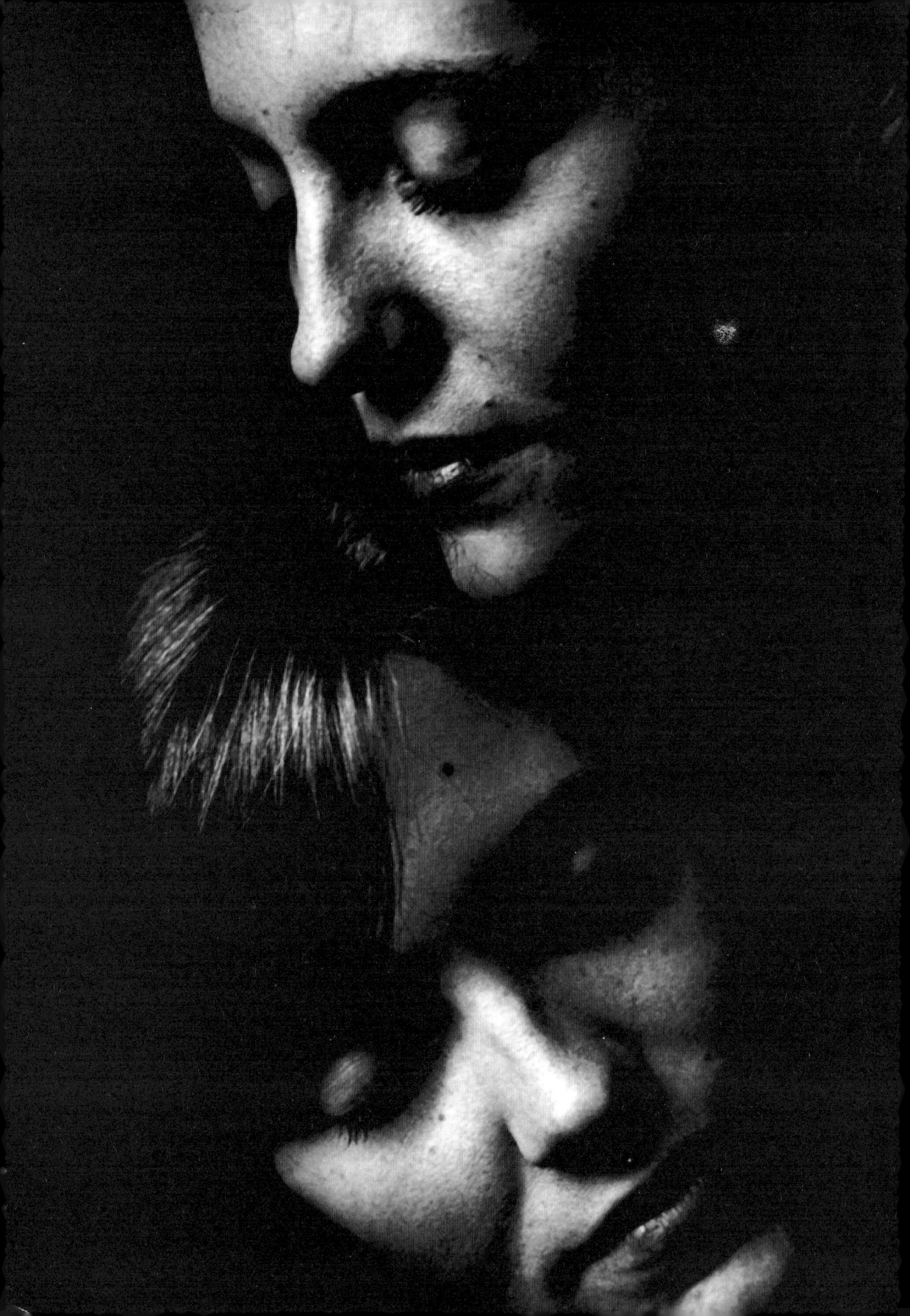

section IX
Parental Concerns

The Bossolt Twins

David Teplica, 1990,
The Collected Image, Evanston, Illinois

The parent–doctor relationship 48

D.M. Keith

Introduction

Generally, by the time a woman first arrives in your office, she already suspects that she is pregnant, wanting to confirm her suspicions, and if correct, to find care for her growing fetus. She is nervous, excited and usually well prepared for the news that she is about to become a parent. However, many mothers, and fathers for that matter, are quite surprised and even shocked to learn that the suspected, single baby is going to be more than just one child.

Because the diagnosis of twins, triplets and higher-order multiples has this paradoxical effect, patients react with any number of emotions, ranging from delight, to apprehension, and often even fear. This spectrum of emotions may begin minutes after your announcement, and can continue as an emotional roller-coaster throughout the pregnancy. Realistic support from the patient's husband is not always available, because he may also be experiencing the same emotional see-saw.

Because of the mother's special needs, women pregnant with multiples may turn to you and rely more heavily on you for a gamut of information than would be the case for mothers pregnant with singletons. This dependence is natural and should not cause alarm or worry. The soon-to-be parents worry about their abilities to cope with the physical, emotional and financial demands associated with multiples. Their questions will seem endless! Will they be able to meet the demands of parenting more than one child? Will the cost of multiples exceed their budget? How will they be able to sleep after the babies arrive? How much additional clothing must be obtained? Are two cribs, two playpens and two of everything needed?

The parents' fears make them see things negatively. Your first reaction may be to respond, 'How do I know the answers to all of these questions? I am a medical doctor, not a financial planner or a nanny'. Remember, however, your patients do not want answers so much as they want reassurance. It is natural, therefore, for expectant mothers of multiples to turn to you for answers to the non-medical questions. Your calm expertise will help them see things positively. Respond generously to both parents with a sense of humor and your best smile.

This chapter provides some old-fashioned common-sense answers for you to meet their special expectations. It is based on the author's extensive experience of talking to mothers of multiples at the Twinsday Festivals in Twinsburg, Ohio, meetings of individual National Organization of Mothers of Twins Clubs and the leadership of COMBO, the Council of Multiple Birth Organizations.

The pregnancy

Most mothers understand that good prenatal care is the single most important factor in the healthy birth of twins and other multiples. Gaining weight is often viewed by many expectant mothers as the most negative aspect of being pregnant. Because you know that healthy weight gain is vital to fetal growth and survival of multiples, stress the importance of a healthy and balanced diet (see Chart in Chapter 21). It may prove helpful to explain that weight gained by a balanced diet is easier to lose after the child's birth than weight gained from diets high in starches and sugars. Also, you can remind your patients that small, frequent meals are easier to digest, especially as the stomach is pushed under the diaphragm.

In addition to increased weight gain, many other physical changes will occur throughout the pregnancy. These changes can have a profound effect on your patients' attitudes toward themselves, their babies and their pregnancy. To minimize stress, explain what changes are occurring and why. For example, rings must be removed if swelling is a problem. Fluid retention may also require expectant mothers to wear flat, comfortable shoes that provide proper support. Stress the fact that, although saddle shoes, tennis shoes, and bedroom slippers are not always fashionable, they are less dangerous than tight shoes, and possibly remind the mothers that no one is going to be looking at their feet anyway.

In addition to experiencing increased physical size, patients carrying twins will probably tire much more easily than their sisters with a single fetus. Whereas this exhaustion is common and perfectly acceptable, it clearly is not a reason to ignore rest and sleep. Advise your patients to lie down and rest whenever they become tired. This advice clearly may precede any reduction of physical activity which you may want to prescribe for medical reasons.

Many patients do not begin worrying about labor and delivery concerns until the third trimester. During the last trimester, however, the patients' questions focus on the pain associated with delivery and the possible complications related to multiple births. Naturally, during this trimester, you probably will feel more comfortable with your patients' questions. Although non-medical questions may be very exasperating, their answers are important to your patients' emotional well-being.

Even if your patient has been pregnant before, chances are she has never delivered twins, and therefore will be uncertain about the labor and delivery. These uncertainties will evoke many questions. Is the discomfort of delivering two babies worse than one? Is the risk of failure in the delivery increased? Can my body handle the stress? Will I be able to deliver the babies naturally or will a Cesarean be necessary? These are all common questions and must be answered.

Before your patient's due dates arrive, have a long, sincere, and heartfelt talk with both parents concerning the delivery and what they should expect. During pregnancy, they probably do not have any idea of what will happen during delivery, and therefore, they are probably more than a little bit frightened. During the actual delivery, you will easily take charge and remain in complete control. Expect your patients to have one thought, and one thought only: *Let's get this over with*! No matter what type of personality your patient demonstrated during the pregnancy, she will almost certainly be a changed woman during the delivery. Be ready for anything! Some patients will declare their eternal love (for you), and others will vow to kill you if you do not do something quickly to relieve their pain. Many mothers will be so exhausted after their delivery that their only desire will be for sleep. A few may remember to thank you, but do not feel rejected if this is not the case. During this euphoric but exhausted state, almost anything, except manners, can be expected from the new mother!

After the birth

Following the birth of multiples, although you may see the new mothers less often, they will continue to ask questions and expect you to provide the answers. You will still be their source of knowledge and this will continue even as the children grow.

Overwhelming exhaustion

During the first few months after the delivery, it is common for the mother to suffer from physical and emotional exhaustion, and possibly believe that something is terribly wrong with her. This exhaustion, and the perfectly normal feelings of postpartum depression which often accompanies it may bring some very perplexed, confused and frightened patients to your office.

Although most new mothers are intellectually aware that their physical and emotional exhaustion is perfectly natural, many are not emotionally equipped to accept this fact. Gently reassure your patients that the exhaustion they are now experiencing results from the increased demand for their time and attention. Let them know that it is difficult enough for a woman to cope with one new baby, let alone the exceptionally enormous task of coping with two or three. It is unreasonable for your patients to think that such a task can, or even should, be handled alone. 'Superwoman' only exists in comic books and in other people's minds; she is not real and neither is 'Supermom'. Therefore, do not let your patients try to live up to the impossible standards held by others. Tell your patients to be realistic about their capabilities and limitations.

Too often, women feel that their inabilities to manage everything smoothly, efficiently, and alone indicates a failure on their part as a wife and mother. This misconception is dangerous. Your patients need to understand and accept that there is little opportunity for daytime rest, and no opportunity for uninterrupted nighttime sleep now that twins have entered their lives. Without proper rest and sleep, however, exhaustion is both inevitable and *permissible*. It is up to you to reassure her, even if all others have stressed this point previously.

Many solutions are available to overcome the physical and emotional exhaustion experienced after birth. Advise your new mothers to make concerted efforts to maintain contact with their old friends and venture out to make new friends. It is important to feel the support and comfort of established relationships; and the challenge and excitement of new friends proves they can still circulate in their ever changing world. Remaining in touch with co-workers is another potential solution. If your patient worked before and during her pregnancy, she should continue to stay in contact with her co-workers during her maternity leave – especially if she plans to return to work. The isolation a new mother endures is often suffocating but not necessary; friends, family, neighbors and adult conversation are only a phone call away.

Advise your patients to join in groups with other mothers of young children like the local Parents of Twins Club (see Chapter 50). Such groups offer new mothers comfort, solace, support and much-needed information about how to cope with raising multiple babies. Indeed, these groups are where the 'veterans of the trench warfare' congregate. The members of these groups also understand the emotional turmoil a new mother experiences after birth, and therefore can provide her with the understanding and support she needs most.

In rare cases where no close relative, friend, or neighbor is available to help with the physical care of the children during their first few weeks at home, it may be necessary to arrange for a home aide to visit the home. The helper's expense is minimal compared to live-in help, and the rewards which the extra hands provide are worth the expense. These care givers allow the mother some much-needed rest by reducing the mother's physical burden and caring for the children. A home aide can also demonstrate proper care for the children to mothers who feel inadequate or unsure of how to tackle such a large task.

Convince your new mothers of multiples of the importance of scheduling weekly personal time, no matter how hectic things seem or become. This invaluable time is great for relieving stress and easing tension. This time need not be extensive . A few hours each week adequately provides the necessary results. Time available to read, write, draw, paint, needlepoint, knit or crochet can do wonders for a new mother's self-esteem and self-worth. Often, something like a trip to the beauty parlor is enough to make a mother again feel good about herself.

Family impact

Without doubt, the introduction of the new babies affects the entire family. Because of the many adjustments that must be made after the birth of multiples, the impact on the family is often overwhelming. New and extensive requirements on time, money, attention and patience often stretch family members beyond their limits. The greater demand for everything may deplete and strain all resources, except love. Families must exercise teamwork now, when it is most valuable.

When family routines are quickly established, the demands of the new burden are lessened. As long as everyone helps with the work, no one family member will have more than he or she can handle. Working together may also bring a family closer together. In particular, older siblings are less likely to feel neglected or rejected when they, too, are given chores which involve them in the lives of the new babies.

Unknown and confusing territories

Many new mothers become frightened when faced by the daily decisions regarding the welfare of their children. Mothers often doubt their ability to make good and effective choices. Many turn to you for answers to their questions. One of the first questions aimed towards your knowledge and expertise is the age-old dilemma: breast or bottle feeding?

Most doctors agree that breast feeding is valuable for babies, not only because it assists the newborn to develop immunity from infections, but also because it provides an intimate and comforting contact between the babies and their mother (see Chapter 41). If, however, bottle feeding is chosen, fathers can become actively involved with the feeding of their children. In addition, it is more convenient when the babies need to be fed in public. Many doctors may fail to remember that the availability of a mother's milk is largely dependent on demand and thus point out the fact that mothers often do not produce enough milk for multiple babies when they start nursing. This initial shortage of milk is nothing for the mother to feel ashamed of or embarrassed about. In any event, the pros and cons on this issue are never-ending. Not all women are comfortable with breastfeeding, and therefore should not be made to feel guilty about their feelings. Convince your new parents to weight all factors carefully before a final decision is made (see Chapter 41). Some families choose to try both options. In these cases, the mother's milk is supplemented by some type of formula. With this method, both the mother and father can become intimate with and bond to the children. This option also relieves the strain on the mother to produce such large quantities of milk, especially if she has more than two infants.

Toilet training also prompts many questions by new mothers. Many women are not sure when to begin toilet training their children. Tell them not to rush, as their children may develop the muscles required to perform this task at different times. Sometimes, multiples become ready for toilet training together; other times one child develops before the other – often by as much as 6 months. When mothers observe their children's behavior, important signs can be discovered. Jumping around may indicate a child's discomfort in trying to hold back the urge to go to the rest room. Sitting down quietly or uncharacteristically can also indicate attempts to hold back urges of the bladder. The easiest way to deal with of these events is to keep the potty close at hand in the room the children occupy.

Mothers may not understand that play is an important activity for their children, because it helps them develop in four very important areas: imagination, adventure, destruction and nature.

Imaginative play helps children familiarize themselves with new things. They dress in white coats and pretend they are doctors or nurses in a hospital. In their play, children can dole out candy pills to sick toys and dolls, and spend hours absorbed in their pretend world. Puppets are good for stimulating the imagination and especially helpful for children who have difficulty communicating. By using a puppet, the child does not have to speak to anyone directly. For some children, communication is quite stressful, and being permitted to play games of pretend gives them the chance to act out their imaginations and not feel responsible for what they say.

Playing adventure games gives children the opportunity to overcome mental and physical obstacles. Adventure games include climbing, running, jumping, crawling and balancing. The older children get, the more challenging the obstacles become. In the beginning, the household sofas, chairs and stairs challenge children. When older, the obstacles expand to include exploring the outdoor world where old tires in the backyard provide hours of healthy, safe play. Swing sets, though popular, are not always advisable. Many children are severely injured each year from accidents incurred on swing sets. Parents may wish to invest in sand boxes instead. These wonderful containers allow the creation of many avenues of imaginative and adventurous play.

Many parents may be stunned to hear a doctor advise the use of destructive play in training children. Parents do not always realize that children, by nature, may need to destroy before they can create. Although these destructive behavioral needs may be necessary for proper development, they must be carefully monitored and channeled into acceptable behavior, without inhibiting activities too much. Sand and clay provide excellent media for destructive play. With clay, a child creates and destroys without causing unmanageable chaos. Crayons and paper are also superb for achieving creative and destructive play.

Finally, natural play encompasses using the elements found in nature as the play activity's focus. As might be expected, water is a perennial favorite of all children. Even when they are opposed to baths, most children will spend many happy hours splashing in a wading pool or running through water spraying from a garden hose.

Twins often play alone when young, which can be very disconcerting for new mothers. When asked, reassure the mothers that such behavior is perfectly normal. The children will begin to play together and share games and toys when they get older. By virtue of being twins, multiples learn to cooperate with other children earlier than their singleton counterparts. However, fighting and squabbles will naturally occur; after all, they are siblings. Fighting is not a problem unless one child continually dominates over the other or unless the threat of physical danger exists. As the children increase the amount of time they spend playing together, they learn to work as a team. This teamwork often leads to mischief, because they develop the habit of egging each other on to greater mischief. Twins also quickly learn to help each other out of trouble when they become too mischievous.

Advise your patients to place utmost emphasis on home safety during their children's early years. The best way to attain home safety is to anticipate dangers and take whatever precautions are necessary to guard against those dangers. Close parental supervision of the children at play is also absolutely essential. Parents should also visit the local hardware store and purchase childproof locks to place on low cabinets and outlet caps to cover all electrical sockets. Also advise your patients to keep breakable objects and valuable treasures out of the children's reach until they are old enough to learn not to touch.

Because the twins often play so closely together, they may develop a special or secret language, understood exclusively by them. (Editor: The medical terms for this are idioglossia or cryptoglossia.) This occurs most often between identical twins, because they are more likely to experience the same visual, auditory, olfactory, tactile and gustatory sensations, causing them to view and judge their environment similarly. Such similar views often negate the need for words and normal language. Mothers often become frightened when children demonstrate this 'babble', because it is not understandable. Reassure them that 'babble' expressed by the twins may be a special means of communication and is not necessarily a sign of retardation. Direct communication with eye-to-eye contact with each child separately allows them to practice their conventional language skills. The babble is often treatable by the parents and, in severe cases, by a speech therapist.

When the children approach school age, your patients may again show signs of nervousness and confusion. A main concern will be whether or not to enroll the children together. The answer to this question must come by studying how each child relates to the world around them. Because children develop at their own rates and not according to specific scales and patterns, some are ready at the normal school age and others are not. (Editor: This may be especially true for children who were born preterm.) Parents need not be alarmed when the twins are not ready to begin school together. In contrast, a forced separation in school can become a traumatic experience for a twin (see Chapter 51). Eventual separation in life is necessary for healthy growth and individuality, even though the children will be somewhat sad and disoriented at first.

Because twins possess different abilities and interests, it is easy for them to fall into patterns of under- or over-achievement. Such developmental problems often depend upon how each views their own personal capabilities. Twins who strongly desire to equal each other usually achieve similar progress. This equality is by no means a problem if the children have fairly equal abilities. However, if the children are unequally endowed with mental and physical capabilities, one child must work extra hard to equal the other's level. The other alternative includes the more endowed child underachieving to wait for the other to catch up. Either option is not healthy for the children and parents need to be alert to the signs. Placing the children with different teachers who have different expectations often helps families achieve a better balance of progress. It is also important for parents to remember that girls tend to develop quicker than boys. No matter what happens, warn the parents never to compare the children against each other or allow others to do so. Careless comparisons often inflict great damage to a child's self-esteem and motivation.

To promote individuality and discourage unwanted comparisons between the twins, both children need to be recognized for who they are as individuals, not for what they represent together. Most twins do not appreciate being compared or fussed over because of their likeness and will go to great lengths to avoid it. Unfortunately, a most effective way to achieve this avoidance is to become disruptive. Twins working together become a powerful force capable of putting their heads together to plan, scheme and connive. Give them a break by treating them as individuals and these problems may be eliminated before they ever start.

Sometimes you will be faced with patients whose child (or children) are handicapped. These families face unique needs and often have difficulty coping with this responsibility. Gently remind these parents of the value of sharing similar experiences, needs and strength with others in support groups. Parents often gain much-needed comfort, courage and information from these interactions.

Death is not a pleasant subject. However, it does happen to twins and there will be those times when your patients face the death of one or both children. This type of loss is a unique and profound for both parents. It also can have a devastating effect on the surviving multiple(s). To assist the parents in coming to grips with their loss, advise them to seek out those who have experienced this kind of loss and who can empathize with them (see Appendix).

When death occurs, warn your patients that unintentionally careless and insensitive remarks by friends, neighbors and acquaintances will be some of the hardest things they will have to face. These harsh comments are well meant, but often come out wrong. Comments like 'This is probably for the best' or 'At least you still have the other one' are especially frustrating and may increase the hurt, confusion, and anger that the parents are trying so desperately to reduce.

For many, tangible memories of the baby or babies provide much comfort. When a child dies at an older age, memories are easy to find, because of the many experiences the parent and child shared. However, the memories of a newborn are hard to find and very difficult to hold onto. You can try talking to your grieving patients about the lost child, but more often than not they simply need you to listen. People, naturally, are afraid to face the pain of the loss, and therefore, often try to avoid mentioning the lost child. However, they must express their feelings if they are ever to get beyond the experience and continue with their lives. Talking about the loss acknowledges its existence and healing begins only after the acknowledgement takes place.

Personal boundaries

As the twins grow older, their individual personalities begin to diverge, much to the delight and confusion of parents. Much is said about the similarities and camaraderie between twins, but little is known about their differences. When differences begin emerging, many parents become frightened. They usually are not prepared for the establishment of personal boundaries between the close siblings. Parents see the extraordinary communication and bonding and naturally expect that it takes precedence over all other emotions. Your patients may come to you in tears, because their once loving children have turned into horrible little monsters toward each other!

Like all humans, twins too have personal boundaries. When these boundaries have been established, it is important that everyone, including the other twin, respect them. Twins who fiercely compete with one another are often at the same time each other's greatest mentors. Twins will cheer each other on while they struggle to outdo each other. Even though they are twins, they are also human. Therefore, no one should expect any more of them.

In fact, twins often have greater struggles over identity than their single birth siblings, friends and contemporaries. They struggle to be separate while the world around them struggles to keep them alike. This conflict causes confusion and resentment. The struggle can even manifest itself into 'alter egos' in which each twin attempts to accomplish what the other desires to do.

The forgotten fathers

Up until now, the father of multiples has been mentioned only peripherally. Indeed, this chapter and other chapters in this Volume have concentrated primarily on the mother. The diagnosis of twins causes many men, like their wives, to feel shocked, delighted, depressed and apprehensive all at one time. Suddenly, the unsuspecting man must face the responsibility of supporting twice the number of children he originally expected. The man's financial future quickly turns bleak. Everything appears to have doubled or halved to the expectant father. The household chores have doubled. The already scare time alone with the spouse will soon be cut in half. In short, the emotional outlook is truly devastating! What will the poor man do? Can the soon-to-be father of twins change his lifestyle to meet all the new demands?

The fathers will, of course, survive. One important condition, however, is that their wives show understanding for their fears and frustrations, cares and concerns. Unfortunately, most men have difficulty voicing their concerns. Be open with the fathers. They will want to know what they can expect from life once the babies arrive. Candidly explain to the father to expect *exhaustion, confusion* and *frustration*. Serious budgeting and some sacrificing will be in order for most families. Financial discipline will be required to stay on top of things, but the task will not be impossible. The entrance of twins will be one of the greatest challenges of the father's life and, in meeting that challenge, he must not be afraid to ask for help.

Having an experienced relative, friend, or care giver stay over the first few days after the new family arrives home from the hospital also benefits the father. Fathers, too, need to learn how to care for the twins. They also need time to establish family and personal routines. Fathers will quickly realize that they will have to accept more of the household chores, because their wives cannot possibly to it all alone. Many times a father's masculine attitude gets in the way of doing what is required of him. As the fathers become accustomed to the idea of helping out, they soon discover that feeding, bathing, dressing, changing, burping and comforting the babies builds wonderful father–child relationships. This bonding is very important to the emotional growth of the family, and gives the father a strong sense of purpose and direction in his life. Most fathers also develop a new sense of respect for their wives when they accept a more active part in the children's care.

The grandparents

Grandparents often are especially delighted by the prospect of having twins in the family. Initially, the news may be shocking, but soon after produces enormous excitement! The grandparents often feel a delightful sense of one-upmanship because few, if any, of their friends and acquaintances can boast the same accomplishment. The idea of twins or triplets, for that matter, is exciting right from the start! Grandparents do not have to worry about bills, diapers, colic and sleepless nights, having finished with those tasks long ago. Grandparents only have to savor the visits and the hugs.

However, getting all the hugs and ignoring all the problems and the bills is not what being a grandparent entails. Grandparents do worry about the children, and the advent of twins can be a terrifying experience for them, too. They may feel bewildered and worried about their abilities to cope with an active set of twins. Commonly grandparents become afraid to commit their help and are embarrassed not to. This situation poses quite a dilemma.

Your patients can relieve some of the tension for their parents by slowly involving the grandparents into the lives of the twins. If the grandparents live far away, they may write and call frequently. Tell the parents to send photographs and audio or video tapes whenever possible, and without being pushy, they can request that the grandparents do the same. This exchange of changing lives, looks and voices helps both the babies and the grandparents continue to know each other and not be too estranged when they come together.

Whether the grandparents can physically help care for the children or not, they will always be quick to shower the twins with love and affection. Grandmas and grandpas can also entertain the other siblings when the mother is too busy with the twins. Grandparents generally have time to listen when mom and dad do not, and there is nothing quite so wonderful as a special cuddle from an adoring grandparent.

Epilogue

This chapter is a condensed version of a layman's common-sense approach to facing the reality of twins. To better prepare yourself for the needs of your patients, send for pamphlets, brochures and booklets listed in the Appendix. Read all you can about twins, and if you have the time, attend a few meetings of a local twins club. Get a feel for what your patients are facing and experiencing. You might be surprised at what you can learn from experienced twin parents.

As hard as you may try, you simply will not know the answers to all questions your patients' questions. As a second source of information, tell them that real life answers to many of their questions can be found at Parents of Twins Clubs (see Chapters 50 and 52). Encourage your patients to seek out the local twins club and join it. Twins clubs are located all over the world, and each provides information, counselling and comfort. New parents are always welcome, because the benefits that are received run in both directions. In addition to drawing from the experiences of other parents, the new parents help others by relating their experiences.

More than support, guidance and friendship are available at Parents of Twins Clubs. Memberships also provides your patients with the opportunity to participate in research programs that focus on multiple-birth families. The final source where information is readily available is the library of the Parents of Twins Clubs or the local library. The answers to many of your patients' questions and even obscure curiosities can be found by reading. Advise your patients to *read*! The city library may also provide addresses where leaflets, pamphlets and booklets are available.

Ethical considerations

M.W. Gallagher

Introduction

The study of ethics is the study of what it means to be a human being involved in various circumstances of life. As such, its subject matter is the entire range of human activity. 'Medical ethics' is not a separate discipline, but rather a branch of ethics that should more accurately be termed 'ethics as applied to medicine'. With this in mind, this chapter will consider ethics as they may be applied to the obstetric management of multifetal pregnancies.

Presuppositions

It is necessary at the outset to establish a framework upon which our considerations will rest, and to explore briefly the meaning of ethics and some of the presuppositions which its study entails. Ethics is primarily concerned with the 'ought' as it is experienced in human life and relationships[1]. This 'ought' is linked with human values, because what a person values determines how he or she will act in specific situations. The discipline of ethics raises questions concerning values and how they are expressed in actions. In so doing, it attempts to encourage reflection on action. This reflection may then reveal incongruence between values and action, or may result in further questioning of the basic values themselves. In this process the notion of what it means to be a human being is constantly refined, in keeping with the observation of Socrates that the unexamined life is not worth living.

Because ethics involves values, it presupposes some source of values. Unfortunately, there is no universal agreement on a single source of values, and anyone interested in the subject must deal with pluralism. For some, this represents an insurmountable obstacle to speaking of a meaningful ethics that can be applied to all human situations. For many individuals the sources of human values are deeply rooted in a particular theological system based on the relationship between God and human beings. For others, these values rest on the nature of human relationships themselves, without reference to a higher order. The ethicist's challenge is to unify the basic principles of ethics so that the 'ought' can be reflected upon from many perspectives, albeit with some common ground. Such reflection encourages questioning of actions and examination of values without reference to source. The ethicist asks, 'Does this action express the desired value?', or 'Is this a value which is worthy of human beings?' The answers will certainly be shaped by the moral background of the responder, but pluralism should never preclude dialogue.

It is important to recognize that the 'ought' of ethics is closely related to obligation imposed by law but is not identical with legal obligation. Whereas law must be informed by ethics, law does not constitute ethics. The purpose of law is order within society. A legal obligation may fall short of a human obligation. On the other hand, a human obligation may be in conflict with a legal obligation, and this conflict may force an individual to make a choice and bear its consequences.

The views expressed in this chapter are those of the author and do not reflect the official policy or position of the Department of the Navy, the Department of Defense, or the United States Government.

Lastly, it should be noted that there are many philosophical perspectives from which ethical questions can proceed[2]. Two of those most commonly encountered in medical ethics are consequentialism (or utilitarianism) and deontology. The former rests on the principle of maximizing the good in each situation. Thus, the 'ought' proceeds from an action's consequences. In contrast, deontological theories hold that factors other than consequences are involved in determining the 'ought' (for example, fidelity to promises, justice, truthfulness). These factors often are given a quasi-absolute status when considering dilemmas. Both viewpoints are developed in detail elsewhere[2,3] and will not be treated fully in this chapter. My personal perspective is grounded in deontologic theory with due consideration of the principle of 'proportionality' (given certain universal principles, where does the greater proportion of good lie?)[4] in resolution of conflict. In this chapter, effort will be made to keep considerations in broad perspective, however, and to address the basic task of raising questions about the 'ought' in particular situations.

Ethics and multifetal pregnancies

Ethics as applied to multifetal pregnancy presupposes the principles of ethics applied to medicine in general. The basic obligations of respect for autonomy, non-maleficence, beneficence and justice, which have been analyzed so well by Engelhardt[5] and Beauchamp and Childress[3] apply in any discussion of the physician/patient relationship involved in the care of multiples. Nonetheless, because these pregnancies are special, they involve additional considerations which at times raise unique questions. Reflection on some of these questions will be the task of the remainder of this chapter.

Preconception counselling

Within many developed nations, the increased incidence of multifetal gestations has been attributed to the impressive advances in the area of assisted reproductive technologies[6–9]. Conception of multiples often is described as a 'complication' which varies in incidence, but which can be as high as 20–30%[10]. Under these circumstances, some of the responsibility for multifetal pregnancy rests with the physicians who treat women and couples for infertility.

The principle of respect for patient autonomy requires that the physician/patient relationship be one of truthfulness from its outset. In particular, the patient has a right to know the risks and benefits of any treatment proposed. These should be explained in a clear, realistic manner, and the physician should undertake all reasonable efforts to ensure that the true implications of the material presented are understood. Only if this is done will the patient be able to give honest, informed consent, free of all reservation. This exchange is the foundation of the trusting relationship upon which all good medicine rests.

The obligation to inform has elicited considerable controversy[3]. To what extent must the physician go to ensure understanding? Is he or she obligated to conduct a short course in medicine for each patient? Obviously, the measures which must be taken to achieve understanding will vary with the situation, but the important point is that efforts to inform be characterized by a genuine intention to convey as much information as possible, in order to enable the patient to make a free and unencumbered decision. This requirement goes beyond a mere recitation of statistical probabilities or the presentation of preprinted pamphlets. While both these methods might afford some legal protection, they can fail to protect the value at risk here, that is, the autonomy of the patient who freely places her trust in the hands of the physician.

The obligation to inform is even more critical in the context of infertility treatment. Many patients have generously participated in long and often unpleasant diagnostic processes which not only have been worrisome but also may have seriously depleted their finances. Despite this, they remain almost desperate to conquer their infertility. Unfortunately, whereas desperation may be an excellent motivator of compliance, it can simultaneously compromise human freedom. Not uncommonly, infertile patients have difficulty 'hearing' the fact that proposed treatments might involve them in decisions for which they are ill prepared. Later on, these same patients may find themselves in the dilemma of having a high-order multiple gestation and facing possibilities of loss of the pregnancy, risk of premature birth and potentially impaired children, or multifetal pregnancy reduction. Understandably, some patients may feel trapped and betrayed by the very physicians who attempted to alleviate their infertility and who had previously been viewed with high esteem.

To avoid creating of such moral dilemmas, infertility specialists as well as those who only occasionally treat infertility must discuss the real possibility of multifetal pregnancy as a result of treatment. The individual or couple seeking treatment should be encouraged seriously to ponder this possibility and to ask questions. The patient's obligation is to be equally honest in trying to grasp the realities of the information being conveyed by the physician. An atmosphere of trust resulting from equal degrees of honesty will benefit all parties involved.

Having considered this, one must not overlook an important principle: a physician must also be free not to treat a patient when he or she thinks that treatment may result in physical or emotional harm. This obligation of nonmaleficence supports the physician who refuses to perform a procedure or treatment on a patient who does not comprehend the risks involved. Whereas proponents of autonomy may view this concept as paternalistic, the physician must retain this option in order to be able to exercise responsible care. Refusal to treat must occur in conjunction with ongoing dialogue and counselling. The physician must express his or her reservations as clearly and honestly as possible. Ultimately, a referral to another caregiver may be necessary.

Diagnosis and early pregnancy

The discovery of a multifetal gestation elicits strong and often mixed emotional responses. The mother frequently is elated at having conceived. Sometimes she is proud and happy that she is carrying twins (or more). Often, however, her elation is tempered by anxiety about the prospect of more than one infant. Occasionally, feelings of anger, fear, or depression are expressed. The physician plays a vital role at this time. After the initial shock has abated, the mother and her partner will turn to the caregiver for answers to numerous questions. The medical advice provided early on is critical in determining the future of the pregnancy.

A multifetal pregnancy is a high-risk pregnancy, requiring specialized care administered by an experienced team in a setting with adequate facilities for provision of full obstetric and neonatal support[11]. It is essential that these facts be communicated to the mother when prenatal care is planned. The mother must be informed that she should plan to be delivered at a center that can accommodate potential complications. Frustrated plans for 'low tech', natural, or even home birth must be addressed in light of the requirements of this type of pregnancy. The obligation for truthfulness and respect for patient autonomy dictates that such information be conveyed in a timely fashion, because advance planning and travel may be required.

These considerations are especially important when a patient's insurance carrier requires delivery at a designated institution. In most cases insurers contract to underwrite appropriate medical care which implies an obligation to take into account the special needs of multifetal gestations. Physicians and parents should address this issue early in the pregnancy, to allow for necessary arrangements. (Editor: If necessary, the physician should communicate the nature of the patient's special needs to the insurance carrier.)

A woman who is newly diagnosed with a multifetal gestation must be made aware of her options. It is clear from the data presented elsewhere in this volume that carrying a multifetal pregnancy to term involves numerous risks to the mother's health. It also involves the real possibility of premature birth of infants with long-term disabilities. At best, it imposes a significant change in the personal and family lifestyle[12]. Although refinements of obstetric and neonatal support have reduced the risks of multifetal pregnancy greatly in the past decade, and although many centers are capable of managing triplet, and even quadruplet, gestations with success, significant risk still exists[13,14] and this fact must be made known to the patient.

Faced with a diagnosis of multifetal pregnancy, a woman may choose termination of the entire pregnancy, reduction of a larger number of fetuses to twins (or occasionally a singleton) to reduce the risks involved, or continuation of the pregnancy to term. The option of elective termination has been a legal reality in the United States since Roe vs. Wade in 1973. Whether this is an acceptable alternative for the woman and her partner depends on personal values and beliefs. This issue will be examined below in conjunction with reduction.

Multifetal pregnancy reduction

The option of fetal reduction became a reality only relatively recently[12,15–17], and has evoked much discussion. Those who offer multifetal pregnancy reduction (MFPR)[18] have presented it as a solution to the tragic dilemma alluded to above in which a woman who has endured much to achieve a pregnancy now finds herself in a situation in which her own health and the health of her fetuses may be at risk (see Chapters 25 and 26). Complete termination (abortion) is abhorrent to many of these parents, because conception has been difficult and future successes are often without guarantee. Yet, the prospect of a high-risk pregnancy with possible poor outcome for the infants is a burden that may exceed the physical, emotional and financial resources of many families. Reduction attempts to salvage a pregnancy and, at the same time, reduce the risks to the mother and remaining fetus(es). This procedure is not without some risk to the pregnancy, and complete loss is possible, although refinements in technique have lessened this possibility[19].

The ethical issues raised by the MFPR have been addressed[12,15,20,21,22]. Arguments in favor of the procedure rest principally on consequentialist reasoning that, faced with a potentially disastrous situation, one must act to bring about the greatest good for the greatest number of people. Thus, killing of some fetuses is justified, so that the pregnancy may result in one or two healthy babies with less risk to the mother. This action is seen by some as morally preferable to complete termination, because it results in preservation, and even enhancement, of the pregnancy instead of its end.

One of the major criticisms of the consequentialist approach states that it represents a 'cold calculation' in which human life is involved, and that no one human life can be said to be worth more than another. It would therefore be immoral, even with good intention, to make a choice for one fetus over another. The right of each fetus to live is inviolable. This argument involves the crux of all questions involving the fetus: what exactly is its status? Although a complete discussion of this question is beyond the scope of the present chapter, some examination of the issue is indicated.

One of the major controversies in the United States today centers on abortion. Proponents and opponents have polarized around the unfortunate slogans of 'pro-life' vs. 'pro-choice'. Like all other slogans, these two obscure more truth than they convey. The current debate has blurred important distinctions and confused many individuals by the indiscriminate use of terms such as 'murder'; which almost invariably assigns a moral intention to individual acts without examination or reflection on the context of these acts. Emotional reaction often replaces clear moral reasoning in approaching what is in reality a tragic human dilemma solved by many women at tremendous emotional expense. At the root of this ethical maelstrom is the question of the status of the fetus in our ethical thought[10,23].

Unfortunately, current obstetric practice contributes to the ambiguity surrounding fetal status. Intervention for termination of a pregnancy is allowed up to 24 weeks from some indications, yet those who practice fetal therapy will treat fetuses at this gestational age as 'patients'[24]. This dichotomy is explained by some with reference to the mother's perception of the status of her fetus and her plans for the continuation of the pregnancy as the determinant of how the fetus is treated[25]. Whereas this argument is philosophically untenable in some systems of thought (notably Roman Catholic theology based on Thomistic scholasticism), it does emphasize a reality which must be considered in the ethical approach to the fetus. Those who feel they must terminate a fetus, for whatever reason, rarely intend to kill another human being *per se*. Rather, a mother most often agrees to the termination of 'the pregnancy'. This neutral terminology conveys an important emotional reality which underlies the intention of the act of termination. Argument can rightly be made as to the 'real' essence of the fetus which is 'human' in the sense that it is a genetically distinct entity which will develop into a human infant. The issue is whether and to what extent the fetus may be regarded as a human being with the same moral status (rights and privileges) as other human beings who are living outside of the uterus. Does the fetus develop in 'humanity' as well as physically? Does mere passage out of the uterus mark a radical change in status[10]?

As recognized by Roe vs. Wade, the determination of the exact moment of becoming human is impossible to establish[26]. We therefore must reflect on how we view the fetus in varying situations and what moral demands this places on us. Tolerance of pregnancy termination is not necessarily incompatible with a view of the fetus as in some manner human. Someone who values human life very highly might at some time be faced with a situation in which the choice to end the life of a fetus is judged to be a tragic necessity in order to promote a good which is more demanding.

Seen in this context, the rationale for MFPR rests not on cold calculation, but on the appreciation that situations may demand painful and tragic choices replete with emotional costs. The practitioner who counsels patients who inquire about MFPR must be aware of the pain experienced in this decision process. A woman sometimes feels trapped into having to make a choice she did not anticipate or desire. She feels pushed to undergo more technological manipulation to solve a problem caused by prior physician-controlled manipulation[27]. If counselling prior to assisted reproduction has not been thorough, the situation may be more bitter. Such a monumental ethical dilemma cannot be adequately handled by set protocols. MFPR cannot and should not be viewed as an easy solution to the 'side effects' of modern reproductive technology, '...but as a provisional approach, appropriate until improved medical care obviates the need for its use'[12].

Reference has been made to the current legal tolerance of abortion on demand to support MFPR with the reasoning that if termination of a fetus in a singleton pregnancy requires no more than maternal desire, then reduction of a multifetal pregnancy should have no greater significance. Employment of this argument as ethical justification for MFPR can be misleading on two accounts. First, that which is legal may not always be ethically sound. Second, the analogy between first-trimester abortion of singletons and MFPR is problematic, and ethical reasoning based on this analogy may be fallacious. There should be no argument that first-trimester MFPR, though not strictly abortion, is legal and in compliance with current abortion legislation in concept. However, MFPR cannot be strictly compared to therapeutic abortion. MFPR is an invasion into the uterus which places the remaining fetus(es) in some danger. Thus, an 'innocent third party' (in ethical terms) is involved and the question of this party's rights, if any, must be addressed. This returns us to the question of fetal status.

Argument can be made that MFPR is aimed at the ultimate benefit and protection of the other fetus(es) and that this justifies any risk. Yet, if some human status is granted to the fetus (and, through the mother's intention to carry the remaining fetus(es) to term, this may be tacitly granted to some degree), one must realize that the remaining fetus is in no position to consent to this risk. Parental proxy consent is deemed sufficient in the case of invasive fetal therapy, but this involves a fetus with some illness who requires a needed treatment. Is this same proxy consent sufficient for the 'bystander' fetus in a multifetal pregnancy who is not ill and who requires no treatment? The answer depends on one's assessment of the risk to this fetus involved in continuation of the original as opposed to the reduced pregnancy. It also rests on the questions of whether the bystander fetus has any rights worthy of consideration.

Realization that the fetuses who will die as a result of MFPR are in many cases totally normal makes the choice of this procedure all the more difficult and necessitates careful consideration of the options before proceeding. Even if one is morally convinced that the fetus is not human at this point, it cannot be denied that many parents consider the entire pregnancy very 'wanted' and therefore might perceive each fetus differently from parents who desire singleton termination because of an undesired pregnancy. The couple may well be convinced that they must proceed with the reduction nonetheless, but will probably have emotional reservations. The decision-making process will be an even greater stress on those whose background or tradition disallows abortion yet who feel that they must act for the good of their present and future family. For these reasons ongoing and follow-up counselling is advisable for all patients for whom MFPR is a possibility.

Although MFPR does offer an important, though imperfect[20], solution to increased maternal and fetal risk in multifetal gestations, its use must be accompanied by careful reflection. MFPR must be viewed as an invasion into a pregnancy which might (depending on the number involved) have a chance of proceeding to term with successful outcome. Viewed as an action to reduce risk and potentially save lives, the proportionate good of MFPR can outweigh the possible harm (loss of the entire pregnancy) which, in recent experience, is often small[19].

Prenatal care in the continuing pregnancy

Whether the mother decides to continue her multifetal pregnancy or elects reduction, she will require specialized care. Data provided elsewhere in this volume demonstrate that maternal and fetal morbidity and mortality are significantly increased in multifetal pregnancies. This prospect can be diminished only by experienced and aggressive antenatal care in a setting which facilitates prompt diagnosis and treatment of complications.

Once the mother is placed in contact with a source of appropriate obstetric care, she must be thoroughly informed of the plan for management of her pregnancy. One cannot assume that she will know what lies ahead, even if she is multiparous or is herself a health professional. The physician and any other caregiver has a duty to inform the mother of what can be expected in future months. The father, or other support person, should be closely involved in strategic planning from the beginning, so that the plan will be clear to all concerned.

Prenatal screening

A vital issue which must be addressed shortly after existence of a multifetal pregnancy is established is prenatal diagnosis. Current standards of care for singleton, and in some cases twin, pregnancy require that a mother be offered certain tests designed to detect physical and/or genetic abnormalities early in pregnancy, so that treatment options or the possibility of termination can be presented if deemed applicable. However, the very nature of a multifetal pregnancy implies that the impact of positive tests will be different. This must be understood from the outset, and a test must not be performed as a matter of routine without reflection on the implication of the various possible results for the pregnancy in question.

One of the screening tests routinely offered at 16–18 weeks' gestation is measurement of maternal serum alpha-fetoprotein (MSAFP). This assay, performed on a sample of maternal blood, was primarily designed to detect possible neural tube defects, but has been found useful in pinpointing other anomalies and defining certain high-risk situations, including genetic anomalies[28–30]. Whereas reliable standards have been worked out for MSAFP values in singleton and twin pregnancies, no reliable standards have yet been proposed for triplet or higher-order gestations. Because of this, automatic MSAFP screening of mothers with higher-order gestations can yield confusing and disturbing information, which cannot be reliably interpreted. This serves to increase parental and physician anxiety without yielding any benefit for the pregnancy. The ethical requirements of MSAFP screening for singletons and twins have been addressed[21], but their application to higher multiples is unclear. Furthermore, the intervention designed to give confirmatory data in patients with elevated or low MSAFP values (especially amniocentesis) might place a higher-order pregnancy at greater risk[29]. Thus, the mother and caregiver might be faced with the dilemma of ignoring the test results as uninterpretable and living with some anxiety or of undergoing invasive diagnostic testing and risking loss of the pregnancy. This dilemma can be avoided by honest, clear discussion of the limitations of MSAFP testing in multifetal gestations.

The patient who has conceived a multifetal pregnancy at what is considered an advanced maternal age, determined by risk for genetic anomalies, presents another difficult situation. Mothers of singletons who will be aged 35 or greater at the birth of their child are usually offered some procedure designed to determine fetal karyotype from cells retrieved from the amniotic fluid (amniocentesis) or the trophoblast (chorionic villus sampling [CVS]). CVS can be performed in the first trimester while amniocentesis is usually offered in the early second trimester. Although reports describe both procedures being successfully performed on higher-order multifetal gestations[31], these situations involve some element of increased risk to the pregnancy[32] (see Chapter 22). Alternatives should be carefully laid out, including clear data on risks of chromosomal anomalies at various maternal ages. Decisions can then be made weighing the risk of having an abnormal fetus(es) vs. the risk of loss from invasive diagnostic procedures. Respect for the mother's autonomous choice requires a clear presentation on the part of the physician, including his or her estimation of the advisability of the procedure. Similar principles apply when the indication for testing is prior pregnancy loss or history of children affected by genetic disease.

Selective termination for medical indication

Should a fetal anomaly be detected in one of the fetuses of a multifetal gestation, the mother is presented with another serious dilemma. The exact nature of the anomaly and the likely prognosis must be determined. Then, depending on the gestational age at which the problem is discovered, a plan for management must be formulated. If the anomaly affecting both fetuses, is lethal, or even moderately debilitating, some patients will elect termination. Whereas abortion of an affected fetus can be performed with little risk in a singleton pregnancy, this obviously is not the case in a multifetal gestation. Clearly, the existence of another fetus or fetuses who may be normal and healthy must be considered before a rational decision can be reached. Is the anomaly likely to affect the other fetus adversely? Should one terminate the entire pregnancy and sacrifice a healthy fetus? Should the pregnancy be continued in the knowledge that the result will be an abnormal infant?

The ethical arguments concerning selective termination of an affected fetus in a multifetal gestation are similar to these described for MFPR above. Some will hold that the greatest good lies in avoidance of the birth of the diseased or anomalous infant even at some risk to the healthy sibling(s). Others will cite the absolute right of every individual to a chance at present and future life without external threat. A position combining these elements appears most useful. The right of the fetus to uninterrupted development (if this is held to exist) should be considered as virtually absolute and should be over-ridden only after careful consideration with a view to a proportionately greater good. This approach gives proper respect to whatever 'humanness' one attributes to the developing fetus, yet takes into account the very real necessities facing parents and caregivers in these situations.

A different dilemma is posed by the discovery of a condition in one fetus which may require immediate treatment (or delivery) at a time when prematurity would seriously threaten the life of the other fetus(es). This dilemma is painful for physicians as well as parents. The parents must choose whether to deliver the pregnancy and subject a normal infant(s) to possible death or impairment or to continue the pregnancy and potentially sacrifice the fetus(es) in need of care. In this case there is no *a priori* correct choice. Consideration must be given to all pertinent facts as an honest prognosis is developed. Parental decisions must then be supported and encouraged with an appreciation of the pain and difficulty involved. The physician must provide guidance through explanation of the options and presentation of realistic recommendations based on his or her assessment of the situation. Mere reporting of the facts followed by subsequent physician 'withdrawal' in order to let the parents decide only serves to promote isolation and place a heavy burden entirely on the parents' shoulders. While patient autonomy is to be respected, it is part of the physician's professional responsibility to express recommendations or at least opinions as part of the counselling process. The physician stands as an expert consulted because of experience and skill. Beneficence requires that this experience be employed to ease the burden of patients in situations such as this.

Final considerations

The material presented in this chapter by no means exhausts the area of ethics as applied to multifetal gestations. As in all areas of human endeavor, we must deal with dynamic situations presenting new challenges. It is hoped that those aspects considered here might serve as a beginning of discussion. Each reader will approach problems from a different background and with different presuppositions. Whatever the perspective, it is vital that care of multifetal pregnancies be constantly re-examined in the light of the basic obligations of medicine to care for and respect human beings. It is often difficult to express this in a practical sense, but the ideal must be sought.

Physicians and society are challenged to provide excellent support for multifetal pregnancies, and at the heart of this excellence lies genuine human care. This is medicine at its best.

References

1. Dyck, A.J. (1977). *On Human Care: An Introduction to Ethics.* (Nashville: Abingdon)
2. Frankena, W.K. (1973). *Ethics.* (Englewood Cliffs: Prentice-Hall)
3. Beauchamp, T.L. and Childress, J.F. (1989). *Principles of Biomedical Ethics.* (New York: Oxford University Press)
4. McCormick, R.A. (1973). *Ambiguity in Moral Choice.* (Milwaukee: Marguette University)
5. Engelhardt, T.H. (1986). *Foundations of Bioethics.* (New York: Oxford University Press)
6. Medical Research International, Society for Assisted Reproductive Technology, and The American Fertility Society. (1989). *In vitro* fertilization–embryo transfer (IVF-ET) in the United States: 1989, results from the IVF-ET registry. *Fertil. Steril.*, **55**, 14
7. Rein, M.S., Barbieri, R.L. and Greene, M.F. (1990). The causes of high-order multiple gestation. *Int. J. Fertil.*, **35**, 154
8. Schenker, J.G., Yarkoni, S. and Granat, M. (1981). Multiple pregnancies following induction of ovulation. *Fertil. Steril.*, **35**, 105
9. Keith, L.G., Ameli, S. and Keith, D.M. (1988). The Northwestern University triplet study I: overview of the international literature. *Acta Genet. Med. Gemellol.*, **37**, 55
10. Poplawski, N. and Gillet, G. (1991). Ethics and embryos. *J. Med. Ethics.*, **17**, 62
11. Gallagher, M.W. and Johnson, T.R.B. (1991). Methods of risk reduction in the delivery of

twins. In Teoh, E.S. (ed.) *Proceedings of 13th World Congress of Gynaecology and Obstetrics, FIGO,* Singapore, September, Vol. 5, *Pregnancy Termination and Labour,* pp. 139–46. (Carnforth, UK: Parthenon Publishing)

12. Evans, M.I., Fletcher, J.C., Zador, I.E. *et al.* (1988). Selective first trimester termination in octuplet and quadruplet pregnancies: clinical and ethical issues. *Obstet. Gynecol.,* **71**, 289

13. Newman, R.B., Hamer, C. and Miller, M.C. (1989). Outpatient triplet management: a contemporary view. *Am. J. Obstet. Gynecol.,* **161**, 547

14. Gonen, R., Heyman, E., Asztalos, E.V. *et al.* (1990). The outcome of triplet, quadruplet, and quintuplet pregnancies managed in a perinatal unit: obstetric, neonatal and follow-up data. *Am. J. Obstet. Gynecol.,* **162**, 454

15. Berkowitz, R.L., Lynch, L., Chitkara, U. *et al.* (1988). Selective reduction of multifetal pregnancies in the first trimester. *N. Engl. J. Med.,* **318**, 1043

16. Lynch, L., Berkowitz, R.L., Chitkara, U. *et al.* (1990). First-trimester transabdominal multifetal pregnancy reductions: a report of 85 cases. *Obstet. Gynecol.,* **75**, 735

17. Tabsh, K.M. (1990). Transabdominal multifetal pregnancy reduction: report of 40 cases. *Obstet. Gynecol.,* **75**, 739

18. Berkowitz, R.L. and Lynch, L. (1990). Selective reduction: an unfortunate misnomer. *Obstet. Gynecol.,* **75**, 873

19. Dumez, Y., Evans, M.I., Wapner, R.J. *et al.* (1991). Efficacy of multifetal pregnancy reduction (MFPR): collaborative experience of the world's largest centers. Abstract presented at *Eleventh Annual Meeting, Society of Perinatal Obstetricians,* January, San Francisco

20. Committee on Ethics, American College of Obstetricians and Gynecologists. (1991). *Multifetal Pregnancy Reduction and Selective Fetal Termination.* ACOG Committee Opinion # 94, April

21. Evans, M.I., Fletcher, J.C., Dixler, A.O. *et al.* (1989). *Fetal Diagnosis and Therapy: Science, Ethics, and the Law.* (Philadelphia: Lippincott)

22. McCullough, L.B. and Chervenak, F.A. (1994). *Ethics in Obstetrics and Gynecology.* (New York: Oxford University Press)

23. Grobstein, C. (1988). *Science and the Unborn: Choosing Human Futures.* (New York: Basic Books)

24. Harrison, M.R., Golbus, M.S. and Filly, R.A. (1990). *The Unborn Patient: Prenatal Diagnosis and Treatment,* 2nd edn. (Philadelphia: Saunders)

25. Chervenak, F.A. and McCullough, L.B. (1992). Ethical issues in perinatology. In Reece, E.A., Hobbins, J.C., Mahoney, M.J. *et al.* (eds.) *Medicine of the Fetus and Mother,* pp. 1308–16. (Philadelphia: Lippincott)

26. Roe vs Wade. 410 U.S. 113, 1973

27. Overall, C. (1990). *Selective Termination of Pregnancy and Women's Reproductive Autonomy.* Hastings Center Report, May/June, pp. 6–11

28. Thomas, R.L. and Blakemore, K.J. (1990). Evaluation of elevations in maternal serum alpha-fetoprotein: a review. *Obstet. Gynecol. Surv.,* **45**, 269

29. American College of Obstetricians and Gynecologists. (1991). *Alpha-fetoprotein.* ACOG Technical Bulletin # 154, April

30. Milunsky, A. (1992). Maternal serum screening for neural tube and other defects. In Milunsky, A. (ed.) *Genetic Disorders and the Fetus: Diagnosis, Prevention and Treatment,* 3rd edn., pp. 502–63. (Baltimore: The Johns Hopkins University Press)

31. King, C.R., Cox, G. and Arthur, T. (1990). Successful chorionic villus sampling of a triplet gestation: a case report. *J. Reprod. Med.,* **35**, 441

32. Pijpers, J., Jahoda, M.G., Vosters, R.P. *et al.* (1988). Genetic amniocentesis in twin pregnancies. *Br. J. Obstet. Gynaecol.,* **95**, 323

National Organization of Mothers of Twins Clubs, Inc.*

M.M. Eicker

Introduction

Since its inception in 1960, the National Organization of Mothers of Twins, Inc. (NOMOTC) has been a grassroots volunteer organization composed of caring and dedicated mothers of multiple birth children. At its heart are the thousands of local club members who meet monthly in each others' homes or community centers. Local club services include speakers, workshops, libraries of twin-related materials, resales of clothing and infant equipment, philanthropic endeavors on behalf of individuals or community organizations, and social activities geared to members and their families. The National Organization draws from this vast pool of members the volunteers who staff its Education, Membership and Research Departments each year. Working from their homes, largely through the mail, the National Committee workers perform a myriad of duties which have, over the years, broadened the support capabilities of local Mothers of Twins Clubs. As the number of multiple birth parents in this country increases, so does the potential of this organization.

The National Organization of Mothers of Twins Clubs, Inc. is a network of approximately 470 local Twins Clubs throughout the United States. Together, these organizations represent 19 000 families of multiples. (Editor: The total number of families of multiples in the United States is unknown.) NOMOTC is a strong advocate for proper attention to the educational and medical needs of multiples and their families. The primary purposes of this voluntary organization are education and research. NOMOTC cooperates with qualified researchers, conducts inter-organizational research, and serves as a clearinghouse of educational information.

The National Organization maintains a Multiple Birth Data Base, an information registry of multiple births across the United States. Data are available to qualified researchers upon request to the Executive Office.

The individual Twins Club functions as a vital source of support for the expectant mother and her family. Increasing numbers of new members join a Mothers of Twins Club (MOTC) during the third trimester of their pregnancy. Local MOTC services run the gamut from providing first-hand information from another mother of twins to providing meals, household help, or babysitting service for older siblings and carpools for trips to the physician's office.

The primary source of communication with new or expectant parents of multiples is through *Your Twins & You*, a NOMOTC informational publication that provides tips for managing a multiple pregnancy as well as information for the postpartum period. The advice for expectant mothers places strong emphasis on the necessity of obtaining good obstetric care; it also helps parents plan for the first hectic weeks after the delivery of their babies. The brochure also includes basic information about multiple births and twin development, because it may be the first educational material parents receive. This publication is

*See Appendix for contact information

provided to physicians and hospitals by local Mothers of Twins Clubs or sent upon request to individuals looking for a support group.

Support services

Disabilities

During the past decade, the National Organization has increased its efforts on behalf of those families who experience medical problems as a result of a multiple pregnancy. About 6% of the respondents to a 1990 survey reported birth defects in one or more of their infants. These parents often face overwhelming challenges in meeting the physical and financial demands of raising disabled or seriously ill children. Local clubs generally strive to provide as much emotional support as possible, drawing upon the experience of members in similar situations. The NOMOTC also has a Pen Pal Program, which provides support for mothers who have a child/children with similar illnesses or disabilities. This program is of special benefit for parents residing in remote areas. The National Organization's Support Service Program maintains comprehensive listings of referral agencies, cope centers, research studies and the like, to help individuals upon request.

Bereavement

Because parents of twins and higher-order multiples face the death of a child more often than do parents of singletons, NOMOTC has recently completed and distributed to its members a fact sheet entitled: *When A Twin Dies*. The National Organization also has a Bereavement Support Referral Program. A Bereavement Brochure and specialized information is sent directly to the bereaved parents who have experienced the loss of a multiple-birth child/ children.

Coping

Regardless of the type of information needed, many parents turn to Mothers of Twins Clubs for educational materials that deal with the care and rearing of their children. NOMOTC, through its Education Department, provides a series of aids designed to help new mothers cope with various facets of infant and early childhood care. *Your Twins & You*, previously mentioned, includes a series of Helpful Hints that are printed separately in French and Spanish. These materials cover topics including new mothers of multiples, feeding multiples, breast feeding/bottle feeding multiples, and selecting a twin/triplet stroller. A feeding schedule especially designed for infant twins is available from the Executive Office. An Annotated Bibliography covers twin care booklets, non-fiction books, poetry, books for children, audiovisual aids, club management and miscellaneous topics. Periodically updated copies are distributed to member clubs to aid in making purchases for their local club libraries.

The National Organization publishes a quarterly newspaper, *MOTC's Notebook*, which is distributed to each of its members across the country. In its theme-oriented issues, this 24-page publication offers national members a wide variety of twin-related articles that are educational as well as inspirational in nature. Regularly appearing columns provide readers with age-appropriate information for raising multiples as well as current research reports, book reviews and items of club concern.

Education

In the fall of 1991, NOMOTC published *Placement of Multiple Birth Children In School: A Guide For Educators*. Findings in this booklet were based on a two-part survey of 62 questions distributed through NOMOTC's members to educators in school districts throughout the United States. Information about educators' experiences and opinions relating to the education of school-age multiples were compiled from 1423 completed surveys. This publication provides educators with a thorough discussion of the issues of separating multiples in school classrooms and provides tips for the teachers of twins. A thorough review of twin-related research and literature is included, along with a bibliography of additional reading material related to this subject. Distribution to local school districts is handled through the National Organization's member clubs.

NOMOTC's Medical Survey, an interorganizational research study, was sent to all member clubs in 1990 to ascertain if the needs of mothers of multiples were being adequately met by the medical community. Over 2400 responses were received.

Using the information gained in this study, NOMOTC published the booklet *Managing Multiple Birth Families (Prenatal-Postpartum): A Guide for Health Care Providers*. This resource provides gynecologists, obstetricians, neonatal specialists, pediatricians and other health-care providers with information specific to the multiple birth experience. It includes comments from survey respondents with specific advice for improving care during and immediately following a multiple pregnancy. This educational aid is available to health-care providers through their local Mothers of Twins Club or upon direct order from the Executive Office.

In the summer of 1995, NOMOTC will have available a video dealing with multiple pregnancy through the first 6 months after delivery. This video will discuss prenatal care, complications and risk of prematurity, labor and delivery, preparations for coming home from the hospital and infant development during the first 6 months of life. Inquiries about the video may be directed to the Executive Office.

Research

Despite the fact that the education of its members and the general public has been a goal of the National Organization since its inception, this has not been its only focus. An ongoing commitment to twin-related research has served to increase the NOMOTC members' knowledge and awareness of issues affecting their children. At the same time, these efforts have expanded the body of medical and scientific knowledge in countless areas. Since NOMOTC was founded, it has worked with professional research workers on a variety of medical, psychological and informational projects. The NOMOTC Data Base provides qualified researchers with access to candidates for specialized studies. Members are encouraged to participate with approved investigators by responding to their requests which are published in the Research Request Column of *MOTC's Notebook*.

The National Organization's Research Department conducts several inter-organizational research projects each year. Past surveys have included such diverse topics as 'Fertility Drug Study' (1986), 'Handedness in Multiples' (1987), 'Similar Responses in Twins' (1989–90) and 'Effects of Multiples on the Family Unit and Marriage' (1990). Inter-organizational studies generally attempt to meet perceived needs of the membership. For example, current on-going studies deal with adoptive parents of multiples and an employment survey of mothers of twins. Five research committee members are responsible for developing and writing NOMOTC's surveys, which are distributed to members in two national mailings. The research tabulator and research interpreter prepare completed survey results for publication in *MOTC's Notebook* and as special mailings for each local club's research file. The Research Librarian maintains a current file of articles and research studies which provide answers to the inquiries she receives from members and other interested parties throughout the year.

International contacts

In order to provide members with the broadest base of current knowledge and research, NOMOTC's International Liaison maintains contact with multiple birth organizations in other countries. An exchange of newsletters provides insight into varied approaches to the parenting of multiples and creates a larger sense of support among mothers who share common interests and concerns. As a collective member of the International Society for Twin Studies, NOMOTC submits its Annual Research Department Summary and a detailed NOMOTC Report for the ISTS Congress.

As NOMOTC's membership has grown over the past 32 years, so have its resources. Today, the National Organization maintains an up-to-date, well-equipped Executive Office in Albuquerque, New Mexico. Staffed by the Organization's Executive Secretary, the office serves as a central clearinghouse for processing official mail, referrals, research, membership, publicity and educational information. Each day the office personnel field inquiries from prospective parents of multiples, media and potential researchers. Referrals of new or prospective members are routinely sent to local Mothers of Twins Clubs. Information is available to assist individuals who are interested in starting a club in an area where none presently exists.

Keeping abreast of the current trends in society is an important part of NOMOTC's agenda. Parents of multiples reflect the same changes in American culture that are in evidence in the general population. The increased use of fertility drugs, the use of *in vitro* fertilization techniques, the prevalence of working mothers and the presence of an economic recession, to cite only a few examples, are topics which should be explored if Mothers of Twins Clubs are to remain viable support systems for parents of multiples. In recent years, NOMOTC has expanded its services to meet the needs of a growing number of single parents within its ranks. Recent National Conventions have featured workshops specifically geared to the needs of its single members. *MOTC's Notebook* contains a column which discusses individual and child-rearing concerns of one-parent families, and local clubs have been provided with a tips sheet that will enable them to be more supportive of single-parent members.

Present activities – future plans

In future decades, NOMOTC will continue to address the concerns which technology and societal change impose upon its members. Parents of twins and higher-order multiples are well aware of the need for improved health care for expectant mothers and at-risk infants. Medical costs and insurance coverage for families of multiple birth children have become increasingly serious problems as the use of fertility drugs and *in vitro* procedures produce higher multiple pregnancy rates. Selective reduction and ethical considerations involving the treatment of severely premature infants will affect our membership profoundly. A growing population of multiple-birth children will cause the medical and educational communities to examine policies and procedures that affect the lives and well-being of these individuals and their families.

NOMOTC will continue its commitment to each parent of multiples in this country who needs information and support during the child-rearing years. That commitment will be best met when the professional medical community becomes fully aware of the support available for parents with multiple pregnancies. Obstetricians, hospital maternity departments and pediatricians, in particular, should be aware of the information and services that can benefit their patients and enhance their own efforts on behalf of maternal and infant well-being. To achieve this goal, NOMOTC educational materials should become an integral part of prenatal instruction and postpartum counselling. Working hand in hand, medical professionals and The National Organization of Mothers of Twins Clubs, Inc. will have an 'extra edge' in promoting an improved standard of health for mothers and infants in the years to come.

Parenting twins: a pediatrician's point of view

E.M. Bryan

Introduction

Although many animal and bird species normally exhibit nurturing behavior to several babies at the same time, it is not normal for a human being to instantly bond with and fall in love with two people at the same time. Yet, this is what a mother and father are asked to do with infant twins. Many parents are disappointed to find how difficult this proves to be, and it is not uncommon for them to find one baby more attractive or more lovable than the other. Sometimes this is just a temporary and superficial attraction. Other times it is not, and neglect of one twin is not unheard of. If babies are of different sizes or if one is sick and the other well, differential bonding may take place and this difference may have long-lasting consequences. Moreover, considerable difficulty may arise if the babies have very different personalities. If one baby is a contented, placid infant who feeds well, enjoys being cuddled and does not cry when left on its own, it is not unreasonable that the mother will find this infant more attractive than its co-twin who is always crying, and who, when offered a feed, fights and resists, but when put down again, continues to cry. Inevitably, the crying infant will require much more time from the mother and she may well resent this when she could be much more happily caring for the other baby. It is important that parents should be aware that this phenomenon is not uncommon and generally works itself out, especially when the roles reverse and the difficult infant becomes a particularly bright and attractive child.

Feeding

Mothers inevitably give thought to how best they will feed their babies, as this activity takes up a great deal of time during the first 6 months. Each couple must decide which is the most appropriate method, either breast or bottle. Not only is it possible to breast feed twins, but this experience can be very rewarding for all concerned. The advantages of bottle feeding are, of course, that someone else can help. The advantages of breast feeding are the same as for singleton babies. Furthermore, the family not only will save more money by breast feeding but, more importantly, it is the only way that both babies can be practically nursed and fed at the same time (see Chapter 41). In view of the fact that most mothers of twins complain that there is not enough time for cuddling, simultaneous breast feeding can be a considerable advantage.

Transport

The problem of transport must be solved, or the mother will become isolated at home. Many types of baby carriages and push-chairs are available, and it is wise to take advice from other mothers of twins before spending a lot of money. Local Twins Clubs often have good quality secondhand carriages for sale as well as other equipment and clothes.

Development

In most respects, twins do as well as singletons (see Chapter 46). The one area in which they tend to fall behind is language. There are several reasons for this developmental delay. First, the mother often has to talk in a threesome and therefore has less one-to-one communication with each child. Second, she is busier than she would otherwise be and therefore may tend to leave the children talking to each other instead of talking to them herself. Third, the primary model for a twin's speech (unlike a single baby who has his mother) is the other twin, that is, someone who talks in the same manner. When one child speaks a word incorrectly, the other often copies it and, furthermore, also reinforces the mistake of the first twin. Not uncommonly, the so-called 'secret language' of twins develops (idioglossia, otherwise known as cryptophasia). Fortunately, this often only represents a 'phase' in the developmental process. In extreme instances, however, this 'secret language' persists. As a general point of caution, however, it is essential that each twin should be spoken to individually as much as possible during the time that they are learning to speak. Clearly, this is a moment for the father and other care givers to help the mother.

Identity and individuality

Parents always plan to treat their children as individuals and to think of them as such. Unfortunately, they forget that other people will hardly be able to do the same if they are unable to tell the children apart. Once children get used to being dressed alike, it may be hard to break the pattern. It may be best to dress twins differently, if only sometimes, right from the start. Dressing in the same style but in different colors is an excellent compromise. This can be started in the maternity unit with different colored hats, mitts or toys, so that each baby can be clearly identified from a distance and called by its name.

Naming

Some parents are tempted to call their children by twin names (e.g. June and Jane or Regina and Reginald). Children have a hard enough time establishing their own individuality and identifying their own desires and needs. They do not always like to be thought of as twins, and often come to resent twin labels, especially as they grow older. Even the same initial can be tiresome at school, let alone for a teenager who is receiving confidential letters.

Opportunity

It is vital that each child be allowed his or her own individual hobbies, excursions and experiences. Whereas it is truly an energetic mother of twins who can manage two separate birthday parties, at least each child should have his own birthday cake and card. From an early age the children should spend time apart. Grandparents and friends often prefer to have one baby or child at a time, and a mother will enjoy having a special time alone with the other child.

To some degree, it is difficult to give twins the same opportunities that single children get quite easily. For example, pastry-making with one child may be a happy experience, but with two it may be chaos. Even so, twins must not be deprived of opportunities essential to their stimulation and development. Like single children, they must learn to feed themselves and to dress themselves, even if this takes more time and causes more mess.

Brothers and sisters

The elder brother or sister of twins may find their arrival especially difficult. Inevitably, the mother will be exceptionally busy, but a more serious issue is the disproportionate amount of attention bestowed on the twins by other people. As a result, the older child may easily feel rejected, isolated and resentful. Such resentments may last a lifetime, especially if one or both twins are sick and require special care. It is not uncommon that an older sibling views the parents as one pair and the twins as another pair and him/herself as being alone. In such a case, it is helpful to find someone like a godparent or a reliable teenager who will give extra, compensating, attention to the older child.

Household help

All families with twins or more deserve special help during the early months, and, for triplets, the early years. The father should be encouraged to play a full part from the start. If there is no grandparent or other relation or friend available on a regular basis, then other sources of help should be explored even before delivery. Church or community organizations of senior citizens are often only too willing to be of assistance, but must be asked in advance as a matter of courtesy. When properly contacted, they may provide invaluable assistance, especially in the case of higher order multiples. It is always better to plan to have help and cancel it if it is not needed, than to have to search it out in an emergency.

Recommendations

Few parents expecting multiples will have any knowledge of what is entailed in the care and upbringing of twin children. It is essential that they should be provided with the necessary information, not least by introducing them to other families with twins.

Special preparation classes run by professionals with experience with multiple births can be helpful to expectant parents and also to others likely to be involved in the care of the children (see Chapters 50 and 52).

Prenatal testing for fetal anomaly in a multiple pregnancy poses special practical and ethical problems. Parents will need informed and sensitive counselling before deciding whether to proceed with the tests (see Chapter 47).

Parents of multiples clubs and clinics: the United Kingdom experience

E.M. Bryan

Introduction

Because society loves twins it tends to assume that parents of twins are privileged and that the care of twins merely involves two of everything. Few outsiders truly appreciate the special and enormous emotional as well as physical stresses that accompany looking after two babies at the same time. Parents need practical tips on how to carry, feed and wash two babies. They also require reassurance that they themselves can survive, regardless of how exhausting the task may seem in the early months.

Twins and Multiple Births Association

Most of the parents of Twins Clubs in the UK belong to the umbrella organization, the Twins and Multiple Births Association (TAMBA). (Editor: Umbrella organizations such as TAMBA exist in many countries, including USA, Canada, Australia, Japan, Germany, Belgium, etc. The reader is referred to the Appendix for a full listing. To our knowledge, none has the advantage of the contained geography of the United Kingdom. The TAMBA model, although appearing unique, could possibly be replicated in other localities.) This national organization was established in 1978 (initially as the Twins Clubs Association), and is now a registered charity. The number of clubs grew from 12 in 1978 to 100 within 2 years. Currently (1994) the total is over 200, with well over 2000 individual members.

In addition to offering support to existing clubs and encouraging and advising on the establishment of new ones, TAMBA publishes leaflets covering a large range of subjects. Among the most popular titles are *Preparing for Twins*, *Language Development in Twins* and *Twins at School*. Leaflets or booklets for particular situations such as bereavement, disability and the parenting of triplets are also available. A number of TAMBA members have written books for parents and for professionals (see list of publications in the Appendix). TAMBA also has a number of advisers from the caring professions who provide an honorary consultancy service and reply to parents' queries.

One of TAMBA's main tasks is to create greater awareness of the special needs of families with multiples among professionals and the general public via the media and through Study Days on all aspects of multiple births. A magazine, *Twins, Triplets and More*, is produced three times a year. This publication is available to press and public as well as TAMBA members. The Supertwins Group, Special Needs Group and Bereavement Support Group produce special newsletters, and one is planned for the Single Parents Group as well.

An annual national conference that is held over a weekend and in different parts of the country allows members to meet each other. It also provides a forum for parents to hear the latest ideas and research from experts in the field of multiple births.

TAMBA is a self-help organization. It is largely self-financing and currently run mostly by volunteers with only one paid member of staff. Many thousands of parents have been helped by TAMBA in material terms, such as being able to buy or exchange secondhand twin baby carriages and other equipment and clothing or being able to get practical advice from other parents of twins at no cost. For many parents, however, the benefits may be much more fundamental and long-lasting, because in such personal non-professional relationships, the receiving and the giving of help frequently enhances personal growth. Advice from professionals on the rearing of twins can be invaluable, but may have the side effect of weakening parents' self-confidence. That other parents have coped with similar problems reassures new parents that they also can cope.

The Twins Clinics

The first 'Twins Clinic' was established by the Multiple Births Foundation in London in 1987; since then, similar clinics have been started in three other centers in the United Kingdom (Birmingham, York and Middlesborough). Most families refer themselves to the clinics. Others are referred by family doctors, pediatricians and health visitors. The clinics are not intended to deal with pediatric illnesses or disabilities *per se*, for which the normal community and hospital services are available; rather, they address family concerns related to the fact that the children are twins. Of the first 137 families referred to the clinic, 38 brought their children for a routine check, 25 for behavioral problems, 21 for sleep problems, 17 because of growth problems, 11 for an opinion on zygosity, and 12 for problems related to speech. The remaining 13 came for reasons such as schooling, nursery placement, financial problems and sources of help[1].

Special Clinics

Special Clinics have been established to facilitate families sharing their particular experiences and problems. Each of the clinics works closely with the respective special TAMBA group, and each is staffed with volunteers whose experiences are similar to those of the clinic's clientele. For example, one mother, herself a pediatrician, with an 18-year-old twin with cerebral palsy, is a great support at the Special Needs Clinic; two mothers of 20-year-old triplets and another with 10-year-old quads help regularly at the Supertwins Clinic. At the Bereavement Clinic, representatives are present from the three TAMBA bereavement support groups (loss of one newborn twin, loss of both twins including miscarriage, loss by sudden infant death). Although all Special Clinics are set up so the families can have an individual appointment with the pediatrician, their particular value is the informal lunchtime meeting where they meet each other.

The Special Needs Clinic

Families with a disabled twin face special problems. The individual needs of the disabled child are usually well met by the programs administered by Health and Social Services, but the healthy twin often suffers unrecognized difficulties. Not only is guilt often present that he/she should have been spared the co-twin's affliction, but jealousy over the considerable extra attention given to the disabled twin often is an additional problem that needs discussion. Severe behavioral disturbances, for which the child and his/her whole family may need help, are not uncommon.

Parents may need help in relinquishing the image of their children as twins when one of them does not share the mental age or the physical attributes of the other. Accepting this circumstance can be extremely painful, but delay of this acceptance can create an added burden for the healthy child as well as the parents.

The Supertwins Clinic

This clinic provides a rare opportunity for families with triplets and higher-order multiples to discuss their problems with other 'supertwin' parents. All concerned enjoy meeting other parents who have shared similar experiences. Some parents also welcome routine developmental checks of their children with the relative luxury of each child being seen individually, and most often with only one child in the room at a time. Other families come with specific problems, such as isolation of one of the triplets, language delay or behavior difficulties in an elder sibling. Occasionally, couples come to this clinic without their children, notably expectant parents who want to meet triplet families, often for the first time. Others cannot manage the journey with all their children, so just bring one or two.

The Supertwins Clinic also provides a supportive setting for the discussion of tensions arising within marriages or other relationships, not least because everyone present understands. Even the most stable of marriages is put under strain through wakeful nights, lack of privacy, and having no time or energy for much except domestic toil and child care. Some parents who otherwise rarely leave the house make heroic efforts to come to this clinic and often gain a new perspective – or at least a reduction of guilt – through spending several hours in the support room with other parents and the volunteers.

The Bereavement Clinic

This clinic is for families who have lost one, both or all members of a multiple pregnancy. When this happens, especially during the perinatal period, unusual problems surface[2]. Not only is their loss underestimated by society in general, but the surviving sibling(s) is (are) a constant reminder of the dead child(ren). All too often, unfortunately, professionals and friends tend to concentrate on the surviving child and encourage the parents to do the same. The exclusion of the memory of the child(ren) that died makes it more difficult for the parents fully to experience and work through their bereavement. Moreover, the focus on the surviving child may make the parents idealize the dead baby to the detriment of the survivor. Parents of newborn multiples also must often experience the extraordinary strain of grieving the death of one (or two) babies as they anxiously watch over their other baby(ies) in intensive care. Other parents have to face the loss of all babies after many long and stressful years of attempting to establish a successful pregnancy.

The loss of the 'twinship' as such can be more painful than most people realize. The pride of parenting twins or more can be enormous, and I have known parents to angrily protest that their 'twins' were really triplets (of whom one had died) and should therefore never be called twins. Bereaved multiples may themselves suffer seriously from the loss of their twin at whatever stage in life. It is not known how much this sense of desolation is due to the effect on a child of grieving parents or to the loss of a close relationship which had developed during intrauterine life. It may well be a combination of both factors.

Apart from getting enormous mutual support from interacting with other parents in similar circumstances, some parents request individual appointments to discuss particular problems. Many seek clarification of the cause of death of their baby. Others need help in creating a memorial, such as an introduction to an artist who will paint a picture or to a clergyman who will conduct a memorial service, possibly some years after the death. Others want to find out the zygosity of their babies. Still others need help coping with their anger against the medical staff, sometimes perhaps justified, sometimes not, but very real in all cases. Help in expressing this anger, even by letter, can be therapeutic. Some parents are so distressed that they require counselling, and introductions to appropriate psychotherapists often are arranged.

References

1. Bendefy, I., Elliman, A.M., Prior, S. and Bryan, E.M. (1994). Is there a role for a Twins Clinic? An evaluation of parents' responses. *Acta Pediatr. Scand.*, **83**, 40–5

2. Lewis, E. and Bryan, E.M. (1988). Management of perinatal loss of a twin. *Br. Med. J.*, **297**, 1321

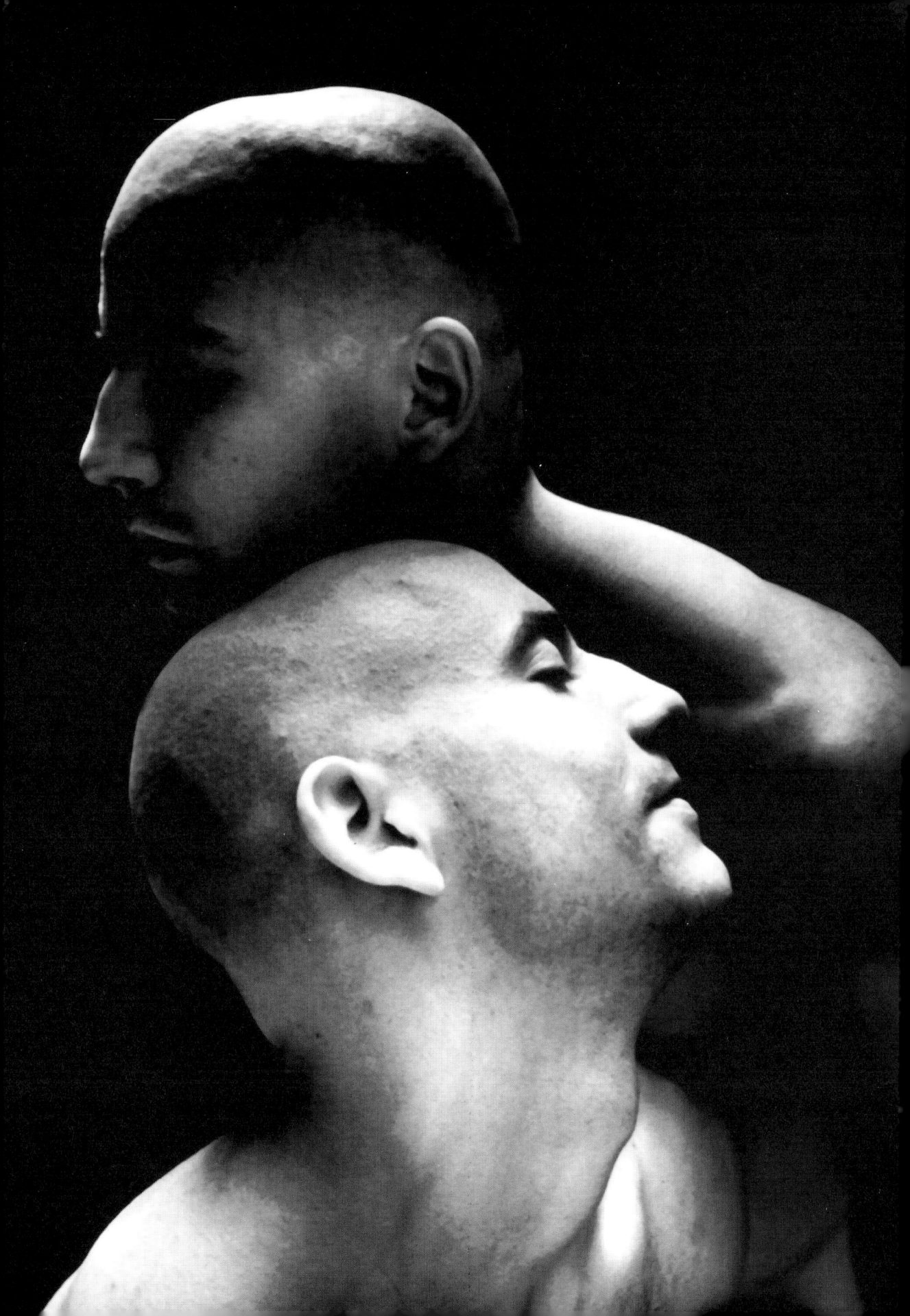

appendix
Resources

Repose

David Teplica, 1990,
The Center for Study of Multiple Birth, Chicago, Illinois

Appendix

Resources

CONTENTS

Associations/groups
- International
  - US-based — 670
  - Non-US-based — 670
- National — 673
- Loss/bereavement — 675
- Single parents — 676

Other resources
- Nutrition in pregnancy — 677
- Psychological counseling, telephone hypnosis — 677
- Vaginal birth after Cesarean — 677

Referrals — 677

Products — 677

Selected readings — 678
- Books
  - General — 678
  - Loss/bereavement — 678
- Booklets, brochures, catalogs, magazines, newsletters — 679

Videos, talk, workshop — 680

ASSOCIATIONS/GROUPS

INTERNATIONAL

US-based

Anchorage Parents of Twins and Multiples Club
PO Box 200-353
Anchorage
Alaska 99520

Combined Organization of Multiple Birth Organizations (COMBO)
c/o Patricia Malmstrom
PO Box 10066
Berkeley, CA 94709
USA
(510) 524-0863

International Society for Twin Studies (ISTS)
c/o Professor Adam P. Matheny, Jr.
Louisville Twin Study
Department of Pediatrics
School of Medicine
University of Louisville
Louisville, KY 40292
(502) 852-1090; FAX (502) 852-1094

International Twins Association, Inc. (ITA)
c/o Lynn Long and Lori Stewart
6898 Channel Road
Minneapolis, MN 55432
(612) 571-3022

The International Twins Foundation (ITF)
PO Box 6043
Providence, RI 02904
(401) 729-1000

La Lèche League International
c/o Lee Ann Deal, Executive Director
1400 N. Meacham
PO Box 4079
Schaumburg, IL 60168-4079
(708) 519-7730; FAX: (708) 519-0035
Hotline (breastfeeding questions)
1-800-LA LECHE

Twinless Twins Support Group, Int'l (see LOSS/BEREAVEMENT)

Twins and Multiple Births Association (TAMBA)
PO Box 30
Litton Sutton
South Wirral L66 1TH
England

Individual

Miss Helen Kirk
Supertwin Statistician
PO Box 254
Galveston, TX 77553-0254

Non-US-based

ABC Club (International organization for triplets and higher multiples and their families)
c/o Helga and Uta Gruetzner
Strohweg 55
D-6100 Darmstadt
Germany 6151
61 515 5430; FAX: 61 515 96388

Association de Soutien à la Recherche Scientifique au Profit des Naissances Multiples (TWINS)
c/o Dr Robert Derom
Kwadenplasstraat 12
B-9070 Destelbergen
Belgium
32 92283655; FAX: 32 92 382287

Association for Parents with Triplets and More
c/o Claudio Heusser
Dorfstr. 16
8175 Windlach
Switzerland
01 858 2655

Association Francophone d'Entraide Pour Naissances Multiples
c/o Madelaine Bouche
1320 Geval
Belgium
02 652 01 81

Association Nationale d'Entraide des Parents à Naissances Multiples (ANEPNM)
26 Boulevard Brune
75014 Paris
France
01 40 44 44 15

Appendix: Resources

Australian Multiple Birth Association, Inc. (AMBA)
   c/o Jenny Noon
   PO Box 105
   Coogee, New South Wales 2034
   Australia
   Phone/FAX: 61 2 665 1061

Australian NHMRC Twin Registry (ATR)
   c/o Dr John Hopper
   The University of Melbourne
   151 Barry Street, Melbourne
   Victoria 3053, Australia
   61 3 347 2983; FAX: 61 3 344 7014

Club for Families of Triplets and More (TRILOGI)
   c/o Irene G. Svela
   Bjaalandsgaten 1
   N-4010 Stavanger
   Norway
   04 582967

Disabled Multiples Parent Registry (see POMBA)

East Flanders Prospective Twin Survey (EFPTS)
   c/o Dr C. Derom
   Katholieke Universiteit Leuvan
   Centre for Human Genetics
   Herestraat 49, B-3000 Leuven
   Belgium
   32 16 345865; FAX: 32 16 345994

Ethiopian Gemini Trust
   c/o Dr Carmela Aabate
   PO Box 3547
   Addis Ababa
   Ethiopia
   151947; Telex: EAWTAA 21263

Gregor Mendel Institute of Medical Genetics and Twin Studies
   c/o Professor Luigi Gedda
   Piazza Galeno 5
   00161 Rome
   Italy
   855 4658; FAX: 855 5179

Japanese Association of Twin Mothers
   c/o Yukiko Aoyama
   5-5-20 Minami Aoyama
   Minatoku, Tokyo
   Japan
   03 400 0838

La Trobe Twin Study
   c/o Dr David Hay
   Department of Psychology
   La Trobe University
   Bundoora, Victoria
   Australia
   03 479 2259; FAX: 03 478 0603

Lone Twin Register (See Multiple Births Foundation)

Maudsley Hospital Psychiatric Twin Register
   c/o Alison Macdonald
   Institute of Psychiatry (Genetics Section)
   De Crespigny Park, Denmark Hill
   London SE5 8AF
   England
   171 703 5411 ext. 3416

Multiple Births Foundation
   c/o Dr Elizabeth Bryan
   Queen Charlotte's and Chelsea Hospital
   Goldhawk Road
   London W6 0XG
   England
   181 740 3519; FAX: 181 740 3041

Nederlands Vereniging Van/Tweeline
   2582 NV 'S-Gravenhage
   Johan V
   Oldernbarneveltlaan 56
   The Netherlands

Netherlands Tweelingen Register
   A.J.M. Jonker
   Vrija Universiteit de Boelelaan 1111
   1081 HV, Amsterdam
   The Netherlands
   020 5483863; FAX: 020 548 4443

New Zealand Multiple Birth Association (NZMBA)
   c/o Carla Wild
   PO Box 1258
   Wellington
   New Zealand
   WGTN 04 769281

Odion Eremionkhale (WIMBA)
   PO Box 8839 Shomolu
   Lagos
   Nigeria

Ottawa Twins' Parents Association
   c/o Lynda P. Haddon
   PO Box 5532, Station F
   Ottawa, Ontario K2C 0A0
   Canada

Parents of Multiple Birth Association of
   Canada (POMBA)
      4981 Highway, 7 East
      Unit 12A, Suite 161
      Markham, Ontario
      Canada L3R 1N1
      (905) 513-7506

South African Multiple Births Association
   (SAMBA)
      PO Box 2590
      Honeyden 2040
      Republic of South Africa

Svensska Tvillingklubben
   c/o L & A Ekelund
   Hennel insvagen 8
   S-433 70 Partille
   Sweden
   031 267083

Swedish Twin Registry
   c/o Dr Nancy Pedersen
   Department of Epidemiology
   Institute of Environmental Medicine
   The Karolinska Institute
   Box 60208
   S-10401 Stockhom
   Sweden

Trilling-foreningen
   c/o Johan Baeckstrom
   Fagelvagen 13
   181 40 Lidingo
   Sweden
   +46 8 723 91 00; FAX: 46 8 10 52 58

Twillingforelddreforeningen (TFF)
   c/o Ingun Ulven Lie
   Abingst 7
   0253 Oslo 2
   Norway
   02 55 92 44

Twine Club "I am You"
   c/o Dr T.B. Morozova
   198052 Russia
   St Petersburg
   Obvodny Kahal 114
   Russia
   812 292 4947; FAX: 812 312 1195

Twins Foundation "Nakula-Sadewa"
   c/o Mr Seto Mulyadi
   J.L. Taman Cirendu Permai No. 13
   Jakarta 15419
   Indonesia
   021 769 4299; FAX: 021 769 4299

The Twins and Multiple Births Association
   (TAMBA)
      PO Box 30
      Little Sutton
      South Wirral L66 1TH
      England
      151 348 0020; FAX: 151 348 0020

Zimbabwe Multiple Births Association
   (ZIMBA)
      c/o C. Goddard
      Charleigh
      3 Hillmorton Road
      Meyrick Park
      Harare
      Zimbabwe

Zwillinge
   c/o Marion von Gratkowski
   Postfach 17 17
   D-8910 Landsberg
   Germany
   08191/5 95 10; FAX: 08191/3 95 07

Zwillingseltern-Club Aagau
   c/o Brigit Brandestini
   Schlierenstrasse 87
   5400 Ennetbaden
   Switzerland
   056 21 21 87

Individuals

   E. and B. Rogers
   33 Mask Drive
   Artane, Dublin 5
   Eire

   Susan de Ferri
   Avenue Cordoba 890
   5.0 Piso
   Buenos Aires
   Argentina

Appendix: Resources

NATIONAL

Adoptive Families of America, Inc.
    c/o Susan Freivalds, Executive Director
    3333 Highway, 100 North
    Minneapolis, MN 55422
    1-800-372-3300; (612) 535-4829;
    FAX: (612) 535-7808

American Academy of Husband-Coached Childbirth
    The Bradley Method®
    c/o Marjorie Hathaway, AAHCC
    PO Box 5224
    Sherman Oaks, CA 91413
    1-800-4A-BIRTH; FAX: (818) 788-1580

Association of Birth Defect Children, Inc.
    c/o Betty Mekdeci, Executive Director
    827 Irma Avenue
    Orlando, FL 32803
    (407) 245-7035; FAX (407) 245-7035

Association of Labor Assistants and Childbirth Educators (ALACE)
    PO Box 382724
    Cambridge, MA 02238
    (617) 441-2500

Breastfeeding National Network
    c/o Debra Kurtz
    c/o Medela, Inc.
    PO Box 660
    4610 Prime Parkway
    McHenry, IL 60051
    1-800/TELL YOU (835-5968);
    FAX: (815) 363-1246

Breastfeeding Support Network
    c/o Peggy Toman, RN, BSN, IBCLC
    330 S. Eagle Street
    Oshkosh, WI 54901-567
    (414) 231-1611

Cesarean Support Education and Concern
    22 Forest Road
    Framingham, MA 01701
    (508) 877-8266

Center for Study of Multiple Birth
    333 East Superior Street
    Suite 464
    Chicago, Il 60611
    (312) 266-9093; FAX: (312) 908-8500

Depression After Delivery
    PO Box 1282
    Morrisville, PA 19067
    (215) 295-3994

Family Care Network (infants requiring special care)
    c/o Karen Streit
    103 William Howard Taft Road
    Cincinnati, OH 45219
    (513) 559-8810; FAX: (513) 281-2664

Health Education Associates
    c/o Ruth Maas
    8 Jan Sebastian Way, #13
    Sandwich, MA 02563
    (505) 888-8044; FAX: (508) 888-8050

Human Growth Foundation
    c/o Kimberly Frye
    777 Leesburg Pike, Suite 2025
    Falls Church, VA 22043
    1-800-451-6434, (703) 883-1773;
    FAX: (713) 883-1776

Hysterectomy Education Resources and Services (HERS) Foundation
    c/o Nora W. Coffey
    422 Bryn Mawr Avenue
    Bala Cynwyd, PA 19004
    (610) 667-7757; FAX: (610) 667-8096

Informed Homebirth/Informed Birth and Parenting
    PO Box 3675
    Ann Arbor, MI 48106
    (313) 662-6857; FAX: (313) 662-9381

Lactation Associates
    c/o Marsha Walker, R.N., I.B.C.L.C.
    254 Conant Road
    Weston, MA 02193
    (617) 893-3553; FAX: (617) 893-8608

Louisville Twin Study
    (See ASSOCIATIONS/GROUPS/INTERNATIONAL, US-based)

Military Parents of Multiples
    c/o Sandra Scott
    PO Box 302
    Henrietta, TX 76365

MULTIPLE PREGNANCY

Minnesota Center for Twin and Adoption Research
c/o Thomas Bouchard, PhD
University of Minnesota
Department of Psychology
75 East River Road
Minneapolis, MN 55455
(612) 625-4067; FAX: (612) 626-2079

Mothers of Supertwins (MOST) (A national non-profit network for families who are expecting to be, or who are parents of triplets, quads or quins)
c/o Maureen Boyle
PO Box 951
Brentwood, NY 11717
(516) 434-MOST; FAX: Same

National Center for Learning Disabilities
c/o Information and Referrals
381 Park Avenue, South
Suite 1420
New York, NY 10016
(212) 545-7510; FAX: (212) 545-9665

National Down Syndrome Congress
c/o Frank Murphy, Executive Director
1605 Chantilly Drive, Suite 250
Atlanta, GA 30324
1-800-232-NDSC; (404) 633-1555;
FAX: (404) 633-2817

National Organization of Mothers of Twins Clubs, Inc. (NOMOTC)
c/o Lois Gallmeyer, Executive Secretary
PO Box 23188
Albuquerque, NM 87192-1188
(shipping address) 12404 Princess Jeanne, N.E.
Albuquerque, NM 87112-4640
(505) 275-0955; FAX: (502) 296-1848

Parent Care, Inc. (Parent support groups in NICU)
c/o Sarah Killion
9041 Colgate Street
Indianapolis, IN 46268-1210
(317) 872-9913; FAX: (317) 872-0795

Parents Helping Parents (support for families of disabled children)
c/o Mary Ellen Peterson, Director
3041 Olcott Street
Santa Clara, CA 95054-2333
(508) 275-5775; FAX: (408) 727-0181

Parents of Prematures (primarily works with families in the Seattle area)
PO Box 3046
Kirkland, WA 98003-3046
(206) 283-7466

PHP - The Family Resource Center
c/o Family Resources: Patti Massey
3041 Alcott Street
Santa Clara, CA 95051-3222
(408) 727-5775; FAX: (408) 727-0182

Spina Bifida Association of America
c/o Information & Referral Coordinator
4590 MacArthur Boulevard, N.W.
Suite 250
Washington, DC 20007-4226
(202) 944-3285; FAX: (202) 944-3295

Spiritual Emergence Network (SEN)
c/o Chris Ann Gordon, Wendy Lees, Craig Turek
603 Mission Street
Santa Cruz, CA 95060
(408) 426-0921; FAX: (408) 429-1614

The Confinement Line (high-risk pregnant women confined to bed)
c/o Sue Johnston (clinical sociologist), Founder
PO Box 1609
Springfield, VA 22151
(703) 237-1896

The Triplet Connection
c/o Janet Bleyl
PO Box 99571
Stockton, CA 95209
(209) 474-0885; FAX: (209) 474-2233

The Twins Foundation
PO Box 6043
Providence, RI 02940-6043
(401) 729-1000

Twins Days Festival Committee, Inc. (also involved in research)
PO Box 29
Twinsburg, OH 44087
(216) 425-3652; FAX: (216) 426-7280

Appendix: Resources

Twin Services, Inc. (a.k.a. Twinline)
(Health and parenting education and referral for providers; technical assistance regarding case management and program development; training; and staff education materials)
   c/o Patricia Malmstrom, Director
   PO Box 10066
   Berkeley, CA 94709
   (510) 524-0863

Twin-to-Twin Transfusion Syndrome Foundation
   c/o Mary Slaman Forsythe, Executive Director
   411 Long Beach Parkway
   Bay Village, Ohio 44140
   (216) 899-0515 or (216) 899-TTTS;
   FAX: (216) 899-1184

LOSS/BEREAVEMENT

AMEND
   c/o Maureen Connelly, Director
   4324 Berrywick Terrace
   St. Louis, MO 63128
   (314) 487-7582

California State University at Fullerton
   c/o Nancy L. Segal, PhD, Director, Twin Studies
   Department of Psychology
   800 N. State College Boulevard
   Fullerton, CA 92634
   (714) 773-2142; FAX: (714) 449-7134

Center for Loss in Multiple Birth (CLIMB, Inc.)
   Jean Kollantai, President
   PO Box 1064
   Palmer, Alaska 99645
   (907) 746-6123

Centering Corporation
   1531 N. Saddle Creek Road
   Omaha, NE 68104
   (402) 553-1200; FAX: (402) 553-0507

Compassionate Friends, Inc.
   PO Box 3696
   Oak Brook, IL 60522-3696
   (708) 990-0010; FAX: (708) 990-0246

Elisabeth Kübler-Ross Center
   c/o Sherry Smith
   South Route 616
   Headwaters, VA 24442
   (703) 396-3441; FAX: (703) 396-6164

HOPING – Helping Other Parents in Normal Grieving
   Sparrow Hospital
   c/o Carolyn Wickham
   1215 E. Michigan Avenue
   PO Box 30480
   Lansing, MI 48090-9986
   (517) 484-3600; FAX: (517) 351-4104

(MIDS) Inc. (Miscarriage, Infant Death, Stillbirth, Ectopic Pregnancy Support Group)
   c/o Janet Tischler, Founder
   16 Crescent Drive
   Parsippary, NJ 07054
   (201) 263-6730

NOMOTC Bereavement Support Services and Cope/Outreach Department (see ORGANIZATIONS/GROUPS/NATIONAL)

Parents of Multiple Birth Association of Canada, Inc. (POMBA) (see ORGANIZATIONS/ GROUPS/ INTERNATIONAL, non-US-based)

Pregnancy and Infant Loss Center
   c/o Charlene Nelson or Donna Roehl
   1421 E. Wayzata Boulevard, #30
   Wayzata, MN 55391
   (612) 473-9372; FAX: (612) 473-8978

RTS Bereavement Services
   c/o Fran Rybarik, RN, MPH, Director
   Gundersen/Lutheran Medical Center
   1910 South Avenue
   La Crosse, WI 54601
   1-800-362-9567, ext. 4947; (608) 791-4747;
   FAX: (608) 791-5137

MULTIPLE PREGNANCY

SHARE – Pregnancy and Infant Loss Support, Inc.
    c/o Catherine Lammert, Executive Director
    St. Joseph Health Center
    200 South Fifth Street
    St. Charles, MO 63301-2893
    (314) 947-6164; FAX: (314) 947-7486

Sudden Infant Death Syndrome Alliance (SIDS Alliance)
    c/o Judith Jacobson
    1314 Bedford Avenue
    Suite 210
    Baltimore, MD 21208
    1-800-221-7437; Local: (410) 653-8226; FAX: (410) 653-8709

Tender Hearts
    c/o Mary Kay Sainsbury
    1302 Aralia Court
    San Luis Obispo, CA 93401
    (805) 544-9766; FAX: (805) 541-2853

The Triplet Connection (see ORGANIZATIONS/GROUPS/NATIONAL)

THEOS (Loss of a Spouse)
    1301 Clark Building
    717 Liberty Avenue
    Pittsburgh, PA 15222-1510
    (412) 471-7779; FAX: (412) 471-7782

Twinless Twins Support Group, Int'l
    c/o Dr Raymond W. Brandt
    11220 St. Joe Road
    Fort Wayne, IN 46835
    (219) 627-5414

Twin Services/Twinline (see ORGANIZATIONS/GROUPS/NATIONAL)

Unite, Inc. Grief Support
    c/o Janis Heil, PhD, Director
    7600 Central Avenue
    Philadelphia, PA 19111-2499
    (215) 728-3777

SINGLE PARENTS

American Association of Retired Persons (AARP) (Widowed Persons Service)
    1909 K Street, NW
    Washington, DC 20049
    (202) 434-2277

Community Church/Synagogue Support Groups
    (See local telephone directories)

Local Community College/University Single Support Groups
    (See local telephone directories)

Local Community College/University

Parents Without Partners
    c/o Kathy M. Bell, CAE, Executive Director
    401 North Michigan Avenue
    Chicago, IL 60611-4267
    (312) 644-6610; FAX: (312) 321-6869

Single Moms of Triplets
    c/o Linda Willis
    308 Rena Drive
    Lafayette, LA 70503
    (318) 981-7933; FAX: (318) 237-2057

Single Mothers by Choice
    c/o Jane Mattes
    PO Box 1642
    Gracie Square Station
    New York, NY 10028
    (212) 988-0993

Single Parent Resource Center
    141 W. 28th Street, Suite 302
    New York, NY 10001
    (212) 947-0221; FAX: (212) 947-0369

Single Triplet Moms Network
    c/o Diana Vincelli
    809 Westover Hills Boulevard
    Richmond, VA 23225-4522
    (804) 233-0099

Appendix: Resources

OTHER RESOURCES

Nutrition in pregnancy (especially multiples)

    Tom Brewer, MD
    64-A High Street
    Exeter, NH 03833
    (603) 778-1476 (Free telephone counseling)

Psychological counseling, telephone hypnosis*

David Cheek, MD
    1140 Bel Air Drive
    Santa Barbara, CA 93105
    (805) 569-7161

Phyllis H. Klaus, MFCC
    657 Creston Road
    Berkeley, CA 94708
    (510) 559-8000

Gayle Peterson, Ph.D.
    1749 Vine
    Berkeley, CA 94708
    (510) 526-5951

Vaginal birth after Cesarean (VBAC)

    c/o Nancy Wainer Cohen
    10 Great Plain Terrace
    Needham, MA 02191
    (617) 449-2490

REFERRALS

American Physical Therapy Association (APTA) Section on Women's Health (formerly Section on Ob/Gyn)
    PO Box 327
    Alexandria, VA 22313
    (703) 684-2782, ext. 3237;
    FAX: (703) 706-3169

International Lactation Consultant Association (local consultant information)
    c/o Jan
    201 Brown Avenue
    Evanston, IL 60202
    (708) 260-8874; FAX: (708) 475-2523

PRODUCTS

Electric breast pumps, shells, etc.

    Ameda-Egnell Corporation
    c/o Customer Service
    755 Industrial Drive
    Cary, IL 60013-1993
    1-800-323-8750; FAX: (708) 639-7897

Medela, Inc.
    c/o Debra Kurtz
    PO Box 660
    McHenry, IL 60051
    1-800-435-8316; FAX: 1-815-363-1246

Twin pillow

Four Dee Products, Inc. 'The Nurse Mate™' (pictures available)
    c/o Denise Duncan
    6014 Lattimer
    Houston, TX 77035
    (713) 728-0389; FAX: Same, call first

---

* These referrals supplied by Elizabeth Noble; not endorsed by The Center for Study of Multiple Birth

SELECTED READINGS

BOOKS

General

Abbe, KM, and Gill, FM. (1980). *Twins on Twins.* (New York: Crown)

Ainslie, R. (1985). *The Psychology of Twinship.* (Lincoln, NE: University of Nebraska Press)

Alexander, T. (1987). *Make Room for Twins.* (New York: Bantam Books)

Brewster, PD. (1979). *You Can Breastfeed Your Baby Even in Special Situations.* (Emmaus, PA: Rodale Press)

Bryan, EM. (1984). *Twins in the Family: A Parent's Guide.* (London: Constable)

Bryan, E. (1992). *Twins, Triplets and More – Their Nature, Development and Care.* (London: St. Martin's Press)

Cassil, K. (1984). *Twins: Nature's Amazing Mystery.* (New York: Atheneum)

Clegg, A, and Woolett, A. (1983). *Twins from Conception to Five Years.* (New York: Van Nostrand Reinhold)

Collier, H. (1980). *The Psychology of Twins* (3rd edn.). (Arizona: O'Sullivan, Woodside)

Friedrich, E, and Rowland, C. (1984). *The Parents' Guide to Raising Twins.* (New York: St. Martin's Press)

Gromada, KK. (1981). *Mothering Multiples.* (Franklin Park, IL: La Lèche League International)

Hagedorn, J, and Kizziar, J. (1983). *Gemini: The Psychology and Phenomena of Twins.* (Chicago: Center for Study of Multiple Birth)

Huggins, K. (1990). *The Nursing Mother's Companion.* (Boston: The Harvard Common Press)

*Keith, DK, McInnes, S, and Keith, LG. (1982). *Breastfeeding Twins, Triplets, and Quadruplets: 195 Practical Hints for Success.* (Chicago: Center for Study of Multiple Birth)

Leigh, G. (1984). *All About Twins: A Handbook for Parents.* (Boston: Routledge and Keegan Paul)

Mattes, J. *Single Mothers by Choice.* (Random House/Times)

Noble, E. (1980). *Having Twins: A Parent's Guide to Pregnancy, Birth, and Early Childhood.* (Boston: Houghton Mifflin)

Noble, E. (1991). *Having Twins.* (Boston: Houghton Mifflin)

Novotny, PP. (1988). *The Joy of Twins.* (New York: Crown)

*Theroux, R, and Tingley, J. (1985). *The Care of Twin Children: A Commonsense Guide for Parents* (2nd edn.). (Chicago: The Center for Study of Multiple Birth)

Loss/bereavement

From MK Sainsbury, and S. Sainsbury, MD (see LOSS/BEREAVEMENT):

    Study of Unique Effects of Multifetal Grief: The Grieving Process in Higher Order Multiple Birth Gestation: The Mother

    Partial Perinatal Loss or Demise in Multiple Birth, a Parental Study

From POMBA of Canada (see ASSOCIATIONS/GROUPS/INTERNATIONAL, non-US-based)
    The Death of a Twin: Miscarriage, Stillbirth, Infancy
    The Death of a Twin: Childhood/Teens
    When a Twin Dies: Role of the Parents of Twins Club

From Pregnancy and Infant Loss Center (see/LOSS/BEREAVEMENT)
    Empty Arms: Coping After Miscarriage, Stillbirth and Infant Death
    Our Baby Died. Why? (for children)
    Sibling Grief: After Miscarriage, Stillbirth or Infant Death

---

* Out of print. May be available in some Mothers of Twins Clubs or libraries.

Appendix: Resources

From Resolve Through Sharing (see LOSS/BEREAVEMENT)
    When a Baby Dies

From Tibbutt Publishing
    Betty Jean Case
    We Are Twins, But Who Am I?
    Living Without Your Twin
    0438 SW Palatine Hill Road
    Portland, OR 97219
    (503) 246-2356; (503) 246-6748;
    1-800-858-9055;
    FAX: (503) 241-7148

Mail Order Bookstore
International Childbirth Education Association (ICEA)
    PO Box 20048
    Minneapolis, MN 55420
    (612) 854-8660; FAX: (612) 854-8772

BOOKLETS, BROCHURES, CATALOGS, MAGAZINES, NEWSLETTERS

AMEND (Aiding a mother and a father experiencing neonatal death (brochure) (see LOSS/BEREAVEMENT)

Association of Labor Assistants and Childbirth Educators (ALACE) (brochure) (see ORGANIZATIONS/GROUPS/NATIONAL)
    Breastfeeding your Premature or Special Care Baby (2nd edn.)
    Lactation Associates, Inc.
    (see ORGANIZATIONS/GROUPS/NATIONAL)

Breastfeeding your Twins
    Health Education Associates
    (see ASSOCIATIONS/GROUPS/NATIONAL)

Caring Concepts (newsletter); Creative Care Package 1994 (catalog)
    Centering Corporation
    (see LOSS/BEREAVEMENT)

Children, A Parent's Guide to Growing (booklet)
    Human Growth Foundation
    (see ORGANIZATIONS/GROUPS/NATIONAL)

Depression After Delivery (brochure); Feelings after Birth, Postpartum Adjustment (brochure)
    From Depression after Delivery
    (see ORGANIZATIONS/GROUPS/NATIONAL)

Double Feature (quarterly newsletter)
    (see POMBA of Canada, ORGANIZATIONS/GROUPS/INTERNATIONAL, non-US-based)

Gemelli and Piu (magazine)
    Alfio Pizzone
    Casella Postale 121
    95100 Catania
    Italy
    039 674192

Informed Homebirth (brochure)
    Informed Homebirth and Parenting
    PO Box 3675
    Ann Arbor, MI 48106
    (313) 662-6857

La Lèche League International (brochure) (see ORGANIZATIONS/GROUPS/INTERNATIONAL, US-based)

MIDS Support Group, Inc. (brochure) (see LOSS/BEREAVEMENT)

NOMOTC (see ORGANIZATIONS/GROUPS/NATIONAL)
    How to organize a Mothers of Twins Club (Booklet)
    MOTC Notebook (Quarterly newspaper)
    Placement of Multiples in School: A Guide for Educators (Booklet)
    Your Twins and You (Brochure)

Nurse Mate™ - "The Nursing Pillow" (brochure)
    Four Dee Products (see PRODUCTS)

Our Newsletter (quarterly)
    From CLIMB, Inc. (see LOSS/BEREAVEMENT)

Pregnancy and Infant Loss Center (brochure)
    1421 East Waytzata Boulevard, #40
    Wayzata, MN 55381
    (612) 473-9372

MULTIPLE PREGNANCY

Single Mothers By Choice (SMS) (brochure)
(see SINGLE PARENTS)

Twinless Twins Support Group International (brochure)
(see LOSS/BEREAVEMENT)

Twins Magazine (bimonthly magazine)
c/o Barbara C. Unell
PO Box 12045
Overland Park, KA 66282-2045
(913) 722-1090; FAX: (913) 722-1767

Twin Services Reporter (semi-annual newsletter)
(see Twin Services: ORGANIZATIONS/GROUPS/NATIONAL)

Zwillinge (magazine)
c/o Marion von Gratkowski
Postfach 17 17
D-8910 Landsberg
Germany
81 191 5 95 10; FAX: 81 191 3 95 07

VIDEOS/TALK/WORKSHOP

Videos

Breastfeeding: Better Beginnings.
Lifecycle Productions, Inc.
PO Box 183
Newton, MA 02165
(617) 964-0047

Breastfeeding Your Baby - "A Mother's Guide"
Breastfeeding National Network (BNN)
(see ORGANIZATIONS/GROUPS/NATIONAL)

Talk

Twins, Triplets and More – A transcript of a talk for expectant parents
Dr Elizabeth Bryan (See Multiple Births Foundation, ORGANIZATION/GROUPS, INTERNATIONAL, Non-US-based)

Workshop

Life, Death and Transition
The Elisabeth Kübler-Ross Center
(see LOSS/BEREAVEMENT)

Index

abdominal circumference (AC) 217
abortion frequency
  in multiple pregnancies 33, 86–87
  monozygotic twins 86
absent end-diastolic velocity (AEDV) 234
acardiac malformation 76–78, 224
  and vascular communications 401–402
  management 78
acceleration of maturation
  brain 585–592
  limitations 591
  lung 592–595
acceptance of multifetal pregnancy 289–291
acid–base status
  and biophysical profile score 232
acoustic stimulation of fetus *see* external stimulation of fetus
actin–myosin interactions
  and uterine contractility 415–416
acute perinatal twin transfusion (APeriTTS) 373
adaptive acceleration, developmental
  brain 585–592
  limitations 591
  lung 592–595
age, gestational *see also* gestational period; pregnancy dating
  and multifetal pregnancy diagnosis 196
  mortality of one twin relationships 409
  ultrasound determination 215–222
age, maternal
  and assisted reproduction 179
  and dizygotic twinning 35, 299–300
  and fetal mortality 63
  multifetal pregnancy relationships 133, 135–138, 146–147, 152–153
    higher order pregnancies 537
agenesis of corpus callosum (ACC)
  fetal diagnosis 245
Allen method 150–151
alpha-fetoprotein (AFP)
  and open neural tube defects 284–286
  indication for prenatal genetic diagnosis 314
  mutifetal pregnancy diagnostic significance 284–286, 300

ambulatory tocolysis 471–488 *see also* labor; preterm delivery; uterine contractility
  agents 474–479
    betamimetics 474–476, 541
    indomethacin 477–478
    magnesium sulfate 476–477
    nifedipine 478–479
  bed rest costs and benefits 472–473
  contradictions for 474
  indications for 473–474
  subcutaneous pump therapy 483–486
amniocentesis 313–318, 321–323
  and twin–twin transfusion syndrome 382
  conjoined twins 106
  genetic outcome 318
  obstetric outcome 316–318
amnionicity 4, 367–368, 626 *see also* diamnionic twins; monoamnionic twins
  ultrasound determination 219–224
amniotic fluid volume (AFV) 230
analgesia during delivery 522–523
anastomoses 118–119, 122, 368–391
  and twin–twin transfusion syndrome 12, 13, 119, 370–391
  obstetric outcome relationships 383–388
  pathological evidence of vanishing twin 51
  types of 369–381
anemia, in higher order multiple pregnancies 540
anencephalus
  fetal diagnosis 240
  incidence in twins 86
anesthesia 504, 517–524
  Cesarean section 508–509, 523–524
  epidural anesthesia 524
  general anesthesia 524
  maternal factors 517–518
  neonatal factors 518
  obstetric considerations 518–519
  vaginal delivery 519–520
aneurysm
  vein of Galen 244–245
  ventricular 253
anomalies, congenital 73–86, 604–605 *see also* conjoined twins

MULTIPLE PREGNANCY

acardiac malformation 76–78, 224
   and vascular communications 401–402
      management 78
chromosome anomalies 5, 81–83, 318, 321, 604
classification of 73–74
definitions 73–74
Ebstein anomaly 252
environmental disorders 83–84
fetal behavior relationships 345–347
fetal diagnosis by ultrasonography 239–264
   central nervous system 239–246
   chest 253–255
   congenital heart disease 246–253
   gastrointestinal tract 255–256
   skeletal 262–264
   urinary tract 256–261
fetus-in-fetu 76
frequency in twins 84–86, 141
   ascertainment biases 84–85
higher order multiple pregnancies 539–540
malformations 30
   Weinberg method applicability 43
monozygotic twins 25, 74–75, 604
surviving twin 78–80
antenatal bias 12–13
antenatal surveillance *see* fetal well-being assessment
antepartum bleeding
   and preterm delivery 421
aorta, coarctation of 250
Apgar score 139–142
appendix displacement during pregnancy 275
arachnoid cyst 245
arterio–arterial anastomoses *see* anastomoses
arterio–venous anastomoses *see* anastomoses
artificial induction of ovulation *see* ovulation induction
asphyxia 606
asplenia syndrome 252
assisted hatching 185
assisted reproduction (ART) *see also in vitro* fertilization and embryo transfer; ovulation induction; tubal embryo transfer
   multifetal pregnancy reduction 185
   multiple gestation relationships 156–158, 175–186
      determining factors 180–181
      maternal age and 179
   multiple oocyte/embryo transfer, risks vs. benefits 179–180
atresia
   duodenal 255
   esophageal 253
atrioventricular septal defects (ASDs) 251–252
attachment 563–570
   case studies 568–569

effects of death of one twin 567
enhancement suggestions 569–570
hospital practices 564–565
individuation processes 566–567

Ballard score 588–589
bed rest 294–295
   and preterm delivery prevention 439–440, 442, 540–541
   with ambulatory tocolysis 472–473
behavior, fetal *see* intrauterine behavior
Bereavement Clinic 665
bereavement support 656
beta-adrenergic receptor stimulators *see* betamimetics
betamimetics
   and preterm delivery prevention 440–441, 474–476, 541
   physiology 474
   precautions 475
   side-effects 474, 540
   therapeutic plan 475
   nursing intervention 475
bi-breech presentation of conjoined twins 107
biases
   antenatal 12–13
   environmental 13–14
   genetic 11–12
   parental 13–14
biliary function during pregnancy 275
biometrics
   ultrasound studies 199–202
      reference curves 200, 202
biophysical profile score (BPS) 230–231, 327
   and acid–base status 232
   conjoined twins 106
   weighted biophysical profile 232–233
biparietal diameter (BPD) 217
   gestational age estimation 219
birth size 613
birth trauma
   mode of delivery relationships 495–496
birth weight *see* weight
bladder
   anomalies 257
   changes during multifetal pregnancy 274
blighted ovum 60, 66
blood
   maternal adaptation to multifetal pregnancy 272
blood groups
   and zygosity determination 14
blood pressure
   maternal adaptation to multifetal pregnancy 269–271

bonding 563–570
  case studies 568–569
  early diagnosis significance 566
  effects of death of one twin 567
  enhancement suggestions 569–570
  hospital practices 564–565
  individuation processes 566–567
  prenatal 291–293, 569
Bonferroni Test of Significance 620, 621
brain
  developmental acceleration 585–592
    clinical data 586–589
    dizygotic twins 586–591
    higher order multiples 592
    monozygotic twins 591–592
  size 615
brain auditory evoked responses (BAERs) 589–590
breast feeding 553–560, 640, 659
  breast pumping 557–558
  higher order multiples 559–560
  home support 558
  maternal nutrition 556–557
  milk supply 554–555, 558
  positioning 555–556
  prenatal preparation 553–554
  psychological aspects 295
  weaning 560
breech delivery 494–498

calcium channel blockers *see* nifedipine
calcium metabolism
  and uterine contractility 416–417
cardiomyopathy 252–252
cardiosplenic syndromes 252
cardiovascular system
  anomalies 76–78
    conjoined twins 104, 106
    incidence in twins 85–86
  maternal adaptation to multifetal pregnancy 269–273, 304
    anesthetic considerations 517
    blood pressure 269–271
    cardiac function 271–272
    hematological profile 272–273
    plasma volume 269, 270
    regional blood flow 271
cat's eye syndrome 5
central nervous system anomalies 239–246
  fetal behavior relationships 346
cephalothoracopagus conjoined twins 96, 100
cerclage
  and preterm delivery prevention 441
cerebral palsy 599–600
cervix 453–466

anatomy and histology 453
antepartum examination 458–459
  preterm delivery prediction 459–464
  safety of 464–466
  term delivery prediction 464
cervical incompetence
  and preterm delivery 421–422
cervical suture
  and preterm delivery prevention 541
dilatation 456–458
  in multifetal pregnancies 428–429, 430, 457–458
maturational changes 453–456
  prostaglandin influence 456
  relaxin influence 456
  steroid hormone influence 456
parity relationships 459
Cesarean section *see also* delivery;
  anesthetic technique 508–509, 523–524
  conjoined twins 107
  prerequisites 504
  prognostic significance 210
  psychological aspects 295
  vertex/non-vertex twin delivery 493–499
chest anomalies
  fetal diagnosis by ultrasonography 253–255
chimeras 30
chorioangiopagus 399–404
chorionic villus sampling (CVS) 313, 315–316, 318–323
  genetic outcome 319–321
  obstetric outcome 318–319, 320
chorionicity 113–117, 367–368, 626 *see also* dichorionic (DC) placentation; monochorionic (MC) placentation
  fetal demise of one twin relationships 408–409
  triplets 117–118, 119
  ultrasound determination 198, 219–224
choroid plexus cyst
  fetal diagnosis 243–244
chromosome anomalies *see* genetic disorders
chronogenetics 5–6
cleft lip 43, 261, 263
cleft palate 43, 261, 263
clomiphene citrate
  and ovular resorption 61
  multiple birth relationships 147, 157, 182–183
cloning 3
co-twin control study 18
coarctation of the aorta 250
cognition studies *see* mental development
collision theory of conjoined twinning 102
common environment 13–14
computed tomography
  conjoined twin diagnosis 104–105, 108

concordance studies 15–16
  birth size 613
  chromosomal anomalies 81–83
  growth
    fetal behavior relationships 346
    placental vascular anatomy relationships 386–388
  intrauterine behavior 337–339
  Mendelian disorders 83
  monozygotic twins 27–28, 83
  sex 82–83
congenital anomalies *see* anomalies, congenital
congenital, definition 74
congenital heart disease *see* heart disease, congenital
conjoined twins 75–76, 93–109
  anatomy 103–104
    associated anomalies 104
  classification 94–101
    diplopagus 94–96
    heteropagus 96–101
  diagnosis of 104–106
  ethical considerations 109
  etiology 93, 101–103
  frequency 25–26, 93
  obstetric management 106–108
    Cesarean section 107
    vaginal delivery 107–108
  separation 108–109
    anesthetic management 109
    operative management 109
    preoperative evaluation 108
    timing 108–109
  sex proportion 94, 159
  survival 108
continuous variable analysis 16–17
  partitioning of variance 16–17
contractility *see* uterine contractility
contraction stress test 327
cord insertion *see* umbilical cord
corpus callosum, agenesis 245
counselling
  and assisted reproduction 185–186
cranial anomalies
  fetal diagnosis 240–245
craniopagus conjoined twins 75, 94, 96
  anatomy 103
cri du chat syndrome 5
critical period in twin pregnancy 171–172
crown–rump length (CRL) 216–217
  gestational age estimation 217–219
cutis aplasia congenita 78–79
cystic hygroma 261
cystic tumors, placental

pathological evidence of vanishing twin 56–58, 69
cytogenetics 5

deformations 74
delivery 491–499, 503–515 *see also* Cesarean section; labor; preterm delivery; vaginal delivery
  complications 513–514
    and developmental outcome 606
    locking 513–514
    twin–twin transfusion syndrome 514
    vasa previa 514
  fetal behavior 344–345
  higher order multiples 511–513, 542, 544
    triplets 511–512
  inter–twin delivery interval 510
  monoamnionic twins 531
  of second twin 509–510
  parental anxiety 514–515
  prerequisites 503–504
    anesthesia 504
    Cesarean section 504
    fetal imaging 504
    fetal monitoring 503–504
    immediate neonatal care 504
  procedures 504–511
    dual-channel monitoring 505
    intrapartum use of ultrasonography 505–506
  route selection 506–509
    birth trauma relationships 495–496
    higher order multiples 511–513
    protocol 507
    vaginal delivery after previous Cesarean section 504–505
    vertex/non-vertex twins 492–499
    vertex/vertex twins 491–492
Denmark
  multifetal pregnancy trends 148–149
dental diameter symmetry 43
depression, postpartum *see* postpartum adjustment
deradelphus conjoined twins 96
developmental outcome 599–608
  cognition 600–601
  brain size 615
  environmental influence 607–608
  genetic factors 602–604
  influences 601–608
    delivery 606
    environment 607–608
    genetic factors 602–604
    hypoxia/asphyxia 606
    intrauterine growth retardation 605–606
    maternal factors 605
    nutrition 614–615
    obstetric factors 605

placental influences 606, 613–614
    prematurity 606–607
  neurological outcome 599–600
diagnosis of multifetal pregnancy 195–197, 279–280
  and preterm delivery prevention 439
  bonding and attachment role 566
  higher order multiple pregnancies 538, 543
  prognostic significance 208–212
diamnionic twins 4
diaphragmatic hernia 255
dicephalus conjoined twins 94, 98, 100
dicephalus dipygus conjoined twins 96
dichorionic (DC) placentation *see also* chorionicity; placentation
  antenatal surveillance 328
  birth weight and 123–126
  dichorionic–diamnionic (DC–DA) 25, 219–223
    separation pattern 26
  fetal growth and 123–125
dietary recommendations during multifetal pregnancy 306–307
  iron sources 304–306
difference method *see* Weinberg method
dilatation, cervical 456–458
  in multifetal pregnancies 428–429, 430, 457–458
diplopagus conjoined twins
  classification 94–96
dipygus conjoined twins 94–96
discordance *see* concordance studies
dispermatic twins 11–12
disruptions 74
dizygotic (DZ) twinning 3, 31–32 *see also* amnionicity; chorionicity; placentation; zygosity determination
  concordance for chromosomal anomalies 81
  mechanisms 10–12
    FSH role 31
  predisposing factors 33–35
    environment 35
    heredity 33–35
    maternal age 35, 299
    maternal height 299
    nutrition 35
    parity 35, 299
    race 33–35
    season 35
  secular trends 147–151
  sex proportion 158–160
  superfecundation 12, 35
  superfetation 12, 35–36
DNA analysis
  zygosity determination 627–632
    DNA fingerprinting 15, 628–629
    new developments 629

doctor–parent relationship 637–644
  after the birth 638–642
  at delivery 638
  during pregnancy 637–638
Doppler sonography 201–202
  fetal well-being assessment 233–235, 327–328
    absent end-diastolic velocity 234
    and electronic testing 234
    and fetal outcome 233–234
    intrauterine growth retardation 234, 327–328
    twin–twin transfusion syndrome 234–235
  umbilical cord study 329
double outlet right ventricle (DORV) 251
Down's syndrome 5, 259
Dubowitz score 588
Duchenne muscular dystrophy 83
duodenal atresia 255
Dutch Twin Register 149, 150

early embryonic size (EES) 216–217
  gestational age estimation 218
East Flanders Prospective Twin Survey 29, 122–127, 150
  infertility treatment statistics 156–159
  sex proportion 159–160
Ebstein anomaly 252
embryo quality
  in assisted reproduction 180
encephalocele
  fetal diagnosis 241
endocardial fibroelastosis 253
England and Wales
  multifetal pregnancy trends 146–149
engorgement during breast feeding 558
entanglement during delivery 211–212
environment
  dizygotic twinning and 35
  environmental biases 13–14
  environmental disorders 83–84
epidural anesthesia 524
esophageal atresia 253
estradiol
  dizygotic twinning and 31
  in superovulation therapy 183
estrogens
  and cervical maturation 456
  and uterine contractility 417–418
  multifetal pregnancy diagnostic significance 283–284
ethics 7–8, 645–652
  fetal reduction 360–362, 364–365, 648–650
  preconception counselling 646–647
  prenatal screening 650–651
  selective termination 651–652

Europe
  twinning rate trends 145–150
exencephalus
  fetal diagnosis 240
exhaustion, postpartum 638–639
external cephalic version 493–494
external stimulation of fetus 231–232, 333
  responses 339–342

fathers 643
femur length (FL) 217
  gestational age estimation 219
fetal acoustic stimulation (FAS) 231–232
fetal behavior see intrauterine behavior
fetal body movement/fetal movement/fetal tone 231
  and intrauterine behavior 332–333
fetal growth see growth
fetal morphology
  ultrasound studies 203
fetal reduction 353–356
  ethical considerations 360–362, 364–365, 648–650
  KCl injection 362–363
  Mount Sinai experience 354–355
  selective termination 353–354, 356, 362–365
    abnormal twin 362
    acardiac twin 78
    and twin–twin transfusion syndrome 382
    KCl injection 362–363
    preterm delivery risks 363
  special concerns 363–364
  subsequence prenatal care 356
  timing 355
    first trimester 354
    second trimester 353–354
fetal weight estimation 226–230
fetal well-being assessment 230–233, 325–329
  biophysical profile score (BPS) 230–231
    and acid–base status 232
    weighted biophysical profile 232–233
  Doppler assessments 233–235
  fetal acoustic stimulation (FAS) 231–232
  recommendations 328–329
fetus papyraceus 59, 61, 66
  anomalies in surviving co-twin 78
fetus-in-fetu 76, 101
Finland
  multifetal pregnancy trends 149, 155
folate requirements during multifetal pregnancy 272, 541
follicle stimulating hormone (FSH)
  dizygotic twinning and 31–34
  multifetal pregnancy relationships 299–300
France
  preterm delivery prevention studies 443–445

gamete intrafallopian transfer (GIFT)
  multiple gestation relationships 157, 178
  maternal age and 179
gap junction formation
  and uterine contractility 418–419
gastrointestinal tract anomalies
  fetal diagnosis by ultrasonography 255–256
  maternal adaptation to multifetal pregnancy 275
general anesthesia 524
genetic bias 11–12
genetic disorders
  chromosomal anomalies 5, 81–83, 318, 321, 604
    discordance 81–83
    monozygotic twins 27–28
    vanishing twin relationships 63–65, 69
  prenatal diagnosis 313–323
    amniocentesis 313–318, 321–323
    chorionic villus sampling (CVS) 313, 315–316, 318–323
    indications for 314
Germany
  multifetal pregnancy trends 148
gestational age see also gestational period
  mortality of one twin relationships 409
  multifetal pregnancy diagnosis and 196
  ultrasound determination 215–222
gestational period 163–164, 437–438 see also preterm delivery
  birth weight relationships 138–141, 164–166, 303
  critical period in twin pregnancy 171–172
  following fetal reduction 360
  higher order multiple pregnancies 544
    and assisted reproduction 538–539
  live birth relationships 137–141
  neonatal and infant mortality relationships 168–170, 172, 173
  perinatal mortality relationships 438
  placental vascular anatomy relationships 386, 387
gonadotropin releasing hormone (GnRH) therapy
  in superovulation therapy 183
  multiple birth relationships 184
grand multifetal pregnancies see multifetal pregnancy
grandparents 644
Grannum classification 202
growth
  discordance
    fetal behavior relationships 346
    placental vascular anatomy relationships 386–388
  fetal
    placentation and zygosity relationships 123–125

race relationships 166
  ultrasound assessment 226–230
  weight estimation 226–230
 postnatal 615–617
  obstetric factors 617
  zygosity influence 616–617
growth retardation 591
 and developmental outcome 605–606
 Doppler studies 234, 327–328
 in higher order multiple pregnancies 539

half-identical twinning 29–30
half-sib method 17
head circumference (HC) 217
 gestational age estimation 219
heart
 maternal adaptation to multifetal pregnancy 271–272
heart disease, congenital
 atrioventricular septal defects (ASDs) 251–252
 cardiosplenic syndromes 252
 coarctation of the aorta 250
 double outlet right ventricle (DORV) 251
 Ebstein anomaly 252
 fetal diagnosis 246–253
 interventricular septum (IVS) 247–250
 left ventricular hypoplasia 250
 placentation relationships 124–125
 right ventricular hypoplasia 250
 tetralogy of Fallot 251
 total anomalous pulmonary venous return 252
 transposition of great arteries (TGA) 251
 truncus arteriosus 251
height, maternal
 multifetal pregnancy relationships 299–300
hematology
 and intrauterine behavior 339
 maternal adaptation to multifetal pregnancy 269–273, 304
hereditary diseases 5
heredity
 cognition and behavior 602–604
 dizygotic twinning and 33–35
 monozygotic twinning 154
 multifetal pregnancy relationships 154–156
  higher order multiple pregnancies 537
heritability estimates
 in concordance studies 16
hermaphroditism
 chimeras 30
heteropagus conjoined twins 96
higher order pregnancies *see* multifetal pregnancy
holoprosencephaly 244
home monitoring
  preterm delivery prevention 441
home support 661
 and breast feeding 558
hormonal stimulation *see* ovulation induction
household help 661
human chorionic gonadotropins (hCG) 31
 in superovulation therapy 183
 multifetal pregnancy relationships 157
  diagnostic signficance 281–283
 vanishing twin relationships 64
human menopausal gonadotropins (hMG)
 multiple birth relationships 157, 182–184
human placental lactogen (hPL)
 multifetal pregnancy diagnostic significance 283
hyaline membrane disease 539
hydramnios
 and higher order multiple pregnancies 540
 placental vascular anatomy relationships 385–386
hydranencephaly 244
hydrocephalus
 fetal diagnosis 241–243
 incidence in twins 86
hydrops 261–262
hyperechogenic bowel 255–256
hypoplasia
 pulmonary 254–255
 ventricular 250
hypoxia 606

identical twins *see* monozygotic (MZ) twinning
identicalness 4–7
 genetic 4–6
 temporal aspects 6
identity 6–8, 643, 660
 bonding and attachment relationships 566–567
idiopathic infantile arterial calcification (IIAC) 253
in vitro fertilization and embryo transfer (IVF-ET)
 monozygotic twinning and 28–30, 184–185
 multiple gestation relationships 157, 175, 177–178, 351
  higher order births 175
  maternal age and 179
  natural cycle IVF 181
individual identity 6–8, 642, 643, 660
 bonding and attachment relationships 566–567
individual twin survival probability 48
individuation processes 566–567
indomethacin
 preterm delivery prevention 441, 477–478
  nursing interventions 478
  physiology 477
  precautions 477–478
  therapeutic plan 478
infantile polycystic kidney disease (IPKD) 260

infection, subclinical
and preterm delivery 420–421
inferior conjunction conjoined twins 101
infertility treatment *see* assisted reproduction
inheritance *see* heredity
iniencephalus
fetal diagnosis 240
intelligence quotient (IQ) differences 13
interfetal communication 342
interfetal vascular anastomoses (IVFA) *see* anastomoses
intermediary twinning 29–30
interventricular septum (IVS) 247–250
intrauterine behavior 331–347
behavior during delivery 344–345
definition of behavioral states 333–336
detection methods 331–333
external stimulation 333
fetal heart rate 332–333
fetal movements 332–333
ultrasound 331–332
zygosity determination 332
diagnostic significance 345–347
hemodynamic considerations 339
individual differences of twins 337–339
interfetal communication 342
maternal influences 342–344
maturation effect 336–337
responses to external stimuli 339–342
intrauterine fetal demise (IUFD) *see* mortality
intrauterine growth retardation (IUGR) 325, 591
and developmental outcome 605–606
Doppler studies 234, 327–328
in higher order multiple pregnancies 539
inverse laterality 4, 6
IQ comparisons 600–601, 606–608, 621
genetic factors 602–603
iron requirements during multifetal pregnancy 272, 304–306, 541
deficiency in higher order multiple pregnancies 540
dietary sources 305
ischiopagus conjoined twins 75, 94, 96
anatomy 104
IVF *see in vitro* fertilization

janiceps conjoined twins 96
Japan
ovulation induction effects on multiple births 34–35

karyotype
early separation evidence 26
vanishing twin relationships 63–65

KCl injection, in selective termination 353–354
kidneys
anomalies, fetal diagnosis 260–261
maternal adaptation to multifetal pregnancy 274–275
Klinefelter's syndrome 5, 31

labor 427–435 *see also* ambulatory tocolysis; delivery; preterm delivery; uterine contractility
cervical dilatation 428–429, 430
duration studies 428
graphic analysis 428–431
influencing factors 427–428
parity 429, 431
univariate and multivariate analysis 431–434
last menstrual period (LMP)
and pregnancy dating 215–219
left ventricular hypoplasia 250
left-handedness
monozygotic twins 25
Linked Birth/Infant Death files, USA 163–166, 171, 173
live-birth order
twinning incidence relationships 135–137
liver
maternal adaptation to multifetal pregnancy 275
locking as complication of delivery 513–514
Louisville Twin Study 12, 618–619
low-amplitude high-frequency contractions (LAHF) 481–483
lung fetal maturation 592–595
luteinizing hormone (LH) 31, 183

macrosomia 230
magnesium sulfate
as tocolytic agent 476–477
nursing interventions 477
physiology 476
precautions 476
therapeutic plans 476–477
magnetic resonance imaging (MRI)
conjoined twin diagnosis 104, 105, 108
malformations *see* anomalies, congenital
maternal adaptation to multifetal pregnancy 269–276
cardiovascular system 269–273, 304
blood pressure 269–271
cardiac function 271–272
hematological profile 272–273
plasma volume 269, 270
regional blood flow 271
endocrine adaptations 300
gastrointestinal tract 275

metabolic adaptations 300
psychological aspects 289–297
   acceptance 289–291
   and preterm delivery 422
   breast feeding 295
   coping with fetal loss 296–297
   education and supportive measures 291–292
   infant hospitalization 296
   journal writing 293–294
   older siblings 296
   postpartum adjustment 296, 573–580
   prenatal bonding 292–293
   the birth 295
pulmonary system 273–274
urinary system 274–275
uterine changes 300
weight gain 300–304
maternal age *see* age
maturation
  fetal brain 585–592
  fetal lung 592–595
megacystis–microcolon–hypoperistalsis syndrome 258
megaureter 257
Mendelian disorders
  concordance 83
meningocele
  fetal diagnosis 241
menstrual dates 215–219, 222
mental development 617–622, 640–642
  cognition studies 600–608
  family factors 619–622
  influences 601–608
    environment 607–608
    genetic factors 602–604
  Louisville Twin Study 618–619
  newborn factors 619
  play 640–641
  retardation 622
  role of play 640–641
microcephalus
  fetal diagnosis 240–241
mid conjunction conjoined twins 101
milk supply 554–555, 558, 640
Minnesota Twin Study 17
miscarriage *see* abortion
monoamnionic twins 4 *see also* amnionicity
  clinical management 527–532
    antepartum diagnosis and care 527–531
    case studies 531–533
    delivery techniques 531
    patient preparation 530
monocephalus conjoined twins 94, 96, 99
  monocephalus diprosopus 94, 97

monochorionic (MC) placentation *see also* amnionicity; chorionicity; placentation
  birth weight and 123–125
  circulation 12
  fetal growth and 123–125
  monitoring of 380
  monochorionic–diamniotic (MC–DA) 25, 116, 221–224
    antenatal surveillance 328
    placental examination 120, 123
  monochorionic–monoamniotic (MC–MA) 25, 221–224
    antenatal surveillance 328
    diagnosis 224
    placental examination 120
    separation pattern 27
    TRAP sequence 224
  sex proportion 126–127
  vascular anatomy 399–402, 404
    acardia 401–402
    anastomoses 118–119, 122, 368–391
    obstetric outcome relationships 383–388
    sirenomelia 402
    twin–twin transfusion syndrome and 12, 13, 370–391
  zygosity 14
monozygotic (MZ) twinning 3, 25–31 *see also* amnionicity; chorionicity; placentation
  assisted reproduction effects 184–185
    in vitro fertilization 184–185
    ovulation induction 156, 158, 184
  congenital anomaly incidence 604
  definition 25–26
  discordance 83
    chromosomal anomalies 81–83
    sex 82–83
  experimental production in mammals 26
  heredity 154
  mechanisms 10
    separation patterns 26–27
  research significance 4
  secular trends 147–151
  sex proportion 158–160
  ultrasound diagnosis 219–224
mortality *see also* vanishing twin syndrome
  feta and gestational age 409
  fetal 41, 407–409
    attachment relationships 567
    bonding relationships 567
    chorionicity significance 408–409
    etiology 407
    management 407–409
    monozygotic co-twin 78–80
    placentation relationships 126

    sex links 30–31
    surviving fetus 409
  in higher order multiple pregnancies 539, 544
  neonatal and infant
    and vaginal delivery 496–497
    birth weight relationships 166–168
    effects on bonding and attachment 567
    gestational period relationships 168–170, 172
    twin sex combination relationships 170–171
  perinatal
    gestational period relationships 438
    placental vascular anatomy relationships 385
    placentation relationships 368, 381, 390
    Swedish study 205
    ultrasound benefits 209–210, 212
mosaicism 30, 83
Mothers of Twins Clubs 655–658
Mount Sinai Medical Center
  experience in fetal reduction 354–355
multicystic, dysplastic kidneys 260–261
multifetal pregnancy
  biochemical parameters 281–286
    alpha-fetoprotein 284
    estrogens 283–284
    human chorionic gonadotropin 281–283
    human placental lactogen 282, 283
    progesterone 284
  clinical parameters 280–281
  early diagnosis 195–197, 279–280
    and preterm delivery prevention 439
    prognostic signficance 208–210
  maternal adaptation *see* maternal adaptation to multifetal pregnancy
  secular trends 145–151
    Europe 145–150
    Sweden 145
    USA 133–135
    zygosity relationships 147–150
  triplet and higher order pregnancies 351–353, 535–544
    complications 538–540, 543–544
    diagnosis 538, 543
    epidemiology 535–538, 542–543
    fetal reduction *see* fetal reduction
    natural course 351–353
    predisposing factors 537
    prevention of 544
multifetal reduction *see* fetal reduction
Multiple Abstract Variance Analysis (MAVA) 16–17
multiple fertilization 10
myometrial contractility *see* uterine contractility

naming 660
National Collaborative Perinatal Project 42, 44

National Natality files, USA 163–166
National Organization of Mothers of Twins Clubs, Inc., USA 655–658
  international contacts 657–658
  research 657
  support services 656–657
    bereavement 656
    coping 656
    disabilities 656
    education 656–657
nervous system anomalies 239–246
  fetal behavior relationships 346
Netherlands
  twinning rate trends 146–149
neural tube defects 27, 43
  and alpha-fetoprotein levels 284–286
  incidence in twins 86
neurological development *see* brain; mental development
neurological scores 588–589
New York, Mount Sinai Medical Center
  experience in fetal reduction 354–355
nifedipine
  as tocolytic agent 478–479
    nursing interventions 479
    physiology 478
    precautions 478
    therapeutic plan 478–479
non-identical twins *see* dizygotic (DZ) twinning
non-immune fetal hydrops 262
non-stress test (NST) 230–231, 325–327
Norway
  multifetal pregnancy trends 148
nutrition
  and breast feeding 556–557
  developmental outcome relationships 614–615
  dizygotic twinning and 35
  maternal requirements during pregnancy 304–307

obstetrics 4
obstructive lesions of gastrointestinal tract 255–256
older siblings 296, 660–661
oligohydramnios 254
omphalocele 256
omphalopagus conjoined twins
  anatomy 103
oocyte aging 29
open neural tube defects 27, 43
  and alpha-fetoprotein levels 284–286
  incidence in twins 86
opposite sex (OS) pairs 14
  as representative of all dizygotic twins 42–43
ovarian stimulation *see* ovulation induction

ovular resorption
  and clomiphene citrate 61
ovulation induction
  monozygotic twinning and 29, 156, 158, 184
  multifetal pregnancy relationships 156–158, 181–184, 351
  in Japan 34–35
  ovarian hyperstimulation 181
  superovulation therapy 182–184
oxygen consumption
  changes during multifetal pregnancy 273
oxytocin sensitivity
  and uterine contractility 418

parasitic conjoined twins 97, 101
  fetus in fetu 76, 101
  teratomas 101
parent–doctor relationship 637–644
  after the birth 638–642
  at delivery 638
  during pregnancy 637–638
parental bias 13–14
parenting considerations 659–661 *see also* postpartum adjustment
  development 660
  feeding 659
  household help 661
  identity and individuality 660
    naming 660
    opportunity 660
  transporting 659–670
parity
  cervical status relationships 459
  labor relationships 429, 431
  multifetal pregnancy relationships 152
    dizygotic twinning 35, 299
    higher order pregnancies 537
partitioning of variance 16–17
personal boundaries *see* identity
photoperiod
  dizygotic twinning and 35
physical condition at birth
  Apgar score 139–142
placenta
  examination of 119–122
    anastomoses 122
    fetal membranes 120–121
    fusion 121
    umbilical cord insertion 122
  hormone synthesis 281–284
    and preterm delivery 422
  influence on developmental outcome 606, 613–614
  pathological evidence of vanishing twin 51–58, 65, 69
  ultrasound studies 202–203
  umbilical cord insertion 118, 122, 126–127
    perinatal outcome relationships 126–127
    velamentous insertion 126, 127, 514
  vascular anatomy 368–391, 399–402
    acardia 401–402
    anastomoses 118–119, 122, 368–391
    and twin–twin transfusion syndrome 12, 13, 370–391, 395–397, 402–404
    obstetric outcome relationships 383–388
    sirenomelia 402
    three-dimensional modelling 395–397
placentation 113–127, 367–368, 626 *see also* amnionicity: chorionicity
  birth weight and 123–126
  determination of 119–121
    ultrasound 219–224
  fetal growth and 123–125
  fetal mortality and 126
  race variation 113, 117
  sex proportion relationships 159–160
  triplets 113, 117–119, 122, 127
  ultrasound observation 198
plasma volume
  maternal adaptation to multifetal pregnancy 269, 270, 304
plasminogen levels during pregnancy 273
platelet counts during pregnancy 273
play, and mental development 640–641
polar body 29, 30
pollution
  dizygotic twinning and 35
polycystic kidney disease 260
polyhydramnios 281
  and preterm delivery 419–420
  conjoined twins 105
polyovulation 10
polysplenia syndrome 252
porencephaly 244
positioning for breast feeding 555–556
posterior fossa
  ultrasonographic imaging 245
posterior urethral valve (PUV) 257–258
postpartum adjustment 296 *see also* parenting considerations
  exhaustion 638–639
  family impact 639–640
    brothers and sisters 660–661
    fathers 643
    grandparents 644
  psychological aspects 575–580
    breast feeding 295
    postpartum depression 576, 638–639

severe postpartum syndromes 576–579
potassium chloride injection
  in selective termination 353–354
pregnancy dating 215–222
pregnancy, multifetal *see* multifetal pregnancy
premature birth *see* preterm delivery
premature rupture of membranes
  and preterm delivery 421, 475
  and twin–twin transfusion syndrome 370
prenatal bonding 291–293
preterm delivery 415–422 *see also* ambulatory tocolysis; labor
  and breast pumping 557–558
  and developmental outcome 606–607
  clinical factors 419–422
    antepartum bleeding 421
    cervical incompetence 421–422
    placental hormone production 422
    polyhydramnios 419–420
    premature rupture of membranes 421
    psychological stress 422
    subclinical infection 420–421
    uterine overdistension 419
  definition 471
  factors affecting uterine contractility 415–419
    actin–myosin interactions 415–416
    estrogen 417–418
    gap junction formation 418–419
    intracellular calcium metabolism 416–417
    local prostaglandin metabolism 417
    oxytocin sensitivity 418
    progesterone 417–418
  higher order multiple pregnancies 352–353, 356, 538–539
    and assisted reproduction 538–539
    prevention 540–541
  home management 479–481
  induced preterm births 447–448
  prediction from antepartum cervical examination 459–464
  recommendations 486–488
  risk reduction 437–442
    bed rest 439–440, 442, 472–473
    betamimetics 440–441
    case studies 442–445
    cerclage 441
    early diagnosis 439
    home monitoring 441
    indomethacin 441
    limitations 446–447
    progestins 441
    reduction of work load 439
    twin clinic 442
  uterine activity monitoring 481–483
    circadian patterns 483
    low-amplitude high-frequency contractions 481–483
progesterone
  and cervical maturation 456
  and uterine contractility 417–418
  multifetal pregnancy diagnostic significance 284
  role in respiratory changes during pregnancy 274
progestins
  preterm delivery prevention 441
prognosis for multifetal pregnancy
  Cesarean section significance 210
  early diagnosis benefits 208–212
pronuclear stage transfer (PROST) *see* tubal embryo transfer
prophylactic bed rest 472–473
prostaglandin synthetase inhibitors *see* indomethacin
prostaglandins
  and cervical maturation 456
  and uterine contractility 417
prune-belly syndrome 258
psychological aspects *see* maternal adaptation to multifetal pregnancy; postpartum adjustment
pulmonary cystic adenomatoid malformation 253–254
pulmonary hypoplasia 254–255
pulmonary system
  lung fetal maturation 592–595
  maternal adaptation to multifetal pregnancy 273–274
pyelectasis 257, 259
pygopagus conjoined twins 94, 95
  anatomy 103–104

quadruplet pregnancies *see* multifetal pregnancy
qualitative analysis 15–16
  partitioning of variance 16–17
quantitative analysis 16–17
quintuplet pregnancies *see* multifetal pregnancy
quintuplets, natural 26–27

race
  birth weight relationships 164–166
  dizygotic twinning and 33–35
  fetal growth relationships 166
  multifetal pregnancy relationships 133–142
    higher order pregnancies 537
  neonatal and infant mortality relationships 166–173
  placentation and 113, 117
radiography
  conjoined twin diagnosis 104, 108
red blood cell volume during pregnancy 272–273,

304
regional blood flow
    maternal adaptation to multifetal pregnancy 271
relaxin
    and cervical maturation 456
renal anomalies 257
    agenesis 260
renal function
    maternal adaptation to multifetal pregnancy 274–275
representativeness 12–13
resorption 63–64, 66
    and clomiphene citrate 61
respiratory changes during multifetal pregnancy 273–274
    anesthetic considerations 518
    role of progesterone 274
right ventricular hypoplasia 250
role switching 567

sacrococcygeal teratoma 261, 262
seasonality
    dizygotic twinning 35
    multifetal pregnancy 154, 155
    twin loss 64, 68–69
seizure disorders 600
selective termination 353–354, 356, 362–365
    abnormal twin 362
    acardiac twin 78
    and twin–twin transfusion syndrome 382
    ethical aspects 651–652
    KCl injection 362–363
    preterm delivery risks 363
separation of conjoined twins 108–109
    anesthetic management 109
    operative management 109
    preoperative evaluation 108
    timing 108–109
separation patterns of monozygotic twins 26–27
sex combination of twins
    infant mortality relationships 170–171
    secular analysis 149
sex discordance
    monozygotic twins 82–83
sex proportion 137–138, 158–160
    placentation relationships 126–127, 159–160
    triplets 160
    zygosity relationships 32–33, 126
sextuplet pregnancies see multifetal pregnancy
shared traits 30–31
Siamese twins see conjoined twins
siblings 296, 660–661
sirenomelia 64, 68, 75–76
    and vascular communications 402

size, birth 613
skeletal anomalies
    fetal diagnosis 262–264
sole survivor frequency 48
sonographic techniques see ultrasound sonography
Special Clinics 664–665
    Bereavement Clinic 665
    Special Needs Clinic 664
    Supertwins Clinic 664–665
speech laterality
    monozygotic twins 25
spina bifida
    fetal diagnosis 245–246
    incidence in twins 86
spontaneous abortion frequency
    in multiple pregnancies 33, 86–87
    monozygotic twins 86
spontaneous premature rupture of membranes see premature rupture of membranes
Standard Certificate of Live Birth
    USA 142
sternopagus conjoined twins 94
    anatomy 103
sternoxiphopagus conjoined twins 94
stillbirth
    conjoined twins 108
    in Sweden 205
stuck twin phenomenon 225
subcutaneous pump therapy 483–486
sudden infant death syndrome (SIDS) 168
superfecundation 12, 35
superfetation 12, 35–36
superior conjunction conjoined twins 101
superovulation therapy 182–184
Supertwins Clinic 664–665
survival following loss of co-twin
    associated anomalies 78–80
        management 80, 409
        pathogenesis 79–80
    monochorionic twins 373, 377
survival to term probability
    twin pregnancies 45–49
        individual twin 48
Sweden
    twinning rate trends 145, 155
    ultrasound program see ultrasound sonography
syncephalus conjoined twins 96

targeted imaging for fetal anomalies (TIFFA) 239
teratomas 101
    acardiac twins 77–78
    sacrococcygeal 261, 262
tetralogy of Fallot 251
third-type twins 11

693

MULTIPLE PREGNANCY

thoracopagus conjoined twins 75, 94, 95
  anatomy 103
tocolytic therapy *see* ambulatory tocolysis
toilet training 640
total anomalous pulmonary venous return 252
toxemia 540
transposition of the great arteries (TGA) 251
TRAP sequence 224
triplet pregnancies *see* multifetal pregnancy
triplets
  delivery of 511–512
  incidence 535–537
    secular trends 150–151, 537–538
  placentation 113, 117–119, 122, 127
  sex proportion 160
  zygosity 32, 117
trisomy 81–82
truncus arteriosus 251
tubal embryo transfer (TET)
  multiple gestation relationships 157, 178–179
Turner's syndrome 5, 31, 83
twin birth incidence 32–32
  influences 151–158
    assisted reproduction *see* assisted reproduction
    genetic factors 154–156
    geographic variation 153–154
    height 153
    live-birth order 135–137, 153
    maternal age 133, 135–138, 152, 153
    parity 152
    race 133–142
    seasonality 154, 155
  secular trends 145–151
    Europe 145–150
    Sweden 145
    USA 133–135
    zygosity relationships 147–150
twin-embolization syndrome 373, 377
twin method 9–18, 80–81
  assumptions 11–14
    antenatal bias and representativeness 12–13
    common environment problem 13–14
    twinning mechanisms and genetic bias 11–12
  data analysis 15–17
    concordance studies 15–16
    continuous variables 16–17
  data ascertainment 14–15
    samples and populations 14
    zygosity determination *see* zygosity
  ethics 7–8
  history 9–10
  research significance 7–8, 10
twin reversed arterial perfusion sequence (TRAP) 224, 373

  management 380–382
twin–twin transfusion syndrome 12, 13, 119, 370–391, 402–404
  and amniocentesis 382
  complications during delivery 514
  diagnosis and prognosis 225
    Doppler applications 234–235
  fetal behavior relationships 345, 346–347
  management 380–383
  monitoring 380
  vascular architecture
    anastomoses 12, 13, 119, 370–391
    three-dimensional modelling 395–397
twinning impetus theory 102
Twins and Multiple Births Association 663–664
Twins Clinics 664
Twins Clubs 655–658

ultrasound sonography 195–204
  and higher order multiple pregnancies 538, 541
  biometric studies 199–201
  causes of error 195–197
    errors related to gestational age 196
    errors related to technique 197
    errors related to type of pregnancy 197
    practitioner errors 197
  chorionicity determination 198
  conjoined twin diagnosis 104–105
  Doppler 201–202
  fetal behavior studies 331–332
  fetal congenital anomaly diagnosis *see* anomalies, congenital
  fetal growth assessment 226–230
    weight estimation 226–230
  fetal morphology 203
  monoamnionic twin monitoring 527–530
  multifetal pregnancy diagnosis 195–197, 280
  placental development 202–203
  placentation determination 198, 219–224
  pregnancy dating 215–222
    choice of measurements 219
  report form 216
  Swedish program 205–212
    development 206–207
    prognostic significance 208–212
    training 207–208
  use during delivery 505–506
vanishing twin 198–199
zygosity determination 219–224
umbilical cord
  complications 606
  Doppler study 329
  insertion 118, 122, 126–127
    pathological evidence of vanishing twin 52–54

perinatal outcome relationships 126–127
velamentous 126, 127, 514
ureteropelvic dilatation and hydronephrosis 257, 258
urinary system
  anomalies
    fetal diagnosis 256–261
    maternal adaptation to multifetal pregnancy 274–275
USA
  demographic trends in twin births 133–142
uterine contractility *see also* ambulatory tocolysis; labor; preterm delivery
  influences 415–419
    actin–myosin interactions 415–416
    estrogen 417–418
    gap junction formation 418–419
    intracellular calcium metabolism 416–417
    local prostaglandin metabolism 417
    oxytocin sensitivity 418
    progesterone 417–418
  monitoring for preterm labor 481–483
    circadian activity 483
    low-amplitude high-frequency contractions 481–483
uterine overdistension
  and preterm delivery 419
uterine receptivity
  in assisted reproduction 180
uterus
  changes in multifetal pregnancy 300
    size as indicator 280

vaginal bleeding
  with fetal wastage 62, 68
vaginal delivery *see also* delivery
  after previous Cesarean section 504–505
  anesthetic considerations 519–520
  conjoined twins 107–108
  neonatal mortality relationships 496–497
  psychological aspects 295
  vertex/non-vertex twin delivery 493–499
  vertex/vertex twins 491–492
vanishing twin syndrome 41, 43, 225–226
  frequency 48, 61–68
  literature review 59–69
  pathological evidence 51–58, 60, 62, 64–65, 69
  prognosis for continuing pregnancy 68
  ultrasound observation 198–199
variable number of tandem repeats (VNTR)
  and zygosity determination 628–629
vasa previa 514
vascular anatomy, placenta 368–391, 399–402 *see also* anastomoses
  and acardiac malformation 401–402
  and twin–twin transfusion syndrome 12, 13, 370–391, 402–404
    three-dimensional modelling 395–397
  obstetric outcome relationships 383–388
vein of Galen, aneurysm 244–245
velamentous cord insertion 126, 127, 514
veno–venous anastomoses *see* anastomoses
ventilatory changes during pregnancy 273–274
  role of progesterone 274
ventral wall defects 256
ventricular aneurysm 253
ventricular hypoplasia 250
vertex/non-vertex twin delivery 492–499
  breech delivery 494–498
  intrapartum external version 493–494
vertex/vertex twin delivery 491–492

weaning 560
weight
  birth 437–438
    gestation period relationships 138–141, 164–166, 303
    higher order multiples 544
    maternal weight gain relationships 302
    neonatal and infant mortality relationships 166–168, 173
    placentation and zygosity relationships 123–126, 368
    race relationships 164–166
    twins vs. singletons 138–139
    umbilical cord insertion relationships 127
  fetal estimation 226–230
    labor relationships 430
  maternal changes during multifetal pregnancy 300–301
    triplets and higher order multiples 301–304
Weinberg method 15, 32–33, 42, 625
  applicability to anomalous twin births 42–43
  secular trend analysis 147–150
well-being of fetus *see* fetal well-being assessment

X chromosome inactivation
  and monozygotic twin discordance 27–28
xiphopagus conjoined twins 94
  anatomy 103

Yoruba tribe 31, 34

zygosity
  birth weight relationships 123–125
  determination 14–15, 122, 124
    and fetal behavior 332
    embryological analysis 626

MULTIPLE PREGNANCY

    genetic analysis 627–632
    postnatal 625–632
    similarity method 626–627
    ultrasound 219–224
fetal growth relationships 123–125

    postnatal growth relationships 616–617
    sex proportion relationships 158–160
    triplets 117
zygote intrafallopian transfer (ZIFT) *see* tubal
    embryo transfer